Textbook of Otitis Media

Marcos V. Goycoolea • Sady Selaimen da Costa
Christopher de Souza • Michael M. Paparella
Editors

Textbook of Otitis Media

The Basics and Beyond

Springer

Editors
Marcos V. Goycoolea
Department of Otolaryngology
Clínica Universidad de Los Andes
Santiago, Chile, USA

Sady Selaimen da Costa
Otolaryngology
Federal University of Rio Grande do Sul
Porto Alegre, Rio Grande do Sul, Brazil

Chris de Souza
Department of Otolaryngology
Tata Memorial Hospital
Mumbai, Maharashtra, India

Michael M. Paparella
Paparella Ear Head & Neck Institute
University of Minnesota
Minneapolis, MN, USA

ISBN 978-3-031-40948-6 ISBN 978-3-031-40949-3 (eBook)
https://doi.org/10.1007/978-3-031-40949-3

This Springer imprint is published by the registered company Springer Nature Switzerland AG
The registered company address is: Gewerbestrasse 11, 6330 Cham, Switzerland

Paper in this product is recyclable.

Preface

The First International Symposium on Recent Advances in Otitis Media was held in May 1975 in Columbus, Ohio. At the time I was a first-year resident—26 years old—in Otolaryngology at the University of Minnesota, with two previous years in General Surgery. I was doing research in otitis media in cats and "my cats made it to the meeting." As a coauthor of Michael Paparella and Steve Juhn, that was my first paper ever. At that symposium I was one of the youngest if not the youngest participant. The meeting in Columbus was organized by Doctors Ben Senturia, Charles Bluestone, David Lim, Michael Paparella, and Steve Juhn, among others. From then on, every 4 years and for many years I participated as a member of the Minnesota team and eventually as a member of the Chilean team. There were many groups at the time. Our group was led by Michael Paparella and Steve Juhn and all of us residents including Tim Jung and myself. Other groups were the Pittsburgh group of Charles Bluestone and Sylvan Stool, the Swedish group of Dr Inglested that included, among others, Sten Hellstrom, Karin Prellner, Margaretha Casselbrandt, and Ann Hermannsonn, the Danish group of Mirko Tos and Jans Thomsen, the Finish group of Tauno Palva and Pekka Karma, the Japanese groups with Drs Mogi, Honjo, Ogra, and many others, including the group in Israel led by Jacob Sadé. All these groups kept participating every 4 years and bonds of friendship developed over time. In between the Swedish group organized the middle inner ear interactions meeting in Umea with unforgettable pre- and post-congress meetings with the leadership of Sten Hellstrom, Jan Wersall, Matti Anniko, Claude Laurent, and others. Over time we became staff, and our fellows became incorporated to the group. That was the case of Marcelo Hueb, Sady Selaimen da Costa, Carlos Ruah, and Chris de Souza, who became prominent otolaryngologists, many of them presidents of their national societies and members of the Collegium.

At the first Symposium in 1975, we were the young members and Doctor Senturia—a wise, kind, and encouraging man—was gradually fading (as heroes often do over time). I will never forget unique moments at these multiple reunions such as the Swedish group dancing and singing "the frog" at a farewell party, Goro Mogi fishing in Tromso, Norway, presenting himself as: "Goro Mogi a great fisherman from Japan," Dr Lars Eric Stenfors talking about the flying penguins of Norway and trying to convince us that the meat we were eating was whale, David Lim in Jukasjarvi (the town of the midnight sun in summer and the Ice Hotel in winter) telling me: "Marcos look how far otitis media has taken you," Ann Hermannson in northern Sweden teaching us about the Hundras and the beliefs of the northern people (I still keep the bone box with the magic power of northern Sweden), Sten Hellstrom organizing a pre-meeting competition of picking berries and mushrooms in the Umea forest, etc.

During these unforgettable meetings we learned a lot about otitis media but more importantly we learned about life and friendship, and my wife and I are thankful and feel privileged to have participated and to have met all of them and consider them our friends. We were scientists but at the same time human beings and friends who enjoyed not only science but, more importantly, friendship. These were meetings that taught us to help and treat people, persons, far beyond thc important use of statistical significance, xi square, and computerized evidence.

The last International Symposium on Recent Advances in Otitis Media was held in June 2021, and there I was, presenting, 46 years later. Only that, this time, the difference was that I was one of the oldest if not the oldest participant, and one of the very few originals of 1975.

However, the difference was that at this last meeting the one that was gradually fading was me, just like Dr Senturia at the first meeting. Many of our mentors and pioneers like Michael Paparella—our honored co-editor and co-author in this book—Steve Juhn and others, just like the old heroes, are fading away. However, although they physically fade away, those that remain and had the privilege to have lived, worked, and learned from them will keep them alive in their hearts and in their concepts because they have become an integral part of the "otitis media family" forever.

At this stage in my professional career, I was not about to edit another book on otitis media; however, I accepted as an exception only to lead this book in honor of our pioneers who so generously encouraged us, taught us, and introduced us to the subject of otitis media. In this spirit, and before fading away myself, I accepted to lead a book in honor of their memory and to give the torch to the young ones on my team and in other teams, who are in the same position that I was in 1975.

God and life have been good to me and my family (it has not been free), and I feel that I should make this last otitis media effort and personally contribute with concepts in structure, function, and pathogenesis which are current and essential for the understanding of this multifactorial disease. At the same time, I wanted to contribute by transmitting the energy that was given to us in 1975 and transmit it modified and improved to the new generations, which will in turn modify and improve it in a constant enrichment that will contain the concepts and the spirits of the "otitis media family" for eternity.

Santiago, MN, USA — Marcos V. Goycoolea
Porto Alegre, Rio Grande do Sul, Brazil — Sady Selaimen da Costa
Mumbai, Maharashtra, India — Chris de Souza
Minneapolis, MN, USA — Michael M. Paparella

Contents

Contributors

José Vicente Boleli Scardini Alves Department of Otolaryngology, Banco de Olhos de Sorocaba Hospital, Sorocaba, Brazil

José Alzerreca Department of Otolaryngology, Clínica Universidad de Los Andes, Santiago, Chile

Aneesa Ansar Department of Otolaryngology, Tarabichi Stammberger Ear and Sinus Institute, Dubai, UAE

Bernard Ars University of Namur, Namur, Belgium

Temporal Bone Foundation, Brussels, Belgium

Douglas Backous Department of Neurotology, Proliance Surgeons, Puget Sound ENT, Edmonds, WA, USA

Margherita Basso Department of Otolaryngology-Head and Neck Surgery, University Hospital of Modena, Modena, Italy

Jefferson André Bauer Hospital de Clinicas de Porto Alegre, Porto Alegre, Brazil

Hospital Mãe de Deus, Porto Alegre, Brazil

Universidade Federal do Rio Grande do Sul, Porto Alegre, Brazil

Instituto Gaúcho de Otorrinolaringologia, Porto Alegre, Brazil

Pierfrancesco Bettini ENT & Audiology Department, University Hospital of Ferrara, Ferrara, Italy

Diane Biju Holy Spirit Hospital, Mumbai, India

Nicola Bisi Department of Otolaryngology-Head and Neck Surgery, University Hospital of Modena, Modena, Italy

Charlotte M. Burford East Kent Hospitals University NHS Foundation Trust, Ashford, Kent, UK

Byanka Cagnacci Buzo Santa Casa de Sao Paulo School of Medical Science Hearing and Speech Science Program, São Paulo, Brazil

Department of Research, Cochlear LATAM, Panamá City, Panamá

Inesangela Canali Department of Otolaryngology, Pontifical Catholic University, Porto Alegre, Rio Grande do Sul, Brazil

Federal University of Rio Grande do Sul, Porto Alegre, Rio Grande do Sul, Brazil

Vlademir Cantarelli Department of Basic Health Sciences, Universidade Federal de Ciencias da Saude de Porto Alegre (UFCSPA), Porto Alegre, RS, Brazil

Jorge Caro Pontificia Universidad Católica de Chile, Santiago, Chile

Antonio Caruso Gruppo Otologico and Mario Sanna Foundation, Piacenza-Rome, Italy

Daniela Carvalho Division of Otolaryngology Head and Neck Surgery, University of California, San Diego, La Jolla, CA, USA

Rady Children's Hospital, San Diego, San Diego, CA, USA

Leandro Guena de Castro Department of Otolaryngology, Head & Neck Surgery, Banco de Olhos de Sorocaba Hospital, Sorocaba, SP, Brazil

Mario Castro Chilean National Museum of Natural History, Santiago, Chile

Department of Morphology, Faculty of Medicine, Clínica Alemana-Universidad del Desarrollo, Santiago, Chile

S. Catherine Catenacci Department of Otolaryngology, Clinica Universidad de Los Andes, Santiago, Chile

Francisco Chiang Department of Radiology, Clínica Universidad de Los Andes, Santiago, Chile

Ana Paula Chornobay Hospital Universitário Cajuru, Curitiba, PR, Brazil

Sara Concha Department of Pediatric Immunology and Infectious Diseases, Pontificia Universidad Católica de Chile, Santiago, Chile

Molly Cooper Department of Surgery/Otolaryngology, UCSD School of Medicine, San Diego, CA, USA

Hannah L. Cornwall Department of Paediatrics, Ysbyty Gwynedd, Bangor, Wales, UK

Sady Selaimen da Costa Department of Otolaryngology, Head and Neck Surgery, School of Medicine, Federal University of Rio Grande do Sul, Porto Alegre, Rio Grande do Sul, Brazil

School of Medicine - Federal University of Rio Grande do Sul, Porto Alegre, Brazil

Otology and Neurotology Division, Hospital de Clínicas de Porto Alegre, Porto Alegre, Rio Grande do Sul, Brazil

Universidade Federal do Rio Grande do Sul, Porto Alegre, Rio Grande do Sul, Brazil

International Hearing Foundation, Minneapolis, MN, USA

American Academy of Otolaryngology and Head & Neck Surgery, Alexandria, VA, USA

Department of Otolaryngology, University of Minnesota, Otopathology Laboratory, Minneapolis, MN, USA

Hospital de Clínicas de Porto Alegre, Porto Alegre, Brazil

Pontifícia Universidade Católica do Rio Grande do Sul, Porto Alegre, Brazil

Otology and Neurotology Division, Sistema Hospitalar Mãe de Deus, Porto Alegre, Brazil

Universidade Federal do Rio Grande do Sul, Porto Alegre, Brazil

Instituto Gaúcho de Otorrinolaringologia, Porto Alegre, Brazil

Felipe da Costa Huve Hospital de Clinicas de Porto Alegre, Porto Alegre, Brazil

Hospital Mãe de Deus, Porto Alegre, Brazil

Universidade Federal do Rio Grande do Sul, Porto Alegre, Brazil

Instituto Gaúcho de Otorrinolaringologia, Porto Alegre, Brazil

Rafael da Costa Monsanto Department of Otolaryngology, Head & Neck Surgery, University of Minnesota, Minneapolis, MN, USA

Department of Otolaryngology, Head and Neck Surgery, Universidade Federal de São Paulo/ Escola Paulista de Medicina (UNIFESP/EPM), São Paulo, Brazil

Department of Otolaryngology, Head & Neck Surgery, Banco de Olhos de Sorocaba Hospital, Sorocaba, SP, Brazil

Sebahattin Cureoglu Otopathology Laboratory, Department of Otolaryngology, University of Minnesota Physicians (UMP), University of Minnesota, Minneapolis, MN, USA

Marcela Lehmkuhl Damiani Hospital de Clínicas de Porto Alegre, Universidade Federal do Rio Grande do Sul, Porto Alegre, Brazil

Hospital de Clínicas de Porto Alegre, Porto Alegre, Brazil

Roland Douglas Eavey Department of Otolaryngology-Head and Neck Surgery, Vanderbilt University Medical Center, Nashville, TN, USA

Caroline Catherine Lacerda Elias Federal University of Rio Grande do Sul, Porto Alegre, Rio Grande do Sul, Brazil

Department of Otolaryngology, Hospital Nossa Senhora da Conceição, de Porto Alegre (GHC), Porto Alegre, Rio Grande do Sul, Brazil

Pilar Epprecht Department of Otolaryngology, Clínica Universidad de Los Andes and Exequiel González Cortés Hospital, Santiago, Chile

Department of Otolaryngology, Exequiel González Cortés Hospital, Santiago, Chile

Dominique Estève Chemin de Sainte-Roustagne, Manosque, France

Matthew R. B. Farr Doncaster Royal Infirmary, Doncaster, UK

Francisco Tocornal J. Department of Otolaryngology, Clínica Universidad de Los Andes, Santiago, Chile

Raimundo José García-Matte Department of Otolaryngology, Clínica Universidad de Los Andes, and Hospital de la Florida, Santiago, Chile

Michael B. Gluth University of Chicago Section of Otolaryngology-Head and Neck Surgery, Chicago, IL, USA

Aditi Govil Lilavati Hospital and Research Centre, Mumbai, India

BJ Medical College, Ahmedabad, India

Marcos V. Goycoolea Department of Otolaryngology, Clínica Universidad de Los Andes, Santiago, Chile

Kanchan Gupta Lilavati Hospital and Research Centre, Mumbai, India

Catalina Gutiérrez Hospital Sótero del Río, Santiago, Chile

Ann Hermansson Department of ENT, Lund University Hospital, Lund, Sweden

María José Herrera J Department of Otolaryngology, Clínica Universidad de Los Andes, Santiago, Chile

Rodrigo Hoyos-Bachiloglu Department of Pediatric Immunology and Infectious Diseases, Pontificia Universidad Católica de Chile, Santiago, Chile

Fernanda Rocha Hueb University of Uberaba, Uberaba, Minas Gerais, Brazil

Marcela Rocha Hueb University Unilago, São Paulo, Brazil

Marcelo Miguel Hueb University of São Paulo, São Paulo, Brazil

ENT Discipline and ENT Service, Federal University of Triângulo Mineiro, Uberaba, Brazil

Hospital Santa Lúcia of Uberaba, Uberaba, Minas Gerais, Brazil

Ryan T. Judd University of Chicago Section of Otolaryngology-Head and Neck Surgery, Chicago, IL, USA

Timothy T. K. Jung Department of Otolaryngology-Head & Neck Surgery, Loma Linda University School of Medicine, Jerry L. Pettis Veterans Medical Center, Loma Linda, CA, USA

Inland Ear Head & Neck Clinic, Riverside, CA, USA

José Carlos Convento Júnior Department of Otolaryngology, Head & Neck Surgery, Banco de Olhos de Sorocaba Hospital, Sorocaba, SP, Brazil

Mustafa Kapadia Department of Otolaryngology, Tarabichi Stammberger Ear and Sinus Institute, Dubai, UAE

Adam C. Kaufman Otorhinolaryngology – Head & Neck Surgery, University of Maryland, Baltimore, Baltimore, MD, USA

Cemil Kayaalp Otopathology Laboratory, Department of Otolaryngology, University of Minnesota, Minneapolis, MN, USA

Suanur M. Kayaalp Otopathology Laboratory, Department of Otolaryngology, University of Minnesota Physicians (UMP), University of Minnesota, Minneapolis, MN, USA

Arwa Kurabi Department of Surgery/Otolaryngology, UCSD School of Medicine, San Diego, CA, USA

Lorenzo Lauda Gruppo Otologico and Mario Sanna Foundation, Piacenza-Rome, Italy

Joel Lavinsky Federal University of Rio Grande do Sul, Porto Alegre, RS, Brazil

Santa Casa de Porto Alegre, Porto Alegre, Brazil

Luiz Lavinsky Federal University of Rio Grande do Sul, School of Medicine, Porto Alegre, Brazil

Sul-Rio-Grandense Academy of Medicine, Porto Alegre, Brazil

Nam K. Lee Department of Otolaryngology-Head and Neck Surgery, School of Medicine, University of Colorado Anschutz Medical Campus, Aurora, CO, USA

Jai-sen F. Leung Pontificia Universidad Católica de Chile, Santiago, Chile

João Pedro Neves Lubianca Federal University of Rio Grande do Sul, Hospital de Clínicas de Porto Alegre, Porto Alegre, RS, Brazil

Marcelo Neves Lubianca Pontifical Catholic University of Rio Grande do Sul, São Lucas Hospital, Porto Alegre, RS, Brazil

Rochane Figini Maciel Chronic Otitis Media Study Group, School of Medicine, Federal University of Rio Grande do Sul (UFRGS), Porto Alegre, RS, Brazil

Daniele Marchioni Department of Otolaryngology-Head and Neck Surgery, University Hospital of Modena, Modena, Italy

Matthew J. Mason Department of Physiology, Development & Neuroscience, University of Cambridge, Cambridge, UK

Rafael C. Monsanto Otopathology Laboratory, Department of Otolaryngology, University of Minnesota, Minnesota, MN, USA

Department of Otolaryngology, Head & Neck Surgery, University of Minnesota, Minnesota, MN, USA

Tiago Isamu Saiguchi Murakami Pontifícia Universidade Católica do Rio Grande do Sul, Porto Alegre, Brazil

José Faibes Lubianca Neto Graduate Program of Pediatrics of Federal University of Health Sciences of Porto Alegre, Porto Alegre, RS, Brazil

Otorhinolaryngology Service at Santa Casa de Misericórdia de Porto Alegre Hospital, Porto Alegre, RS, Brazil

Pediatric Otorhinolaryngology Service at Santo Antonio Children's Hospital, Porto Alegre, RS, Brazil

Carrie L. Nieman Department of Otolaryngology-Head and Neck Surgery, Johns Hopkins University School of Medicine, Baltimore, MD, USA

Wiquinylson França de Oliveira Universidade Federal do Rio Grande do Sul, Porto Alegre, Brazil

Norma de Oliveira Penido Department of Otolaryngology, Head and Neck Surgery, Universidade Federal de São Paulo/Escola Paulista de Medicina (UNIFESP/EPM), São Paulo, Brazil

Letícia A. Oyama Hospital Universitário Cajuru, Curitiba, PR, Brazil

Michael M. Paparella Department of Otolaryngology, University of Minnesota and Paparella Clinic, Minneapolis, MN, USA

Otopathology Laboratory, Department of Otolaryngology, University of Minnesota and Paparella Clinic, Minneapolis, MN, USA

American Academy of Otolaryngology and Head & Neck Surgery, Alexandria, VA, USA

Department of Otolaryngology, Head & Neck Surgery, University of Minnesota, Minnesota, MN, USA

Javiera Pardo Otolaryngologist Department of Otolaryngology, Clínica Universidad de Los Andes, Santiago, Chile

Aishan Patil Vascular Surgery, Borders General Hospital, Melrose, Scotland, UK

Henrique Furlan Pauna Hospital Universitário Cajuru, Curitiba, PR, Brazil

Hospital IPO, Curitiba, Paraná, Brazil

Department of Otolaryngology, Hospital Universitario Cajuru, Curitiba, Paraná, Brazil

Denise Rotta Ruttkay Pereira Department of Otolaryngology and Head and Neck Surgery, Hospital de Clinicas de Porto Alegre, Universidade Federal do Rio Grande do Sul (UFRGS), Porto Alegre, RS, Brazil

Manuel Ruttkay Pereira Department of Pediatrics, School of Medicine, Pontificia Universidade Católica do Rio Grande do Sul (PUCRS), Porto Alegre, RS, Brazil

Department of Pediatrics, School of Medicine, Universidade Federal do Rio Grande do Sul (UFRGS), Porto Alegre, RS, Brazil

Maria Beatriz Rotta Pereira Department of Otolaryngology and Head and Neck Surgery, Hospital Sao Lucas, Pontificia Universidade Católica do Rio Grande do Sul (PUCRS), Porto Alegre, RS, Brazil

Gianluca Piras Gruppo Otologico and Mario Sanna Foundation, Piacenza-Rome, Italy

Dennis S. Poe Department of Otolaryngology-Head and Neck Surgery, Boston Children's Hospital, Boston, MA, USA

Berenice Dias Ramos Phoniatrics, Department of Ophthalmology and Otorhinolaryngology, Faculty of Medicine, Federal University of Rio Grande do Sul, Porto Alegre, RS, Brazil

Otorhinolaryngology & Head and Neck Surgery Service, Hospital de Clínicas de Porto Alegre, Porto Alegre, RS, Brazil

Phoniatrics, DERDIC—PUCSP, São Paulo, SP, Brazil

Phoebe H. Ramos Pontificia Universidad Católica de Chile, Santiago, Chile

G. Raquel Levy Department of Otolaryngology, Clinica Universidad de Los Andes, Santiago, Chile

Douglas K. Reinhardt Hospital São Lucas da PUCRS, Porto Alegre, Brazil

Leandro Rodríguez Department of Otolaryngology, Clínica Universidad de Los Andes, and Hospital del Salvador, Santiago, Chile

Letícia Petersen Schmidt Rosito School of Medicine - Federal Universityof Rio Grande do Sul, Porto Alegre, Brazil

Hospital de Clínicas de Porto Alegre, Porto Alegre, Brazil

International Hearing Foundation, Minneapolis, MN, USA

Department of Otolaryngology—Head and Neck Surgery, Porto Alegre Clinica's Hospital, Porto Alegre, Rio Grande do Sul, Brazil

Alessia Rubini Department of Otolaryngology-Head and Neck Surgery, University Hospital of Modena, Modena, Italy

Allen F. Ryan Department of Surgery/Otolaryngology, UCSD School of Medicine, San Diego, CA, USA

Department of Neurosciences, UCSD School of Medicine, San Diego, CA, USA

San Diego VA Healthcare System, La Jolla, CA, USA

Matheus Saito Department of Otolaryngology, Head & Neck Surgery, Banco de Olhos de Sorocaba Hospital, Sorocaba, SP, Brazil

Hamed Sajjadi Stanford University, School of Medicine, San Jose Ear & Sinus Medical Center, Los Gatos, CA, USA

Karina Salvi Department of Otolaryngology, Banco de Olhos de Sorocaba Hospital, Sorocaba, SP, Brazil

Mario Sanna Gruppo Otologico and Mario Sanna Foundation, Piacenza-Rome, Italy

Peter L. Santa Maria Otolaryngology, Head & Neck Surgery, Stanford University, Stanford, CA, USA

Claudia M. Santoni School of Clinical Medicine, University of Cambridge, Cambridge, UK

Regie Lyn P. Santos-Cortez Department of Otolaryngology-Head and Neck Surgery, School of Medicine, University of Colorado Anschutz Medical Campus, Aurora, CO, USA

Livia Tamie T. Sassaki Department of Otolaryngology, Banco de Olhos de Sorocaba Hospital, Sorocaba, SP, Brazil

M. Schürmann Department of Otorhinolaryngology, Head and Neck Surgery, Klinikum Bielefeld, Medical Faculty OWL, Bielefeld University, Bielefeld, Germany

Fabio Andre Selaimen Hospital de Clínicas de Porto Alegre, Porto Alegre, Brazil

Instituto Gaúcho de Otorrinolaringologia, Porto Alegre, Brazil

Fábio André Selaimen Hospital de Clínicas de Porto Alegre, Porto Alegre, Brazil

Instituto Gaúcho de Otorrinolaringologia, Porto Alegre, Brazil

Emily Sereno Department of Surgery/Otolaryngology, UCSD School of Medicine, San Diego, CA, USA

Shaila Sidam All India Institute of Medical Sciences, Bhopal, Madhya Pradesh, India

Alice Lang Silva Instituto Gaúcho de Otorrinolaringologia, Porto Alegre, Brazil

Mauricio Noschang Lopes da Silva Hospital de Clínicas de Porto Alegre, Porto Alegre, Brazil

Instituto Gaúcho de Otorrinolaringologia, Porto Alegre, Brazil

Hospital de Clínicas de Porto Alegre, Universidade Federal do Rio Grande do Sul, Porto Alegre, Brazil

Otology and Neurotology Division, Sistema Hospitalar Mãe de Deus, Porto Alegre, Brazil

Service of Otolaryngology, Head & Neck Surgery, Hospital de Clínicas de Porto Alegre, Porto Alegre, Brazil

Vagner Antonio Rodrigues da Silva State University of Campinas (Unicamp), Campinas, Brazil

Faculty of Medical Sciences—UNICAMP, Campinas, Brazil

Chris de Souza Lilavati Hospital, Mumbai, India

Holy Family Hospital, Mumbai, India

Otolaryngology—Head and Neck Surgery, SUNY Brooklyn, New York, NY, USA

Otolaryngology—Head and Neck Surgery, LUSHSC, Shreveport, LA, USA

Faculty SUNY, Brooklyn, NY, USA

LSUHSC, Shreveport, LA, USA

Lilavati Hospital, Holy Family Hospital, Holy Spirit Hospital, Mumbai, India

Rosemarie de Souza Internal Medicine, BYL Nair Hospital and TNM College, Mumbai, India

Joshua A. Stramielo Division of Otolaryngology Head and Neck Surgery, University of California, San Diego, La Jolla, CA, USA

H. Sudhoff Department of Otorhinolaryngology, Head and Neck Surgery, Klinikum Bielefeld, Medical Faculty OWL, Bielefeld University, Bielefeld, Germany

Abdelkader Taibah Gruppo Otologico and Mario Sanna Foundation, Piacenza-Rome, Italy

Alex Joseph Fejta Tampio Department of Neurotology, Proliance Surgeons, Puget Sound ENT, Edmonds, WA, USA

Wenlong Tang Gruppo Otologico and Mario Sanna Foundation, Piacenza-Rome, Italy

Muaaz Tarabichi Department of Otolaryngology, Tarabichi Stammberger Ear and Sinus Institute, Dubai, UAE

Vishal Tyagi Holy Family Hospital, Holy Spirit Hospital, Mumbai, India

Department of ENT, VN Desai Hospital, Mumbai, India

Bryan K. Ward Department of Otolaryngology-Head and Neck Surgery, Johns Hopkins University School of Medicine, Baltimore, MD, USA

Stephanie J. Wong Pediatric Otolaryngology, Mount Sinai, NY, USA

1 Definitions, Terminology, and Classification

Marcos V. Goycoolea, Sady Selaimen da Costa, Chris de Souza, and Michael M. Paparella

Otitis media (OM) is a multifactorial, multifaceted disease that manifests as an inflammatory process in the middle ear, mastoid, and Eustachian tube. It is the result of prevailing aggression against the body's immunological defense system, the degree of which depends on the interactions between the two opposing forces (aggressive and defensive). It is a dynamic disease, often used to describe a continuum of related diseases [1], in which some forms lead to others (Figs. 1.1 and 1.2), resulting at times in complications and sequelae (Table 1.1). In addition to local factors, this process is directly influenced not only by the neighboring anatomical structures but also by the host's relationship with the environment.

The term "otitis media (OM)" itself describes an inflammation of the middle ear and includes not only the middle ear cavity but also the Eustachian tube and the mastoid.

This disease can be classified on a clinical or histopathological basis [3].

M. V. Goycoolea (✉)
Department of Otolaryngology, Clínica Universidad de Los Andes, Santiago, Chile

S. S. da Costa
Department of Otolaryngology, Head and Neck Surgery, School of Medicine, Federal University of Rio Grande do Sul, Porto Alegre, Rio Grande do Sul, Brazil

Otology and Neurotology Division, Hospital de Clínicas de Porto Alegre, Porto Alegre, Rio Grande do Sul, Brazil

C. de Souza
Lilavati Hospital, Mumbai, India

Holy Family Hospital, Mumbai, India

Otolaryngology—Head and Neck Surgery, SUNY Brooklyn, New York, NY, USA

Otolaryngology—Head and Neck Surgery, LUSHSC, Shreveport, LA, USA

M. M. Paparella
Department of Otolaryngology, University of Minnesota and Paparella Clinic, Minneapolis, MN, USA
e-mail: papar001@umn.edu

M. V. Goycoolea et al. (eds.), *Textbook of Otitis Media*, https://doi.org/10.1007/978-3-031-40949-3_1

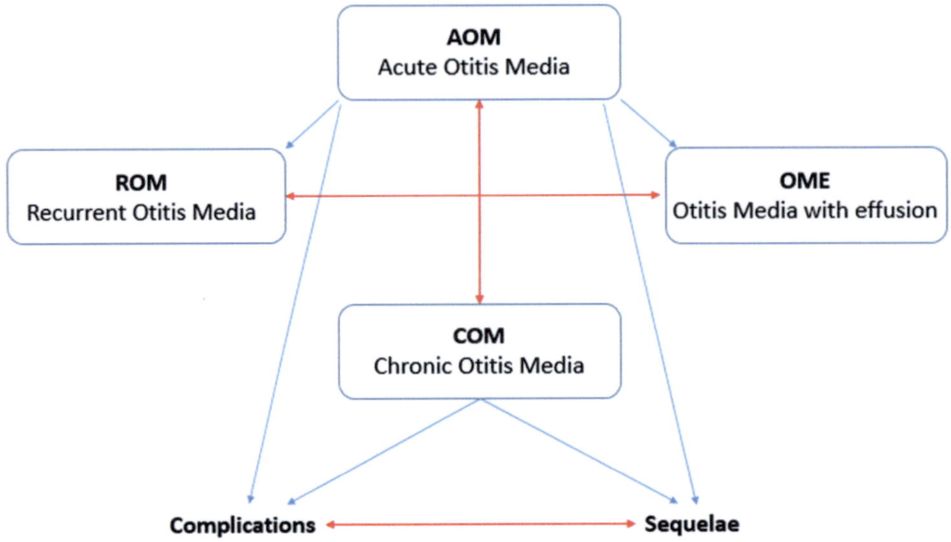

Fig. 1.1 The continuum of otitis media (Copyright Marcos Y. Goycoolea 2023; all rights reserved)

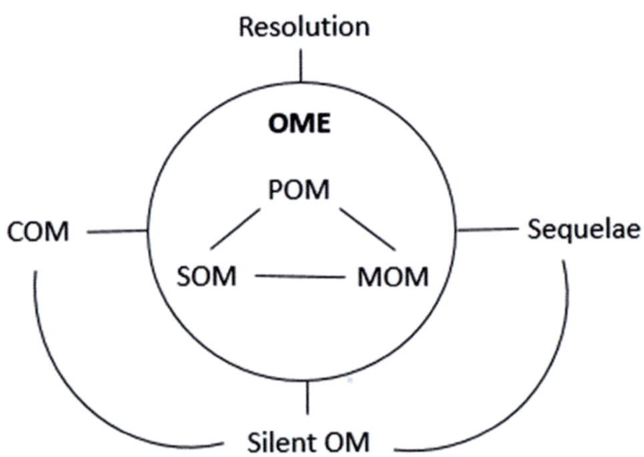

Fig. 1.2 Classification and continuum of otitis media. (Copyright Marcos Y. Goycoolea 2023; all rights reserved). Classification and continuum of otitis media with effusion (OME). *POM* purulent otitis media, *SOM* serous otitis media, *MOM* mucoid otitis media, *COM* chronic otitis media, *OM* otitis media

Table 1.1 Complications and sequelae of otitis media (from Goycoolea and Jung 1991 [2])

Complications	
Temporal bone	**Extratemporal**
Middle ear	*Intracranial*
Facial nerve paralysis	Extradural abscess
Ossicular lesions	Subdural abscess
Perforations of the TM[a]	Brain abscess
	Meningitis
Mastoid	Lateral sinus thrombophlebitis
Reduced pneumatization	Otitis hydrocephalus
Coalescent mastoiditis	
	Extracranial
Inner ear	Bezold's abscess
Labyrinthitis	Zygomatic abscess
Sensorineural hearing loss	Postauricular abscess
	Others
	Developmental
	Behavioral
Sequelae	
Active	
Recurrent attacks of otitis media	
Chronic otitis media with effusion	
Silent otitis media	
Masked mastoiditis	
Continuum of POM-SOM-MOM-COM[b]	
Inactive	
Atelectasis	
Tympanosclerosis	
Adhesive otitis media	

[a] Tympanic membrane
[b] *POM* purulent otitis media, *SOM* serous otitis media, *MOM* mucoid otitis media, *COM* chronic otitis media

Clinical Classification

The Task Force of the Fourth International Symposium of Otitis Media, held in June 1987, at Bal Harbor, Florida, classified otitis on clinical grounds [4], as did the Task Force of the Seventh Symposium in 1999 [5].

For purposes of communication and uniform reporting, we have followed this classification, with a clear understanding, however, that it is a working classification that allows a "common language" in the subject. It is important to mention that this is more than just a "final classification" written in stone; it has represented, over the years, a "consensus or working agreement" between different clinicians and investigators who have different viewpoints and perspectives. In other words, as Cicero stated centuries ago: "Every rational discussion of anything whatsoever should begin with a definition in order to make clear what is the subject of dispute."

The classification is as follows:

1. **Myringitis**, which is an inflammation of the tympanic membrane that occurs alone or in association with external otitis or otitis media
2. **Acute suppurative otitis media** (acute purulent otitis media (POM) or acute otitis media), which refers to a clinically identifiable infection of the middle ear with sudden onset and short duration
3. **Otitis media with effusion or secretory otitis media** (chronic otitis media with effusion, otitis media with effusion, nonsuppurative otitis media, catarrh, serous otitis media (SOM), serotympanum, mucoid otitis media (MOM), mucositis, or mucotympanum), which refers to the presence of middle ear effusion (MEE) behind an intact tympanic membrane without any acute signs or symptoms. This broad term includes nonsuppurative or clinically noninfectious forms of OM. However, evidence suggests that effusions are, for the most part, infectious. Cultures of serous effusions yield between 22% and 52% positively, percentages that increase to 77.3% if PCR is used [6].
4. **Chronic suppurative otitis media** (chronic otitis media), which refers to a chronic discharge from the middle ear through a perforation of the tympanic membrane. Suppurative refers to an active clinical infection. A perforation without discharge can be an inactive stage of the infection (but not of the underlying histopathological process).

   Over time, a new entity was incorporated:
5. **Recurrent otitis media**, which refers to repeated episodes of acute otitis media in between periods of "apparent remission" (three episodes in 6 months or four episodes in 1 year)

In addition, the definition of "chronic" can also be applied to otitis with an intact tympanic membrane, as in the cases of **masked mastoiditis** [7] and **silent otitis media** [8, 9].

Based on its duration, this disease can be divided into acute (up to 3 weeks), subacute (from 3 weeks to 3 months), and chronic (more than 3 months) [10].

Middle Ear Effusions

Otitis media is associated with the presence of middle ear fluid (effusion). Basically, three types of effusions are found: (1) serous otitis media (SOM), (2) mucoid otitis media (MOM), and (3) purulent otitis media (POM).

Two other types can be added: hemorrhagic and any combination of the previously mentioned effusions. In practice, it is unusual to see a pure effusion because effusions reflect a dynamic process in which some forms evolve into others. This will depend on the interaction between defensive and aggressive forces (e.g., the aggressive forces prevail in the more infectious phases, whereas the defensive forces prevail in the noninfectious phases). Moreover, fluid composition represents what is going on in the underlying mucoperiosteum, as will be described in Chap. 5.

Histopathological Classification

Histopathologically an infiltration by polymorphonuclear cells is a sign of acute inflammmation, and an infiltration by round cells is a sign of chronic inflammation. The term "chronic" implies infiltration of the mucoperiosteum by round cells or the cells of chronic inflammation. However, studies of the histopathological process of otitis media provide much more comprehensive knowledge and understanding that goes much further than the practical clinical terms "acute" and "chronic." These histopathological changes are described in Chap. 5.

Complications and Sequelae

In addition to the acute and chronic involvement of the mucoperiosteum by the otitis media process, there are potential complications and sequelae. A complication occurs when the inflammatory process extends beyond the mucoperiosteum. Sequelae refer to histopathological changes that are secondary to the otitis media process that remain within the mucoperiosteum and have the capacity or potential to develop a complication [11]. For example, the granulation tissue is a sequela (active sequela), but erosion of bone and fistula by the granulation tissue is a complication. In addition, the overall consequences of a localized problem (e.g., ossicular disruption causing conductive hearing loss) can have significant effects on a person and their relationship with others (lack of communication, isolation, learning problems, and so forth). Complications and sequelae are described in Table 1.1.

The Concept of Overall Involvement

An essential concept in otitis media is that the otitis media process involves not only the middle ear cavity but also the Eustachian tube and the mastoid. This manifests by changes in the whole mucoperiosteum covering these cavities—including osteitis of the underlying bone—(Fig. 1.3) and in the fluids that the cavities contain (middle ear effusions). In addition, effusions are not stagnant spillage but are dynamic

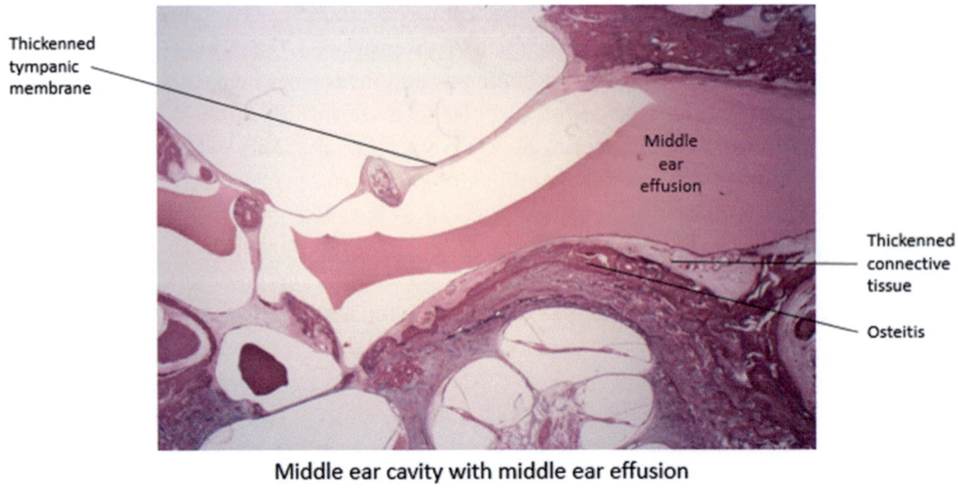

Fig. 1.3 Middle ear cavity with middle ear effusion (Copyright Marcos Y Goycoolea 2023; all rights reserved). The inflammatory process involves all the walls, cavities, and anatomical structures that these contain as well as the mucoperiosteum that lines these cavities and structures

forms that evolve and change in response to and as part of the overall mucoperiosteal changes [11, 12]. We see the inflammatory changes as a continuum, with some forms evolving or resolving into other forms and, at times, resulting in complications and sequelae, depending on the multiple factors involved. Viewed from this perspective, it becomes obvious that otitis media implies much more than fluid behind the tympanic membrane.

References

1. Paparella MM, Goycoolea MV, Jung TK. Otitis media with effusion. In: Paparella MM, Shumrick DA, Gluckman JL, Meyerhoff WL, editors. Otolaryngology, vol. II. Philadelphia: WB Saunders; 1991. p. 1317–42.
2. Goycoolea MV, Jung TK. Complications of suppurative otitis media. In: Paparella MM, Shumrick DA, Gluckman JL, Meyerhoff WL, editors. Otolaryngology, vol. II. Philadelphia: Saunders; 1991. p. 1381–403.
3. Goycoolea MV, Hueb MM, Ruah CB. Otitis Media. Definitions and terminology. In: Goycoolea MV, editor. Otitis media. The pathogenesis approach, The otolaryngologic clinics of NA, vol. 24. Philadelphia: WB Saunders; 1991. p. 757–61.
4. Klein JO, Tos M, Hussl B, et al. Definition and classification. Ann Otol Rhinol Laryngol. 1989;98(Suppl 139):10.
5. Bluestone C, Ogra P, Paparella M, et al. Definitions, terminology and classification of otitis media. In: Lim DJ, editor. Recent advances in otitis media. Report of the Seventh Research Conference. Ann Otol Rhinol Laryngol 2002; 111 (suppl.111): 8–18.
6. Liu YS, Lim DJ, Lang R, et al. Microorganisms in chronic otitis media with effusion. Ann Otol Rhinol Laryngol. 1976;85(Suppl 25):245.
7. Mawson SR. Latent mastoiditis. In: Mawson SR, editor. Diseases of the ear. Baltimore: Williams and Wilkins; 1963. p. 286, 344.
8. Paparella MM, Bluestone CD, Arnold W, et al. Definition and classification. Ann Otol Rhinol Laryngol. 1985;94(Suppl 116):8.
9. Paparella MM, Goycoolea MV, Bassiouni M, et al. Silent otitis media: clinical applications. Laryngoscope. 1986;96:978.
10. Paparella MM, Senturia BH, Bluestone CD, Lim DJ, et al. Report of the ad hoc committee on definition and classification of otitis media and otitis media with effusion. Ann Otol Rhinol Laryngol. 1980;89(Suppl 68):3–4.
11. Goycoolea MV, Paparella MM, Juhn SK, Carpenter AM. The cells involved in the middle ear defense system. Ann Otol Rhinol Laryngol. 1980;89(Suppl. 68):121–1980.
12. Goycoolea MV. Surgical procedures in different forms of otitis media. Summary of concepts. In: Goycoolea MV, et al., editors. Atlas of otologic surgery, vol. 1. New Delhi: Jaypee Brothers Medical Publishers Ltd; 2012. p. 463–89.

Otitis Media: Basic Concepts and Fundamentals

2

Sady Selaimen da Costa and Rafael da Costa Monsanto

"Acute pain of the ear, with continued strong fever, is to be dreaded, for there is danger that man may become delirious and die." **Hippocrates**

Introduction

The term "otitis media (OM)" describes a multifactorial inflammatory process that involves not only the middle ear but also the Eustachian tube and the mastoid. It is one of the most prevalent infectious diseases, being considered a worldwide public health problem [1–6]. In the United States alone, more than 5 billion dollars are spent annually to treat OM. It is estimated that 30 million dollars are spent toward antibiotic treatment of OM. In 2006, OM-related expenditure with outpatients alone in the United States was around 2.8 billion dollars [7]. The **National Ambulatory Medical Care Survey** and the **National Hospital Ambulatory Medical Care Survey** in the USA indicated that—in 2019 only—more than one million emergency department visits were patients with OM. In Germany (2014–2019), the population under 16 years of age only represented more than 900,000 episodes of OM, 15% of which were identified as recurrent [8, 9]. A study in Boston showed that, out of 17,000 pediatric outpatient consultations performed during the first year of life, acute otitis media (AOM) constituted one-third of them [10]. According to Lanphear et al. [11], the number of outpatient consultations due to OM in preschoolers, which has always been traditionally high, increased even more in the past decade. In the United States, half a million patients undergo tympanostomy tube surgery every year, either for OM with effusion (OME) or recurrent acute OM (AOM) that is refractory to conventional clinical treatments [12]. Tympanostomy tube insertion is the most frequent surgical procedure performed under general anesthesia in American children [13].

OM is a dynamic disease in which some forms lead to others, resulting at times in complications and sequelae. The progression of middle ear inflammation and tissue changes is influenced by many factors, including the anatomy and physiology of the middle ear, mastoid, and Eustachian tube, and the host's immunological response to environmental factors. In addition to local factors, this process is directly influenced not only by the neighboring anatomical structures but also by the host's relationship with the environment.

Classification and Definitions

Otitis media can be classified on a clinical or histopathological basis. Although these elements have been already addressed in Chap. 1, they will be duplicated here in order to stress their importance in the understanding of many concepts that will be discussed in the next paragraphs.

Clinical Classification

OM was classified on the clinical basis by both the "Task Force of the Fourth International Symposium of Otitis Media" (June 1987, Bal Harbor, Florida) and the "Task Force of the Seventh Symposium in 1999" [14]. For purposes of

S. S. da Costa (✉)
Otolaryngology and Head and Neck Surgery, School of Medicine, Federal University of Rio Grande do Sul, Porto Alegre, Rio Grande do Sul, Brazil

Service of Otolaryngology and Head and Neck Surgery, Hospital de Clínicas, Porto Alegre, Rio Grande do Sul, Brazil

Brazilian Association of Otorhinolaryngology and Cervico-Facial Surgery, São Paulo, SP, Brazil

Brazilian Society of Otology, São Paulo, SP, Brazil

International Hearing Foundation, Minneapolis, MN, USA

International Advisory Board—American Academy of Otolaryngology and Head & Neck Surgery, Alexandria, VA, USA

Collegium Oto-Rhino-Laryngologicum Amicitiae Sacrum, Helsinki, Finland

R. da Costa Monsanto
Department of Otolaryngology, Head & Neck Surgery, University of Minnesota, Minneapolis, MN, USA
e-mail: rdacosta@umn.edu

M. V. Goycoolea et al. (eds.), *Textbook of Otitis Media*, https://doi.org/10.1007/978-3-031-40949-3_2

consistency, we have followed this classification throughout this chapter. However, it is important to highlight that this is a working classification that allows a "common language" in the subject. These definitions represent a "consensus or working agreement" between different clinicians and investigators who have different viewpoints and perspectives. In other words, as Cicero stated centuries ago: "Every rational discussion of anything whatsoever should begin with a definition in order to make clear what is the subject of dispute."

The classification is as follows:

- Myringitis: Inflammation of the tympanic membrane that occurs alone or in association with external otitis or otitis media
- Acute suppurative otitis media (acute purulent otitis media, acute otitis media): A clinically identifiable infection of the middle ear with sudden onset and short duration
- Secretory otitis media (chronic otitis media (COM) with effusion, otitis media with effusion, nonsuppurative otitis media, catarrh, serous otitis media, serotympanum, mucoid otitis media, mucositis, mucotympanum): The presence of middle ear effusion (MEE) behind an intact tympanic membrane without any acute signs or symptoms. This broad term includes nonsuppurative or clinically noninfectious forms of OM. However, evidence suggests that effusions are, for the most part, infectious. Cultures of serous effusions yield between 22% and 52% positively, percentages that increase to 77.3% if PCR is used [15].
- Chronic suppurative otitis media (CSOM) (chronic otitis media): Chronic discharge from the middle ear through a perforation of the tympanic membrane. Suppurative refers to an active clinical infection. A perforation without discharge can be an inactive stage of the infection (but not of the underlying histopathological process).

Later, other terms were incorporated into this classification:

- Recurrent otitis media: Repeated episodes of acute otitis media in between periods of "apparent remission" (three episodes in 6 months or four episodes in 1 year)
- Silent (or "masked") otitis media: The presence of a chronic inflammatory process affecting the middle ear and the mastoid behind an intact tympanic membrane [16]

Additionally, OM can be classified based on its duration into acute (up to 3 weeks), subacute (from 3 weeks to 3 months), and chronic (more than 3 months) [17].

Middle Ear Effusions

Otitis media is associated with the presence of middle ear effusion. Three types of effusions can be found in OM cases: (1) serous, which comprises a thin, pale transudate; (2) mucoid, which is a thick exudate that is the result of goblet cells present in the metaplastic epithelium; and (3) purulent, which is characterized by the presence of inflammatory cells. In addition, two other types can be included: hemorrhagic, when red blood cells are present, and middle ear effusions that can appear as a combination of any of these.

Histopathological Classification

Histopathologically, the term "acute" refers to infiltration by polymorphonuclear cells, characterized by classic signs of acute inflammation. The term "chronic" implies the presence of clinically intractable tissue changes affecting the middle ear and/or the mastoid. Histopathological changes secondary to OM are described in Chap. 5.

Basic Concepts

Otitis media is a multifaceted pathology, and, therefore, its complete understanding can only be achieved through analysis and meticulous study of each of its small facets. These studies will have to be skilled enough to dissect the individual aspects of this disease without, however, denying the fact that they are organically and evolutionarily interconnected. Analogously, it would be as if we tried to understand a chain by examining only one of its links and extrapolating that to include every form of the disease. For this reason, we will dedicate the next paragraphs to dive deeper into the basic concepts that we consider essential for addressing issues relevant to the etiology, classification, pathogenesis, and treatment of this prevalent disease.

As mentioned in the "Introduction" section, OM is defined as the presence of an inflammatory process (which may or may not be infectious) affecting the middle ear and the mastoid. However, before navigating through the more specific aspects of this disease, it is important to further discuss definitions. To do so, it is necessary to review foundations related to general pathology and primary anatomy and physiology, which is critical to the global understanding of this entire fascinating process.

Inflammation is a nonspecific biological process that is inherent to organisms, which occurs in response to pathogenic stimuli of different nature. These stimuli include chemical, physical, or biological agents. Although inflammation is essentially a defense mechanism, it can sometimes result in damage to the body. In clinical practice, it is more frequently associated with trauma, infections, deposits of crystals, or antigen–antibody complexes.

The first description of inflammation, an important milestone in the history of medicine, is attributed to Celsus in the first century AD, who described four cardinal signs: **heat, redness, pain, and tumor**. A century later, Galen added another sign: loss of function. The inflammatory process begins with a more or less intense nonspecific tissue injury. As a result, there is local activation of the complement system, which is an enzymatic cascade, constituted by several elements endowed with biological activity [18].

At the histopathological level, two different stages of inflammation occur, namely, acute and chronic. The first is characterized by arteriolar and venular vasodilation, with increased hydrostatic pressure in the microcirculation and fluid leakage into the interstitial tissues (edema); increased permeability in microvascularization, by cell contraction in the venular endothelium (fenestration), with protein escape that decreases vascular oncotic pressure and favors the formation of inflammatory exudates in the tissue; migration of polymorphonuclear cells (chemotaxis), initially; and accumulation of macrophages at the injury site, approximately 24 h later. The chronic phase of inflammation begins 36–48 h after the inflammatory stimulus, where leukocyte migration continues, with a predominance of monocytes, lymphocytes, plasmocytes, and fibroblasts and signs of regeneration and reconstruction of the connective matrix. At the molecular level, there is protein denaturation, from lytic enzymes, released by the rupture of the lysosome membrane, due to the action of phagocytes. Protein alteration is the starting point for the activation of a series of systems that synthesize and release substances such as histamine, serotonin, bradykinin, prostaglandins, leukotrienes, and various chemotactic factors, which are responsible for vasodilation, increased vascular permeability, leukocyte migration, and platelet aggregation, in addition to other manifestations of the acute inflammatory process.

One of several characteristics that differentiate inflammation from infection is that the latter only exists in the presence of biological agents and microorganisms, which include bacteria, viruses, and fungi. The infectious process includes an inflammatory response of the body, but as seen, not every inflammatory process is caused by an infectious agent. An infection can be defined through Koch's principles, which establish criteria for relating a specific microorganism to a given disease: (1) the organism is regularly found in disease lesions, (2) the organism can be isolated in colonies on a solid medium, (3) inoculation of this culture causes lesions in an experimental animal, and (4) the organism can be recovered from lesions in the animals. In the last 10 years, advances in molecular biology have led to a change in Koch's postulates that link a particular characteristic of an organism to a particular disease: (1) the phenotype or characteristic should be associated with virulent strains of the microorganism and not with strains that are not virulent; (2) the specific inactivation of the gene associated with virulence, replacing the wild-type gene with a mutant, can lead to a measurable decrease in the pathogenicity of the microorganism; and (3) replacing the mutant gene with the wild-type gene can restore the pathogenicity of the organism.

The infectious process can be didactically divided into the following stages:

(a) *Interactions between the agent and the host*: The infectious agent can be exogenous, such as the flu virus or *Pseudomonas* bacteria, or endogenous, colonizing agents of the organism, which, for some reason, become pathogenic.
(b) *Tissue invasion*: Penetration of the microorganism can occur through a rupture of the epithelial barrier or, in some situations, through the intact epithelium. The microorganism can also enter through inhalation and ingestion.
(c) *Dissemination*: The microorganism propagates from the original site of entry to the adjacent or distant tissues. In any case, microorganisms only disseminate and proliferate if they overcome the host's defenses. Dissemination depends on the anatomical factors of the host and also on the characteristics of the invading agent.
(d) *Tissue damage*: The degree of tissue damage mainly depends on the pathogenicity of the invading agent. Damage due to the infectious process may be due to mechanical causes, cell death, pharmacological changes in metabolism, and exaggerated host responses.
(e) *Outcome*: This is the end result of the entire process. It can culminate in elimination of the infectious agent, death, or chronic colonization of the host [19].

In COM, the bacterial flora found in the middle ear is mixed, deriving either from the upper aerodigestive tract and/or through tympanic perforation. The Gram-negative bacteria *Pseudomonas aeruginosa* and *Hemophilus influenzae* are the most frequently identified bacteria in patients with COM, whereas the Gram-positive bacteria *Streptococcus pneumoniae* and *Staphylococcus aureus* and anaerobic microorganisms are less frequent [20].

There is a correlation between the strain of bacteria present in the middle ear during an episode of infection and those found in the nasopharynx. In children with upper airway infections, the microbiota of the upper aerodigestive tract seems to be less biodiverse as compared with to that in children without infections. The presence of lower airway disease (asthma, for example) is also correlated with lower biodiversity of the middle ear microbiota. After an episode of AOM, the bacteria in the middle ear cleft and nasopharynx can form a biofilm, thus passing to a saprophytic state in the local mucosa. A few days after the initial infection, the biofilm matrix is matured by the pathogen. The formation of biofilms protects bacterial colonies and also increases their defense against host immunity and antibiotic treatments. Thus, it seems to play a role in the chronicity of otitis media [6, 21].

This imbalance in the local bacterial flora plays a decisive role in the pathophysiology and perpetuation of COM. More recently, vaccinations against *Hemophilus influenzae* and *Streptococcus pneumoniae* seem to have increased the relevance of other bacteria in this process. *Alloiococcus otitidis* and *Turicella otitidis*, previously considered normal participants of the middle ear flora, have now been detected as possible pathogens in COM, including helping in the formation of biofilms.

Some bacteria seem to have the means of bypassing the host's immune pathways. The presence of intracellular Gram-positive cocci in the middle ear of children with OME has already been verified, which could imply greater bacterial resistance and perpetuation of inflammatory cascades. Innate immunity is the first line of defense against these microorganisms. It consists of nonspecific barriers (that is, not directed at specific pathogens) that range from mucociliary flow to proinflammatory molecules. Among these, we highlight the role of lysozymes, defensins, complement factors, cytokines, and chemokines in the middle ear. Bacteria and viruses act as triggers for the activation of inflammatory mediators in the nasopharynx, auditory tube, and middle ear cleft. Cellular receptors, such as Toll-like receptors (TLRs), detect the presence of pathogenic antigens, triggering an immunoinflammatory cascade. Adding certain bacterial biofilms (mainly *Pseudomonas aeruginosa* and *Staphylococcus aureus*) to the innate immune system receptors that are in a state of upregulation results in the middle ear being in a constant inflammatory state. The clinical effects of this prolonged inflammation translate into what we call chronic otitis media [6, 22, 23].

As for humoral immunity, its role in fighting middle ear infection is mainly through immunoglobulin (Ig)A (present in the mucous membranes) and IgG (found in tissue plasmocytes). These molecules act by adhering to the bacterial wall, in a process called "coating." One factor that could explain the colonization of *P. aeruginosa* in the middle ear clefts in COM is that this pathogen easily prevents the "coating" of immunoglobulins. Children with secretory COM seem to have deficiency in the local production of IgA, whose role in the defense of the middle ear mucosa is reduction of adherence and colonization of potentially pathogenic microorganisms. IgG facilitates the phagocytosis of microorganisms and stimulates the complement system. Some children with recurrent respiratory tract infections may also be deficient in specific IgGs, such as IgG2.

However, an individual's immune response and susceptibility to the chronicity of otitis media does not exclusively depend on the presence of microorganisms. Several other genetic and molecular factors as well as environmental exposure to pollution and cigarette smoke are well-established as an integral part of this process. External factors trigger the onset of an immune-mediated inflammatory cascade in the middle ear cleft. Models in rats also suggest that alterations in the recruitment of neutrophils and macrophages, as well as a deficient phagocytic function, seem to be linked to the prolongation of the inflammatory process in the middle ear. Deficiencies in the tympanic membrane plasminogen, in these specimens, lead to a deficient regeneration after an episode of tympanic perforation. On the other hand, inflammatory pathways that act in local protection against microorganisms, when overexpressed, lead to a high secretion of cytokines that can also lead to tissue damage and chronicity of the otitis media process.

Molecular biology techniques have identified several genes that act in the process of perpetuating the inflammation that occurs in AOM and its subsequent progression to COM. Middle ear inflammation caused by AOM reduces the availability of oxygen to the middle ear mucosa, perpetuating the inflammatory process through production of reactive oxygen species. Hypoxia is a trigger to the nuclear factor kappa B (NF-κB) pathway, releasing further inflammatory mediators such as vascular endothelial growth factor (VEGF), which increases neoangiogenesis, propagates inflammation, and results in production of exudates. This further results in the upregulation of inflammatory gene expression, propagating the inflammatory process and increasing the risks of development of COM. Individual variations in inflammatory response and gene expression also play a role in this process. Polymorphisms of the *FBX011* and *TGIF1* genes, for example, modulate transforming growth factor beta (TGF-β) expression during inflammatory processes. Interleukin (IL) regulatory genes have also been identified as participants in this process. In COM, polymorphisms of receptor regulatory genes, such as Toll-like and Nod-like, are also found in the middle ear mucosa that is in a state of upregulation. Overexpression of the inflammasome NLRP3 (nucleotide-binding domain, leucine-rich-containing family, pyrin domain–containing-3), a subtype of the Nod-like receptor, results in alterations in the inflammatory pathway of IL-1β and IL-18. The IL-17 inflammatory pathway also appears to be more active in the mucosa of patients with COM and sinusitis. Its deregulation can lead to overexpression of cytokines and chronic inflammation in chronic mucosal diseases. IL-17 also appears to be increased in the effusions and peripheral blood samples from children with OME. The Toll-like receptor (TLR)-2 is capable of recognizing lipoproteins from Gram-positive bacteria and mediating the inflammatory immune response. TLR-4, on the other hand, recognizes lipopolysaccharides, a cell membrane component of Gram-negative-bacteria present in the middle ear of patients with otitis media. It has been shown that the transtympanic injection of lipopolysaccharides into rat ears generates IL-1β production [24–26].

Conversely, some genes that mediate host innate immunity and signaling pathways, have anti-inflammatory properties and mediate middle ear regeneration after an acute inflammatory episode. The TGF-β pathway, for example, helps minimize a possible exaggerated inflammatory process, modulating the action of these proteins. The balance of molecular forces seems to be at the core of links that are still not well-understood in the pathogenesis of COM [27]. Mucins, which are highly glycosylated glycoproteins that are present in the granules of mucus-producing cells, can also prevent bacterial invasion in mouse ear models. Exposure of the human middle ear to live bacteria or bacterial lysates from *S. pneumonia*, non-typeable *H. influenzae*, and *Moraxella catarrhalis* induces regulation of mucin production via messenger RNA. These pathways are responsible for epithelial metaplasia that transforms the middle ear epithelium into mucus-producing cells. Pollution particles seem to have the same effect on the middle ear epithelium.

In acute otitis media, the ossicles undergo an initial reabsorption and posterior remodeling process, which can alter their sound conduction capacity. The activity of osteoclasts responsible for bone remodeling seems to be mediated by lipopolysaccharides. Ossicular destruction in the middle ear of rats is much more strong when the osteoprotegerin cytokine receptor is absent. Some pathogens have the ability to bypass the round window barrier and cause migration of inflammatory cells to the scala tympani. Pneumococcus, for example, when producing the pneumolysin enzyme, caused tissue damage in the inner ear of examined rats [28, 29].

Development, Anatomy, and Physiology of the Middle Ear

Phylogenetic Evolution of the Middle Ear

Communication is a key factor in the interrelationship between numerous animal groups. This ability came about as the demands for survival in the environment led to the emergence and improvement of structures adapted for the production and capture of sound energy. Thousands of years of evolution have made this exchange of information indissoluble, at first rudimentary, but largely responsible for the perpetuation of these animals in the biosphere. The structures responsible for sound production and capture show a wide range of variations across species.

Regarding the capture of sounds from the environment, the crucial moment in the refinement of the auditory system occurs when life-forms born in water start to inhabit the terrestrial environment. Thus, the sound waves previously captured through vibrations in the aquatic environment must overcome the resistance of a different medium, such as air, to be perceived. It was with the intention of improving this process that the evolution occurred from purely sensory structures in aquatic beings to those with much more elaborate auditory functions.

Among fish, the sense of hearing is demonstrably more evolved in the teleost group, including carp, catfish, and goldfish, which have auditory structures somewhat similar to those of tetrapods [30]. These fish have developed the so-called swim bladder, which works as a hydrophone that captures sound waves transmitted by the water [31]. From the anterior portion of this organ arises pairs of bones derived from the ribs, called the Weberian ossicles, which transmit and amplify vibrations to the perilymphatic space adjacent to the sensory epithelium of the saccule, a rudimentary hearing organ, in addition to its role in maintaining the vestibular balance [30, 32, 33]. This ingenious primitive mechanism of transmission of sound vibrations to a sensorial epithelium through a true bone bridge finds an analogy with the tympanic membrane and middle ear ossicles found in tetrapods. Conversely, other fish have openings called spiracles, which open into the mouth to transport oxygen from the external environment, in addition to the hyomandibular bone, which is adjacent to the inner ear and participates in sound transmission from the aquatic environment [32]. Theoretically, during the evolutionary process, the spiracles gave way to the middle ear and the hyomandibular bone was modified in the columella found in amphibians [34].

Even in the most primitive amphibians, a tympanic membrane is found on the outer surface of the head. In the middle ear, a single bone ("columella") connects the tympanic membrane to the inner ear. This bone is interposed between the superficial region of the head and the inner ear, and its most proximal portion has already been called stapes by some authors [35]. Similar to the eardrums of amphibians, in fish, communication takes place between the throat and the external environment through the spiracle, an orifice that is located adjacent to the hyomandibular bone and that transmits sound from the cranial vault to the inner ear [34]. This topographic location allows us to deduce the evolution of the spiracle into the auditory tube and middle ear chamber and the hyomandibular bone into the columella, as we find in most modern amphibians. In the most primitive reptiles, for example, lizards, some modifications have been observed. We observed that the columella remains isolated while communicating sounds to the inner ear, with no further involvement of the mandible bones. In addition, the columella can become complicated in its most external portion in the extracolumella when it becomes cartilaginous and adapts to the eardrum, thus playing the role of a sound-capturing organ. A small external depression is also observed, which would be an outline of the external acoustic meatus, compared to that found in more evolved vertebrates.

In addition to a well-developed cochlea, mammals as a whole also have particularities in the middle ear. In this chamber, there are three typical ossicles, namely, the malleus, the anvil, and the stirrup, whose basic function is to conduct and amplify many times the vibrations captured from the air environment. Much was debated about the phylogenetic origin of such structures, until a joint study between comparative anatomy and paleontology clarified the issue. As already mentioned, primitive reptiles had two bones forming the mandibular joint: the quadrate and the articular. It seems that the first mammals developed other bones of their own for articulation, with which such elements were relegated to exclusive functions in the middle ear. The quadrate, conserving its connection with the eardrum, became the malleus, whereas the articulation placed between it and the stapes was modified into the incus [32]. The biggest stimulus for these changes seems to have been improving hearing in order to capture prey and escape from predators not in the direct line of sight. This was especially striking for the first mammals that survived the tyranny of reptiles in the Mesozoic era, when nocturnal behavior emphasized auditory and olfactory perception [36].

Embryology

The Middle Ear Cleft

Between the third and seventh months of gestation, four endothelial pouches evaginate from the first branchial arch to form the tympanic cavity. At the points where these bags come into contact, mucous folds and suspensory ligaments of the ossicles are formed, thus generating compartmentalization of the middle ear [37].

The middle sac, occasionally with a contribution from the anterior sac, forms the epitympanum, as described by Jackler [38]. It is divided into three saccules: anterior, middle, and posterior. The middle saccule forms Prussak's space—bounded by Shrapnell's membrane, the neck, and the lateral process of the malleus and the lateral malleolar fold—and the superior incudal space (laterosuperior to the malleus head and body of the incus) [38].

The posterior saccule pneumatizes the petrous portion of the mastoid cell system. The anterior saccule often gives rise to the anterior compartment of the epitympanum. At these times, the anterior and posterior epitympanic compartments are confluent and separated from the anterior mesotympanum by the tensor tympani fold. The anterior epitympanum can also derive from the saccus anticus when the anterior saccule delays its expansion in this direction. When this occurs, the saccus anticus—which is already responsible for the formation of the anterior mesotympanum and the anterior space of Von Trölscht—also forms the so-called supratubal recess that freely communicates with the protympanum, since the tympanic tensor fold is incomplete in these cases. The saccus superior forms the inferior incudal space (below the body of the incus) and proceeds to pneumatize the squamous portion of the temporal bone. The limit of mastoid pneumatization proceeding from the superior saccus—squamous—and from the saccus medius—petrous—may become evident as a bone plate known as the petrosquamous plate or Körner's septum, a reference point in the posterior approach to the antrum. The saccus posticus forms the posterior mesotympanum and hypotympanum.

The Otic Capsule

The embryological development of the otic capsule is no less complex, being unique in several aspects. In all bones of the human body, the ossification process takes place concomitantly with the deposition of new cartilage plates. In the otic capsule, however, this pattern is not followed since ossification takes place only after the cartilaginous matrix has reached its definitive stage. By the time the ossification of the otic capsule is complete, all inner ear structures must have reached their adult size since the bony framework thus formed does not allow for further growth. The other peculiarity of this region (and of the ossicles) is that the endochondral bone initially formed will never be removed and replaced by the Haversian periosteal bone, as occurs in other bones. In this way, it will continue throughout life as a relatively avascular bone, of stony consistency, poor in osteogenic responses and exhibiting discreet remodeling activity [39].

The first ossification center appears around the cochlea when it reaches the adult state around the 16th week. The last center appears around the semicircular canals in the 20th week of intrauterine life. Once initiated, ossification progresses at an accelerated pace until the 23rd week when it should be complete, except for a small area over the posterior semicircular canal and a reniform area around the oval window and the ante fenestram fissula [40].

The Ossicles

In an 8-week-old embryo, the tympanic cavity corresponds to only the lower half of the future middle ear, and its upper half is completely filled with the mesenchymal tissue. The ossicles originate from small cartilaginous condensations found in the mesenchyme of the first and second branchial arches (hammer and incus predominantly of the first and stapes of the second branchial arch). Initially, the malleus, incus, and cartilaginous mandible are interconnected as the Meckel's cartilage of the first branchial arch, whereas the styloid process, hyoid bone, stapes, lenticular process of the incus, and malleus handle make up the so-called cartilage of the incus. Reichert's cartilage is formed in the second branchial arch. The primitive ossicles quickly separate from the cartilages from which they originated and begin independent development. The ossicles, as well as the otic capsule and the labyrinth, grow only until the first half of intrauterine life when, then, they ossify each one from a single ossification center that appears in the 16th week in the incus, between the 16th and 17th weeks in the malleus, and in the 18th week of intrauterine life in the stapes. Interestingly, the hammer and anvil remain solid and structurally constant after the ossification process. The stapes, on the other hand, develops a curious process of erosion and remodeling right after its ossification. The result of this process is the less robust and a much more delicate appearance of the adult stirrup when compared to the fetal one.

Anatomy

At the beginning of this chapter, we defined otitis media as an inflammatory process, infectious or noninfectious, located in the middle ear cleft. It is important to state that the term "middle ear cleft" should be preferred over "middle ear." As we will discuss below, this deliberate substitution has precise clinicopathological reasons, echoing modern concepts of classification and pathogenesis of otitis, not constituting, therefore, just a semantic caprice. This concern makes sense when we verify that the dimensions of the middle ear have been inadequately compressed to the region subjected to otomicroscopic inspection. In other words, the universe of inflammatory and infectious alterations that are characteristic of this disease would be limited to the mesotympanum, which is clearly exposed through the transparency or even the absence of the tympanic membrane. It is clear that the middle ear is multi-compartmental and that the mesotympanum represents only one of these compartments; however, we note that the conception of this scope is facilitated with the introduction of a new concept, namely, the middle ear cleft, which includes the bony portion of the auditory tube in all its extension as well as its opening next to the protympanum. This association, which may even be debatable from a strictly anatomical point of view, makes sense insofar as this entire complex reacts en bloc when it is subjected to an insult of an inflammatory nature.

The Middle Ear Cleft

When reviewing and summarizing the anatomy of this region, it is convenient to remember that it is represented by two aerated cavities, an anterior cuboid—the middle ear cleft with its three floors, epitympanum or attic, mesotympanum, and hypotympanum, and the tympanic portion of the auditory tube—and a grossly posterior pyramidal—the cell complex of the mastoid with its largest cell: the mastoid antrum. These cavities are continuous and are joined by a small triangular opening called an adyte. The upper boundary of the tympanic cavity is the tegmen tympani, a thin bony roof that separates it from the dura of the middle fossa, communicates inferiorly with another bony lamina in close relationship with the jugular gulf, anteriorly with the tympanic orifice of the Eustachian tube, which connects the middle ear with the nasopharynx, anteromedially with the vertical segment of the petrous portion of the internal carotid artery, posteriorly with the aditus, a passage that connects the upper floor of the tympanic cavity (the epitympanum or attic) with the cells of the mastoid, laterally with the tympanic membrane that separates it from the external auditory canal, and medially with the otic capsule that protects the inner ear and its two windows, oval and round, filled, respectively, by the footplate of the stapes and the membrane of the round window. In addition, the tympanic cavity has a set of small articulated bones, the ossicular chain, constituted by the malleus, incus, and stapes, which, attached to muscles and ligaments, transmits and amplifies the sounds that reach the tympanic membrane and are conducted to the eardrum through the oval window [41]. All the structures described above are covered by the respiratory epithelium, which modifies its ciliary and glandular histological structure according to the region it covers or the pathological alterations to which it adapts [41].

The Eustachian Tube

The Eustachian tube consists of a canal comprised part by bone and part by fibrocartilaginous tissue that runs from the nasopharynx to the middle ear. The bony part and the fibrocartilaginous part are connected at the level of the isthmus, which is the narrowest part of the Eustachian tube, with an approximate diameter of 1.5 mm. Thus, the Eustachian tube has an hourglass shape, with its tympanic and nasopharyngeal orifices being much larger than the isthmus. In adults, the Eustachian tube is longer, more inclined, and narrower than in children, which seems to indicate one of the reasons why AOM is more frequent in childhood, when there would be less protection against infected nasopharyngeal secretions. While the bony part of the Eustachian tube is, under normal conditions, permanently open, the fibrocartilaginous portion is closed most of the times. The fibrocartilaginous portion opening mechanism involves a complex muscular contraction in which the tensor and levator palate muscles play a preponderant role [42, 43]. These muscles contract during physiological actions such as swallowing, which happens every minute when the individual is awake and every 5 min when sleeping, by reflex arc, as well as the act of yawning. This dilation causes air to pass from the nasopharynx to the middle ear cleft, renewing its air content and balancing its pressure with atmospheric pressure, thus keeping the tympanic membrane and ossicular chain in a balanced position, with minimum impedance. The fibrocartilaginous portion of the Eustachian tube can also be passively dilated, as in the act of sneezing or in the Valsalva maneuver when, regardless of muscle action, air is forced into the middle ear cleft. The Eustachian tube has three main functions (ventilation, drainage, and protection) that will be discussed below.

Tubal Physiology

Ventilation of the Middle Ear and the Mastoid

As previously mentioned, the middle ear ossicles originated in vertebrates when they became terrestrial in order to recover the loss of energy resulting from the passage of sound from an air medium to a liquid medium or, in other words, to overcome the so-called interface of air–bone impedances [34]. To fulfill this function properly, the tympanic–ossicular system requires minimal friction between its various components and the presence of a physically inert environment. Such an environment is provided by the middle ear cleft, which is a structure analogous to a gas bag. Biological gas sacs are not rare in the animal world, as they are present in a multitude of forms and with the most varied functions: birds have respiratory air sacs that can extend to the bones in order to facilitate flight, fish have swim bladders with the function of floating, and mammals have intestines, paranasal sinuses, and tympanic cavities [34]. In fact, the middle ear cleft and the Eustachian tube can be roughly compared to the lower airways, with the former representing a sort of a "mini lung." All these air bags face a common problem, which is the possibility of collapsing if they fail to compensate for pressure variations verified inside them caused by the continuous gaseous exchanges carried out with the adjacent circulation. A second problem characteristic of these structures is the absolute need to maintain their self-cleaning properties. These two attributions, namely, ventilation and drainage, and the overlapping function of protection, are carried out in the middle ear by the Eustachian tube [44].

There are some general principles that regulate the so-called **gaseous economy** of the middle ear or any other bag of biological gas. The presence of a certain gas in a gaseous environment is expressed in terms of its partial pressure (PP). The sum of all the partial pressures of the gases that make up this mixture corresponds to the total pressure (TP) of this environment. Under normal conditions of temperature and pressure, ambient air is composed of a combination of five gases: nitrogen (N_2), argon (Ar), oxygen (O_2), carbon dioxide (CO_2), and water vapor. The same gases are found in different dilutions in blood, tissues and, obviously, in the tympanic cavity. Thus, the TP of ambient air at sea level is 10,000 mm of water (H_2O) or 760 mm of mercury (Hg), and its composition at a temperature of 37 °C (when saturated by water vapor) is 150 mmHg of O_2, practically zero CO_2, and approximately 563 mmHg N_2. The amount of water vapor present in one or another environment will dilute or concentrate the other gases in direct dependence on its degree of saturation and also on the function of the temperature where this system is found. The PP of gases present in the alveoli and the TP of inspired air are practically identical and in balance with those found in the arterial blood leaving the alveolar capillaries. As the blood transits the circulation toward the tissues, several changes occur in the composition of these gases. Thus, volumetrically speaking, O_2 is consumed more proportionally at the cellular level than CO_2 is produced [44]. This difference can be expressed through a typical equation or as the CO_2/O_2 respiratory quotient less than one (0.85). The PP of CO_2 is also influenced by the lower solubility of this gas in tissues and blood when compared to O_2. This asymmetry between the solubility and the shape of the O_2 and CO_2 saturation curves in the blood results in a sharp drop in O_2 levels and, on the other hand, in only a slight increase in the CO_2 concentration in the transition from the arterial to the venous compartment. For example, partial pressure of oxygen (PO_2) decreases from 102 mmHg in the alveoli to approximately 93 mmHg in arterial blood, plummeting to 38 mmHg in venous blood. On the other hand, partial pressure of carbon dioxide (PCO_2) has a slight increase from 39 mmHg in the alveoli to only 44 mmHg in the venous level. Thus, while the metabolic consumption of oxygen causes the PO_2 to decrease by 55 mmHg, the tissue production of carbon dioxide raises the PCO_2 by only 5 mmHg. This difference corresponds to a gaseous pressure deficit found in the venous blood that circulates in the tympanic cavity and with which this structure has to adapt. These PO_2 and PCO_2 variations between arterial and venous blood are not accompanied by corresponding changes in N_2 levels since this gas hardly participates in metabolic processes. As an example, the partial pressure of nitrogen (PN_2) of alveolar air is 572 mmHg, whereas in the venous system, this number rises by only 3 mmHg (575 mmHg). Thus, the behavior of the gases in the transition from alveolar air to the arterial and then venous system will show a considerable drop in PO_2, a slight increase in PCO_2, and maintenance of PN_2. Consequently, the venous environment surrounding the middle ear has, at sea level, a TP lower than the atmospheric pressure found in the light of the tympanic cavity [44].

The particles of a gas have the tendency to transfer from an environment of high pressure to that of low pressure until the balance between these two systems is reached. This transfer occurs in any permeable medium at rates specific to fluids, tissues, blood walls, and epithelial surfaces. In this way, the gases that fill the tympanic cavity "strive" to find a balance with the corresponding pressures in the adjacent venous capillaries, which effectively happens in relation to water vapor, O_2, and CO_2 in the middle ear cleft. Under these conditions, when we provoke a perforation in the tympanic membrane, the gaseous content of the middle ear quickly becomes similar to atmospheric air. Just a few moments after the closure of this perforation, the middle ear's gaseous concentration returns to find its balance point with the venous capillary system that surrounds it [44]. Assuming that the venous blood draining the middle ear has a gaseous PP and TP composition similar to that of the venous system, a steady state of equilibrium will finally be reached at slightly subatmospheric levels or around 56 mmHg (760 − 704 = 56). This theoretical composition would result in a pressure difference acting on the tympanic membrane (with an excess of 56 Hg external to it), which would be absolutely undesirable for the perfect functioning of the tympanic-ossicular mechanism. Thus, for the middle ear to obtain a TP equal to the atmospheric pressure, some physiological mechanism must be put into action, which effectively happens in the form of periodic openings of the Eustachian tube, causing the entry of an air bolus into the middle ear from the nasopharynx. As we discussed earlier, water and CO_2 moving from the mucosa into the tympanic cavity lumen and diffusing in the opposite direction of O_2 quickly equilibrate, leaving it to N_2 (which diffuses poorly and remains longer in the CT light) to partially offset this pressure deficit of 56 mmHg. Due to its diffusion and solubility characteristics, N_2 tends to present a higher PP in the middle ear than in blood, thus compensating for the discrepancy produced by the negative O_2/CO_2 equation. This extra dose of air that fills the middle ear and balances the extra- and intratympanic pressures is a direct consequence of the ventilatory function of the Eustachian tube. The amount of gas admitted (which occurs mainly during swallowing) is so proportionally small, when compared with the total amount of gas present in the light of the middle ear cleft, that the alterations in the PP of H_2O, O_2, and CO_2 resulting from it are practically imperceptible. In other words, the act of swallowing does not significantly modify the PP of these gases in the middle ear cleft [44]. On the other hand, the gas that penetrates the middle ear in this way is not exactly the same as the atmospheric one (since it is slightly modified by expiration) presenting in its composition: 99 mmHg of O_2, 36 mmHg of CO_2, 47 mm of H_2O, and 578 mmHg of N_2. Thus, the main gas inhaled by the middle ear at each swallow is N_2, which slowly diffuses into the adjacent circulation. As a result, a difference in the PP of N_2 is consistently maintained between the middle ear cleft and the circulation with an excess of around 56 mmHg for the former. This PP difference (light × circulation) systematically transfers N_2 molecules from the middle ear lumen to the circulation, consequently reducing the middle ear PN_2 until a new gush of air penetrates via the Eustachian tube, fulfilling what we call the ventilatory cycle of the middle ear cleft [44].

Normally, this process repeats itself periodically at a rate directly proportional to the diffusion of N_2. Even today, much is discussed in relation to the factors that positively or negatively modulate this rhythm. It has been suggested that the ventilatory function of the Eustachian tube is controlled by neuronal feedback circuits with sensory components capable of detecting both TP and PP alterations of the gases present in the middle ear and effector components that modulate the activities responsible for the opening of the Eustachian tube or the variation of peritubal pressures. Consubstantiating this hypothesis, a series of possible chemoreceptors and baroreceptors have been identified to be dispersed in the middle ear cleft. Likewise, afferent and efferent nerve pathways between the tympanic plexus and the respiratory subnucleus of the solitary tract, trigeminal motor nucleus, nucleus ambiguus, and peritubal musculature have been described in rabbits, cats, and chimpanzees [15, 45, 46]. Cantekin et al. [47] demonstrated that stimulation of the tympanic nerve in the middle ear of monkeys increased the electrical activity verified in the muscle fibers of the palate tensor in these animals. Shupak et al. [48], using animal models, confirmed these findings and showed that this electrical activity could be modified according to the concentration of different gases present in a gaseous mixture offered experimentally to these animals. Without the possibility of periodically renewing the air dispersed inside, all biological air pockets would definitely be doomed to collapse. In the middle ear cleft, a situation of negative pressure would imply, at first, a more dramatic repercussion on its only nonosseous wall: the tympanic membrane. In the tympanic membrane, these pressure deficiencies affect its dimer composition portion or the tympanic **pars flaccida** (Shrapnell's membrane) more strongly. Thus, this small triangular fraction of the tympanic membrane in opposition to the rest of the eardrum, which is highly inelastic under normal conditions, would function as a legitimate mirror of intratympanic pressure variations.

Even today, we have little information regarding the laws that govern the quantitative and qualitative physiological parameters of gas transfer from the nasopharynx to the middle ear. This lack of knowledge becomes critical as we wish to identify and compare operational ventilatory parameters in healthy and diseased ears. The volume of gas admitted in the middle ear cleft (which could be defined as the ventilatory coefficient) is equivalent to the product of the inhaled volume by the number of gaseous admissions per unit of time [44]. In humans, the Eustachian tube has a total length of around 4 cm and roughly resembles two conical portions joined by a narrow ring called the isthmus. The anterior and medial cone is formed by an elastic cartilage, which is collapsed most of the time. The posterior portion is bony and, therefore, rigid, when considered from a physiological point of view as an extension of the middle ear. These two portions meet at the isthmus, which is an annular structure 1–2 mm long and 0.6–1.2 mm in diameter. The cartilaginous portion is actively opened through contraction of the tensor palatini muscle during swallowing, yawning, or lateral movements of the mandible. This opening is in the order of 0.2 ms every 1 or 2 min (for a total of 3–4 min over 24 h). In general, a gas moves from one environment to another according to the difference in pressure between these two environments. During its course through the Eustachian tube, the air column coming from the nasopharynx finds its point of maximum obstruction next to the tubal isthmus. For practical purposes, once the air passes the isthmic region, it is already inside the middle ear. As we will see later, the geometry of the Eustachian tube is peculiar in the sense that its ventilatory and drainage functions do not interfere with each other. Drainage is carried out through the ciliary beat that generates a current of mucus that follows from the tympanic cavity to the nasopharynx through the floor of the Eustachian tube, whereas ventilation is processed in the opposite direction and in the middle and upper floors of the Eustachian tube (unless they meet—if blocked by mucus due to acute or subacute inflammatory events). The amount of gas that passes through the isthmus is a direct function of the pressure difference existing between the nasopharyngeal and tympanic ends of the Eustachian tube, the time this channel opens, and its dimensions (length × diameter). Elner [49] calculated that, under physiological and stable conditions, around 1–2 mL of gas penetrates the middle ear cleft every 24 h, a volume that would correspond to the daily gaseous loss from the middle ear lumen to the circulation. Even though there are small pressure fluctuations in the nasopharynx when we breathe, these variations are practically insignificant during swallowing and the consequent tube opening (1 mm H_2O). Thus, the main, if not the only, difference in pressure between the Eustachian tube and the nasopharynx is due to the continuous loss of gas from the middle ear to the adjacent circulation. As seen, if the middle ear transfers between 1 and 2 mL of gas into the circulation daily, and around 1000 swallows are performed every 24 h, it is calculated that 1–2 μL of gas diffuses into the circulation at intervals of 1–2 min and that the same volume is retrieved from the nasopharynx with each swallow. It is worth mentioning that not all swallows open the Eustachian tube, and, likewise, even if this occurs, there are occasions when this opening does not transfer air to the CT. The magnitude of the difference in pressure between the middle ear and the nasopharynx (due to the loss of gas by diffusion, as already mentioned) is also directly proportional to the total dimension of the middle ear cleft (Eustachian tube orifice, meso-, hypo-, and epitympanum, aditus, antrum, and, mainly, the mastoid cell complex). In a system with the mastoid normally pneumatized (12 cm^3), the difference in negative pressure resulting from the subtraction of 1–2 μL of gas due to diffusion is in the order of only 1–2 mm H_2O. This difference is so small that it provides the ability to passively move an air current across the tubal isthmus (1 mm in diameter × 2 mm in length for a total volume of 1–3 μL) in a time interval of only 0.2 ms [44]. From these considerations, it is suggested that this transfer of air from the nasopharynx to the middle ear should not be an exclusive consequence of passive events but that active mechanisms may also play a role (supporting or even the main) in this scenario. Sadé [44] even proposed a theoretical model in this sense: when the palate tensor muscle contracts during swallowing or yawning, the cartilaginous portion of the Eustachian tube opens, thus creating a new volume with a pressure lower than that found in the nasopharynx or middle ear, and the air coming from the nasopharynx quickly occupies this new volume. In the second phase, the tubal walls, after muscle contraction, tend to return to their resting state and do so by practically pushing this new air pocket toward the isthmus. Another force that could help in this regard would be the contraction that happens just milliseconds after the palate elevator muscle. In this sense, this muscle (whose function is not yet fully elucidated) is larger than the tensor palate. Furthermore, it is located on the Eustachian tube floor and contracts for a much longer period of time (0.45 s).

The existence of more than one operational mechanism in the equalization and maintenance of intra- and extratympanic pressures increases the degree of complexity of these functions. A logical and expected side effect of this refinement is the possibility of pathological phenomena interfering in several phases of these operations [2]. In other words, there is a need to identify and test a series of etiological variants (anatomical and/or functional) that are still little explored in the pathophysiology of the Eustachian tube and its most relevant consequences: **otitis media**.

Drainage

The drainage function allows the flow of middle ear secretions toward the nasopharynx through the Eustachian tube. It is basically exercised by three factors, namely, the mucociliary flow from the middle ear to the nasopharynx, the air renewal mechanism of the ventilatory function that can mobilize secretions in the same direction, and the surface tension of the secretions themselves [41].

All living surfaces of an organism are covered by an epithelium whose purpose is to offer protection to the deeper tissues. The epithelium that is in contact with the outside world is our skin; those that cover the internal organs are the mucous membranes or their analogues. The inner surface of organs such as the intestines and lungs are lined by a modified mucosa with flat cells. The life span of the cells that form part of this protective lining is limited, and, when dead, they are automatically removed from the organ in question. In order to keep this epithelial mantle intact, the cells of the deeper layers begin to divide, replacing the first ones, until they themselves mature and descend in a monotonously repetitive cycle. The anterior portion of the middle ear is covered by the respiratory epithelium whose cells live for a short time. Under inflammatory conditions, the epithelium differentiates with increased numbers of mucus-producing cells and hair cells. This occurs throughout the respiratory tract: nose, trachea, bronchi, etc. The excess of dead and desquamated cells must be constantly eliminated, otherwise it will accumulate and fill the cavity from where it originated. Nature has conveniently provided the middle ear cleft with a cleansing organ: the Eustachian tube. Both the middle ear cleft and the Eustachian tube are lined by a mucociliary system similar to that found in the trachea and bronchi. A thin layer of mucus produced by the secretory cells remains as a film on the surface of the cilia. These move synchronously, removing any middle ear debris similarly to a conveyor belt that travels through the Eustachian tube from the middle ear to the nasopharynx. The composition and consistency of this mucus layer is critical to the functioning of this entire self-cleaning mechanism. As an example, if a small particle of charcoal is placed in the anteroinferior part of the headland, through a perforation in the tympanic membrane, one can observe this particle being propelled toward the opening of the Eustachian tube.

Although this mucociliary "belt" system transports mucus unidirectionally from the middle ear via the Eustachian tube to the nasopharynx, some microorganisms can travel in the opposite direction and reach the middle ear cleft from the nasopharynx. The mechanism used by these microorganisms to reach the middle ear is one of the many issues that needs to be completely elucidated in the pathogenesis of otitis media. The resulting inflammatory reaction, otitis media, leads to the formation of an inflammatory exudate and usually causes cells to synthesize more mucus than usual. Again, this phenomenon is analogous to tracheobronchitis, or nasal secretions, produced during a common cold.

Long-lasting inflammation induces the middle ear mucosa to differentiate, through metaplastic processes, into a typically secretory epithelium (cylindrical, ciliated, pseudostratified, rich in goblet cells and submucosal glands), which, in turn, synthesizes greater amounts of mucus than under normal physiological conditions. In fact, some of these histopathological findings are found even in healthy ears since, at some point in life, they have been subjected to inflammatory insults. Only animals reared in germ-free conditions are completely devoid of such glands, cysts, or previous evidence of inflammation. This metaplastic alteration, with the consequent increase in mucus production, may cause it to completely fill the middle ear. The excessive presence of mucus in the respiratory tree can be easily eliminated by coughing or, in the case of the nasal cavity, by sneezing. However, through the narrow Eustachian tube, it is not possible to cough or sneeze, and, so, these secretions can accumulate inside the AF for several months. Why large amounts of mucus are not rapidly cleared from the middle ear by ciliary beating is still an intriguing question today, especially since cilia, although microscopic in size, are biologically quite robust organelles. Mechanical (adenoid) and functional tubal obstructions, changes in the rheological characteristics of secretions, primary or secondary ciliary dysfunction, mucus plugging, negative pressure, and vacuum are some of the hypotheses already tested in this regard. It is our conviction that the course developed by middle ear inflammatory processes from their most incipient phases to chronification can be compared to a theatrical play with a few main actors, several supporting characters, and countless extras. The latter, when analyzed separately, lack greater importance, but as a whole they acquire significance and are absolutely essential in triggering the entire process.

Protection

The protective function comprises defending the middle ear from sounds, especially from contaminated secretions from the nasopharynx. This objective is achieved by the fact that the Eustachian tube remains closed, opening only quickly during swallowing. On the other hand, it has an ascending path, making contamination in this direction difficult due to gravity, and a narrow isthmus that by capillarity protects the passage of secretions in the ascending direction. In addition, the air column inside it also makes it difficult for secretions to pass through. As its direction is from the middle ear to the nasopharynx, the mucociliary flow contributes to the protective function. This protective mechanism, however, can be overcome in some circumstances, such as positive pressure in the nasopharynx, which occurs when blowing your nose, sneezing, and crying. It should be remembered that swallowing, in the presence of severe nasal obstruction, also creates positive pressure in the nasopharynx when the palate contracts. Minor Eustachian tube obstructions that create moderately and slowly progressive negative pressure in the middle ear can lead to aspiration of nasopharyngeal secretions into this cavity. This does not happen when the obstruction is complete and of sudden installation because then the negative pressure contributes even more to aggravate the obstruction that caused it. In children, because they have a wider, more horizontal, and shorter Eustachian tube, the protective function is less effective. The fact that children spend more time lying down and younger ones eat in this posture facilitates the reflux of secretions and food into the middle ear. The vulnerability of the Eustachian tube in children has been identified as one of the factors responsible for the high incidence of AOM in this age group [41].

Aeration of the Middle Ear Cleft

Proctor [50] demonstrated that despite the fact that the middle ear cleft has its aeration ensured by the Eustachian tube, the paths taken by the air currents inside the tympanic cavity are narrow and sinuous. A series of mucous folds, ligaments, and parts of the ossicles make up the so-called tympanic diaphragm, practically separating the mesotympanum from the epitympanum and mastoid. This diaphragm comprises the head of the malleus, the body of the incus, the lateral and medial incudal folds, the anterior and lateral malleolar folds, and the tensor tympani fold. Only two narrow passages—the anterior and posterior tympanic isthmuses—pass through this diaphragm. The anterior isthmus is larger and more consistent, lying medially to the body of the incus, passing between the states and the tendon of the tensor tympani. When the medial incudal fold is present, a small posterior isthmus appears between this fold and the posterior tympanic wall. As previously mentioned, in less than 10% of individuals, the anterior epitympanum can be formed from the saccus anticus, opening a second air channel between the two compartments. From the point of view of embryological anatomy, the tympanic isthmus corresponds to an area where the structures of the first and second branchial arches come together, through which the first pharyngeal pouch extends to the extrabranchial region.

Epidemiology

AOM has an annual incidence rate of 10.8 episodes per 100 people per year. There are a number of factors that influence the incidence patterns among different locations, with the most critical one being socioeconomic conditions: developed regions (such as central Europe) have an average AOM incidence of 3.6 episodes per 100 people/year, whereas in less developed areas (such as sub-Saharan West Africa and Central Africa), the incidence rises up to 43.4/100 people/year [4]. Although AOM can affect people of all age groups, the peak of maximum prevalence occurs at the age of 4 years. Children are the most at risk in the first year of life, with an incidence of 45.3 episodes of AOM per 100 children per year [4].

The incidence and prevalence of otitis media with effusion (OME) might be even higher than those of AOM. Studies have shown that by the age of 3 years, virtually all children will have had experienced at least one episode of OME [6, 51, 52]. The peak of incidence/prevalence of chronic suppurative otitis media (CSOM), differently from than AOM and OME, has a less clear pattern: children <5 years represent only 22% of new cases every year. The average estimated global rate of new CSOM cases is 4.8 episodes per 1000 people or 31 million new cases every year [4].

In the last few decades, there has been a decrease in the global rates of OM due to two mains factors: the use (and abuse) of antibiotics and the development of strict treatment guidelines for OM, in addition to the introduction of pneumococcal conjugate vaccinations. Before these vaccinations were introduced in the United States, it was estimated that 95% of all children have had one or more middle ear infections before reaching the age of 5 [53]. Even if the overall rates of OM seemed to decrease, the prevalence of CSOM and the rates of complications arising from either AOM and CSOM have not changed significantly [6], suggesting that other factors may be involved in the pathogenesis of CSOM and the risks of developing such complications.

The first prevalence peak of AOM and OME (early childhood) is probably explained by the intrinsic aspects of the infant, such as its **immunological immaturity** and the anatomical and physiological characteristics of the **Eustachian tube**, which are typical for this age group (smaller, more horizontal and patent). Between the ages of 4 and 7, however, a series of events that are extraneous to the child and specific to the environment are responsible for causing a second peak in prevalence. At these ages, children are introduced to the community, increasing exposure to microbes and bacteria. Among all these circumstances, the most disastrous is **socialization** in day-care centers, kindergartens, and schools. Not only do children begin to share closed spaces but they also tend to share bottles, pacifiers, toys, and others; consequently, the risks of developing **recurrent cycles of infections of the upper airways** arise. Children with **immunodeficiencies** [54] and **adenoid hypertrophy** are also at an increased risk of developing OM.

Recent studies have confirmed the classical estimative of a higher frequency of OM in boys: MacIntyre et al. [55], in a cohort that followed more than 50,000 children in Canada from birth to the age of 3 years, found that 51.5% of AOM episodes occurred in **male** children. Around 20 months of age, the difference of prevalence between boys and girls seemed to become less evident. Moreover, the study found that children **born in the winter and spring seasons**, and those with **older siblings**, were at an increased risk of developing OM in their first year of life.

There is seasonal variation in the prevalence of OM, with an increase in incidence in winter and early spring. It is believed that the incidence of OM during winter is four times greater than in summer, coinciding with the increased incidence of respiratory viral infections. Uhari et al. [56], in a case–control study, found an association between respiratory syncytial virus infection in children and a higher risk of developing AOM.

Craniofacial malformations (Pierre Robin sequence, Treacher Collins syndrome, Crouzon's disease and, especially, cleft palate) are also associated with a higher risk of OM due to a malfunctioning ET [57]. According to Bluestone (1997), virtually all children with cleft palates have chronic effusion in the middle ear, which persists even after surgical reconstitution of the palate. Histopathological studies have shown that tubal dysfunction in these cases is due to functional dysfunction rather than an anatomical obstruction. Abnormalities in the constitution of the tubal cartilage, erratic insertion of the palate tensor muscle into the lateral layer of the Eustachian Tube, and deficiency in the amount of elastin can all compromise the tubal opening mechanism.

Children with **Down syndrome** are also at a risk of OM. In these situations, it seems that a decrease in the total length of the Eustachian tube when compared to those of normal individuals would facilitate the access of germs to the middle ear [57].

Ciliary diseases (Kartagener's syndrome) or diseases that affect the natural composition of the mucus (mucoviscidosis) can cause accumulation and stasis, and subsequent contamination of secretions, also predisposing to OM. O'Reilly et al. [58] studied 129 pediatric patients undergoing myringotomy for ventilation tubes. Among them, 50% had pepsin A in their middle ear fluid. This suggests that **extraesophageal reflux** may play a role in the complex process of the OM pathophysiology.

The social factors that may increase the risk of developing OM are low socioeconomic status, secondhand tobacco smoking, and the use of a pacifier. Conversely, breastfeeding is considered a protection factor, as it provides adequate nourishment and transmits acquired immunity from the mother [6].

A meta-analysis by Zhang et al. [59] evaluated the **risk factors for recurrent OM and COM**: Allergy or atopy (may be associated with Eustachian tube disfunction); upper respiratory tract infection; snoring (possibly related to adenoid hypertrophy); and previous history of recurrent OM or chronic OM. Schilder also listed social factors such as malnutrition, contaminated water, poor hygiene, overcrowding, human immunodeficiency virus (HIV) infection, tuberculosis, malaria and poor access to healthcare, which seem to increase the risk of chronicity and complications of OM in children [6]. Conversely, sex, breastfeeding, and the number of siblings did not result in increased risks of developing OM or chronic OM.

In adults, OM tends to affect people who have allergies [60], recurrent infections of the upper airways [60], nasopharyngeal tumors [61], and tobacco dependence [62]. Finkelstein et al. [63], in a study carried out in Israel, found a considerable number of adults with OME, which was mostly associated with the presence of recurrent sinus infections. Head and neck tumors, located especially at the nasopharynx, should be actively searched for in adult patients with OME, especially ones with unilateral disease [64]. Besides, patients with head and neck tumors treated with radiotherapy may develop temporary Eustachian tube dysfunction [65].

References

1. Brown OE, Meyerhoff WL. Complications and sequelae of chronic suppurative otitis media. Ann Otol Rhinol Laryngol. 1988;97(131):38–40.
2. Costa SS. Contribution to the study of chronic otitis media. Masters dissertation, Faculty of Medicine of Ribeirão Preto, USP. 1991.
3. Meyerhoff WL, Kim CG, Paparella MM. Pathology of chronic otitis media. Ann Otol Rhinol Laryngol. 1978;87(6):749–61.
4. Monasta L, Ronfani L, Marchetti F, Montico M, Vecchi Brumatti L, Bavcar A, Grasso D, Barbiero C, Tamburlini G. Burden of disease caused by otitis media: systematic review and global estimates. PLoS One. 2012;7(4):e36226. https://doi.org/10.1371/journal.pone.0036226. Epub 2012 Apr 30. PMID: 22558393; PMCID: PMC3340347.
5. Ohashi Y, Nakai Y, Ikeoka H, Esaki Y, Koshimo H, Onoyama Y. Mucosal pathology of an experimental otitis media with effusion after x-ray irradiation. Am J Otol. 1987;8:223–35.
6. Schilder AG, Chonmaitree T, Cripps AW, Rosenfeld RM, Casselbrant ML, Haggard MP, Venekamp RP. Otitis media. Nat Rev Dis Primers. 2016;2(1):16063. https://doi.org/10.1038/nrdp.2016.63. PMID: 27604644; PMCID: PMC7097351.
7. Hoffman HJ, Daly KA, Bainbridge KE, Casselbrant ML, Homøe P, Kvestad E, Kvaerner KJ, Vernacchio L. Panel 1: Epidemiology, natural history, and risk factors. Otolaryngol Head Neck Surg. 2013;148(4 Suppl):E1–E25. https://doi.org/10.1177/0194599812460984. PMID: 23536527.
8. Hu T, Done N, Petigara T, Mohanty S, Song Y, Liu Q, Lemus-Wirtz E, Signorovitch J, Sarpong E, Weiss T. Incidence of acute otitis media in children in the United States before and after the introduction of 7- and 13-valent pneumococcal conjugate vaccines during 1998–2018. BMC Infect Dis. 2022;22(1):294. https://doi.org/10.1186/s12879-022-07275-9. PMID: 35346092; PMCID: PMC8962537.
9. Hu T, Podmore B, Barnett R, Beier D, Galetzka W, Qizilbash N, Haeckl D, Weaver J, Boellinger T, Mihm S, Petigara T. Incidence of acute otitis media in children <6 years old in Germany during 2014–2019. BMC Pediatr. 2022;22(1):204. https://doi.org/10.1186/s12887-022-03270-w. PMID: 35418046; PMCID: PMC9006409.
10. Kvaerner KJ, Tambs K, Harris JR, Magnus P. Distribution and heritability of recurrent ear infections. Ann Otol Rhinol Laryngol. 1997;106(8):624–32.
11. Lanphear BP, Byrd RS, Auinger P, Hall CB. Increasing prevalence of recurrent otitis media among children in the United States. Pediatrics. 1997;99(3):E1.
12. Jefferson ND, Hunter LL. Contemporary guidelines for tympanostomy tube placement. Curr Treat Options Pediatr. 2016;2:224–35. https://doi.org/10.1007/s40746-016-0055-7.
13. Cullen KA, Hall MJ, Golosinskiy A. Ambulatory surgery in the United States, 2006. Natl Health Stat Report. 2009;11:1–25.
14. Bluestone CD, Gates GA, Klein JO, et al. Definitions, terminology, and classification of otitis media. Ann Otol Rhinol Laryngol. 2002;111(3_suppl):8–18. https://doi.org/10.1177/00034894021110S304.
15. Lim D, Jackson D, Bennet J. Human middle ear corpuscles: a light and electron microscopic study. Laryngoscope. 1975;85:1725–37.
16. Paparella MM, Goycoolea MV, Bassiouni M, Koutroupas S. Silent otitis media. Clinical applications. Laryngoscope. 1986;96(9):978–85.
17. Senturia BH, Bluestone CD, Lim DJ, Klein JO, Paradise JL. Report of the AD HOC Committee on definition and classification of otitis media and otitis media with effusion. Ann Otol Rhinol Laryngol. 1980;89(3_suppl):3–4. https://doi.org/10.1177/00034894800890S303.
18. Contran RS, Kumar V, Robbins. Robbins pathologic basis of disease. 5th ed. Saunders; 1994.
19. Schaechter M. Establishment of infectious diseases. In: Johnson JT, Yu VL, editors. Infections diseases and antimicrobial therapy of the ears, nose and throat, Chap 3. Saunders; 1997. p. 3–8.
20. Rovers MM, Schilder AG, Zielhuis GA, Rosenfeld RM. Otitis media. Lancet. 2004;363(9407):465–73. https://doi.org/10.1016/s0140-6736(04)15495-0.

21. Homøe P. Recurrent otorrhea in chronic suppurative otitis media: is biofilm the missing link? Eur Arch Otorhinolaryngology. 2017;274(7):2741–7. https://doi.org/10.1007/s00405-017-4586-8.
22. Cayé-Thomasen P, Hermansson A, Bakaletz L, Hellstrøm S, Kanzaki S, Kerschner J, et al. Panel 3. Otolaryngol Head Neck Surg. 2013;148(4_Suppl):E37–51. https://doi.org/10.1177/0194599813476257.
23. Mittal R, Lisi CV, Gerring R, Mittal J, Mathee K, Narasimhan G, Azad RK, Yao Q, Grati M, Yan D, Eshraghi AA, Angeli SI, Telischi FF, Liu XZ. Current concepts in the pathogenesis and treatment of chronic suppurative otitis media. J Med Microbiol. 2015;64(10):1103–16. https://doi.org/10.1099/jmm.0.000155. Epub 2015 Aug 5. PMID: 26248613; PMCID: PMC4835974.
24. Jotic A, Jesic S, Zivkovic M, Tomanovic N, Kuveljic J, Stankovic A. Polymorphisms in Toll-like receptors 2 and 4 genes and their expression in chronic suppurative otitis media. Auris Nasus Larynx. 2015;42(6):431–7. https://doi.org/10.1016/Jan.anl.2015.04.010. Epub 2015 Jun 6. PMID: 26055429.
25. Santos-Cortez RLP, Ehrlich GD, Ryan AF. Editorial: Otitis media genomics and the middle ear microbiome. Front Genet. 2021;12:763688. https://doi.org/10.3389/fgene.2021.763688. PMID: 34712274; PMCID: PMC8546293
26. Thornton RB, Hakansson A, Hood DW, Nokso-Koivisto J, Preciado D, Riesbeck K, Richmond PC, Su YC, Swords WE, Brockman KL. Panel 7 - Pathogenesis of otitis media - a review of the literature between 2015 and 2019. Int J Pediatr Otorhinolaryngol. 2020;130(Suppl 1):109838. https://doi.org/10.1016/j.ijporl.2019.109838. Epub 2019 Dec 19. PMID: 31879085; PMCID: PMC7062565.
27. Kariya S, Okano M, Zhao P, Maeda Y, Kataoka Y, Higaki T, Nishizaki K. NLRP3 inflammasome expression in lipopolysaccharide-induced otitis media. Acta Oto-Laryngologica. 2019; https://doi.org/10.1080/00016489.2018.1515499.
28. Lin S, Zhang W, Xu Y, Liu Q, Zhang W, Shao L. Gene expression analysis reveals immune and metabolic candidate pathways in the pathogenesis of chronic otitis media. Am J Transl Res. 2022;14(1):264–74. PMID: 35173843; PMCID: PMC8829611.
29. Preciado D, Granath A, Lin J, Val S, Kurabi A, Johnston N, Vijayasekaran S, Valdez T, Depireux D, Hermansson A. Panel 8: Report on recent advances in molecular and cellular biochemistry. Otolaryngol Head Neck Surg. 2017;156(4_Suppl):S106–13. https://doi.org/10.1177/0194599816658290. PMID: 28372528.
30. Kent GC. Comparative anatomy of the vertebrates. Saint Louis: The CV Mosby Co.; 1973. 414p
31. Baer JG. Cours d'anatomie comparée. Paris: Du Griffon, Neuchatel, Masson & CIE Editeurs; 1958. 206p
32. Romer AS, Parsons TS. The vertebrate body. Philadelphia: Sauders College Publishing; 1986. p. 679p.
33. Quay WB, Müller-Schwarze D. Functional histology of integumentary glandular regions in black-tailed deer (Odocoileus hemionus columbianus). J Mammal. 1970;51(4):675–94. https://doi.org/10.2307/1378294.
34. Costa SS, Souza M, Silva DB. Compared anatomy of the hearing organs and their phylogeny. RBM-ORL. 1996;3(3):135–43.
35. Adams JG. LXXXI tuberculosis of the middle ear and the temporal bone. Ann Otol Rhinol Laryngol. 1948;57(4):980–3. https://doi.org/10.1177/000348944805700404.
36. Strickberger MW. Evolution. Saint Louis: Jones and Bartlett Publishers; 1989. 569p
37. Levenson MJ, Michaels L, Parisier SC, Juarbe C. Congenital cholesteatomas in children: an embryologic correlation. Laryngoscope. 1988;98(9):949–55. https://doi.org/10.1288/00005537-198809000-00008.
38. Jackler RK. The surgical anatomy of cholesteatoma. Otolaryngol Clin North Am. 1989;22(5):883–96.
39. Gulya, A. J. Developmental anatomy of the ear. In Surgery of the ear, 4th edn., eds. Glasscock, M. E. & Shambaugh, G. E.. 1990; Philadelphia, PA: W. B. Saunders, pp. 5–33.
40. Bast TH, Anson BJ. The temporal bone and the ear. By Theodore H. Bast and Barry J. Anson. 1949. xviii + 478 pages, 165 figures. $12.00. Charles C. Thomas, Springfield, Illinois. Anat Rec. 1950;106:115–7. https://doi.org/10.1002/ar.1091060110.
41. Caldas N, Caldas S. Acute otitis media. In: Costa SS, et al., editors. Otorhinolaryngology: principles and practice. Porto Alegre: Artes Médicas; 1994.
42. Misurya VK, Shrivastava PK. Functional eustachian tuboplasty: a new surgical technique. Arch Otolaryngol. 1976;102(6):330–3. https://doi.org/10.1001/archotol.1976.00780110042003.
43. Ross MA. Functional anatomy of the tensor palati. Its relevance in cleft palate surgery. Arch Otolaryngol. 1971;93(1):1–3passim. https://doi.org/10.1001/archotol.1971.00770060033001.
44. Sadé J. Middle ear and auditory tube: middle ear clearance, gas exchange, and pressure regulation. Otolaryngol Head Neck Surg. 1997;116:499–524.
45. Nagai T, Tono T. Encapsulated nerve corpuscles in the human tympanic membrane. Arch Otorhinolaryngol. 1989;246:169–72.
46. Ylikoski J, Panula P. Neuropeptides in the middle ear mucosa. ORL J Report Spec. 1988;50:176–82.
47. Cantekin EI, Doyle WJ, Reichert TJ, et al. Dilation of the eustachian tube by electrical stimulation of the mandibular nerve. Ann Otol Rhinol Laryngol. 1979;88:40–51.
48. Shupak A, Tabari R. Effects of middle ear oxygen and carbon dioxide tensions on eustachian tube ventilatory function. Laryngoscope. 1996;106:221–4.
49. Elner A. Normal gas change in human middle ear. Ann Otol Rhinol Laryngol. 1976;85:161–4.
50. Proctor B. The development of the middle ear spaces and their surgical significance. J Laryngol Otol. 1964;78:631–47.
51. Tos M. Epidemiology and natural history of secretory otitis. Am J Otol. 1984;5(6):459–62. PMID: 6542752.
52. Williamson IG, et al. The natural history of otitis media with effusion—a three-year study of the incidence and prevalence of abnormal tympanograms in four South West Hampshire infant and first schools. J Laryngol Otol. 1994;108(11):930–4. https://doi.org/10.1017/s0022215100128567. PMID: 7829943.
53. Bluestone CD. Recent advances in the pathogenesis, diagnosis and management of otitis media. Pediatr Clin North Am. 1981;28(4):727–55.
54. Wilson NW, Hogan MB. Otitis media as a presenting complaint in childhood immunodeficiency diseases. Curr Allergy Asthma Rep. 2008;8(6):519–24. https://doi.org/10.1007/s11882-008-0095-6. PMID: 18940144.
55. Macintyre EA, Karr CJ, Koehoorn M, Demers P, Tamburic L, Lencar C, Brauer M. Otitis media incidence and risk factors in a population-based birth cohort. Paediatr Child Health. 2010;15(7):437–42. https://doi.org/10.1093/pch/15.7.437. PMID: 21886448; PMCID: PMC2948776
56. Uhari M, Hietala J, Tuokko H. Risk of acute otitis media in relation to the viral etiology of infections in children. Clin Infect Dis. 1995;20(3):521–4.
57. Austeng ME, Akre H, Øverland B, Abdelnoor M, Falkenberg ES, Kværner KJ. Otitis media with effusion in children with in Down syndrome. Int J Pediatr Otorhinolaryngol. 2013;77(8):1329–32. https://doi.org/10.1016/j.ijporl.2013.05.027. Epub 2013 Jun 20. PMID: 23790958.
58. O'Reilly RC, Soundar S, Tonb D, Bolling L, Yoo E, Nadal T, Grindle C, Field E, He Z. The role of gastric pepsin in the inflammatory cascade of pediatric otitis media. JAMA Otolaryngol Head Neck Surg. 2015;141(4):350–7. https://doi.org/10.1001/jamaoto.2014.3581. PMID: 25633964.

59. Zhang Y, Xu M, Zhang J, Zeng L, Wang Y, Zheng QY. Risk factors for chronic and recurrent otitis media-a meta-analysis. PLoS One. 2014;9(1):e86397. https://doi.org/10.1371/journal.pone.0086397. PMID: 24466073; PMCID: PMC3900534.
60. Tos M. Etiologic factors in secretory otitis. Adv Otorrhinolaryngol. 1988;40:57–64.
61. Wei WI. Serous otitis media in malignancies of the nasopharynx and maxilla. J Laryngol Otol. 1988;102(2):129–32.
62. Richardson MA. Upper airway complications of cigarette smoking. J Allergy Clin Immunol. 1988;81(5):1032–5.
63. Finkelstein Y, Ophir D, Talmi YP, et al. Adult-onset otitis media with effusion. Arch Otolaryngol Head Neck Surg. 1994;120:517–27.
64. Qureishi A, Lee Y, Belfield K, Birchall JP, Daniel M. Update on otitis media – prevention and treatment. Infect Drug Resist. 2014;7:15–24. https://doi.org/10.2147/IDR.S39637.
65. Hamd AA, Behiry EAEW, Atallah AT, et al. Effect of head and neck radiotherapy on the Eustachian tube functions. Egypt J Otolaryngol. 2020;36:39. https://doi.org/10.1186/s43163-020-00038-w.

Otitis Media and Human Efforts to Deal with It Through Time

3

Marcos V. Goycoolea and Mario Castro

Introduction

The study of diseases with a historical perspective strengthens scientific knowledge. When reviewing the prevalence, clinical manifestations, and complications of specific diseases through the centuries, the clever way in which physicians approached problems in spite of the scant knowledge available at a particular time often amazes us. While evaluating the different treatments used over the years, it is interesting to learn about them and the procedures involved, which, at times, were rediscovered and described as new. Some rediscoveries that were once considered a contribution, soon thereafter were discredited. Therefore, it is important to review the history in order to understand the present clinical approaches and why and how some treatments have failed and why they have been discarded. In addition, the study of significant changes in approaches and treatments over time has shown us that, what at one moment seems to be the final truth is eventually surpassed by new information, and the mistake of being strict and dogmatic in the approach to multifactorial diseases repeats itself in history, over and over again. This is the case of otitis media, which is a multifactorial, multifaceted disease that manifests in the middle ear, mastoid, and auditory (Eustachian) tube. It is the result of prevailing aggression against the body's defense system, the degree of which depends on the balance between these two opposing forces: the disease against the immunological defense system.

M. V. Goycoolea (✉)
Department of Otolaryngology, Clínica Universidad de Los Andes, Santiago, Chile

M. Castro
Chilean National Museum of Natural History, Santiago, Chile

Department of Morphology, Faculty of Medicine, Clínica Alemana-Universidad del Desarrollo, Santiago, Chile

Early Descriptions

The earliest written reports of otitis media and its complications can be traced to the Egyptians and Assyrians [1]. In the Ebers Papyrus (dating to the New Kingdom, circa 1550 BC), it is suggested that "For an ear that is suppurating, olive oil, frankincense and sea salt syringed into the ear" [2, 3]. In the Brugsch Papyrus (written "shortly" after), otitis is characterized as "fire in the heart of the ear" and the use of verdigris (copper sulfate) paste is recommended for its treatment [4]. In India's oldest available medical works, the Vedas (circa between 1500 and 500 BC), purulent discharge of the ear is described and, as in other cultures, ointments and powders are prescribed [5].

Hippocrates (460–370 BC) was well aware of otitis media and its consequences: "Children suffer from ear discharge, adults from deafness." Likewise, he was also aware of brain abscesses but not as caused by otitis media [6]. In fact, it was not until 1736 that Morgagni demonstrated that some brain abscesses were, in many cases, secondary to middle ear infection [7]. The Babylonian Talmud (352–427 AD) also refers to this subject [4, 5, 8].

The earliest Chinese written records of middle ear disease date to the Warring States period, 475–221 BC. In the *Inner Cannon of Huangdi*, two conditions analogous to complications of mastoiditis and cholesteatoma are described [9]. Likewise, in tractate Avodah Zarah (in the Talmud on page 28) when Rabbi Abahu suffered from earache, Rabbi Jochanan prescribed the following: "Otitis is to be treated by roasting upon embers the kidney of a goat collecting the juice and instilling it into the ear in a lukewarm state, not cold and not hot" [4, 5]. Paul of Aegina (625–690 AD), the great Byzantine Greek physician, recommended that: "Watery discharges of the ears may be dried up by applying to them wool with alum, or wine and honey" [4]. On the other hand, ancient Japanese texts also referred to otitis media. A text dating to about 982 AD, refers to "Te-ro," the chronic form of suppurative otitis media, whereas in the book *Sen-kin-po* (1315 AD), chronic otitis media with nasal polyposis is mentioned [5].

M. V. Goycoolea et al. (eds.), *Textbook of Otitis Media*, https://doi.org/10.1007/978-3-031-40949-3_3

Paleopathological Evidence of Otitis Media

The antiquity of infectious middle ear disease and its complications has been documented through different methodological approaches in several regions of the world. In 1909, Derry [10] reported two cases of mastoid infection in Egyptian skulls of the Predynastic/Early Dynastic and Coptic periods, whereas Elliot-Smith and Wood-Jones [11] described a perforation of the suprameatal triangle caused by a mastoid abscess in an Egyptian adult female skull of the New Empire period. In addition, in the Middle East, a probable case of chronic middle ear disease was reported in an early modern *Homo sapiens* skull found at Qafzeh, Israel. In this specimen, the extremity of the manubrium of the malleus and the long crus of the incus showed erosion, possibly because of chronic otitis media [12]. In 1973, Ziv et al. [13] reported an unusual bony mass obstruction of the right jugular bulb in a 2000-year-old temporal bone of an adult male found near Jerusalem. According to the authors, the most probable cause of the bony formation was thrombophlebitis of the internal jugular vein in the area of the jugular formation followed by calcification and ossification of the thrombus, all of which occurred as a complication of acute otitis media. Recently, Floreanova et al. [14] have examined the promontory of the tympanic cavity to check for either the presence or absence of bone remodeling in 229 individuals from 6 prehistoric and historic populations of the southern Levant (14,900 cal BP–1917 AD). They concluded that otitis media was highly prevalent in protohistoric populations (80%), followed by prehistoric populations (60.6%), and, finally, historic groups (50.4%). Furthermore, they attribute these fluctuations to lifestyle and climatic conditions.

In 1974, Lynn and Benitez [15] described perforated tympanic membranes in a 2600-year-old Egyptian male mummy, which they attribute to the sequelae of otitis media; later histological studies have confirmed this diagnosis [15, 16]. Additionally, Horne et al. [17] examined decalcified histological sections of a 4000-year-old Egyptian mummy's head and found sclerotic changes within the mastoid process, suggesting that the individual suffered from acute and probably chronic otitis media. At Dinkha Tepe, Iran (1300–300 BC), Rathbun and Mallin [18] found that 40% of the temporal bones studied had evidence of otitis media and mastoiditis.

In North America, Gregg et al. [19] carried out a comprehensive longitudinal radiological study of mastoid development in prehistoric Native Americans from the South Dakota area and found altered mastoids in 44% of Arikara burials and in 51.8% of Middle Plains Woodland people (Sioux and others). Additionally, Titche et al. [20] evaluated the prevalence of mastoid infection in ancient populations (Late Mogollon Pueblo) from Arizona (950–1450 AD) and reported that 17.3% of the skulls examined had decreased pneumatization (a reflection of having had otitis media during childhood). Gregg and Steele [21] studied the effects of otitis media on the human mastoid process by comparing present-day and four pre-Columbian populations from North America. Based on pneumatization patterns, they suggested that otitis media and its complications were more common and virulent in Native Americans who lived in the interval after contact with Europeans. In a more recent study (2018), Ochi et al. [22] have assessed mastoid development in Puebloan groups (850–1300 AD) using computed tomography (CT) scanning and found that 25% of the individuals examined showed arrested mastoid pneumatization. Homoe et al. [23] examined pneumatization in ancient Greenlandic Inuit temporal bones and found low frequencies of decreased pneumatization in the crania from the pre-European colonization period (before 1721 AD).

Studies in South America have also reported a high prevalence of decreased pneumatization in prehistoric and historic populations. Goycoolea et al. [24] estimated a 53.7% occurrence of infectious middle ear disease in prehistoric coastal groups (400–1450 AD) and a 47.9% in highland groups (400–1000 AD) from northern Chile. Besides, the skulls of historic (1500–1800 AD) coastal populations from southern Chile evaluated by Castro et al. [25] also showed a high prevalence of decreased pneumatization.

Among populations of European ancestry, Bruitjes [26] examined the auditory ossicles of 89 individuals from a leper cemetery in Chichester, England, dating from the twelfth century to about the mid-seventeenth century, and found erosive changes attributable to middle ear disease in 51% of them. Flohr et al. [27] used light microscopy and backscattered electron imaging to examine mastoid hypocellularity in 151 temporal bones from 99 individuals from an early medieval cemetery from Germany and found that 33.8% showed some type of mastoid alteration most probably due to middle ear infection. Krenz-Niedbala and Lukasik [28] examined 169 ear ossicles of children from an early medieval urban site (1000–1400 AD) and a postmedieval (1400–1700 AD) rural site located in Poland and found that 33.9% of them showed pathological changes, with a significantly higher frequency of altered bones at the early urban site. Likewise, the majority of the mastoid processes of children with pathological ear ossicles showed decreased pneumatization.

Recently (2021), Olivé-Busom et al. [29] have reported evidence of middle ear disease in an Islamic adolescent skull (10–15 years) from Castellón, Spain, dating to the Middle Ages (between the tenth and sixteenth centuries). The right temporal bone presents a perforation with relative smooth margins located superior to the mastoid process as well as abnormal pneumatization. According to the authors, the individual suffered from acute otitis media, which resulted in mastoiditis, and possibly received medical treatment for this condition [29].

There are sparse reports of complications of suppurative otitis media in ancient populations both in the clinical and anthropological literature. Singer [30] described a probable case of cholesteatoma in a skull from Boskop, South Africa (Late Stone Age), which eroded through the roof of the antrum and then produced a subdural abscess. Armentano et al. [31] described a unilateral cholesteatoma in a prehistoric skeleton found at La Cova des Pas (800–900 BC) on the island of Minorca, in the western Mediterranean Sea. Mays and Holst [32] documented the existence of cholesteatoma in a skull from Lincolnshire, England (late fifth to sixth centuries). Based on gross examination, low-power microscopy, and radiology, they suggest middle ear cholesteatoma because of chronic otitis media. Goycoolea et al. [24] described a case of mastoiditis with a temporal bone fistula in a prehistoric skull from the highlands of northern Chile (400–1000 AD). This case is described in Figs. 3.1, 3.2, and 3.3. The skull had a visible fistula above the entrance of the external ear canal and CT scans confirmed the fistula and showed signs of mastoiditis. It is of interest to mention that in this study, the data provided by the CT images were used to generate three-dimensional (3D) reconstructions with the specific characteristics of this individual skull [24]. On the other hand, facial reconstruction techniques were used to reconstruct the face of this individual [33, 34] to study how it looked.

In short, these reports from different times and different geographic locations confirm the high prevalence of this disease worldwide over the centuries. Moreover, Bluestone and Swarts [35] suggested that otitis media is primarily a human condition, which results from two evolutionary adaptations: being born too soon due to the development of a large fetal brain and the loss of facial prognathism due to speech.

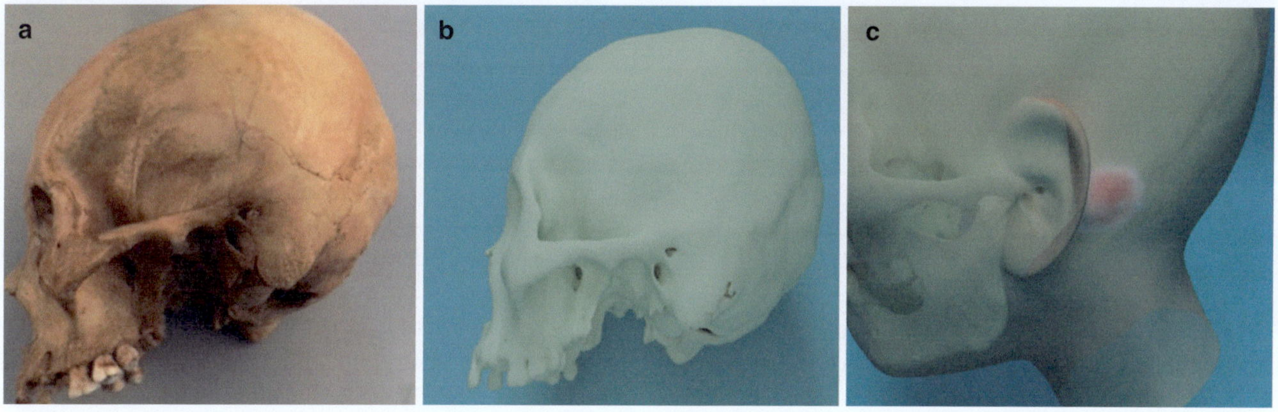

Fig. 3.1 (**a**) An ancient skull with a temporal bone fistula. (**b**) A model of the skull after 3D reconstruction. (**c**) 3D reconstruction of the skull with mastoiditis and abscess. (From: Goycoolea MV, Castro M, Galvez M, Montoya C, Fuentes J, Silva-Pinto V. Otitis media and mastoiditis in temporal bones of prehistoric Chilean populations. A paleopathological and paleoepidemiological study. *Acta Otolaryngol.* 2019;139:340–344 [24])

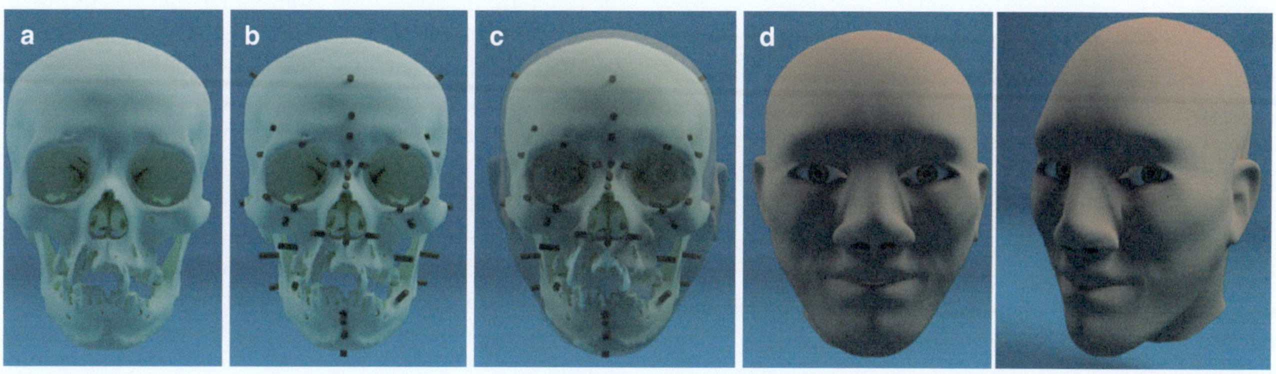

Fig. 3.2 Facial reconstruction of the skull with a temporal bone fistula. (**a**) 3D skull reconstruction from CT images. (**b**) Fiducial positioning for face reconstruction using forensic anthropological techniques. (**c**) Face reconstruction (transparency) allowing see-through. (**d**) Face reconstruction using forensic anthropological techniques [34]. (From: Goycoolea MV, Castro M, Galvez M, Montoya C, Fuentes J, Silva-Pinto V. Otitis media and mastoiditis in temporal bones of prehistoric Chilean populations. A paleopathological and paleoepidemiological study. *Acta Otolaryngol.* 2019;139:340–344 [24])

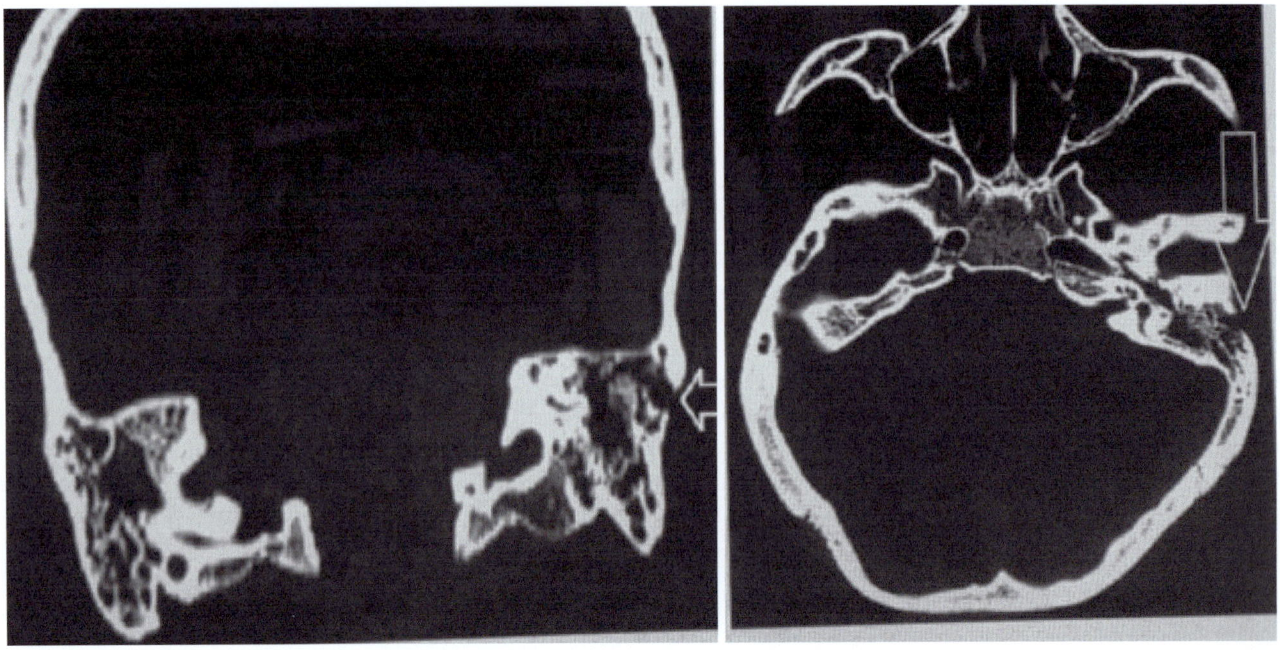

Fig. 3.3 Coronal and transaxial CT views showing fistula (arrows) and signs of mastoiditis. (From: Goycoolea MV, Castro M, Galvez M, Montoya C, Fuentes J, Silva-Pinto V. Otitis media and mastoiditis in temporal bones of prehistoric Chilean populations. A paleopathological and paleoepidemiological study. *Acta Otolaryngol.* 2019;139:340–344 [24])

Early Surgical Approaches

The following paragraph was the initial paragraph of my PhD thesis in the Department of Anatomy (major in histology) at the University of Minnesota in 1978. It was also my initial paragraph in our chapter "Complications of Suppurative Otitis Media" in Michael Paparella's textbook *Otolaryngology* in 1991 [8]. "Man's efforts to treat and control otitis media and its complications go far back into history. Ear surgery proper, or surgery for ear complications may have started as early as the Neolithic age [36], in which there is evidence that trephining was performed in skulls." Since then, we have studied different skeletal remains and trephinations in Chile and in Perú, and, to date, we have never found a skull in which trephination was seemingly performed for relief from suppuration. We found evidence of mastoiditis and even mastoid fistula (as described earlier), but although we looked purposefully we never found evidence of even a mastoidectomy procedure. It was not until 2022 when Sonia Díaz-Navarro and a team from the University of Valladolid [37] reported the discovery of a skull with evidence of otitis media and mastoiditis and also with two bilateral perforations, suggestive of mastoidectomy procedures. Moreover, the findings suggest that the individual survived both procedures. The skull was found at the El Pendón site in northern Spain and dates to the fourth millennium BC. This would be not only the first mastoidectomy but also the earliest surgical ear intervention in the history of mankind.

The earliest evidence of trepanation, according to Díaz-Navarro [38], is documented during the Mesolithic period in Europe and Northern Africa; however, most cases are dated to the Late Neolithic and the Bronze Age [38]. Again, whether trepanation was for relief from suppuration in the mastoid region or from intracranial conditions is unknown [39]. Trephining was also practiced in Peru over a long period of time by various cultural groups from circa 400 BC through the emergence of the Inca Empire, circa 1400 AD [40].

Except for the possibility of trephination as a treatment for relief from suppuration from either the mastoid or the brain, and the case of the possible mastoidectomy that has been described, ancient treatments, up to the early eighteenth century, were local treatments with different agents, some of which have been described previously. Although "seemingly of little use" and limited to local treatment, it is interesting to note that compounds such as alum (acidic and astringent), copper (a natural antimicrobial), sea salt (antimicrobial, antifungal), virgin olive oil and wine (strong bactericidal activity [41]), and frankincense (antimicrobial activity) have all been demonstrated to have antimicrobial and/or antifungal activities.

From the Greeks to the Middle Ages, descriptions of otitis media and local remedies persisted and no significant modifications occurred until the seventeenth century when therapy changes began to establish the basis for significant treatment developments in the eighteenth century.

The Greek physician Claudius Galenus (Pergamon, Asia Minor, 131 AD) recognized the importance of draining an infected ear [42]. Nevertheless, Jean Riolanus the Younger [4, 42] published the first documented recommendation of mastoidectomy. In 1649, he advocated perforation of the mastoid process in cases of Eustachian tube obstruction and when inflammatory pulsating pain occupied the back of the ear [39, 43]. By the eighteenth century, clinical and surgical treatments began to improve and concepts like Eustachian tube function and aeration of the middle ear and mastoid cavities brought about new treatments. Valsalva advocated evacuating pus from the middle ear by performing "Valsalva's experiment" [7]. In 1724, Edmé-Gilles Guyot, a French postmaster, physician, and inventor, described the catheterization of the Eustachian tube through the mouth and behind the palate [7]. In 1741, Archibald Cleland described catheterization of the Eustachian tube by way of the nose [39].

As early as 1720, Eli, a French ear surgeon, employed myringotomy [7]. However, Sir Astley Cooper (1768–1841) was the first to propose clear indications for this procedure and practiced it on a large scale (an opening to permit a free passage of air to and from the tympanum, perhaps a substitute for the Eustachian tube) [43]. Given that the procedure was also used for other pathological conditions not related to drainage of middle ear effusions, and since the opening tended to heal, the application of myringotomy fluctuated in terms of indications and usage. It was not until 1954 when Beverly Armstrong developed the pressure equalization (PE) tube that maintained the myringotomy puncture open.

In 1736, Jean-Louis Petit (1674–1750) adapted the process of trephining the infected mastoid cavity with a chisel (simple mastoidectomy) [7]. He suggested not only opening the infected tract but also actively opening the bone in order to evacuate the pus [42]. Drainage of mastoid infections through a retroauricular incision were inaugurated by William Wilde (1815–1876), father of the writer Oscar Wilde, and Toynbee (1815–1866), "to give an early exit to imprisoned fluid," and "for a thorough evacuation of the contents of the mastoid," respectively [39, 42]. By 1873, Herman Schwartze (1837–1900) established mastoid surgery proper (as we know it today) for relief from suppuration by drilling the mastoid cortex and reaching the antrum using chisels, gouges, and curettes [7, 42].

Ernst Kuster (1838–1930) described radical mastoidectomy in order to promote complete drainage. He removed the "infected focuses" and posterior wall [39]. Ernst von Bergmann (1836–1907) went even further and converted the antrum, attic, middle ear, and external canal into one cavity [39]. The next step was mastoidectomy with radical surgery while preserving the middle ear ossicles and tympanic membrane by Janssen (1893), Korner and Scheide (1894), and Bondy (1910), thus promoting modified mastoidectomy with preservation of the tense part of the tympanic membrane and ossicles. German otologists Wullstein and Zollner pioneered rehabilitation surgery for deafness due to chronic middle ear and mastoid disease. Wullstein pioneered tympanoplasty to improve hearing in 1953 [7], but PE tubes were developed by Beverly Armstrong in 1954 [43].

What followed medically and surgically to the present—including the revolutionary developments of microscopic and endoscopic surgery, audiology, imagenology, immunology, vaccines, bacteriology, and virology—is described throughout both volumes of this book.

An additional important point to mention here is the improvements in diagnosis that came along in the first half of the nineteenth century, such as the inventions of the ear speculum, the ear mirror, and the otoscope. According to Politzer [5]: "Neuburg deserves the credit for having developed the first unslit speculum, though its invention is usually attributed to Ignaz Gruber. Hoffman of Burgsteinfurt deserves credit for introducing a light source in the form of a centrally pierced concave mirror. And the otoscope was invented by Toynbee." A direct observation made a significant improvement in diagnostic capabilities.

The greatest and most radical and dramatic change in the history of treatment of otitis media was the advent of antimicrobials. In 1869, Politzer (published in 1909) [44] stated that " the temporal bone has four sides: the outside is bounded by life, from which there comes the opening of the auditory canal, one form of our appreciation of what life means; on the other three sides it is bounded by death" (Lederer [6]). This statement attests the potential seriousness of otitis media in the pre-antibiotic era, based on its anatomic location and boundaries with vital structures.

It was the advent of antimicrobials in the mid-twentieth century, an increasing awareness on the part of physicians and the public regarding the seriousness of the disease, and diagnostic methods yielding earlier identification and treatment that immensely reduced the incidence of otitis media's lethal complications. Prior to the antibiotic era, intracranial complications occurred in 2.3% of cases of acute or chronic otitis media [45] and acute otitis media resulted in mastoiditis in 25–50% of cases [46]. Antibiotics reduced these figures to 0.15% in 1962 [47], to 0.02% in 1985 [48], and 0.04% [49] and that of coalescent mastoiditis to 0.4% in 1959 [50]. However, we must keep in mind that despite this dramatic decline, the complication rate in acute mastoiditis still fluctuates between 8% and 12% [51, 52].

An example of the dramatic decline in mortality is the Couville report [53] (from Los Angeles County Hospital in 1955). At this institution, between 1928 and 1933 (in the pre-antibiotic era), 25 out of every 1000 deaths were due to intracranial complications of otitis media; between 1949 and 1954 (in the antibiotic era), only 25 of every 10,000 deaths were due to such complications. This represents a 90% decrease in mortality. Despite this overall decline in the incidence of intracranial complications of otitis media with significant mortality, complications and/or sequelae of otitis media in the temporal bone still occur [8] and may have devastating effects both physiologically and psychologically, resulting in behavioral complications. Unfortunately, severe complications still exist, and this cannot be emphasized enough. Although statistical figures have shown a dramatic decrease in the absolute number of cases, those cases that still occur represent a significant medical problem. This is in part because physicians confronted with such uncommon cases are obviously less experienced and may underestimate or misinterpret the symptoms. In many cases, not even the best treatment available will prevent sequelae. The important factors in the development of complications include the infecting agent, the adequacy and timing of treatment, and the resistance of the infected individual.

In 1986, Samuel et al. [54] reported their experience in South Africa with 224 otogenic intracranial complications occurring between 1978 and 1983. Their patient population comprised of African Blacks with neglected otitis media, who were reluctant to seek medical attention. Their study described a prevalent problem at the time in many areas of the world, which was earlier overlooked. This, in part, reflects the contrast between the incidence and prevalence of complications in a group of low socioeconomic status (analogous to patients in the pre-antibiotic era) and the results of the same group when subsequently exposed to modern medicine. Of the 85,000 patients attending the ear, nose, and throat clinic, Samuel et al. reported that 335 had otogenic complications, of which 224 presented with intracranial complications. Meningitis occurred in 83 patients, brain abscesses in 53, extradural abscesses in 49, and lateral sinus thrombosis in 39. Of these patients, 74% were children and young adults (under 15 years of age), which reflects conditions of the pre-antibiotic era. The current trend is that of an increasing number of complications in older individuals with chronic otitis. With modern-day evaluation and treatment, the overall mortality of 14% reported by these investigators compares highly favorably with the more current reports of European and American groups. Although both prevention and early diagnosis are crucial, this study, most importantly, reflects the difference that modern-day medicine can make and is supportive of arguments for the existence of sophisticated facilities.

Going back to our previous considerations about antimicrobials and their dramatic effect on otitis media, even if otitis media continued to have a high incidence and prevalence, antimicrobials have changed the predominance of mortality toward morbidity. The success of antibiotics has been such that they are used on a massive scale to treat all forms of otitis media, and, since the 1960s [55], different forms of "prophylactic treatments" have appeared. These consist of low doses once a day for a prolonged length of time and have been prescribed for recurrent and serous otitis media [56–59]. This view coincided with the emergence of "evidence-based medicine," which supported these successful results.

The exaggerated use of antimicrobials, in detriment to other reasonable alternatives, has led some authors to argue that in many cases it could suffice to remove the effusions and that low-dose antimicrobials could attenuate and not eradicate the underlying inflammatory process [60]. The fact that antimicrobials would achieve maintained therapeutic tissue levels was also pointed out [61] as was the importance of individualizing the patients rather than fitting them into rigid forms of treatment that would not cover all factors of a multifactorial disease such as otitis media [62].

Notwithstanding these considerations, "statistical evidence" indicated that the use of antimicrobials in low or high doses for prolonged periods was effective. A large part of the medical community proceeded accordingly, and, literally, millions of children all over the world were treated with antimicrobials on a massive scale. No too long after new resistant strains of bacteria began making their appearance, together with studies that suggested that antimicrobial usefulness was only marginal, statistical evidence shifted to support such observations, and the same medical community proceeded accordingly and millions of children around the world with bacterial otitis media were treated without antibiotics. When new evidence suggested that a middle point was the solution, there arose the need to define in which individuals antimicrobials would work and in which they would not [62].

Finally, the invention of the ear speculum, the ear mirror, and the otoscope made a significant improvement in our diagnostic capabilities, although they have been far from ideal. Authors in the United States reported the reexamination of children diagnosed with acute otitis media and found a 50% diagnostic error [63]. The same situation occurred in Chile with children over 3 months of age referred to the otolaryngologist for otitis media evaluation. Of 522 patients referred, only in 41.9% of them was the diagnosis of otitis media confirmed [64]. If we extrapolate these findings, one wonders about the validity of statistical studies conducted by data collectors who do not see patients.

Currently, there is a more holistic approach, as pathogenesis has become relevant, examination skills are improving, patients are evaluated as individuals and not as numbers, and bacteriology and virology have made great improvements. A significant advance is vaccine development, discussed at length in this book. Moreover, pronicity factors, immunological status, environmental factors (day-care center conditions etc.) are better defined, and our aims are toward awareness, timely intervention, and prevention. We believe that this approach will produce substantial results and become a new revolutionary change. As far as the future is concerned, we expect the definition of genetic factors and a shift from a preventive to a predictive medical intervention (before things happen), with treatments based on pathogenesis and drug therapy based on pharmacogenomics.

Summary

Here, the history of otitis media has been briefly reviewed. In ancient times, middle ear disease was seemingly limited to identification and local treatments of its complications and approaches used. By the eighteenth century, human understanding evolved in terms of the concepts of aeration and the need for drainage either via the Eustachian tube or myringotomy and, if needed, mastoidectomy. Initially developed as a method for drilling the bone with the intent of removing the infection, mastoidectomy was followed by conservative and reconstructive surgery. The profound change that occurred with antimicrobials is examined, and changes from mortality to morbidity are described, with the understanding that complications still occur. A point is delivered about the risk of rigid and dogmatic treatments in multifactorial diseases. Advances in vaccines, a pathogenesis approach, individualization, awareness, and knowledge of environmental and inherent factors are expected to spark a new revolution in the comprehension of otitis media. Finally, as far as the future is concerned, we expect the definition of genetic factors and a shift from a preventive to a predictive medical intervention (before things happen), with treatments based on pathogenesis and drug therapy on pharmacogenomics.

References

1. Thompson RC. Assyrian prescriptions for diseases of the ear. J R Asiat Soc Great Br Irel. 1931;1:1–25.
2. Ebbell B. The Papyrus Ebers: the greatest Egyptian medical document. Copenhagen: Levin & Munksgaard; 1937.
3. Pahor AL. Ear, nose and throat in ancient Egypt. Part II. J Laryngol Otol. 1992;106:773–9.
4. Stevenson RS, Guthrie D. A history of otolaryngology. London: E & S Livingstone; 1949.
5. Politzer A. History of otology. Phoenix, AZ: Collumella Press; 1981. (Translation of the original German edition of 1907, Stuttgart, Enke Verlag).
6. Lederer FL. The development of otorhinolaryngology and bronchoesophagology. Int Coll Surg. 1960;33:83–97.
7. Hanckel R. History of otology. J South Carolina Med Assoc. 1962;58:11–6.
8. Goycoolea MV, Jung TK. Complications of suppurative otitis media. In: Paparella MM, Shumrick DA, Gluckman JL, Meyerhoff WL, editors. Otolaryngology, vol. II. Philadelphia: Saunders; 1991. p. 1381–403.
9. Zhang X, Zhao Y, Niu Y, Wang Z, Zeng W. Two probable cases of mastoiditis in a cemetery from the Warring States to Han Dynasty (475 BCE–220 CE) in Qufu, Shandong Province, China. Int J Paleopathol. 2020;30:77–84.
10. Derry DE. Anatomical report. Bull Archaeol Survey Nubia. 1909;3:29–52.
11. Elliot-Smith G, Woodjones, F. Report on the human remains. Archaeol. Survey Nubia. Report 1907–1908. Volume II. Ministry of Finance, Survey Department, Cairo 1910.
12. Arensburg B, Nathan H. A propos de deux osselets de l'oreille moyenne d'un Neandertaloide trouves a Qafzeh (Israel). Anthropologie. 1972;76:301–8.
13. Ziv M, Arensburg B, Leventon G, Nathan H. Ossification in the jugular foramen in an ancient skull. Arch Otolaryngol. 1973;97:406–9.
14. Floreanova K, Gilat E, Koren I, May H. Ear infection prevalence in prehistoric and historic populations of the southern Levant: a new diagnostic method. Int J Osteoarchaeol. 2020;30:449–57.
15. Lynn GE, Benítez JT. Temporal bone preservation in a 2,600-year-old Egyptian mummy. Science. 1974;183:200–2.
16. Benitez JT. Otopathology of Egyptian mummy Pum II: final report. J Laryngol Otol. 1988;102:485–90.
17. Horne PD, MacKay A, Jahn AF, Hawke M. Histologic processing and examination of a 4,000-year-old human temporal bone. Arch Otolaryngol. 1976;102:713–5.
18. Ratbun TA, Mallin R. Middle ear disease in a prehistoric Iranian population. Bull N Y Acad Med. 1977;53:901–5.
19. Gregg JB, Steele JP, Holzhueter A. Roentgenographic evaluation of temporal bones from South Dakota Indian Burials. Am J Phys Anthropol. 1965;23:51–62.
20. Titche LL, Coulthard SW, Wachter RD, Thies AC, Harries LL. Prevalence of mastoid infection in prehistoric Arizona Indians. Am J Phys Anthropol. 1981;56:269–73.
21. Gregg JB, Steele JP. Mastoid development in ancient and modern populations. JAMA. 1982;248(4):459–64.
22. Ochi JW, Wheelbarger L, Dautenhahn LW. Chronic otitis media in ancient American Indians. Pediatrics. 2018;141:e20172308.
23. Homoe P, Rasmussen N, Lynnerup N, Skovgaard LT. Statistical model estimating the occurrence of otitis media from temporal bone pneumatization. Ann Otol Rhinol Laryngol. 1994;103:469–73.
24. Goycoolea MV, Castro M, Galvez M, Montoya C, Fuentes J, Silva-Pinto V. Otitis media and mastoiditis in temporal bones of prehistoric Chilean populations. A paleopathological and paleoepidemiological study. Acta Otolaryngol. 2019;139:340–4.
25. Castro M, Goycoolea MV, Silva-Pinto V. External ear canal exostosis and otitis media in temporal bones of prehistoric and historic Chilean populations. A paleopathological and paleoepidemiological study. Acta Otolaryngol. 2017;137:365–9.
26. Bruitjes TD. The auditory ossicles in human skeletal remains from a leper cemetery in Chichester, England. J Archaeol Sci. 1990;17:627–33.
27. Flohr S, Hartmann AK, Kierdorf H, Schultz M, Kierdorf U. Histomorphological study on hypocellularity in mastoid processes from archaeological human skeletons. Int J Paleopathol. 2019;26:27–36.
28. Krenz-Niedbala M, Lukasik S. Skeletal evidence for otitis media in Mediaeval and post-Mediaeval children from Poland, Central Europe. Int J Ostearchaeol. 2017;27:375–86.
29. Olivé-Busom J, López-Costas O, Quer-Agustí M, Márquez-Grant N, Kirchner H. Evidence of otitis media and mastoiditis in a Medieval Islamic skeleton from Spain and possible implications for ancient surgical treatment of the condition. Int J Paleopathol. 2021;32:17–22.
30. Singer R. Pathology in the temporal bone of the Boskop skull. S Afr Archaeol Bull. 1961;16:103–4.
31. Armentano N, Malgosa A, Martínez B, Abelló P, Delago M, Prats-Muñoz G, Isidro A. Unilateral cholesteatoma in the first millenium BC. Otol Neurotol. 2013;35:561–4.
32. Mays S, Holst M. Palaeo-otology of cholesteatoma. Int J Osteoarchaeol. 2006;16:1–15.

33. Grant GT. Craniomaxillofacial reconstruction based on 3D modeling. In: Greenberg AM, editor. Digital technologics in craniomaxillofacial surgey. New York: Springer; 2018. p. 55–65.
34. Cebellin MS. Reconstrucción del rostro con técnicas de antropología forense. Rev Chungara. 1983;11:173–82.
35. Bluestone CD, Swarts JD. Human evolutionary history: consequences for the pathogenesis of otitis media. Otolaryngol Head Neck Surg. 2010;143:739–44.
36. Parry NT. Prehistoric man and his early efforts to combat disease, vol. 8 and 15. The Medical Press and Circular; 1914. p. 1–8.
37. Díaz-Navarro S, Tejedor-Rodríguez C, Arcusa-Magallón H, Pastor-Vazquez JF, et al. The first otologic surgery in a skull from El Pendón site (Reinoso, Northern Spain). Sci Rep. 2022;12:2537. www.nature.com/scientificreports.
38. Díaz-Navarro S. A new case of prehistoric trepanation and scalping in the Iberian Peninsula: the tomb of La Saga (Cáseda, Navarre). Int J Osteoarchaeol. 2021;31:88–98.
39. Sonnenschein R. A brief consideration of the history of the development of mastoidectomy. Ann Med Hist. 1935;8:500–10.
40. Andrushko VA, Verano JW. Prehistoric trepanation in the Cuzco region of Peru: a view into an ancient Andean practice. Am J Phys Anthropol. 2008;137:4–13.
41. Medina E, Romero C, Brenes M, De Castro A. Antimicrobial activity of oil, vinegar, and various beverages against foodborne pathogens. J Food Prot. 2007;70:1194–9.
42. Ferreira Bento R, de Oliveira Fonseca AC. A brief history of mastoidectomy. Int Arch Otorhinolaryngol. 2013;17:168–78.
43. Rimmer J, Giddings CE, Weir N. The history of myringotomy and grommets. Ear Nose Throat J. 2020;99(IS):2s–7s.
44. Politzer A. Diseases of the ear. 5th ed. London: Baillere, Tindall and Cox; 1909.
45. Dowes JD. Complications of infections of the middle ear. In: Scott-Brown WG, Ballantyle J, Groves J, editors. Diseases of the ear, nose, and throat, vol. 2. London: Butterworths; 1965. p. 478–554.
46. Boies L. Acute mastoiditis: 1931–1941. Trans Laryngol Rhinol Otol. 1942;48:97.
47. Jeanes A. Otogenic intracranial suppuration. J Laryngol Otol. 1962;76:388–402.
48. Prellner K, Rydell R. Acute mastoiditis. Influence of antibiotic treatment on the bacterial spectrum. Acta Otolaryngol (Stockh). 1985;99:293–7.
49. Palva T, Virtanen H, Mäkinen J. Acute and latent mastoiditis in children. J Laryngol Otol. 1985;99:127–36.
50. Palva T, Pulkinen K. Mastoiditis. J Laryngol Otol. 1959;73:573–88.
51. Ginsburg CM, Rudoy R, Nelson JD. Acute mastoiditis in infants and children. Clin Pediatr. 1980;19:549–53.
52. Pfaltz CR, Griesemer C. Complications of acute middle ear infections. Ann Otol Rhinol Laryngol Suppl. 1984;112:133–6.
53. Couville CB. Symposium: Intracranial complications of otitis media and mastoiditis in the antibiotic era. Laryngoscope. 1955;65:31–46.
54. Samuel J, Fernandes CM, Steinberg JL. Intracranial otogenic complications: a persisting problem. Laryngoscope. 1986;96:272–8.
55. Ensign PR, Urbanich EM, Moran M. Prophylaxis for otitis media in an Indian population. Am J Public Health. 1960;50:195–9.
56. Maynard JE, Fleshman JK, Tschopp CF. Otitis media in Alaska Eskimo children: prospective evaluation of chemoprophylaxis. JAMA. 1972;219:597–9.
57. Perrin J, Charney E, MacWhinney JB, McInerny TK, Miller RL, Nazarian LF. Sulfisoxazole as chemoprophylaxis for recurrent otitis media. A double-blind crossover study in pediatric practice. N Engl J Med. 1974;291:664–7.
58. Klein JO. Antimicrobial prophylaxis for recurrent acute otitis media. Pediatr Ann. 1984;13:398–403.
59. Bluestone CD. Antimicrobial therapy for otitis media with effusion ("secretory" otitis media). Pediatr Ann. 1984;13:405–10.
60. Paparella MM, Jung TK, Goycoolea MV. Otitis media with effusion. In: Paparella MM, Shumrick DA, Gluckman JL, Meyerhoff WL, editors. Otolaryngology, vol. II. Philadelphia: Saunders; 1991. p. 1317–42.
61. Canafax DM, Giebink GS. Clinical and pharmacokinetic basis for the antimicrobial treatment of otitis media. In: Goycoolea MV, editor. Otitis media, Otolaryngologic Clinics of North America, vol. 24. Philadelphia: Saunders; 1991. p. 957–66.
62. Goycoolea MV. Otitis media and evidence-based medicine. What acute otitis media? What medicine and which evidence? (Article in Spanish. Summary in English). Consideraciones sobre la otitis media aguda y la medicina basada en evidencias. ¿Cuál otitis media aguda; cual medicina y cuales evidencias? Rev Med Clin Condes. 2009;20(4):395–9.
63. Pichichero ME, Poole MD. Assesing diagnostic accuracy and tympanocentesis skills in the management of otitis media. Arch Pediatr Adolesc Med. 2001;155:1137–42.
64. Rosenblut A, Santolaya ME, González P, Corbalán V, Avendaño LF, Martínez MA, Hormazabal JC. Bacterial and viral etiology of acute otitis media in Chilean children. Pediatr Infect Dis J. 2001;20:501–7.

Development and Anatomy of the Human Middle Ear

4

Charlotte M. Burford, Hannah L. Cornwall, Matthew R. B. Farr, Claudia M. Santoni, and Matthew J. Mason

Introduction

Contained within the temporal bone of the skull, the human middle ear (Fig. 4.1) comprises a system of air-filled cavities, communicating with the nasopharynx via the Eustachian tube (ET). The tympanic membrane, which separates the external meatus from the middle ear cavity, is connected to the malleus, the first of the three auditory ossicles that cross the cavity to communicate acoustic vibrations through to the inner ear. Two small muscles insert on these ossicles, and several nerves and arteries pass through or near the middle ear region. The embryology and adult anatomy of this region is complex and is often covered only briefly in textbooks and undergraduate medical courses. However, a knowledge of the structural relationships between the middle ear components and how they come to develop is essential for understanding the function of the middle ear and necessary for the provision of safe surgical care. In this chapter, we shall first review middle ear development before providing an overview of adult anatomy.

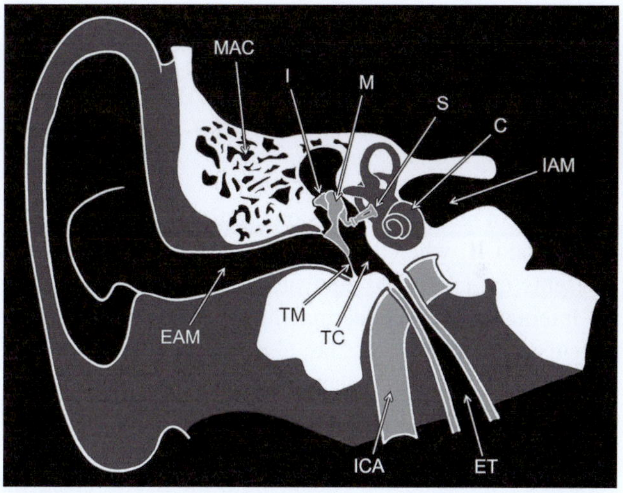

Fig. 4.1 Diagrammatic representation of the human peripheral auditory system (right ear, anterior view). *C*, cochlea; *EAM*, external auditory meatus; *ET*, Eustachian tube; *I*, incus; *IAM*, internal auditory meatus; *ICA*, internal carotid artery; *M*, malleus; *MAC*, mastoid air cells; *S*, stapes; *TC*, tympanic cavity; *TM*, tympanic membrane

Part 1: Development of the Middle Ear

Many of the structures in the head and neck, including the middle ear, arise from the pharyngeal apparatus of the embryo (Fig. 4.2). The development of the pharyngeal apparatus and its derivatives has been extensively studied in humans and model organisms [1, 2]. In humans, this apparatus consists of five pairs of arches (I–IV and VI), which form on either side of the developing foregut. Although it is sometimes said that arch V appears transiently but then regresses, it has recently been argued that it does not exist at all in amniotes and the other arches should be renumbered accordingly [3]. The arches appear between the second and fourth weeks of gestation [4]. Externally, the pharyngeal arches are covered with ectoderm, which invaginates to form pharyn-

C. M. Burford
East Kent Hospitals University NHS Foundation Trust, Ashford, Kent, UK
e-mail: charlotte.burford1@nhs.net

H. L. Cornwall
Department of Paediatrics, Ysbyty Gwynedd, Bangor, Wales, UK

M. R. B. Farr
Doncaster Royal Infirmary, Doncaster, S Yorks, UK

C. M. Santoni
School of Clinical Medicine, University of Cambridge, Cambridge, Cambridgeshire, UK
e-mail: cms208@cantab.ac.uk

M. J. Mason (✉)
Department of Physiology, Development & Neuroscience, University of Cambridge, Cambridge, Cambridgeshire, UK
e-mail: mjm68@cam.ac.uk

M. V. Goycoolea et al. (eds.), *Textbook of Otitis Media*, https://doi.org/10.1007/978-3-031-40949-3_4

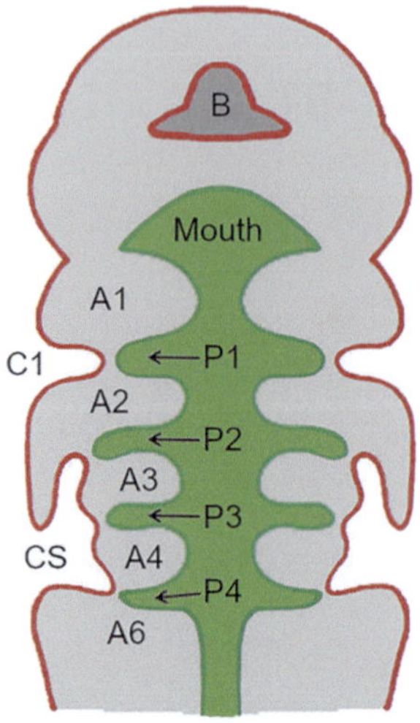

Fig. 4.2 Schematic representation of the pharyngeal apparatus in the early human embryo, demonstrating the contribution of the three germ cell layers (ectoderm = red; mesoderm = grey; endoderm = green). *A1–6*, pharyngeal arches I–VI (there is no arch V); *B*, developing brain; *C1*, pharyngeal cleft I; *CS*, cervical sinus; *P1–4*, pharyngeal pouches I–IV

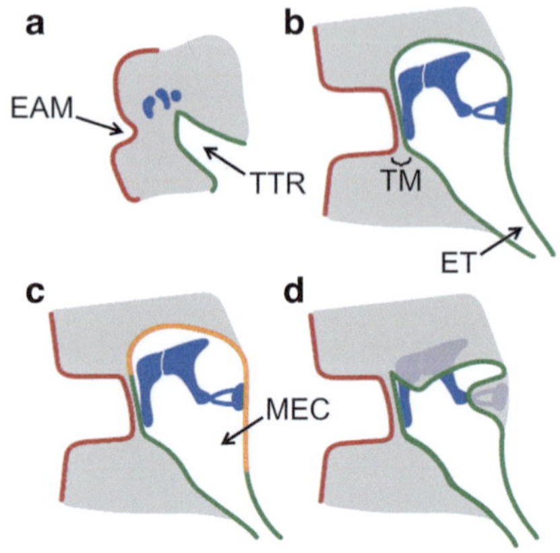

Fig. 4.3 Development of the middle ear cavity. (**a**) Middle ear ossicles condensing between the developing external auditory meatus and the tubotympanic recess. (**b**) The 'endodermal model' in which the epithelium covering the middle ear cavity is entirely endodermal in origin. (**c**) The 'mesenchymal model' in which the epithelium of the dorsal wall and the majority of the lateral wall of the middle ear cavity is mesenchymal in origin, whereas the medial and ventral walls are endodermal. (**d**) Schematic representation of the findings of van Waegeningh et al. [7] in a 25-week fetus, which these authors argue support the 'endodermal model'. They demonstrated cavitation to the level of the ossicles, with the loose connective tissue remaining in the attic, and a continuous epithelium. Both models agree that the tympanic membrane is composed of thin layers of ectoderm, endoderm and mesoderm. *EAM*, external auditory meatus; *ET*, Eustachian tube; *MEC*, middle ear cavity; *TM*, tympanic membrane; *TTR*, tubotympanic recess. Red = ectoderm; green = endoderm; grey = mesoderm; blue = auditory ossicles; orange = middle ear cavity lining that has undergone a mesenchymal-to-epithelial transition

geal clefts. In humans, there is one distinct cleft (I) between arches I and II, whereas a cavity called the cervical sinus represents the combined equivalent of clefts II, III and IV [1]. Internally, the endodermal lining invaginates to form pharyngeal pouches. As the clefts and pouches extend towards one another, they separate the intervening tissue into individual pharyngeal arches.

The mesodermal core of the pharyngeal arches is surrounded by mesenchyme arising from the neural crest, the cells of which migrate from the nearby regions on the dorsal surface of the developing neural tube. The mesodermal core gives rise to the skeletal muscles, whereas the neural crest-derived cells give rise to bony and cartilaginous structures, including the ossicles. The arches are innervated by particular cranial nerves, for example V_3 to the first arch and VII to the second: this has been used to establish muscle origins. The pharyngeal arches grow at differing rates during embryogenesis, leading to arches I and II becoming larger in volume than the others. These two arches and their intervening structures will form the components of the external and middle ears, discussed in more detail in the following sections.

Congenital abnormalities of pharyngeal arch development are well-documented in the literature. They can include complete fistulae arising from the first or second pharyngeal cleft and pouch contact, persisting into postnatal life [5].

The Middle Ear Cavity

Using the chick as a model of ear development, studies have shown that the endodermal cells of the pharyngeal pouches contain a web of actin fibres, just underneath their apical plasma membranes, which appear to constrain pouch morphology and direct their expansion [6]. The first pharyngeal pouch in humans begins to expand outwards in the fourth week of gestation [4]. It forms the tubotympanic recess, a wing-like evagination of the pharynx, which will ultimately form the middle ear cavity and Eustachian tube (ET; Figs. 4.3a and 4.4). The second pharyngeal pouch may contribute to the posterior part of the recess, at least initially [8–10]. The recess reaches the middle ear region at around 8 weeks of gestation and reaches the antrum by 29 weeks [11].

The middle ear region is originally entirely cellular in the embryo. As it develops, an epithelium-lined cavity forms, filled with fluid in utero, which contains the auditory ossicles and the inserting tendons of the two middle ear muscles. This process by which the mesenchymal cells surrounding the ossicles and developing muscle tendons are cleared is referred to as 'cavitation'. In humans, cavitation begins in the third month and is normally complete prior to birth [12], although residual mesenchyme is frequently found in both children and adults (see later).

How exactly cavitation happens is linked to the origins of the epithelial lining of the middle ear cavity. There are two main theories describing the origins of the middle ear cavity epithelium: the 'endodermal model' and the 'mesenchymal model' [13]. The endodermal model, originally proposed by

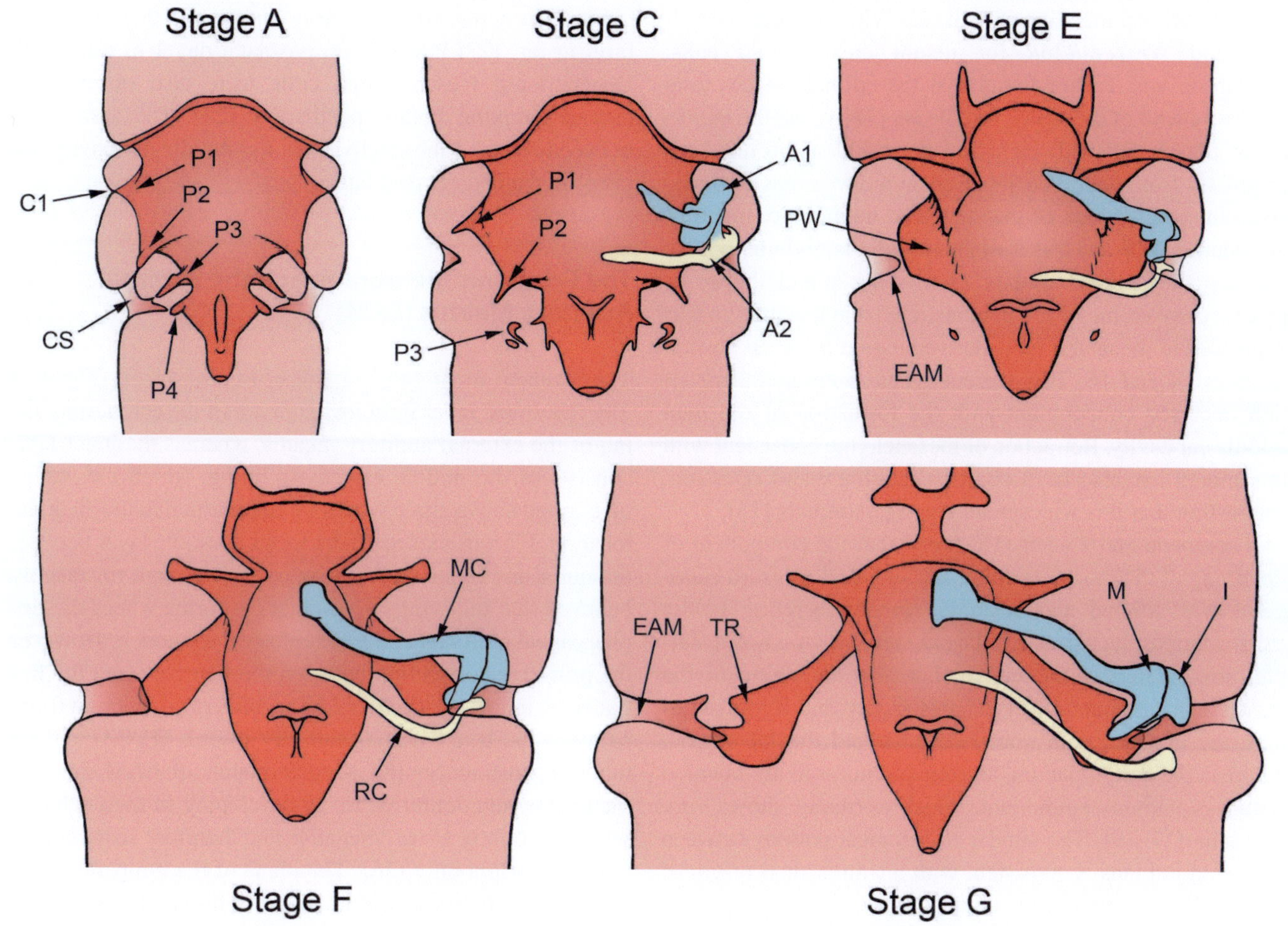

Fig. 4.4 Diagrammatic rostral views of five stages of pharyngeal development in human embryos, based on WinSurf reconstructions; not to scale. The pharynges are curved in these embryos: each opens into the oral and nasal cavities towards the top of the diagram, while at the bottom, it tapers into the oesophagus. Derivatives of the first pharyngeal arch mesenchyme are colour-coded blue, derivatives of second pharyngeal arch mesenchyme cream. These are shown, where apparent, on each embryo's left side only. The first and second pharyngeal arch mesenchyme is beginning to condense into ossicular precursors in stage C; just in front of the first pouch, the two mesenchymal populations cannot be separated. The developing stapes is hidden behind the first pouch and first-arch derivatives, and hence is not visible in the figures. The original contact between pouch I and the caudodorsal end of pharyngeal cleft I is visible in the stage A embryo but later disappears. The external auditory meatus develops as a separate invagination from the rostroventral end of cleft I. (Reprinted with the permission of John Wiley & Sons, Inc. from Burford, C.M. & Mason, M.J. (2016) Early development of the malleus and incus in humans. *Journal of Anatomy* 229:857–870. ©2016 Anatomical Society). Key: *A1–2* mesenchymal condensations within pharyngeal arches I–II; *C1* pharyngeal cleft I; *CS* lateral cervical sinus from which pharyngeal clefts II–IV originate; *EAM* external auditory meatus; *I* incus; *M* malleus; *MC* Meckel's cartilage; *PW* pharyngeal 'wing' (precursor of tubotympanic recess); *P1–4* pharyngeal pouches I–IV; *RC* Reichert's cartilage; *TR* tubotympanic recess. Stage A, 7–9 mm crown-rump length (CRL); Stage C, 10–15 mm CRL; Stage E, 14–18 mm CRL; Stage F, 20–22 mm CRL; Stage G, 24–28 mm CRL

Wittmaack [14], states that the expanding tubotympanic recess invades the middle ear region and envelopes the developing middle ear structures. In this model, the entire middle ear cavity is lined with an epithelium which is wholly endodermal in origin (Fig. 4.3b). How the endoderm might come to enwrap the ossicles is unclear, but it might potentially rupture at some point, continue to migrate around the cavity and later reunite to create a complete lining [13]. The mesenchymal model was first proposed by Schwarzbart [15] after histological examination of more than 100 human temporal regions, aged from four fetal months to adulthood. According to this model, the endoderm of the tubotympanic recess ruptures and the lining of much of the middle ear cavity is instead formed from the mesenchyme, which migrates and retracts to the edges of the cavities (Fig. 4.3c).

These competing theories were put to the test by Thompson and Tucker [16]. Immunostaining for E-cadherin in a mouse model showed that the intact endodermal lining of the first pharyngeal pouch on embryonic day 15.5 breaks down to allow an influx of mesenchyme by day 17.5. Transgenic mouse lines were used to investigate the origin of the cells ultimately lining the middle ear cavity: *Sox17-*

2AicreR26R reporter lines for tissues with endodermal origins and *Wnt1creR26R* for neural crest-derived cells. Thompson and Tucker found that the epithelium covering the dorsal wall of the mouse middle ear cavity, and the majority of the medial wall including the cochlear promontory, originates from neural crest mesenchyme, whereas that covering the medial side of the tympanic membrane, much of the ventral wall and the Eustachian tube is endodermal. In addition, they studied the expression of the epithelial-specific protein cytokeratin 14 and demonstrated that this protein was expressed in the neural crest-derived region between postnatal days 14 and 16. This mesenchymal-to-epithelial transition occurred concomitant with the formation of the final middle ear cavity. Retraction of mesenchyme consistent with this model has also been observed in shrew and opossum, suggesting that it is widespread among mammals [13].

Thompson and Tucker [16] found that the component of the lining of the mouse middle ear cavity derived from endoderm was ciliated and contained mucus-secreting goblet cells, whereas the part derived from mesenchyme was a simple, non-ciliated epithelium. In humans, the lining of the Eustachian tube, anterior tympanic cavity and hypotympanum are ciliated, with goblet cells around the ET region, whereas the epitympanum, antrum and mastoid are covered with a squamous epithelium, which normally shows very few cilia [17–19]. The similar histological pattern between mice and humans is consistent with a similar dual origin of the middle ear epithelium in humans.

However, the 'mesenchymal model' of the human middle ear cavity epithelium is not universally supported. van Waegeningh et al. [7] carefully examined the epithelial lining of the middle ear cavity using immunohistological sections from one 25-week gestation fetus. The process of cavitation had only just passed the level of the ossicles in their specimen, as the loose mesenchyme remained around the attic. Significantly, the whole cavitated region was covered by an intact epithelium, which, these authors argued, could represent endoderm, which had expanded to enwrap the ossicles without rupturing (Fig. 4.3d).

Irrespective of whether the epithelium of the human middle ear is derived entirely from endoderm, or from both endoderm and mesenchyme, the mesenchyme that fills the middle ear cavity prenatally must somehow be replaced with fluid and, later, air. Based on observations and measurements made from postnatal human temporal bones, Piza et al. [20, 21] suggest that the mesenchyme recedes as the middle ear cavity expands, thinning as it does so and thus contributing to the submucosal lining of the cavity, from which it is not easily distinguished. Other studies suggest that mesenchymal cells disintegrate. Terminal deoxynucleotidyl transferase dUTP nick end labelling (TUNEL) assays, which detect DNA fragmentation, have been used to demonstrate apoptosis of the middle ear mesenchyme, thus contributing to cavitation in rodents, from the 16th embryonic day until after birth in rats [22] but only on postnatal day 1 in mice [23]. Degenerating mesenchymal cells were also observed in human temporal bones, postnatally [24]. The association between retained mesenchyme in the middle ear cavity and otitis media is discussed later.

The Tympanic Membrane and the External Auditory Meatus (EAM)

The tympanic membrane is made up of three layers (Fig. 4.3). The outermost layer is an invagination of the ectodermal lining of the external auditory meatus, whereas the inner layer consists of the middle ear cavity lining, which the studies mentioned above agree would be endodermal in origin at this location. Fibrous mesenchyme forms a middle layer between the outer and inner layers. It is often, although mistakenly, believed that the tympanic membrane forms where the first pharyngeal cleft meets the first pharyngeal pouch. However, the primitive connection between the first cleft and the first pouch is, in fact, lost [25], and a secondary connection forms between the true external auditory meatus (EAM) and the tubotympanic recess [8]. Mouse models of EAM development show the definitive EAM developing in mesenchyme, which is entirely *Hoxa2*-negative and therefore seemingly of first-arch origin only [26]. The plane of the tympanic membrane is nearly horizontal in the early human fetus, becoming more vertical throughout fetal life and also increasingly inflected at the umbo [27].

It was suggested that the formation of the middle ear cavity and tympanic membrane is coordinated by an 'epidermoid formation', identified at the primitive connection where pouch I meets cleft I [28, 29] and persisting in some specimens postnatally, at the junction between the middle ear and the ET epithelia, just anterior to the tympanic membrane [30]. Later molecular studies have focused instead on the role of the tympanic ring, which undergoes intramembranous ossification to provide a frame for the tympanic membrane and will go on to form part of the temporal bone (see later). Mouse molecular genetic investigations have strongly suggested that tympanic ring development is necessary for the invagination of the external meatus and for the development of the tympanic membrane [31]. For example, mice deficient in expression of *Goosecoid* (*Gsc*) fail to develop a tympanic ring, a tympanic membrane and an EAM and also have other craniofacial defects [32–34]. Defects, including bilateral EAM atresia, have been linked to the human syndrome SAMS (a syndrome of short stature, auditory canal atresia, mandibular hypoplasia and skeletal abnormalities), which is also caused by *Gsc* genetic mutations [35]. Experimental evidence in mice suggests that the development of the manubrium of the malleus, which is attached to the interior surface of the tympanic membrane, depends on the normal development of the external meatus [36], and this appears to be the case in humans too [37]. In one study, 98% of those with severely defective external ear development were found to have ossicular dysplasias, and other middle ear defects were also commonly observed [38].

Eustachian Tube Development

The Eustachian tube (ET), named after the sixteenth century Italian anatomist Bartolomeo Eustachi (1500–1574) [39], is also known as the auditory tube or pharyngotympanic tube. Beginning as an expansion from the first pharyngeal pouch around the fourth week of gestation [4], the tube is transformed by epithelial differentiation and the development of cartilage and muscle from around the ninth week [40]. The development of the ET is of specific clinical interest due to its postulated links to pathologies such as otitis media [41–43].

The cartilage of the ET develops between about the 12th and 20th weeks of gestation, beginning at the pharyngeal end and progressing towards the middle ear [40]. The tube increases in length throughout gestation [40], with the main period of extension of the cartilaginous part occurring between weeks 16 and 28 [44]. Mouse models have shown that most of the ET cartilage is mesodermal in origin, but there is a small, dorsal component derived from the neural crest [45]. The bony portion of the Eustachian tube undergoes upward expansion in the late fetal stage, and this continues through childhood, thus contributing to the supratubal recess [46]. The lumen of the tube begins as round in cross section, becoming oval, and then, from around the 27th week, slit-shaped [40], but it is said to remain patent throughout prenatal life [47].

In neonates, the ET has a narrower diameter than in adults, especially the cartilaginous region [48, 49]. A child's ET has a rather uniform cross section along much of its length, whereas in an adult, it is more gradually tapering from a large pharyngeal orifice towards the narrowest portion, which is near the tympanic end of the cartilaginous zone [50]. The tube is also shorter in absolute length in children, with a relatively shorter bony section, and it is straighter than that of adults [51]. At 6 months' gestation, the ET is horizontal; by 6 months of age, it forms an angle of around 10° to the skull base [52]. Although the ET is shorter and more horizontally inclined in children under the ages of around 7, compared to adults, the fact that older children are more similar in these respects to adults, and that no difference was found between children with and without otitis media, suggests that the length and inclination of the tube may not contribute to susceptibility to this disease [53]. Other studies, however, have suggested that such a link might exist [54].

Muscles of the Eustachian Tube

Derived from the first pharyngeal arch, the tensor veli palatini (TVP) is first seen around week 6 in the human embryo, arising with the medial blastema of the muscles of mastication, together with the medial pterygoid and tensor tympani muscles [55]. All were found to be innervated by the medial root of the mandibular nerve (V). By week 7, the TVP is differentiated and related to the pterygoid hamulus, and it becomes continuous with the palatine aponeurosis by week 9. At week 13, there is a connective tissue link between the TVP and the goniale of the malleus. By birth the TVP has reached its adult relationship with the ET mesenchyme at one end, and at the other end with the palatine aponeurosis. The pterygoid hamulus, around which the TVP tendon glides, chondrifies around week 8 [55] and ossifies around week 16 [40]. The TVP remains in mesenchymal and later tendinous connection with the tensor tympani muscle throughout its development [56].

The levator veli palatini (LVP) is first seen around week 8, just ventromedial to the pharyngeal aperture of the ET; by week 9, it is found to run along the full length of the ET [57]. Kishimoto et al. found the LVP to receive innervation from the lesser palatine nerve, a branch of VII. Although innervated via the pharyngeal plexus [58] and classically believed to derive from pharyngeal arches IV–VI, Kishimoto et al. [57] suggest that the LVP may actually originate from pharyngeal arch II, based on its anatomical relationship with the ET and the component of its innervation from the facial nerve. Both *Tbx1*$^{+/-}$ and *Df1*/+ mice, used as models of DiGeorge syndrome in humans, were found to have smaller LVP muscles than wild-type mice, and this was associated with an increased incidence of otitis media [59].

Very little is known about the development of the salpingopharyngeus muscle. It is closely associated with the other longitudinal pharyngeal muscles, representing part of the palatopharyngeus complex [60, 61]. As such, its innervation and pharyngeal arch origin are probably similar to those of the LVP. The salpingopharyngeus muscle was not found to be present by week 8 of development [62].

Middle Ear Ossicle Development

The three middle ear ossicles, found in all mammals, are the malleus, incus and stapes. These are the Latin terms for a hammer, anvil and stirrup, respectively, reflecting their shape.

The pharyngeal arch origins of the ossicles have been much debated [63, 64]. The currently favoured theory, initially proposed by Reichert [65], states that the malleus and incus develop from the caudal end of Meckel's cartilage, which arises within pharyngeal arch I, whereas the stapes develops from the cartilage of pharyngeal arch II (Reichert's cartilage: Figs. 4.4 and 4.5). Meckel's cartilage, a long rod which forms the lower jaw in embryonic life, separates from the malleus during later development [66]. The anterior process of the malleus develops as a separate, intramembranous ossification referred to in the embryo as the goniale [67–69].

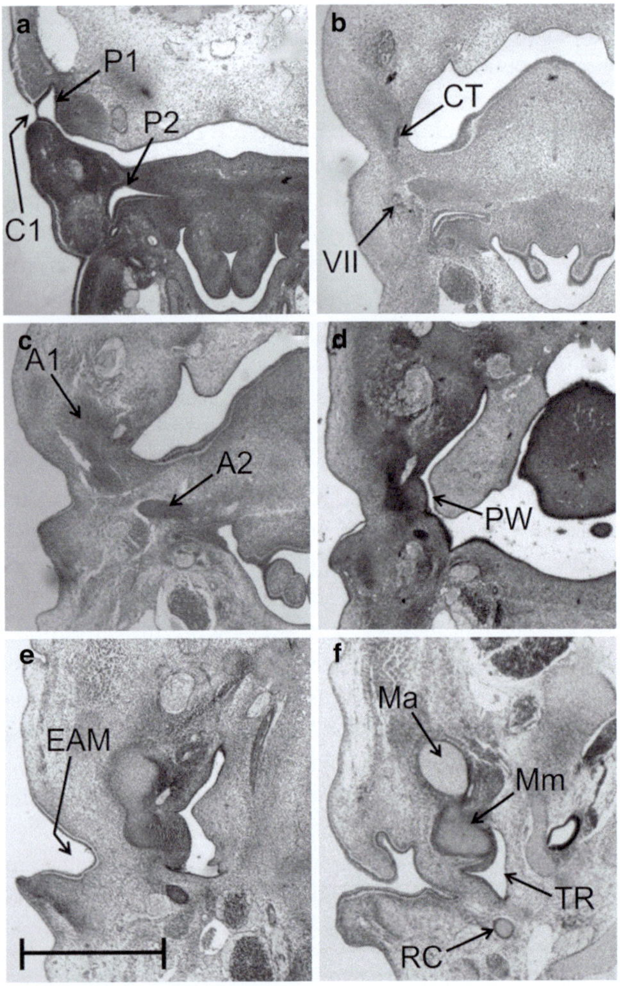

Fig. 4.5 Photomicrographs of sections through the left ear region of six human embryos, between around 5.5 and 8 weeks of gestation, from the Boyd Collection, University of Cambridge. (**a**) 9.5-mm crown-rump length (CRL); (**b**) 13.5-mm CRL; (**c**) 14.5-mm CRL; (**d**) 17 mm-CRL; (**e**) 20-mm CRL; (**f**) 24-mm CRL. In the early embryo, the first pharyngeal pouch meets the first cleft, visible in panel (**a**), but this transient spiracular union soon disappears. Sections **b–f** are rostroventral to this, where the true external auditory meatus is developing. In panel (**b**), the incipient meatus is visible as the indentation to the left of the chorda tympani nerve. The meatus converges on the extension of the pharynx that will become the tubotympanic recess, leaving the manubrium of the malleus sandwiched in between (**c–f**). The tissue between the meatus and recess will continue to narrow and the tympanic membrane will develop here. *A1, A2*, mesenchyme condensing in pharyngeal arches I and II, respectively; *C1*, pharyngeal cleft I; *CT*, chorda tympani nerve; *EAM*, external auditory meatus; *Ma*, body of the malleus; *Mm*, manubrium of the malleus; *P1, P2*, pharyngeal pouches I and II, respectively; *PW*, pharyngeal 'wing' (precursor of the tubotympanic recess); *RC*, Reichert's cartilage; *TR*, tubotympanic recess; *VII*, facial nerve. Scale bar for all photomicrographs = 1 mm

The view that the bulk of the malleus and all of the incus are derived from pharyngeal arch I has been supported by more recent evidence from mouse genetic models. Mice with homozygous mutations in *Hoxa2*, a gene expressed in arch II which is known to play a role in early embryonic facial development, show duplication of first-arch structures, including the malleus and incus, but lack a stapes [70, 71].

However, others have argued for a 'dual-arch' origin of the malleus and incus in humans, claiming that whilst the bodies of the incus and malleus are derived from the first pharyngeal arch, the manubrium of the malleus and the long process of the incus are actually second-arch structures. The earliest evidence supporting this theory comes from Hanson et al. [72], who examined human embryonic specimens between approximately 6 and 9.5 weeks of gestational age. They described the primitive blastemal mass, which will later form the malleus and incus, extending across the first pharyngeal cleft into the second pharyngeal arch region. Tracing the development of this blastemal mass suggested that the manubrium of the malleus and the long process of the incus actually developed from the region of pharyngeal arch II. This finding was corroborated by Louryan [73], who independently examined embryonic specimens of a similar age. Whyte et al. [74] also supported the dual-arch origin theory but described the long process and the manubrium fusing with the ossicular bodies at a later stage, around 9.5 weeks in their series. Further support for this theory came from observations that the stapedius muscle tendon can have a small insertion onto the long process of the incus as well as the stapes [72, 75], the stapedius being of second-arch origin. This 'dual-arch' theory was presented in the form of a figure in the 37th, 38th and 39th editions of *Gray's Anatomy* [76–78].

More recent histological examinations of human embryonic specimens have failed to find any clear evidence to support the dual-arch hypothesis [8, 79]. In mouse *Hoxa2* mutants, the long process of the incus was duplicated with the undisputed first-arch structures and was fused with its counterpart distally; the duplicated malleus shared one manubrium, which was longer than that in the wild-type [71]. O'Gorman [80] used lineage tracing to determine the second-arch contributions to the middle ear in mice. The manubrium was found to be only first arch, but O'Gorman did identify a short process near the manubrium of the malleus that was a second-arch derivative. Although this process was referred to as the '*processus brevis*', an alternative term for the lateral process of the malleus, it was subsequently identified as the orbicular apophysis [81]. The orbicular apophysis is a process of the mouse malleus, which is not found in the human ossicle and which is not homologous with the human lateral process. Louryan et al. [82] showed that Hox-A2 immunostaining, for second-arch derivatives, labelled the orbicular apophysis and Reichert's cartilage of mice very strongly, as expected. However, the rest of the ossicular chain, including the stapes, picked up diffuse labelling. This result is difficult to interpret, but Louryan et al. argued that it keeps alive the possibility of a second-arch contribution to the malleus and incus bodies.

The stapes is believed to largely arise from the pharyngeal arch II cartilage. A contribution of the human otic capsule to the stapes footplate had been suggested, based on histological observation [72, 83], but this was denied by Rodríguez-Vázquez [84]. However, O'Gorman [80] found that the peripheral footplate and the annular ligament did not label as second-arch neural crest derivatives, in mice. These portions were later shown to be mesodermally derived [85]. Thompson et al. found that the neural crest component is necessary for the normal formation of the mesodermal component, and the oval window.

Ossicular Embryology in More Detail

The loose, mesodermal condensations representing the first signs of the malleus and incus appear at around 5.5 weeks of gestation [72]. The malleus becomes precartilaginous by the seventh week and separates from the incus [67]. It begins to ossify around 15–16 weeks and reaches its maximum size at around 17–21 weeks, after which point Meckel's cartilage degenerates into fibrous tissues contributing to the anterior ligament. Meanwhile, the goniale appears at around 8.5 weeks and fuses with the rest of the malleus between around 18 and 21 weeks [11, 67].

Studies in rodents [86] and humans [8, 72, 87] suggest that the malleus and incus are part of a single mesenchymal condensation, with a joint forming between the two ossicles later. In humans, the articular cavity starts to form in the ninth week of gestation and the capsular ligament becomes visible in the following week [88]. In patients with Treacher Collins syndrome (TCS), the malleus and incus are often fused together, hypothesised to occur as the result of disruption to this joint formation process [89, 90]. A more recent study has suggested that the earliest trace of the incus forms independently of Meckel's cartilage within the first arch, appearing as a separate mesenchymal condensation to that of the malleus at 6 weeks' gestation and only joining the malleus shortly afterwards [79]. Rodríguez-Vázquez et al. [91] found that a transient cartilaginous union between what will become the short process of the incus and the otic capsule forms from week 8 onwards. Having passed through a stage where there is a narrow joint cavity between the short process and the otic capsule, laterally, the articulation becomes fully fibrous from 17 weeks onwards. The incus begins to ossify just before the malleus, at around 16 weeks [11, 92].

The incudostapedial joint starts as densely-packed mesenchyme between the distal long process and what will become the stapes head, at 7–8 weeks' gestation [88]. The lenticular apophysis of the incus forms at around 9 weeks, and the incipient incudostapedial joint cavity first appears at 13 weeks. The cavity is completed by around 16 weeks [88].

A variable amount of remodelling of both the malleus and incus occurs in postnatal life [67]. Yokoyama et al. [93] described bone marrow spaces persisting in the malleus and incus until 25 months of age, after which point they are replaced by narrow, vascular channels. Vestiges of embryonic cartilage have been described within the adult malleus and incus [94], and cartilage is found around the periphery of the manubrium [95] and lateral process [96]. The anterior process of the malleus appears to shorten slightly, postnatally [97].

The stapedial anlage, first visible at around 4.5 weeks' gestation [72], begins as an ovoid, mesenchymal condensation, which is connected to Reichert's cartilage through a separate condensation representing the interhyale [84]. The developing stapes is penetrated by the stapedial artery. This artery degenerates at around 7 weeks, during which time the stapes chondrifies, but the ossicle is left with its characteristic intercrural foramen [84]. Rarely, a stapedial artery passing through the stapes may persist through to adulthood in humans: variations in its morphology and its pharyngeal arch origins have been reviewed by Hitier et al. [98].

The developing stapes footplate is juxtaposed to the otic capsule by the end of the embryonic period, during which time the stapes takes the form of a bulky ring. The annular ligament begins as a mesenchymal condensation between the footplate and the otic capsule, visible at around 9 weeks, completing its differentiation into fibrous tissue by week 12 [88]. Stapes ossification begins at around 19 weeks [83]. Unlike the malleus and incus, which thicken over the course of prenatal development, the stapes undergoes considerable thinning. Attaining its maximum size at around 5 months' gestation, it subsequently develops into a much more delicate ossicle with internally hollowed crura and a wider intercrural foramen, reaching near-adult morphology after around 7 months. However, the vestibular aspect of the footplate remains cartilaginous even in children [83].

Middle Ear Muscle Development

The two smallest skeletal muscles in the human body, the tensor tympani and stapedius, lie in the middle ear and insert on the malleus and stapes, respectively. The tensor tympani is derived from pharyngeal arch I and is hence innervated by the mandibular branch of the trigeminal nerve (V_3), whereas the stapedius is from arch II and is innervated by the stapedial branch of the facial nerve (VII).

The developing tensor tympani is already connected to the malleus at 6 weeks; its anlage is in communication with that of the tensor veli palatini via a mesenchymal connection

[56]. The *processus cochleariformis* develops at around 15–16 weeks' gestation [56]. Like the levator veli palatini, the tensor tympani was found to be smaller in heterozygous *Tbx1*$^{+/-}$ mice than in wild-type [59].

The stapedius muscle develops from two initially separate parts. The tendon is derived from the interhyale, which develops as a mesenchymal condensation between the stapes and Reichert's cartilage around week 6 [84, 99]. The belly forms as a separate anlage, medial to the facial nerve, which joins with the interhyale around week 8; the external portion of the interhyale disappears by around 9 weeks, detaching the muscle and its tendon from Reichert's cartilage. The stapedius tendon is of variable length and angle in adults, which may depend on the position of attachment of the belly of the muscle to the interhyale during development [100]. The pyramidal eminence appears between 12 and 14 weeks [99].

Temporal Bone Development

The human temporal bone is a composite structure comprising petromastoid, styloid, tympanic and squamous components. It houses the bony external meatus, middle ear cavity and inner ear. The cartilaginous otic capsule, containing the inner ear, contributes to the petromastoid component of the temporal bone. It has been shown to be mesodermally derived in mice [85], except for a small component derived from second-arch neural crest [80]. The styloid process, which is joined to the otic capsule in the embryo, is derived from the cranial segment of Reichert's cartilage and so is of second-arch neural crest origin [85, 101]. The tympanic and squamous components of the temporal bone are also derived from the neural crest [102] but ossify directly in mesenchyme [91, 103].

From around 11 weeks' gestation, the tympanosquamous fissure begins to close and the tegmen tympani forms [104]. The tegmen tympani, which forms on the roof of the middle ear cavity, is considered part of the petromastoid component of the temporal bone. It initially forms as an independent cartilage, becoming almost fully ossified by 17 weeks [104]. The petromastoid, squamous and tympanic components of the temporal bone remain separate in the fetus, fusing only postnatally [105]. The development of the hypotympanum is considered in detail by Spector and Ge [106] and that of the facial recess and associated structures by Eby [107].

The Otic Capsule

The inner ear arises from the otic placode, a non-neural ectodermal thickening near the hindbrain region, associated with cranial nerve VIII [108, 109]. At 5–6 weeks, the otocyst, which will develop into the membranous labyrinth, is surrounded by mesenchyme, which has developed into the cartilaginous otic capsule by 8.5 weeks [108]. This becomes increasingly complex in shape as the labyrinth develops within it. The otic capsule ossifies from a large number of separate centres, which first appear between around 16 and 21 weeks of gestation, and it reaches adult size in the fetus [11, 110]. The first signs of ossification in the otic capsule visible by computed tomography were seen at the age of 18.5 weeks [111].

The Tympanic Ring

The tympanic ring is an intramembranous ossification, developing from pharyngeal arch I [31]. Representing the border between the outer and middle ears, it contains a groove, the tympanic sulcus, to which the tympanic membrane attaches circumferentially. The tympanic ring appears as a distinct mesenchymal condensation in the eighth week of gestation [103]. It then begins to ossify without any cartilaginous precursor and increases in diameter. By 10 weeks, it is C-shaped, lying between Meckel's and Reichert's cartilages and lateral to a region which will later become the tympanic cavity. By 19 weeks, it forms an almost complete annulus but for a gap in its upper part known as the notch of Rivinus (*incisura tympanica*). Its rostral free end expands in the region of the anterior process of the malleus, where Meckel's cartilage begins to degenerate and the goniale fuses with the rest of the malleus [103].

Fetal tympanic rings are located below the auricle and are more horizontally inclined than they are in adults [112]. The ring nearly reaches adult diameter by around 34 weeks and begins to fuse with the otic capsule [103]. The orientation of the sulcus tympanicus, supporting the tympanic membrane, gradually becomes more vertical in later fetal and early postnatal life [27]. The ring remains open but is incorporated into the temporal bone near term [103]; lateral growth later leads to the formation of the bony external meatus [27, 113].

Molecular studies have found evidence of a role of the *Gsc* gene in condensation of the tympanic ring in the first-arch tissue: this fails in *Gsc*-null mice [114]. *Hoxa2* expression in pharyngeal arch II seems to inhibit the *Gsc*-expressing mesenchymal cells in that arch from developing a second tympanic ring [31].

The Mastoid

The small rodents most often used as model species in ear development studies lack cellular mastoid processes like those of humans [115], so what we know about mastoid development has had to come directly from observations on human specimens.

The connective tissue extending from the middle ear reaches the antral region at around 22 weeks' gestation; by 29 weeks, the epithelium of the tympanic cavity has arrived and begins to invade the diploic bone from there, resulting in the development of a cavity [116]. The future air cells begin to extend outwards from the antral region into the mastoid before birth [116]. At birth, the antrum is well-pneumatised; most of the mastoid pneumatisation occurs from then until around 6 years of age, with continued expansion until the age of puberty, taking the air cells all the way to the petrous apex in some [117]. The possible pathways for the pneumatisation of the mastoid are illustrated by Halewyck et al. [118]. The overall extent of pneumatisation is highly variable between individuals, following a normal distribution [119]. The growth of the mastoid process of the temporal bone, which is largely independent of its internal excavation, occurs fastest in the first postnatal year but continues until puberty [117].

Mastoiditis in children may result in the formation of new bone and sclerosis, leading to failure of pneumatisation even after the infection is resolved; an infection can also obliterate pre-existing air cells [120].

Middle Ear Development and Otitis Media

Although it is generally held that the mesenchyme within the middle ear cavity should disappear within about a year of birth, its presence has been well-documented in some children and even in adults [12, 121, 122]. One study found mesenchyme in 2% of 1404 temporal bones of patients aged 5–81 years [123]. It has been suggested that this mesenchyme might block the aeration routes through to the rest of the middle ear cavity [122]. If this interferes with the drainage of exudate from the middle ear through the ET into the pharynx, then this may explain the association between retained mesenchyme in the middle ear and the development of otitis media [122–125]. Retained mesenchyme in the middle ear cavity has also been cited as a possible cause of conductive hearing loss in Down syndrome patients [126, 127]. Given this evidence, it has been suggested that cases of recurrent suppurative otitis media in young children could be better treated with tympanic paracentesis than with antibiotics [128]. Mesenchymal remnants may adversely affect the tympanic membrane and ossicular chain function and may also play a role in the formation of cholesteatoma [129].

Retained mesenchyme in the middle ear cavity seems to be most commonly found in the epitympanum/mastoid region [122, 123]. A poorly pneumatised mastoid is associated with a blocked tympanic isthmus [130], which may restrict aeration and drainage of the epitympanum and mastoid. This may help explain why underdevelopment of the mastoid air cells, a condition that has a hereditary element, is associated with more frequent presentations of acute otitis media [131]. However, what represents cause and what represents effect in these associations remains unclear.

Underdevelopment of the ET can result in fluid accumulating in the tympanic cavity, and this is considered to be an important cause of otitis media with effusion in children [132]. It has been proposed that the evolution of larger brain volumes leading to the requirement for earlier birth in humans, alongside the flattening of the face and adaptations of the palate and its musculature associated with speech, may have reduced the functionality of the ET, predisposing humans to develop this condition [133]. As an experimental model of this condition, mice with mutations of *Eya4* have been found to have an narrower, malpositioned ET and inflammation of the middle ear cavity, and they also suffer from middle ear effusion and hearing loss [134].

Part 2: Anatomy of the Adult Middle Ear

The Tympanic Cavity

The Eustachian tube, tympanic cavity and mastoid complex (Fig. 4.6) are collectively described as the 'middle ear cleft'. Of these, the tympanic cavity contains the key structures involved in sound transmission from the external to inner ears. The human tympanic cavity is commonly subdivided into three compartments. The epitympanum (epitympanic recess) contains the head of the malleus and the dorsal incus. It is separated from the mesotympanum below by the ossicles and the lateral incudal and tensor mucosal folds that surround them, but remains in communication with the mesotympanum by means of the narrow tympanic isthmus in the posteromedial quadrant [135]. The mesotympanum is

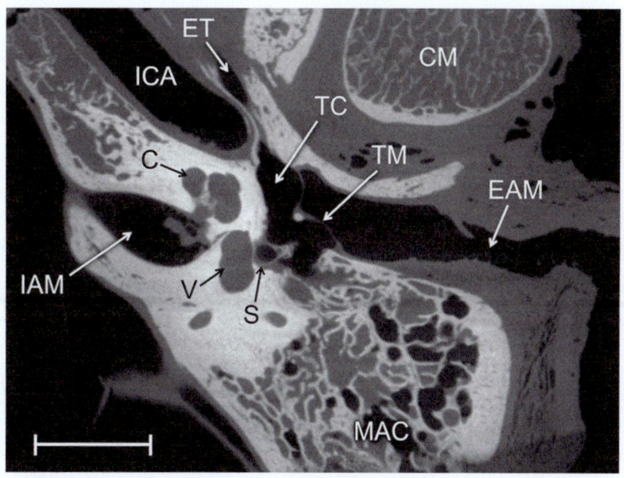

Fig. 4.6 Computed tomographic image of a preserved human temporal bone, in an approximately horizontal plane. The bone is white, the soft tissue and fluid are grey and air is black. The internal carotid artery and internal auditory meatus are both empty in this specimen but would not be in real life. *C*, cochlea; *CM*, condyle of the mandible; *EAM*, external auditory meatus; *ET*, Eustachian tube; *IAM*, internal auditory meatus; *ICA*, internal carotid artery; *MAC*, mastoid air cells, some of which are filled with fluid; *S*, stapes; *TC*, tympanic cavity; *TM*, tympanic membrane (the manubrium of the malleus is visible centrally); *V*, vestibule. Scale bar = 10 mm

that part of the middle ear cavity at the level of the tympanic membrane, and the hypotympanum is the region below the inferior extent of the tympanic sulcus.

The anterior wall of the tympanic cavity is superiorly comprised of the bony portion of the Eustachian tube, separated by a thin plate of bone from the tensor tympani muscle. Inferior to these structures runs the internal carotid artery (Fig. 4.6), which enters the temporal bone medial to the styloid process and initially runs vertically, anteroinferior to the cochlea. It then turns anteromedially and runs under the Eustachian tube towards the foramen lacerum, whence it enters the cranial fossa. Knowledge of the normal and aberrant courses of the carotid artery is essential for safe middle ear surgery.

The posterior wall of the middle ear cleft is penetrated superiorly by the *aditus ad antrum*, the opening that connects the epitympanum and the mastoid antrum (discussed later). Below the *aditus* is the pyramidal eminence, the bony prominence that contains the stapedius muscle belly; the tendon projects anteriorly and inserts on the stapes. The lower portion of the posterior wall of the tympanic cavity may be subdivided into two. 'Facial recess' is the term for the groove between the facial nerve and the tympanic annulus, whereas the *sinus tympani* is an extension of air cells into the posterior wall, deep to the facial nerve.

The bony medial wall of the tympanic cavity (Fig. 4.7) features the rounded elevation of the cochlear promontory, which is crossed by the tympanic branch of the glossopharyngeal nerve (IX). Posterosuperior to the promontory lies the oval window (*fenestra vestibuli*), which contains the stapes footplate held in place by the annular ligament. Inferior to this lies the round window niche, separated from the oval window by the subiculum. The round window niche is a small channel containing at its base the 'secondary tympanic membrane', which covers the round window itself, separating the middle ear cavity from the perilymph [136]. The round window (*fenestra cochleae*), accessed via a posterior tympanotomy into the facial recess from the mastoid antrum, is a common insertion point during cochlear implantation [137].

A large portion of cranial nerve VII, the facial nerve, runs in an anterior to posterior direction along the medial aspect of the tympanic cavity, prior to its descent through the mastoid. The nerve travels within the Fallopian canal, just superior to the oval window. The *processus cochleariformis*, a bony projection over which the tendon of the tensor tympani muscle runs, is a landmark for the anterior portion of the Fallopian canal. Posterosuperior to the Fallopian canal, the bone covering the lateral semicircular canal forms the medial part of the epitympanum.

The lateral boundary of the tympanic cavity consists of the tympanic membrane and bony walls of the epitympanum and hypotympanum, located superior and inferior to the membrane, respectively. The wedge-shaped bony lateral wall of the epitympanum, termed the 'scutum', may be eroded by cholesteatoma.

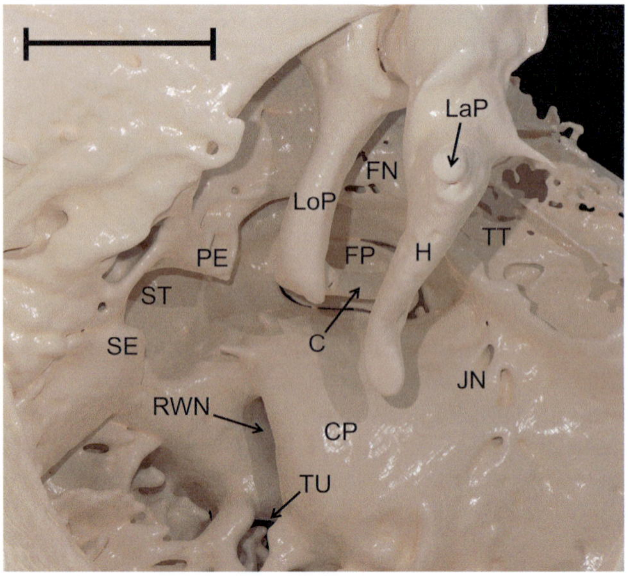

Fig. 4.7 Micro-CT reconstruction of the medial wall of the middle ear cleft, right ear. Scale bar = 3 mm. *C*, stapedial anterior crus; *CP*, cochlear promontory; *FN*, bony impression of the facial nerve; *FP*, footplate of stapes in the oval window; *H*, handle of the malleus (manubrium); *JN*, bony impression of Jacobson's nerve; *LaP*, lateral process of the malleus; *LoP*, long process of the incus; *PE*, pyramidal eminence; *RWN*, round window niche; *SE*, styloid eminence; *ST*, sinus tympani, *TT*, bony canal of the tensor tympani muscle; *TU*, subcochlear tunnel

The Tympanic Membrane

The tympanic membrane separates the external auditory meatus from the tympanic cavity (Fig. 4.6). In adults, this is a thin membrane about 9–10 mm in diameter, attached around its circumference to the sulcus of the tympanic bone. The taut *pars tensa* is connected to the sulcus by means of the tympanic annulus (*annulus fibrosus tympanicus*), the thickened rim of the membrane [138]. The smaller, thicker but more flexible *pars flaccida* fills the notch of Rivinus superiorly.

The tympanic membrane appears as a semi-transparent, oval structure when examined from the external ear canal. From the lateral aspect, the division between *pars tensa* and *pars flaccida* is demarcated by the lateral process of the malleus, which forms a bulge in the membrane known as the malleolar prominence. The manubrium of the malleus extends from here to the centre of the *pars tensa*, attaching to its medial side. From the medial aspect, the division between the *pars tensa* and the *pars flaccida* is demarcated by the ligamentous anterior and posterior malleolar folds, which hold the lateral process of the malleus in place. Within these folds lies the chorda tympani nerve, as it passes medial to the tympanic membrane.

The *pars tensa* takes the shape of a shallow cone, and the apex of this cone as seen from the ear canal is known as the umbo. Although the umbo is indented into the middle ear cavity, the membrane surrounding this bulges outwards, except where it is connected to the manubrium. The outer circumference of the tympanic membrane is oriented at an angle to the external auditory meatus, such that the surface area of the *pars tensa* is increased relative to the perpendicular meatus cross section [139].

Incoming sound waves cause vibration of the *pars tensa*, with the energy being transmitted to the inner ear by the coupling of the membrane to the ossicular chain via the manubrium. Vibratory amplitude can be modulated by contraction of the tensor tympani, which pulls the manubrium medially, increasing the tension of the *pars tensa* [140]. The *pars flaccida* is believed to play only a minor acoustic role in humans [141].

The Eustachian Tube

The Eustachian tube (Fig. 4.8a) comprises three anatomical parts: a bony lateral third, a fibrocartilaginous anteromedial portion and a junctional region where the bone and cartilage overlap over 3–4 mm [144]. Surrounded by soft tissue and muscles, it connects the tympanic orifice in the anterior wall of the middle ear to the nasopharyngeal orifice, which is posterior to the inferior nasal concha and lateral to the adenoid pad. The Eustachian tube is predominantly lined by a ciliated, pseudostratified, columnar epithelium, with nonciliated and goblet cells being more crowded at the bone–cartilage junction [17, 145]. The cilia assist in secretion clearance by sweeping the mucus and debris towards the nasopharynx.

In a study of 286 non-cadaveric Eustachian tubes imaged with cone beam computed tomography (143 subjects), the shortest measured adult tube was 34.5 mm and the longest 47.2 mm [146]. The average length was 40.3 mm. The bony portion was approximately 1 mm longer in males than in females, and the cartilaginous portion was 1.5 mm longer [146]. The narrow ET descends anteromedially, with the cartilaginous part at an angle of approximately 35° in adults [146]. The slope of the fibrocartilaginous portion of the Eustachian tube relative to the horizontal plane was approximately 2° shallower on the right side, with a corresponding increase of 0.5 mm in the length of the right bony portion, explained by the lower *fossa cranii media* on the right [146].

The 12-mm-long bony portion [146] passes through the petrous temporal bone where it is crossed by the horizontal segment of the internal carotid artery passing medially in its carotid canal [147]. Bone rigidity prevents tubal occlusion by external pressure along this portion. The fibrocartilaginous portion is comprised of a flanged plate of cartilage posteromedially, with fibrous tissue making up the anterolateral wall [148].

The pharyngeal and tympanic ends of the ET are both wider than the central section. In the nasopharynx, the ostium is visible as the tubal elevation known as the *torus tubarius*, where the mucosa is lifted by the end of the cartilage [146]. Posterior to this lies the fossa of Rosenmüller, a common site for nasopharyngeal carcinoma. The narrowest

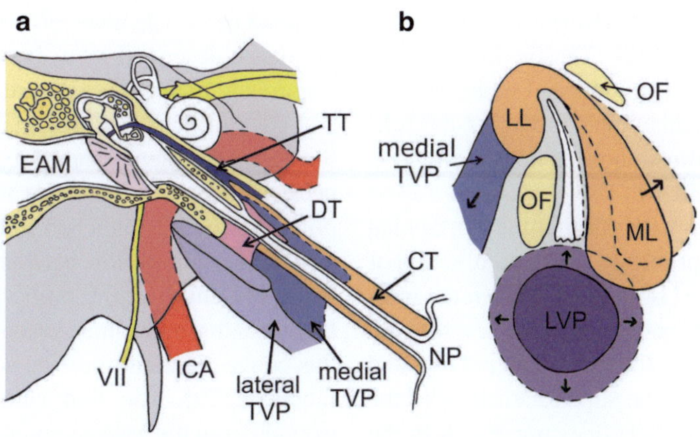

Fig. 4.8 (**a**) Schematic cross section of the Eustachian tube. Dilatator tubae adjoins the membranous Eustachian tube at the isthmus. The medial tensor veli palatini attaches to the lateral lamina of the cartilaginous Eustachian tube. The levator veli palatini is not pictured. (**b**) Dilatation of the Eustachian tube lumen (central white space) by the contraction of associated muscles, based in part on the studies by Ishijima et al. [142] and Smith et al. [143]. The tensor veli palatini acts on the superior and medial portions of the Eustachian tube, whereas the levator veli palatini predominantly acts on the inferior portion. *CT*, cartilaginous portion of the Eustachian tube; *DT*, dilatator tubae; *EAM*, external auditory meatus; *ICA*, internal carotid artery; *LL*, lateral lamina of the tubal cartilage; *LVP*, levator veli palatini; *ML*, medial lamina of the tubal cartilage; *OF*, Ostmann fat pads (medial and lateral); *TVP*, tensor veli palatini

part of the Eustachian tube lumen, known as the isthmus, usually lies within the cartilaginous part of the tube, near the junctional region [50, 144]. In a study of nine temporal bones, the narrowest part of the tube measured 0.65 mm^2 ± 0.22 mm^2 in cross-sectional area and lay 3.1 mm ± 1.6 mm from the pharyngeal margin of the junctional region [144].

Functions of the Eustachian Tube

The Eustachian tube has three main functions in adults: (1) periodic ventilation of the middle ear cavity to equalise pressure with ambient atmospheric pressure, a requirement for appropriate impedance matching across the middle ear, (2) unidirectional mucociliary drainage of middle ear secretions and (3) protection of the middle ear from ascending nasopharyngeal microorganisms and sound.

At rest, the fibrocartilaginous part of the tube in the parapharyngeal space is passively closed by elastic recoil of the elastin hinge found between the lateral and medial cartilaginous laminae [149] and pressure from the adjacent Ostmann fat pads [150]. It opens actively for brief periods (around 200 ms: [151]) on swallowing and yawning and passively with high nasopharyngeal pressures such as those achieved by the Valsalva manoeuvre. Three muscles are generally believed to be involved in active Eustachian tube functions: the tensor veli palatini, levator veli palatini and salpingopharyngeus. Their innervation was considered in the earlier section on their development.

The medial bundle of the tensor veli palatini typically arises from the middle to superior lateral lamina of the fibrocartilaginous portion of the Eustachian tube [142]. Where it attaches to and dilates the isthmus it is known as the dilatator tubae muscle [152]. It joins the lateral bundle of the tensor veli palatini to wrap around the hamulus of the medial pterygoid, before inserting into the palatal aponeurosis and posterior edge of the hard palate [142]. Tensor veli palatini contraction is believed to open the middle and superior cartilaginous portions of the Eustachian tube, including the isthmus [142]. A diagrammatic illustration of how the tube is opened is presented in Fig. 4.8b.

The most inferior cartilaginous portion of the Eustachian tube is believed to be opened primarily by the contraction of the levator veli palatini muscle [142]. Arising from the inferior aspect of the petrous temporal bone, the levator veli palatini descends to pass between the tensor veli palatini and salpingopharyngeus to attach to the superior surface of the soft palate aponeurosis. This muscle does not attach to the Eustachian tube but forms a sling, passing in close proximity to the medial cartilaginous lamina [142]. By increasing its cross-sectional area, levator veli palatini contraction is believed to displace the medial lamina, elevating and rotating it to open the inferior lumen of the cartilaginous Eustachian tube [142].

The salpingopharyngeus muscle originates from the cartilaginous portion of the Eustachian tube and courses inferiorly to form the salpingopharyngeal fold, eventually attaching to the lateral pharyngeal wall. The size and presence of this muscle has been reported to be variable across individuals [153], leading to the suggestion that it lacks any significant role in Eustachian tube function. However, salpingopharyngeus dysfunction has been implicated in myogenic tinnitus associated with palatal tremor [154].

Two additional muscles have been implicated in normal Eustachian tube function: the medial and lateral pterygoid muscles. Innervated by V_3 [155], contraction of these muscles appears to enhance Eustachian tube dilatation achieved by the tensor veli palatini and levator veli palatini, but it is not necessary or sufficient to achieve Eustachian tube opening [156]. In fact, the exact mechanism by which muscular contraction results in middle ear aeration remains disputed.

The Ossicular Chain

As in all mammals, the human ossicular chain consists of three tiny bones suspended within the tympanic cavity. These bones conduct sound from the tympanic membrane to the fluid-filled inner ear, via the oval window. Although largely made of compact bone, there are vascular channels and cavities within the ossicles, which are in communication with the external supplying vessels, as described and illustrated by Manoharan et al. [157].

The adult human malleus (Figs. 4.7 and 4.9a) measures approximately 8 mm along its longest axis, from the manubrial tip to the top of the head, and typically weighs around 25 mg [158]. The malleus is likened to a hammer because of its long, tapering manubrium ('handle'), above which is a rounded head. The head has a posterior articulation facet for the incus, described later; between the head and the manubrium is a more constricted region called the neck. The lateral edge of the manubrium is attached to the *pars tensa* of the tympanic membrane; dorsally, it projects out from the neck of the malleus to form the lateral process ('*processus brevis*'), which is attached to the dorsal margin of the *pars tensa*. The connection between the manubrium and membrane is tightest at the umbo and lateral process, although there is substantial inter-individual variability in the size of this connection that must be accounted for in finite element models [159]. The thin anterior process of the malleus extends from the neck region to form an articulation with the anterior wall of the tympanic cavity, by means of the anterior malleal ligament [97]. The smaller lateral and superior ligaments attach to the lateral process and malleus head, respectively, whereas the tensor tympani tendon inserts on the manubrial base, medially [160, 161]. The positions of these attachments vary significantly between individuals.

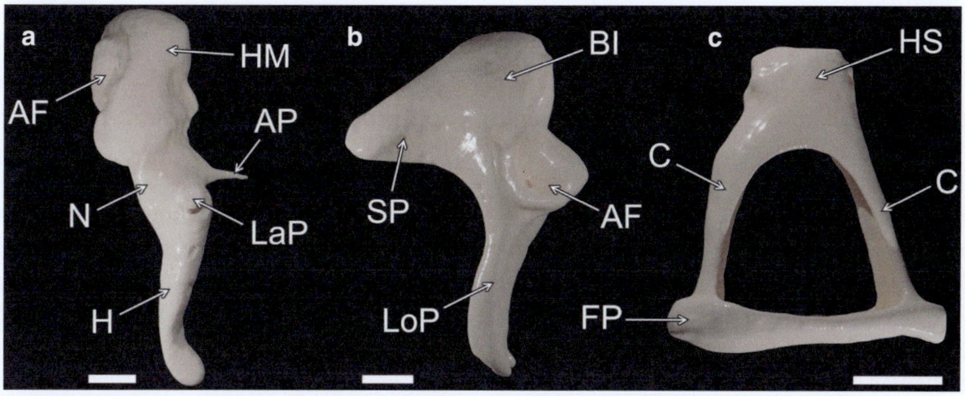

Fig. 4.9 Micro-CT reconstructions of the human ossicular chain. (**a**) Right malleus, lateral view; (**b**) right incus, lateral view; (**c**) right stapes, ventral view. Scale bars = 1 mm. *AF*, articulation facet (of the malleus or incus); *AP*, anterior process; *BI*, body of the incus (*corpus incudis*); *C*, stapedial crus (anterior and posterior); *FP*, footplate (*basis stapedis*); *H*, handle (*manubrium mallei*); *HM*, head of the malleus (*caput mallei*); *HS*, head of the stapes (*caput stapedis*); *LaP*, lateral process; *LoP*, long process (*crus longum*); *N*, neck (*collum mallei*); *SP*, short process (*crus brevis*)

The second bone of the ossicular chain, the incus (Figs. 4.7 and 4.9b), measures roughly 6.5 mm along the axis of the long process and has a mass of around 27–28 mg [158]. The bulky body of the incus has an anterior articulation facet for the malleus and two processes extending from it. The long process is narrow, extending ventrally and bending medially at its tip, where it tapers into a narrow pedicle that supports the lenticular apophysis for articulation with the stapes. The tiny, disc-shaped lenticular apophysis was once believed to represent a fourth ossicle [162], but a thin pedicle connecting it to the incus was confirmed in 97% of 270 human specimens [163]. The blood supply to this region comes from intraosseous vessels running down the incudal long process as well as from mucosal vessels [164]. Erosion of the long process can disrupt the internal vessels, potentially making the distal part of the process more vulnerable to surgical insults [157]. The short process of the incus is stout and conical, extending posteriorly from the body. The main ligamentous attachment of the incus is its posterior ligament, which connects the end of the short process to the *fossa incudis* in the posterior tympanic cavity. This ligament extends both laterally and medially to the short process and is thicker laterally [161]. A thin superior ligament of the incus is also described [160]. Additional support is provided by the incudomalleolar articulation as well as the articulation between the lenticular apophysis and the head of the stapes.

The smallest bone of the ossicular chain is the stapes (Figs. 4.7 and 4.9c). The head is little more than a flattened, oval articulation facet for the lenticular apophysis of the incus. It is attached to a neck region, which, on its posterior aspect, provides the insertion point for the stapedius muscle. The neck diverges medially to form the two crura, which attach to either end of the footplate. The crura and neck are internally hollowed by a sulcus, which opens into the intercrural foramen. The stapes footplate itself fits snugly within the oval window (Fig. 4.7); its thickened rim is anchored to the rim of the oval window by means of an annular ligament. Although usually regarded as a fibrous connection, small joint cavities were found in 70% of human stapediovestibular joints [165]. The perpendicular distance from the footplate to the most distant point of the stapes head is approximately 3.3 mm, whereas the length of the long axis of the footplate averages around 2.8 mm [166]. The mass of the entire ossicle is approximately 3 mg [158]. The stapes provides input to the cochlea through motion of the footplate within the oval window.

Two joints separate the bones of the ossicular chain. The malleus head and incus body within the epitympanum have been likened in shape to 'two lovers kissing in a small closet' [167]. More prosaically, the malleoincudal articulation is a diarthrodial joint with saddle-shaped articular surfaces covered by a layer of hyaline cartilage [168]. Another diarthrodial joint, the incudostapedial articulation, connects the lenticular apophysis of the incus and the head of the stapes. A narrow space lined by synovium is located between these two cartilaginous joint surfaces, which are enveloped by a substantial joint capsule [163]. Whilst modelling suggests that these flexible joints will reduce the transmission of sound energy through the ossicular chain, they may protect the inner ear from high-amplitude static pressure changes [169].

Middle Ear Muscles

The tensor tympani muscle, around 25 mm long, attaches medially to the greater wing of the sphenoid, passes around the cochleariform process and inserts on the medial side of the malleus, where the manubrium meets the neck. Recent work has confirmed the anatomical connection by means of a common tendon between the tensor tympani and tensor veli palatini muscles in adult humans [170, 171], reflecting the embryonic connection mentioned earlier. The functional significance of this connection remains unclear, as indeed is the function of the tensor tympani itself [172, 173].

The 6-mm-long stapedius muscle inserts on the neck of the stapes after arising from the pyramidal eminence of the posterosuperior mesotympanum (Fig. 4.7). Reflex contraction in response to intense acoustic stimulation results in stiffening of the annular ligament, which connects the stapes footplate to the rim of the oval window, which should serve to reduce low-frequency sound transmission [174]. Evidence suggests that this protects the inner ear from noise damage, minimises the masking of speech frequencies by loud background noise and reduces self-stimulation from vocalisation [175].

The Nerves of the Middle Ear

Four cranial nerves provide innervation to the structures of the middle ear. These are the trigeminal nerve (V), facial nerve (VII), glossopharyngeal nerve (IX) and vagus nerve (X).

The lateral surface of the tympanic membrane receives sensory innervation from the auriculotemporal branch of the trigeminal nerve, the glossopharyngeal nerve and the auricular branches of the facial and vagus nerves. The medial surface of the tympanic membrane is innervated by the tympanic nerve (a branch of the glossopharyngeal nerve also named Jacobson's nerve), which also provides general sensory innervation to the tympanic cavity via the tympanic plexus. Motor function is provided by the medial pterygoid branch of the trigeminal nerve to the tensor tympani and the stapedial branch of the facial nerve to the stapedius muscle. Sympathetic innervation is provided by the caroticotympanic nerve, which arises from the internal carotid sympathetic plexus to join the tympanic plexus.

The motor root of the facial nerve and *nervus intermedius* (containing sensory and parasympathetic fibres) pass through the internal auditory meatus to enter the Z-shaped facial (Fallopian) canal, wherein they fuse to form the facial nerve. The facial canal passes between the cochlea and vestibule, turning posteriorly at the geniculate ganglion. Within this part of the facial canal, the labyrinthine segment of the facial nerve gives off three branches: the greater superficial petrosal nerve (carrying parasympathetic innervation to the lacrimal gland and taste sensation from the palate), the lesser petrosal nerve and the external petrosal nerve. The facial nerve then traverses the medial wall of the middle ear cavity within the facial canal, directly inferior to the lateral semicircular canal, as the tympanic segment. In the facial canal between the pyramidal eminence and stylomastoid foramen, the facial nerve is termed the 'mastoid segment', giving off three further branches:

- The motor nerve to the stapedius muscle
- The chorda tympani, which provides taste sensation to the anterior two-thirds of the tongue and parasympathetic innervation to the submandibular and sublingual salivary glands [176]
- A sensory branch that joins the auricular branch of the vagus nerve, conveying sensation from the pinna and ear canal

The facial nerve leaves the facial canal at the stylomastoid foramen, providing motor function to the *m. digastricus*, *m. stylohyoideus* and muscles of facial expression [177]. Dehiscence of the canal of the facial nerve can occur, resulting in an exposed facial nerve.

When originating from the lateral side of the facial nerve, the chorda tympani ascends and courses anteriorly into the middle ear [178]. However, when originating from the posterolateral side, the chorda tympani forms a posteriorly convex curve on ascending, before passing anteriorly into the middle ear, thus bulging into the anterior portion of the mastoid complex [178]. Occasionally, the chorda tympani originates inferior to the stylomastoid foramen, outside the facial canal [178]. The chorda tympani enters the tympanic cavity via the posterior canaliculus, on a level with the handle of the malleus and round window. It arches upwards and forwards to cross the *pars flaccida*, passing medially to the neck of the malleus and just dorsally to the insertion of the tensor tympani tendon, before exiting the tympanic cavity through the anterior canaliculus [176].

As the first branch arising from the petrous ganglion of the glossopharyngeal nerve, the tympanic nerve ascends through the tympanic canaliculus to emerge onto the cochlear promontory, where it branches and coalesces with branches of the caroticotympanic nerve to form the tympanic plexus. The plexus is variably located in submucosal open grooves and bony canals over the promontory, supplying sensation and autonomic innervation [179] to the tympanic cavity and medial surface of the tympanic membrane. Tympanic plexus somatic fibres are postulated to provide the afferent pathway by which middle ear aeration could be regulated [180]. However, evidence in humans is inconclusive [181]. The tympanic nerve exits the middle ear through or near the canal for the tensor tympani muscle as the lesser superficial petrosal nerve [182], conveying presynaptic parasympathetic fibres to the otic ganglion. Post-ganglionic fibres travel with the auriculotemporal nerve (a branch of V_3) to provide parasympathetic secretomotor innervation to the parotid gland. Tympanic neurectomy has been used in the management of Frey's syndrome [183].

The Mastoid Complex

Lying within the mastoid process of the temporal bone, the mastoid complex (Figs. 4.1 and 4.6) is a collection of interconnected, air-filled spaces lined by a thin, flat epithelium with a dense underlying capillary network [184]. These air-filled spaces are in communication with the epitympanum via the *aditus ad antrum*. This connection allows unrestricted movement of gas between the mastoid complex and middle ear cavity.

As mentioned earlier, the extent of pneumatisation of the mastoid can vary greatly between individuals, from well-pneumatised to acellular or sclerotic. The well-pneumatised adult mastoid cavity can be subdivided into two areas: the mastoid antrum (and central tract) and the peripheral area [119]. Lying at the same level as the spine of Henle in the external ear canal, the mastoid antrum is a cave-like space that extends inferiorly and laterally to form the oblong central tract. It is surrounded by smaller, thin-walled cavities known as the peripheral air cells that can be subdivided by location but are variable in size, number and distribution [119]. As a result, the total gaseous volume of the pneumatised mastoid complex can vary greatly. A recent high-resolution micro-computed tomography (micro-CT) study has produced volumes of 2.7–13.6 cm^3, with a corresponding mucosal surface area of 81–326 cm^2 [185].

The tegmen tympani forms the roof of the mastoid complex, separating the mastoid air cells from the middle cranial fossa [186]. On the surface, this margin is approximated by the temporal line at the inferior limit of the temporal muscle [186]. The anterior boundary of the mastoid complex comprises the *aditus ad antrum* superiorly and the bony canal for the descending facial nerve inferiorly. A thin plate of bone separates the mastoid antrum from the descending sigmoid sinus, marking the posterior limit of the mastoid complex. However, pneumatisation can occur throughout the temporal bone. Thereby, peripheral air cells can be present outside the boundaries of the mastoid complex.

On the medial wall of the mastoid complex, the bony prominence demarcating the lateral semicircular canal can be located near the *aditus ad antrum*. The posterior semicircular canal lies deep to the remainder of the medial wall of the mastoid complex. The medial wall itself is defined as the thin plates of bone overlying these semicircular canals. The lateral wall is a thick, bony layer identifiable as the squamous part of the temporal bone inferior to the supramastoid crest. Towards the occiput, up to four mastoid emissary veins may perforate the superficial petromastoid surface, on average 35 mm along a line drawn from the mastoid tip to the asterion [187]. In some subjects, these vessels may be absent [187].

Within the mastoid, a bony plate dividing the superficial squamous air cells from the petrous air cells and mastoid antrum may be present in some individuals. Known as Körner's septum, this structure results from the incomplete fusion and obliteration of the fetal petrosquamosal suture. This is believed to contribute to attic blockage and has been correlated with the presence of chronic otitis media and its complications [188]. It has surgical relevance during mastoidectomy, as failure to remove Körner's septum results in failure to locate the mastoid antrum. MacEwen's (suprameatal) triangle [189] is used to locate the mastoid antrum from surface anatomy.

The mastoid cavities are widely believed to contribute to middle ear pressure regulation via membrane gas exchange [190, 191] and passive 'air buffering' [192]. Gas exchange and aeration of the mastoid complex are dependent on an intact mastoid mucosa [193]. The mucosa has two characteristics supporting this function: (1) a short diffusion distance provided by the flattened epithelial cells and proximity to the underlying capillaries and (2) a high surface area generated by cellular pneumatisation. Through its communication with the middle ear cavity, gas exchange across the mastoid mucosa can produce gradual pressure changes within the middle ear cavity [191]. This pressure regulation activity may complement that of the Eustachian tube, which acts to produce larger and more rapid changes in pressure [191], and the mastoid cavities have been postulated to slow down the decline of middle ear pressure during periods of Eustachian tube dysfunction [190]. However, a mastoid cavity is not required to achieve normal middle ear pressure in the context of a functioning Eustachian tube [194], and some mathematical modelling has opposed the postulated function of the mastoid complex as a gas reserve [195].

Alternative or additional functions of the mastoid cavities, which have been proposed, include frequency-dependent impedance modulation affected by the anatomical layout of air cell networks [196], middle and inner ear temperature regulation [197], protection of intracranial structures from lateral trauma [198] and reduction of skull density [199]. However, the variability in development of the mastoid cavities among individuals shows that a well-defined morphology and volume of the mastoid complex is not vital to function; indeed, cellular mastoid cavities are lacking in most non-primates, including all common laboratory mammals. Some authors have suggested that the mastoid complex in humans has no adaptive function [200].

Conclusions

Our current knowledge of middle ear development comes from nearly two centuries of research, with much of it based on the detailed comparison of wax-embedded, serial sections. What we know about postnatal middle ear anatomy in humans comes largely from surgical observations and temporal bone dissections, again dating back centuries. However, the advent of molecular biology techniques has led, over the last 30 years, to a revolution in our understanding of the mechanisms of middle ear development while the increased availability and resolution of micro-computed tomography allows us to explore the anatomy in even more detail. This work is not yet finished. Questions remain regarding how appropriate mice are as models for human middle ear development, given the many differences in ear structure between the two species. Although adult human middle ear morphology is extremely well-described, the functions of some of its prominent features, including the tensor tympani, mastoid complex and *pars flaccida* of the tympanic membrane, are still very poorly understood. More detailed studies of how anatomical variations correlate with middle ear pathologies may help address this. After a long period of relative stasis, our knowledge of the human middle ear is now increasing exponentially; we very much expect that there will be many changes to be made in the future editions of this book!

Acknowledgements Temporal bone specimens from which CT reconstructions were made were obtained from the Human Anatomy Centre, Department of Physiology, Development & Neuroscience, University of Cambridge. Prior to decease, all donors had provided consent for the use of their bodies for anatomical research, in compliance with the Human Tissue Act 2004. The authors thank Will Ashley-Fenn, Darren Broadhurst, Sue Jones, Prabhvir Marway and Maria Wright for preparation of the temporal bone specimens that we used and Cecilia Brassett and Richard Lloyd for their help with project logistics and permissions. CT scans were conducted at the Cambridge Biotomography Centre.

References

1. Grevellec A, Tucker AS. The pharyngeal pouches and clefts: development, evolution, structure and derivatives. Semin Cell Dev Biol. 2010;21:325–32.
2. Mallo M. Formation of the middle ear: recent progress on the developmental and molecular mechanisms. Dev Biol. 2001;231:410–9.
3. Graham A, Poopalasundaram S, Shone V, Kiecker C. A reappraisal and revision of the numbering of the pharyngeal arches. J Anat. 2019;235:1019–23.
4. Sudler MT. The development of the nose, and of the pharynx and its derivatives in man. Am J Anat. 1902;1:391–416.
5. Benson MT, Dalen K, Mancuso AA, Kerr HH, Cacciarelli AA, Mafee MF. Congenital anomalies of the branchial apparatus: embryology and pathologic anatomy. Radiographics. 1992;12:943–60.
6. Quinlan R, Martin P, Graham A. The role of actin cables in directing the morphogenesis of the pharyngeal pouches. Development. 2004;131:593–9.
7. van Waegeningh HF, Ebbens FA, van Spronsen E, Oostra R-J. Single origin of the epithelium of the human middle ear. Mech Dev. 2019;158:103556.
8. Burford CM, Mason MJ. Early development of the malleus and incus in humans. J Anat. 2016;229:857–70.
9. Frazer JE. The second visceral arch and groove in the tubo-tympanic region. J Anat Physiol. 1914;48:391–408.
10. Kanagasuntheram R. A note on the development of the tubotympanic recess in the human embryo. J Anat. 1967;101:731–41.
11. Anson BJ, Bast TH, Cauldwell EW. The development of the auditory ossicles, the otic capsule and the extracapsular tissues. Ann Otol Rhinol Laryngol. 1948;57:603–32.
12. Guggenheim P, Clements L, Schlesinger A. The significance and fate of the mesenchyme of the middle ear. Laryngoscope. 1956;66:1303–26.
13. Tucker AS. Major evolutionary transitions and innovations: the tympanic middle ear. Philos Trans Royal Soc B Biol Sci. 2017;372:20150483.
14. Wittmaack K. Über die normale end die pathologische Pneumatisation des Schlafenbeines einschliesslich ihrer Beziehungen zu den Mittelohrerkrankungen. Jena: Verlag von Gustav Fischer; 1918.
15. Schwarzbart A. The pneumatization of the temporal bone: a new concept. J Laryngol Otol. 1959;73:45–7.
16. Thompson H, Tucker AS. Dual origin of the epithelium of the mammalian middle ear. Science. 2013;339:1453–6.
17. Akaan-Penttilä E. Middle ear mucosa in newborn infants. A topographical and microanatomical study. Acta Otolaryngol. 1982;93:251–9.
18. Lim DJ. Normal and pathological mucosa of the middle ear and eustachian tube. Clin Otolaryngol Allied Sci. 1979;4:213–32.
19. Sade J. Middle ear mucosa. Arch Otolaryngol. 1966;84:137–43.
20. Piza J, Northrop C, Eavey RD. Embryonic middle ear mesenchyme disappears by redistribution. Laryngoscope. 1998;108:1378–81.
21. Piza JE, Northrop CC, Eavey RD. Neonatal mesenchyme temporal bone study: typical receding pattern versus increase in Potter's sequence. Laryngoscope. 1996;106:856–64.
22. Nikolic P, Järlebark LE, Billett TE, Thorne PR. Apoptosis in the developing rat cochlea and its related structures. Brain Res Dev Brain Res. 2000;119:75–83.
23. Roberts DS, Miller SA. Apoptosis in cavitation of middle ear space. Anat Rec. 1998;251:286–9.
24. Palva T, Ramsay H. Fate of the mesenchyme in the process of pneumatization. Otol Neurotol. 2002;23:192–9.
25. Presley R. Lizards, mammals and the primitive tetrapod tympanic membrane. Symp Zool Soc Lond. 1984;52:127–52.
26. Minoux M, Kratochwil CF, Ducret S, Amin S, Kitazawa T, Kurihara H, Bobola N, Vilain N, Rijli FM. Mouse Hoxa2 mutations provide a model for microtia and auricle duplication. Development. 2013;140:4386–97.
27. Ars B. Organogenesis of the middle ear structures. J Laryngol Otol. 1989;103:16–21.
28. Michaels L. Evolution of the epidermoid formation and its role in the development of the middle ear and tympanic membrane during the first trimester. J Otolaryngol. 1988a;17:22–8.
29. Michaels L. Origin of congenital cholesteatoma from a normally occurring epidermoid rest in the developing middle ear. Int J Pediatr Otorhinolaryngol. 1988b;15:51–65.
30. Lee TS, Liang JN, Michaels L, Wright A. The epidermoid formation and its affinity to congenital cholesteatoma. Clin Otolaryngol Allied Sci. 1998;23:449–54.

31. Mallo M, Gridley T. Development of the mammalian ear: coordinate regulation of formation of the tympanic ring and the external acoustic meatus. Development. 1996;122:173–9.
32. Rivera-Pérez JA, Mallo M, Gendron-Maguire M, Gridley T, Behringer RR. *Goosecoid* is not an essential component of the mouse gastrula organizer but is required for craniofacial and rib development. Development. 1995;121:3005–12.
33. Yamada G, Mansouri A, Torres M, Stuart ET, Blum M, Schultz M, De Robertis EM, Gruss P. Targeted mutation of the murine *goosecoid* gene results in craniofacial defects and neonatal death. Development. 1995;121:2917–22.
34. Yamada G, Ueno K, Nakamura S, Hanamure Y, Yasui K, Uemura M, Eizuru Y, Mansouri A, Blum M, Sugimura K. Nasal and pharyngeal abnormalities caused by the mouse goosecoid gene mutation. Biochem Biophys Res Commun. 1997;233:161–5.
35. Parry DA, Logan CV, Stegmann AP, Abdelhamed ZA, Calder A, Khan S, Bonthron DT, Clowes V, Sheridan E, Ghali N, Chudley AE, Dobbie A, Stumpel CT, Johnson CA. SAMS, a syndrome of short stature, auditory-canal atresia, mandibular hypoplasia, and skeletal abnormalities is a unique neurocristopathy caused by mutations in Goosecoid. Am J Hum Genet. 2013;93:1135–42.
36. Mallo M, Schrewe H, Martin JF, Olson EN, Ohnemus S. Assembling a functional tympanic membrane: signals from the external acoustic meatus coordinate development of the malleal manubrium. Development. 2000;127:4127–36.
37. Ishimoto S, Ito K, Kondo K, Yamasoba T, Kaga K. The role of the external auditory canal in the development of the malleal manubrium in humans. Arch Otolaryngol Head Neck Surg. 2004;130:913–6.
38. Mayer TE, Brueckmann H, Siegert R, Witt A, Weerda H. High-resolution CT of the temporal bone in dysplasia of the auricle and external auditory canal. AJNR Am J Neuroradiol. 1997;18:53–65.
39. Adanır SS, Bahşi İ. The giant anatomist, whose value is later understood: Bartolomeo Eustachi. Childs Nerv Syst. 2021;37:1–4.
40. Tos M. Growth of the foetal Eustachian tube and its dimensions. Archiv Fur Klinische Und Experimentelle Ohren- Nasen- Und Kehlkopfheilkunde. 1971;198:177–86.
41. Church MW, Gerkin KP. Hearing disorders in children with fetal alcohol syndrome: findings from case reports. Pediatrics. 1988;82:147–54.
42. Magnuson B, Falk B. Diagnosis and management of eustachian tube malfunction. Otolaryngol Clin N Am. 1984;17:659–71.
43. Todd NW. Otitis media and eustachian tube caliber. Acta Otolaryngol Suppl. 1983;404:1–17.
44. Swarts JD, Rood SR, Doyle WJ. Fetal development of the auditory tube and paratubal musculature. Cleft Palate J. 1986;23:289–311.
45. Anthwal N, Thompson H. The development of the mammalian outer and middle ear. J Anat. 2016;228:217–32.
46. Tono T, Schachern PA, Morizono T, Paparella MM, Morimitsu T. Developmental anatomy of the supratubal recess in temporal bones from fetuses and children. Am J Otol. 1996;17:99–107.
47. Tamari MJ. Auditory tube and tympanic cavity during embryonal, fetal, and prenatal life; histologic study. AMA Arch Otolaryngol. 1953;57:627–47.
48. Kitajiri M, Sando I, Takahara T. Postnatal development of the eustachian tube and its surrounding structures. Preliminary study. Ann Otol Rhinol Laryngol. 1987;96:191–8.
49. Luntz M, Sadé J. Growth of the eustachian tube lumen with age. Am J Otolaryngol. 1988;9:195–8.
50. Suzuki C, Balaban C, Sando I, Sudo M, Ganbo T, Kitagawa M. Postnatal development of Eustachian tube: a computer-aided 3-D reconstruction and measurement study. Acta Otolaryngol. 1998;118:837–43.
51. Ishijima K, Sando I, Balaban C, Suzuki C, Takasaki K. Length of the eustachian tube and its postnatal development: computer-aided three-dimensional reconstruction and measurement study. Ann Otol Rhinol Laryngol. 2000;109:542–8.
52. Oberascher G, Grobovschek M. The eustachian tube in HR computerized tomography. Imaging in the fetus, newborn infant and infant. HNO. 1987;35:455–61.
53. Takasaki K, Takahashi H, Miyamoto I, Yoshida H, Yamamoto-Fukuda T, Enatsu K, Kumagami H. Measurement of angle and length of the eustachian tube on computed tomography using the multiplanar reconstruction technique. Laryngoscope. 2007;117:1251–4.
54. Dinç AE, Damar M, Uğur MB, Öz II, Eliçora S, Bişkin S, Tutar H. Do the angle and length of the eustachian tube influence the development of chronic otitis media? Laryngoscope. 2015;125:2187–92.
55. De la Cuadra Blanco C, Peces Peña MD, Rodríguez-Vázquez JF, Mérida-Velasco JA, Mérida-Velasco JR. Development of the human tensor veli palatini: specimens measuring 13.6–137 mm greatest length; weeks 6–16 of development. Cells Tissues Organs. 2012;195:392–9.
56. Rodríguez-Vázquez JF, Sakiyama K, Abe H, Amano O, Murakami G. Fetal tendinous connection between the tensor tympani and tensor veli palatini muscles: a single digastric muscle acting for morphogenesis of the cranial base. Anat Record (Hoboken). 2016;299:474–83.
57. Kishimoto H, Yamada S, Kanahashi T, Yoneyama A, Imai H, Matsuda T, Takeda T, Kawai K, Suzuki S. Three-dimensional imaging of palatal muscles in the human embryo and fetus: development of levator veli palatini and clinical importance of the lesser palatine nerve. Dev Dyn. 2016;245:123–31.
58. Logjes RJ, Bleys RL, Breugem CC. The innervation of the soft palate muscles involved in cleft palate: a review of the literature. Clin Oral Investig. 2016;20:895–901.
59. Fuchs JC, Linden JF, Baldini A, Tucker AS. A defect in early myogenesis causes otitis media in two mouse models of 22q11.2 deletion syndrome. Hum Mol Genet. 2015;24:1869–82.
60. Diogo R, Abdala V, Lonergan N, Wood BA. From fish to modern humans—comparative anatomy, homologies and evolution of the head and neck musculature. J Anat. 2008;213:391–424.
61. McMyn JK. The anatomy of the salpingo-pharyngeus muscle. J Laryngol Otol. 1940;55:1–22.
62. Warmbrunn MV, de Bakker BS, Hagoort J, Alefs-de Bakker PB, Oostra R-J. Hitherto unknown detailed muscle anatomy in an 8-week-old embryo. J Anat. 2018;233:243–54.
63. Gaupp E. Die Reichertsche Theorie (Hammer-, Amboss- und Kieferfrage). Archiv für Anatomie und Entwickelungsgeschichte (suppl). 1913;1912:1–416.
64. Strickland EM, Hanson JR, Anson BJ. Branchial sources of auditory ossicles in man. I. Literature. Arch Otolaryngol. 1962;76:100–22.
65. Reichert C. Ueber die Visceralbogen der Wirbelthiere im Allgemeinen und deren Metamorphosen bei den Vögeln und Säugethieren. Archiv für Anatomie, Physiologie und Wissenschaftliche Medicin. 1837;1837:120–222.
66. Wyganowska-Świątkowska M, Przystańska A. The Meckel's cartilage in human embryonic and early fetal periods. Anat Sci Int. 2011;86:98–107.
67. Hanson JR, Anson BJ. Development of the malleus of the human ear. Illustrated in atlas series. Q Bull Northwest Univ Med Sch. 1962;36:119–37.
68. Rodríguez-Vázquez JF, Mérida-Velasco JR, Jiménez-Collado J. A study of the os goniale in man. Cells Tissues Organs. 1991;142:188–92.
69. Tucker AS, Watson RP, Lettice LA, Yamada G, Hill RE. Bapx1 regulates patterning in the middle ear: altered regulatory role in the transition from the proximal jaw during vertebrate evolution. Development. 2004;131:1235–45.

70. Gendron-Maguire M, Mallo M, Zhang M, Gridley T. Hoxa-2 mutant mice exhibit homeotic transformation of skeletal elements derived from cranial neural crest. Cell. 1993;75:1317–31.
71. Rijli FM, Mark M, Lakkaraju S, Dierich A, Dollé P, Chambon P. A homeotic transformation is generated in the rostral branchial region of the head by disruption of Hoxa-2, which acts as a selector gene. Cell. 1993;75:1333–49.
72. Hanson JR, Anson BJ, Strickland EM. Branchial sources of the auditory ossicles in man. II. Observations of embryonic stages from 7 mm to 28 mm (CR length). Arch Otolaryngol. 1962;76:200–15.
73. Louryan S. Le développement des osselets de l'ouie chez l'embryon humain: corrélations avec les données recueillies chez la souris. Bull Assoc Anat. 1993;77:29–32.
74. Whyte J, Cisneros A, Yus C, Fraile J, Obón J, Vera A. Tympanic ossicles and pharyngeal arches. Anat Histol Embryol. 2009;38:31–3.
75. Harrison MS, Leeming R. Preservation of the stapedius tendon in surgery of the stapes. Br J Audiol. 1971;5:78–84.
76. Standring S, Ellis H, Healy JC, Johnson D, Williams A, editors. Gray's anatomy: the anatomical basis of clinical practice. 39th ed. Edinburgh: Elsevier Churchill Livingstone; 2005.
77. Williams PL, Bannister LH, Berry MM, Collins P, Dyson M, Dussek JE, Ferguson MWJ, editors. Gray's Anatomy. 38th ed. Edinburgh: Churchill Livingstone; 1995.
78. Williams PL, Warwick R, Dyson M, Bannister LH, editors. Gray's anatomy. 37th ed. Edinburgh: Churchill Livingstone; 1989.
79. Rodríguez-Vázquez JF, Yamamoto M, Abe S, Katori Y, Murakami G. Development of the human incus with special reference to the detachment from the chondrocranium to be transferred into the middle ear. Anat Record (Hoboken). 2018;301:1405–15.
80. O'Gorman S. Second branchial arch lineages of the middle ear of wild-type and Hoxa2 mutant mice. Dev Dyn. 2005;234:124–31.
81. Mason MJ. Of mice, moles and Guinea pigs: functional morphology of the middle ear in living mammals. Hear Res. 2013;301:4–18.
82. Louryan S, Lejong M, Choa-Duterre M, Vanmuylder N. Hox-A2 protein expression in mouse embryo middle ear ossicles. Morphologie. 2018;102:243–9.
83. Anson BJ, Cauldwell EW. The developmental anatomy of the human stapes. Ann Otol Rhinol Laryngol. 1942;51:891–904.
84. Rodríguez-Vázquez JF. Development of the stapes and associated structures in human embryos. J Anat. 2005;207:165–73.
85. Thompson H, Ohazama A, Sharpe PT, Tucker AS. The origin of the stapes and relationship to the otic capsule and oval window. Dev Dyn. 2012;241:1396–404.
86. Amin S, Tucker AS. Joint formation in the middle ear: lessons from the mouse and guinea pig. Dev Dyn. 2006;235:1326–33.
87. Anson BJ, Bast TH. The development of the auditory ossicles and associated structures in man. Ann Otol Rhinol Laryngol. 1946;55:467–94.
88. Whyte JR, González L, Cisneros AI, Yus C, Torres A, Sarrat R. Fetal development of the human tympanic ossicular chain articulations. Cells Tissues Organs. 2002;171:241–9.
89. Jahrsdoerfer RA, Aguilar EA, Yeakley JW, Cole RR. Treacher Collins syndrome: an otologic challenge. Ann Otol Rhinol Laryngol. 1989;98:807–12.
90. Phelps PD, Poswillo D, Lloyd GA. The ear deformities in mandibulofacial dysostosis (Treacher Collins syndrome). Clin Otolaryngol Allied Sci. 1981;6:15–28.
91. Rodríguez-Vázquez JF, Yamamoto M, Kim JH, Jin Z-W, Katori Y, Murakami G. The incudopetrosal joint of the human middle ear: a transient morphology in fetuses. J Anat. 2020;237:176–87.
92. Anson BJ, Bast TH. Development of the incus of the human ear; illustrated in atlas series. Q Bull Northwest Univ Med Sch. 1959;33:110–9.
93. Yokoyama T, Iino Y, Kakizaki K, Murakami Y. Human temporal bone study on the postnatal ossification process of auditory ossicles. Laryngoscope. 1999;109:927–30.
94. Oesterle F. Über den Feinbau der Gehörknöchelchen und seine Entstehung. Arch Ohren Nasen Kehlkopfheilkd. 1933;135:311–27.
95. Anson BJ, Winch TR. Vascular channels in the auditory ossicles in man. Ann Otol Rhinol Laryngol. 1974;83:142–58.
96. Michaelides E, Kansal A, Rutter S, Schutt C. The malleus cap: anatomic description of cartilage of the lateral process of the malleus. Am J Otolaryngol. 2018;39:208–11.
97. Proops D, Hawke M, Berger G, MacKay A. The anterior process of the malleus. J Otolaryngol. 1984;13:39–43.
98. Hitier M, Zhang M, Labrousse M, Barbier C, Patron V, Moreau S. Persistent stapedial arteries in human: from phylogeny to surgical consequences. Surg Radiol Anat. 2013;35:883–91.
99. Rodríguez-Vázquez JF, Mérida-Velasco JR, Verdugo-López S. Development of the stapedius muscle and unilateral agenesia of the tendon of the stapedius muscle in a human fetus. Anat Record (Hoboken). 2010;293:25–31.
100. Rodríguez-Vázquez JF. Development of the stapedius muscle and pyramidal eminence in humans. J Anat. 2009;215:292–9.
101. Rodríguez-Vázquez JF, Mérida-Velasco JR, Verdugo-López S, Sánchez-Montesinos I, Mérida-Velasco JA. Morphogenesis of the second pharyngeal arch cartilage (Reichert's cartilage) in human embryos. J Anat. 2006;208:179–89.
102. Noden DM, Trainor PA. Relations and interactions between cranial mesoderm and neural crest populations. J Anat. 2005;207:575–601.
103. Anson BJ, Bast TH, Richany SF. The fetal development of the tympanic ring, and related structures in man. Q Bull Northwest Univ Med Sch. 1955;29:21–36.
104. Rodríguez-Vázquez JF, Murakami G, Verdugo-López S, Abe S-I, Fujimiya M. Closure of the middle ear with special reference to the development of the tegmen tympani of the temporal bone. J Anat. 2011;218:690–8.
105. Bowden RE. Development of the middle and external ear in man. Proc R Soc Med. 1977;70:807–15.
106. Spector GJ, Ge XX. Development of the hypotympanum in the human fetus and neonate. Ann Otol Rhinol Laryngol Suppl. 1981;90:1–20.
107. Eby TL. Development of the facial recess: implications for cochlear implantation. Laryngoscope. 1996;106:1–7.
108. Anson BJ, Bast TH. Development of the otic capsule of the human ear; illustrated in atlas series. Q Bull Northwest Univ Med Sch. 1958;32:157–72.
109. Sai X, Ladher RK. Early steps in inner ear development: induction and morphogenesis of the otic placode. Front Pharmacol. 2015;6:19.
110. Anson BJ, Bast TH. The development of the otic capsule in the region of surgical fenestration. Q Bull Northwest Univ Med School. 1949;23:465–77.
111. Nemzek WR, Brodie HA, Chong BW, Babcook CJ, Hecht ST, Salamat S, Ellis WG, Seibert JA. Imaging findings of the developing temporal bone in fetal specimens. AJNR Am J Neuroradiol. 1996;17:1467–77.
112. Leibovitz Z, Egenburg S, Bronshtein M, Shapiro I, Tepper R, Malinger G, Ohel G. Sonographic imaging of fetal tympanic rings. Ultrasound Obstet Gynecol. 2013;42:536–44.
113. Humphrey LT, Scheuer L. Age of closure of the foramen of Huschke: an osteological study. Int J Osteoarchaeol. 2006;16:47–60.
114. Rivera-Pérez JA, Wakamiya M, Behringer RR. Goosecoid acts cell autonomously in mesenchyme-derived tissues during craniofacial development. Development. 1999;126:3811–21.
115. Mason MJ. Functional morphology of rodent middle ears. In: Hautier L, Cox PG, editors. Evolution of the rodents: advances

in phylogeny, functional morphology and development, vol. 5. Cambridge: Cambridge University Press; 2015. p. 373–404.
116. Bast TH, Forester HB. Origin and distribution of air cells in the temporal bone. Arch Otolaryngol. 1939;30:183–205.
117. Cinamon U. The growth rate and size of the mastoid air cell system and mastoid bone: a review and reference. Eur Arch Otorhinolaryngol. 2009;266:781–6.
118. Halewyck S, Louryan S, Van Der Veken P, Gordts F. Craniofacial embryology and postnatal development of relevant parts of the upper respiratory system. B-ENT. 2012;8(Suppl 19):5–11.
119. Virapongse C, Sarwar M, Bhimani S, Sasaki C, Shapiro R. Computed tomography of temporal bone pneumatization: 1. Normal pattern and morphology. AJR Am J Roentgenol. 1985;145:473–81.
120. Palva T, Palva A. Size of the human mastoid air cell system. Acta Otolaryngol. 1966;62:237–51.
121. Crowe SJ, Polvogt LM. Embryonic tissue in the middle ear and mastoid: report of two cases. Arch Otolaryngol. 1930;12:151–61.
122. Kasemsuwan L, Schachern P, Paparella MM, Le CT. Residual mesenchyme in temporal bones of children. Laryngoscope. 1996;106:1040–3.
123. Jaisinghani VJ, Paparella MM, Schachern PA, Schneider DS, Le CT. Residual mesenchyme persisting into adulthood. Am J Otolaryngol. 1999;20:363–70.
124. Paparella MM, Shea D, Meyerhoff WL, Goycoolea MV. Silent otitis media. Laryngoscope. 1980;90:1089–98.
125. Sánchez Fernandez JM, Yarnoz J. Study of the mesenchymal clearance factor and its importance in the middle ear pneumatization process in rat and in man. Acta Otolaryngol. 1981;91:557–65.
126. Bilgin H, Kasemsuwan L, Schachern PA, Paparella MM, Le CT. Temporal bone study of Down's syndrome. Arch Otolaryngol Head Neck Surg. 1996;122:271–5.
127. Harada T, Sando I. Temporal bone histopathologic findings in Down's syndrome. Arch Otolaryngol. 1981;107:96–103.
128. Zavadskiĭ NV, Zavadskiĭ AV, Ntutumu AN. Controversial issues in the treatment of recurrent purulent otitis media in young children. Vestn Otorinolaringol. 1990;1990:3–7.
129. Rauchfuss A. Myxomatous remnants in the human middle ear. Histologic studies of their regression and microtopography. Laryngol Rhinol Otol. 1985;64:441–5.
130. Shewel Y, Bassiouny M, Ebrahim M. Endoscopic assessment of the isthmus tympanicum and tensor tympani fold and their relationship with mastoid pneumatization in chronic otitis media. J Int Adv Otol. 2020;16:227–33.
131. Dahlberg G, Diamant M. Inheritance of pneumatisation of the mastoid bone. Hereditas. 1945;31:441–56.
132. Lazaridis E, Saunders JC. Can you hear me now? A genetic model of otitis media with effusion. J Clin Investig. 2008;118:471–4.
133. Bluestone CD, Swarts JD. Human evolutionary history: consequences for the pathogenesis of otitis media. Otolaryngol Head Neck Surg. 2010;143:739–44.
134. Depreux FF, Darrow K, Conner DA, Eavey RD, Liberman MC, Seidman CE, Seidman JG. Eya4-deficient mice are a model for heritable otitis media. J Clin Investig. 2008;118:651–8.
135. Aimi K. The tympanic isthmus: its anatomy and clinical significance. Laryngoscope. 1978;88:1067–81.
136. Tóth M, Alpár A, Patonay L, Oláh I. Development and surgical anatomy of the round window niche. Ann Anat. 2006;188:93–101.
137. Franz BK, Clark GM, Bloom DM. Surgical anatomy of the round window with special reference to cochlear implantation. J Laryngol Otol. 1987;101:97–102.
138. Kassem F, Ophir D, Bernheim J, Berger G. Morphology of the human tympanic membrane annulus. Otolaryngol Head Neck Surg. 2010;142:682–7.
139. Decraemer WF, Dirckx JJ, Funnell WR. Shape and derived geometrical parameters of the adult, human tympanic membrane measured with a phase-shift moiré interferometer. Hear Res. 1991;51:107–21.
140. Djupesland G. Middle ear muscle reflexes elicited by acoustic and nonacoustic stimulation. Acta Otolaryngol Suppl. 1964;188:287–92.
141. Aritomo H, Goode RL, Gonzalez J. The role of pars flaccida in human middle ear sound transmission. Otolaryngol Head Neck Surg. 1988;98:310–4.
142. Ishijima K, Sando I, Balaban CD, Miura M, Takasaki K. Functional anatomy of levator veli palatini muscle and tensor veli palatini muscle in association with eustachian tube cartilage. Ann Otol Rhinol Laryngol. 2002;111:530–6.
143. Smith ME, Scoffings DJ, Tysome JR. Imaging of the Eustachian tube and its function: a systematic review. Neuroradiology. 2016;58:543–56.
144. Sudo M, Sando I, Ikui A, Suzuki C. Narrowest (isthmus) portion of Eustachian tube: a computer-aided three-dimensional reconstruction and measurement study. Ann Otol Rhinol Laryngol. 1997;106:583–8.
145. Hiraide F, Inouye T. The fine surface view of the human adult eustachian tube. J Laryngol Otol. 1983;97:149–57.
146. Janzen-Senn I, Schuon RA, Tavassol F, Lenarz T, Paasche G. Dimensions and position of the Eustachian tube in humans. PLoS One. 2020;15:e0232655.
147. Liu J, Pinheiro-Neto CD, Fernandez-Miranda JC, Snyderman CH, Gardner PA, Hirsch BE, Wang E. Eustachian tube and internal carotid artery in skull base surgery: an anatomical study. Laryngoscope. 2014;124:2655–64.
148. Bluestone CD, Doyle WJ. Anatomy and physiology of eustachian tube and middle ear related to otitis media. J Allergy Clin Immunol. 1988;81:997–1003.
149. Matsune S, Sando I, Takahashi H. Elastin at the hinge portion of the eustachian tube cartilage in specimens from normal subjects and those with cleft palate. Ann Otol Rhinol Laryngol. 1992;101:163–7.
150. Aoki H, Sando I, Takahashi H. Anatomic relationships between Ostmann's fatty tissue and eustachian tube. Ann Otol Rhinol Laryngol. 1994;103:211–4.
151. Alper CM, Swarts JD, Singla A, Banks J, Doyle WJ. Relationship between the electromyographic activity of the paratubal muscles and eustachian tube opening assessed by sonotubometry and videoendoscopy. Arch Otolaryngol Head Neck Surg. 2012;138:741–6.
152. Rood SR, Doyle WJ. Morphology of tensor veli palatini, tensor tympani, and dilatator tubae muscles. Ann Otol Rhinol Laryngol. 1978;87:202–10.
153. Dickson DR, Dickson WM. Velopharyngeal anatomy. J Speech Hear Res. 1972;15:372–81.
154. Chien HF, Sanchez TG, Sennes LU, Barbosa ER. Endonasal approach of salpingopharyngeus muscle for the treatment of ear click related to palatal tremor. Parkinsonism Relat Disord. 2007;13:254–6.
155. Akita K, Sakaguchi-Kuma T, Fukino K, Ono T. Masticatory muscles and branches of mandibular nerve: positional relationships between various muscle bundles and their innervating branches. Anat Record (Hoboken). 2019;302:609–19.
156. McDonald MH, Hoffman MR, Gentry LR, Jiang JJ. New insights into mechanism of Eustachian tube ventilation based on cine computed tomography images. Eur Arch Otorhinolaryngol. 2012;269:1901–7.
157. Manoharan SM, Gray R, Hamilton J, Mason MJ. Internal vascular channel architecture in human auditory ossicles. J Anat. 2022;241:245–58.
158. Kamrava B, Roehm PC. Systematic review of ossicular chain anatomy: strategic planning for development of novel middle ear prostheses. Otolaryngol Head Neck Surg. 2017;157:190–200.

159. De Greef D, Goyens J, Pintelon I, Bogers JP, Van Rompaey V, Hamans E, Van de Heyning P, Dirckx JJJ. On the connection between the tympanic membrane and the malleus. Hear Res. 2016;340:50–9.
160. Gan RZ, Sun Q, Dyer RK, Chang K-H, Dormer KJ. Three-dimensional modeling of middle ear biomechanics and its applications. Otol Neurotol. 2002;23:271–80.
161. Sim JH, Puria S. Soft tissue morphometry of the malleus–Incus complex from micro-CT imaging. J Assoc Res Otolaryngol. 2008;9:5.
162. Graboyes EM, Hullar TE, Chole RA. The lenticular process of the incus. Otol Neurotol. 2011;32:1600–4.
163. Chien W, Northrop C, Levine S, Pilch BZ, Peake WT, Rosowski JJ, Merchant SN. Anatomy of the distal incus in humans. J Assoc Res Otolaryngol. 2009;10:485–96.
164. Enghag S, Strömbäck K, Li H, Rohani SA, Ladak HM, Rask-Andersen H, Agrawal S. Incus necrosis and blood supply: a micro-CT and synchrotron imaging study. Otol Neurotol. 2019;40:e713–22.
165. Bolz EA, Lim DJ. Morphology of the stapediovestibular joint. Acta Otolaryngol. 1972;73:10–7.
166. Sim JH, Röösli C, Chatzimichalis M, Eiber A, Huber AM. Characterization of stapes anatomy: investigation of human and guinea pig. J Assoc Res Otolaryngol. 2013;14:159–73.
167. Guggenheim P. Mesenchyme in the middle ear. Laryngoscope. 1971;81:1665–70.
168. Marquet J. The incudo-malleal joint. J Laryngol Otol. 1981;95:543–65.
169. Mason MJ, Farr MRB. Flexibility within the middle ears of vertebrates. J Laryngol Otol. 2013;127:2–14.
170. Kierner AC, Mayer R, v Kirschhofer, K. Do the tensor tympani and tensor veli palatini muscles of man form a functional unit? A histochemical investigation of their putative connections. Hear Res. 2002;165:48–52.
171. Ramirez Aristeguieta LM, Ballesteros Acuña LE, Sandoval Ortiz GP. Tensor veli palatini and tensor tympani muscles: anatomical, functional and symptomatic links. Acta Otorrinolaringol Espanola. 2010;61:26–33.
172. Howell P. Are two muscles needed for the normal functioning of the mammalian middle ear? Acta Otolaryngol. 1984;98:204–7.
173. Jones SE, Mason MJ, Sunkaraneni VS, Baguley DM. The effect of auditory stimulation on the tensor tympani in patients following stapedectomy. Acta Otolaryngol. 2008;128:250–4.
174. Pang XD, Peake WT. *How* do contractions of the stapedius muscle alter the acoustic properties of the ear? In: Allen JB, Hall JL, Hubbard A, Neely ST, Tubis A, editors. Peripheral auditory mechanisms. New York: Springer; 1986. p. 36–43.
175. Mukerji S, Windsor AM, Lee DJ. Auditory brainstem circuits that mediate the middle ear muscle reflex. Trends Amplif. 2010;14:170–91.
176. McManus LJ, Dawes PJ, Stringer MD. Clinical anatomy of the chorda tympani: a systematic review. J Laryngol Otol. 2011;125:1101–8.
177. Monkhouse WS. The anatomy of the facial nerve. Ear Nose Throat J. 1990;69:677–83, 686–7.
178. Shin KJ, Gil YC, Lee JY, Kim JN, Song WC, Koh KS. Three-dimensional study of the facial canal using microcomputed tomography for improved anatomical comprehension. Anat Record (Hoboken). 2014;297:1808–16.
179. Ito J, Oyagi S, Honjo I. Autonomic innervations in the middle ear and pharynx. Acta Otolaryngol Suppl. 1993;506:90–3.
180. Eden AR, Gannon PJ. Neural control of middle ear aeration. Arch Otolaryngol Head Neck Surg. 1987;113:133–7.
181. Songu M, Aslan A, Unlu HH, Celik O. Neural control of eustachian tube function. Laryngoscope. 2009;119:1198–202.
182. Kanzara T, Hall A, Virk JS, Leung B, Singh A. Clinical anatomy of the tympanic nerve: a review. World J Otorhinolaryngol. 2014;4:17–22.
183. Ross JA. The function of the tympanic plexus as related to Frey's syndrome. Laryngoscope. 1970;80:1816–33.
184. Padurariu S, Röösli C, Røge R, Stensballe A, Vyberg M, Huber A, Gaihede M. On the functional compartmentalization of the normal middle ear. Morpho-histological modelling parameters of its mucosa. Hear Res. 2019;378:176–84.
185. Cros O, Knutsson H, Andersson M, Pawels E, Borga M, Gaihede M. Determination of the mastoid surface area and volume based on micro-CT scanning of human temporal bones. Geometrical parameters depend on scanning resolutions. Hear Res. 2016;340:127–34.
186. Singh A, Thakur R, Kumar R, Verma H, Irugu DVK. Grading of the position of the mastoid tegmen in human temporal bones—a surgeon's perspective. J Int Adv Otol. 2020;16:63–6.
187. Louis RG Jr, Loukas M, Wartmann CT, Tubbs RS, Apaydin N, Gupta AA, Spentzouris G, Ysique JR. Clinical anatomy of the mastoid and occipital emissary veins in a large series. Surg Radiol Anat. 2009;31:139–44.
188. Ozer E, Bayazit YA, Kara C, Mumbuç S, Kanlikama M, Gümüşburun E. Körner's septum (petrosquamosal lamina) and chronic ear disease. Surg Radiol Anat. 2004;26:118–21.
189. MacEwen W. Pyogenic and infective diseases of the brain and spinal cord: meningitis, abscess of brain, infective sinus thrombosis. Glasgow Med J. 1893;41:57–63.
190. Doyle WJ. The mastoid as a functional rate-limiter of middle ear pressure change. Int J Pediatr Otorhinolaryngol. 2007;71:393–402.
191. Gaihede M, Dirckx JJ, Jacobsen H, Aernouts J, Søvsø M, Tveterås K. Middle ear pressure regulation—complementary active actions of the mastoid and the Eustachian tube. Otol Neurotol. 2010;31:603–11.
192. Cinamon U, Sadé J. Mastoid and tympanic membrane as pressure buffers: a quantitative study in a middle ear cleft model. Otol Neurotol. 2003;24:839–42.
193. Takahashi H, Honjo I, Naito Y, Miura M, Tanabe M, Hasebe S, Toda H. Gas exchange function through the mastoid mucosa in ears after surgery. Laryngoscope. 1997;107:1117–21.
194. Belyea J, Wickens B, Bance M. Middle ear ventilation status postoperatively after translabyrinthine resection of vestibular schwannoma with mastoid obliteration and Eustachian tube occlusion: is the Eustachian tube enough to ventilate the middle ear without the mastoid air cell system? J Otolaryngol Head Neck Surg. 2016;45:44.
195. Swarts JD, Cullen Doyle BM, Alper CM, Doyle WJ. Surface area-volume relationships for the mastoid air cell system and tympanum in adult humans: implications for mastoid function. Acta Otolaryngol. 2010;130:1230–6.
196. Stepp CE, Voss SE. Acoustics of the human middle-ear air space. J Acoust Soc Am. 2005;118:861–71.
197. Magnuson B. Functions of the mastoid cell system: auto-regulation of temperature and gas pressure. J Laryngol Otol. 2003;117:99–103.
198. Ilea A, Butnaru A, Sfrângeu SA, Hedeşiu M, Dudescu CM, Berce P, Chezan H, Hurubeanu L, Trombiţaş VE, Câmpian RS, Albu S. Role of mastoid pneumatization in temporal bone fractures. AJNR Am J Neuroradiol. 2014;35:1398–404.
199. Proetz AW. Observations upon the formation and function of the accessory nasal sinuses and the mastoid cells. Ann Otol Rhinol Laryngol. 1922;31:1083–99.
200. Alicandri-Ciufelli M, Gioacchini FM, Marchioni D, Genovese E, Monzani D, Presutti L. Mastoid: a vestigial function in humans? Med Hypotheses. 2012;78:364–6.

Normal Histology of the Eustachian Tube, Middle Ear, and Mastoid Complex: The Mucoperiosteum Concept

5

Marcos V. Goycoolea, Raimundo José García-Matte, and Catalina Gutiérrez

Introduction

The middle ear, mastoid, and Eustachian tube constitute a continuous, irregular, three-dimensional pneumatic cavity located within the temporal bone, between the tympanic membrane laterally and the petrous portion of the temporal bone medially. It is in this pneumatic space that otitis media occurs.

The middle ear, mastoid, and Eustachian tube are lined by a continuous mucosa of endodermal origin that originates in the nasopharynx. Through the opening of the Eustachian tube, this complex is exposed to the nasopharyngeal space and, in turn, to the environment. The purpose of the mucosa is to maintain an air-filled cavity so that the middle ear can perform its function of sound transmission and amplification. This mucosal lining consists of an epithelium and an underlying connective tissue. In addition, in the bony cavities (middle ear and mastoid), it has a periosteal layer (Fig. 5.1).

M. V. Goycoolea (✉) · R. J. García-Matte
Department of Otolaryngology, Clínica Universidad de Los Andes, Santiago, Chile

C. Gutiérrez
Hospital Sótero del Río, Santiago, Chile

M. V. Goycoolea et al. (eds.), *Textbook of Otitis Media*, https://doi.org/10.1007/978-3-031-40949-3_5

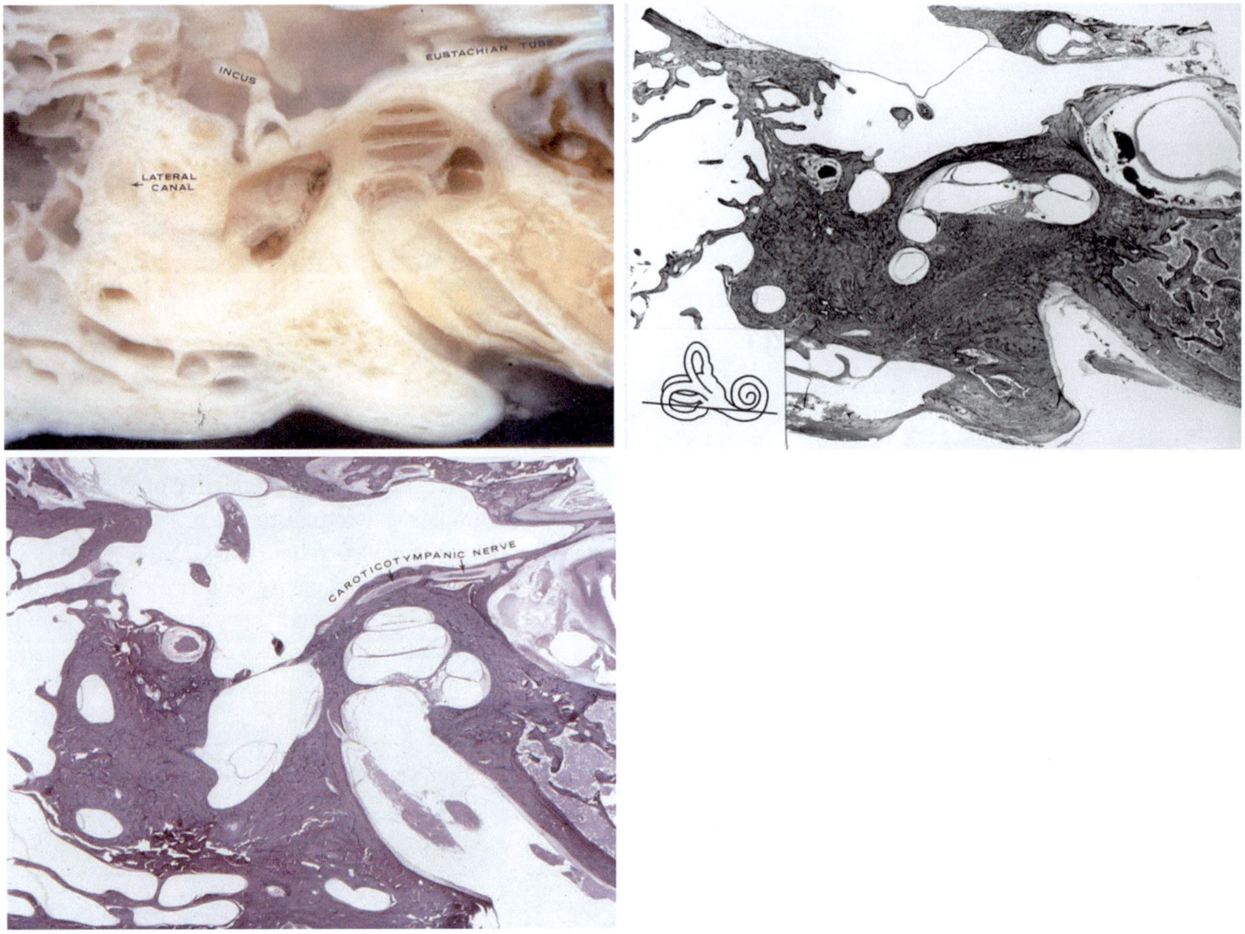

Fig. 5.1 Horizontal section of a temporal bone used as orientation to the different sites of the mucosal lining to be described in the middle ear, mastoid, and Eustachian tube. The Eustachian tube is located in the anterior wall and the mastoid cavity is posterior. The caroticotympanic nerve is over the promontory. (© Marcos Y. Goycoolea 2023; all rights reserved)

The Epithelium

The epithelium is continuous, and the types of cells will depend on their location in the mucosal lining of the middle ear and mastoid. Anteriorly, toward the Eustachian tube opening, there is a respiratory epithelium (Fig. 5.2). As it turns back toward the promontory, it gradually becomes cuboidal, with occasional glands (Fig. 5.3). The hypotympanum has tall ciliated columnar cells with some goblet cells and underlying basal cells, whereas toward the epitympanum, it has cuboidal ciliated cells with interposed small numbers of non-ciliated cells. As it extends towards the posterior wall and towards the aditus and antrum there is a gradual (Fig. 5.4a, b) flattening of epithelial cells with occasional ciliated cells toward the antrum initially, to become a simple squamous epithelium toward the mastoid (Fig. 5.5). In the mastoid the epithelium consists of flat non-ciliated cells devoid of glands and goblet cells. In other words, the mas-

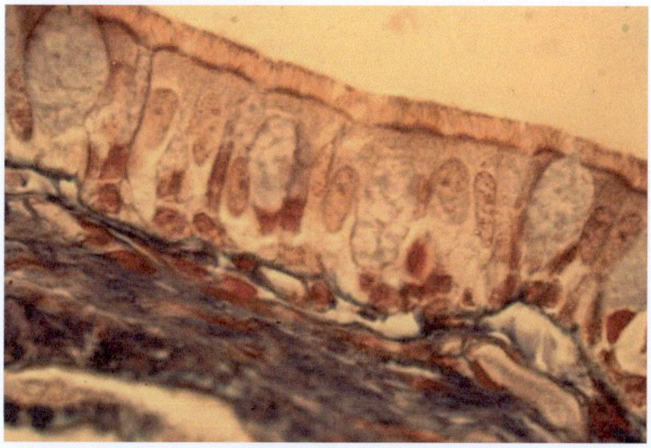

Fig. 5.2 A light micrograph of the Eustachian tube. A respiratory epithelium. Collagen fibers are stained blue with Azan stain. (© Marcos Y. Goycoolea 2023; all rights reserved)

toid cavity is covered by a simple squamous epithelium with occasionally scattered ciliated cells (Fig. 5.5). The ossicles are almost entirely lined by flat non-ciliated cells.

A respiratory epithelium refers to a ciliated, pseudostratified columnar epithelium with goblet cells. Pseudostratified means that all cells are in contact with the basal lamina. The epithelium provides a moist surface because of mucus production that is constantly moving toward the nasopharynx by the beating of the cilia of the ciliated cells. This has been termed "the mucociliary transport system" of the ear. The cells that form this epithelium are ciliated cells, goblet cells (mucus-secreting cells), intermediate cells, and basal cells. Basal cells are stem cells from which the other cells develop (Figs. 5.6 and 5.7).

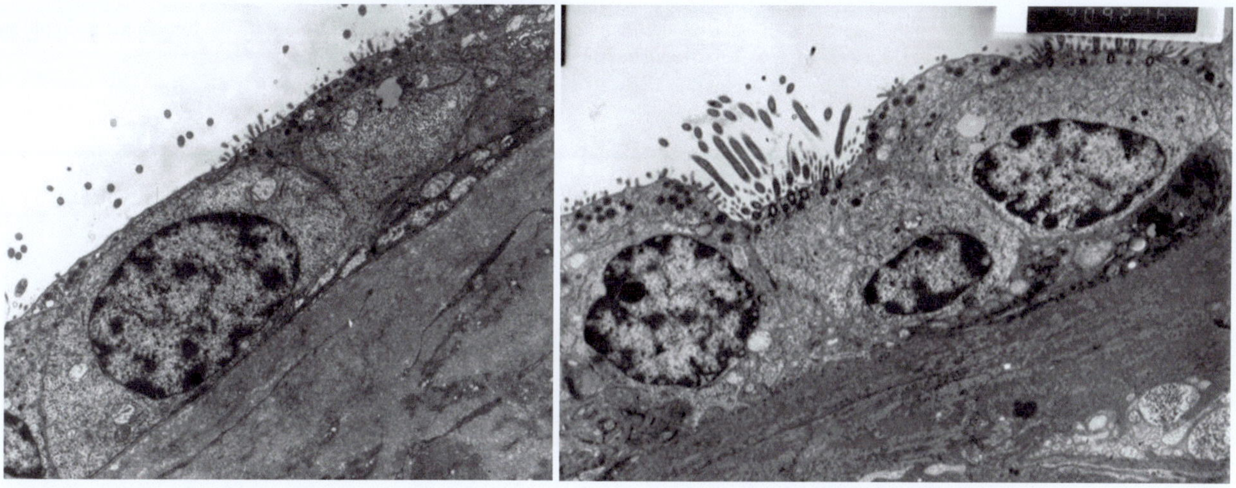

Fig. 5.3 A cuboidal ciliated epithelium at the promontory level. (© Marcos Y. Goycoolea 2023; all rights reserved)

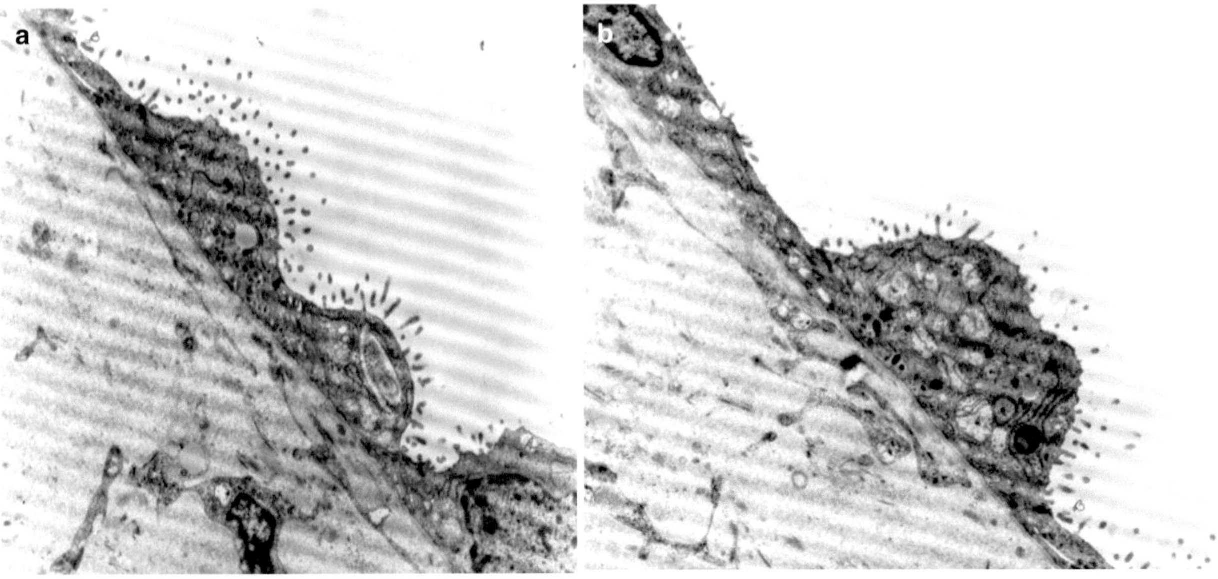

Fig. 5.4 (**a**, **b**) Gradual flattening of epithelial cells with occasional ciliated cells toward the aditus ad antrum initially, to become a simple squamous epithelium toward the mastoid (Fig. 5.5). (© Marcos Y. Goycoolea 2023; all rights reserved)

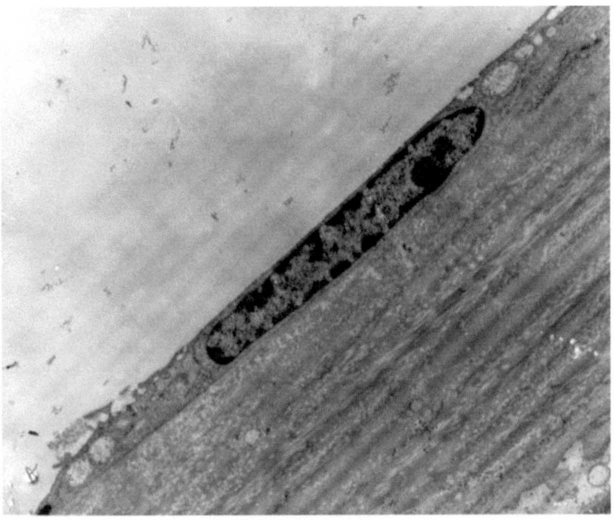

Fig. 5.5 A simple squamous epithelium in the mastoid. (© Marcos Y. Goycoolea 2023; all rights reserved)

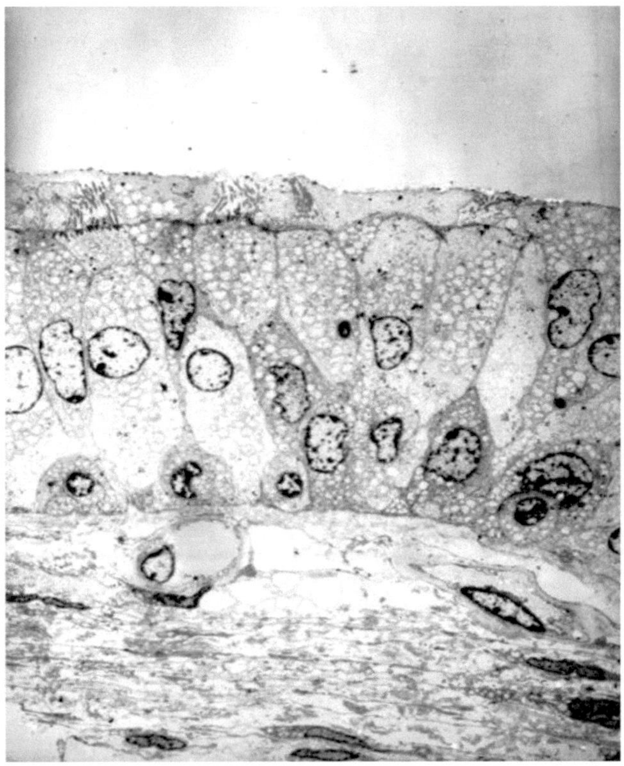

Fig. 5.6 An electron micrograph of a respiratory epithelium. (© Marcos Y. Goycoolea 2023; all rights reserved)

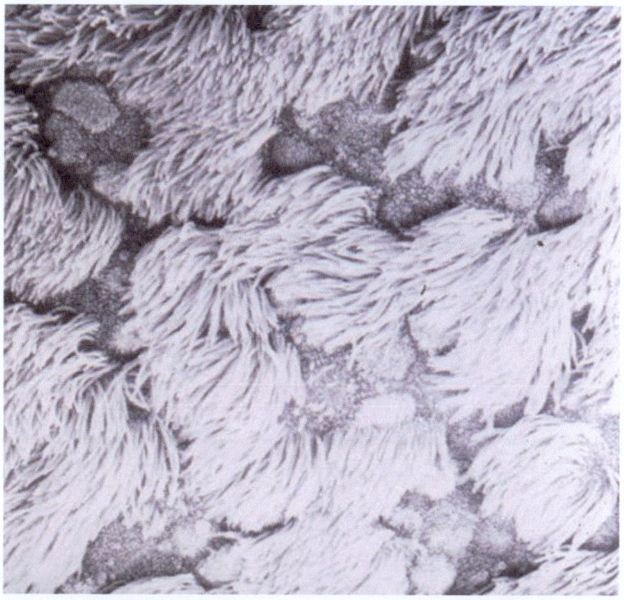

Fig. 5.7 A scanning electron micrograph of the cilia of the mucociliary transport system. (© Marcos Y. Goycoolea 2023; all rights reserved)

The Connective Tissue

The connective tissue of the middle ear and mastoid is continuous. In fact, the connective tissue of the entire body is continuous. Being of mesodermal origin, the connective tissue mechanically joins the different elements of the mucoperiosteum, establishes a fluid space, and contains vessels, nerves, and cells (Figs. 5.2 and 5.8). The most common cells are the fibroblasts that maintain the fiber system and are seemingly capable of performing other functions. Most other cells are those of the defense system such as neutrophils, macrophages, lymphocytes, and plasma cells. Mast cells containing histamine and serotonin are also found. Capillaries are also found in this layer. Forming a definite layer around the endothelium are the basement membrane and pericytes. There are also nerve fibers (myelinated and unmyelinated).

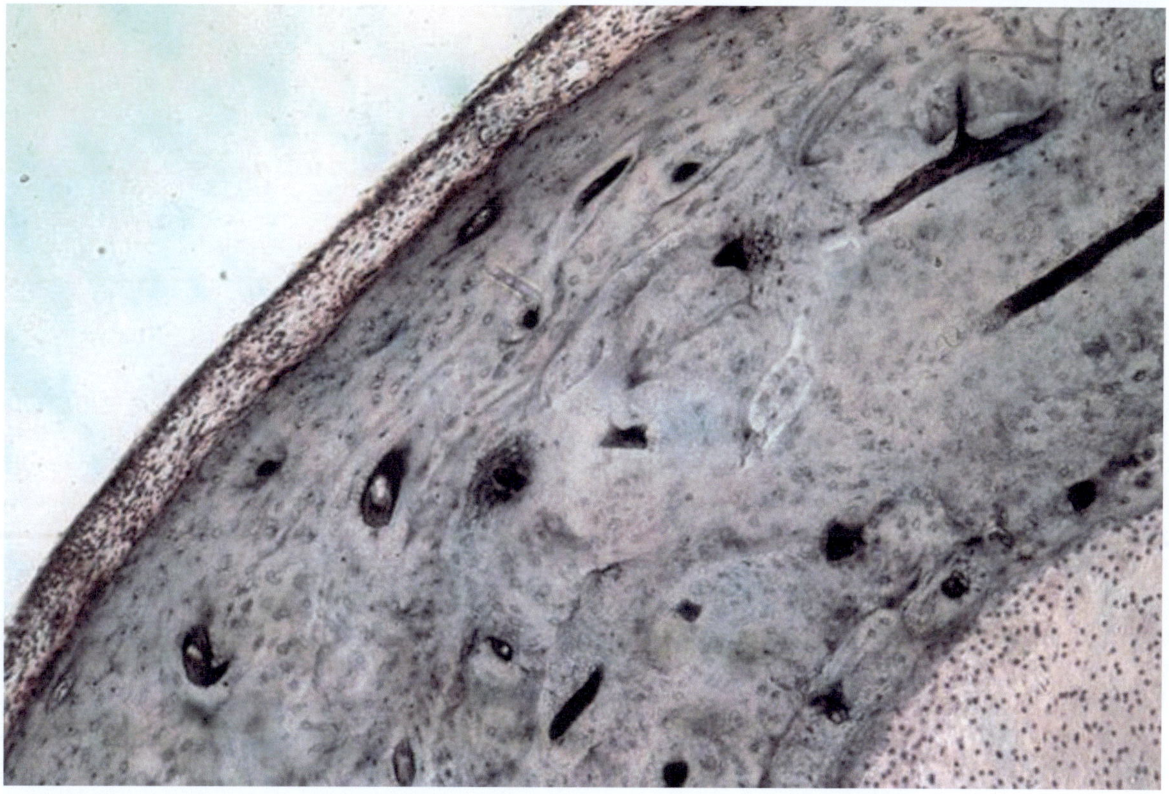

Fig. 5.8 A light micrograph of the promontory lined by the mucoperiosteum. (© Marcos Y. Goycoolea 2023; all rights reserved)

The Periosteum

With the exception of the tympanic membrane, Eustachian tube, and round-window membrane, the middle ear and mastoid are surrounded by a bone with its periosteum facing the connective tissue layer (Figs. 5.3, 5.5, and 5.8).

The Tympanic Membrane

The tympanic membrane is a thin, elliptically shaped membrane situated between the medial end of the external meatus and the middle ear cavity. Structurally, the membrane consists of three layers that are approximately 0.1 mm thick (combined): These layers include:

1. An outer cutaneous layer of thin skin, which is continuous with the skin of the external canal
2. A middle layer of connective tissue consisting of the following:
   (a) A radiate fibrous layer, made up of fibers radiating peripherally from the umbo and manubrium of the malleus
   (b) A circular fibrous layer, made up of concentrically arranged fibers that are most prominent peripherally, where they thicken to form a fibrocartilage ring or annulus, attaching the membrane to the tympanic sulcus of the temporal bone
3. An inner layer of the mucous membrane continuous with that of the middle ear cavity

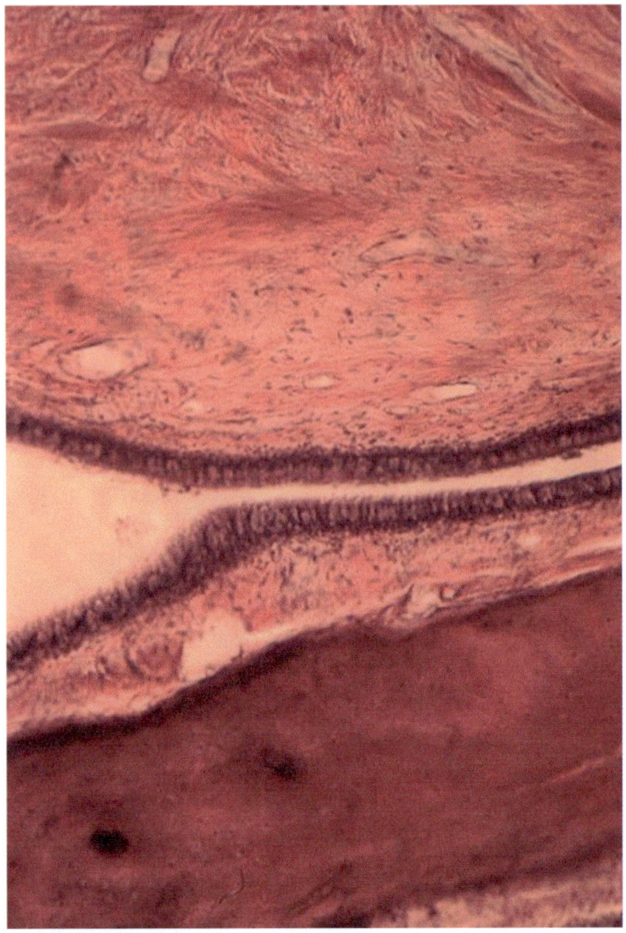

Fig. 5.9 Middle ear opening of the Eustachian tube. (© Marcos Y. Goycoolea 2023; all rights reserved)

The Eustachian Tube

The Eustachian tube extends from the anterior wall of the tympanic cavity to its nasopharyngeal opening just posterior to the dorsal end of the inferior nasal concha. Structurally, the auditory tube consists of both cartilaginous and bony components. The bony portion makes up approximately two-thirds of the tube; it is widest at the tympanic orifice and gradually narrows throughout its length, with its anterior extremity (the isthmus) being the most constricted portion of the entire tube. The cartilaginous portion of the tube extends from the isthmus to the nasopharynx. It is not totally cartilaginous. Its lower lateral and inferior walls consist of a fibrous connective tissue overlying the tensor veli and levator veli palatini muscles.

The lumen of the auditory tube, in the resting state, is a closed, slit-like cavity. The pharyngeal end of the tube strongly resists passage of air from the pharynx to the middle ear. Passage from the tympanic cavity to the pharynx is much easier.

The Eustachian tube is lined by a respiratory epithelium, and, in addition to the opening function of the tensor veli palatini muscle, there is seemingly some role of a surfactant. The respiratory epithelium with its cilia and mucus secretion are the basis of the mucociliary transport system of the middle ear (Figs. 5.6, 5.7, and 5.9).

The Round-Window Membrane

The round-window membrane is located in the medial wall of the middle ear, within the round-window niche. It consists of three layers: an outer epithelium facing the middle ear, a core of connective tissue, and an inner ear epithelium bordering the inner ear. The outer epithelium consists of a single layer of cells that are continuous with that of the promontory. The cells are low cuboidal. Tight junctions are present near the surface, and there is a continuous underlying basement membrane. The connective tissue layer contains fibroblasts, collagen, and elastic fibers as well as blood and lymph vessels and nerve fibers. The inner epithelium is lined by squamous cells with long lateral extensions that overlap each other. Histological descriptions of the round-window membrane are provided in this chapter of this book that discusses the use of topical treatment and middle inner ear interaction (Chap. 31).

The Otitis Media Process

Once aggression occurs, the ear responds with histopathological defensive factors that are gradual, systematic and universal, and have variations, which are adaptations to the different forms of insults. Their forms of presentation and severity will depend on the balance between the aggression and defense, with a direct influence of the environment, the genetic predisposition of the host, and the general defensive conditions at the time of occurrence.

The result of the response of the ear to aggression is the universal reaction of inflammation. This is the starting point of the sequential steps to be described. This inflammatory process involves all the walls, cavities, and anatomical structures that these contain as well as the mucoperiosteum that lines these cavities and structures (Fig. 5.10). With the understanding that the reaction is simultaneous at all levels, for practical reasons, the epithelial changes will be initially described.

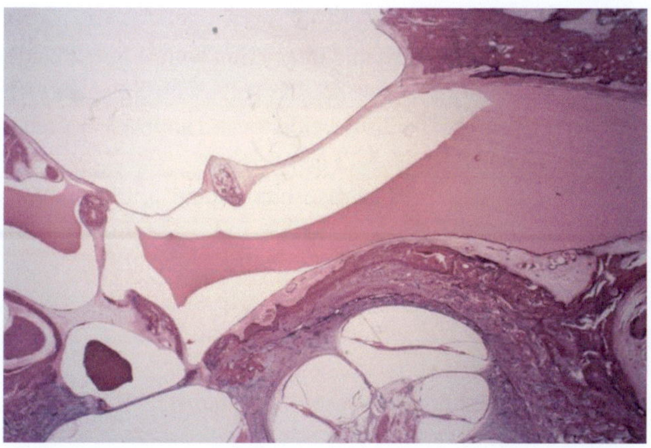

Fig. 5.10 Middle ear cavity with middle ear effusion. The inflammatory process involves all the walls, cavities, and anatomical structures that these contain as well as the mucoperiosteum that lines these cavities and structures. (© Marcos Y. Goycoolea 2023; all rights reserved)

Epithelial Changes

The epithelial cells participate in the inflammatory reaction by themselves and also as part of the mucociliary system. The cells become taller and have increased secretion (Figs. 5.11 and 5.12). There is also new gland formation and an increase in goblet cells.

Cells secrete different defensive substances such as lysozymes. The epithelial cells also have the capacity to synthesize the secretory piece of immunoglobulin (Ig)A (secretory IgA) just like the intestine since both epithelia are of the endodermal origin (Fig. 5.13).

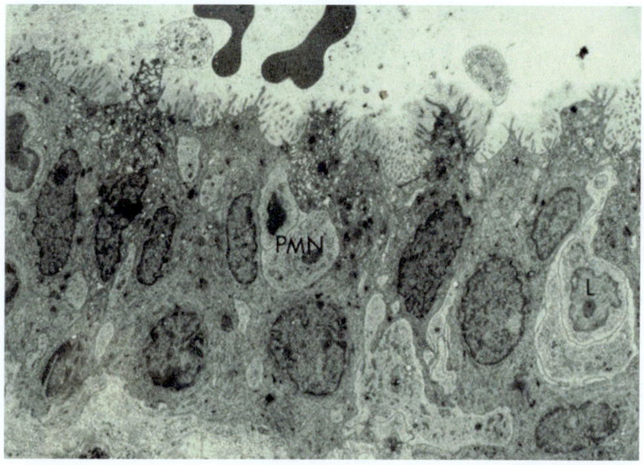

Fig. 5.11 An electron micrograph of the respiratory epithelium in acute otitis media. Secretory granules and migration of polymorphonuclear cells toward the middle ear cavity. (© Marcos Y. Goycoolea 2023; all rights reserved)

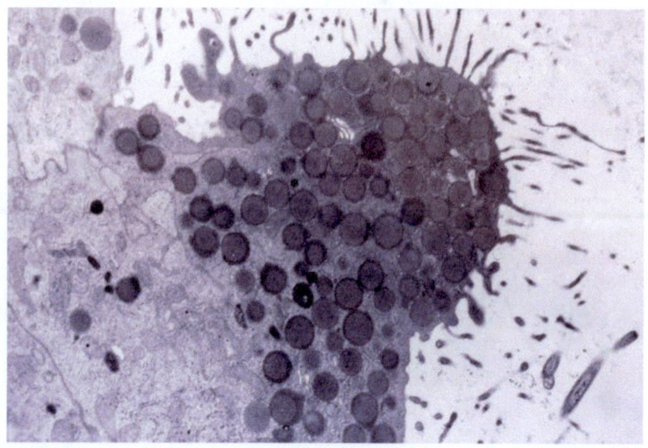

Fig. 5.12 An epithelial cell full of secretory granules and secreting toward the middle ear cavity. (© Marcos Y. Goycoolea 2023; all rights reserved)

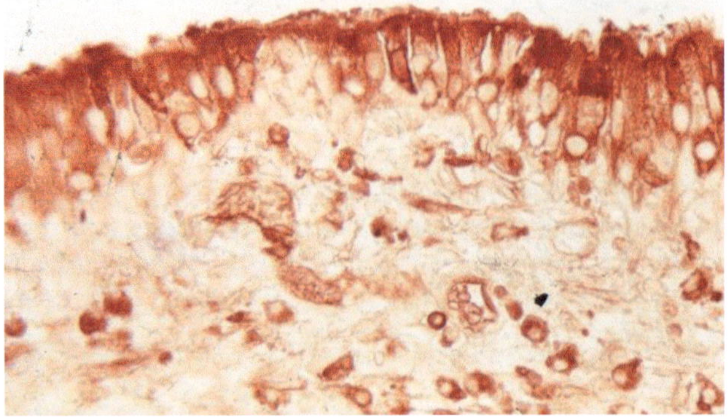

Fig. 5.13 Plasma and epithelial cells staining positive for IgA. (© Marcos Y. Goycoolea 2023; all rights reserved)

All these secretions plus the cellular elements in the middle ear cavity develop middle ear effusion. In some areas and depending on the degree of aggression, epithelial ruptures occur. Cholesteatomas seem likely to develop because of migration of the squamous epithelium of the tympanic membrane (and/or ear canal) rather than as a result of metaplastic changes of the inflamed epithelium (Goycoolea et al. 1999).

The Connective Tissue and Periosteal Changes

These are characterized as (Fig. 5.10) follows:

1. Thickening, edema, and increased vascularity
2. Cellular changes: Gradual cellular infiltration, changes in the types and numbers of cells
3. Changes in the shape and numbers of fibers
4. Inflammatory reaction of the periosteum
5. Inflammatory reaction of the underlying bone (osteitis)

In the early stages of the inflammatory process, the initial infiltration is based on polymorphonuclears that respond rapidly and traverse the capillaries toward the connective tissue (Fig. 5.14). From there, some migrate through the epithelium to the middle ear cavity (Fig. 5.11). Their primary function is engulfment of particles and microorganisms. The majority are neutrophils, but there are occasional eosinophils. The second cells to appear active are macrophages (Fig. 5.15) and abundant and active fibroblasts. Macrophages, despite being nonspecific, mark the starting point toward a specific immunological reaction mediated by T and B lymphocytes. Macrophages play a role in processing antigens and interacting with B lymphocytes (humoral immunity), which are the cells with a capacity for specific recognition. B cells develop toward antibody-secreting cells (plasma cells) (Figs. 5.13 and 5.16).

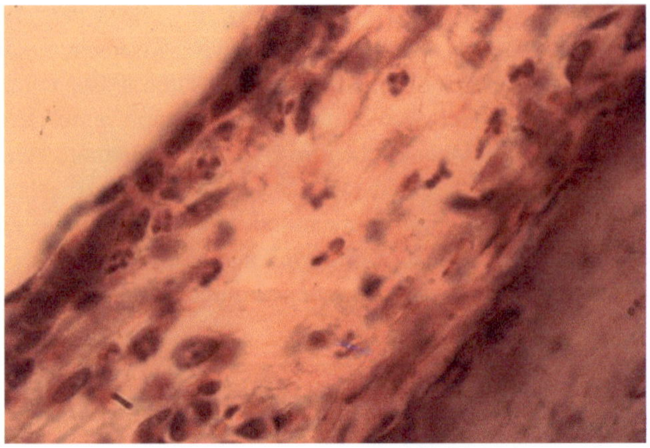

Fig. 5.14 Polymorphonuclears in the connective tissue of the promontory. (© Marcos Y. Goycoolea 2023; all rights reserved)

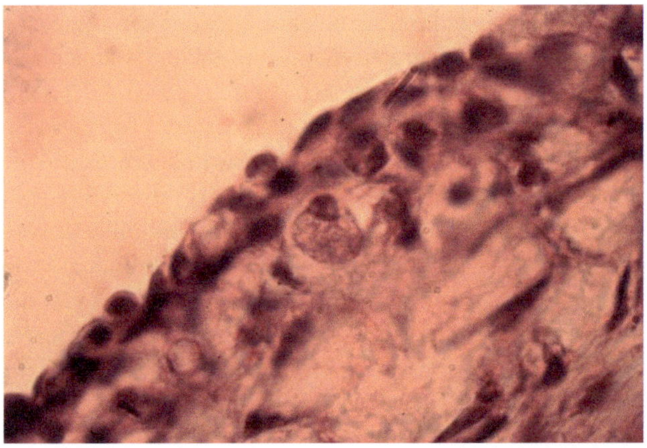

Fig. 5.15 Macrophages and active fibroblasts in the connective tissue of the promontory. (© Marcos Y. Goycoolea 2023; all rights reserved)

The middle ear mucosa also has a local immunological system via secretory IgA in which IgA is secreted by the plasma cells (B cells) and the epithelial cells add the secretory piece. Both IgG and IgM are also synthesized by the plasma cells and are secreted toward the mucosal surface. Fibroblasts are also active since the early stages.

The middle ear defense system consists of:

1. An epithelium that is continuous, regenerative, and constitutes a mechanical barrier
2. A mucociliary transport system (mucus, lysozymes, ciliated and secretory cells)

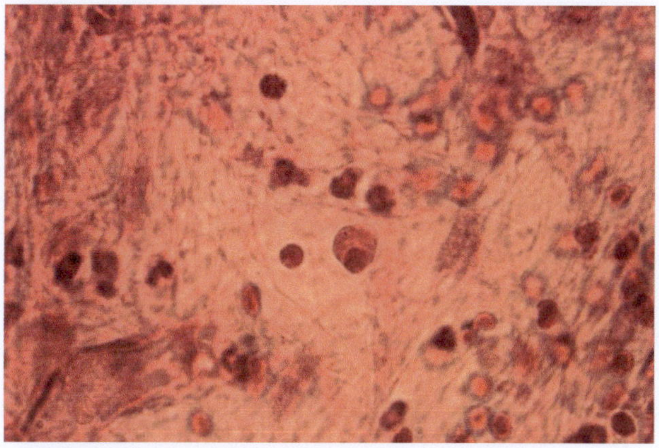

Fig. 5.16 Plasma cells in the connective tissue. (© Marcos Y. Goycoolea 2023; all rights reserved)

3. A patent and functional Eustachian tube
4. An inflammatory reaction of the connective tissue
5. Edema
6. Fibroblasts, collagen, and amorphous substance
7. Polymorphonuclear cells
8. Lymphocytes (small and large T and B cells, respectively).
9. Plasma cells: immunoglobulins (IgA, IgG, IgE, IgM)
10. A complement system.

Effusion Formation

Effusion formation is dynamic and reflects what is going on in the mucoperiosteum in terms of the phase and type of an inflammatory process. Samples will eventually be helpful for deciding treatments accordingly.

Changes in the Mucosa as a Whole

The middle ear develops polypoidal changes with areas that are prominent and areas that are depressed. Gland and blood vessel formation occur.

All structures are involved in the inflammatory process. The inflammatory process is dynamic and so is the middle ear effusion that tends to follow the histopathological changes that occur in the middle ear mucosa. The different forms of presentation of the otitis media process are therefore moments or instants of this dynamic process.

If otitis media is understood in this manner, it is much more than classifications and/or middle ear fluid and an inflammatory process. The changes described are in reality a reflection of the stage of confrontation between the aggression and the defensive factors. Thus, one form may lead to others in a dynamic way (Tables 5.1 and 5.2).

Table 5.1 Forms of otitis media

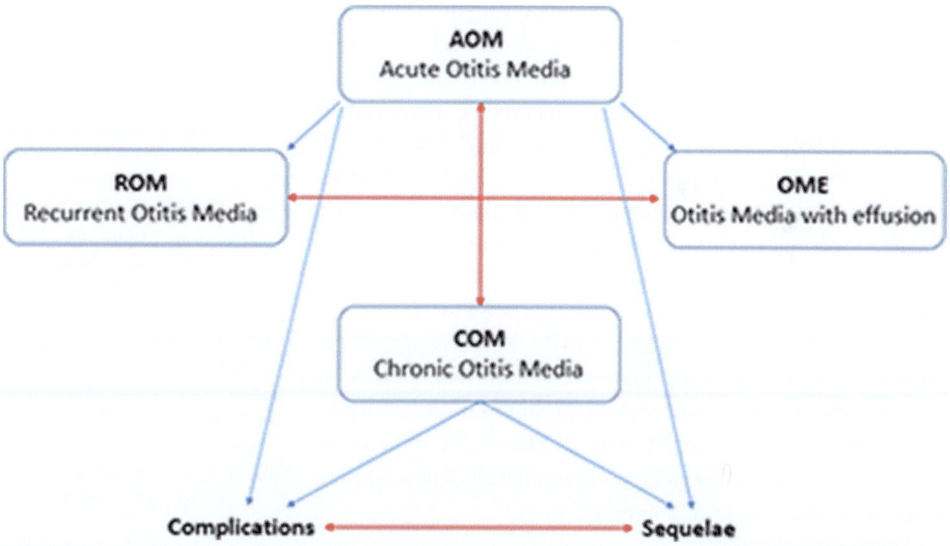

The form of presentation described in this table and the severity of the otitis media process will depend on the balance between two opposing forces, namely, the aggressive factors and the defensive factors of the middle ear. These are directly influenced by environmental factors, genetic predisposition, and the status of the defensive system of the host at the moment of aggression

Table 5.2 Classification and continuum of otitis media with effusion (OME)

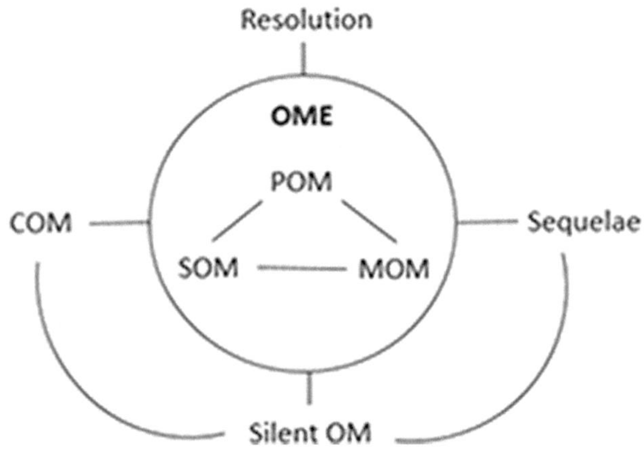

POM, purulent otitis media; *SOM*, serous otitis media; *MOM*, mucoid otitis media; *COM*, chronic otitis media; *OM*, otitis media

Complications and Sequelae

In addition to the involvement of the mucoperiosteum of the middle ear and mastoid as well as the Eustachian tube, there are potential complications and sequelae in this disease process. A complication is a secondary disease or condition developing in the course of a primary disease without being part of it. It occurs when the inflammatory process extends beyond the mucoperiosteum. A sequela is an after effect of a disease or injury. Herein, the term "sequela" refers to processes that remain within the mucoperiosteum (mucoperiosteal changes) and that have the capacity or potential to develop a complication (Goycoolea and Jung 1991) [1, 2]. The line between complications and sequelae is at times extremely tenuous. For example, the granulation tissue is a sequela (active sequela), but erosion of bone by the granulation tissue is a complication. In addition, the overall consequences of a localized problem (e.g., ossicular disruption causing conductive hearing loss) can have significant effects on a person and on their relationships with others (lack of communication, isolation, learning problems, and so forth).

At the level of the epithelium, ruptures occur in some areas of the mucosa (the degree of which will depend on the magnitude and type of aggression).

These ruptures allow:

Pockets with serous content

The inflamed connective tissue without epithelial covering (granulation tissue) can migrate through these openings. This tissue can persist or disappear. When it persists, it can erode the neighboring bone (with or without an associated cholesteatoma) and cause complications. It can disappear or be covered with an epithelium and cause adherences, which at times can serve as bridges for cellular migration as is the case of cholesteatomas (Goycoolea et al. 1999).

References[1]

1. Goycoolea M. Middle ear and mastoid. Chapter 1.4. In: Goycoolea M, et al., editors. Atlas of otologic surgery and magic otology. New Delhi: Jaypee Brothers Medical Publishers Ltd.; 2012. p. 21–57.
2. Goycoolea M. Surgical procedures in different forms of otitis media. Summary of concepts. Chapter 5.2.1. In: Goycoolea M, et al., editors. . New Delhi: Jaypee Brothers Medical Publishers Ltd; 2012. p. 463–89.

Further Reading[2]

Friedmann I. The pathology of acute and chronic infections in the middle ear cleft. Ann Otol Rhinol Laryngol. 1971;80:390–6.

Goycoolea MV. Pathogenesis of otitis media. Dissertations Abstr Int. 1978;39(6):132–210.

Goycoolea MV, Jung TK. Complications of suppurative otitis media. In: Paparella MM, Shumrick DA, Gluckman JL, Meyerhoff WL, editors. Otolaryngology, vol. II. Philadelphia: Saunders; 1991. p. 1381–403.

Goycoolea MV, Paparella MM, Carpenter AM, Juhn SK. A longitudinal study of cellular changes in experimental otitis media. Otolaryngol Head Neck Surg. 1979;87:685–700.

Goycoolea MV, Paparella MM, Juhn SK, Carpenter AM. The cells involved in the middle ear defense system. Ann Otol. 1980;68(Suppl 89):121–8.

Goycoolea MV, Hueb MM, Muchow D, Paparella MM. The theory of the trigger, the bridge and the transmigration in the pathogenesis of acquired cholesteatoma. Acta Otolaryngol. 1999;119(2):244–8.

Hentzer E. Ultrastructure of the middle ear mucosa. Ann Otol Rhinol Laryngol. 1976;85(Suppl 25):30–5.

Lim DJ. Functional morphology of the mucosa of the middle ear and Eustachian tube. Ann Otol. 1976;85(Suppl 25):36–43.

Lim DJ, Klamer A. Cellular reactions in acute otitis media. Scanning and transmission electron microscopy. Laryngoscope. 1971;81:1772–86.

Lim DJ, Shimada T. Secretory activity of normal middle ear epithelium. Ann Otol. 1971;80:319–29.

Mogi G. Secretory IgA and antibody activities in middle ear effusions. Ann Otol. 1976;85(Suppl 25):36–43.

Paparella MM, Sipila P, Jun SK, Jung TTK. Subepithelial space in otitis media. Laryngoscope. 1985;95:414–20.

Paparella MM, Goycoolea MV, Jung TK. Otitis media with effusion. In: Paparella MM, Shumrick DA, Gluckman JL, Meyerhoff WL, editors. Otolaryngology, vol. II. Philadelphia: Saunders; 1991. p. 1317–42.

Sadé J. Ciliary activity and middle ear clearance. Arch Otol. 1967;86:128–35.

Sadé J, Alufa I. Middle ear mucosa. Arch Otol. 1966;84:137–43.

Tos M. Production of mucus in the middle ear and Eustachian tube. Ann Otol. 1974;83:44–58.

Tos M, Bak-Pedersen K. Goblet cell density in Eustachian tube of children. Arch Otol. 1976;102:20–6.

[1]This chapter is a summary of many of our previous reports that are concentrated in two chapters of our *Atlas of Surgical Otology*.

[2]All the figures are my own and represent some of my best in more than 40 years of histological studies of temporal bones.

The references include some of the classic reports of the otitis media leaders, who, together with Michael Paparella and Steve Juhn, inspired my work. I had the privilege of knowing those whose reports are quoted and of learning from all of them—initially as a resident—and then in many symposia of otitis media through the years.

My coauthors are young staff members who have contributed—as I did initially—and, hopefully, they will also become inspired and improve by far these studies to which all of us have contributed.

Understanding the Aeration Avenues of the Middle Ear with the Aid of the Endoscope

6

Alessia Rubini, Margherita Basso, Nicola Bisi, Pierfrancesco Bettini, and Daniele Marchioni

Introduction

The study of the ventilation pathways of the middle ear, in particular of the epitympanic diaphragm, has long been one of the main interests of otologists, as, in the early 40s, it was first understood how its structure can affect the pathology of the middle ear. The inter-attico-tympanic diaphragm, later renamed the epitympanic diaphragm, was first identified in a histological study in newborns by Chatellier and Lemoine [1]. They described a set of membranous structures that, along with the incus and the malleus, shaped the floor of the epitympanum. Their study was based on the previous histological description of the development of middle ear spaces in fetuses at different stages of development by Hammar [2] and on anatomical treatises, like the one by Prussak [3]. Palva et al. further defined this structure through studies of microdissection of both healthy and diseased specimens, focusing on the ventilation pathways and their implication in the pathological processes of the middle ear. The epitympanic diaphragm divides the middle ear into two compartments: the epitympanum and the medial tympanum. It was Palva et al. who underlined the association between the blockage of the aeration pathways and the lesions of the upper compartment, due to dysventilation [4, 5].

During the last 10 years, the endoscope has gained increasing importance, first as a support to traditional microscopic surgery [6, 7] and then as a tool of its own, to carry out surgical procedures [8, 9].

The endoscopic approach to the middle ear has provided a unique way of evaluating its anatomy and disease, as it has made spaces, which cannot be reached with the use of traditional microscopes, easily accessible; in fact, 30°, 40°, and 75° endoscopes enable the surgeon to reach blind spaces in the middle ear, without disrupting any anatomical structures. While traditional approaches with a microscopic postauricular tympanomastoidectomy provide a limited access to the attic, especially to its anterior portion, the endoscope allows the surgeon to assess the integrity of the whole epitympanic diaphragm [10].

Since 2009, Marchioni et al. have published several studies on the endoscopic anatomy of the middle ear and have developed a nomenclature of the structures they identified. This classification has made it possible to standardize surgical approaches to lesions that require careful exploration of all the compartments of the middle ear, such as acquired or congenital cholesteatoma [11].

Ventilation Pathways

Anatomy of the Epitympanic Diaphragm (Fig. 6.1)

The epitympanic diaphragm, along with the malleus and the incus, forms the floor of the epitympanum, and it consists of the following folds (Fig. 6.2):

- Anterior, posterior, and lateral malleal ligament folds
- Posterior incudal ligament fold
- Tensor fold
- Lateral incudomalleal fold [12]

The anterior malleal ligament fold defines the anterior limit of Prussak space, as it extends from the anterior portion of the malleus neck to the anterior attic bony wall.

The posterior malleal ligament fold inserts into the posterior portion of the malleus neck and extends into the posterior tympanic spine. von Tröltsch's pouch is medially bounded by the posterior malleal ligament fold.

The lateral malleal ligament extends from the lateral wall of the malleus head to the medial wall of the scutum. It pos-

A. Rubini · M. Basso · N. Bisi (✉) · D. Marchioni
Department of Otolaryngology-Head and Neck Surgery, University Hospital of Modena, Modena, Italy

P. Bettini
ENT & Audiology Department, University Hospital of Ferrara, Ferrara, Italy

M. V. Goycoolea et al. (eds.), *Textbook of Otitis Media*, https://doi.org/10.1007/978-3-031-40949-3_6

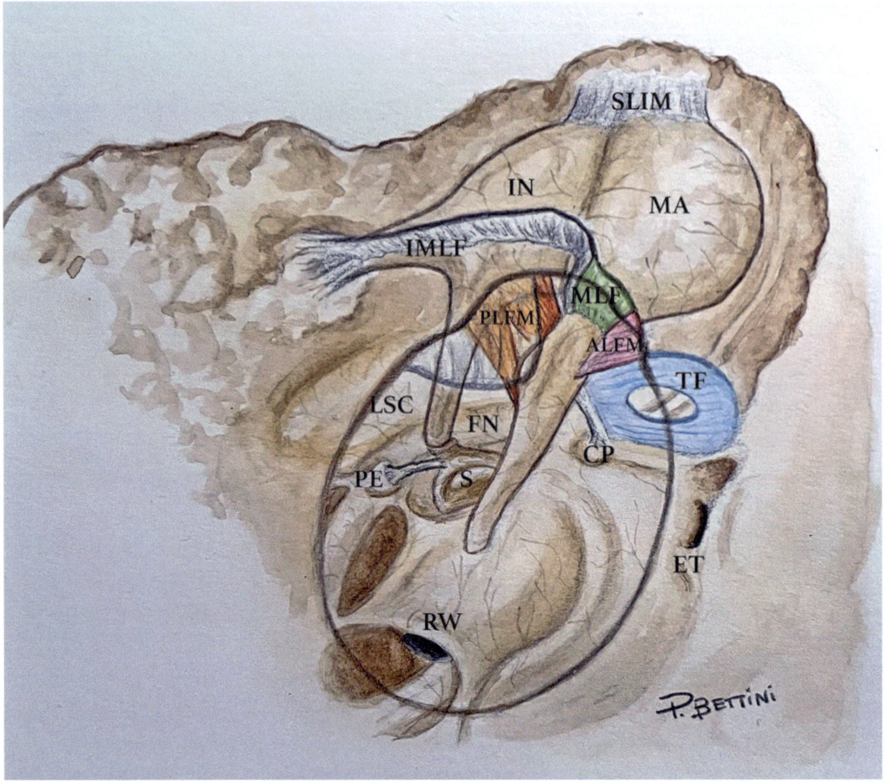

Fig. 6.1 The right ear. A drawing showing the epitympanic diaphragm seen in a caudal-to-cranial orientation and from a lateral to a medial one. The tensor fold is incomplete, showing a possible further ventilation pathway of the anterior epitympanum. *SLIM*, superior malleal ligament; *IN*, incus; *MA*, malleus; *IMLF*, lateral incudomalleal fold; *MLF*, lateral malleal fold; *PLFM*, posterior ligament of the malleus; *ALFM*, anterior malleal ligamental fold; *TF*, tensor fold; *LCS*, lateral semicircular canal; *FN*, facial nerve; *PE*, pyramidal eminence; *S*, stapes; *RW*, round window; *CP*, cochleariform process; *ET*, Eustachian tube

teriorly turns downward and merges with the anterior portion of the posterior incudal fold, whereas it anteriorly converges with the posterior portion of the anterior malleal fold.

The incudomalleal lateral fold is superior to the lateral malleal ligament fold, and it separates into two more compartments: the upper and lower lateral attic spaces. This fold has its insertion in the body of the incus and in the incudomalleal joint; it runs horizontally and extends to the medial wall of the scutum. Anteriorly, this structure bends and merges with the posterior margin of the lateral malleal ligament. During an endoscopic approach to the middle ear, the lateral incudomalleal fold must be disinserted from the body of the incus, to fully expose the upper lateral attic.

The anatomy of the tensor fold was defined owing to the introduction of the endoscope; in fact, its orientation and location make it undetectable through traditional retroarticular approaches. The tensor fold separates the supratubal recess in the protympanum from the anterior epitympanum, which is the space between the head of the malleus and the anterior bony wall of the scutum [12]. The tensor fold can appear as either complete or incomplete and can have three different orientations: vertical, horizontal, or oblique [13].

The relationship between the tensor fold and the cog (transverse crest) is important. The latter is a bony septum that cranially detaches from the tegmen tympani and vertically descends just anterior to the cochleariform process; it usually defines two compartments of the epitympanum: the anterior epitympanic space and the posterior epitympanic space. When the tensor fold has a vertical orientation, it is inserted into the cog, thus leading to a large supratubal recess. In this case, the cog does not separate the anterior from the posterior epitympanic space, rather, it represents the bony boundary between the supratubal recess and the epitympanic space. In the majority of cases, the tensor fold has an oblique orientation and attaches to the anterior tegmen tympani; therefore, the cog represents the division between the anterior and the posterior epitympanic spaces. When the tensor fold has a horizontal orientation and attaches to the tensor tympani semicanal, the supratubal recess is small or nonexistent. Thus, the anterior epitympanic space is large, and it is divided from the posterior epitympanic space by the transverse crest. As it is, the more vertical the tensor fold is, the wider the supratubal recess becomes.

Ventilation of the Upper Unit

It is known that three main factors influence the ventilation of the middle ear: the Eustachian tube function, the buffer mechanism provided by the mastoid, and the mucosal gas exchange.

The Eustachian tube plays a role in providing equalization of the pressure between the middle ear and the outside air. When the Eustachian tube fails, the pressure in the tympanic cavity becomes negative, causing a retraction of the tympanic membrane. The pressure in the middle ear is also related to the transmucosal gas exchange through the mas-

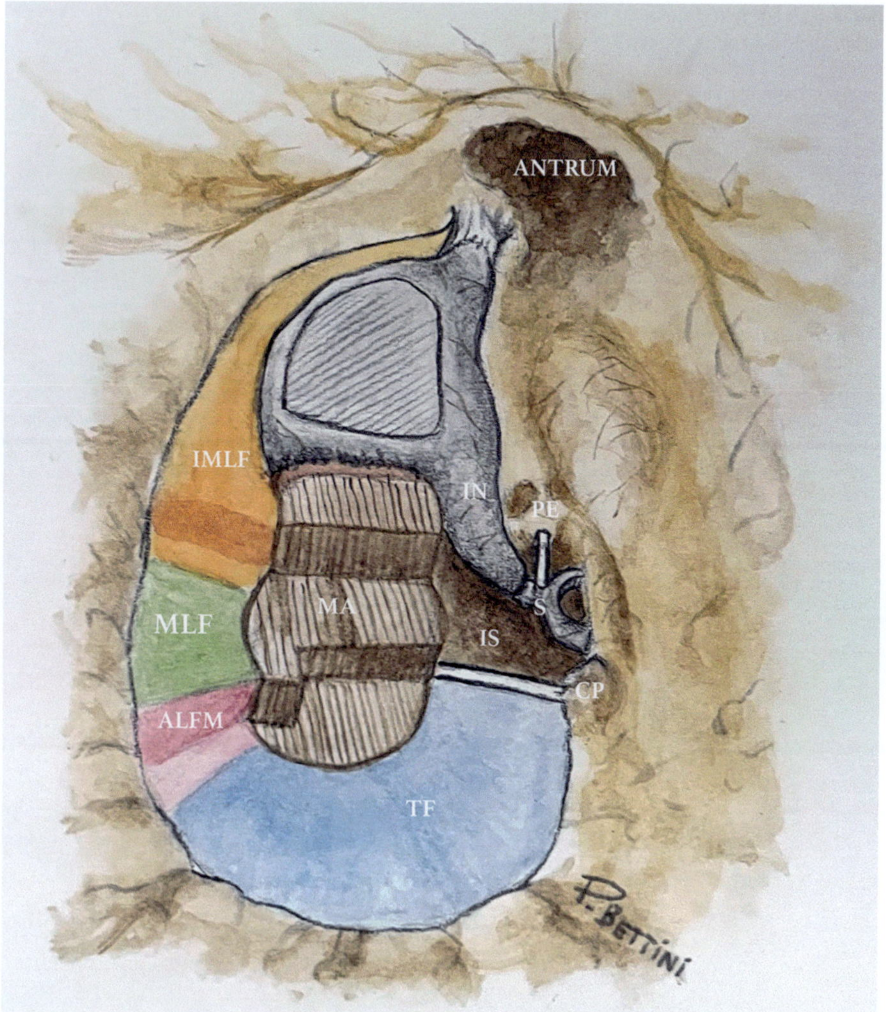

Fig. 6.2 The right ear. An epitympanic diaphragm from a superior view. The malleus is severed at different heights to show the attachment levels of the epitympanic diaphragm. The incus is sectioned at the level of its upper body. *IMLF*, lateral incudomalleal fold; *MLF*, lateral malleal fold; *ALFM*, anterior malleal ligamental fold; *TF*, tensor fold; *MA*, malleus; *IN*, incus; *IS*, tympanic isthmus; *S*, stapes; *PE*, pyramidal eminence; *CP*, cochleariform process

toid mucosa. These two systems achieve a balance if the ventilation pathways in the middle ear are open [14].

Two separate areas can be identified for what concerns the ventilation: an upper unit and a lower unit. The upper unit is made up of the superior lateral attic, along with the medial attic, and is connected to the mastoid. In case of a complete tensor fold, the upper unit is only aerated through two narrow spaces called the anterior and posterior isthmus, as the epitympanic diaphragm separates the epitympanum from the mesotympanum. The inferior lateral attic, which is divided from the superior one by the lateral incudomalleal fold, by contrast, is the only compartment of the epitympanum, which is aerated by the mesotympanic region [12].

The tympanic isthmus (Fig. 6.3) was first described by Chatellier and Lemoine; it was then outlined by Aimi as a narrow passage between the upper tubotympanic cavity and the atticomastoid space [15].

It is laterally bounded by the short process of the incus and the malleus head, anteriorly by the tensor tympani tendon and posteriorly by the posterior incudal ligament. The isthmus is divided into an anterior isthmus, which is the space defined by the incudostapedial joint and the tensor tympani tendon, and a variable posterior isthmus, which is just behind the incudostapedial joint.

The tensor fold plays a key role in the ventilation of the upper unit (Fig. 6.4), as it provides a separation between the anterior epitympanum and the protympanum. When the tensor fold is complete, the only ventilation pathway is through the tympanic isthmus, whereas in case of an incomplete tensor fold, additional ventilation is created between the protympanum and the anterior epitympanum.

Ventilation of the Lower Unit

The lower unit is represented by Prussak space; it is located below the epitympanic diaphragm, since its roof corresponds to the lateral malleal ligament fold. Prussak space is inferiorly defined by the short process of the malleus and medially by the malleus neck. The area is anteriorly bounded by the membranous anterior malleal ligamental fold, and its lateral wall is represented by Shrapnell's membrane, whereas the

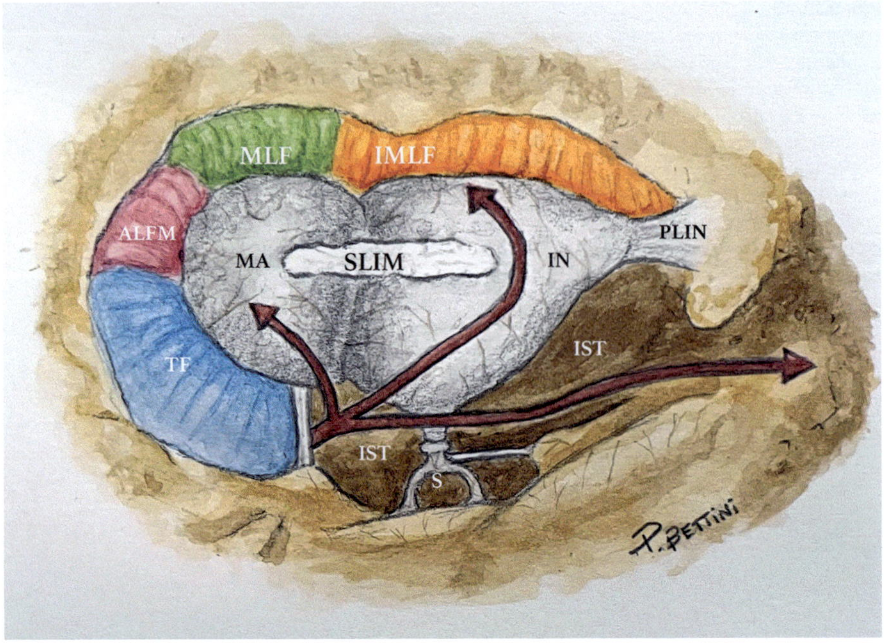

Fig. 6.3 The right ear. An epitympanic diaphragm seen from above. The arrows indicate the main ventilation of the epitympanum through the tympanic isthmus (one arrow is for the anterior epitympanum and the others are for the posterior epitympanum and mastoid). *ALFM*, anterior malleal ligamental fold; *MLF*, lateral malleal fold; *IMLF*, lateral incudomalleal fold; *TF*, tensor fold; *MA*, malleus; *SLIM*, superior malleal ligament; *IN*, incus; *IST*, tympanic isthmus; *S*, stapes; *PLIN*, lateral and medial posterior incudal ligaments

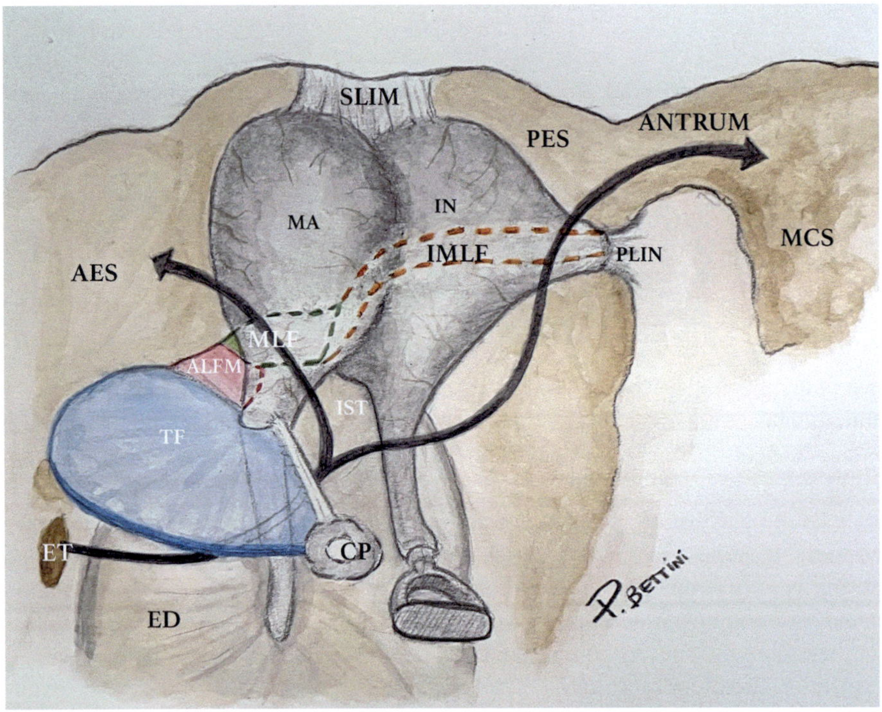

Fig. 6.4 The right ear. View of a complete tensor fold from a medial to a lateral direction and the main ventilation pathway of the epitympanum, through the tympanic isthmus. The epitympanic diaphragm is also seen in transparency as lateral to the incus and the malleus (dashed line). The black arrows show the ventilation of the anterior and posterior epitympanum. *AES*, anterior epitympanic space; *ET*, Eustachian tube; *TF*, tensor fold; *ALFM*, anterior malleal ligamental fold; *MLF*, lateral malleal fold; *MA*, malleus; *SLIM*, superior malleal ligament; *IN*, incus; *IMLF*, lateral incudomalleal fold; *IST*, tympanic isthmus; *ED*, eardrum; *PES*, posterior epitympanic space; *PLIN*, lateral and medial posterior incudal ligaments; *MCS*, mastoid cell; *CP*, cochleariform process

posterior wall corresponds to the posterior pouch of von Tröltsch.

The ventilation of Prussak space occurs through communication with the mesotympanum, represented by von Tröltsch's pouch, which is posteroinferiorly open, at the level of the most cranial portion of the mesotympanum, and it is laterally bordered by the pars tensa and the pars flaccida of the eardrum and medially by the posterior malleal ligament

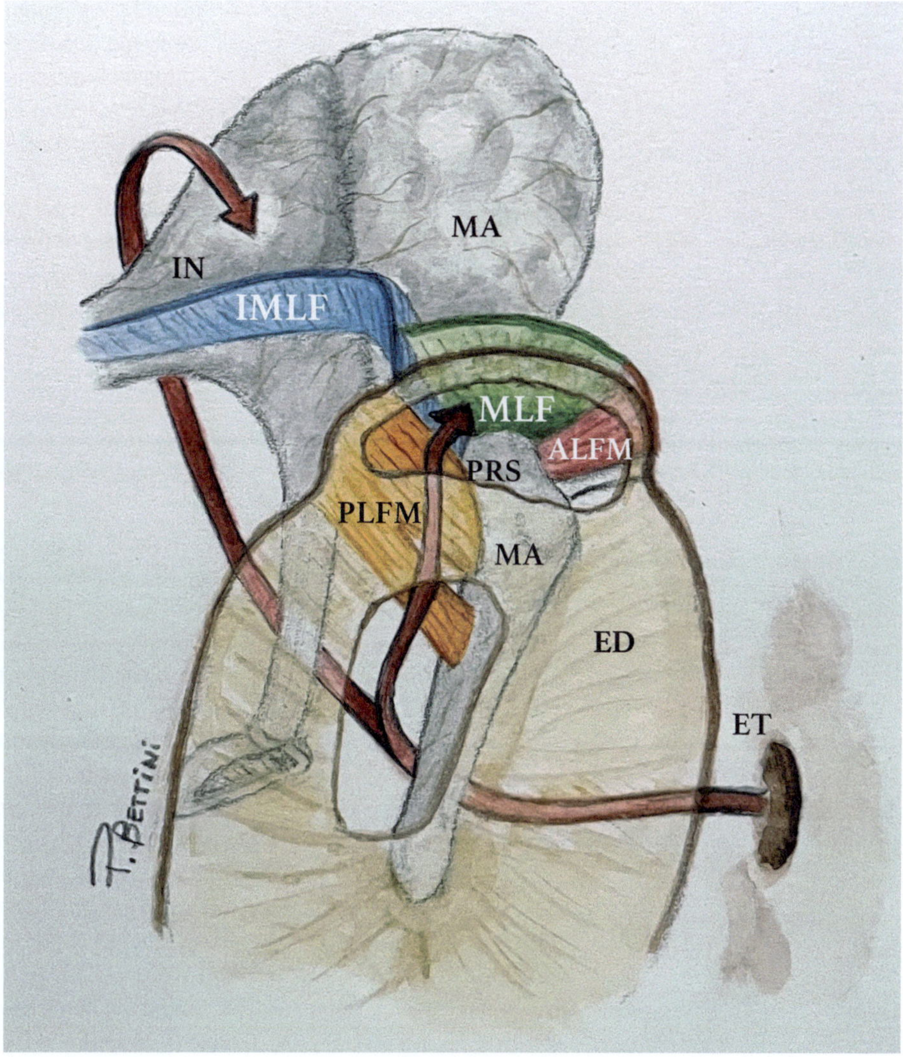

Fig. 6.5 The right ear. Lower and upper unit ventilation and epitympanic diaphragm. The tympanic membrane has been partially removed both in the pars flaccida (showing Prussak space) and in the pars tensa. The red arrows indicate the main ventilation pathway for the upper unit through the isthmus and for the lower unit (Prussak space) through von Tröltsch's pouch. *IN*, incus; *MA*, malleus; *IMLF*, lateral incudomalleal fold; *MLF*, lateral malleal fold; *ALFM*, anterior malleal ligamental fold; *PRS*, Prussak space; *PLFM*, posterior ligament of the malleus; *MA*, malleus; *ED*, eardrum; *ET*, Eustachian tube

(Fig. 6.5). The ventilation path of Prussak space is narrow and can easily tighten until it completely closes [16].

Even if the lower unit is an important component of the epitympanum, its aeration pathway can be blocked without affecting the function of the compartments, which lie superior to the epitympanic diaphragm or the one of other middle ear structures and the mastoid air system.

The Role of the Mastoid and Transmucosal Gas Exchange

The aerated mastoid is one of the three main factors influencing the ventilation of the middle ear.

Sadé and Ar [17] observed that the mastoid plays the role of an air reservoir to buffer rapid pressure changes within the middle ear (Fig. 6.6). Since volume and pressure are inversely proportional, a small, poorly aerated mastoid does not grant an optimal buffer function, allowing for wider pressure variations in the tympanic cavity (Fig. 6.7). Consequently, a largely aerated mastoid requires great changes in volume to achieve the same pressure as a small mastoid [12].

Another buffer mechanism is performed by the tympanic membrane since, and, if it is mobile enough, it has the possibility of bending inward and outward according to the pressure changes of the middle ear. Conversely, if the tympanic membrane is rigid and cannot bend properly, then the dilution of the pressure changes entirely depends on the aerated areas of the mastoid.

Since a small mastoid is most vulnerable to pressure changes, compensatory buffering mechanisms may develop, such as additional tympanic membrane retraction or middle ear volume reduction through fluid accumulation. A correlation exists between a poorly pneumatized mastoid and pars flaccida retraction, with a wider risk of atelectasis and subsequent cholesteatoma formation [18]. In the same way, it has been observed that children with recurrent otitis media, also complicated with cholesteatoma formation, usually have more sclerotic (less pneumatized) mastoids than do healthy children [19]. These examples provide further evidence of

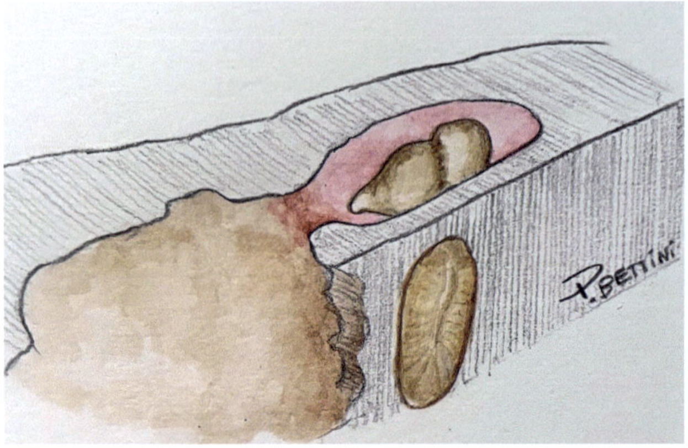

Fig. 6.6 The right ear. Regular buffer function of the mastoid. Sagittal section at the level of the tympanic membrane. Pink: middle ear; red: mastoid antrum; brown: mastoid

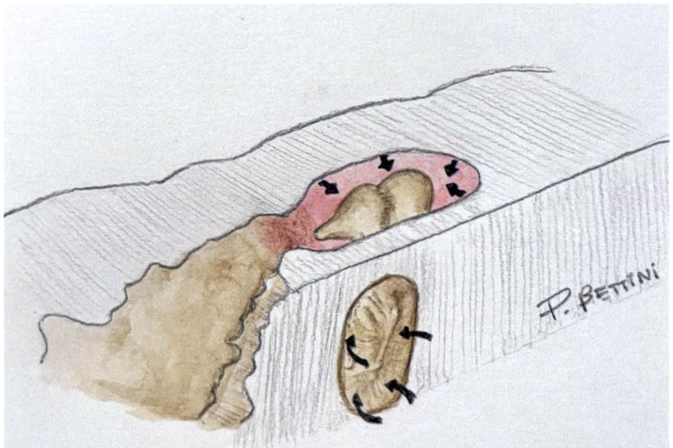

Fig. 6.7 The right ear. Sagittal section at the level of the tympanic membrane. Worse buffer function of a small mastoid that leads to wider pressure variations in the tympanic cavity, with a consequent retraction of the tympanic membrane (arrows) and a reduction of volume in the middle ear (arrows)

the fact that the mastoid plays an important buffering role in regulating the pressure of the middle ear [20].

As previously stated, the pressure balance is the result of the interaction between gas exchange in the mastoid air cells' mucosa, directly related to the degree of mastoid pneumatization, and a functioning Eustachian tube. Since these two mechanisms are interdependent, an isthmus blockage, even with a working Eustachian tube, could prevent mastoid cells' ventilation, leading to sclerotization of the mastoid itself. Görür et al. [21] classified the degree of radiological mastoid pneumatization shown in computed tomography (CT) scans as follows:

- Type 1 (normal pneumatization): The aerated mastoid cells reach the mastoid tip and the zygomatic, perisigmoid, and periantral regions and the aditus ad antrum is open.
- Type 2 (hypopneumatization): The aerated mastoid cells are found only in the antral and periantral regions and the aditus ad antrum is open.
- Type 3 (sclerotic): Mastoid pneumatization is absent and the aditus ad antrum is blocked.

Marchioni et al. ran CT scans on a group of subjects with an impairment of the middle ear aeration pathways. The vast majority of this group (18 out of 22) presented a hypopneumatized or scleroid mastoid. The degree of mastoid pneumatization was worse in the pathological ear, when compared to the contralateral one [22].

Blockage of the Ventilation Pathways

A primarily acquired cholesteatoma is morphologically characterized by epithelial cell proliferation. Unfortunately, despite a large number of studies, our understanding of the mechanisms underlying the pathogenesis of cholesteatoma is still limited. In the past, Bezold and Young suggested that the etiology of attic cholesteatoma could be attributed to an Eustachian tube dysfunction, resulting in an increased negative pressure in the tympanic cavity [19, 23]. On the other hand, Palva et al. observed how an attic retraction pocket could occur even in the case of a regular Eustachian tube function. Therefore, there must be other factors that affect the pathogenesis of attic cholesteatoma. The group led by Palva studied children with a blockage of the isthmus, who had undergone a tympanostomy tube placement, and they observed the persistence of inflammatory materials and cholesterol granuloma in the superior attic, despite the tympanostomy tube. They believed that an epitympanic diaphragm obstruction might be the origin of an attical cholesteatoma, stemming from an attical retraction. In contrast, children with an incomplete or absent tensor fold showed good ventilation of the anterior attic [24].

The theory that the obstruction of the aeration route between the mesotympanum and the attic is a contributing factor in the pathogenesis of attic retraction and cholesteatoma was severely challenged years ago by Yamasoba [25] and Kobayashi [26]. Yamasoba pointed out that it is possible for a cholesteatoma to stem from an attic retraction pocket despite the aeration of the mesotympanum in the middle ear. However, the importance of tensor fold removal during the surgical treatment of middle ear attic cholesteatoma remains of paramount importance, to restore the ventilation route from the protympanum to the anterior epitympanum, thus preventing the development of an attic cholesteatoma.

In microscopic ear surgery, since it is difficult to visualize the tensor fold due to its anterior position, some authors proposed different surgical approaches to microscopically visualize that fold. Morimitsu et al. [27] proposed an "anterior tympanotomy;" they removed the bone from the lateral attic to the zygoma, allowing for a possible drilling in front of the malleus head to remove the tensor fold. Palva et al. [28] suggested a tensor fold excision to create a large, new attic aeration pathway during cholesteatoma surgery through an endaural atticotomy extending to the supratubal recess.

With the introduction of an endoscope during middle ear surgery, it has become possible to study the anatomical variations and the ventilation pathways in pathological patients, owing to the magnification of critical areas such as the tensor fold and tympanic isthmus [16]. The exclusive transcanal endoscopic approach allows for a wide exposure of the anterior epitympanic compartment, especially the tensor fold and its inclination and its complete or incomplete structure, also granting the possibility of tensor fold removal with an angled instrument, thus restoring the ventilation of the upper unit.

The endoscopic approach to the tensor fold and to the anterior epitympanic compartment mainly depends on the dimensions of the anterior epitympanic space [29]. In most cases, it is wide, and the inferior endoscopic approach to the tensor fold area provides a good exposure to the inferior edge of the tensor fold, allowing for its removal and restoring direct ventilation from the protympanic space to the anterior epitympanic space.

In subjects with an extremely narrow anterior epitympanic space, associated with a vertical orientation of the tensor fold, it is only possible to explore the fold component close to the cochleariform process. In this case, a removal of the incus and the head of the malleus is necessary to obtain a good visualization of the superior edge of the tensor fold.

Selective Epitympanic Dysventilation Syndrome

As stated above, a physiological middle ear pressure seems to be connected to a functioning Eustachian tube and to the transmucosal gas exchange through the mastoid mucosa, which is directly related to the degree of pneumatization. An inflammatory middle ear chronic disease may thus be due to an Eustachian tube dysfunction and subsequent poor tympanic ventilation, which is often associated with the hypopneumatization or sclerotization of the mastoid cells [15, 16]. Conversely, in subjects with an excellent Eustachian tube function, two different conditions could give rise to an epitympanic selective dysventilation. The first condition is an obstruction of the posterior pouch of von Tröltsch, which closes the gap between the tympanic membrane and the posterior malleal ligamental fold, creating a selective dysventilation of the lower unit (Prussak space) [24]. The second state is an obstruction of the isthmus associated with a complete tensor fold, determining a selective dysventilation of the upper unit [30]. Several factors may obstruct the tympanic isthmus or von Tröltsch's pouch, such as mucosal fold variations, inflammatory webs, a retracted tympanic membrane, a pathological attic mucosa, and a cholesteatoma. In the two abovementioned conditions, a limited disease in the respective areas, possibly associated with an attical retraction, might occur [14]. As a confirmation of this, a tympanic isthmus obstruction is a consistent finding in patients with a limited attic cholesteatoma (Fig. 6.8).

A selective epitympanic dysventilation syndrome thus appears with four simultaneous distinctive features: an attic retraction pocket or cholesteatoma, a type A tympanogram or a regular tubal function test, a complete epitympanic diaphragm, and an isthmus blockage. In patients with this syndrome, while the epitympanum is poorly ventilated, with a subsequent decreased pressure that also extends to the mastoid, the mesotympanum is well-aerated, receiving air directly from a functioning Eustachian tube. In clinical practice, it is not uncommon to find an isolated retraction pocket of the pars flaccida and/or a cholesteatoma in this region, with a normal pars tensa and mesotympanum. Conversely, when the Eustachian tube function is impaired, the middle ear mucosa is usually widely involved in the inflammation process, and the tympanic membrane is completely retracted.

So, in patients with a selective epitympanic dysventilation, it is usually possible to intraoperatively appreciate an open Eustachian tube, a good protympanic and mesotympanic mucosa, and a partial or complete isthmus blockage that could alone explain it, thus strengthening the preoperative evaluation of a working Eustachian tube [14, 31]. From this, we can understand the importance of a surgical approach that can completely visualize the epitympanic diaphragm and surgically restore the ventilation pathways.

Selective Dysventilation of the Mesotympanum

Pars tensa cholesteatoma is a primarily acquired (retraction pocket) cholesteatoma that has a different pathogenesis from that of the attic, and it is associated with a negative middle ear pressure, due to a chronic Eustachian tube dysfunction. However, a ventilation dysfunction in the mesotympanum could also be attributed to fibrous or mucous webs between the medial wall of the tympanic cavity and the tympanic membrane that can exclude the tubal orifice and can create selective dysventilation areas in the anterior or posterior mesotympanum. This often leads to selective mesotympanic retraction pockets rather than the whole mesotympanum [32].

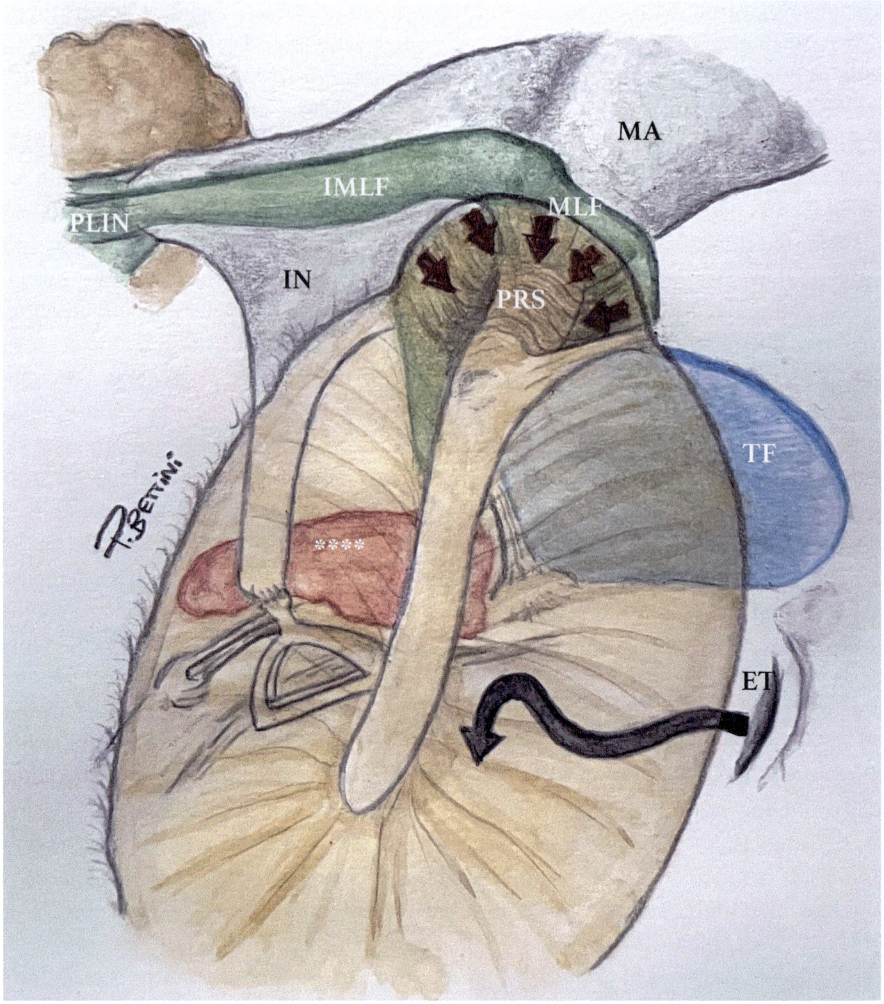

Fig. 6.8 The right ear. Lateral-to-medial view with a slight anterior rotation. Selective epitympanic dysventilation syndrome: blockage of the tympanic isthmus with a complete tensor fold. The arrow indicates the ventilation of the mesotympanum, through the Eustachian tube. The epitympanum is not properly ventilated due to the tympanic isthmus blockage. Prussak space is regularly aerated through von Tröltsch's pouch. ****: blockage of the tympanic isthmus. *PLIN*, lateral and medial posterior incudal ligaments; *IMLF*, lateral incudomalleal fold; *IN*, incus; *MA*, malleus; *MLF*, lateral malleal fold; *PRS*, Prussak space; *TF*, tensor fold; *ET*, Eustachian tube

References

1. Chatellier HP, Lemoine J. Le diaphragme interatticotympanique du nouveau-ne. Ann Otolaryngol Chir Cervicofac. 1946;13:534–66.
2. Hammar JA. Studien über die Entwicklung des Vorder-darms und einiger angrenzenden Organe. Archiv f Mikrosk Anat. 1902;61:404–58. https://doi.org/10.1007/BF02977928.
3. Prussak A. Zur Anatomie des menschlichen Trommelfells. Arch Augenheilkd. 1867;3:255–80. https://doi.org/10.1007/BF01804289.
4. Palva T, Ramsay H. Aeration of Prussak's space is independent of the supradiaphragmatic epitympanic compartments. Otol Neurotol. 2007;28(2):264–8. https://doi.org/10.1097/01.mao.0000247822.06022.07.
5. Palva T, Ramsay H. Epitympanic diaphragm in the new-born. Int J Pediatr Otorhinolaryngol. 1998;43(3):261–9. https://doi.org/10.1016/s0165-5876(98)00018-4.
6. McKennan KX. Endoscopic 'second look' mastoidoscopy to rule out residual epitympanic/mastoid cholesteatoma. Laryngoscope. 1993;103(7):810–4. https://doi.org/10.1288/00005537-199307000-00016.
7. Thomassin JM, Korchia D, Doris JM. Endoscopic-guided otosurgery in the prevention of residual cholesteatomas. Laryngoscope. 1993;103(8):939–43. https://doi.org/10.1288/00005537-199308000-00021.
8. Tarabichi M. Endoscopic management of acquired cholesteatoma. Am J Otol. 1997;18(5):544–9.
9. Tarabichi M. Endoscopic middle ear surgery. Ann Otol Rhinol Laryngol. 1999;108(1):39–46. https://doi.org/10.1177/000348949910800106.
10. Tarabichi M, Marchioni D, Kapadia M. The Epitympanum revisited: endoscopic anatomy. Indian J Otolaryngol Head Neck Surg. 2016;68(4):490–5. https://doi.org/10.1007/s12070-016-1000-6.
11. Marchioni D, Piccinini A, Alicandri-Ciufelli M, Presutti L. Endoscopic anatomy and ventilation of the epitympanum. Otolaryngol Clin N Am. 2013;46(2):165–78. https://doi.org/10.1016/j.otc.2012.10.002.
12. Marchioni D, Alicandri-Ciufelli M, Piccinini A, Presutti L. Ventilation and physiopathology of the middle ear. In: Presutti L, Marchioni D, editors. Endoscopic ear surgery: principles, indications, and techniques. Thieme; 2015. p. 66–85.
13. Li B, Doan P, Gruhl RR, Rubini A, Marchioni D, Fina M. Endoscopic anatomy of the tensor fold and anterior attic. Otolaryngol Head Neck Surg. 2018;158(2):358–63. https://doi.org/10.1177/0194599817739295.
14. Marchioni D, Alicandri-Ciufelli M, Molteni G, Artioli FL, Genovese E, Presutti L. Selective epitympanic dysventilation syndrome. Laryngoscope. 2010;120(5):1028–33. https://doi.org/10.1002/lary.20841.

15. Aimi K. The tympanic isthmus: its anatomy and clinical significance. Laryngoscope. 1978;88(7 Pt 1):1067–81. https://doi.org/10.1002/lary.1978.88.7.1067.
16. Marchioni D, Mattioli F, Alicandri-Ciufelli M, Presutti L. Endoscopic approach to tensor fold in patients with attic cholesteatoma. Acta Otolaryngol. 2009;129(9):946–54. https://doi.org/10.1080/00016480802468187.
17. Sadé J, Ar A. Middle ear and auditory tube: middle ear clearance, gas exchange, and pressure regulation. Otolaryngol Head Neck Surg. 1997;116(4):499–524. https://doi.org/10.1016/s0194-5998(97)70302-4.
18. Sadé J, Fuchs C, Luntz M. Shrapnell membrane and mastoid pneumatization. Arch Otolaryngol Head Neck Surg. 1997;123(6):584–8. https://doi.org/10.1001/archotol.1997.01900060026004.
19. Young N, Chole RA. Retraction pocket cholesteatoma. Curr Opin Otolaryngol Head Neck Surg. 2002;10:355–9. https://doi.org/10.1097/00020840-200210000-00004.
20. Marchioni D, Mattioli F, Cobelli M, Todeschini A, Alicandri-Ciufelli M, Presutti L. CT morphological evaluation of anterior epitympanic recess in patients with attic cholesteatoma. Eur Arch Otorhinolaryngol. 2009;266(8):1183–9. https://doi.org/10.1007/s00405-008-0871-x.
21. Görür K, Ozcan C, Talas DU. The computed tomographical and tympanometrical evaluation of mastoid pneumatization and attic blockage in patients with chronic otitis media with effusion. Int J Pediatr Otorhinolaryngol. 2006;70(3):481–5. https://doi.org/10.1016/j.ijporl.2005.07.023.
22. Marchioni D, Mattioli F, Alicandri-Ciufelli M, Molteni G, Masoni F, Presutti L. Endoscopic evaluation of middle ear ventilation route blockage. Am J Otolaryngol. 2010;31(6):453–66. https://doi.org/10.1016/j.amjoto.2009.08.010.
23. Bezold F. Uber des cholesteatom des mittelohres. Z Orenhk. 1891;21:252–63.
24. Palva T, Johnsson LG, Ramsay H. Attic aeration in temporal bones from children with recurring otitis media: tympanostomy tubes did not cure disease in Prussak's space. Am J Otol. 2000;21(4):485–93.
25. Yamasoba T, Kikuchi S. Is an isthmus block a prerequisite for the development of an attic retraction cholesteatoma? Eur Arch Otorhinolaryngol. 1993;250(5):300–3. https://doi.org/10.1007/BF00186231.
26. Kobayashi T, Toshima M, Yaginuma Y, Ishidoya M, Suetake M, Takasaka T. Pathogenesis of attic retraction pocket and cholesteatoma as studied by computed tomography. Am J Otol. 1994;15(5):658–62.
27. Morimitsu T, Tono T, Makino K, Miyanaga S, Ushisako Y. Improvement of the surgical technique of anterior tympanoplasty in cholesteatoma. Rev Laryngol Otol Rhinol (Bord). 1995;116(5):369–71.
28. Palva T, Ramsay H, Böhling T. Lateral and anterior view to tensor fold and supratubal recess. Am J Otol. 1998;19(4):405–14.
29. Marchioni D, Alicandri-Ciufelli M, Grammatica A, Mattioli F, Genovese E, Presutti L. Lateral endoscopic approach to epitympanic diaphragm and Prussak's space: a dissection study. Surg Radiol Anat. 2010;32(9):843–52. https://doi.org/10.1007/s00276-010-0691-8.
30. Palva T, Johnsson LG. Epitympanic compartment surgical considerations: reevaluation. Am J Otol. 1995;16(4):505–13.
31. Marchioni D, Mattioli F, Alicandri-Ciufelli M, Presutti L. Prevalence of ventilation blockages in patients affected by attic pathology: a case-control study. Laryngoscope. 2013;123(11):2845–53. https://doi.org/10.1002/lary.24165.
32. Marchioni D, Bisi N, Rubini A. Endoscopic transcanal surgery of pars tensa cholesteatoma: preliminary results. Acta Otorrinolaringol Esp. 2022;74:101. https://doi.org/10.1016/j.otorri.2022.03.003.

Regulated Balance of Pressure Variations in the Temporal Pneumatic Spaces

7

Bernard Ars and Dominique Estève

Brief Basic and Morpho-Functional Quotes

From a quantitative point of view, gaseous spaces of the middle ear cleft embody the largest part of the pneumatic spaces of the temporal bone. It consists of interconnected gas cells lined with the same respiratory mucosa.

The middle ear cleft consists of both the mastoid gas cell system and the tympanic cavity. The latter includes the tympanum and four annexes: the epi- and hypo-tympanum and the retro- and pro-tympanum that corresponds to the bony Eustachian tube. The fibrocartilaginous Eustachian tube is part of contiguous organs, including the nose, palate, and rhinopharynx, and is connected to the middle ear cleft. It is not a simple tube but is rather a complex organ consisting of a dynamic conduit with an innervated and vascularized mucosa, cartilage, surrounding soft tissue, peritubal muscles (i.e., the tensor and elevator veli palatini, salpingopharyngeus, and tensor tympani), and the superior bony support, namely, the sphenoid sulcus.

The middle ear cleft, in the tympanic cavity, is constricted in its superior third by the inter-attico-tympanic diaphragm, a bony membranous barrier perforated by two small permanent openings: the anterior tympanic isthmus, which is located between the tensor tympani tendon and the stapes, and the posterior tympanic isthmus, which is located between the double posterior ligament of the incus and the bony posterior tympanic wall.

This barrier divides the middle ear cleft into two separate compartments: an anteroinferior one and a posterosuperior one [1, 2]. The anteroinferior compartment of the middle ear cleft, located under the diaphragm, includes the pro-, meso-, and hypo-tympanum and is mainly covered by secretory or non-secretory ciliated cells performing mucociliary clearance. It consists of a flexible chamber due to the presence of the eardrum. Because of the fibrocartilaginous Eustachian tube, it consists of an gas pocket with intermittent gas transfers. It communicates with the posterosuperior compartment by both the anterior and posterior tympanic isthmi.

The posterosuperior compartment of the middle ear cleft, located above the diaphragm, includes the epi- and retro-tympanum, aditus ad antrum, antrum, and the mastoid gas cell system. It is mainly covered by a richly vascularized cuboidal epithelium primarily devoted to gas exchanges. It consists of a rigid chamber and an open gas pocket that communicates with the anteroinferior compartment via both openings. The middle ear cleft is essentially a non-collapsible gas pocket with poor gas exchanges, through which sound wave energy is transported to the inner ear.

The gas must be contained in a three-dimensional container with volume V. The pressure of the gas P is created by the molecules of the gas striking the walls of the container. It is defined as force per unit area. The physical characteristics of the gas are linked together by the ideal gas law: $PV = nRT$, where n is the mass expressed in molecule grams, R is the universal gas constant, and T is the absolute temperature. The middle ear cleft is subjected to physiological variations in volume and pressure. It has the capacity to maintain steady-state volume and pressure; this is achieved by different regulatory mechanisms, which neutralize or minimize pressure and volume variations. This is performed by adjusting either the quantity of gas, its diffusion, and/or the volume of the middle ear cleft.

Gas Exchanges

Morphological Structures

The gas content of the middle ear cleft is constituted and maintained due to gas exchanges between the middle ear cleft and the neighboring structures, including the environ-

B. Ars (✉)
University of Namur, Brussels, Belgium

Temporal Bone Foundation, Brussels, Belgium; http://www.arsbernard.com

D. Estève
Chemin de Sainte-Roustagne, Manosque, France

M. V. Goycoolea et al. (eds.), *Textbook of Otitis Media*, https://doi.org/10.1007/978-3-031-40949-3_7

ment across the tympanic membrane, the inner ear via the round-window membrane, the blood compartment via the mucosa, and the rhinopharynx through the fibrocartilaginous Eustachian tube [3, 4].

What Happens in the Mucosa?

The gases present in the middle ear cleft are identical to those found in the blood and in the atmosphere: oxygen (O_2), carbon dioxide (CO_2), nitrogen (N_2), argon (Ar), and water vapor (H_2O). Their relative amounts may be expressed as their partial pressure $P(x)$. Nitrogen is neither produced nor consumed in the middle ear cleft. $P(O_2)$ in the middle ear cleft is slightly lower, and $P(CO_2)$ is slightly higher than in venous blood. This means that there is modest O_2 consumption and CO_2 production in the middle ear cleft. Oxygen and nitrogen are absorbed from the middle ear cleft through the mucosa into the blood compartment. CO_2 and water vapor diffuse from the blood compartment, through the mucosa, into the middle ear cleft.

The steady exchange of gas through the mucosa depends on the functional properties of the cells of the mucosa, the specific diffusion rate of the gas, which is a constant value, characteristic of a particular gas, and the behavior of the vascular system [5, 6]. The primary purpose of the mucosa is to facilitate gas exchanges between the middle ear cleft and the blood compartment through a constitutive tissular barrier.

Middle ear cleft gas exchange is an ongoing process that continually generates a net absorption of gases, resulting in an increasingly negative pressure between tubal dilations. There is a gradient of partial pressures of gases between the middle ear cleft gases and the venous capillary soluble gases that drives the net flow of gas toward the circulation over time. CO_2 has the highest diffusion coefficient and is most rapidly exchanged with the net exchange passing from the venous blood to the middle ear cleft. The next fasted diffusion is that of O_2, passing from the middle ear cleft into the blood. N_2, the predominant partial pressure in both air and blood and the source of the largest gradient, diffuses much more slowly into the circulation. It is the slow absorption of N_2 that causes the increasing relative vacuum between ambient air and the middle ear cleft over time.

In the Eustachian tube, the proximal third of the tubal tent is a bony funnel-shaped extension of the middle ear cleft, the "protympanum," which narrows down at the isthmus. The distal third of the tubal length is the pharyngeal portion, which is made up of a cartilaginous skeleton to which is attached a complex arrangement of peritubal muscles, capable of a wide range of dynamic movements [7].

This cartilaginous portion is normally closed in the resting position due to apposition of the mucosal walls. Closure occurs over a variable length (a 5–10-mm segment), just a few millimeters distal to the bony isthmus where the cartilaginous skeleton becomes flexible. This portion that intermittently dilates to the open position is termed the "functional valve" because it serves such a purpose.

Contraction of the elevator veli palatini muscle raises the soft palate and rotates the medial cartilaginous lamina medially. Contraction of the tensor veli palatini muscle tenses the anterolateral membranous wall and pulls it laterally to dilate the tubal valve to the open position. Intermittent brief tubal dilation is most likely the principal mechanism of equalizing the middle ear cleft pressure with the ambient atmosphere.

Involuntary dilatation of the fibrocartilaginous Eustachian tube occurs throughout the day, typically during swallowing or yawning, but it does not accompany every swallow or yawn.

Tubal dilation occurs in normal subjects approximately 1.4 times per minute during daytime with an average duration of opening of 0.4 s. During sleep, the frequency of tubal opening is substantially reduced. Sequential muscular contractions initiate rotational movements of the cartilaginous framework and create tension within the anterolateral wall, causing the effacement of its resting bulge. This effacement is the primary action that opens the lumen to the middle ear cleft.

Tubal dilation begins with the action of the elevator veli palatini muscle to medially rotate the cartilaginous skeleton, primarily its mobile distal half of the medial cartilaginous lamina. Tensor veli palatini muscle contraction follows, causing the resting convexity of the anterolateral wall to become effaced or even concave as the final step to transiently open the lumen.

Intermittent brief dilation of the tube is the principal mechanism for equalizing the middle ear cleft pressure with the ambient atmosphere, regulating the nitrogen balance. Tubal dilation is likely facilitated by the presence of surface tension-lowering substances that are found in its mucus. Surfactants are produced within the tubal mucosa and probably help reduce the surface tension of the lumen, which reduces the work required to dilate the tube.

1. The in situ adaptation and local control systems of gas exchanges in the middle ear cleft mainly consist of the compliance of the tympanic membrane lamina propria, the fibrocartilaginous Eustachian tube function, and the behavior of the vascular system of the middle ear cleft mucosa, especially that of the mastoid.
   (a) The compliance of the tympanic membrane lamina propria [8] is used in the case of sudden pressure changes (altitude, diving, flight, explosion, etc.). This is largely due to the viscoelastic properties of the lamina propria and the flexibility of the incudomallear joint, which acts as a static pressure receptor for the tympanic membrane, ensuring three-dimensional movement into the malleus. Distortion of the eardrum causes a volume change of the semirigid mid-

dle ear cleft and can therefore partially compensate for fast pressure changes. The tympanic membrane's lamina propria is not only an active pressure buffer but also a passive pressure victim.

(b) The fibrocartilaginous Eustachian tube does not function as a ventilation hole, which keeps pressure inside the middle ear cleft equal to the outside pressure. Only at large pressure differences, above 2 kPa, will the fibrocartilaginous Eustachian tube open spontaneously [9]. Changes in position seem to affect the function of the fibrocartilaginous Eustachian tube. The mean volume of gas passing through the tube in the upright position is reduced by a third when the body raised at 20° with respect to the horizontal position. It is reduced by two-thirds in the horizontal position. This is the result of an increase in the venous tissular pressure around the fibrocartilaginous Eustachian tube.

(c) The vascular system, in combination with the mastoid gas cell system, plays an important regulatory role in the physiological balance of pressure variations in the middle ear cleft. Variations in the middle ear cleft blood flow, associated with variations in the permeability of the vessels, allow ample adaptation to normal gas pressure fluctuations [10–13].

The normal extensive variations observed in the middle ear cleft pressure over a 24-h period, which appear regularly, are related to the vascular adaptations required by body position and sleep.

The mastoid gas cell system constitutes the most important volume of the middle ear cleft, and, therefore, it represents the largest part of the area of the middle ear cleft mucosa, accessible to the vascular network, further increased by a large number of mucosal folds. The extent of mastoid gas exchanges is important for regulating middle ear cleft pressure variations for two reasons.

First, the physical and anatomical properties of mastoid volume affect compliance: the larger the volume, the more compliant the system.

Second, the mucosal surface area affects mucosal gas exchanges: the larger the surface area, the more efficient the middle ear cleft gas exchanges.

The mastoid carries out the function of a passive pressure buffer as a gas reservoir for pressure variation regulations, obtained by its volume. However, it also carries out an active pressure buffer function. Cros demonstrated retroauricular microchannels connecting the outer cortical bone surface directly to the underlying mastoid gas cells. Gaheide showed the presence of a separate vascular supply for the mucosa lining the mastoid gas cell system, in these microchannels. If a certain number of such channels run in parallel, as some of the pictures of the authors seem to demonstrate, there must exist a mechanism of counter-current exchange that maintains the two compartments with a stable difference of composition. We may conclude that the mastoid also carries out an active buffer function.

The size of the mastoid gas cell system varies to a large extent between individuals. Irrespective of the cause, genetically determined growth, or environmental factors, there is unanimous agreement that a small mastoid gas cell system has a pathophysiological association. The smaller the system, the faster the deviation from normal pressures. However, nature is a matter of balance. It is not a single question of determining the volume of the mastoid in order to predict its clinical potential.

In normal conditions, with a healthy mucosa, a small mastoid in an adult is normal in so far as it constitutes the complete outcome of normal and standard development, i.e., the individual simply has the morphological particularity of being "small." A small mastoid in an adult is normal, in that it is sufficient for the physiological balance of pressure variations in the middle ear cleft. However, this small mastoid is not more likely to particularly develop a pathology. However, when the mucosa undergoes an inflammatory process, a small mastoid in an adult, e.g., resulting from a disturbed or failed development, is certainly at a disadvantage when it is exposed to excessive pressure variations. This mastoid is "too small" compared to the rest of the middle ear cleft. If the expansion reservoir is too small, then it cannot adequately play its role.

In normal conditions, with a healthy mucosa, a "normal," small, negative pressure is present in the middle ear cleft compared to the outside air, created by exchanges of gas between the cleft and the blood compartment. Gas exchanges through the mucosa of the middle ear cleft are driven by the gradient of partial pressure of gases between the cleft and the capillaries of the submucosal connective tissue.

Given the capacity of gas diffusion in the middle ear cleft, partial pressures of these gases aim at balancing both sides of the mucosal barrier of the middle ear cleft.

The progressive diffusion of gases is capable of modifying the gas composition in the middle ear cleft and in the circulating blood. The gas, which penetrates into the middle ear cleft from the rhinopharynx, is not outside air. Its composition is rather close to that of exhaled gas.

Quantitatively, the main gas entering the middle ear cleft is nitrogen. N_2 diffuses much more slowly in the blood than do other gases (35 times more slowly than CO_2 and 1.8 times less than O_2). Considering this nitrogen in steady state, there is a difference in partial pressure between the middle ear cleft and the blood flow around the middle ear cleft. This steady state corresponds more or less to the total amount of pressure difference (54–56 mmHg) between the middle ear cleft and blood. In the steady state, oxygen, carbon dioxide, and water vapor have nearly the same partial pressures in the middle ear cleft as in the blood compartment.

Consequently, an increase in blood flow in the middle ear cleft has little effect on gas exchanges, except perhaps during the night, when CO_2 increases and O_2 is reduced in the blood flow. On the other hand, N_2 always maintains a higher partial pressure in the middle ear cleft as compared with the blood. Therefore, there is a clear and continuous elimination of N_2 from the middle ear cleft in the direction of the blood compartment. This leads to a slight negative pressure in the middle ear cleft.

The innervation of the mucosa of the middle ear cleft originates from the autonomic nervous system, which sends and receives information from both the sympathetic and parasympathetic networks at the same time. Adrenergic nerve endings have been detected, most of them in the vicinity of vessels. They probably control their muscle tonus. The peptidergic system would also play a role. It has been established that the presence of peptide mediators such as P substance, vasoactive intestinal peptide (VIP), or calcitonin gene-related peptide (CGRP) lead to vasodilatation and an increase in vascular permeability.

In the middle ear cleft, chemosensors located in the glomic tissue of the mucosa respond to variations in the gas composition and send impulses to reflexes of gas transfer from the rhinopharynx toward the middle ear cleft. In normal conditions, under the control of the isobaric system, the elimination of nitrogen from the middle ear cleft to the blood compartment is regularly compensated for by the gas contribution originating from the rhinopharynx. Inflammatory processes increase both the number and diameter of the blood vessels, thus increasing blood supply to the mucosa. The middle ear cleft is 210 times more perfused than ventilated under normal conditions and is 251 times more perfused than ventilated under inflammatory conditions. The result of this increased blood perfusion is a larger diffusion of nitrogen from the middle ear cleft toward the blood. This explains the apparent contradiction between the increase in thickness and the barrier of the mucosa and the increase in gas elimination in inflammatory conditions. The negative pressure of the "normally" slightly balanced middle ear cleft thus increases.

Higher nitrogen absorption would normally be sufficiently compensated through the fibrocartilaginous Eustachian tube but could now generate pathological negative pressure in the middle ear cleft compared with the atmospheric pressure. This conditions carries a "gas deficit," and therefore a negative pressure, which could constitute a mutual physical–pathological support to the development of chronic otitis media.

The Neural Regulating System: The Isobaric System of the Middle Ear Cleft

The principle of the isobaric system of the middle ear cleft is based not only on the presence of pressure-sensitive mechanoreceptors, i.e., barosensors, which are able to collect the middle ear cleft pressure, but also on the atmospheric pressure in the upper airway.

Barosensors Located in the Middle Ear Cleft

Gussen's report [14] indicate that the human tympanic cavity and antrum contained Pacinian corpuscles. Lim et al. [15] located these sensors in the mucosa, most commonly in the epitympanum and the epitympanic recess. Nagai and Tono [16] identified encapsulated nerve endings in the subepidermal connective tissue and the lamina propria of the second quadrant of the pars tensa of the tympanic membrane. The structure of the corpuscles was round or oval with diameters that were about 40 µm and contained a number of axon terminals with the mitochondria, Schwann cell processes, and amorphous materials in the intercellular space. These features appear to be at work in transmitting mechanical forces (stretching of the tympanic membrane) and are comparable to the function of mechanoreceptors that could detect middle ear cleft pressure [17]. Based on the studies by Nagai et al. [18], showing that the tubal function changed following topical anesthesia of the eardrum, Estève [19] pointed out that opening of the tube occurs when a pressure imbalance occurs between the two sides of the tympanic membrane.

After anesthesia of the drum, many subjects felt some dull sensation on external ear pressures or stated that they could not detect the gas coming into the tympanic cavity during the Valsalva maneuver. Out of 20 subjects, 13 ears needed more than 2 swallows and 4 ears failed to equalize middle ear cleft pressure in spite of repeated swallows.

The mechanoreceptors, located in the middle ear cleft, might possibly play an effective role in tubal function where the mechanoreceptors on the drum seem to have a minor effect.

With different elasticity and histological structures from the rest of the membrane, the pars flaccida has been suggested as a highly sensitive and fast reacting part of the tympanic membrane, providing pressure balance with the middle ear cleft in the range of natural levels of atmospheric pressure fluctuations. The pars flaccida could act as a barosensor, initiating the physiological reactions in the body in the course of adaptation to atmospheric pressure fluctuations.

Barosensors Located in the Rhinopharynx

In a study of the human rhinopharyngeal innervation, Kanagasuntheram et al. [20] reported a predominance of free nerve endings and a few organized non-encapsulated endings, with the latter only in the subepithelial tissue. From patients undergoing adenoidectomy or biopsy examination of the postnasal space for the exclusion of neoplasia, Guindi [21] identified free nerve endings in the rhinopharynx and encapsulated receptors in the subepithelial tissue of the pharyngeal recess. In the histological study by Salburgo et al. [17], Ruffini corpuscles were accurately identified in the rhinopharynx, with a higher concentration in the pharyngeal recess and the posterior rhinopharyngeal wall.

The "Neuronal Reflex Arc" of the Isobaric System of the Middle Ear Cleft (Fig. 7.1)

Owing, above all, to the stretch receptors of the pars flaccida, sensitive to extremely weak horizontal changes in Patm (atmospheric pressure) (>0.1 mbar), and owing to the Ruffini corpuscles of the pharyngeal recess, sensitive to vertical changes in Patm (>10 mbar), the neurosensory reflex loop implements gas exchanges essentially at the level of the mastoid and of the opening of the fibrocartilaginous Eustachian tube, depending on the intensity of the initial stimulus. There is a true specialization of the sensors as well as of the effectors.

In this isobaric system, the fibrocartilaginous Eustachian tube and the mastoid are capable of active counter-regulation of the middle ear cleft pressure variations and function in a complementary way where the tube is related to the intermittent regulation of higher pressures (it is a security valve) and where the mastoid is related to the continuous regulation of smaller pressures, especially of climatic origin. In the isobaric system of the middle ear cleft, the key point is the "neuronal reflex arc," based on a mechanism that is highly sensitive to a pressure gradient between the middle ear cleft and the ambient environment, on the one hand, and on an effector process of pressure balancing, on the other hand—a neural feedback control similar to the respiratory control and related to similar central centers in the nucleus of the solitary tract of the brainstem [22–24].

The afferent plexus of the "neuronal reflex arc" are the mechanoreceptors, barosensors, located in the epitympanum and antrum, the pars flaccida, and those located in the pharyngeal recess and the posterior rhino pharyngeal wall. The efferent plexus of the "neuronal reflex arc" are the tubal muscles, resulting in tube opening, and the blood vessels of the mastoid mucosa, regulating middle ear cleft gas exchanges.

In normal conditions, i.e., in a healthy mucosa, when a pressure gradient between the middle ear cleft and the ambient environment is detected, two distinct and combined patterns contribute to maintain near-ambient pressures in the middle ear cleft, namely, the tubal opening with steep intermittent changes in pressure against 0 Pa and mastoid-related changes in pressure, which are gradual and appear in both negative and positive directions and which could transverse 0 Pa into opposite pressures. These gradual pressure changes by gas exchanges are related to the perfusion of the mastoid mucosa (Table 7.1).

The "neuronal reflex arc" of the isobaric system of the middle ear cleft can be reeducated, an extremely important property in the clinical management of gas and pressure disorders in the middle ear cleft [25, 26].

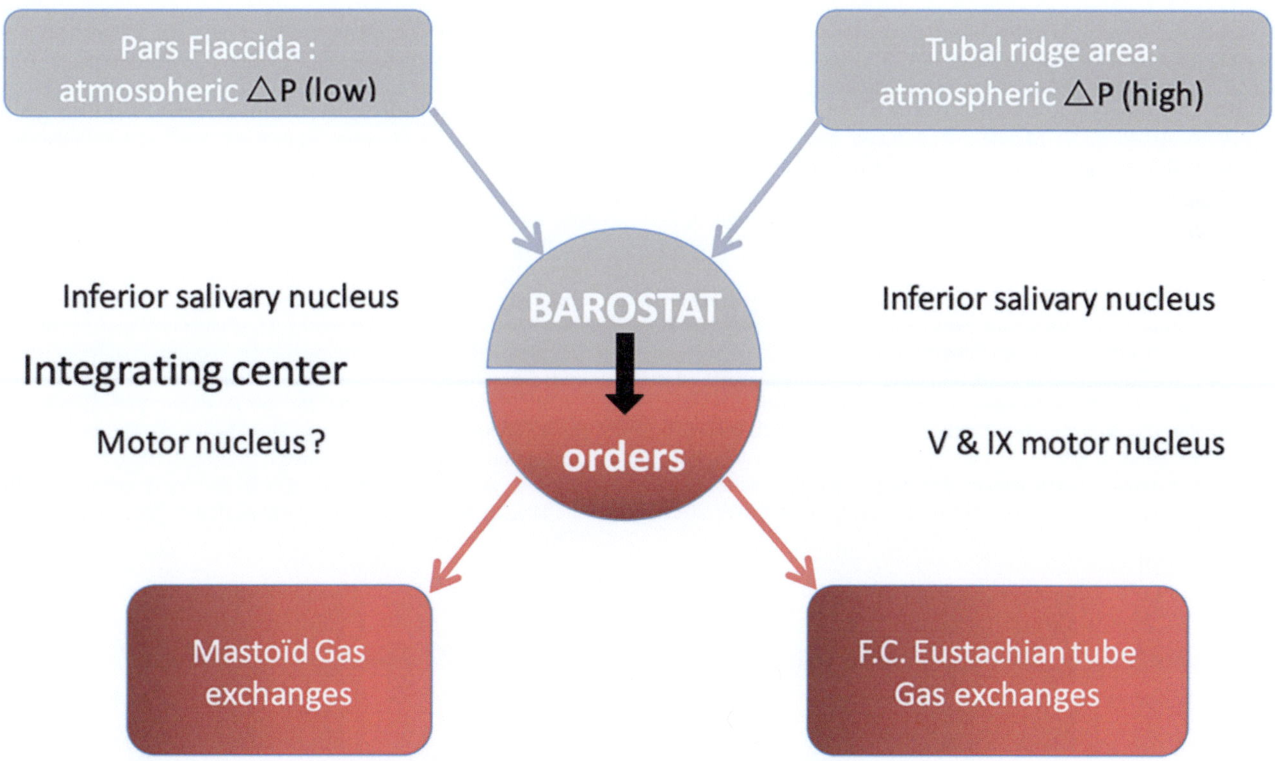

Fig. 7.1 Schematic representation of the middle ear cleft isobaric system

Table 7.1 Schematic characterization of the middle ear cleft isobaric system effectors

	Gas exchanges	Isobaric function
System type	Sensory reflex loop then neuro-muscular and neuro-vascular with common barostatic integrating center	
Starting point Baroreceptor sensitivity (innate character)	**Pars flaccida** of the tympanic membrane (TM) Stretch receptors $\Delta P > 0.1$ mbar and low pressure rise slope	**Tubal ridge area** Ruffini corpuscles $\Delta P \geq 10$ mbar and high pressure rise slope
Center	**Inferior salivary nucleus**	
Level of intervention	**Immediate**	Tubal opening: **early**, **late**, or **absent** (areflexia)
Type of response after implementation	Slow	Fast
Effects on middle Ear/blood gas concentration	Maintained balance	Imbalance
Circumstances of implementation	Works permanently	Only if there is middle ear cleft barotrauma risk

Acknowledgment We thank Professor Jean Lebacq for thoroughly reviewing this chapter.

References

1. Ars B, Ars-Piret N. Morpho-functional partition of the middle ear cleft. Acta Otorhinolaryngol Belg. 1997;51:181–4.
2. Ars B, Ars-Piret N. Morpho-functional partition of the middle ear cleft. Mediterranean J Otol. 2007;3:31–9.
3. Ars B, Ars-Piret N. Middle ear pressure balance under normal conditions. Specific role of the middle ear structures. Acta Otorhinolaryngol Belg. 1994;48(4):339–42.
4. Ars B. Physiology of Eustachian tube dysfunction. In: Suddhoff H, editor. Eustachian tube dysfunction. 2nd ed. Bremen: UNI-MED Verlag; 2017. p. 23–33.
5. Tideholm B. Middle ear cleft pressure. In: Ars B, editor. Fibrocartilaginous Eustachian tube—middle ear cleft. The Hague, The Netherlands: Kugler Publications; 2003. p. 99–112.
6. Kania R. Modélisation expérimentale et mathématique des échanges gazeux transmuqueux de l'oreille moyenne en conditions normales et inflammatoires. Thèse de doctorat de l'Université de Paris VI; 2006. p. 155.
7. Poe D. Pathophysiology and surgical treatment of Eustachian tube dysfunction. Academic dissertation, University of Helsinki; 2011. p. 74.
8. Ars B, Decraemer W, Ars-Piret N. The lamina propria and cholesteatoma. Clin Otolaryngol. 1989;14:471–5.
9. Estève D. Tubomanometry and pathology. In: Ars B, editor. Fibrocartilaginous Eustachian tube-middle ear cleft. The Hague, The Netherlands: Kugler Publications; 2003. p. 159–17.
10. Ars B, Wuyts F, Van de Heyning P. Histomorphometric study of the normal middle ear mucosa. Preliminary results supporting the gas exchange function in the postero-superior part of the middle ear cleft. Acta Otolaryngol (Stockh). 1997;117:704–7.
11. Matanda R, Van de Henning P, Bogers J, Ars B. Behaviour of middle ear cleft mucosa during inflammation: histomorphometric study. Acta Otolaryngol (Stockh). 2006;126:905–9.
12. Ars B, Dirckx J, Ars-Piret N, Buytaert J. Insights in the physiology of the human mastoid: message to the surgeon. Int Adv Otol. 2012;8(2):296–310.
13. Padurariu S, Röösli C, Røge R, Stenshalle A, Vyberg M, Huber A, Gaihede M. On the functional compartmentalization of the normal middle ear. Morpho-histological modeling parameters of its mucosa. Hear Res. 2019;378:176–84.
14. Gussen R. Pacinian corpuscules in the middle ear. J Laryngol Otol. 1970;84:71–6.
15. Lim DJ. Human tympanic membrane. An ultrastructural observation. Acta Otolaryngol. 1970;70:176–86.
16. Nagai T, Tono T. Encapsuled nerve corpuscules in the human tympanic membrane. Arch Otolrhinolaryngol. 1989;246:169–72.
17. Salburgo F, Garcia S, Lagier A, Estève D, Lavieille JP, Montava M. Histological identification of nasopharyngeal mechanoreceptors. Eur Arch Otorhinolaryngol. 2016;273:4127–33.
18. Nagai T, Nagai M, Nagata Y, Morimitsu T. The effects of anesthesia of the tympanic membrane on Eustachian tube function. Arch Otorhinolaryngol. 1989;246:210–2.
19. Estève D, Dubreuil C, Vella Vedova C, Normand B, Laveille JP, Martin C. Physiology and physiopathologie of the Eustachian tube opening function: interest of tubomanometry. J F ORL. 2001;50:233–41.
20. Kanagasuntheram R, Wong WC, Chan HL. Some observations on the innervation of the human nasopharynx. J Anat. 1969;104:361–76.
21. Guindi GM. Nasopharyngeal mechanoreceptors and their role in auto regulation of endotympanic pressure. ORL J Otorhinolaryngol Relat Spec. 1981;43:56–60.
22. Eden AR. Neural connections between the middle ear, Eustachian tube and brain. Implications for the reflex control of middle ear aeration. Ann Otol Rhino Laryngol. 1981;90:566–9.
23. Eden AR, Gannon PJ. Neural control of middle ear aeration. Arch Otolaryngol Head Neck Surg. 1987;113:133–7.
24. Eden AR, Laitman JT, Gannon PJ. Mechanisms of middle ear aeration: anatomic and physiologic evidence in primates. Laryngoscope. 1990;100:67–75.
25. Ars B. Chronic otitis media. In: Ars B, editor. Pathogenesis oriented therapeutic management. The Hague, Amsterdam: Kugler Publications; 2008. p. 355. ISBN13: 978 6299 216 4.
26. Kania R, Ars B. In: Kania R, Ars B, editors. Biofilms in otitis. The Hague, Amsterdam: Kugler Publications; 2015. p. 363. ISBN 978-90-6299-243-0.

The Role of Immunity in the Development of Otitis Media

8

Sara Concha and Rodrigo Hoyos-Bachiloglu

Part I: The Role of Innate and Adaptive Immunity in Otitis Media

The term "immunity" comes from the Latin word *immunitas*, which refers to the protection from legal prosecution offered to Roman senators during their tenures in office. The immune system is responsible for protecting an organism against foreign substances, especially infectious microbes, and also products of damaged cells [1].

A normal immune response against microbes involves sequential and coordinated responses by different branches of the immune system (Table 8.1). Innate immunity is essential for the defense against microbes during the first few hours or days after infection, is mediated by mechanisms that are in place even before an infection occurs, facilitates rapid responses to the invading microbes, and stimulates adaptive immunity. Innate immunity detects microbial infections using pattern recognition receptors (PRRs) that are specific to molecules shared by groups of related microbes (pathogen-associated molecular patterns (PAMPs)). Adaptative immunity is stimulated by exposure to infectious agents and generates pathogen-specific immune responses, and it also has significant receptor diversity and memory. Immunological memory allows the adaptive system to increase in magnitude and defensive capabilities with each successive exposure to a particular agent.

Innate Immunity

The innate system is composed of cellular and chemical barriers such as the skin, mucosal epithelia, antimicrobial peptides, blood proteins, including the complement system, and cells like macrophages and neutrophils.

Table 8.1 Components of innate and adaptive immunity

	Innate	Adaptive
Epithelial and chemical barriers	• Mucociliary apparatus • Mucous glycoproteins • Surfactants • Defensins, interferons, lactoferrin, and nitric oxide • Middle ear epithelial cells	Epithelial lymphocytes and antibodies
Blood proteins	Complement	Antibodies
Cells	• Neutrophils • Macrophages • Mast cells • Dendritic cells	• Lymphocytes T – CD4 Th1 Th2 Th17 – CD8 • Lymphocytes B

Epithelial and Chemical Barriers

Mucosal immunity constitutes the first line of defense against respiratory pathogens in the respiratory tract. Epithelial cells of the middle ear contain several key defense mechanisms such as the mucociliary apparatus, the trapping function of mucous glycoproteins and surfactants, and the ability to secrete innate defense molecules such as defensins, interferons, lactoferrin, and nitric oxide [2].

Mucins are high-molecular-weight glycoproteins responsible for the viscous properties of middle ear effusion [3]. Although mucins are important components of innate immunity in the respiratory tract, they can also play a pathological role. Abnormally high levels of mucins have been demonstrated in middle ear effusions of chronic suppurative otitis media (OM) patients, preventing the transmission of sound waves and leading to conductive hearing loss. The upregulation of some mucin genes such as *MUC2*, *MUC5AC*, and *MUC5B* plays an important role in the pathogenesis of otitis media [2].

Surfactant proteins (SPs) such as SP-A are expressed in the middle ear and Eustachian tube and play an important role in innate responses through opsonization and comple-

S. Concha (✉) · R. Hoyos-Bachiloglu
Department of Pediatric Immunology and Infectious Diseases, Pontificia Universidad Católica de Chile, Santiago, Chile
e-mail: sconcha1@uc.cl; rhoyos@med.puc.cl

M. V. Goycoolea et al. (eds.), *Textbook of Otitis Media*, https://doi.org/10.1007/978-3-031-40949-3_8

ment activation. SP-A opsonizes Gram-negative bacteria and modulates the expression of pro-inflammatory cytokines like interleukin (IL)-1β, IL-6, and tumor necrosis alpha (TNF-α). The immune function of SP-A in vivo has been studied using mouse models of otitis media, which demonstrated its role in enhancing bacterial phagocytosis and modulating middle ear inflammation [4].

Defensins are cationic proteins, whose main antimicrobial mechanisms are forming a pore in the microbial membrane and stimulating the production of pro-inflammatory cytokines and chemokines. Human B-defensin 2 and 3 are upregulated in the middle ear in response to bacteria and play a critical role in eliminating *Haemophilus influenzae* (*Hi*) [5, 6].

Middle ear epithelial cells express PRRs such as Toll-like receptors (TLRs) that detect infections by recognizing PAMPs and activate the innate immune response. Peptidoglycans such as those on the surface of *Haemophilus influenzae* (*Hi*) are recognized by TLR2; upon biding to its ligand, TLR2 initiates nuclear factor kappa B (NF-κB)-dependent cascades that activate the immune response and upregulate TLR2 expression in a positive feedback loop [7, 8]. Polymorphisms of the *TLR4* gene are associated with recurrent acute OM. When infected with *Hi*, TLR4 knockout mice had a worse mucosal immune response, with impairment of phagocytosis and phagosome maturation of polymorphonuclear cells as compared to wild-type mice [9]. Additional genes involved in the innate immunity have been found to be differentially regulated in acute otitis media (AOM)-prone children compared to healthy-age appropriate controls. Downregulation of TLR adaptor molecule 2 was found in middle ear fluid of 24 children with acute otitis media [10]. TLRs are not the only PRRs involved in the pathogenesis and recovery of otitis media; Nod-like receptors (NLRs) have also been shown to initiate and support robust immune responses through the production of inflammatory cytokines and recruitment of leukocytes to the middle ear [11].

Finally, impairment of epithelial and chemical barriers in otitis-prone children has been observed. They have lower capacity for epithelial repair, lower pro-inflammatory neutrophil chemoattractants such as macrophage inflammatory protein-1β (MIP-1β), IL-8, and CXCL5 [12], and pro-inflammatory cytokines of higher levels such as IL-2 and lower levels such as IL-7, IL-6, and IL-10 in nasal washes, thus showing that middle ear cytokine responses mirror those of the nasal mucosa versus the peripheral blood and suggesting that proximal mucosal sites may better predict the quality of middle ear responses compared to peripheral blood [13].

The Complement System

The complement system consists of several plasma proteins that work together to opsonize microbes, promote recruitment of phagocytes to the sites of infection, and, in some cases, directly kill the microbes [1]. There are three pathways of complement activation, among which the most important for responding to capsulated bacteria is the classical pathway, which is one of the major effector mechanisms of the humoral arm of adaptive immune responses.

Cells

Neutrophils are the most abundant leukocytes and the first line of defense against invading pathogens in the middle ear, experiencing roughly a 600-fold increase during acute otitis media [14]. They express multiple TLRs and play a crucial role in eradicating middle ear infections [2]. Upon activation, they form neutrophil extracellular traps (NETs) that are positively correlated with higher bacterial loads within middle ear fluids and surface-attached bacteria and contribute to effusion viscosity, thus leading to chronic suppurative otitis media [15].

Macrophages are also present in middle ear effusions, and their role in infection depends on the causative agent. *Streptococcus pneumoniae* serotypes 14 and 19F were found to be resistant to phagocytosis that can lead to bacterial antigens being trapped in the middle ear, thus promoting effusion [2]. *Haemophilus influenzae* utilizes a system of phase-variable epigenetic regulation, to facilitate adaptation and survival by evading opsonization, the process by which it is marked for destruction by macrophages [16].

Mast cells are distributed throughout the tubotympanum, predominantly in the pars flaccida, and can trigger allergic rhinitis, thus causing persistent inflammation that can lead to tube dysfunction and also impediment of mucociliary function that can lead to recurrent otitis media with effusion [17]. A possible role of mast cells and their cytokines in the pathogenesis of chronic serous otitis media has been suggested as these cells are increased in the patient's adenoid tissue and in thymic stromal lymphopoietin [18].

A normal tympanic membrane also contains abundant dendritic cells that have the potential to migrate and activate T cells. A significant increase in the number of these cells has been found in tubotympanic disease and in atticoantral disease, with the difference being more pronounced in the latter form of otitis media [19].

Adaptive Immune Responses

The adaptive immune system is composed of T and B lymphocytes and their products. There are two branches of adaptive immunity, namely, humoral immunity, which is mediated by antibodies and B cells, and cell-mediated or cellular immunity mediated by T cells.

Humoral Immunity

A humoral immune response combats microbes in many ways. Antibodies bind to microbes and prevent them from infecting cells, thus neutralizing the microbes. In fact, antibody-mediated neutralization is the only mechanism of adaptive immunity that stops an infection before it is established; this is why eliciting the production of potent antibodies is the key goal of vaccination. Immunoglobulin (Ig)G antibodies coat microbes and target them for phagocytosis because phagocytes (neutrophils and macrophages) express receptors for parts of IgG molecules. Both IgG and IgM activate the complement system, and complement products promote phagocytosis and destruction of microbes. IgA is secreted from mucosal epithelia and neutralizes microbes in the lumens of mucosal tissues, such as the respiratory and gastrointestinal tracts, thus preventing inhaled and ingested microbes from infecting the host [1].

There are differences between children and adult's humoral immunity, and the susceptibility of infants to AOM wanes with age due to immunological maturation. During pregnancy, IgG antibodies are passively transferred to the infant and progressively decrease during extrauterine life, reaching their lowest point at 6 months of life. The production of IgM and IgA begins progressively from birth. The capacity to respond to protein antigens is approximately 80% at birth and achieves levels like those of adults around 3 months of life. The ability to respond to polysaccharide antigens is not optimal until 2 years of life due to the absence of B cells in the marginal zone of the spleen [1].

For the normal development of humoral immunity, a correct development of B cells and a normal interaction of these with circulating T lymphocytes is necessary. Developing antibody-mediated immunity to *Streptococcus pneumoniae* and non-typeable *Hi* (NT*Hi*), the two most common pathogens causing AOM, is a cardinal step in preventing recurrent infections in young children. Upon receiving T cell help, B lymphocytes that recognized an antigen proliferate and differentiate into plasma cells that secrete different classes of antibodies with distinct functions. Polysaccharides and lipids stimulate secretion mainly of the antibody class called immunoglobulin M (IgM). Protein antigens induce the production of antibodies of different classes (IgG, IgA, IgE) from a single clone of B cells.

Otitis prone children have lower serum bactericidal antibody titers against pneumococcal proteins: histidine triad protein D (PhtD), pneumococcal choline binding protein A (PcpA) and pneumolysin (PlyD1) compared with nonotitis prone children after nasopharyngeal colonization and acute otitis media [20]. This may be due to poor memory B-cell and T-helper cell generation associated with reduced levels of pneumococcal-specific IgG in the serum after the infection [21].

Comparing acute to convalescent antibody titers after AOM, otitis-prone children had no significant change in total IgG responses to three *Hi* proteins (protein D, P6, and OMP26), whereas non-otitis-prone children had significant increases in protein D. Anti-protein D, P6, and OMP26 antibody levels measured longitudinally during *Hi* colonization between the ages of 6 and 24 months demonstrated subtle anti-protein D IgG increases over time in otitis-prone children compared to more than fourfold increases in non-otitis-prone children [22]. The raise in the antibody's levels in non-otitis-prone children probably prevents them from having recurrent otitis.

Cellular Immunity

T lymphocytes consist of two functionally distinct populations: helper T cells or $CD4^+$ cells and cytotoxic T lymphocytes (CTLs) or $CD8^+$ cells. The functions of helper T cells are mainly mediated by secreted cytokines, whereas CTLs produce molecules that directly kill other cells. $CD4^+$ T cells comprise functionally distinct populations characterized by specific transcription factors and cytokine profiles; T helper 1 (Th1), Th2, and Th17 [1].

Antigen-specific $CD4^+$ T cells have been shown to reduce *Streptococcus pneumoniae* nasopharyngeal colonization. An effective pathogen-specific T-cell response in adults has been associated with protection from invasive *Streptococcus pneumoniae* disease (invasive pneumococcal disease, IPD) and chronic obstructive pulmonary disease (COPD) caused by *Streptococcus pneumoniae* and NT*Hi*, respectively. More recently, Th17 cells have been described to mediate antibody-independent protection in a mouse model of pneumococcal infection. Moreover, $CD4^+$ T cells in samples collected from the adenoids and tonsils of traditionally defined otitis-prone children showed no proliferation in response to NT*Hi* protein P6, which led the authors to conclude that otitis-prone children lack pathogen-specific T cells. [23] Other authors have shown that adenoids have a reduced capacity to produce interferon-gamma (IFN-γ) and speculate that this alteration could cause susceptibility to recurrent acute otitis media [24].

For several decades, Pichichero et al. studied the underlying pathogenesis of AOM in children and also why the risk of AOM decreases over time. They observed that this susceptibility is not only due to a Eustachian tube dysfunction but also due to immune factors [13]. Peripheral blood mononuclear cells (PBMCs) from otitis-prone children between the ages of 6 and 12 months display a general skewing away from Th1 and Th17 immunity and toward Th2 and regulatory T cell (Treg) dominance [25]. This abnormality was largely outgrown by 3 years of age, coinciding with the epidemiological observation of diminishing AOM at that age [13]. They also showed that otitis-prone children are more frequently diagnosed with viral upper respiratory infections possibly due to deficient antiviral responses at the nasopharynx with decreased production of pro-inflammatory cytokines and chemokines like IL-6, IL-10, and TNF-α [26].

Part II: The Ear Microbiota

The microbiota plays critical roles in the regulation and development of the major components of the host's immune system, whereas the immune system orchestrates the maintenance of the key features of the host–microbe symbiosis [27].

The human microbiota consists of ecological communities of commensal, symbiotic, and pathogenic microorganisms that colonize several body sites and play a critical role in the regulation of many homeostatic processes, including inflammation and defense against pathogens, to inhibit the colonization and growth of otopathogens [28]. Immediately after birth, the respiratory tract becomes colonized, and, in the first week of life, there is a predominance of *Staphylococcus* spp., *Corynebacterium*, *Dolosigranulum*, and *Moraxella*. This early bacterial colonization plays a pivotal role in the stability of microbial communities: profiles dominated by *Moraxella* and *Dolosigranulum/Corynebacterium* are associated with a stable microbiota and with lower rates of respiratory infections in later stages of life, whereas the less stable profiles are associated with a high abundance of *Hi* and *Streptococcus* [29].

Several environmental factors can influence the shaping of the microbiota's composition in the first years of life. Children born by vaginal delivery have predominance of bacteria previously associated with microbiome stability and respiratory health, but some authors suggest that this impact disappears at 6 weeks of age. Breastfed infants develop a bacterial profile enriched by *Dolosigranulum* and *Corynebacterium* at 6 weeks of age in comparison with formula-fed infants; however, this effect also disappears around 6 months of age. In children with AOM, recent antibiotic therapy induces a reduction of beneficial bacteria such as *Streptococcaceae* and *Corynebacteriaceae* and an increased abundance of *Enterobacteriaceae* and *Pasteurellaceae* in the upper respiratory tract. The effect of the conjugated pneumococcal vaccines in the microbiome is controversial and it seems to vary by ethnicity; Swiss vaccinated children have an increase in beneficial bacteria and in bacterial diversity, whereas in children from Gambia, vaccination reduced the nasopharyngeal carriage of vaccine serotypes, but pneumococcal carriage remained high among vaccinated infants, probably because of an immediate expansion of non-vaccine serotypes [30].

According to the pathogen reservoir hypothesis (PRH), the adenoid pad serves as a source of pathogens that can grow in this region and further spread to the respiratory system and middle ear, leading to infections and diseases [31]. Owing to the introduction of culture-independent techniques such as gene analysis with a polymerase chain reaction (PCR) using primers that target a segment of the *16SrRNA* gene, microbiological investigations now allow the knowledge of entire bacterial communities. There are keystone species that maintain the balance and function of the bacterial community such as *Dolosigranulum* spp. and *Corynebacterium* spp. In children, a diverse microbiota and a higher relative abundance of *Corynebacterium*, *Dolosigranulum*, *Propionibacterium*, *Lactococcus*, and *Staphylococcus* were associated with a lower incidence of *S. pneumoniae*, *H. influenzae*, and *Moraxella catarrhalis* colonization, lower AOM, a shorter course of AOM, and a better clinical outcome [30]. An unstable microbiota during an acute respiratory tract infection episode with the predominance of otopathogens is associated with the occurrence of a symptomatic viral infection and with a higher risk of transition to otitis, whereas children with asymptomatic viral infections had no predominance of otopathogens [32]. There are several trials of probiotic administration for prevention of middle ear diseases in children, but there is lack of evidence for their use [33].

References

1. Abbas A, Lichtman A, Pillai S. Cellular and molecular immunology, vol. 1. Elsevier; 2019. p. 1–2.
2. Mittai R, Kodiyan J, Gerring R, Mathee K, Li J-D, Grati M, et al. Role of innate immunity in the pathogenesis of otitis media. Int J Infect Dis. 2014;0:29–267.
3. Mittal R, Grati M, Gerring R, Blackwelder P, Yan D, Li JD, et al. In vitro interaction of Pseudomonas aeruginosa with human middle ear epithelial cells. PLoS One. 2014;9(3):1–11.
4. Abdel-Razek O, Ni L, Yang F, Wang G. Innate immunity of surfactant protein A in experimental otitis media. Innate Immun. 2019;25(7):391–400.
5. Jones EA, McGillivary G, Bakaletz LO. Extracellular DNA within a nontypeable Haemophilus influenzae-induced biofilm binds human beta defensin-3 and reduces its antimicrobial activity. J Innate Immun. 2013;5(1):24–38.
6. Lee HY, Takeshita T, Shimada J, Akopyan A, Woo JI, Pan H, et al. Induction of beta defensin 2 by NTHi requires TLR2 mediated MyD88 and IRAK-TRAF6-p38MAPK signaling pathway in human middle ear epithelial cells. BMC Infect Dis. 2008;8:87.
7. Chen R, Lim JH, Jono H, Gu XX, Kim YS, Basbaum CB, et al. Nontypeable Haemophilus influenzae lipoprotein P6 induces MUC5AC mucin transcription via TLR2-TAK1-dependent p38 MAPK-AP1 and IKKβ-IκBα-NF-κB signaling pathways. Biochem Biophys Res Commun. 2004;324(3):1087–94.
8. Shuto T, Imasato A, Jono H, Sakai A, Xu H, Watanabe T, et al. Glucocorticoids synergistically enhance nontypeable Haemophilus

influenzae-induced toll-like receptor 2 expression via a negative cross-talk with p38 MAP kinase. J Biol Chem. 2002;277(19):17263–70. https://doi.org/10.1074/jbc.M112190200.
9. Hirano T, Kodama S, Fujita K, Maeda K, Suzuki M. Role of Toll-like receptor 4 in innate immune responses in a mouse model of acute otitis media. FEMS Immunol Med Microbiol. 2007;49(1):75–83.
10. Kaur R, Casey J, Pichichero M. Differences in innate immune response gene regulation in the middle ear of children who are otitis prone and in those not otitis prone. Am J Rhinol Allergy. 2016;30(6):e218–23.
11. Lee J, Leichtle A, Zuckerman E, Pak K, Spriggs M, Wasserman SI, et al. NOD1/NOD2-mediated recognition of non-typeable Haemophilus influenzae activates innate immunity during otitis media. Innate Immun. 2019;25(8):503–12.
12. Verhoeven D, Nesselbuch M, Pichichero M. Lower nasopharyngeal epithelial cell repair and diminished innate inflammation responses contribute to the onset of acute otitis media in otitis-prone children. Med Microbiol Immunol. 2013;202(4):295–302.
13. Pichichero M. Immunologic dysfunction contributes to the otitis prone condition. J Infect. 2020;80(6):614–22.
14. Morris MC, Pichichero ME. Streptococcus pneumoniae burden and nasopharyngeal inflammation during acute otitis media. Innate Immun. 2017;23(8):667–77.
15. Simon D, Simon HU, Yousefi S. Extracellular DNA traps in allergic, infectious, and autoimmune diseases. Allergy Eur J Allergy Clin Immunol. 2013;68(4):409–16.
16. Robledo-Avila FH, Ruiz-Rosado JD, Partida-Sanchez S, Brockman KL. A bacterial epigenetic switch in non-typeable Haemophilus influenzae modifies host immune response during otitis media. Front Cell Infect Microbiol. 2020;10(October):1–15.
17. Quaranta N, Iannuzzi L, Gelardi M. Does the type of rhinitis influence development of otitis media with effusion in children? Curr Allergy Asthma Rep. 2014;14(11):1–5.
18. Kumral TL, Dikker O, Yıldırım G, Karaketir S, Altındağ C, Çakın MC, et al. The role of thymic stromal lymphopoietin in the development of chronic otitis media with effusion. Eur Arch Otorhinolaryngol. 2021;279:1937. https://doi.org/10.1007/s00405-021-06995-z.
19. Jacob TM, Indrasingh I, Yadav BK, Rupa V. Langerhans cells in the human tympanic membrane in health and disease: a morphometric analysis. Otol Neurotol. 2013;34(2):325–30.
20. Xu Q, Casey JR, Newman E, Pichichero ME. Otitis-prone children have immunologic deficiencies in naturally acquired nasopharyngeal mucosal antibody response after streptococcus pneumoniae colonization. Pediatr Infect Dis J. 2016;35(1):54–60.
21. Sharma SK, Casey JR, Pichichero ME. Reduced serum IgG responses to pneumococcal antigens in otitis-prone children may be due to poor memory B-cell generation. J Infect Dis. 2012;205(8):1225–9.
22. Kaur R, Casey J, Pichichero M. Serum antibody response to three non-typeable Haemophilus influenzae outer membrane proteins during acute otitis media and nasopharyngeal colonization in otitis prone and non-otitis prone children. Vaccine. 2011;29(5):1023–8. https://www.ncbi.nlm.nih.gov/pmc/articles/PMC3624763/pdf/nihms412728.pdf.
23. Sharma S, Pichichero M. Cellular immune response in young children accounts for recurrent acute otitis media. Curr Allergy Asthma Rep. 2013;13(5):495.
24. Avanzini AM, Castellazzi AM, Marconi M, Valsecchi C, Marseglia A, Ciprandi G, et al. Children with recurrent otitis show defective IFNγ-producing cells in adenoids. Pediatr Allergy Immunol. 2008;19(6):523–6.
25. Surendran N, Nicolosi T, Kaur R, Pichichero ME. Peripheral blood antigen presenting cell responses in otitis-prone and non-otitis-prone infants. Innate Immun. 2016;22(1):63–71.
26. Ren D, Xu Q, Almudevar AL, Pichichero ME. Impaired pro-inflammatory response in stringently defined otitis-prone children during viral upper respiratory infections. Clin Infect Dis. 2019;68(9):1566–74.
27. Zheng D, Liwinski T, Elinav E. Interaction between microbiota and immunity in health and disease. Cell Res. 2020;30(6):492–506. https://doi.org/10.1038/s41422-020-0332-7.
28. Peterson J, Garges S, Giovanni M, McInnes P, Wang L, Schloss JA, et al. The NIH Human Microbiome Project. Genome Res. 2009;19(12):2317–23.
29. Paradise JL, Rockette HE, Colborn DK, Bernard BS, Smith CG, Kurs-Lasky M, et al. Otitis media in 2253 Pittsburgh-area infants: prevalence and risk factors during the first two years of life. Pediatrics. 1997;14(1):121–8.
30. Folino F, Ruggiero L, Capaccio P, Coro I, Aliberti S, Drago L, et al. Upper respiratory tract microbiome and otitis media intertalk: lessons from the literature. J Clin Med. 2020;9(9):1–27.
31. Nistico L, Kreft R, Gieseke A, Coticchia JM, Burrows A, Khampang P, et al. Adenoid reservoir for pathogenic biofilm bacteria. J Clin Microbiol. 2011;49(4):1411–20.
32. Lappan R, Imbrogno K, Sikazwe C, Anderson D, Mok D, Coates H, et al. A microbiome case-control study of recurrent acute otitis media identified potentially protective bacterial genera. BMC Microbiol. 2018;18(1):1–20.
33. Scott AM, Clark J, Julien B, Islam F, Roos K, Grimwood K, et al. Probiotics for preventing acute otitis media in children. Cochrane Database Syst Rev. 2019;2019(6):CD012941.

When to Suspect and How to Evaluate Immune Deficiencies in Otitis Media

9

Sara Concha and Rodrigo Hoyos-Bachiloglu

Part I: General Features of Inborn Errors of Immunity (IEI)

Immunodeficiencies are clinical situations where there is a quantitative or functional deficiency of the immune system. They can be divided into two main groups based on their ontogeny. Secondary immunodeficiencies include conditions such as surgical asplenia, prematurity, human immunodeficiency virus (HIV) infection, malnutrition, hematological diseases, autoimmune diseases, and metabolic diseases such as diabetes and can result from various immunosuppressive drugs. Inborn errors of immunity (IEI), also referred to as primary immunodeficiencies (PIDs), are caused by mutations affecting genes involved in the normal functioning of the immune system. Although recurrent infections are the main symptoms of such conditions, PIDs have a broad spectrum of clinical presentations even for the same genetic defect (Table 9.1). An underlying immunodeficiency should be considered not only in patients presenting with frequent infections but also in those with infections lasting for a longer duration than usual, severe infections, infections with a poor response to antibiotic treatment, complicated infections, and infections due to unusual, multiple, or opportunistic microorganisms (Table 9.2). Noninfectious manifestations of an underlying PID can be extremely broad and include severe allergic diseases like eczema and food allergies, recurrent skin inflammation, oral ulcers, autoimmunity (most frequently autoimmune cytopenias), and lymphoproliferative diseases amongst others [1]. IEI are caused by monogenic germline mutations that result in loss of expression and/or loss of function or gain of function of the encoded protein. This results in aberrant immunity due to the critical roles that these proteins play in the development, maintenance, and function of cells of the immune system or cells other than leukocytes that contribute to immunity, during homeostasis and in response to external (e.g., infectious agents or environmental antigens) and internal (e.g., cytokines, self-antigens, and cancer cells) stimuli [2]. For a long time, IEI were consider rare diseases, but with the technological advances in genetics leading to improved diagnostic capabilities, the number of IEI has increased in more than 200 new conditions over the past 10 years and their incidence is now estimated to be around 1:1000 to 1:5000 in newborns [3]. In the last International Union of Immunological Societies (IUIS) classification of 2019, 404 phenotypes with 430 known genetic defects were included and they were separated into 10 groups (Table 9.1) [2].

In the last few years, there has been great advances in the development of new methods to expedite the identification of defects of the immune system and the cellular, molecular, and genetic aberrations underlying these conditions. Sequencing in general and next-generation sequencing (NGS) techniques are becoming technically more accurate, fast, and affordable and are therefore widely available to researchers and physicians [1]. A new insight into the pathogenesis of IEI has introduced targeted treatments next to substitution and symptomatic therapy (immunoglobulin replacement, antimicrobial and anti-inflammatory or immunosuppressive treatments), on one side, and replacement of the flawed immune system by hematopoietic stem cell trans-

Table 9.1 Inborn errors of immunity: International Union of Immunological Societies (IUIS) classification of 2019

1. Immunodeficiencies affecting cellular and humoral immunity
2. Combined immunodeficiencies with associated or syndromic features
3. Predominantly antibody deficiencies
4. Diseases of immune dysregulation
5. Congenital defects of phagocyte number or function
6. Defects in intrinsic and innate immunity
7. Autoinflammatory disorders
8. Complement deficiencies
9. Bone marrow failure
10. Phenocopies of inborn errors of immunity

S. Concha (✉) · R. Hoyos-Bachiloglu
Department of Pediatric Immunology and Infectious Diseases, Pontificia Universidad Católica de Chile, Santiago, Chile
e-mail: sconcha1@uc.cl; rhoyos@med.puc.cl

M. V. Goycoolea et al. (eds.), *Textbook of Otitis Media*, https://doi.org/10.1007/978-3-031-40949-3_9

plantation (HSCT) or gene therapy, on the other [4]. This has improved not only the survival rate but also the quality of life of these patients.

Part II: When to Suspect IEI in Patients with Recurrent Otitis Media

Otitis media is one of the most common diseases in young children. The decrease in the occurrence of otitis with age is explained by the transitioning of the Eustachian tube's anatomy by 3–5 years of age to a more "adult-like" structure and also by the maturation of the immune system [5]. In most children, otitis will not reveal a deficient immune system beyond physiological immaturity; however, it can be the first sign of a congenital disorder and unrecognized immunodeficiencies can lead to severe and potentially fatal infections. Recurrent otitis, with more than 4 episodes in a year, has been established as the first of the 10 warning signs of EIE in children by the Jeffrey Modell Foundation and the American Red Cross (Table 9.2). In adults, the European Society for Immunodeficiencies (ESID) advise suspecting IEI in case of four or more infections treated with antibiotics in 1 year (otitis, bronchitis, sinusitis, pneumonia) and recurrent infections needing prolonged therapy with antibiotics [6]. Although the number of infections is an important warning sign, the most important red flag is a family history of IEI. This feature has proven to be the key warning sign suggesting the presence of IEI and, as such, should be actively investigated when evaluating a patient with recurrent infections, including patients with recurrent otitis media [7]. Bardou et al. have proposed four warning signs for underlying IEI in otitis media: progressing infections leading to mastoiditis, associated abscesses or systemic infections, lack of responsiveness to adequate antibiotic treatment, and occurrence of unusual, severe, or frequently relapsing infections in other sites [6] (Table 9.3).

Table 9.2 Warning signs of primary immunodeficiency

1. Four or more new ear infections within 1 year
2. Two or more serious sinus infections within 1 year
3. Two or more months on antibiotics with little effect
4. Two or more pneumonias within 1 year
5. Failure of an infant to gain weight or grow normally
6. Recurrent, deep skin or organ abscesses
7. Persistent thrush in the mouth or fungal infection on the skin
8. Need for intravenous antibiotics to clear infections
9. Two or more deep-seated infections, including septicemia
10. A family history of primary immunodeficiency

Table 9.3 Warning signs to investigate inborn errors of immunity in otitis

1. Otitis media evolving with mastoiditis, abscesses or systemic infections
2. No response to appropriate antibiotic therapy
3. Otitis media associated with other infections
4. Recurrent otitis, leading to failure to thrive and general developmental delay
5. Family history of primary immunodeficiency and/or consanguinity

Part III: IEI Presenting with Otitis Media

Otitis media and pneumonia are the main infectious manifestations of IEI, with up to 57% of patients reporting having otitis media [8]. We will detail those IEI most frequently associated with otitis media.

Antibody Deficiencies

Antibodies are antigen-specific proteins produced by B cells and are synthesized and secreted by plasma cells, which arise from terminally differentiated B cells. They neutralize toxins and viruses, prevent colonization by pathogenic organisms, opsonize bacteria and fungi, activate the complement cascade, which enhances opsonization, and may directly lyse Gram-negative bacteria. Most patients with primary antibody deficiencies present with recurrent, severe, or persistent bacterial infections of the sinopulmonary tract, including recurrent otitis media, sinusitis, and pneumonia most commonly secondary to *Streptococcus pneumoniae*, *Hemophilus influenzae*, *Staphylococcus*, and *Pseudomonas*. Diarrhea affects up to 25% of these patients, often caused by *Giardia lamblia* infection [9]. Of the nine IEI categories, predominantly, antibody deficiency has the highest prevalence (1:25,000), but, despite advances in genomics, utilizing the current gold standard of whole exome sequencing for diagnosis, pathogenic gene variants are only identified in less than 20% of patients, especially in nonconsanguineous populations [10].

They are classified into four groups:

1. *Severe reduction in all serum immunoglobulin isotypes with profoundly decreased or absent B cells, agammaglobulinemia*

   Agammaglobulinemia is defined by the complete or near absence of B cells (less than 1%) and severe reduction of all major serum immunoglobulin isotypes (immunoglobulin (Ig)G, IgM, IgA). Clinical onset is typically within the first year(s) of life and is characterized by recurrent infections, mainly by encapsulated bacteria, which may affect the respiratory and gastrointestinal tracts, the skin, the joints, and the central nervous system [11]. The most common IEI in this group is X-linked agammaglobulinemia (XLA) due to Bruton's tyrosine kinase (BTK) deficiency, which plays a critical role in precursor B-cell development in the bone marrow [12]. The incidence of XLA is around 1:100,000 to 1:200,000 depending on ethnicity [11]. Clinical symptoms in affected patients initiate between the age of 6 and 12 months, when the maternal IgGs are catabolized; however, some patients may remain asymptomatic in the first years of life. Recurrent bacterial respiratory and/or gastrointestinal infections are the hallmarks of this disorder. The most frequent type of upper respiratory tract infection in large cohorts of XLA patients is otitis media (70%), followed by sinusitis (almost 60%). Recurrent otitis media may be the only infectious manifestation prior to diagnosis in XLA patients and should therefore always be considered as an alarm sign for immune deficiency during routine clinical practice [13]. Other frequent infections are pneumonia and gastrointestinal infections due to *Giardia lamblia*, the mycoplasma species, and enteroviruses. They also present with autoimmunity and up to 20% may develop arthritis. In a limited number of cases, gross deletions encompassing BTK and TIMM8A (translocase of inner mitochondrial membrane 8A) have been associated with sensorineural hearing loss in the first year of life, even though the underlying pathogenic mechanisms are not known [14]. Immunoglobulin replacement therapy is fundamental in XLA as in all humoral immunodeficiencies. Maintaining pre-infusion IgG levels >500 mg/dL assures a notable reduction in the number of infections. Using a dose of 400 mg/kg/dose every 3–4 weeks (in the case of intravenous immunoglobulin (IVIG)) or 100 mg/kg/dose every week (in the case of subcutaneous immunoglobulin) is usually sufficient to maintain such levels [15]. Frequently, antibiotic prophylaxis is necessary in order to control the number of infections even when IVIG therapy is adequate [11].

2. *Severe reduction in at least two serum immunoglobulin isotypes with a normal or low number of B cells, common variable immunodeficiency (CVID) phenotype*

CVID is a heterogeneous condition in which there is reduction of serum IgG by two or more standard deviations (SDs) below the mean age, along with a reduction of at least one of the other two isotypes (IgA or IgM) and with poor-to-absent specific antibody responses to an infection or vaccination [11]. Bonilla and coworkers, in an international consensus document in 2016, proposed that the main diagnostic criteria should also include the onset of immune deficiency after 2 years of age and that the defined causes of hypogammaglobulinemia must be excluded to establish a diagnosis of CVID [16]. In 2019, the European Society for Immunodeficiencies (ESID) added that there should be no evidence of profound T-cell deficiency, based on T cell and naive T cell numbers and T cell proliferative capacity in children older than 4 years [17] (Table 9.4). The prevalence of CVID is estimated at 1:25,000 in Europeans, but there are regional differences, with CVID being less commonly diagnosed in Asians and Afro-Americans [18]. The percentage of patients with monogenic defects associated with CVID is only about 20–25%. Although the first genes to be identified were autosomal recessive mutations, increasing numbers of autosomal dominant defects, with variable penetrance, have been discovered and now constitute the majority of genetic defects identified in CVID patients [19]. The onset of symptoms may be at any age but is generally between the ages of 15 and 40 years. The history of severe or recurrent bacterial infections of the upper and/or lower respiratory tract is commonly the reason an immune defect is first suspected. Pneumonia, usually due to *Streptococcus pneumoniae*, *H. influenzae*, or mycoplasma species is found in up to 70% of patients. Almost 50% of patients present noninfectious complications such as

Table 9.4 Diagnostic criteria for probable common variable immunodeficiency (CVID)

International consensus document CVID	European Society for Immunodeficiencies (ESID) criteria for CVID
Male or female patient who has a marked decrease of IgG (at least 2 SD below the mean age), a marked decrease in either IgM or IgA, and fulfills all of the following criteria: 1. Onset of immune deficiency at greater than 2 years of age 2. Absent isohemagglutinins and/or poor response to vaccines 3. Defined causes of hypogammaglobulinemia have been excluded	Male or female patient older than 4 years with at least one of the following: increased susceptibility to infection, autoimmunity, granulomatous disease, unexplained polyclonal lymphoproliferation, and/or affected family member with antibody deficiency AND marked decrease of IgG and marked decrease of IgA with or without low IgM levels (measured at least twice; <2 SD of the normal levels for their age) AND at least one of the following: poor antibody response to vaccines (and/or absent isohemagglutinins), i.e., the absence of protective levels despite vaccination where defined and/or low switched memory B cells (<70% of the age-related normal value) AND secondary causes of hypogammaglobulinemia have been excluded AND no evidence of profound T-cell deficiency, based on T cell and naive T cell numbers and T cell proliferative capacity

autoimmunity (most frequently autoimmune cytopenias), allergy, chronic pulmonary disease, granulomatous disease, and lymphoproliferation. The treatment goal for patients with CVID is to prevent infections and control additional secondary complications when present and clinically relevant and mainly consists of immunoglobulin replacement therapy and antibiotics [11].

3. *Severe reduction in serum IgG and IgA with normal/elevated IgM and normal numbers of B cells, hyper-IgM*

   The presence of elevated or normal serum IgM levels and low or null serum levels of the switched isotypes (IgG, IgA, and IgE) is called hyper-IgM syndrome. Defective production of IgG, IgA, and IgE and normal IgM production result from abnormal class switch recombination, a process that is essential for antibody maturation [20]. Although IgM antibodies have been shown to be protective against bacteria (such as non-typable *Haemophilus influenzae*), the production of switched isotypes is required for a fully efficient humoral response [21]. The estimated frequency of hyper-IgM syndrome is around 1 in 500,000 births. These patients suffer from recurrent bacterial infections that predominantly affect the respiratory tract and lead to severe sinusitis and bronchiectasis if left untreated. The clinical features and treatment depend on the precise nature of the molecular defect [11].

4. *Isotype, light chain, or functional deficiencies with generally normal numbers of B cells*

   Patients with recurrent respiratory infections may have defects in the amount or function of immunoglobulins. Those with a defect in the quantity can have reduced IgG in the context of normal IgA and IgM, and are defined as hypogammaglobulinemia, can have low quantity of IgG subclasses, or y can have low quantity of IgA or IgM. The most common functional defect is specific antibody deficiency (SAD) with a normal Ig level and normal B cells.

Quantity Defects

- Hypogammaglobulinemia: The age of the patient first needs to be considered as transient hypogammaglobulinemia of infancy presents in children, usually under the age of 3 years. Secondary causes, such as drug-induced hypogammaglobulinemia (steroids, immunosuppressants, certain biologicals and small molecules, selected anticonvulsants, and others), protein loss due to renal, gastrointestinal disease or potentially less well-defined third space, and lymphoma, must be considered. Patients with hypogammaglobulinemia of unknown significance and origin need to be referred for regular follow-up and further diagnostic testing [11].
- IgA deficiency: This is frequently asymptomatic, but affected patients can have a minor risk of allergy, autoimmunity, and bacterial infections. The genetic defect is commonly unknown. There is no specific treatment, but prophylactic antibiotics can be used in case of recurrent infections.
- IgG subclasses deficiency: This is defined as a level of IgG subclasses less than 2 SDs below the mean age with normal total IgG levels [22]. Up to 20% of the population has a subnormal IgG subclass level for one or more subclasses. Most IgG subclass-deficient subjects are asymptomatic, particularly those with an IgG4 deficiency. Thus, IgG subclass deficiency does not define a disease; instead, it defines a clinical laboratory finding [11]. A clinically significant IgG subclass deficiency occurs when the IgG subclass deficiency is associated with recurrent infections, a significant defect in functional antibody response, or is part of another IEI.

Functional Defects: Specific Antibody Deficiency

Polysaccharide antigens are repetitive molecular structures present in the outer capsule of bacteria, against which B cells can mount a T cell-independent immune response. The difference with a T cell-dependent response is that without the help of activated T cells, B cells do not experience a germinal center reaction, leading to the production of high-affinity antibodies and memory cells and immunoglobulin class switching [20]. The immunological responsiveness to polysaccharide antigens matures during the first years of life so that children below 2 years of age can have deficient antibody responses to those types of antigens. The consequence of this immaturity is an increased susceptibility to infections with encapsulated bacteria such as pneumococcus [23].

In order to bypass the poor immunological responses to polysaccharide antigens during the first 2 years of life and elicit protective humoral responses using vaccines, these antigens must be conjugated to a protein. These conjugated antigens can generate a T cell-dependent anti-polysaccharide response with a T cell–B cell interaction, resulting in adequate protection against disease [24]. The Centers for Disease Control and Prevention recommends four doses of a 13-valent pneumococcal conjugate vaccine for children under 2 years of age and a 23-valent pneumococcal polysaccharide vaccine for all adults 65 years or older. Vaccine indications and timings depend on age, previous vaccinations, and the presence of high-risk conditions, including congenital immunodeficiency [25].

Specific antibody deficiency (SAD) is defined as the inability to mount an antibody response to *Streptococcus pneumoniae* capsular polysaccharide antigens in the presence of normal immunoglobulin concentrations and normal antibody responses to protein antigens [26]. Patients with SAD generally present with recurrent, chronic, or/and severe rhinosinusitis, otitis and bronchopulmonary infections due to capsulated bacteria such as *Streptococcus pneumoniae*, *Haemophilus influenzae*, and *Moraxella catarrhalis*; however, they can also be asymptomatic [11].

The estimated incidence of SAD is unclear, and studies reporting prevalence should be evaluated with caution as they are based on reports from different centers, use different definitions, and normal values can differ between referral populations. Nevertheless, SAD is estimated to one of the most common IEI [27], with a reported prevalence of 6–14% in children with recurrent respiratory infections, 11–24% in adults with chronic rhinosinusitis, and 8% in adults with recurrent pneumonia.

Response to pneumococcal vaccines is usually determined by assessing the levels of serotype-specific IgG by multiplex bead immunoassays or enzyme-linked immunosorbent assays [23]. In order to stablish the diagnosis, serotype-specific IgG levels must be measured before and 4–8 weeks after receiving a pneumococcal polysaccharide vaccine in children older than 2 years of age. In patients exclusively vaccinated with pneumococcal conjugate vaccines, serotype-specific antibody levels ≥0.35 μg/mL are considered protective. In patients who have received the polysaccharide vaccine, a normal response is defined as serotype-specific antibody levels ≥1.3 μg/mL and/or increases in antibody levels between two and four times postimmunization with the polysaccharide vaccine with respect to basal levels in at least 50% of the serotypes tested in patients aged 2–5 years and in at least 70% in patients aged 6 years and over.

Treatment recommendations by the American Academy and the American College of Allergy, Asthma and Immunology are defined according to the severity of the disease. Most patients with mild-to-moderate disease might benefit from the use of prophylactic antibiotics, whereas unresponsive patients might benefit from a period of IgG replacement [3].

Inborn Errors of the Complement System

The complement system is composed of serum and cell surface proteins that play a major role in host defense, inflammation, immune complex clearance, induction of a normal humoral immune response and clearance of apoptotic cells. This system can be activated by IgM or IgG antibodies bound to a pathogen (classical pathway) or by the spontaneous hydrolysis of C3 and its attachment to a cell surface (alternative pathway). Each activation pathway requires a subgroup of complement proteins, but both use the same terminal components. As a group, defects of the complement system are infrequent, but, in specific groups of patients, such as those with systemic infections with encapsulated organisms, their frequency can be up to 11% [28].

Defects in different proteins of the complement system present with susceptibility to different kinds of microbes, depending on the biological function of the affected component. Patients with C3 deficiencies have an increased susceptibility to encapsulated bacteria for which opsonization is the primary host defense. Patients with deficiencies of C1, C4, or C2 have a lower prevalence of infection compared to C3-deficient patients because their alternative pathway is intact and therefore are able to activate C3. The terminal components, C5–C9, form a membrane attack complex required for the bactericidal/bacteriolytic functions of the complement system. Patients with C5–C9 deficiencies are susceptible to Neisserial infections [11].

During the initial evaluation of patients with a suspected defect in the complement system, it is recommended to functionally evaluate the classic pathway using a test known as CH50. The CH50 evaluates the time in which 50% of sensitized sheep erythrocytes are lysed in the presence of functional C1–C9 proteins. A similar test exists for the alternative pathway, namely, the AH50. Almost all complement deficiencies are associated with either a CH50 or AH50 near zero. Moderately low CH50, C3, or C4 levels are a common finding and are most frequently due to inadequate sample handling.

Treatment of patients with recurrent capsulated bacteria due to complement deficiency is mostly with prophylactic antibiotics.

Phagocytic Defects

Defects of the phagocytes most frequently associated with recurrent otitis media can be classified into those due to a numerical defect, such as congenital neutropenia, and those due to functional defects, like chronic granulomatous disease (CGD).

Congenital Neutropenia

Neutropenia is defined as an absolute neutrophil count of less than 1500 cells/μL in individuals over 1 year of age and less than 2000 cells/μL during the first year of life. Severe neutropenia is defined as a neutrophil count less than 500 cells/μL; these patients are usually symptomatic and present with severe bacterial infections. The temporal course of neutropenia may vary and can be classified as persistent, intermittent, or cyclic. Persistent neutropenia, also referred to as chronic neutropenia, is defined as a low neutrophil count lasting at least 3 months. Cyclic neutropenia is characterized by fluctuating neutrophil counts, with a decreased number of neutrophils every 2–3 weeks and normal counts between episodes [11].

The risk of infections in neutropenia patients correlates with the severity and duration of neutropenia. Patients with severe neutropenia are at risk of sepsis, periodontitis, gingivitis, and oral aphthae, whereas those with less profound neutropenia are at risk of infections due to the *Staphylococcus* and *Streptococcus* species [6].

Chronic Granulomatous Disease (CGD)

This is a genetically heterogeneous disease characterized by recurrent life-threatening bacterial and fungal infections and dysregulated granuloma formation caused by the absence, low expression, or malfunction of one of the phagocyte nicotinamide adenine dinucleotide phosphate hydrogen (NADPH) oxidase components, resulting in a defect of the phagocyte respiratory burst and the generation of phagocyte superoxide used to destroy microbes [29].

The clinical manifestations of this disease depend on the underlying genetic defect. Most patients with the X-linked form present infections early in life and have a more severe clinical course and have an increased mortality compared to patients with the autosomal-recessive disease. These individuals are most affected by infections due to catalase-positive bacteria such as *Staphylococcus aureus*, *Burkholderia cepacia*, and *Klebsiella*, *Aerobacter*, and *Serratia* spp. Fungal infections are also extremely common in these patients, mostly due to *Aspergillus*. The most infected sites in CGD are the skin, soft tissue, bone, sinus, gut, and lungs, although complicated acute otitis media has been reported as the first sign of the disease [30].

The diagnosis of CGD is made by an absent or significantly decreased respiratory burst in stimulated neutrophils by means of a dihydrorhodamine (DHR)-123 test. This test measures the production of superoxide by phagocytes after stimulation with phorbol myristate acetate (PMA) by flow cytometry using fluorescent probes like DHR-123. In stimulated neutrophils, DHR is oxidized by hydrogen peroxide (produced in the presence of normal NADPH oxidase and myeloperoxidase) to rhodamine-123 that emits fluorescence [31].

Treatment is based on the management of infections and on the use of antibiotic and antifungal prophylaxis, with or without the use of interferon-gamma. The only known cure for this disease is hematopoietic stem cell transplantation (HSCT) [32].

Combined Immunodeficiencies (CIDs)

Combined T- and B-cell immunodeficiencies are also associated with otitis media, although patients affected by these conditions usually present with opportunistic infections and recurrent bacterial, viral, fungal, and parasitic infections. Combined immunodeficiencies with defective control of viral infections may have an increased risk of malignancy, especially Epstein–Barr virus lymphoma, and can present autoimmune disease, allergy, and autoinflammation. They can also have nonimmune manifestations and manifest with a syndromic presentation [11].

Severe combined immunodeficiencies are characterized by profound impairment of T-cell development and/or function, so children will present in the first months of life with severe opportunistic infections, and, in the absence of definitive therapy, patients inevitably die within the first year of life [33].

Other less profound combined immunodeficiencies have also been associated with recurrent sinopulmonary infections. CD40 ligand deficiency, also known as X-linked hyper-IgM (X-HIGM) syndrome, results in the absence or non-function of molecules involved in immunoglobulin class switch recombination, a critical process in the production and maturation of antibodies triggered by the T cell–B cell interaction. Patients with hyper-IgM syndrome present with infections early in life, most frequently pneumonia (86%) and upper respiratory tract infections like otitis media and tonsillitis (70%). They can also present with neutropenia and gastrointestinal manifestations like sclerosing cholangitis [34]. Laboratory tests show normal or elevated IgM levels associated with low IgG and IgA in most patients. Diagnosis is made by CD40L expression on activated $CD4^+$ T cells by flow cytometry and genetic test. Treatment usually includes IVIG replacement and antimicrobial prophylaxis; however, the only curative treatment is HSCT [35].

Combined immunodeficiencies with associated or syndromic features can also present recurrent otitis media. Such conditions include Wiskott–Aldrich syndrome, ataxia-telangiectasia, chromosome 22q11.2 deletion syndrome, and hyper-IgE syndrome.

Children with Wiskott–Aldrich syndrome usually present with thrombocytopenia with small platelets, eczema, bloody diarrhea, and bacterial infections. They experience a progressive decline in T cell number and low IgM and low antibody responses to polysaccharides [36].

Ataxia-telangiectasia presents with decreasing T cell numbers, associated with low IgG and IgA, increased alpha-fetoprotein, increased radiosensitivity, and malignancies due to chromosomal instability [37].

Patients with thymic defects like chromosome 22q11.2 deletion syndrome or DiGeorge/velocardiofacial syndrome present with hypoparathyroidism, conotruncal cardiac malformations, and thymic defect determined either by a small or absent thymus and low T-cell counts. They frequently present with otitis media mainly due to anatomical defects of the upper respiratory tract like palatal anomalies [38].

Hyper-IgE syndromes are an heterogeneous CID group of different genetic defects like STAT3 (signal transducer and activator of transcription 3) deficiency and DOCK8 (dedicator of cytokinesis 8) deficiency that manifest as eczema, high IgE, infections like recurrent ear and sinopulmonary infections, skin abscesses due to *Staphylococcus*, mucocutaneous candidiasis, cutaneous viral infections, atopy, and malignancies [39].

Part IV: How to Evaluate IEI in Recurrent Otitis Media Cases

An accurate and prompt diagnosis of patients with IEI is critical for timely initiation of therapeutic measures and to provide the patients and their families with appropriate genetic counseling. Given the diversity of IEI that can present with recurrent ear and sinopulmonary infections, laboratory evaluation must be rational and guided by the patient's infection history.

The nature of pathogens causing the ear infection provides relevant diagnostic information (Table 9.5). Increased susceptibility to pyogenic encapsulated bacteria such as *Streptococcus pneumoniae* and *Haemophilus influenzae* is seen in defects of the antibody and/or complement system. Infections due to a virus like *Cytomegalovirus* and fungi like *Candida* and *Pneumocystis jirovecii* are frequent in patients with T-cell defects. Patients with *Staphylococcus aureus*, *Serratia marcescens*, *Burkholderia cepacian*, and *Aspergillus* infections must be screened for phagocytic defects [9].

As IEI can alter not only the number of its components but also their functionality, it is important not only to perform quantitative laboratory tests but also qualitative tests (Table 9.6).

When a humoral defect is suspected, immunoglobulin levels must be evaluated and testing results compared to age-adjusted reference values. Hypogammaglobulinemia is defined as a value below two standard deviations for age, and agammaglobulinemia is defined as an IgG level less than 100 mg/dL. Functional evaluation of the humoral response can be done by evaluating serum titers to common vaccines, protein-based vaccines such as tetanus and diphtheria, and polysaccharide-based vaccines such as pneumococcus. If serum vaccination titers are below normal, revaccination and assessment of titers 4–6 weeks later are warranted.

When a B- or T-cell defect is suspected, a complete blood count study should be requested to evaluate the number of lymphocytes and lymphocyte subsets by flow cytometry to enumerate them. It can be observed that lymphocyte count varies with age; in newborns, the normal value is considered over $2.0 \times 10^3/mm^3$, but, in adults, a normal value is over $1.0 \times 10^3/mm^3$ [40]. Functional tests that evaluate the T-cell compartment are meant to quantify their ability to proliferate in response to different stimuli; this can be done using nonspecific agents known as mitogens or specific antigens [41].

The evaluation of patients with suspected phagocytic defects must include a total blood count to measure neutrophil count and chemotaxis, phagocytosis, or respiratory burst testing to evaluate their functionality.

Table 9.6 Laboratory tests for the qualitative and quantitative study of inborn errors of immunity

Immunity	Quantitative	Qualitative
Humoral	Total immunoglobulin count	Specific antibody production (pneumococcus, tetanus)
Cellular	Total blood count (lymphocytes) Lymphocyte subsets	Lymphoproliferation
Phagocyte	Total blood count (neutrophils)	Chemotaxis, phagocytosis, respiratory burst
Complement	C2, C3, C4, etc.	CH50, AH50

Table 9.5 Pathogens associated with the underlying inborn errors of immunity

Agent	Antibody defects	Combined defects	Phagocytic defects	Complement defects
Viruses	Enterovirus	Cytomegalovirus Epstein–Barr virus	No	No
Bacteria	*S. pneumoniae* *H. influenzae* *M. catarrhalis* *P. aeruginosa* *S. aureus* *N. meningitidis* *Mycoplasma*	*S. pneumoniae* *H. influenzae* *M. catarrhalis* *P. aeruginosa* *S. aureus* *N. meningitidis Mycoplasma* *S. typhi* *L. monocytogenes*	*S. aureus* *P. aeruginosa* *S. typhi Nocardia*	*S. pneumoniae* *H. influenzae* *M. catarrhalis* *P. aeruginosa* *S. aureus* *N. meningitidis* *Mycoplasma*
Mycobacteria	No	Non-tuberculous, including Bacillus Calmette-Guérin (BCG)	Non-tuberculous, including BCG	No
Fungi	No	*Candida* species *Aspergillus* species *Cryptococcus neoformans* *Histoplasma capsulatum*	*Candida* sp., *Aspergillus* sp.	No
Protozoa	*Giardia lamblia*	*P. jirovecii* *Toxoplasma gondii* *Cryptosporidium*	No	No

Evaluation of a patient with a suspected defect in the complement pathway should start with a functional evaluation of the classic pathway by CH50. This test can be coupled with an AH50 to complete the functional evaluation of the complement system. The next step in the evaluation of such patients consists of the quantification of different complement components based on functional testing results, most commonly by nephelometry or enzyme-linked immunoassay (ELISA) variations [20]. Patients with C1, C2, or C4 deficiency will have a low CH50 but normal AH50. Patients with a low AH50 but normal CH50 have a deficiency of factor B, factor D, or properdin. A decrease in both CH50 and AH50 suggests a deficiency in a shared complement component, C3 or C5–C9 [41].

References

1. Bucciol G, Meyts I. Recent advances in primary immunodeficiency: from molecular diagnosis to treatment. F1000Research. 2020;9:F1000 Faculty Rev-194.
2. Tangye SG, Al-Herz W, Bousfiha A, Chatila T, Cunningham-Rundles C, Etzioni A, et al. Human inborn errors of immunity: 2019 update on the classification from the International Union of Immunological Societies Expert Committee. J Clin Immunol. 2020;40(1):24–64.
3. Bonilla FA, Khan DA, Ballas ZK, Chinen J, Frank MM, Hsu JT, et al. Practice parameter for the diagnosis and management of primary immunodeficiency. J Allergy Clin Immunol. 2014;136(5):1186–1205.e78. https://doi.org/10.1016/j.jaci.2015.04.049.
4. Delmonte OM, Notarangelo LD. Targeted therapy with biologicals and small molecules in primary immunodeficiencies. Med Princ Pract. 2020;29(2):101–12.
5. Pichichero M. Immunologic dysfunction contributes to the otitis prone condition. J Infect. 2020;80(6):614–22.
6. Bardou MLD, Pontarolli D, Grumach AS. Otitis media and inborn errors of immunity. Curr Allergy Asthma Rep. 2020;20(10):1–5.
7. Subbarayan A, Colarusso G, Hughes SM, Gennery AR, Slatter M, Cant AJ, et al. Clinical features that identify children with primary immunodeficiency diseases. Pediatrics. 2011;127(5):810–6.
8. Bazregari S, Azizi G, Tavakol M, Asgardoon MH, Kiaee F, Tavakolinia N, et al. Evaluation of infectious and non-infectious complications in patients with primary immunodeficiency. Cent Eur J Immunol. 2017;42(4):336–41.
9. Oliveira JB, Fleisher TA. Laboratory evaluation of primary immunodeficiencies. J Allergy Clin Immunol. 2010;125(2 Suppl. 2):297–305.
10. Edwards ESJ, Bosco JJ, Ojaimi S, O'Hehir RE, van Zelm MC. Beyond monogenetic rare variants: tackling the low rate of genetic diagnoses in predominantly antibody deficiency. Cell Mol Immunol. 2021;18(3):588–603. https://doi.org/10.1038/s41423-020-00520-8.
11. Sullivan KE, Stiehm ER. Stiehm's immune deficiencies inborn errors of immunity. 2nd ed. Elsevier; 2020. p. 443–64.
12. Block H, Zarbock A. The role of the Tec kinase Bruton's tyrosine kinase (Btk) in leukocyte recruitment. Int Rev Immunol. 2012;31(2):104–18. https://doi.org/10.3109/08830185.2012.668982.
13. Conley ME, Howard V. Clinical findings leading to the diagnosis of X-linked agammaglobulinemia. J Pediatr. 2002;141(4):566–71.
14. Šedivá A, Smith CIE, Asplund AC, Hadač J, Janda A, Zeman J, et al. Contiguous X-chromosome deletion syndrome encompassing the BTK, TIMM8A, TAF7L, and DRP2 genes. J Clin Immunol. 2007;27(6):640–6.
15. Quinti I, Soresina A, Guerra A, Rondelli R, Spadaro G, Agostini C, et al. Effectiveness of immunoglobulin replacement therapy on clinical outcome in patients with primary antibody deficiencies: results from a multicenter prospective cohort study. J Clin Immunol. 2011;31(3):315–22.
16. Bonilla FA, Barlan I, Chapel H, Costa-Carvalho BT, Charlotte Cunningham-Rundles M, de la Morena T, Espinosa-Rosales FJ, Hammarström L, Shigeaki NM. International Consensus Document (ICON): common variable immunodeficiency disorders. J Allergy Clin Immunol Pract. 2016;4(1):38–59.
17. Seidel MG, Kindle G, Gathmann B, Quinti I, Buckland M, van Montfrans J, et al. The European Society for Immunodeficiencies (ESID) registry working definitions for the clinical diagnosis of inborn errors of immunity. J Allergy Clin Immunol Pract. 2019;7(6):1763–70.
18. Odnoletkova I, Kindle G, Quinti I, Grimbacher B, Knerr V, Gathmann B, et al. The burden of common variable immunodeficiency disorders: a retrospective analysis of the European Society for Immunodeficiency (ESID) registry data 11 Medical and Health Sciences 1117 Public Health and Health Services. Orphanet J Rare Dis. 2018;13(1):1–17.
19. Maffucci P, Filion CA, Boisson B, Itan Y, Shang L, Casanova JL, et al. Genetic diagnosis using whole exomesequencing in common variable immunodeficiency. Front Immunol. 2016;7:220.
20. Abbas A, Lichtman A, Pillai S. Cellular and molecular immunology, vol. 1. Elsevier; 2019. p. 1–2.
21. Micol R, Kayal S, Mahlaoui N, Beauté J, Brosselin P, Dudoit Y, et al. Protective effect of IgM against colonization of the respiratory tract by nontypeable Haemophilus influenzae in patients with hypogammaglobulinemia. J Allergy Clin Immunol. 2012;129(3):770–7.
22. Wahn V, von Bernuth H. IgG subclass deficiencies in children: facts and fiction. Pediatr Allergy Immunol. 2017;28(6):521–4.
23. Perez E, Bonilla FA, Orange JS, Ballow M. Specific antibody deficiency: controversies in diagnosis and management. Front Immunol. 2017;8(May):1–11.
24. O'Brien KL, Santosham M. Potential impact of conjugate pneumococcal vaccines on pediatric pneumococcal diseases. Am J Epidemiol. 2004;159(7):634–44.
25. https://www.cdc.gov/vaccines/vpd/pneumo/hcp/who-when-to-vaccinate.html.
26. Sorensen RU, Edgar D. Specific antibody deficiencies in clinical practice. J Allergy Clin Immunol Pract. 2019;7(3):801–8. https://doi.org/10.1016/j.jaip.2019.01.024.
27. Modell V, Knaus M, Modell F, Roifman C, Orange J, Notarangelo LD. Global overview of primary immunodeficiencies: a report from Jeffrey Modell Centers worldwide focused on diagnosis, treatment, and discovery. Immunol Res. 2014;60(1):132–44.
28. Ingels H, Schejbel L, Lundstedt AC, Jensen L, Laursen IA, Ryder LP, et al. Immunodeficiency among children with recurrent invasive pneumococcal disease. Pediatr Infect Dis J. 2015;34(6):644–51.
29. Yu HH, Yang YH, Chiang BL. Chronic granulomatous disease: a comprehensive review. Clin Rev Allergy Immunol. 2021;61(2):101–13.
30. Wilson R, Bhuta T, Haydon R. Multiple simultaneous complications of acute otitis media in a child diagnosed with chronic granulomatous disease: a case report. Ear Nose Throat J. 2008;87(5):271–9.
31. Roos D, de Boer M. Molecular diagnosis of chronic granulomatous disease. Clin Exp Immunol. 2014;175(2):139–49.
32. Chiesa R, Wang J, Blok HJ, Hazelaar S, Neven B, Moshous D, et al. Hematopoietic cell transplantation in chronic granulomatous disease: a study of 712 children and adults. Blood. 2020;136(10):1201–11.

33. Bustamante Ogando JC, Partida Gaytán A, Aldave Becerra JC, Álvarez Cardona A, Bezrodnik L, Borzutzky A, et al. Latin American consensus on the supportive management of patients with severe combined immunodeficiency. J Allergy Clin Immunol. 2019;144(4):897–905.
34. França TT, Barreiros LA, Salgado RC, Napoleão SMS, Gomes LN, Ferreira JFS, et al. CD40 ligand deficiency in Latin America: clinical, immunological, and genetic characteristics. J Clin Immunol. 2022;42(3):514–26. https://doi.org/10.1007/s10875-021-01182-5.
35. Castagnoli R, Delmonte OM, Calzoni E, Notarangelo LD. Hematopoietic stem cell transplantation in primary immunodeficiency diseases: current status and future perspectives. Front Pediatr. 2019;7(August):1–25.
36. Massaad MJ, Ramesh N, Geha RS. Wiskott-Aldrich syndrome: a comprehensive review. Ann N Y Acad Sci. 2013;1285(1):26–43.
37. van Os NJH, Haaxma CA, van der Flier M, Merkus PJFM, van Deuren M, de Groot IJM, et al. Ataxia-telangiectasia: recommendations for multidisciplinary treatment. Dev Med Child Neurol. 2017;59(7):680–9.
38. Sullivan KE. Chromosome 22q11.2 deletion syndrome and DiGeorge syndrome. Immunol Rev. 2019;287(1):186–201.
39. Bergerson JRE, Freeman AF. An update on syndromes with a hyper-IgE phenotype. Immunol Allergy Clin N Am. 2019;39(1):49–61.
40. Ding Y, Zhou L, Xia Y, Wang W, Wang Y, Li L, et al. Reference values for peripheral blood lymphocyte subsets of healthy children in China. J Allergy Clin Immunol. 2018;142(3):970–973.e8.
41. Locke BA, Dasu T, Verbsky JW. Laboratory diagnosis of primary immunodeficiencies. Clin Rev Allergy Immunol. 2014;46(2):154–68.

Genetics and Otitis Media

10

Nam K. Lee and Regie Lyn P. Santos-Cortez

Introduction

Otitis media (OM) is a complex disease with various risk factors for its development, chronicity, and recurrence as well as a multifactorial etiology that is yet to be fully understood. An intricate interplay among environmental, genetic, microbial, anatomic, and immunological factors contributes to the pathogenesis of OM. Within this context, young age, lack of breastfeeding, use of pacifiers, day-care attendance or overcrowding at home, and exposure to tobacco smoke and particulate matter, to name a few, have been identified as environmental risk factors for the development of OM [1–3].

Within the otolaryngology practice, the presence of family history remains one of the most important inquiries made during an evaluation of a child with OM. Inherited or genetic factors were found to influence the early onset and development of OM, with a higher incidence observed in certain populations [4–7]. For example, the frequency of OM is increased in children with chromosomal abnormalities such as Down syndrome (MIM 190685) and Turner syndrome (MIM 300082), in which the affected chromosomes often contain numerous genes of various functions [8, 9]. Chromosome 21, which is affected in Down syndrome, contains many genes that are involved in the immune system, particularly those that play a role in interferon signaling, thereby causing a predisposition to viral and bacterial infections [10–15]. Compounded by distinct craniofacial structures of Down syndrome and its associated dysfunctions, such as small middle ear compartments, poor palatal tone, and maldeveloped Eustachian tubes, individuals with Down syndrome often experience OM that does not resolve easily, requiring multiple tympanostomy tube procedures, and subsequent persistent tympanic membrane perforation and hearing loss [16–19]. Turner syndrome is similar in its clinical manifestation with immune alterations found in T cells and immunoglobulins (Igs) along with craniofacial abnormalities of the palate, jaw, and ears that range from the external to inner ear system [20–22]. As a result, affected individuals are predisposed to a range of otologic problems from recurrent or chronic OM to conductive or sensorineural hearing loss and tympanic membrane pathology [9, 23].

The socioeconomic impact of health-care costs and delay in speech and language for OM-affected individuals underline the need for further research in OM. Although our current understanding of the main contributors of genetic susceptibility to OM remains scant compared to our overall genetic knowledge of other common diseases, such as cardiovascular disorders and cancer, continued efforts toward the identification of the determinants of human susceptibility and host genomic responses to OM will help elucidate its multifactorial etiology. Recent advances in genomic databases, sequencing, and analytic techniques will benefit the ongoing genetic investigation into OM and ultimately lead to a better understanding of its pathogenesis, which, in turn, can improve strategies for its prevention and treatment.

Human DNA Studies

Heritability

Heritability, in the narrow sense, is an estimate of the proportion of the variance in phenotypic or trait values under study (in this case, OM), which is due to genetic factors [24]. Because OM is a complex trait, heritability has been estimated using data from related individuals as was done in twin studies performed in three cohorts from Norway, the United States, and the United Kingdom (UK). The initial twin study from Norway in 1997 consisted of 2850 twins, which was then followed up in 2004 with an enlarged cohort of 4247 twins [25, 26]. In the initial study, gender differences

N. K. Lee · R. L. P. Santos-Cortez (✉)
Department of Otolaryngology-Head and Neck Surgery, School of Medicine, University of Colorado Anschutz Medical Campus, Aurora, CO, USA
e-mail: nam.lee@cuanschutz.edu; regie.santos-cortez@cuanschutz.edu

M. V. Goycoolea et al. (eds.), *Textbook of Otitis Media*, https://doi.org/10.1007/978-3-031-40949-3_10

were detected in female twins who had higher heritability for OM at 74% compared to males with 45% heritability [25]. In the follow-up study that included an additional 1397 twins, gender-based differences for heritability estimates were not observed, although the overall heritability for OM remained high at 61–72% [26].

In Pittsburgh, a prospective cohort study of 168 same-sex twins and 7 same-sex triplets was conducted to determine the heritability of time or duration of middle ear effusion (MEE) [27]. The same cohort was reassessed after 5 years, and it was determined that the heritability of the time with MEE as a phenotype remained consistent [28]. Heritability was 73% in the initial study and 72% in the follow-up study, and both had $p < 0.001$ [27, 28].

Rovers et al. (2002) assessed the heritability of both OM and chronic airway blockage in a prospective study of 1373 twins from the UK [29]. The heritability of acute OM was estimated to be 57%. For both OM and chronic airway blockade, an increasing genetic contribution to the phenotypic variance was observed at ages 2 years (49%), 3 years (66%), and 4 years (71%). However, no gender differences were observed [29].

Valuable information can also be gleaned from familial studies with multiple OM-affected siblings as in the study by Hafrén [30]. Heritability estimates of recurrent acute and chronic OM were determined in their survey of 2436 children, who underwent surgery for OM, and their relatives from 590 Finnish families. Chronic OM had lower heritability (22%) compared to recurrent acute OM (38%), and the overall heritability of all types of OM was estimated at 48% [30]. As expected, heritability estimates are higher in identical twins than in other familial relations due to the greater similarity in both genetic makeup and environmental background of twins. Nonetheless, these heritability studies, albeit with various heritability estimates, phenotypic definitions, ethnic background, and cohort composition, confirm the significant contribution of genetic factors to OM susceptibility.

Genetic Linkage Studies

Genetic linkage studies test whether a pattern of inheritance of a disease or trait coincides with the genotypes of families: genetic linkage is therefore a test of co-segregation of a variant or variants inherited together (e.g., a haplotype) with the known disease status of family members. The main metric for linkage is the logarithm of odds (LOD) score, which is usually considered statistically significant if a LOD score of 3.3 or greater is obtained for a variant or haplotype within pedigrees that co-segregate a disease or a trait [31]. To obtain a significant LOD score, either a large enough pedigree or a consanguineous family with multiple affected individuals is needed. Alternatively, smaller families that each on its own cannot obtain linkage but, when analyzed together, can lead to mapping of significant loci may be used. Before the advent of next-generation sequencing, genetic variants that are distributed across the genome were genotyped and then tested for linkage in order to identify a genomic region where the pathogenic variant is statistically the most likely to occur. Early linkage studies using different cohorts of families identified multiple loci in various regions of the human genome, most significantly on chromosome 10q (Table 10.1). It should be noted, however, that in many of the mapped loci,

Table 10.1 Genomic loci mapped for otitis media susceptibility in linkage studies using family data

Loci	Studies	LOD score	Significance and candidate genes within the loci
19q13.42–q13.43	Daly et al. [32]	LOD 2.61 ($p = 5.3 \times 10^{-4}$)	Leukocyte receptor cluster (*LRC*)—cluster of genes with polymorphic functions; mainly prevents immune cell activation [38]
	Chen et al. [35]	LOD 3.75 ($p = 1.6 \times 10^{-5}$)	Zinc finger and zinc finger-related genes (*ZNF71, ZNF8, ANF304*) Inflammasome protein complex (*NLRP13, NLRP5, NLRP8*)
10q26.3	Daly et al. [32]	LOD 3.78 ($p = 3.0 \times 10^{-5}$)	*ADAM8*—identified in allergen-induced asthma, expressed in leukocytes [193, 194]
	Rye et al. [33]	Z_{lr} 2.69 ($p = 3.6 \times 10^{-3}$)	*ADAM12*—involved in the epidermal growth factor receptor signaling pathway [41, 194] Dedicator of cytokinesis 1 (*DOCK1*)—phagocytosis of apoptotic cells, skeletal and respiratory muscle tissue development in embryogenesis [42] *TCERG1L* and *PPP2R2D*—an intergenic region Transcription elongation regulator-like protein (*TCERG1L*)—suggested in fasting insulin, attention deficit disorder Protein phosphatase 2A (*PPP2R2D*)—a modulator of the TGF-β/Activin/Nodal pathway [33, 43]

Table 10.1 (continued)

Loci	Studies	LOD score	Significance and candidate genes within the loci
3p25.3	Daly et al. [32]	Unconditional: LOD 0.60 Conditional: 10q LOD 2.43 19q LOD 1.84	Presumed to be involved in the gene–gene interaction between 19q13.42 and 10q26.3 *HRH1*—an inflammatory mediator [195] *IRAK2*—mediates inflammatory gene expression via NF-κB [196]
17q12	Casselbrant et al. [197]	LOD 2.83 ($p = 7.0x10^{-5}$)	Adaptor-related protein complex2, beta 1 subunit (*AP2B1*)—CD8⁺ downregulation [198]Chemokine C–C motif ligand (*CCL*)—recruitment of eosinophils [199]
10q22.3	Casselbrant et al. [197]	LOD > 2 ($p = 1.8 \times 10^{-3}$)	*SFTPA2*—part of surfactant protein A, which regulates the phagocytosis of pathogens; expressed in the Eustachian tube [45]
	Rye et al. [33]	Z_{lr} 1.64 ($p = 0.05$)	–
7q33	Casselbrant et al. [197]	LOD > 2 ($p = 1.0 \times 10^{-3}$)	–
6p25.1	Casselbrant et al. [197]	LOD > 2 ($p = 2.6 \times 10^{-3}$)	–
4p15.2	Casselbrant et al. [197]	LOD > 2 ($p = 3.0 \times 10^{-3}$)	–
15q26.1	Allen et al. [59]	$p = 9.1 \times 10^{-7}$	*KIF7*—the region is related to the splice site; regulates sonic hedgehog [200] and Indian hedgehog [64] via protein trafficking *TICRR*—initiation of DNA replication [65]
5p15.33	Allen et al. [59]	$p = 0.045$	Tubulin polymerization-promoting protein (*TPPP*)—located at the intron; affects microtubule function [63]
2q31.1	Allen et al. [59]	$p = 1.3 \times 10^{-5}$	Non-coding region: possible role in the regulation of LDLR (ch19), which is expressed in ciliated airway epithelial cells [201]

the pathogenic variants responsible for OM susceptibility remain unknown. This is partly due to the lack of genetic studies performed in families with OM and potentially due to genetic heterogeneity for OM where families carry variants within multiple genes that are mostly rare or private variants, such that current family cohorts lack the power to detect significant OM loci. Below is a review of loci that have been mapped using families with OM.

19q13.42–q13.43

Daly et al. (2004) first identified the 19q13.42–q13.43 region as a suggestive susceptibility locus (LOD 2.61, $p = 5.3 \times 10^{-4}$) using genotype data from Minnesotan families with OM [32]. Approximately 100 annotated genes are present in this region, but many of their functions remain unknown. The leukocyte receptor cluster (*LRC*) genes were suggested as potential candidate genes within the 10q locus. Within this region are genes encoding the leukocyte Ig-like receptor (*LIR*; also known as Ig-like transcripts) and the killer cell immunoglobulin-like receptor (*KIR*), which are transmembrane proteins expressed on cells of immune function for various protein activation or inhibition [33]. Such proteins include tyrosine phosphatases Src homology region 2 domain-containing phosphatase (SHP)-1 and/or SHP-2 [34]. This region was replicated by Chen et al. (2011), who fine-mapped the locus to chromosome 19q13.43 using additional single nucleotide variant genotypes (LOD 3.75, $p = 1.6 \times 10^{-5}$) [35]. The additional candidate genes identified within the 19q locus include genes related to zinc fingers, the tumor necrosis factor-alpha (TNFα), bone morphogenetic protein (BMP), and fibroblast growth factor-beta (FGFβ) pathways, lymphocyte activation, and the inflammasome protein complex, all of which regulate innate immunity in response to harmful stimuli [35–37].

10q26.3

In an initial linkage study for OM using the Minnesota family cohort, the 10q26.3 locus was identified with a LOD score of 3.78 ($p = 3.0 \times 10^{-5}$) and was replicated in another cohort of Western Australia-based trios by Rye et al. in 2014 (Z_{lr} 2.69, $p = 3.6 \times 10^{-3}$) [32, 33]. Herein, trios are composed of the OM-affected individual (proband) and both parents, without affected or unaffected siblings. Within the 10q26.3 locus, the Minnesotan and Australian studies identified candidate genes encoding a disintegrin and metalloproteinase (ADAM) domain. ADAM8 is found in leukocytes in response to allergen exposure in asthma and is also upregulated in epithelial cells of the airway during allergic inflammation [38, 39]. The function of ADAM12 is most strongly associated with cell adhesion and fusion, extracellular matrix restructuring, and cell signaling [40]. It has been found to be upregulated in the middle ear in response to tobacco smoke [41]. Other genes implicated in this region include *DOCK1* (MIM 601403), which is involved in phagocytosis; *TCERG1L* encoding transcription elongation regulator-like protein, and *PPP2R2D* (MIM 613992), which modulates the modulator of the transforming growth factor (TGF)/Activin/Nodal pathway [33, 42, 43].

10q22.3

Chromosomal region 10q22.3 has also been identified (LOD >2, $p = 1.81 \times 10^{-3}$) and replicated with suggestive evidence (Z_{lr} 1.64, $p = 0.05$), though not reaching statistical significance [2, 33]. *SFTPA1* (MIM 178630) and *SFTPA2* (MIM 178642) are genes within this region that together encode the human surfactant protein (SP-A) and have previously been implicated in OM [44]. SP-A haplotype and genotype variations have been observed in children with the first episode of OM before 6 months, and common variants in these genes were associated with protection against OM in infants at risk of asthma [45, 46]. SP-A is expressed in the middle ear mucosa and in the Eustachian tube and is known to contribute to innate immune responses by increasing the phagocytosis of otopathogens [45–48].

Candidate Gene Association Studies

Using a gene of interest, candidate gene association studies estimate the frequency with which the minor allele, or the less prevalent allele in the background population, is found in OM-affected patients in comparison to a control group. Healthy or unaffected individuals that are related to the OM-affected patients within the same families, or unrelated healthy individuals with no previous history of OM, may be used as controls (case–control study). Numerous studies have been conducted, particularly using candidate genes, relating to inflammation and innate immune responses, but many candidate gene studies will not lead to a significant association when a more stringent threshold for genome-wide significance is applied. Nonetheless, some genes that were initially identified in smaller case–control association studies, such as the *HLA* and *ABO* (MIM 110300) genes, were also deemed significant loci in genome-wide association studies (GWASs) for OM [49–56].

Genome-Wide Association Studies (GWASs)

A GWAS is currently the starting point in identifying the loci of interest. It assesses the association of variants spread throughout the genome with the trait or disease under investigation and, in contrast to candidate gene association studies, does not assume an association between a locus of interest and the trait. Instead, a GWAS employs an agnostic approach to identifying the loci of interest, which may be a regulatory variant often found in the non-coding region, a haplotype encompassing variants that are inherited together, or a gene harboring multiple rare variants associated with the trait. For OM, a series of GWASs have been conducted using common variant genotypes from microarrays, with each describing independent findings (Table 10.2). With advances

Table 10.2 Otitis media susceptibility genes identified from genome-wide association studies

Study	SNP	Cases	Controls	Cohort	Significant associations[a]	Candidate genes
Rye et al. 2012 [33]	2,524,817	416	1075	Western Australian Pregnancy Cohort (Raine) Study	rs6755194 ($p = 8.3 \times 10^{-7}$) rs1862981 ($p = 2.2 \times 10^{-5}$)	*CAPN14* *GALNT14* *BPIFA* gene cluster
Allen et al. 2013 [59]	324,748	373	229	University of Minnesota [20] University of Pittsburgh [24]	rs1110060 ($p = 9.1 \times 10^{-7}$) **rs10497394 ($p = 1.5 \times 10^{-8}$)** rs10775247 ($p = 6.3 \times 10^{-5}$)	*KIF7* *TICRR* *TPPP*
Einarsdottir et al. 2016 [66]	964,193	829	2118	Finnish	**rs16974263 ($p = 1.8 \times 10^{-7}$)** rs268662 ($p = 1.6 \times 10^{-6}$) rs4150992 ($p = 3.4 \times 10^{-6}$)	*PLD3* *SERTAD1* *SERTAD3* *HIPK4* *PRX* *BLVRB*
van Ingen et al. 2016 [70]	460,000	825	7936	European-descent Americans	**rs2932989 ($p = 4.4 \times 10^{-8}$)** rs3767498 ($p = 1.25 \times 10^{-6}$) rs12725646 ($p = 4.3 \times 10^{-5}$) rs255142 ($p = 1.9 \times 10^{-6}$) rs9514552 ($p = 2.1 \times 10^{-5}$) rs12888576 ($p = 7.8 \times 10^{-6}$) rs2809139 ($p = 3.2 \times 10^{-6}$) rs8036951 ($p = 3.8 \times 10^{-5}$) rs10409140 ($p = 4.4 \times 10^{-5}$)	*FNDC1* *KIF21B* *CACNA1S* *ASCL5* Intergenic region near *MIR205HG* *CRHR2* *INMT* *ARGLU1* *BDKRB2* Intergenic region near *C14orf177* *FAM189A1* *TPM4*

Table 10.2 (continued)

Study	SNP	Cases	Controls	Cohort	Significant associations[a]	Candidate genes
Pickrell et al. 2016 [49]; Tian et al. 2017 [53]	560,000–950,000	46,936	74,874	European-descent Americans	**rs681343 ($p = 3.5 \times 10^{-30}$)** **rs1978060 ($p = 1.2 \times 10^{-19}$)** **rs2808290 ($p = 5.1 \times 10^{-16}$)** **rs7174062 ($p = 3.5 \times 10^{-14}$)** **rs4329147 ($p = 9.6 \times 10^{-12}$)** **rs8176643 ($p = 3.7 \times 10^{-11}$)** **rs1802575 ($p = 1.5 \times 10^{-10}$)** **rs5829676 ($p = 1.8 \times 10^{-10}$)** **rs72931768 ($p = 2.6 \times 10^{-9}$)** **rs35213789 ($p = 3.8 \times 10^{-9}$)** **rs114947103 ($p = 5.4 \times 10^{-9}$)** **rs13281988 ($p = 9.8 \times 10^{-9}$)** **rs67035515 ($p = 1.6 \times 10^{-8}$)** **rs73015965 ($p = 3.8 \times 10^{-8}$)**	HLA genes Several intergenic regions *FUT2* *ABO* *TBX1* *MKX* *AUTS2* *CDHR3* *PLG*

[a] *p*-values in bold font indicate those that passed the genome-wide significant thresholds of the study

in computational efficiency, continuous decline in the cost of sequencing, and increasing availability of large-scale biobank data with genotypes and OM phenotypes, the discovery of additional novel findings from GWASs, which include both common and rare variants, is possible in the near future.

In the first GWAS on OM, Rye et al. (2012) used data from Australian trios and identified three novel candidate genes/gene clusters, namely, (1) rs6755194 within chromosome 2p23.1, which is either upstream of or intronic to two isoforms of *CAPN14* (MIM 610229); (2) rs1862981, also located on 2p23.1, intronic to *GALNT14* (MIM 60822) and proximal to *CAPN14*; and (3) *BPIFA* clusters, including *BPIFA1* (MIM 607412), *BPIFA2*, and *BPIFA3* on the genomic region 20q11.21 [57]. However, these findings could not be replicated in an independent cohort [58]. Other genes identified in this study with trends toward association were linked to the TGF-β pathway [57].

In the Minnesota-based cohort, Allen et al. (2013) identified an intergenic locus rs10497394 between the genes *CDCA7* (MIM 609937) and *SP3* (MIM 601804) on 2q31.1, which was subsequently replicated in an independent Pittsburgh-based US cohort as being associated with both chronic OM with effusion and recurrent acute OM [59]. This locus was found to regulate the expression of *LDLR* (MIM 606945) on chromosome 19, a gene that is expressed in ciliated epithelial cells of the airway with its transcribed protein predicted to be a binding site for human rhinovirus C, a known pathogen for upper respiratory tract infections and OM [60]. Newer data from the Genotype-Tissue Expression (GTEx) database showed that the rs10497394 variant significantly regulates RNA levels of *CDCA7* in thyroid and arterial tissues; however, GTEx does not include data from middle ear tissues [61]. *CDCA7* mutations cause immunodeficiency, centromeric instability, and facial anomalies syndrome (MIM 616910), wherein hypo- or agammaglobulinemia leads to recurrent life-threatening infections [62]. Additional loci on chromosomes 5 and 15 (rs386057, rs1110060, and rs10775247) were also identified but did not reach genome-wide significance in the replication study [59]. The genes affected by these three variants are involved in microtubule function, regulation of mammalian sonic hedgehog and Indian hedgehog pathways, and DNA replication [63–65].

Einarsdottir et al. (2016) found three variants, all on chromosome 19, to be associated with childhood OM in the Finnish population [66]. None of the identified regions overlapped with those previously found in association with OM on chromosome 19. Genome-wide significance was established for rs16974263, a variant intronic to the *PRX* (MIM 605725) gene, which was found in association with chronic OM with effusion in a UK cohort, albeit with opposite directions of effect [66]. Out of the several genes identified within this region are three candidate genes, *PLD3* (MIM 615698), *SERTAD1* (MIM 617850), and *BLVRB* (MIM 600941), which are previously known to be associated with immune function with expression found in macrophages [67, 68]. In the GTEx database, the rs16974263 variant regulates either the RNA levels or splicing of isoforms for *SERTAD3*, *HIPK4* (MIM 611712), *PLD3*, and *PRX* in various tissues [61]. In particular, *SERTAD3* is expressed in the mucosal tissue and its protein inhibits the replication of influenza A virus upon induction by type I interferon responses during an infection [61, 69].

Additional studies in Americans of European-descent identified genome-wide significance for a variant on chromosome 6 (rs2932989) that alters the methylation status of the gene encoding fibronectin type III domain containing 1 (*FNDC1*, MIM 609991) [70]. Although its function is not clearly elucidated, the study found an upregulation of this gene in the middle ear tissue under pro-inflammatory conditions [70]. Other candidate genes from suggestive loci largely contained those related to immune responses.

Finally, 14 genome-wide significant loci were identified by Pickrell et al. (2016) and Tian et al. (2017) using GWAS data from 23&Me [49, 53]. Among these loci, the OM-associated genes included *FUT2* (MIM 182100) and *ABO*, both involved in glycosphingolipid biosynthesis, as well as *TBX1* (MIM 602054) and *MKX* (MIM 601332), which encode transcription factors. Genes important for embryogenesis and neurodevelopment (*FGF3* (MIM 164950) and *AUTS2* (MIM 607270)), as well as those implicated in asthma (*CDHR3* (MIM 615610)), and spontaneous chronic OM in mice (*PLG* (MIM 173350)) were also found in association with OM [71–73]. To date, only 4 of these 14 loci, *FUT2*, *TBX1*, *ABO*, and *CDHR3*, have been replicated in independent human cohorts with additional evidence from functional or multi-omics studies performed for *FUT2* and *CDHR3* [49–52, 74–78].

To identify pathways that are potentially important for OM susceptibility, 21 genes with $p < 5 \times 10^{-5}$ available in the literature were selected from candidate gene association studies and GWAS results. Using NetworkAnalyst software [79–81], these genes were then used as an input for defining protein–protein interaction networks. Within these networks exist subnetworks that are involved in significant pathways, highlighting the underlying pathophysiology and serving as potential targets for novel therapeutics (Fig. 10.1). The major pathways identified included a rhythmic process, a viral process, negative regulation of an? apoptotic process, transcription, transcription by RNA polymerase II, chromatin remodeling, regulation of cell cycle, and circadian rhythm (Table 10.3). These identified pathways suggest that basic

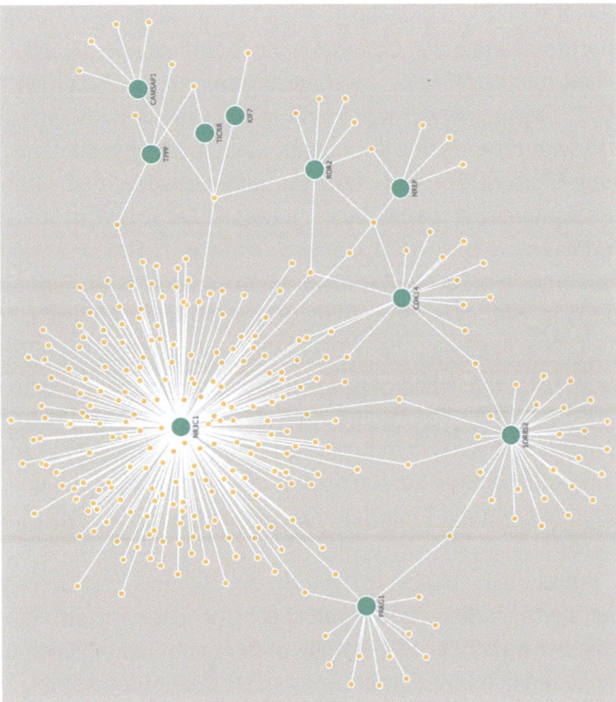

Fig. 10.1 Protein–protein interactions in the network analysis of genes implicated in otitis media from exome sequencing and genome-wide association studies. The green nodes represent proteins encoded by input or seed genes with a $p < 5 \times 10^{-5}$ from exome sequencing and genome-wide association studies. The orange nodes represent proteins that are found in association with the seed proteins within a significant cellular process

Table 10.3 Significant pathways identified from network analysis of genes implicated in otitis media from exome sequencing and genome-wide association studies

Significant pathways	*p*-value	Genes	
Rhythmic process	7.9×10^{-17}	*PPARG*	*TOP1*
		NCOA2	*CREB1*
		CREBBP	*DDX5*
		TP53	*SFPQ*
		PRKDC	*KDM5A*
		UBE3A	*GNB2L1*
		PML	*NFKB2*
		EP300	*HNRNPU*
		NRIP1	*MLL*
		PPARGC1A	*HDAC1*
		SP1	*HDAC2*
		MAGED1	*THRAP3*
Viral process	1.99×10^{-16}	*MDM2*	*LCK*
		YWHAE	*RB1*
		COPS6	*HSPD1*
		KAT5	*TOP1*
		CREBBP	*SRC*
		TP53	*CREB1*
		STAT3	*TBP*
		CD4	*YWHAB*
		TSG101	*CEBPA*
		NEDD4L	*RAN*
		UBE3A	*RBX1*
		PML	*SUMO1*
		HNRNPA1	*GNB2L1*
		EP300	*SET*
		FYN	*PAK2*
		SP1	*TRIM28*
		STAT1	*CUL1*
		IRAK1	*CUL2*
		RELA	*EIF4A2*
		MAP3K7	*DAXX*
		MMP1	*IKBKG*
Negative regulation of the apoptotic process	2.95×10^{-13}	*ROR2*	*ADA*
		MDM2	*WNT1*
		AKT1	*JUN*
		EGFR	*HSPA1A*
		YWHAZ	*HSP90AB1*
		PTK2B	*HSPD1*
		STAT5B	*SRC*
		IL6	*MIF*
		TMF1	*CBL*
		TP53	*DUSP1*
		RAF1	*AKT2*
		PRKDC	*MSX2*
		CD38	*SNCA*
		STAT3	*CDKN1A*
		SMAD3	*BCL6*
		NFKB1	*PPID*
		MED1	*PAK2*
		IRAK1	*HDAC1*
		RELA	*NTRK2*
		IL10	*HDAC2*
		UBC	*BAG1*
		COPS5	

Table 10.3 (continued)

Significant pathways	*p*-value	Genes	
Transcription, DNA-templated	6.0×10^{-13}	*NR3C1*	*RELA*
		PPARG	*GTF2I*
		NCOA1	*JUN*
		NR3C2	*POU2F2*
		IRF1	*POU2F1*
		IRF8	*RXRB*
		POU1F1	*CEBPA*
		NR4A1	*PPP5C*
		NR1H3	*NR1H2*
		TCF3	*NR1I3*
		POLR1D	*ASXL1*
		IRF2	*PHF3*
		IRF5	*ARHGAP35*
Transcription by RNA polymerase II	6.9×10^{-11}	*NR3C1*	*NR4A1*
		STAT5B	*NR1H3*
		TMF1	*SMAD3*
		TADA2A	*EP300*
		ONECUT1	*IRF2*
		TP53	*NCOR1*
		TGFB1I1	*NFKB1*
		IRF1	*CEBPB*
		STAT3	*PBX1*
		POU1F1	*IRF5*
		MAFF	*NFATC2*
		TAF6	*NFATC1*
		TRIM24	*GTF2I*
Chromatin remodeling	5.96×10^{-9}	*TADA2A*	*SMARCA2*
		SMARCE1	*RB1*
		SMARCD1	*MYB*
		HMGB1	*TOP1*
		SMARCC1	*HDAC1*
		SMARCA4	*HDAC2*
		HMGB2	*DAXX*
Regulation of cell cycle	1.3×10^{-8}	*CDK11A*	*DTL*
		IRF1	*ABL1*
		STAT3	*JUN*
		EP300	*RB1*
		SRSF5	*SFPQ*
		MED1	*CCND3*
		CDK14	*SFN*
		COPS5	*GNB2L1*
		USP16	
Circadian rhythm	4.6×10^{-8}	*EGFR*	*JUN*
		NCOA2	*TOP1*
		EP300	*CREB1*
		NRIP1	*HDAC1*
		PPARGC1A	*NTRK2*
		NCOR1	*THRAP3*
		HNRNPR	

cellular processes are involved in OM susceptibility with viral infection as a primary target for OM prevention and treatment.

Exome Sequencing

The coding regions or exome, i.e., all the exons comprising the parts of all genes that are transcribed and translated into proteins, only make up approximately 1% of the human genome. With growing knowledge and advancements in technology, exome sequencing allows for the assessment of variants within all coding regions of the genome and has become a cheaper alternative for identifying pathogenic variants for various diseases, particularly for rare variants with strong phenotypic effects. Using exome sequence data, rare pathogenic variants in three genes, *A2ML1* (MIM 610627), *FUT2*, and *SPINK5* (MIM 605010), were found in association with OM in an Indigenous Filipino pedigree and has since been replicated in various OM cohorts of different ethnicities [74, 82–84].

The *A2ML1* gene encodes a protease inhibitor that is specifically expressed in the middle ear [83]. It is similar to alpha-2-macroglobulin (A2M), also a protease found in the middle ear that is associated with recurrent acute OM [85]. Two loss-of-function *A2ML1* variants, i.e., a frameshift variant and a splice variant, were identified in a cohort of Indigenous Filipino population with an estimated 50% prevalence of OM [83]. The same frameshift variant in *A2ML1* was identified in US-based otitis-prone children with early-onset severe OM ($p = 3.34 \times 10^{-14}$) [83]. An additional 25 variants of the same gene were found in probands with OM from different cohorts [82, 83]. Moreover, differential expression analysis of RNA sequence data from Coloradan children with OM revealed co-upregulation of *A2ML1* with genes (e.g., *SPINK5*) that are involved in several pathways, including keratinocyte differentiation [82]. Follow-up microbiota studies showed a significantly higher relative abundance of the *Leptotrichia* spp. in the middle ears of individuals with *A2ML1* variants [84, 86]. In contrast, for a rare pathogenic *SPINK5* variant that was also identified in the Indigenous Filipino population through exome sequencing and linkage analysis, a greater biodiversity in the oral cavity and increased relative abundance of *Microbacteriaceae* were observed [84]. Notably, *A2ML1* is expressed in the middle ear mucosa, whereas *SPINK5* is faintly localized to the mucosal tissues but strongly localized to the outer ear and tympanic membrane in mouse middle ears [83, 84].

FUT2, located on chromosome 19, encodes 2-fucosyltransferase and is involved in the synthesis of blood group H antigens and the regulation of its expression on various mucosal surfaces [87]. Several common and rare variants within *FUT2* were associated with an increased risk for OM in US trios and various ethnic cohorts [74]. These include two stop variants, p.Trp154* and p.Arg202*, and two missense variants, p.Ala104Val and p.Arg138Cys [74]. For these four *FUT2* variants, levels of A antigen, a common binding spot for potential otopathogens and commensal bacteria, were reduced on the cell surface of mutant epithelial cells [74]. *FUT2* variants also affect gene transcription and alter the mucosal microbiome in the setting of OM. Differential expression analysis revealed downregulation of *FN1*, *KMT2D*, *MUC16*, and *NBPF20* and upregulation of *MTAP* in individuals with the *FUT2* p.Trp154* variant [75]. Changes in regulation of these four genes were also seen in the middle ears of mice inoculated with the human otopathogen non-typeable *Haemophilus influenzae* (NTHi), except upregulation of *Fn1* found in the inoculated mice [75]. Additionally, the *FUT2* variant was associated with an increased load of otopathogens within the middle ear with concordant decrease in relative taxa abundance of commensal bacteria in the nasopharynx [75].

Also utilizing exome sequencing, Jamieson et al. reported two genes, *NR3C1* (MIM 138040) and *NREP* (MIM 607332), as candidates for severe OM in a cohort from the Australian Aboriginal population [88]. Although these genes failed to attain genome-wide significance, *NR3C1* and *NREP* implicate a role of gene–environment interaction in the expression of inflammatory modulators due to environmental stress and shifts in the microbiome, respectively [89–93].

Mouse DNA Studies

A critical limitation to human studies is the inability to adequately control for genetic or environmental factors due to variability and heterogeneity across human subjects. Animal models present an alternative method in the exploration of the genetics of OM through the control of genetic and environmental factors and have led to a growing number of genes identified in association with OM [94]. Despite the availability of numerous animal models in the study of OM, the murine model has been largely favored in genetic studies. In all, 99% of mouse genes are homologous to human genes and, consequently, mice and humans share similar physiology and development of many basic functions [95]. Owing to the early mapping of the mouse genome, tools to manipulate mouse genes for phenotyping and susceptibility studies are widely available, along with a growing number of knockout and transgenic mouse models [96].

Gene-driven models and phenotype-driven *N*-ethyl-*N*-nitrosourea (ENU) mutagenesis methods have been used to understand the genes involved in OM in mice. In the gene-driven method, a growing availability of transgenic and knockout mouse strains through efforts such as the Knockout Mouse Phenotyping Program (KOMP2) is harnessed to assess the effect of mutations on OM susceptibility [97]. In the phenotype-driven model, ENU is used as a mutagen to induce random nucleotide changes [95]. This is then followed by screening of the phenotype of interest (e.g., increased OM prevalence), allowing for the discovery of novel genes. Genetically altered mice from either method may express the desired phenotypes, for example, by developing spontaneous OM, or in other studies, changes in OM expression after inoculation of otopathogens through transbullar injection or pressure-induced translocation of microbes to the middle ear from the nasopharynx [98, 99]. The genes identified thus far mainly involve craniofacial development or innate immune responses. Here, we will discuss a number of genes with a distinctive expression of OM phenotypes, illustrating the key points.

Mice with Craniofacial Abnormalities

Mice with impaired craniofacial development from DNA modifications often develop chronic OM with effusion and are frequently associated with congenital syndromes. Gene-driven models have led to the implication of numerous genes in knockout mice with similar phenotypic observations. *E2f4* is a key transcription factor that interacts with pRB during cell cycle progression [100]. Many $E2f4^{-/-}$ mice die early on, but the surviving mice develop OM due to craniofacial defects that increase their susceptibility to opportunistic infections [101]. In humans, mutations in the *EYA* gene family, comprised of nuclear phosphatases that act as transcriptional coactivators, are known to cause branchiootorenal syndrome 1 (MIM 113650) from variants in *EYA1* (MIM 601653) and sensorineural hearing loss (MIM 601316) from variants in *EYA4* (MIM 603550) [102–106]. In mice, deficiency of *Eya4* caused middle ear and Eustachian tube abnormalities, ultimately leading to OM with effusion [107]. Similar findings were observed in haploinsufficient *Ets1* and *Fli1* mice that developed OM and had craniofacial abnormalities consistent with those of the small middle ear cavity, short nasal bone, and malformation of the nasal bony-cartilaginous junction [108]. Specific to the middle ear, anatomical abnormalities, including ossicular fusion to the middle ear wall and stapedial malformations, were observed. The genes *ETS1* (MIM 164720) and *FLI1* (MIM 193067) lie within a genomic region of the human genome on the long arm of chromosome 11, which is deleted in Jacobsen syndrome (MIM 147791); Jacobsen syndrome includes craniofacial dysmorphisms and isoimmune thrombocytopenia among its clinical features [109]. These genes are E26 transformation-specific (ETS) transcription factors that are expressed in neural crest cells during embryogenesis [110–112].

ENU-derived *edison* and *Jeff* variants both lead to spontaneous chronic OM and mild craniofacial defects in mice [113, 114]. In both *edison* and *Jeff* variants, their respective mutations in the mouse genes *Nisch* and *Fbxo11* are also associated with faulty innate immune responses (further described below) [115]. *Eya4* is another gene with a possible regulatory role in the immune system [116].

Studies of Innate Immune Responses in Mice

An innate immune response is broad and encompasses cellular functions of macrophages and neutrophils to mucosal integrity and ciliary function. As such, the genetic findings related to innate immunity are accordingly diverse. Toll-like receptors (Tlrs) are a class of pattern recognition receptors involved in innate immunity at the cellular level. Numerous *Tlr* mutations have been identified through knockout mouse models (gene-driven) as causing or prolonging otitis media in mice. *Tlr4* deletion caused a delay in immune responses, leading to an early development of OM, which was often chronic [117, 118]. Knockout of *Tlr2* and *Tlr9* also resulted in similar findings with prolonged or severe infections [119, 120]. A similar phenotype was observed with the deletion of *Myd88*, which encodes an adaptor protein recruited in response to Tlr and interleukin (IL)-1 for activation of downstream signaling pathways [121, 122]. After *Myd88* knockout, a delay in macrophage and neutrophil recruitment resulted in chronic OM and prolonged mucosal thickening, which were more severe than those found with *Tlr* mutations [123].

In response to TLR activation, the NF-κB pathway is triggered downstream to initiate an inflammatory response [124]. Through phenotype-driven models, a number of genes have been associated with the NF-κB pathway and OM. As described above, the *edison* mouse variant displayed disruption in immune response in addition to the observed craniofacial abnormalities. The deletion of the *Nisch* gene further impacted the downstream signaling of the NF-κB pathway as well as the LIMK1 pathway, which is associated with vascular permeability and perturbation that lead to middle ear effusion and mucoperiosteal inflammation [113, 125, 126]. Another ENU-derived mouse strain is *Junbo*, which has a deletion of the *Evi1* gene and demonstrated spontaneous acute OM and chronic OM [127]. *Evi1* encodes a transcription factor that is known to be involved in multiple pathways [128, 129]. In the NF-κB pathway, *Evi1* binds to a subunit of NF-κB, preventing its interaction with DNA, thereby downregulating inflammation [130].

In the TGF-β pathway, the activation of TGF-β causes a cell signaling cascade with SMAD proteins, leading to transcription of target genes, RNA processing, translation of messenger RNA (mRNA), and protein regulation for numerous cellular processes, including craniofacial development and inflammation [131–134]. The genes implicated in association with the TGF-β pathway include *Tgif1*, *Fbxo11*, and *Evi1*. As previously mentioned, the phenotypic changes observed in *Jeff* mice were attributed to a mutation in the *Fbxo11* gene, which encodes for a ubiquitination protein involved in tumor suppression [135, 136]. *Jeff* mice displayed nuclear accumulation of the Smad2 protein, which mediates transcription of target genes within the TGF-β pathway [137]. Evi1, defects in which are responsible for the OM observed in *Junbo* mice, interacts with Smad3 proteins, resulting in the suppression of the growth-inhibiting mechanism of the TGF-β pathway [127, 129, 138]. Based on the mutagenesis studies that implicated the TGF-β pathway in OM in these gene-based mouse models, TGIF1, a homeodomain protein that acts as a negative regulator of the TGF-β pathway, binds to Smad2 to recruit a co-repressor and subsequently recruits histone deacetylases, leading to inhibition of transcription [132, 139, 140]. In *Tgif1*-knockout mice, conductive hearing loss was associated with chronic effusion, middle ear mucosal thickening, and an increase in goblet cells [141].

Other pathways and functions presumed to be associated with OM include the c-Jun N-terminal kinase (JNK) pathway, mucociliary clearance, mitogen-activated protein kinase (MAPK) pathway, and bony development [76, 129, 142–145]. Despite the vast expansion of genetic knowledge gained from these mouse studies, there are a number of limitations that prevent rapid application of knowledge from mouse models to application in the management of OM in humans. Because the otopathogens in humans differ from those in mice, these mouse models require inoculation of human otopathogens into the middle ear, which often cause a shorter course of OM in mice. There are also immunological and anatomical differences. The lymphocyte-rich immune system of mice versus the neutrophil-rich immune system in humans as well as the lack of mastoid air cells in mice require additional consideration [146]. At the genetic level, alternative splicing and innumerable factors contributing to complex disease processes like OM require additional complementary studies in humans.

RNA Studies

There are various types of RNAs, each serving numerous functions beyond protein translation to the regulation of gene expression. Examination of RNA profiles can thus provide a more accurate and detailed picture of the cellular mechanisms at play for various disease processes. A messenger RNA (mRNA) is a single-stranded RNA, complementary to the DNA, used as codes for protein synthesis. In contrast, a microRNA (miR) provides insights into gene expression. A microRNA is a 23 nucleotide-long RNA that functions to control gene expression posttranscriptionally by binding to the 3′ untranslated region (UTR) of a target mRNA [147]. Accordingly, investigators have studied mRNAs and miRNAs in order to understand OM pathophysiology.

mRNAs

mRNA expression in OM has been studied through the assessment of single gene transcription or whole transcriptome of various cells within the middle ear. Single-gene studies performed on human samples showed differential expression of aquaporins, C-type lectin receptors, mucins, beta-defensins, and cytokines in different types of OM, implicating the roles of cellular homeostatic and inflammatory responses in OM pathogenesis [148–152]. Differential expression of the protooncogene C/EBP-homologous protein (*DDIT3*, MIM 126337) was observed in otitis-prone children, associating the frequency of OM with the endoplasmic reticulum stress response through the PERK (protein kinase RNA-like endoplasmic reticulum kinase) signaling pathway [153].

Various methods of genetic expression analysis, including reverse transcription PCR (RT-PCR), microarray, and RNA sequencing (RNA-seq), have been used to profile the genetic expression of middle ear epithelial cells (MEECs) in association with OM. The types of information that can be gathered from these studies are wide-ranging. Inoculation of murine models with a common human otopathogen, NTHi, helped identify differential expression of 3657 genes, most of which are involved in innate immune response modulation, cell marker variation, and recruitment of neutrophils and macrophages [154]. The substantial role that innate immunity plays in OM was reinforced in the study by Ryan et al. (2020) with single-cell transcriptome analysis in mice [155]. Considerable cellular diversity in the mouse middle ear mucosa was observed with identification of 17 distinct cell types, all with expression of innate immune genes [155]. The cellular diversity of the middle ear mucosal tissue is further demonstrated in the variable types of MEECs identified [156, 157]. In the process of MEEC differentiation, approximately 500 genes that are associated with secretory proteins and ciliogenesis were upregulated [158]. Such findings provide a pathway for improving the characterization of the unrestrained responses of MEECs with the cellular remodeling that occurs in OM. Stabenau et al. (2021) studied human MEECs in OM with effusion in comparison with normal mucosal cells and identified 1282 differentially expressed genes [159]. The functions of identified genes encompassed inflammation, bacterial immunity, mucociliary clearance, cellular proliferation and transformation, and auditory cell differentiation. Of these functions, the most upregulated genes involved mucin production, immunity, and cell cycle regulation.

MicroRNAs (miRs)

miRs have diverse actions and targets that are context-specific. Most commonly, miRs bind to the 3′UTR of an mRNA in perfect pairs or with imperfect complementation but with additional base pairings at the 5′ of the mRNA [160]. miRs have also been observed to bind to 5′UTRs, the coding region of RNA, or directly to gene promoters [161–163]. The complexity in understanding the mechanism of miRs is also due to the ability of one miR to bind to numerous distinct mRNAs. Furthermore, one mRNA can be bound by different miRs, with each pairing leading to a distinct outcome [161]. As a result of miR binding to mRNA and 3′UTR, translational suppression can occur as deadenylases and decapping factors are recruited [164]. With its protective ends exposed, the resulting mRNA strand will be prone to degradation. Binding of miR to 5′UTR and the coding region causes silencing of expression, but its interaction with a promotor region has been observed to lead to transcription [165, 166]. The presence of miRs in various cellular compartments, the abundance of miRs, mRNAs, and their various combinations, and the miRNA-induced silencing complex mediating translational inhibition make the function of miRs dynamic [162].

The role of miRs in OM is increasingly being examined. In vitro analysis of human MEECs revealed differential expression of 15 genes as a result of both up- and downregulating functions of miRs. These changes ultimately led to an increase in cell differentiation, endocytosis, cellular communication, IκBK/NF-κB cascade, developmental process, complement activation, innate immune response, and cell adhesion [167]. miR-146 has been implicated in numerous inflammatory diseases owing to its negative regulatory role in activating TLRs and its ability to fine-tune signaling cascades. In OM, miR-146 expression increased in response to in vitro exposure to pro-inflammatory cytokines, which, in turn, was correlated with middle ear mucosal thickness and observed decline in the expression of tumor necrosis factor receptor (TNFR)-associated factor 6 (TRAF6), a modulator in the TLR pathway [168].

Exosomal release of endocytic vesicles leads to extracellular release of mRNAs, miRs, and proteins to be then transported between cells [169, 170]. Particularly, exosomal miRs have been found to influence expressions of distant cells and promote positive or negative effects on pro-inflammatory signaling of the receiving cell [171–174]. Human MEECs produce a baseline level of extracellular miR, the microRNAome, which is composed of 110 different miRs during in vitro stimulation [175]. For example, stimulation by NTHi induces elevation in the levels of five distinct miRs, namely, miR-378a-3p + miR-378i, miR-200a-3p, miR-378g, miR30d-5p, and miR-222-3p, all known to target genes related to innate immunity [175–180]. The targeted mRNAs are involved in apoptosis, cancer, cell growth, and the IL-8 pathway mediated by CXCR1/2 that activates NF-κB, oxidative stress, inflammation, chemotaxis, angiogenesis, and neutrophil functions [175]. Of the miRs, miR-320e has been further associated with the presence of allergies in children with OM [181]. In an exosomal miR analysis in patients with middle ear effusion, 17 miRs unique to middle ear effusions compared to serum controls were identified, with the most abundant being miR-223-3p [170]. These exosomal miRs regulate a total of 442 target genes, most of which were involved in the IL-8 signaling process and were also mediated by CXCR1/2. miR-223 regulates innate immune response, protease activity, and a few key functions of neutrophils [182, 183].

Another form of RNA that plays a role similar to miR is long non-coding RNA (lncRNA). As the name suggests, it is longer than miR with its length greater than 200 nucleotides and does not code any proteins [184, 185]. It has the ability to interact with DNA, RNA, and proteins and modulate transcription, epigenetic changes, RNA and protein stabilization, translation, and posttranslational modifications [186–189]. Interestingly, it can also interact with miR to modulate cellular function. In OM, the lncRNA nuclear-enriched abundant transcript 1 (NEAT1) targets miR-495 to activate p38 MAPK, allowing the release of inflammatory cytokines and promoting the expression of genes involved in acute inflammatory responses [190–192].

The extent of miR interactions and their functions are still in the process of discovery with much to uncover. Understanding the role of RNA in the expression of final protein products helps delineate complex and dynamic disease processes such as OM.

Future Directions

Although prevention and diagnostic and treatment strategies are available for OM patients, we still lack the understanding of the progression of OM from acute to chronic forms. This lack of knowledge undermines efforts to develop novel therapies and fine-tune the current management protocols, particularly for patients with undiscovered genetic susceptibility to OM. To reduce the massive burden on global healthcare due to OM, ongoing investigations furthering our understanding of the genetic component of OM susceptibility are important to ultimately deliver effective therapeutic solutions to patients. We must continue to identify OM-pathogenic variants within different populations, especially to include underrepresented groups across the world. Advancements in technology bring about efficiency and speed in our ability to sequence genetic materials, which must be harnessed in studying complex diseases with multifactorial contributors at play such as OM. Currently, many human studies involve patients of European descent. A few available studies on minority groups focus on populations with an especially high incidence of OM; however, it is equally as important to study underrepresented groups without such context. Using bioinformatics, we can glean the genetic networks at play in various types of OM. The influence of pathogens on gene expression requires an in-depth understanding of the microbiome and gene expression responses to different pathogens. Genetic variations from splicing, epigenetic modifications, and different factors that influence production of proteins are especially important. It is essential to continue harnessing the availability of animal models, especially in studying therapeutic solutions, but even more important is the application of the findings from animal models to treating OM in humans.

Acknowledgments This work was supported by the National Institutes of Health (NIH)—the National Institute on Deafness and Other Communication Disorders (NIDCD) via grants R01 DC015004 and R01 DC019642 (to RS-C). NKL was supported by the T32 DC012280 grant from NIH-NIDCD (to Sue C. Kinnamon and Herman A. Jenkins). The contents of this chapter are solely the responsibility of the authors and do not necessarily represent the official views of the NIH.

References

1. Swanson JA, Hoecker JL. Concise review for primary-care physicians. Mayo Clin Proc. 1996;71:179–83.
2. Neto JFL, Hemb L, Silva DB, et al. Systematic literature review of modifiable risk factors for recurrent acute otitis media in childhood. J Pediatr. 2006;82:87–96. http://www.jped.com.br/conteudo/Ing_resumo.asp?varArtigo=1453&cod=&idSecao=3.
3. Uhari M, Mäntysaari K, Niemelä M. A meta-analytic review of the risk factors for acute otitis media. Clin Infect Dis. 1996;22:1079–83.
4. Hudson HM, Rockett IR. An environmental and demographic analysis of otitis media in rural Australian aborigines. Int J Epidemiol. 1984;13:73–82.
5. Daly KA, Hoffman HJ, Kvaerner KJ, Kvestad E, Casselbrant ML, Homoe P, et al. Epidemiology, natural history, and risk factors: panel report from the Ninth International Research Conference on Otitis Media. Int J Pediatr Otorhinolaryngol. 2010;74:231–40.
6. Gunasekera H, Haysom L, Morris P, Craig J. The global burden of childhood otitis media and hearing impairment: a Systematic review. Pediatrics. 2008;121:S107. https://doi.org/10.1542/peds.2007-2022QQ.
7. Santos-Cortez RLP, Reyes-Quintos MRT, Tantoco MLC, Abbe I, Llanes EGV, Ajami NJ, et al. Genetic and environmental determinants of otitis media in an indigenous Filipino population. Otolaryngol Head Neck Surg. 2016;155:856–62. https://www.ncbi.nlm.nih.gov/pmc/articles/PMC5093071/.
8. Austeng ME, Akre H, Øverland B, Abdelnoor M, Falkenberg E-S, Kværner KJ. Otitis media with effusion in children with in Down syndrome. Int J Pediatr Otorhinolaryngol. 2013;77:1329–32. https://linkinghub.elsevier.com/retrieve/pii/S0165587613002644.
9. Bois E, Nassar M, Zenaty D, Léger J, Van Den Abbeele T, Teissier N. Otologic disorders in Turner syndrome. Eur Ann Otorhinolaryngol Head Neck Dis. 2018;135:21–4. https://linkinghub.elsevier.com/retrieve/pii/S1879729617301291.
10. Ram G, Chinen J. Infections and immunodeficiency in Down syndrome: immunodeficiency in Down syndrome. Clin Exp Immunol. 2011;164:9–16. https://doi.org/10.1111/j.1365-2249.2011.04335.x.
11. Chung H, Green PHR, Wang TC, Kong X-F. Interferon-driven immune dysregulation in Down syndrome: a review of the evi-

dence. J Inflamm Res. 2021;14:5187–200. https://www.ncbi.nlm.nih.gov/pmc/articles/PMC8504936/.
12. Kong AM, Hurley D, Evans KA, Brixner D, Csoboth C, Visootsak J. A retrospective, longitudinal, claims-based comparison of concomitant diagnoses between individuals with and without Down syndrome. J Manag Care Spec Pharm. 2017;23:761–70. https://doi.org/10.18553/jmcp.2017.23.7.761.
13. Sullivan KD, Evans D, Pandey A, Hraha TH, Smith KP, Markham N, et al. Trisomy 21 causes changes in the circulating proteome indicative of chronic autoinflammation. Sci Rep. 2017;7:14818.
14. Kong X-F, Worley L, Rinchai D, Bondet V, Jithesh PV, Goulet M, et al. Three copies of four interferon receptor genes underlie a mild type I interferonopathy in Down syndrome. J Clin Immunol. 2020;40:807–19. https://www.ncbi.nlm.nih.gov/pmc/articles/PMC7418179/.
15. Hüls A, Costa ACS, Dierssen M, Baksh RA, Bargagna S, Baumer NT, et al. Medical vulnerability of individuals with Down syndrome to severe COVID-19–data from the Trisomy 21 Research Society and the UK ISARIC4C survey. EClinicalMedicine. 2021;33:100769. https://www.ncbi.nlm.nih.gov/pmc/articles/PMC7897934/.
16. Nogaki T, Paparella MM, Cureoglu S. A structural analysis of tympanic compartments of the middle ear in patients with Down's syndrome: a temporal bone study. Otol Neurotol. 2020;41:1149–57.
17. Omar M, McCoy JL, McCormick AA, Vellody K, Chi DH. Repeat tympanostomy tubes in children with Down syndrome. Int J Pediatr Otorhinolaryngol. 2021;148:110811.
18. Ghadersohi S, Ida JB, Bhushan B, Billings KR. Outcomes of tympanoplasty in children with Down syndrome. Int J Pediatr Otorhinolaryngol. 2017;103:36–40.
19. Kreicher KL, Weir FW, Nguyen SA, Meyer TA. Characteristics and progression of hearing loss in children with Down syndrome. J Pediatr. 2018;193:27–33.e2.
20. Mock, Markert UR, Vogelsang H, Jäger L. Selective T-cell deficiency in Turner's syndrome. J Investig Allergol Clin Immunol. 2000;10:312–3.
21. Cacciari E, Masi M, Fantini MP, Licastro F, Cicognani A, Pirazzoli P, et al. Serum immunoglobulins and lymphocyte subpopulations derangement in Turner's syndrome. J Immunogenet. 1981;8:337–44.
22. Makishima T, King K, Brewer CC, Zalewski CK, Butman J, Bakalov VK, et al. Otolaryngologic markers for the early diagnosis of Turner syndrome. Int J Pediatr Otorhinolaryngol. 2009;73:1564–7. https://www.ncbi.nlm.nih.gov/pmc/articles/PMC2757481/.
23. Stenberg AE, Nylén O, Windh M, Hultcrantz M. Otological problems in children with Turner's syndrome. Hear Res. 1998;124:85–90.
24. Balding DJ, et al., editors. Handbook of statistical genetics, vol. 1 and 2. Somerset, NJ: John Wiley and Sons Ltd; 2003. https://www.biblio.com/book/handbook-statistical-genetics-volumes-1-2/d/1465841857.
25. Kvaerner KJ, Tambs K, Harris JR, Magnus P. Distribution and heritability of recurrent ear infections. Ann Otol Rhinol Laryngol. 1997;106:624–32.
26. Kvestad E, Kvaerner KJ, Røysamb E, Tambs K, Harris JR, Magnus P. Otitis media: genetic factors and sex differences. Twin Res. 2004;7:239–44.
27. Casselbrant ML, Mandel EM, Fall PA, Rockette HE, Kurs-Lasky M, Bluestone CD, et al. The heritability of otitis media: a twin and triplet study. JAMA. 1999;282:2125–30.
28. Casselbrant ML, Mandel EM, Rockette HE, Kurs-Lasky M, Fall PA, Bluestone CD, et al. The genetic component of middle ear disease in the first 5 years of life. Arch Otolaryngol Head Neck Surg. 2004;130:273–8.
29. Rovers M, Haggard M, Gannon M, Koeppen-Schomerus G, Plomin R. Heritability of symptom domains in otitis media: a longitudinal study of 1,373 twin pairs. Am J Epidemiol. 2002;155:958–64.
30. Hafrén L. Genetic background and the risk of otitis media. Int J Pediatr Otorhinolaryngol. 2012;76(1):41–4.
31. Risch N, Merikangas K. The future of genetic studies of complex human diseases. Science. 1996;273:1516–7.
32. Daly KA, Brown WM, Segade F, Bowden DW, Keats BJ, Lindgren BR, et al. Chronic and recurrent otitis media: a genome scan for susceptibility loci. Am J Hum Genet. 2004;75:988–97.
33. Rye MS, Scaman ESH, Thornton RB, Vijayasekaran S, Coates HL, Francis RW, et al. Genetic and functional evidence for a locus controlling otitis media at chromosome 10q26.3. BMC Med Genet. 2014;15:18.
34. Lanier LL. NK cell receptors. Annu Rev Immunol. 1998;16:359–93.
35. Chen W-M, Allen EK, Mychaleckyj JC, Chen F, Hou X, Rich SS, et al. Significant linkage at chromosome 19q for otitis media with effusion and/or recurrent otitis media (COME/ROM). BMC Med Genet. 2011;12:124.
36. Mataki C, Murakami T, Umetani M, Wada Y, Ishii M, Tsutsumi S, et al. A novel zinc finger protein mRNA in human umbilical vein endothelial cells is profoundly induced by tumor necrosis factor alpha. J Atheroscler Thromb. 2000;7:97–103.
37. Sabater L, Ashhab Y, Caro P, Kolkowski EC, Pujol-Borrell R, Domínguez O. Identification of a KRAB-containing zinc finger protein, ZNF304, by AU-motif-directed display method and initial characterization in lymphocyte activation. Biochem Biophys Res Commun. 2002;293:1066–72.
38. André P, Biassoni R, Colonna M, Cosman D, Lanier LL, Long EO, et al. New nomenclature for MHC receptors. Nat Immunol. 2001;2:661.
39. Schroder K, Tschopp J. The inflammasomes. Cell. 2010;140:821–32.
40. Nyren-Erickson EK, Jones JM, Srivastava DK, Mallik S. A disintegrin and metalloproteinase-12 (ADAM12): function, roles in disease progression, and clinical implications. Biochim Biophys Acta. 2013;1830:4445–55.
41. Cho J-G, Woo J-S, Lee H-M, Jung HH, Hwang S-J, Chae S. Effects of cigarette smoking on mucin production in human middle ear epithelial cells. Int J Pediatr Otorhinolaryngol. 2009;73:1447–51.
42. Hasegawa H, Kiyokawa E, Tanaka S, Nagashima K, Gotoh N, Shibuya M, et al. DOCK180, a major CRK-binding protein, alters cell morphology upon translocation to the cell membrane. Mol Cell Biol. 1996;16:1770–6.
43. Batut J, Schmierer B, Cao J, Raftery LA, Hill CS, Howell M. Two highly related regulatory subunits of PP2A exert opposite effects on TGF-beta/Activin/Nodal signalling. Dev Camb Engl. 2008;135:2927–37.
44. Floros J, DiAngelo S, Koptides M, Karinch AM, Rogan PK, Nielsen H, et al. Human SP-A locus: allele frequencies and linkage disequilibrium between the two surfactant protein A genes. Am J Respir Cell Mol Biol. 1996;15:489–98.
45. Rämet M, Löfgren J, Alho O-P, Hallman M. Surfactant protein-A gene locus associated with recurrent otitis media. J Pediatr. 2001;138:266–8. https://linkinghub.elsevier.com/retrieve/pii/S0022347601576544.
46. Pettigrew MM, Gent JF, Zhu Y, Triche EW, Belanger KD, Holford TR, et al. Association of surfactant protein A polymorphisms with otitis media in infants at risk for asthma. BMC Med Genet. 2006;7:68.
47. Abdel-Razek O, Ni L, Yang F, Wang G. Innate immunity of surfactant protein A in experimental otitis media. Innate Immun. 2019;25:391–400.

48. McNeely TB, Coonrod JD. Aggregation and opsonization of type A but not type B Hemophilus influenzae by surfactant protein A. Am J Respir Cell Mol Biol. 1994;11:114–22.
49. Pickrell JK, Berisa T, Liu JZ, Segurel L, Tung JY, Hinds D. Detection and interpretation of shared genetic influences on 42 human traits. Nat Genet. 2016;48:709–17. https://www.ncbi.nlm.nih.gov/pmc/articles/PMC5207801/.
50. Mortensen EH, Lildholdt T, Gammelgård NP, Christensen PH. Distribution of ABO blood groups in secretory otitis media and cholesteatoma. Clin Otolaryngol Allied Sci. 1983;8:263–5.
51. Apostolopoulos K, Labropoulou E, Konstantinos B, Rhageed S, Ferekidis E. Blood group in otitis media with effusion. ORL J Otorhinolaryngol Relat Spec. 2002;64:433–5.
52. Wiesen BM, Hafrén L, Einarsdottir E, Kere J, Mattila PS, Santos-Cortez RLP. ABO genotype and blood type are associated with otitis media. Genet Test Mol Biomark. 2019;23:823–7. https://www.ncbi.nlm.nih.gov/pmc/articles/PMC6857544/.
53. Tian C, Hromatka BS, Kiefer AK, Eriksson N, Noble SM, Tung JY, et al. Genome-wide association and HLA region fine-mapping studies identify susceptibility loci for multiple common infections. Nat Commun. 2017;8:599.
54. Kalm O, Johnson U, Prellner K. HLA frequency in patients with chronic secretory otitis media. Int J Pediatr Otorhinolaryngol. 1994;30:151–7.
55. Kalm O, Johnson U, Prellner K, Ninn K. HLA frequency in patients with recurrent acute otitis media. Arch Otolaryngol Head Neck Surg. 1991;117:1296–9.
56. Kalm O, Johnson U, Prellner K, Ninn K. HLA antigens and recurrent acute otitis media. Acta Otolaryngol Suppl. 1992;492:107–9.
57. Rye MS, Warrington NM, Scaman ESH, Vijayasekaran S, Coates HL, Anderson D, et al. Genome-wide association study to identify the genetic determinants of otitis media susceptibility in childhood. PLoS One. 2012;7:e48215.
58. Allen EK, Manichaikul A, Chen W-M, Rich SS, Daly KA, Sale MM. Evaluation of replication of variants associated with genetic risk of otitis media. PLoS One. 2014;9:e104212.
59. Allen EK, Chen W-M, Weeks DE, Chen F, Hou X, Mattos JL, et al. A genome-wide association study of chronic otitis media with effusion and recurrent otitis media identifies a novel susceptibility locus on chromosome 2. J Assoc Res Otolaryngol. 2013;14:791–800. https://www.ncbi.nlm.nih.gov/pmc/articles/PMC3825021/.
60. Bochkov YA, Palmenberg AC, Lee W-M, Rathe JA, Amineva SP, Sun X, et al. Molecular modeling, organ culture and reverse genetics for a newly identified human rhinovirus C. Nat Med. 2011;17:627–32.
61. GTEx Consortium. The Genotype-Tissue Expression (GTEx) project. Nat Genet. 2013;45:580–5.
62. Thijssen PE, Ito Y, Grillo G, Wang J, Velasco G, Nitta H, et al. Mutations in CDCA7 and HELLS cause immunodeficiency–centromeric instability–facial anomalies syndrome. Nat Commun. 2015;6:7870. https://www.ncbi.nlm.nih.gov/pmc/articles/PMC4519989/.
63. Ovádi J, Orosz F. An unstructured protein with destructive potential: TPPP/p25 in neurodegeneration. BioEssays News Rev Mol Cell Dev Biol. 2009;31:676–86.
64. Hsu S-HC, Zhang X, Yu C, Li ZJ, Wunder JS, Hui C-C, et al. Kif7 promotes hedgehog signaling in growth plate chondrocytes by restricting the inhibitory function of Sufu. Dev Camb Engl. 2011;138:3791–801.
65. Kumagai A, Shevchenko A, Shevchenko A, Dunphy WG. Treslin collaborates with TopBP1 in triggering the initiation of DNA replication. Cell. 2010;140:349–59.
66. Einarsdottir E, Hafrén L, Leinonen E, Bhutta MF, Kentala E, Kere J, et al. Genome-wide association analysis reveals variants on chromosome 19 that contribute to childhood risk of chronic otitis media with effusion. Sci Rep. 2016;6:33240.
67. Hammarén-Malmi S, Tarkkanen J, Mattila PS. Analysis of risk factors for childhood persistent middle ear effusion. Acta Otolaryngol (Stockh). 2005;125:1051–4.
68. Jasenosky LD, Scriba TJ, Hanekom WA, Goldfeld AE. T cells and adaptive immunity to Mycobacterium tuberculosis in humans. Immunol Rev. 2015;264:74–87.
69. Sun N, Li C, Li X-F, Deng Y-Q, Jiang T, Zhang N-N, et al. Type-I interferon-inducible SERTAD3 inhibits influenza A virus replication by blocking the assembly of viral RNA polymerase complex. Cell Rep. 2020;33:108342.
70. van Ingen G, Li J, Goedegebure A, Pandey R, Li YR, March ME, et al. Genome-wide association study for acute otitis media in children identifies FNDC1 as disease contributing gene. Nat Commun. 2016;7:12792.
71. Bønnelykke K, Sleiman P, Nielsen K, Kreiner-Møller E, Mercader JM, Belgrave D, et al. A genome-wide association study identifies CDHR3 as a susceptibility locus for early childhood asthma with severe exacerbations. Nat Genet. 2014;46:51–5.
72. Eriksson P-O, Li J, Ny T, Hellström S. Spontaneous development of otitis media in plasminogen-deficient mice. Int J Med Microbiol. 2006;296:501–9.
73. Jolley A, Corbett M, McGregor L, Waters W, Brown S, Nicholl J, et al. De novo intragenic deletion of the autism susceptibility candidate 2 (AUTS2) gene in a patient with developmental delay: a case report and literature review. Am J Med Genet A. 2013;161A:1508–12.
74. Santos-Cortez RLP, Chiong CM, Frank DN, Ryan AF, Giese APJ, Bootpetch Roberts T, et al. FUT2 variants confer susceptibility to familial otitis media. Am J Hum Genet. 2018;103:679–90. https://www.ncbi.nlm.nih.gov/pmc/articles/PMC6217759/.
75. Elling CL, Scholes MA, Streubel S-O, Larson ED, Wine TM, Bootpetch TC, et al. The FUT2 variant c.461G>A (p.Trp154*) is associated with differentially expressed genes and nasopharyngeal microbiota shifts in patients with otitis media. Front Cell Infect Microbiol. 2021;11:798246.
76. Tian C, Harris BS, Johnson KR. Ectopic mineralization and conductive hearing loss in Enpp1asj mutant mice, a new model for otitis media and tympanosclerosis. PLoS One. 2016;11:e0168159.
77. Hirsch SD, Elling CL, Bootpetch TC, Scholes MA, Hafrén L, Streubel S-O, et al. The role of CDHR3 in susceptibility to otitis media. J Mol Med. 2021;99:1571–83. https://doi.org/10.1007/s00109-021-02118-7.
78. Everman JL, Sajuthi S, Saef B, Rios C, Stoner AM, Numata M, et al. Functional genomics of CDHR3 confirms its role in HRV-C infection and childhood asthma exacerbations. J Allergy Clin Immunol. 2019;144:962–71.
79. Xia J, Benner MJ, Hancock REW. NetworkAnalyst—integrative approaches for protein–protein interaction network analysis and visual exploration. Nucleic Acids Res. 2014;42:W167–74. https://doi.org/10.1093/nar/gku443.
80. Xia J, Gill EE, Hancock REW. NetworkAnalyst for statistical, visual and network-based meta-analysis of gene expression data. Nat Protoc. 2015;10:823–44.
81. Zhou G, Soufan O, Ewald J, Hancock REW, Basu N, Xia J. NetworkAnalyst 3.0: a visual analytics platform for comprehensive gene expression profiling and meta-analysis. Nucleic Acids Res. 2019;47:W234–41.
82. Larson ED, Magno JPM, Steritz MJ, Llanes EGV, Cardwell J, Pedro M, et al. A2ML1 and otitis media: novel variants, differential expression and relevant pathways. Hum Mutat. 2019;40:1156–71. https://www.ncbi.nlm.nih.gov/pmc/articles/PMC6711784/.
83. Santos-Cortez RLP, Chiong CM, Reyes-Quintos MRT, Tantoco MLC, Wang X, Acharya A, et al. Rare A2ML1 variants confer

susceptibility to otitis media. Nat Genet. 2015;47:917–20. https://www.ncbi.nlm.nih.gov/pmc/articles/PMC4528370/.
84. Frank DN, Giese APJ, Hafren L, Bootpetch TC, Yarza TKL, Steritz MJ, et al. Otitis media susceptibility and shifts in the head and neck microbiome due to SPINK5 variants. J Med Genet. 2021;58:442–52.
85. Bondestam M, Foucard T, Gebre-Medhin M. Serum albumin, retinol-binding protein, thyroxin-binding prealbumin and acute phase reactants as indicators of undernutrition in children with undue susceptibility to acute infections. Acta Paediatr Scand. 1988;77:94–8.
86. Santos-Cortez RLP, Hutchinson DS, Ajami NJ, Reyes-Quintos MRT, Tantoco MLC, Labra PJ, et al. Middle ear microbiome differences in indigenous Filipinos with chronic otitis media due to a duplication in the A2ML1 gene. Infect Dis Poverty. 2016;5:97. https://www.ncbi.nlm.nih.gov/pmc/articles/PMC5088646/.
87. Ravn V, Dabelsteen E. Tissue distribution of histo-blood group antigens. Acta Pathol Microbiol Immunol Scand. 2000;108:1–28.
88. Jamieson SE, Fakiola M, Tang D, Scaman E, Syn G, Francis RW, et al. Common and rare genetic variants that could contribute to severe otitis media in an Australian Aboriginal Population. Clin Infect Dis. 2021;73:1860–70. https://www.ncbi.nlm.nih.gov/pmc/articles/PMC8599203/.
89. Barnes PJ. Corticosteroid effects on cell signalling. Eur Respir J. 2006;27:413–26.
90. Yue MM, Lv K, Meredith SC, Martindale JL, Gorospe M, Schuger L. Novel RNA-binding protein P311 binds eukaryotic translation initiation factor 3 subunit b (eIF3b) to promote translation of transforming growth factor β1-3 (TGF-β1-3). J Biol Chem. 2014;289:33971–83.
91. Mulligan CJ, D'Errico NC, Stees J, Hughes DA. Methylation changes at NR3C1 in newborns associate with maternal prenatal stress exposure and newborn birth weight. Epigenetics. 2012;7:853–7.
92. Lewis CR, Breitenstein RS, Henderson A, Sowards HA, Piras IS, Huentelman MJ, et al. Harsh parenting predicts novel HPA receptor gene methylation and NR3C1 methylation predicts cortisol daily slope in middle childhood. Cell Mol Neurobiol. 2021;41:783–93.
93. Deshpande NP, Riordan SM, Castaño-Rodríguez N, Wilkins MR, Kaakoush NO. Signatures within the esophageal microbiome are associated with host genetics, age, and disease. Microbiome. 2018;6:227.
94. Santos-Cortez RLP, Bhutta MF, Earl JP, Hafrén L, Jennings M, Mell JC, et al. Panel 3: Genomics, precision medicine and targeted therapies. Int J Pediatr Otorhinolaryngol. 2020;130:109835. https://www.ncbi.nlm.nih.gov/pmc/articles/PMC7155947/.
95. Justice MJ, Noveroske JK, Weber JS, Zheng B, Bradley A. Mouse ENU mutagenesis. Hum Mol Genet. 1999;8:1955–63.
96. Ringwald M, Iyer V, Mason JC, Stone KR, Tadepally HD, Kadin JA, et al. The IKMC web portal: a central point of entry to data and resources from the International Knockout Mouse Consortium. Nucleic Acids Res. 2011;39:D849–55. https://www.ncbi.nlm.nih.gov/pmc/articles/PMC3013768/.
97. Knockout Mouse Phenotyping. 2013. https://commonfund.nih.gov/komp2.
98. Ryan AF, Ebmeyer J, Furukawa M, Pak K, Melhus A, Wasserman SI, et al. Mouse models of induced otitis media. Brain Res. 2006;1091:3–8. https://linkinghub.elsevier.com/retrieve/pii/S0006899306003799.
99. Stol K, van Selm S, van den Berg S, Bootsma HJ, Blokx WAM, Graamans K, et al. Development of a non-invasive murine infection model for acute otitis media. Microbiology. 2009;155:4135–44.
100. Brehm A, Kouzarides T. Retinoblastoma protein meets chromatin. Trends Biochem Sci. 1999;24:142–5.
101. Humbert PO, Rogers C, Ganiatsas S, Landsberg RL, Trimarchi JM, Dandapani S, et al. E2F4 is essential for normal erythrocyte maturation and neonatal viability. Mol Cell. 2000;6:281–91.
102. Ohto H, Kamada S, Tago K, Tominaga SI, Ozaki H, Sato S, et al. Cooperation of six and eya in activation of their target genes through nuclear translocation of Eya. Mol Cell Biol. 1999;19:6815–24.
103. Rayapureddi JP, Kattamuri C, Steinmetz BD, Frankfort BJ, Ostrin EJ, Mardon G, et al. Eyes absent represents a class of protein tyrosine phosphatases. Nature. 2003;426:295–8.
104. Tootle TL, Silver SJ, Davies EL, Newman V, Latek RR, Mills IA, et al. The transcription factor Eyes absent is a protein tyrosine phosphatase. Nature. 2003;426:299–302.
105. Krug P, Morinière V, Marlin S, Koubi V, Gabriel HD, Colin E, et al. Mutation screening of the EYA1, SIX1, and SIX5 genes in a large cohort of patients harboring branchio-oto-renal syndrome calls into question the pathogenic role of SIX5 mutations. Hum Mutat. 2011;32:183–90. https://doi.org/10.1002/humu.21402.
106. Pfister M, Tóth T, Thiele H, Haack B, Blin N, Zenner H-P, et al. A 4-bp insertion in the eya-homologous region (eyaHR) of EYA4 causes hearing impairment in a Hungarian family linked to DFNA10. Mol Med Camb Mass. 2002;8:607–11.
107. Depreux FFS, Darrow K, Conner DA, Eavey RD, Liberman MC, Seidman CE, et al. Eya4-deficient mice are a model for heritable otitis media. J Clin Invest. 2008;118:651–8. https://www.ncbi.nlm.nih.gov/pmc/articles/PMC2213371/.
108. Carpinelli MR, Kruse EA, Arhatari BD, Debrincat MA, Ogier JM, Bories J-C, et al. Mice haploinsufficient for Ets1 and Fli1 display middle ear abnormalities and model aspects of Jacobsen syndrome. Am J Pathol. 2015;185:1867–76.
109. Jones C, Slijepcevic P, Marsh S, Baker E, Langdon WY, Richards RI, et al. Physical linkage of the fragile site FRA11B and a Jacobsen syndrome chromosome deletion breakpoint in 11q23.3. Hum Mol Genet. 1994;3:2123–30.
110. Hollenhorst PC, McIntosh LP, Graves BJ. Genomic and biochemical insights into the specificity of ETS transcription factors. Annu Rev Biochem. 2011;80:437–71.
111. Kola I, Brookes S, Green AR, Garber R, Tymms M, Papas TS, et al. The Ets1 transcription factor is widely expressed during murine embryo development and is associated with mesodermal cells involved in morphogenetic processes such as organ formation. Proc Natl Acad Sci U S A. 1993;90:7588–92.
112. Mélet F, Motro B, Rossi DJ, Zhang L, Bernstein A. Generation of a novel Fli-1 protein by gene targeting leads to a defect in thymus development and a delay in Friend virus-induced erythroleukemia. Mol Cell Biol. 1996;16:2708–18.
113. Crompton M, Purnell T, Tyrer HE, Parker A, Ball G, Hardisty-Hughes RE, et al. A mutation in Nischarin causes otitis media via LIMK1 and NF-κB pathways. PLoS Genet. 2017;13:e1006969.
114. Hardisty RE, Erven A, Logan K, Morse S, Guionaud S, Sancho-Oliver S, et al. The deaf mouse mutant Jeff (Jf) is a single gene model of otitis media. J Assoc Res Otolaryngol. 2003;4:130–8. https://www.ncbi.nlm.nih.gov/pmc/articles/PMC3202714/.
115. Hardisty-Hughes RE, Tateossian H, Morse SA, Romero MR, Middleton A, Tymowska-Lalanne Z, et al. A mutation in the F-box gene, Fbxo11, causes otitis media in the Jeff mouse. Hum Mol Genet. 2006;15:3273–9. http://academic.oup.com/hmg/article/15/22/3273/713947/A-mutation-in-the-Fbox-gene-Fbxo11-causes-otitis.
116. Okabe Y, Sano T, Nagata S. Regulation of the innate immune response by threonine-phosphatase of Eyes absent. Nature. 2009;460:520–4.
117. MacArthur CJ, Hefeneider SH, Kempton JB, Trune DR. C3H/HeJ mouse model for spontaneous chronic otitis media. Laryngoscope. 2006;116:1071–9.

118. Hirano T, Kodama S, Fujita K, Maeda K, Suzuki M. Role of Toll-like receptor 4 in innate immune responses in a mouse model of acute otitis media. FEMS Immunol Med Microbiol. 2007;49:75–83.
119. Leichtle A, Hernandez M, Pak K, Yamasaki K, Cheng C-F, Webster NJ, et al. TLR4-mediated induction of TLR2 signaling is critical in the pathogenesis and resolution of otitis media. Innate Immun. 2009;15:205–15.
120. Leichtle A, Hernandez M, Lee J, Pak K, Webster NJ, Wollenberg B, et al. The role of DNA sensing and innate immune receptor TLR9 in otitis media. Innate Immun. 2012;18:3–13.
121. Akira S, Takeda K. Toll-like receptor signalling. Nat Rev Immunol. 2004;4:499–511.
122. Fritz JH, Girardin SE. How Toll-like receptors and Nod-like receptors contribute to innate immunity in mammals. J Endotoxin Res. 2005;11:390–4. https://doi.org/10.1177/09680519050110060301.
123. Hernandez M, Leichtle A, Pak K, Ebmeyer J, Euteneuer S, Obonyo M, et al. Myeloid differentiation primary response gene 88 is required for the resolution of otitis media. J Infect Dis. 2008;198:1862–9.
124. Kawai T, Akira S. TLR signaling. Semin Immunol. 2007;19:24–32.
125. Gorovoy M, Han J, Pan H, Welch E, Neamu R, Jia Z, et al. LIM kinase 1 promotes endothelial barrier disruption and neutrophil infiltration in mouse lungs. Circ Res. 2009;105:549–56.
126. Rothwarf DM, Karin M. The NF-kappa B activation pathway: a paradigm in information transfer from membrane to nucleus. Sci STKE Signal Transduct Knowl Environ. 1999;1999:RE1.
127. Parkinson N, Hardisty-Hughes RE, Tateossian H, Tsai H-T, Brooker D, Morse S, et al. Mutation at the Evi1 locus in Junbo mice causes susceptibility to otitis media. PLoS Genet. 2006;2:e149.
128. Alliston T, Ko TC, Cao Y, Liang Y-Y, Feng X-H, Chang C, et al. Repression of bone morphogenetic protein and activin-inducible transcription by Evi-1. J Biol Chem. 2005;280:24227–37.
129. Kurokawa M, Mitani K, Yamagata T, Takahashi T, Izutsu K, Ogawa S, et al. The evi-1 oncoprotein inhibits c-Jun N-terminal kinase and prevents stress-induced cell death. EMBO J. 2000;19:2958–68.
130. Xu X, Woo C-H, Steere RR, Lee BC, Huang Y, Wu J, et al. EVI1 acts as an inducible negative feedback regulator of NF-κB by inhibiting p65 acetylation. J Immunol. 1950;2012(188):6371–80. https://www.ncbi.nlm.nih.gov/pmc/articles/PMC3370108/.
131. Tzavlaki K, Moustakas A. TGF-β signaling. Biomol Ther. 2020;10:487. https://www.ncbi.nlm.nih.gov/pmc/articles/PMC7175140/.
132. Massagué J, Chen YG. Controlling TGF-beta signaling. Genes Dev. 2000;14:627–44.
133. Shi Y, Massagué J. Mechanisms of TGF-beta signaling from cell membrane to the nucleus. Cell. 2003;113:685–700.
134. Kouskoura T, Fragou N, Alexiou M, John N, Sommer L, Graf D, et al. The genetic basis of craniofacial and dental abnormalities. Schweiz Monatsschrift Zahnmed Rev Mens Suisse Odonto-Stomatol Riv Mens Svizzera Odontol E Stomatol. 2011;121:636–46.
135. Kipreos ET, Pagano M. The F-box protein family. Genome Biol. 2000;1:REVIEWS3002.
136. Duan S, Cermak L, Pagan JK, Rossi M, Martinengo C, di Celle PF, et al. FBXO11 targets BCL6 for degradation and is inactivated in diffuse large B-cell lymphomas. Nature. 2012;481:90–3. https://www.ncbi.nlm.nih.gov/pmc/articles/PMC3344385/.
137. Tateossian H, Hardisty-Hughes RE, Morse S, Romero MR, Hilton H, Dean C, et al. Regulation of TGF-β signalling by Fbxo11, the gene mutated in the Jeff otitis media mouse mutant. PathoGenetics. 2009;2:5. https://www.ncbi.nlm.nih.gov/pmc/articles/PMC2714483/.
138. Mitani K. Molecular mechanisms of leukemogenesis by AML1/EVI-1. Oncogene. 2004;23:4263–9.
139. Bertolino E, Reimund B, Wildt-Perinic D, Clerc RG. A novel homeobox protein which recognizes a TGT core and functionally interferes with a retinoid-responsive motif. J Biol Chem. 1995;270:31178–88.
140. Massagué J, Wotton D. New EMBO member's review. EMBO J. 2000;19:1745–54. https://www.ncbi.nlm.nih.gov/pmc/articles/PMC302010/.
141. Tateossian H, Morse S, Parker A, Mburu P, Warr N, Acevedo-Arozena A, et al. Otitis media in the Tgif knockout mouse implicates TGFβ signalling in chronic middle ear inflammatory disease. Hum Mol Genet. 2013;22:2553–65. https://www.ncbi.nlm.nih.gov/pmc/articles/PMC3674796/.
142. Yao W, Frie M, Pan J, Pak K, Webster N, Wasserman SI, et al. C-Jun N-terminal kinase (JNK) isoforms play differing roles in otitis media. BMC Immunol. 2014;15:46.
143. Azar A, Piccinelli C, Brown H, Headon D, Cheeseman M. Ectodysplasin signalling deficiency in mouse models of hypohidrotic ectodermal dysplasia leads to middle ear and nasal pathology. Hum Mol Genet. 2016;25:3564–77. https://www.ncbi.nlm.nih.gov/pmc/articles/PMC5179950/.
144. Li X, Xu L, Li J, Li B, Bai X, Strauss JF, et al. Otitis media in sperm-associated antigen 6 (Spag6)-deficient mice. PLoS One. 2014;9:e112879.
145. Konduru AS, Matsuyama S, Lee B-C, Komatsu K, Li J-D. Curcumin inhibits NTHi-induced MUC5AC mucin overproduction in otitis media via upregulation of MAPK phosphatase MKP-1. Int J Inflamm. 2017;2017:4525309.
146. Mestas J, Hughes CCW. Of mice and not men: differences between mouse and human immunology. J Immunol Baltim Md 1950. 2004;172:2731–8.
147. Bartel DP. MicroRNA target recognition and regulatory functions. Cell. 2009;136:215–33. https://www.ncbi.nlm.nih.gov/pmc/articles/PMC3794896/.
148. Doo JG, Kim YI, Shim HS, Kim DJ, Park JW, Dong SH, et al. Expression of C-type lectin receptor mRNA in otitis media with effusion and chronic otitis media with and without cholesteatoma. Auris Nasus Larynx. 2019;46:672–80. https://linkinghub.elsevier.com/retrieve/pii/S0385814618306680.
149. Jung SY, Kim SS, Kim YI, Kim H-S, Kim SH, Yeo SG. Expression of aquaporins mRNAs in patients with otitis media. Acta Otolaryngol (Stockh). 2018;138:701–7.
150. Kerschner JE, Tripathi S, Khampang P, Papsin BC. MUC5AC expression in human middle ear epithelium of patients with otitis media. Arch Otolaryngol Head Neck Surg. 2010;136:819–24.
151. Jin Shin D, Gan-Undram S, Jin Kim S, Joon Jun Y, Jung Im G, Hyun Jung H. Expression of β-defensins in the tubotympanum of experimental otitis media. Acta Otolaryngol (Stockh). 2006;126:1040–5. https://doi.org/10.1080/00016480600672626.
152. Trune DR, Kempton B, Hausman FA, Larrain BE, MacArthur CJ. Correlative mRNA and protein expression of middle and inner ear inflammatory cytokines during mouse acute otitis media. Hear Res. 2015;326:49–58. https://www.ncbi.nlm.nih.gov/pmc/articles/PMC4492826/.
153. Kang DW, Dong SH, Kim SH, Kim YI, Park DC, Yeo SG. Expression of endoplasmic reticulum stress-related mRNA in otitis media with effusion. Int J Pediatr Otorhinolaryngol. 2019;121:109–13. https://linkinghub.elsevier.com/retrieve/pii/S0165587619301272.
154. Hernandez M, Leichtle A, Pak K, Webster NJ, Wasserman SI, Ryan AF. The transcriptome of a complete episode of acute otitis media. BMC Genomics. 2015;16:259.
155. Ryan AF, Nasamran CA, Pak K, Draf C, Fisch KM, Webster N, et al. Single-cell transcriptomes reveal a complex cellular landscape in the middle ear and differential capacities for acute response to infection. Front Genet. 2020;11:358. https://www.ncbi.nlm.nih.gov/pmc/articles/PMC7174727/.

156. Luo W, Yi H, Taylor J, Li J, Chi F, Todd NW, et al. Cilia distribution and polarity in the epithelial lining of the mouse middle ear cavity. Sci Rep. 2017;7:45870. http://www.nature.com/articles/srep45870.
157. Tucker AS, Dyer CJ, Romero JMF, Teshima THN, Fuchs JC, Thompson H. Mapping the distribution of stem/progenitor cells across the middle ear during homeostasis and inflammation. Development. 2017;145:dev.154393. https://doi.org/10.1242/dev.154393/264412/Mapping-the-distribution-of-stem-progenitor-cells.
158. Mulay A, Chowdhury MMK, James CT, Bingle L, Bingle CD. The transcriptional landscape of the cultured murine middle ear epithelium in vitro. Biol Open. 2021;10:bio056564.
159. Stabenau KA, Zimmermann MT, Mathison A, Zeighami A, Samuels TL, Chun RH, et al. RNA sequencing and pathways analyses of middle ear epithelia from patients with otitis media. Laryngoscope. 2021;131:2590–7. https://doi.org/10.1002/lary.29551.
160. Liu B, Li J, Cairns MJ. Identifying miRNAs, targets and functions. Brief Bioinform. 2014;15:1–19. https://www.ncbi.nlm.nih.gov/pmc/articles/PMC3896928/.
161. Correia de Sousa M, Gjorgjieva M, Dolicka D, Sobolewski C, Foti M. Deciphering miRNAs' action through miRNA editing. Int J Mol Sci. 2019;20:6249. https://www.ncbi.nlm.nih.gov/pmc/articles/PMC6941098/.
162. O'Brien J, Hayder H, Zayed Y, Peng C. Overview of microRNA biogenesis, mechanisms of actions, and circulation. Front Endocrinol. 2018;9:402.
163. Place RF, Li L-C, Pookot D, Noonan EJ, Dahiya R. MicroRNA-373 induces expression of genes with complementary promoter sequences. Proc Natl Acad Sci U S A. 2008;105:1608–13.
164. Martin HC, Wani S, Steptoe AL, Krishnan K, Nones K, Nourbakhsh E, et al. Imperfect centered miRNA binding sites are common and can mediate repression of target mRNAs. Genome Biol. 2014;15:R51.
165. Zhang J, Zhou W, Liu Y, Liu T, Li C, Wang L. Oncogenic role of microRNA-532-5p in human colorectal cancer via targeting of the 5′UTR of RUNX3. Oncol Lett. 2018;15:7215. https://doi.org/10.3892/ol.2018.8217.
166. Dharap A, Pokrzywa C, Murali S, Pandi G, Vemuganti R. MicroRNA miR-324-3p induces promoter-mediated expression of RelA gene. PLoS One. 2013;8:e79467. https://doi.org/10.1371/journal.pone.0079467.
167. Song J-J, Kwon SK, Cho CG, Park S-W, Chae S-W. Microarray analysis of microRNA expression in LPS induced inflammation of human middle ear epithelial cells (HMEECs). Int J Pediatr Otorhinolaryngol. 2011;75:648–51. https://linkinghub.elsevier.com/retrieve/pii/S0165587611000668.
168. Samuels TL, Yan J, Khampang P, MacKinnon A, Hong W, Johnston N, et al. Association of microRNA 146 with middle ear hyperplasia in pediatric otitis media. Int J Pediatr Otorhinolaryngol. 2016;88:104–8.
169. Janas T, Janas MM, Sapoń K, Janas T. Mechanisms of RNA loading into exosomes. FEBS Lett. 2015;589:1391–8.
170. Val S, Jeong S, Poley M, Krueger A, Nino G, Brown K, et al. Purification and characterization of microRNAs within middle ear fluid exosomes: implication in otitis media pathophysiology. Pediatr Res. 2017;81:911–8. http://www.nature.com/articles/pr201725.
171. O'Neill LA, Sheedy FJ, McCoy CE. MicroRNAs: the fine-tuners of Toll-like receptor signalling. Nat Rev Immunol. 2011;11:163–75.
172. Camussi G, Deregibus MC, Bruno S, Cantaluppi V, Biancone L. Exosomes/microvesicles as a mechanism of cell-to-cell communication. Kidney Int. 2010;78:838–48.
173. Moon S-K, Moon S-K, Park R, Moon S-K, Park R, Lee H-Y, et al. Spiral ligament fibrocytes release chemokines in response to otitis media pathogens. Acta Otolaryngol (Stockh). 2006;126:564–9. https://doi.org/10.1080/00016480500452525.
174. Watanabe T, Jono H, Han J, Lim DJ, Li J-D. Synergistic activation of NF-kappaB by nontypeable Haemophilus influenzae and tumor necrosis factor alpha. Proc Natl Acad Sci U S A. 2004;101:3563–8.
175. Val S, Krueger A, Poley M, Cohen A, Brown K, Panigrahi A, et al. Nontypeable Haemophilus influenzae lysates increase heterogeneous nuclear ribonucleoprotein secretion and exosome release in human middle-ear epithelial cells. FASEB J. 2018;32:1855–67. https://www.ncbi.nlm.nih.gov/pmc/articles/PMC5893168/.
176. Li H-G, Zhao L-H, Bao X-B, Sun P-C, Zhai B-P. Meta-analysis of the differentially expressed colorectal cancer-related microRNA expression profiles. Eur Rev Med Pharmacol Sci. 2014;18:2048–57.
177. Pellatt DF, Stevens JR, Wolff RK, Mullany LE, Herrick JS, Samowitz W, et al. Expression profiles of miRNA subsets distinguish human colorectal carcinoma and normal colonic mucosa. Clin Transl Gastroenterol. 2016;7:e152. https://www.ncbi.nlm.nih.gov/pmc/articles/PMC4822091/.
178. Lin J, Wang Y, Zou Y-Q, Chen X, Huang B, Liu J, et al. Differential miRNA expression in pleural effusions derived from extracellular vesicles of patients with lung cancer, pulmonary tuberculosis, or pneumonia. Tumour Biol. 2016;37:15835.
179. Bracken CP, Li X, Wright JA, Lawrence DM, Pillman KA, Salmanidis M, et al. Genome-wide identification of miR-200 targets reveals a regulatory network controlling cell invasion. EMBO J. 2014;33:2040–56. https://www.ncbi.nlm.nih.gov/pmc/articles/PMC4195771/.
180. Inamura K, Ishikawa Y. MicroRNA in lung cancer: novel biomarkers and potential tools for treatment. J Clin Med. 2016;5:36. https://www.ncbi.nlm.nih.gov/pmc/articles/PMC4810107/.
181. Adamczyk P, Narożna B, Szczepankiewicz A, Bręborowicz A, Pucher B, Kotowski M, et al. Decreased miRNA-320e correlates with allergy in children with otitis media with effusion. Auris Nasus Larynx. 2021;48:1061–6.
182. Gantier MP. The not-so-neutral role of microRNAs in neutrophil biology. J Leukoc Biol. 2013;94:575–83.
183. Baek D, Villén J, Shin C, Camargo FD, Gygi SP, Bartel DP. The impact of microRNAs on protein output. Nature. 2008;455:64–71.
184. Hangauer MJ, Vaughn IW, McManus MT. Pervasive transcription of the human genome produces thousands of previously unidentified long intergenic noncoding RNAs. PLoS Genet. 2013;9:e1003569.
185. St Laurent G, Wahlestedt C, Kapranov P. The landscape of long noncoding RNA classification. Trends Genet. 2015;31:239–51.
186. Arora R, Lee Y, Wischnewski H, Brun CM, Schwarz T, Azzalin CM. RNaseH1 regulates TERRA-telomeric DNA hybrids and telomere maintenance in ALT tumour cells. Nat Commun. 2014;5:5220.
187. Kleaveland B, Shi CY, Stefano J, Bartel DP. A network of noncoding regulatory RNAs acts in the mammalian brain. Cell. 2018;174:350–362.e17.
188. Ahn J-H, Lee H-S, Lee J-S, Lee Y-S, Park J-L, Kim S-Y, et al. nc886 is induced by TGF-β and suppresses the microRNA pathway in ovarian cancer. Nat Commun. 2018;9:1166.
189. Bridges MC, Daulagala AC, Kourtidis A. LNCcation: lncRNA localization and function. J Cell Biol. 2021;220:e202009045. https://www.ncbi.nlm.nih.gov/pmc/articles/PMC7816648/.
190. Hu Y, Dong H, Huang J, Huang J, Tao D, Huang C, et al. Long non-coding RNA (lncRNA) nuclear enriched abundant transcript 1 (NEAT1) promotes the inflammation and apoptosis of otitis media with effusion through targeting microRNA (miR)-495

and activation of p38 MAPK signaling pathway. Bioengineered. 2021;12:8080–8.
191. Kraatz J, Clair L, Rodriguez JL, West MA. Macrophage TNF secretion in endotoxin tolerance: role of SAPK, p38, and MAPK. J Surg Res. 1999;83:158–64.
192. Shames BD, Selzman CH, Pulido EJ, Meng X, Meldrum DR, McIntyre RC, et al. LPS-induced NF-kappaB activation and TNF-alpha release in human monocytes are protein tyrosine kinase dependent and protein kinase C independent. J Surg Res. 1999;83:69–74.
193. King NE, Zimmermann N, Pope SM, Fulkerson PC, Nikolaidis NM, Mishra A, et al. Expression and regulation of a disintegrin and metalloproteinase (ADAM) 8 in experimental asthma. Am J Respir Cell Mol Biol. 2004;31:257–65.
194. Knolle MD, Owen CA. ADAM8: a new therapeutic target for asthma. Expert Opin Ther Targets. 2009;13:523–40.
195. Yamashita M, Fukui H, Sugama K, Horio Y, Ito S, Mizuguchi H, et al. Expression cloning of a cDNA encoding the bovine histamine H1 receptor. Proc Natl Acad Sci U S A. 1991;88:11515–9.
196. Janssens S, Beyaert R. Functional diversity and regulation of different interleukin-1 receptor-associated kinase (IRAK) family members. Mol Cell. 2003;11:293–302.
197. Casselbrant ML, Mandel EM, Jung J, Ferrell RE, Tekely K, Szatkiewicz JP, et al. Otitis media: a genome-wide linkage scan with evidence of susceptibility loci within the 17q12 and 10q22.3 regions. BMC Med Genet. 2009;10:85.
198. Stove V, Van de Walle I, Naessens E, Coene E, Stove C, Plum J, et al. Human immunodeficiency virus Nef induces rapid internalization of the T-cell coreceptor CD8alphabeta. J Virol. 2005;79:11422–33.
199. Iino Y, Kakizaki K, Katano H, Saigusa H, Kanegasaki S. Eosinophil chemoattractants in the middle ear of patients with eosinophilic otitis media. Clin Exp Allergy. 2005;35:1370–6.
200. Ingham PW, McMahon AP. Hedgehog signalling: Kif7 is not that fishy after all. Curr Biol. 2009;19:R729–31.
201. Jia L, Landan G, Pomerantz M, Jaschek R, Herman P, Reich D, et al. Functional enhancers at the gene-poor 8q24 cancer-linked locus. PLoS Genet. 2009;5:e1000597.

Predictive Medicine in Otitis Media

11

Raimundo José García-Matte, María José Herrera J, and Marcos V. Goycoolea

Introduction

Otitis media (OM) is a multifactorial, multifaceted disease that manifests as an inflammatory process in the middle ear (ME), mastoid, and Eustachian tube (ET). It is the result of prevailing aggression against the body's defense system, the degree of which depends on the interactions between these two opposing forces, i.e., the disease against the immunological defense system [1].

Selecting a rational therapy is essential to understand the anatomy, function, and pathology of the organs involved and the disease mechanisms. Understanding the mechanisms of disease allows for the most critical concept of timing. At the right time, insertion of a ventilating tube might be all that is needed, whereas, at the wrong time, a tube will not suffice. The ultimate goal is to prevent OM (e.g., through environmental factors, vaccines, innate immunity) and, if unsuccessful, treat it medically, reserving surgery only to restore function rather than to eradicate the disease [1].

Precision medicine (PM) is a relatively new concept to understand and face these disease mechanisms, which involves "treatments targeted to the needs of individual patients based on genetic, biomarker, phenotypic, or psychosocial characteristics that distinguish a given patient from other patients with similar clinical presentations. Inherent in this definition is the goal of improving clinical outcomes for individual patients and minimizing unnecessary side effects for those less likely to have a response to a particular treatment" [2].

To provide each patient with the right treatment at the right dose and at the right time, considering all available information, is the philosophy behind PM. Predictive, preventive, personalized, and participatory (P4) are the four core values that guide its implementation and highlight the importance of overall individual wellness rather than the disease [3].

As "all the available information" can be a broad and unspecific term, it must be classified to retrieve such information in an orderly and helpful manner. Individual features are the result of the integration of internal and external information. Internal information corresponds to the genetic makeup or **genome**, and external information refers to the cumulative environmental exposures that individuals encounter throughout life or **exposome**. Interactions between the genome and the exposome result in each individual's phenotype "through **networks of biological pathways** that capture, transmit, and integrate signals and, finally, send instructions to the molecular machines that execute the functions of life" [3].

The same processes are valid in diseases, as the interactions between a genome and an exposome result in an observable clinical phenotype of a given disease. However, this concept of phenotype fell short under the PM prism as it did not acknowledge the mechanisms underlying the same phenotype with diagnostic and treatment implications. Accordingly, the phenotype definition was modified to "a single or combination of disease attributes that describe differences between individuals as they relate to clinically meaningful outcomes" [4], and the term "endophenotype" was resurfaced from the psychiatric literature, contracted to **endotype** and defined as "subtype of disease defined functionally and pathologically by a molecular mechanism or by treatment response" [5] Endotypes and phenotypes can be detected by appropriately validated **biomarkers**, which are objectively measurable indicators that can be evaluated to gauge a particular biological or pathogenic process or response to treatment (Biomarkers Definitions Working Group 2001) (see Fig. 11.1).

R. J. García-Matte (✉)
Department of Otolaryngology, Clínica Universidad de Los Andes, and Hospital de la Florida, Santiago, Chile

M. J. Herrera J
Department of Otolaryngology, Clínica Universidad de Los Andes, and Hospital Luis Calvo Mackenna, Santiago, Chile

M. V. Goycoolea
Department of Otolaryngology, Clínica Universidad de Los Andes, Santiago, Chile

M. V. Goycoolea et al. (eds.), *Textbook of Otitis Media*, https://doi.org/10.1007/978-3-031-40949-3_11

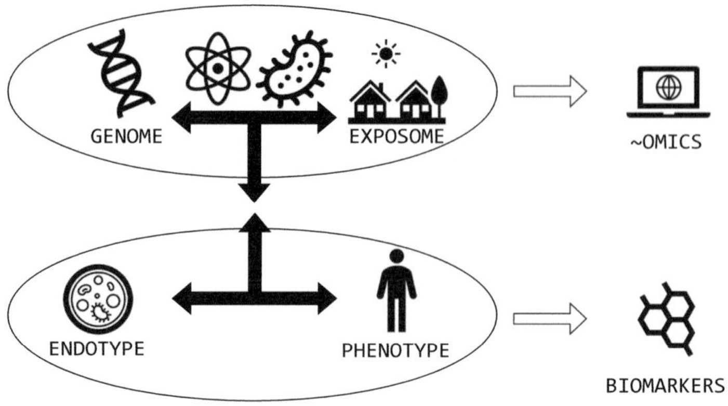

Fig. 11.1 Graphical representation of the different components involved in the precision medicine disease model

PM requires and stimulates the creation of tons of data. As more information is generated exponentially every year, new complex forms and fields of study have surged, which are collectively referred to as "omics." Each "-omics" studies an "-ome" (e.g., proteomics studies the proteome), focusing on the collective characterization and quantification of large numbers of biological molecules that translate into the structure, function, and dynamics of an organism (CDC NIOSH2). Genomics studies the genome and exposomics the exposome, but there are many interrelated omics in between, such as epigenomics, transcriptomics, and proteomics. Moreover, omics that could be considered a part of the exposome are studied apart, like microbiomics.

The PM approach has been gaining traction, and recent models on cronic rhinosinusitis (CRS) and obstructive sleep apnea syndrome (OSAS) have been developed in otolaryngology [6, 7]. Although there have been efforts in OM toward PM, highlighting the importance of patterns in acute otitis media (AOM) to approximate individualized care [8, 9], there are no current formal models for this clinical entity. Despite the lack of OM precision models, its research has not been away from omics, and, so, in the next part, we review the different omics approaches to the study of OM.

Otitis Media Omics

Genomics

As the oldest and the most advanced omics, most OM studies focus on this area. Early observations of the heritability of OM prompted additional and specific studies to understand its pathophysiology and, ultimately, find new strategies for its prevention and treatment. There are many different approaches to clinical human genetic studies. However, all share the definition of a phenotype, in this case, OM, to which genetic data are compared. Therefore, it is crucial to carefully characterize the phenotypes in genetic studies to avoid biases induced by an inconsistent or poorly defined disease status. Regretfully, an accurate diagnosis is a known problem in OM, with frequent misdiagnosis, as addressed by the latest clinical practice guidelines [10, 11], so studies must acknowledge and avoid this problem.

Heritability Studies

Heritability is the proportion of observed variation in a particular trait that can be attributed to inherited genetic factors in contrast to environmental ones. Several studies have confirmed evidence for a heritable component in OM, some of which are exposed below.

AOM: One cohort study of 1279 Finnish children and their parents showed that the heritability to recurrent acute otitis media (RAOM) was 38.5% [12].

Otitis media with effusion (OME): Twin and triplet studies have shown robust evidence of genetic susceptibility to OME. In the prospective twin and triplet Pittsburgh study, the estimated heritability of OM at the 2-year end point was 0.79 in girls and 0.64 in boys [13]. The correlation between twins' middle ear effusion (MEE) duration was significantly higher in monozygotic than in dizygotic twins. A second study that extended the observation period estimated the same heritability to be 0.72 [14].

Chronic suppurative otitis media (CSOM): A 2013 study conducted among Australian aboriginal communities found that 12% of young children presented with CSOM, with a 50% and 37% prevalence of OME and AOM, respectively [15].

Approaches to Studying the Genetics of a Common Disease

Two general approaches have been widely used to study the genetics of OM that differ in terms of dependence on a previous pathophysiological hypothesis. First, candidate gene association studies evaluate genetic variations in a determined number of genes (candidates) that are selected based on the current knowledge of the disease's pathogenesis. In contrast, genome-wide studies do not require a prior hypothesis as they explore the whole genome of the researched group either in families through linkage studies or in large case–control population cohorts known as genome-wide association studies (GWASs).

Candidate Gene Association Studies in OM

As stated above, in candidate gene association studies, the frequencies of a determined genetic marker are compared between subjects presenting the phenotype of interest (cases) and control subjects that do not present such a phenotype. The control subjects can be unrelated healthy controls (case–control study) or healthy relatives (family study).

These candidate genes were previously determined mainly through animal models (generally mice) and assumed biology. In concordance with known pathophysiology, most candidate gene-association studies on OM have focused on inflammation and immunity genes, as has been highlighted by a recent, thorough review [16] (see Table 11.1).

Linkage Studies in Families

Linkage genome-wide family studies examine DNA from all the available family members (or series of families) and compare it with the phenotype of interest to assess the statistical linkage between them. A few chromosomes were associated with OM through this method, but the complex genetics and causative factors of this condition make linkage studies a not-so-effective tool.

Genome-Wide Association Studies

A GWAS compares the general population's genetic profiles to individuals with phenotypic traits of interest to identify genetic variants that may be related to said traits. A catalog of the most published GWASs (https://www.ebi.ac.uk/gwas) shows that 5 studies and 11 associations are related to OM. The most recent study, an independent GWAS on European ancestry individuals, has studied genetic association with childhood ear infections and myringotomy in 121,810 and 89,227 subjects, respectively. They reported a significant ($p < 5 \times 10^{-8}$) association in 13 genomic regions for infections and in 1 for myringotomy. The strongest associations for ear infections were FUT2 and TBX1, with the latter also being related to myringotomy [17].

Table 11.1 The principal genes involved in OM pathogenesis according to the immune pathway and their roles

Immunity	Pathway	Gene	Gene function
Innate	Immune response and inflammation	MBL2	COMPLEMENT ACTIVATION
		TLR2	PRRR WIDE
		TLR4	PRRR LPS
		CD14	TLR4 CORECEPTOR
	Tissue clearance	SFPTA	GOBLET CELL SURFACTANT
		SFTPA1	GOBLET CELL SURFACTANT
		SFTPD	GOBLET CELL SURFACTANT
		SLC11A1	PATHOGEN CLEARANCE
		MUC2	GOBLET CELL MUCUS
		MUC5AC	GOBLET CELL MUCUS
		MUC5B	GOBLET CELL MUCUS
	Microbe adhesion	ABO	BACTERIAL ADHESION
		FUT2	BACTERIAL ADHESION
	Anatomy	TBX1	ET FUNCTION
Adaptative	Cytokines	IL6	CYTOKIN
		IL10	CYTOKIN
		IL1A	CYTOKIN
		IL1B	CYTOKIN
		TNFA	CYTOKIN
		IFNG	CYTOKIN
		TGFB1	ANTIGEN BINDING
	Transcriptional modulation	SMAD2	TRANSCRIPTION MODULATOR
		SMAD4	TRANSCRIPTION MODULATOR
	Extracellular matrix	A2ML1	PROTEASE INHIBITOR
		PAI1	PROTEASE REGULATOR
	Protein modification	CPT1A	FATTY ACID OXIDATION
		FBXO11	PROTEIN UBIQUITINATION
	Channel activity	SCN1B	ION CHANNEL BINDING

Epigenomics

Epigenomics refers to the study of epigenetics, the biochemical and functionally relevant changes of DNA without altering its sequence. Epigenetic mechanisms include DNA methylation, a gene expression suppressor, and histone modification, considered a protein production modifier. These processes can result from intrinsic regulation factors or extrinsic stimuli (exposures), such as tobacco smoke and viral infections, and are tissue-type- and time-specific, although hindering the epigenetic study.

The fibronectin type III domain-containing protein 1 gene (*FNDC1*), believed to be an activator of G protein, was significantly associated with AOM through a GWAS. In the same study, *FNDC1* variants were positively correlated with *FNDC1* expression levels but negatively correlated with the methylation status of *FNDC1*, indicating the epigenetic nature of the alteration [18].

Histone modifications, which control T-cell differentiation and memory formation, have also been associated with OM. One study showed that UTX, a histone demethylase, played a role in antibody generation in chronic infections and presented reduced expression in the immune cells of patients with Turner syndrome, a genetic disorder of partial or complete loss of chromosome X in females [19]. Previous studies described a greater prevalence and longer duration of middle ear pathologies in Turner syndrome [16]. Although the immunological status has been studied in these patients, the results are contradictory.

Transcriptomics

The study of gene expression through RNA sequencing (RNA-Seq) is known as transcriptomics. As gene expression is highly dynamic and has multiple influences, its study must account for the specific conditions and cell/tissue types on which it is performed. RNA will not have the same status in a healthy tissue as in a sick tissue (what transcriptomics wants to portray). The transcriptome has mainly been described using microarrays, but with the recent technological advances that allow whole transcriptome analysis, next-generation RNA sequencing (RNA-Seq) studies have flourished. Given the transcriptome's variability, tissue selection is of the highest importance to accurately describe how the disease affects gene expression. Cells directly affected by disease must be studied, and, in the case of OM, transcriptomes from the middle ear epithelium (MEE) and middle ear effusions (MEEFs) have been described.

Two recent studies of MEE transcriptomes have been conducted. In one, RNA-Seq demonstrated differential gene expression in MEE cells between pediatric OME patients and children with a healthy ME. Genes with differences in expression were involved in inflammation, immune responses to bacterial OM pathogens, mucociliary clearance, regulation of proliferation and transformation, and auditory cell differentiation. Pathway analysis revealed an association with auditory development nicotine degradation genes [20]. In the other study, the RNA expression of six "candidate" molecules (tumor necrosis factor-alpha (TNF-α), interleukin (IL)-1B, IL-6, IL-8, IL-10, and mucin 5B (MUC5B)) was assessed in MEE cell cultures from children with RAOM, OME, and no ME pathology and an immortalized MEE adult cell line (HMEEC-1). The reported expressions were frequently higher in all pediatric lines compared to the adult line, and, within the pediatric lines, OME lines were often more responsive than were RAOM lines. Noting the difference among age groups, the researchers concluded that pediatric MEE cultures are needed to improve the OM research [21].

Other human investigations regarding the OM transcriptome have focused on MEEFs, reporting a hypoxic inflammatory environment in the genome-wide transcript of white blood cells in the effusions of OME [22]. Furthermore, the study of MEEF microRNAs in exosomes as a distant cell genetic communication system opens the door to new pathways in the intricate OM pathophysiology [23]. MicroRNAs are small RNA molecules that can negatively control their target gene expression posttranscriptionally. There are two types relevant to OM, miR-378 and miR-146, associated with mucogenic responses and mucosal inflammation, respectively [24, 25].

Proteomics, Lipidomics, and Glycomics

Although genes contain "life's instructions," life's actual building blocks are three other molecule groups: proteins, lipids, and carbohydrates (glycans). Moreover, though disease research has mainly concentrated on genomics, new technologies, and more significant data processing capacity, studies on these molecules have gained terrain.

The omics approach to these molecules can be defined as the qualitative and quantitative analysis of the collection of protein, lipid, or glycan constituents in a biological sample. Polyacrylamide gel electrophoresis (PAGE), matrix-assisted laser desorption/ionization (MALDI), and liquid chromatography-tandem mass spectrometry (LC-MS) are some of the techniques used to study proteins and lipids. These methods provide measures of their types and abundance in biological samples.

So far, proteomics is the only one of these omics approaches with promising publications. In 2010, LC-MS allowed the identification of the MUC5B protein as the predominant mucin in mucoid MEEF [26]. A more extensive analysis of mucoid samples from MEEFs of children undergoing grommet surgery showed the presence of abundant innate immunity products, leukocytes, neutrophil extracellular traps (NETs), epithelial/glandular antimicrobial proteins, and mucins such as MUC5B [27].

Proteomic analysis has also differentiated MEEF compositions and biological signatures between mucoid and serous effusions. For example, mucoid MEEF showed a neutrophilic signature associated with MUC5B presence and extracellular DNA, confirming the implication of NETs in OME. On the other hand, serous MEEFs contained a much lower number of mucins and neutrophil markers but a higher amount of early innate immunity markers (complement and immunoglobulin proteins) and serum proteins. It can be suggested that this difference could be due to the MEE propensity to remodel in patients exhibiting mucoid MEEFs [24].

Microbiomics

Microbiomics, the characterization of the microbes that reside in an individual (or a determined anatomical site), is another omics type that has exponentially increased in the last two decades, especially since the National Institutes of

Health (NIH) launched the Human Microbiome Project (HMP) in 2008. There are ten times more bacteria than human cells in our bodies, so studying them seems appropriate. Moreover, the human microbiome is dynamic and changeable, making it an attractive target for therapy in highly diverse pathologies such as cancer, autism, inflammatory bowel disease, and infectious diseases.

The microbiota plays a beneficial role in the host's immunity. It protects the host from pathogenic bacterial colonization by different methods like competing for adherence to epithelial cells and by immune response regulation. There is also evidence of an interaction between the upper airway microbiome and the host's genes and innate mucosal immunity [28], with a role in the modulation of inflammatory processes [29].

The microbiome of the upper respiratory tract (URT) is present since birth, varies over time, and depends on several factors. The delivery and feeding modes are the most critical factors in the initial months of life. In addition, environmental and host factors can modify the microbiota from a balanced and resilient one (remains healthy even when exposed to stress) to an unstable community that predisposes the host to an infection or inflammation. Currently, the identified factors are host genetics, seasons, siblings, antibiotic use, daycare attendance, and tobacco exposure. There is also evidence of the beneficial role of vaccines and probiotics [30, 31].

Microbiome study was initially conducted through culture, a slow and inefficient method. However, the development of new sequencing techniques, such as 16S ribosomal RNA (16S rRNA), has led to more extensive population studies and the discovery of new microorganisms that did not appear in previous culture research.

OM microbiomics focuses on studying the middle ear (ME) and nasopharynx (NP) microbiota, communicated through the Eustachian tube (ET). According to the pathogen reservoir hypothesis (PRH), the adenoids, a lymphatic tissue mass in the NP, serve as a source of pathogens that can grow in this region and further spread to the respiratory system and ME, thus resulting in different infections like OM.

Healthy microbiome: Healthy (without OM) human NP and ME microbiomes are diverse [32] and change with age. Some bacterial genera, namely, *Corynebacterium* and *Dolosigranulum*, can be considered commensals of a healthy nasopharynx [33].

AOM

The ME: The primary bacterial pathogens contributing to AOM are *Streptococcus pneumoniae*, *Haemophilus influenzae*, and *Moraxella catarrhalis*. However, newer studies suggest a pathogenic role for other taxa, such as *Turicella* (*T. otitidis*) and *Alloiococcus* (*A. otitidis*) [34].

Regarding these new bacteria, a 2020 review found that there was currently insufficient evidence available to determine whether these organisms are pathogens, commensals, or contribute indirectly to the pathogenesis of OM. They also remarked that their closest relatives are the NP commensals *Dolosigranulum* and *Corynebacterium*, thus proposing that they may have a commensal, homologous role in the ME, generated by developing specialized and highly different interactions with the dominant pathogens in their respective niches [33].

The NP: As discussed above, evidence is available on the commensal role of *Dolosigranulum* and *Corynebacterium* in the NP. They have been associated with a healthy status and a lower colonization rate of otopathogens such as *S. pneumoniae* [35]. Moreover, the risk of developing AOM after a viral URT infection has been related to the number of otopathogens colonizing the nasopharynx. Half of the children carrying all the three primary AOM pathogens develop AOM after a viral URT infection, compared to only 10% if none of these pathogens is present [36].

A different global microbiome profile and reduced alpha diversity were observed in the NP microbiome of otitis-prone children compared to healthy controls at 6 months of age. This difference was resolved when both groups were compared at 12 months of age. The same study showed that dysbiosis occurs in the NP microbiome of otitis-prone children at an early age, even when healthy [37].

OME

The ME: The dominant bacteria in the MEEFs of OME patients appears to be *H. influenzae*, as different systematic reviews have reported. The addition of PCR techniques increases the detection of known otopathogens (mostly *M. catarrhalis*). The newest sequencing techniques have added several bacteria to the OME microbiome, with *A. otitidis* standing out [34, 38, 39]. Many of these new MEEF bacteria are usually found in the external auditory canal (EAC) but not in the NP. By definition, OME occurs with an intact tympanic membrane (TM), which has led to consider the EAC microbiome's role in OM. This colonization could occur in previous asymptomatic perforations or through inflammation-mediated TM microlesions that allow bacterial translocation to the ME. Both theories are plausible as OME frequently occurs after a suppurated AOM and TM substance transport has been previously demonstrated [11, 40].

Biofilms also seem to play a role in OME pathogenesis, as a case–control study reported a significant difference regarding biofilm presence in the middle ear mucosa (84% in OME patients and 0% in controls (p-value <0.001*)) [41].

The NP

There are differences between the NP microbiome of patients with and without OME. In addition, the NP microbiome is less diverse in children suffering from OME than in controls [42, 43].

There is no strong correlation between the NP microbiome and the MEEFs in patients with OME. Several studies have shown that OME patients' MEEF microbiome is dissimilar to the NP with diversity analyses [44–46]. One case–control study showed that although the three main otopathogens were highly prevalent in the NP of children, only *S. pneumoniae* and *M. catarrhalis* were significantly related to OME [47].

The NP microbiome undoubtedly plays a role in OME, but it seems more complex than just a pathogen reservoir.

CSOM

The ME: There is scarce recent evidence regarding the ME microbiome and CSOM. A 2017 study characterized the microbiomes with cultures and 16S rRNA sequence of 155 subjects with no ME pathology, dry CSOM, and wet CSOM. The main findings were a significant change in the normal ME microbiota with age. The healthy ME and dry CSOM microbiome did not present significant differences but did differ from wet CSOM [48].

The penetration of microorganisms residing in the EAC into the ME has been considered in the pathogenesis of active inflammation in CSOM, but further studies are needed to define this aspect better.

The NP: The NP microbiome has not been studied in CSOM patients to the best of our knowledge.

Exposomics

The exposome is the sum of exposures that an individual encounters over a period of time. These may include nutrients, foods, toxins, stresses, exercise, vaccinations, medications, and other exposures. The exposome is highly dynamic and malleable over an individual's life.

The exposome attempts to measure, integrate, and interpret the complex exposures faced throughout life. Furthermore, it measures how these complex exposures impact our biological systems and provides a connection to health and disease outcomes.

High-resolution metabolomics (HRM), which uses gas or liquid chromatography with ultrahigh-accuracy mass spectrometry, is the most promising analytical technology for an exposome platform for precision medicine.

A recent meta-analysis of OM risk factors has shown that passive smoke and low social status significantly increased the risk of chronic otitis media/recurrent otitis media (COM/ROM) in children [49]. Similar results regarding social status were reported in a Latin American study of adults with CSOM, in which a higher socioeconomic status was found to be a protective factor [50].

Regarding air pollution and OM, it has been determined that an increase in the concentration of air particulate matter is directly associated with the incidence of AOM [51].

Other exposome risk factors for OM in children include day-care attendance for AOM [52–54] and the use of pacifiers for AOM and RAOM if used after 6 months of age [55, 56].

On the other hand, breastfeeding has been proven to protect children against AOM until 2 years of age, with a more significant effect observed in exclusive and more prolonged-duration breastfeeding [57].

Otitis Media Impact

While the omics approach can help us understand OM risks factors, disease severity, biological activity, and treatment response, an essential part of the PM domain is the personalized approach to the impact of the disease on the patient's life.

There are many instruments designed to measure this impact on the quality of life (QoL) of the patient or the family, with the Otitis Media 6 (OM-6) being one of the most used ones. This validated questionnaire consists of six items that assess physical suffering, hearing loss, speech impairment, emotional distress, activity limitations, and caregiver concerns [58].

As OM encompasses different diseases with their own clinical manifestations, it is only logical to think that the burden of each disease is also specific to it. AOM negatively affected the QoL of the caregivers and children in varying degrees. When AOM occurs in younger patients, the episode is more severe (as perceived by the parents), or in cases of RAOM, the caregivers' QoL is more affected [59]. Parents of children with RAOM also have a poorer QoL when compared with parents of children with OME and those without OM [60–62]. In COM/OME patients, it seems that hearing level improvement is correlated with QoL after surgery (tympanomastoidectomy/grommets) [60, 63].

Clinical Application

Current

PM can help us deliver better medicine to our patients, but there is a risk of getting lost within the vast amount of growing available information. As there is no point in collecting millions of gigabytes of OM omics data if we cannot use it with our patients, we need to develop PM application instruments. These instruments must allow us to apply the PM principles in our daily activity without

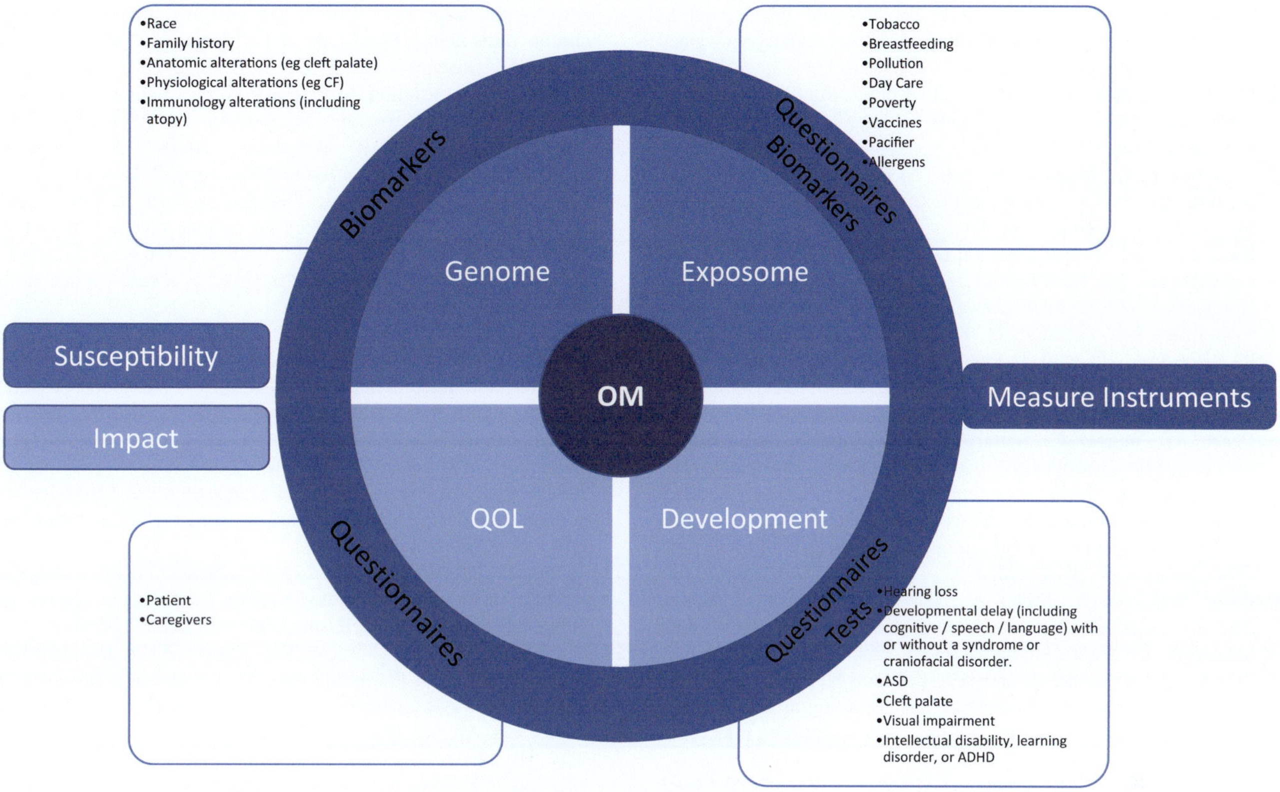

Fig. 11.2 The proposed model for clinical application of precision medicine on otitis media. *OM* otitis media, *QoL* quality of life, *ASD* autistic spectrum disorder, *ADHD* attention-deficit/hyperactivity disorder, *CF* cystic fibrosis

interfering with patient care. The model proposed by Ruben [8] is a step in the right direction under the PM prism but needs to be updated as it was created more than 10 years ago. Acknowledging the current information reviewed here, we propose this update, as can be seen in detail in Fig. 11.2.

Future

Using the PM approach in OM could help us identify different endotypes, with their respective biomarkers linked to the existing phenotypes. For example, RAOM, one of the OM phenotypes, has multiple causes, including anatomical alterations, NP otopathogens, and immune deficiencies. These causes could represent a different endotype with a specific biomarker waiting to be discovered. Taken to practice, when faced with a patient with RAOM, some tests should be conducted (biomarkers) to determine its endotype with the corresponding best treatment strategy. For example, children with NP-altered microbiome RAOM would have a different therapeutic approach than would children with innate immune deficiency RAOM. One could hypothesize that the former could be treated with probiotics, whereas the latter with biological therapy.

References

1. Marcos G. In: Goycoolea M, de Souza C, editors. Atlas of otologic surgery and magic otology, vols. 1 and 2. 2nd ed. Jaypee Brothers Medical Publishers; 2012. 1664 p.
2. Jameson JL, Longo DL. Sounding board precision medicine-personalized, problematic, and promising, vol. 372. 2015. p. 2229.
3. Hood L, Friend SH. Predictive, personalized, preventive, participatory (P4) cancer medicine. Nat Rev Clin Oncol. 2011;8(3):184–7.
4. Agustí A, Bafadhel M, Beasley R, Bel EH, Faner R, Gibson PG, et al. Precision medicine in airway diseases: moving to clinical practice. Eur Respir J. 2017;50(4):1701655.
5. Anderson GP. Endotyping asthma: new insights into key pathogenic mechanisms in a complex, heterogeneous disease, vol. 372. Lancet; 2008. p. 1107–19.
6. Martinez-Garcia MA, Campos-Rodriguez F, Barbé F, Gozal D, Agustí A. Precision medicine in obstructive sleep apnoea, vol. 7. Lancet Respir Med; 2019. p. 456–64.
7. Hellings PW, Fokkens WJ, Bachert C, Akdis CA, Bieber T, Agache I, et al. Positioning the principles of precision medicine in care pathways for allergic rhinitis and chronic rhinosinusitis—a EUFOREA-ARIA-EPOS-AIRWAYS ICP statement. Allergy. 2017;72(9):1297–305.
8. Ruben RJ. Otitis media: the application of personalized medicine. Otolaryngol Head Neck Surg. 2011;145:707–12.
9. Sibbald AD. Acute otitis media in infants: the disease and the illness. Clinical distinctions for the new treatment paradigm. Otolaryngol Head Neck Surg. 2012;147(4):606–10.
10. Lieberthal AS, Carroll AE, Chonmaitree T, Ganiats TG, Hoberman A, Jackson MA, et al. The diagnosis and management of acute otitis media. Pediatrics. 2013;131:e964.

11. Rosenfeld RM, Shin JJ, Schwartz SR, Coggins R, Gagnon L, Hackell JM, et al. Clinical practice guideline. Otolaryngol Head Neck Surg. 2016;154:S1–S41.
12. Hafrén L, Kentala E, Einarsdottir E, Kere J, Mattila PS. Current knowledge of the genetics of otitis media. Curr Allergy Asthma Rep. 2012;12(6):582–9.
13. Casselbrant ML, Mandel EM, Fall PA, Rockette HE, Kurs-Lasky M, Bluestone CD, et al. The heritability of otitis media a twin and triplet study's hospital of Pittsburgh (Drs Casselbrant, Mandel, and Bluestone, and Ms Fall); and the Departments of Biostatistics (Dr Rockette and Ms Kurs-Lasky) and Human Genetics (Dr Ferrell) [Internet]. JAMA. 1999;282. www.jama.com.
14. Casselbrant ML, Mandel EM, Rockette HE, Kurs-Lasky M, Fall PA, Bluestone CD, et al. The genetic component of middle ear disease in the first 5 years of life [internet]. Arch Otolaryngol Head Neck Surg. 2004;130:273. http://archotol.jamanetwork.com/.
15. Leach AJ, Wigger C, Beissbarth J, Woltring D, Andrews R, Chatfield MD, et al. General health, otitis media, nasopharyngeal carriage and middle ear microbiology in northern territory aboriginal children vaccinated during consecutive periods of 10-valent or 13-valent pneumococcal conjugate vaccines. Int J Pediatr Otorhinolaryngol. 2016;86:224–32.
16. Giese APJ, Ali S, Isaiah A, Aziz I, Riazuddin S, Ahmed ZM. Genomics of otitis media (OM): molecular genetics approaches to characterize disease pathophysiology. Front Genet. 2020;11:313.
17. Tian C, Hromatka BS, Kiefer AK, Eriksson N, Noble SM, Tung JY, et al. Genome-wide association and HLA region fine-mapping studies identify susceptibility loci for multiple common infections. Nat Commun. 2017;8(1):599.
18. van Ingen G, Li J, Goedegebure A, Pandey R, Rose Li Y, March ME, et al. Genome-wide association study for acute otitis media in children identifies FNDC1 as disease contributing gene. Nat Commun. 2016;7:12792.
19. Cook KD, Shpargel KB, Starmer J, Whitfield-Larry F, Conley B, Allard DE, et al. T follicular helper cell-dependent clearance of a persistent virus infection requires T cell expression of the histone demethylase UTX. Immunity. 2015;43(4):703–14.
20. Stabenau KA, Zimmermann MT, Mathison A, Zeighami A, Samuels TL, Chun RH, et al. RNA sequencing and pathways analyses of middle ear epithelia from patients with otitis media. Laryngoscope. 2021;131(11):2590–7.
21. Espahbodi M, Samuels TL, McCormick C, Khampang P, Yan K, Marshall S, et al. Analysis of inflammatory signaling in human middle ear cell culture models of pediatric otitis media. Laryngoscope. 2021;131(2):410–6.
22. Bhutta MF, Lambie J, Hobson L, Williams D, Tyrer HE, Nicholson G, et al. Transcript analysis reveals a hypoxic inflammatory environment in human chronic otitis media with effusion. Front Genet. 2020;10:1327.
23. Val S, Jeong S, Poley M, Krueger A, Nino G, Brown K, et al. Purification and characterization of microRNAs within middle ear fluid exosomes: implication in otitis media pathophysiology. Pediatr Res. 2017;81(6):911–8.
24. Val S, Poley M, Anna K, Nino G, Brown K, Pérez-Losada M, et al. Characterization of mucoid and serous middle ear effusions from patients with chronic otitis media: implication of different biological mechanisms? Pediatr Res. 2018;84(2):296–305.
25. Samuels TL, Yan J, Khampang P, MacKinnon A, Hong W, Johnston N, et al. Association of microRNA 146 with middle ear hyperplasia in pediatric otitis media. Int J Pediatr Otorhinolaryngol. 2016;(88):104–8.
26. Preciado D, Goyal S, Rahimi M, Watson AM, Brown KJ, Hathout Y, et al. MUC5B is the predominant mucin glycoprotein in chronic otitis media fluid [internet]. 2010. www.pedresearch.org.
27. Val S, Poley M, Brown K, Choi R, Jeong S, Colberg-Poley A, et al. Proteomic characterization of middle ear fluid confirms neutrophil extracellular traps as a predominant innate immune response in chronic otitis media. PLoS One. 2016;11(4):e0152865.
28. Igartua C, Davenport ER, Gilad Y, Nicolae DL, Pinto J, Ober C. Host genetic variation in mucosal immunity pathways influences the upper airway microbiome. Microbiome. 2017;5(1):16.
29. Sokolowska M, Frei R, Lunjani N, Akdis CA, O'Mahony L. Microbiome and asthma. Asthma Res Pract. 2018;4(1):1.
30. Mika M, Maurer J, Korten I, Allemann A, Aebi S, Brugger SD, et al. Influence of the pneumococcal conjugate vaccines on the temporal variation of pneumococcal carriage and the nasal microbiota in healthy infants: a longitudinal analysis of a case-control study. Microbiome. 2017;5(1):85.
31. Glück U, Gebbers J-O. Ingested probiotics reduce nasal colonization with pathogenic bacteria (Staphylococcus aureus, Streptococcus pneumoniae, and B-hemolytic streptococci [internet]. Am J Clin Nutr. 2003;77:517. https://academic.oup.com/ajcn/article-abstract/77/2/517/4689718.
32. Kalcioglu MT, Durmaz R, Ari O, Celik S, Karabudak S. Microbiological investigation of samples collected from healthy middle ears during cochlear implant surgery. Diagn Microbiol Infect Dis. 2021;100(4):115390.
33. Lappan R, Jamieson SE, Peacock CS. Reviewing the pathogenic potential of the otitis-associated bacteria Alloiococcus otitidis and Turicella otitidis. Front Cell Infect Microbiol. 2020;10:51.
34. Ngo CC, Massa HM, Thornton RB, Cripps AW. Predominant bacteria detected from the middle ear fluid of children experiencing otitis media: a systematic review. PLoS One. 2016;11(3):e0150949.
35. Laufer AS, Metlay JP, Gent JF, Fennie KP, Kong Y, Pettigrewa MM. Microbial communities of the upper respiratory tract and otitis media in children. mBio. 2011;2(1):e00245.
36. Revai K, Mamidi D, Chonmaitree T. Association of nasopharyngeal bacterial colonization during upper respiratory tract infection and the development of acute otitis media. Clin Infect Dis. 2008;46(4):e34.
37. Xu L, Earl J, Bajorski P, Gonzalez E, Pichichero ME. Nasopharyngeal microbiome analyses in otitis-prone and otitis-free children. Int J Pediatr Otorhinolaryngol. 2021;143:110629.
38. Coleman A, Wood A, Bialasiewicz S, Ware RS, Marsh RL, Cervin A. The unsolved problem of otitis media in indigenous populations: a systematic review of upper respiratory and middle ear microbiology in indigenous children with otitis media. Microbiome. 2018;6:199.
39. Jörissen J, van den Broek MFL, de Boeck I, van Beeck W, Wittouck S, Boudewyns A, et al. Case-control microbiome study of chronic otitis media with effusion in children points at Streptococcus salivarius as a pathobiont-inhibiting species. mSystems. 2021;6(2):e00056–21. https://doi.org/10.1128/mSystems.
40. Santos-Cortez RLP, Bhutta MF, Earl JP, Hafrén L, Jennings M, Mell JC, et al. Panel 3: genomics, precision medicine and targeted therapies. Int J Pediatr Otorhinolaryngol. 2020;130 Suppl 1(Suppl 1):109835.
41. Elzayat S, Nosair N, Ghazy AA, Abdulghaffar IA. Otitis media with effusion is not a sterile inflammatory process: scanning electron microscope evidence. Eur Arch Otorhinolaryngol. 2021;278(8):2713–21.
42. Kim SK, Hong SJ, Pak KH, Hong SM. Analysis of the microbiome in the adenoids of Korean children with otitis media with effusion. J Int Adv Otol. 2019;15(3):379–85.
43. Walker RE, Walker CG, Camargo CA, Bartley J, Flint D, Thompson JMD, et al. Nasal microbial composition and chronic otitis media with effusion: a case-control study. PLoS One. 2019;14(2):e0212473.
44. Xu J, Dai W, Liang Q, Ren D. The microbiomes of adenoid and middle ear in children with otitis media with effusion and hypertrophy from a tertiary hospital in China. Int J Pediatr Otorhinolaryngol. 2020;134:110058.

45. Chan CL, Wabnitz D, Bardy JJ, Bassiouni A, Wormald PJ, Vreugde S, et al. The microbiome of otitis media with effusion. Laryngoscope. 2016;126(12):2844–51.
46. Ari O, Karabudak S, Kalcioglu MT, Gunduz AY, Durmaz R. The bacteriome of otitis media with effusion: does it originate from the adenoid? Int J Pediatr Otorhinolaryngol. 2019;126:109624.
47. Binks MJ, Cheng AC, Smith-Vaughan H, Sloots T, Nissen M, Whiley D, et al. Viral-bacterial co-infection in Australian indigenous children with acute otitis media. BMC Infect Dis. 2011;11:161.
48. Minami SB, Mutai H, Suzuki T, Horii A, Oishi N, Wasano K, et al. Microbiomes of the normal middle ear and ears with chronic otitis media. Laryngoscope. 2017;127(10):E371–7.
49. Zhang Y, Xu M, Zhang J, Zeng L, Wang Y, Zheng QY. Risk factors for chronic and recurrent otitis media—a meta-analysis. PLoS One. 2014;9(1):e86397.
50. Pérez-Herrera LC, Peñaranda D, Moreno-López S, Otoya-Tono AM, Gutiérrez-Velasco L, García JM, et al. Associated factors, health-related quality of life, and reported costs of chronic otitis media in adults at two otologic referral centers in a middle-income country. PLoS One. 2020;15(12):e0244797.
51. Oh J, Lee S, Kim MH, Kwag Y, Kim HS, Kim S, et al. The impact of PM2.5 on acute otitis media in children (aged 0–3): a time series study. Environ Int. 2020;145:106133.
52. Kaur R, Morris M, Pichichero ME. Epidemiology of acute otitis media in the postpneumococcal conjugate vaccine era. Pediatrics. 2017;140(3):e20170181.
53. Ladomenou F, Kafatos A, Tselentis Y, Galanakis E. Predisposing factors for acute otitis media in infancy. J Infect. 2010;61(1):49–53.
54. Prins-Van Ginkel AC, Bruijning-Verhagen PCJ, Uiterwaal CSPM, van der Ent CK, Smit HA, de Hoog MLA. Acute otitis media during infancy: parent-reported incidence and modifiable risk factors. Pediatr Infect Dis J. 2017;36(3):245–9.
55. Uhari M, Mantysaari K, Niemela M. A meta-analytic review of the risk factors for acute otitis media [internet]. 1996. http://cid.oxfordjournals.org/.
56. Rovers MM, Numans ME, Langenbach E, Grobbee DE, Verheij TJM, Schilder AGM. Is pacifier use a risk factor for acute otitis media? A dynamic cohort study. Fam Pract. 2008;25(4):233–6.
57. Bowatte G, Tham R, Allen K, Tan D, Lau M, Dai X, et al. Breastfeeding and childhood acute otitis media: a systematic review and meta-analysis. Acta Paediatr. 2015;104:85–95.
58. Rosenfeld RM, Goldsmith AJ, Tetlus L, Balzano A. Quality of life for children with otitis media. Arch Otolaryngol Head Neck Surg [Internet]. 1997;123. http://archotol.jamanetwork.com/.
59. Holl K, Rosenlund M, Giaquinto C, Silfverdal SA, Carmona A, Larcombe J, et al. The impact of childhood acute otitis media on parental quality of life in a prospective observational cohort study. Clin Drug Investig. 2015;35(10):613–24.
60. van Brink J, Gisselsson-Solen M. Quality of life in Swedish children receiving grommets—an analysis of pre- and postoperative results based on a national quality register. Int J Pediatr Otorhinolaryngol. 2019;120:44–50.
61. Kujala T, Alho OP, Kristo A, Uhari M, Renko M, Pokka T, et al. Recurrent acute otitis media detracts from health-related quality of life. J Laryngol Otol. 2017;131(2):128–37.
62. Heidemann CH, Lauridsen HH, Kjeldsen AD, Faber CE, Johansen ECJ, Godballe C. Quality-of-life differences among diagnostic subgroups of children receiving ventilating tubes for otitis media. Otolaryngol Head Neck Surg. 2015;153(4):636–43.
63. Lucidi D, de Corso E, Paludetti G, Sergi B. Quality of life and functional results in canal wall down vs canal wall up mastoidectomy. Acta Otorhinolaryngol Ital. 2019;39(1):53–60.

Importance of Animal Studies in the Understanding of Otitis Media

12

Marcelo Miguel Hueb, Fernanda Rocha Hueb, Marcela Rocha Hueb, and Michael M. Paparella

Introduction

According to biological data, after life on Earth has gone through 4.5 billion years of evolution, our planet has an estimated 8.7 million species, taxonomically classified under the five kingdoms of Fungi, Protista, Monera, Plantae, and Animalia [1, 2], of which 80% live in tropical forests [3]. Recently, Cavalier-Smith's group [4] added three more kingdoms to this taxonomic classification: Archaebacteria, Chromista, and Archezoa. A breakdown of the kingdoms' classification shows seven sequential levels, namely kingdom, phylum, class, order, family, genus, and species.

On top of the kingdoms' classification, Woese and Fox [5] proposed a higher level of three domains on the basis of ribosomal RNA signatures, namely Archaea, Bacteria, and Eukaryotes. Human beings, belonging to the Eukarya domain in the Animalia kingdom, have been subjected to an extensive list of infectious diseases. The UNEP [3] has estimated that about 60% of all infectious diseases known to affect humans are zoonotic, and the number of emerging diseases points to an increasing trend (e.g., coronavirus disease 2019, or COVID-19).

M. M. Hueb (✉)
University of São Paulo, São Paulo, Brazil

ENT Discipline and ENT Service, Federal University of Triângulo Mineiro, Uberaba, Brazil

Hospital Santa Lúcia of Uberaba, Uberaba, Brazil

F. R. Hueb
University of Uberaba, Uberaba, Brazil

M. R. Hueb
University Unilago, São Paulo, Brazil

M. M. Paparella
Department of Otolaryngology, University of Minnesota, Minneapolis, MN, USA

Otopathology Laboratory, University of Minnesota, Minneapolis, MN, USA

The International Hearing Foundation, Minneapolis, MN, USA
e-mail: papar001@umn.edu

Otitis media and its various forms are known to spontaneously affect humans largely through infections by bacterial, viral, or fungal agents. Although a multifaceted disease, otitis media is generally classified, on a clinical or anatomical/histopathological basis, as acute, subacute, or chronic and affects the middle ear cleft, Eustachian tube, and mastoid [6].

Humans, as a part of the vertebrate and placental mammalian class of the Animalia kingdom, share some anatomical, functional, and immunological characteristics with dogs, cats, rats, mice, chinchillas, guinea pigs, monkeys, and so on. On the other hand, in humans, the common bacteria associated with otitis media are not necessarily associated with middle ear infections in other animals; many nonhuman animal models colonized with these bacteria contract middle ear infection through a direct bullae injection or nasopharyngeal inoculation in an unnatural development of the disease. On top of that, these animals experience significantly fewer spontaneous episodes of this disease, with the exception of spontaneous or induced genetic knockout in animal models, where otitis media episodes are far too common.

Although using animal models for otitis media is subject to criticism from political and animal protection groups and to strict legislation, they are relevant sources of valid, focused, and consistent information on an all-too-common disease and have significant health, social, education, labor, and economic implications. Although the findings of these kinds of studies cannot be entirely extrapolated to humans, they do provide undeniably helpful data despite the ethical challenges, especially because such procedures may not be carried out on humans.

Legislation and Ethics in Animal Studies

Animal studies and animal experiments have long been performed in many areas, such as human medicine, dentistry, animal science, veterinary medicine, pharmacology, cosmetics, biotechnology, and agrochemistry, among others. Basic studies on anatomy, physiology, drug responses, behavior,

M. V. Goycoolea et al. (eds.), *Textbook of Otitis Media*, https://doi.org/10.1007/978-3-031-40949-3_12

and so on are used for teaching even today. Other than these, the development of surgical skills and surgical techniques, disease models, drugs and testing, drug interactions, drug tolerance levels, vaccines and testing, induced serum antibodies, and many others have made undeniable contributions to the current state of the art in many fields.

Animal studies in the context of otitis media generally use rodents as living subjects for experimentation because of their known anatomical, genomic, and functional similarities to humans. These animals are small and easy to care for and have high reproduction rates and genetic stability, making them cost-effective and easy to keep in good hygiene and health conditions, as determined by related legislation.

Legislation drawn from ethics committees, welfare acts, and local and federal rules ([7–9] and others) generally advise that any experimental study must have previous ethical approval and adequate documentation for checking, reporting and reproducibility. Animal studies should have minimal time spans to reach their objectives; no animal should be subject to simultaneous or sequential experiments; sedation or anesthesia should be used when pain is possible; and deep anesthesia is needed or recommended when they are sacrificed.

Experimental Models

Many experimental models designed for studying the various forms of otitis media and have been proposed, especially by the Otitis Media Research Group at the University of Minnesota in Minneapolis, United States, focusing on the histology, histopathology, cellular and functional dynamics, immunology, disease induction, biochemistry, and treatment of otitis media.

As a fellow, the main author Marcelo Miguel Hueb (MMH) had the opportunity to work with that group under the guidance of Marcos Goycoolea, the senior author of this book, and also at other University of Minnesota facilities, including the Otopathology Laboratory, under Michael Paparella's guidance. I become acquainted with or participated in experimental studies on the continuum of otitis media after Eustachian tube obstructions [10], acute otitis media induced by microorganisms inoculated into the middle ear [11–14], round window membrane permeability [15–17], inner ear damage caused by otitis media [18–20], the dynamics of microspheres in the middle ear mucosa of Eustachian tube–obstructed animals [21, 22], the efficacy of drug-delivery systems through absorbable membranes [23–25], experimental cholesteatoma induced by a tympanic membrane perforation with epithelial migration through a scaffold and inflammatory process [26–28], studies on cholesterol granuloma [29] and granulation tissues [30], interventions in mucoid otitis media [31], and many others by different authors.

Mimicking the infectious process in humans, some of these studies used bacteria such as *S. pneumoniae*, non-typeable *H. influenzai*, and *M. catharralis* and viruses such as influenza A and respiratory syncytial virus (RSV). As a major etiopathogenetic factor for otitis media, Eustachian tube disfunction was induced in some experiments, also mimicking what happens in humans; this can be achieved through cauterization, mechanical occlusion, ligation, radiation, microorganism inoculation, and mucosa irritation.

It generally leads to an initial stage of subepithelial edema and polymorphonuclear cell infiltration, followed by serous fluid that passively and hydrostatically occupies the middle ear space thanks to negative pressure (serous stage). Later on, chronic inflammatory cells infiltrate the subepithelial layer, and epithelial metaplasia and pseudoglandular formation ensue, along with active effusion production (mucoid stage). In these studies, latex microspheres of different sizes were shown to be phagocyted, to traverse the mucosa, or to traverse the round window membrane into the inner ear. According to these studies, infection and inflammation can be controlled through the use of antibiotics (e.g., ampicillin) delivered via biodegradable membranes.

Eventually, viral or bacterial proliferation occurs in acute cases and in cases of exacerbation in chronic disease. Epithelial breaks due to subepithelial edema or inflammation have led to granulation tissue formation—at the initial stages, they are immature, without an epithelial cover, whereas at later stages, they are mature, with an epithelial cover. Mature granulation tissues and cholesterol granulomas are associated with tissue and bone destruction, which is evident in cases of experimental cholesteatoma. Effusion and the inflammatory process have been shown to act as triggers for epithelial migration to occur through mechanical bridges (e.g., absorbable membranes and mucoid effusion), leading to cholesteatoma formation.

Evolving from this broad and fundamental knowledge, current experimental research has been focused, as it should be, on the safety and efficacy of prevention and also on different treatment alternatives for otitis media. Vaccines, probiotic use, transtympanic injections aiming to elicit topical antimicrobial effects, inflammation control, and biofilm disruption are some of the foci of ongoing studies.

In one study, chinchillas parentally immunized with *H. influenza* type b (Hib) conjugate vaccines were each challenged with an intranasal inoculation of adenovirus and were shown to transudate antibodies into the middle ear effusion [32]. These authors chose the chinchilla animal model for their studies [33] and were able to show efficacy and disease control even when using a transcutaneous route for vaccination in single or polymicrobial models [34–37]. Similar results have been achieved for efficacy and disease control in a mice model with a monovalent (e.g., histidine triad protein D, choline binding protein A, or detoxified pneumolysin) or trivalent pneumococcal protein recombinant vaccine administered intramuscularly [38].

On another study, emerging pathogens in the microbiota of the middle ear in acute otitis media have recently been shown, and studies on its full relevance in the development of or protection against the infectious process are on the way [39]. These authors mentioned several possible probiotic actions (e.g., competition, production of molecules, stimulation of epithelial cells, enhancement of epithelial barriers, modulation of immune system), and according to their study, some of these emerging pathogens could be used for the prevention or treatment of otitis media. The experimental induction of otitis media with effusion has been achieved through intratympanic histamine injection in rats [40]; the authors of that study divided the animals into four groups, and after sacrificing them, the group that received probiotics before and after the histamine injection had the highest mucosa healing, as determined by the presence of effusion and by submucosa neutrophil leukocyte counts.

In another study, transtympanic injections of *Lactobacillus plantarum* in chinchillas have been shown not to affect the inner ear in an animal model, as measured by auditory brainstem responses evaluated before, 7–10 days after, and 28 days after injection [41]. This probiotic is known to decrease *S. aureus* and *P. aeruginosa* growth in mice wounds [42] and therefore seems a promising option for the treatment of chronic suppurative otitis media.

Other than that, even the relationship, population expansion, and infection kinetics between bacterial pathogens can be influenced when wild-type bacteria are replaced by isogenic mutant strains in the transbullar inoculation mixtures of an induced co-infection model of experimental otitis media in chinchillas using nontypeable *H. influenzae* and *M. catarrhalis* and its mutant strains [43]. Another chinchilla study using inoculations of nontypeable *H. influenza* showed that bacterial populations that were able use a phasevarion (phase-variable regulon) induced a more severe disease in this animal model, showing that controlling the bacteria's gene expression could be a promising way to control infection [44].

Maintaining vitamin D levels is also a promising way to control otitis media, as suggested by a rat model that induced otitis media via nontypeable *H. influenza* inoculation, where animals on a vitamin D–deficient diet showed greater mucosal changes, increased expressions of interleukin 6, tumor necrosis factors, and decreased interleukin 10 expression compared to nondeficient rats [45]. These studies substantiate the claim that inducing microbiota competition, gene-expression control, and adequate vitamin D levels can be powerful treatment modalities for otitis media.

Other treatment modalities aiming to control inflammation, as observed in adjuvant therapies with alpha-lipoic acid in a guinea pig model for acute otitis media [46] and surfactant protein D in a mouse model for acute otitis media induced by nontypeable *H. influenza* [47], have shown good control of inflammatory changes. This research group showed in another mouse acute otitis media model induced by nontypeable *H. influenza* inoculation that animals knocked out with surfactant protein A exhibited greater mucosal changes and higher interleukin levels when compared to wild-type mice [48]. Inflammation control was also achieved with caffeic acid phenethyl ester and thymoquinone in a rat model for otitis media with effusion [49]. These studies suggest that inflammation control plays an important role in otitis media treatment.

Also, regarding otitis media treatment models, biofilm formation caused by the most common bacterial pathogens involved in its etiopathogenesis must be taken into consideration. Microbiota competition in this scenario should also be relevant, as it is in coinfections and biofilm disruptions. A recent study using a chinchilla otitis media model has shown the clearance of *H. parainfluenza* from biofilm colonies that had already been establishe when challenged with *H. influenza* [50]. In a recent study, chinchillas immunized with a biofilm-disrupting nontypeable *H. influenza* vaccine antigen were shown to have disrupted biofilms that had previously been formed or prevented their formation from nontypeable *H. influenza* [51]. In another chinchilla model of chronic otitis media with nontypeable *H. influenza*, biofilm formation happened after middle ear inoculation; tympanostomy tubes were placed, and ofloxacin, monoclonal antibodies against DNABII bacterial proteins, or a combination of both were introduced in the middle ears [52]. The animals that received the mixture performed better against biofilm disruption and on bacterial clearance when compared to the single-drug animals.

These experimental studies suggest that modern treatment modalities, or combinations of them, have enormous potential improve quality of life for humans and even other animals afflicted by otitis media in all its forms, and they demonstrate the importance of continuing these kinds of studies in a controlled manner, optimizing or even replacing traditional treatment modalities (e.g., antibiotics).

Future of Animal Studies

The use of animals in teaching, experimentation, and research has decreased over time, although it is still necessary in many areas and situations, as demonstrated above. This need should be carefully considered because animals have been exploited and abused since prehistoric times as sources of food, for sports (e.g., hunting and fights), for labor, sometimes as pets, and so on.

Animal studies provide known/controlled conditions, different groupings for comparisons, and possibilities for longitudinal analysis; however, a large database of previous animal experiments exists, and computer science simulations based on mathematical models can help reduce this need for using animal. Modern laboratory equipment, developments in biology, the genetic sequencing of microorganisms, in vitro studies on cell cultures that can be evaluated even at the molecular level, and bioluminescence for in vivo analyses of infections [53] can be leveraged or conducted. These in turn will lead to more-focused research and will eventually reduce the need for animal sacrifice.

Prioritizing **reduction** and **replacement** when possible and prioritizing **refinement** and **respect** at all times should pave the way for an ethical future in animal studies. A fourth R, for the word **respect**, should be added to the 3R principle of reduction, replacement and refinement (Arouca law: law no. 11.749 in Brazil [8, 9]), such that it would be renamed as the **4R principle** that guide experimental animal studies.

References

1. Whittaker RH. On the broad classification of organisms. Q Rev Biol. 1959;34(3):210–26.
2. Whittaker RH. New concepts of kingdoms or organisms. Evolutionary relations are better represented by new classifications than by the traditional two kingdoms. Science. 1969;163:150–94.
3. UNEP and Biodiversity | UNEP—UN Environment Programme. Accessed 28 Feb 2021.
4. Ruggiero MA, Gordon DP, Orrell TM, et al. A higher level classification of all living organisms. PLoS One. 2015;10(4):e0119248.
5. Woese CR, Fox GE. Phylogenetic structure of the prokaryotic domain: the primary kingdoms. Proc Natl Acad Sci U S A. 1977;74:5088–90.
6. Goycoolea MV, Hueb MM, Ruah CB. Otitis media: the pathogenesis approach. Definitions and terminology. Otolaryngol Clin North Am. 1991;24(4):757–61.
7. Animal Welfare Act, 1966. https://www.nal.usda.gov/awic/animal-welfare-act-public-law-89-544-act-august-24-1966. Accessed 20 Mar 2021.
8. Arouca law, 2008. http://www.planalto.gov.br/ccivil_03/_ato2007-2010/2008/lei/l11794.htm. Accessed 20 Mar 2021.
9. Directive of the European Parliament and of the Council, 2010. https://eur-lex.europa.eu/legal-content/PT/TXT/PDF/?uri=CELEX:32010L0063&from=PT. Accessed 20 Mar 2021.
10. Goycoolea MV, Paparella MM, Carpenter AM, Juhn SK. A longitudinal study of cellular changes in experimental otitis media. Otolaryngol Head Neck Surg. 1979;87:685–700.
11. Giebink GS, Pyne EE, Mills EL, Juhn SK, Quie PG. Experimental otitis media due to Streptococcus pneumoniae: immunopathogenic response in the chinchilla. J Infect Dis. 1976;134:595–604.
12. Giebink GS. Otitis media: the chinchilla model. Microb Drug Resist. 1999;1999(5):57–72.
13. Antonelli PJ, Juhn SK, Goycoolea MV, Giebink GS. Pseudomonas otitis media after eustachian tube obstruction. Otolaryngol Head Neck Surg. 1992;107:511–5.
14. Antonelli PJ, Juhn SK, Goycoolea MV, Giebink GS. Middle ear susceptibility to pseudomonas infection during acute otitis media. Ann Otol Rhinol Laryngol. 1993;102:531–6.
15. Goldberg B, Goycoolea MV, Schleivert PM, Shea D, Schachern P, Paparella MM, Carpenter AM. Passage of albumin from the middle ear to the inner ear in otitis media in the chinchilla. Am J Otolaryngol. 1981;2:210–4.
16. Goycoolea MV, Carpenter AM, Muchow D. Ultrastructural studies of the round-window membrane of the cat. Arch Otolaryngol Head Neck Surg. 1987;113:617–24.
17. Goycoolea MV, Muchow D, Schachern P. Experimental studies on round window structure: function and permeability. Laryngoscope. 1988;98:1–20.
18. Morizono T, Giebink GS, Paparella MM, Sikora MA, Shea D. Sensorineural hearing loss in experimental purulent otitis media due to Streptococcus pneumoniae. Arch Otolaryngol. 1985;111:794–8.
19. Juhn SK, Hamaguchi Y, Jung TTK. Biochemistry of middle ear effusion. In: Bernstein JM, Ogra PL, editors. Immunology of the ear. New York: Raven Press; 1987. p. 319–29.
20. Juhn SK, Hamaguchim Y, Goycoolea MV. Review of round window membrane permeability. Acta Otolaryngol. 1989;475:43–8.
21. Hueb MM, Goycoolea MV, Ruah CB, Muchow D. Dynamics of micro spheres in the inflamed middle ear mucosa. In: Lim DJ, editor. Recent advances in otitis media. Hamilton: BC Decker; 1993. p. 340–2.
22. Hueb MM, Goycoolea MV, Ruah CB, Muchow DC. Permeability of the mucoperiosteum in otitis media. An experimental study in the cat. Braz J Otolaryngol. 1993;59:17–24.
23. Goycoolea MV, Muchow DC, Sirvio LM, Winandy RM, Canafax D, Hueb MM. Extended middle ear drug delivery. A new concept; a new device. Acta Otolaryngol. 1992;493:119–26.
24. Hueb MM, Goycoolea MV, Muchow DC, Ruah CB. Efficacy of middle ear drug delivery systems. A comparative study on poly-l-lactic acid and collagen-based biomaterial membranes. Braz J Otolaryngol. 1992;58:198–204.
25. Goycoolea MV, Muchow D, Hueb MM, Ruah CB. Sustained release of ampicillin in the middle ear using a reconstituted collagen membrane. An experimental study in the cat. In: Lim DJ, editor. Recent advances in otitis media. Hamilton: BC Decker; 1993. p. 277–9.
26. Hueb MM, Goycoolea MV, Muchow DC, Duvall AJ, Paparella MM, Sheridan C. In search of missing links in otology III. Development of a new animal model for cholesteatoma. Laryngoscope. 1993;103:774–84.
27. Hueb MM, Goycoolea MV, Muchow D. Padrões de migração epitelial em colesteatoma adquirido: um estudo experimental. Braz J Otolaryngol. 1994;60:186–94.
28. Goycoolea MV, Hueb MM, Muchow D, Paparella MM. The theory of the trigger, the bridge and the transmigration in the pathogenesis of acquired cholesteatoma. Acta Otolaryngol. 1999;119:244–8.
29. Ruah CB, Hueb MM, Goycoolea MV, Muchow DC, Paparella MM. Cholesterol granuloma: insights on pathogenesis. In: Lim DJ, editor. Recent advances in otitis media. Hamilton: BC Decker; 1993. p. 348–52.
30. Hueb MM, Goycoolea MV, Paparella MM, Muchow DC. Experimental studies of the pathogenesis of granulation tissue in the middle ear. In: Lim DJ, editor. Recent advances in otitis media. Hamilton: BC Decker; 1996. p. 451–7.
31. Hueb MM, Goycoolea MV. Experimental evidence for early intervention in mucoid otitis media. Acta Otolaryngol. 2009;129:444–8.
32. Bakaletz LO, Holmes KA. Evidence for transudation of specific antibody into the middle ears of parenterally immunized chinchillas after an upper respiratory tract infection with adenovirus. Clin Diagn Lab Immunol. 1997;4:223–5.
33. Bakaletz LO. Chinchilla as a robust, reproducible and polymicrobial model of otitis media and its prevention. Expert Rev Vaccines. 2009;8:1063–82.
34. Novotny LA, Clements JD, Bakaletz LO. Transcutaneous immunization as preventative and therapeutic regimens to protect against experimental otitis media due to nontypeable *Haemophilus influenzae*. Mucosal Immunol. 2011;4:456–67.

35. Novotny LA, Clements JD, Bakaletz LO. Kinetic analysis and evaluation of the mechanisms involved in the resolution of experimental nontypeable *Haemophilus influenzae*-induced otitis media after transcutaneous immunization. Vaccine. 2013;31:3417–26.
36. Novotny LA, Clements JD, Bakaletz LO. Therapeutic transcutaneous immunization with a band-aid vaccine resolves experimental otitis media. Clin Vaccine Immunol. 2015;22:867–74.
37. Novotny LA, Clements JD, Goodman SD, Bakaletz LO. Transcutaneous immunization with a band-aid prevents experimental otitis media in a polymicrobial model. Clin Vaccine Immunol. 2017;24:6.
38. Xu Q, Pryharski K, Pichichero ME. Trivalent pneumococcal protein vaccine protects against experimental acute otitis media caused by Streptococcus pneumoniae in an infant murine model. Vaccine. 2017;35:337–44.
39. van den Broek MFL, De Boeck I, Kiekens F, Boudewyns A, Vanderveken OM, Lebeer S. Translating recent microbiome insights in otitis media into probiotic strategies. Clin Microbiol Rev. 2019;32:1–33.
40. Kaytez SK, Ocal R, Yumusak N, Celik H, Arslan N, Ibas M. Effect of probiotics in experimental otitis media with effusion. Int J Pediatr Otorhinolaryngol. 2020;132:109922.
41. Nhan C, Bezdjian A, Saha S, Prakash S, Nguyen LHP, Daniel SJ. Safety of transtympanic application of probiotics in a chinchilla animal model. J Otolaryngol Head Neck Surg. 2017;46:63.
42. Al-Mathkury HJF, Al-Aubeidi HJR. Probiotic effect of lactobacilli on mice in wound infections. J Al-Nahrain Univ. 2008;11:111–6.
43. Lakhani V, Tan L, Mukherjee S, Stewart WCL, Swords WE, Das J. Mutations in bacterial genes induce unanticipated changes in the relationship between bacterial pathogens in experimental otitis media. R Soc Open Sci. 2018;5(11):180810.
44. Brockman KL, Jurcisek JA, Atack JM, Srikhanta YN, Jennings MP, Bakaletz LO. ModA2 Phasevarion switching in nontypeable Haemophilus influenzae increases the severity of experimental otitis media. J Infect Dis. 2016;214(5):817–24.
45. Kim HB, Lim SH, Cho CG, Choi HS. Influence of vitamin D deficiency on progression of experimental otitis media in rats. Endocrinol Metab. 2018;33:296–304.
46. Tatar A, Korkmaz M, Yayla M, Gozeler MS, Mutlu V, Halici Z, Uslu H, Korkmaz H, Selli J. Anti-inflammatory and anti-oxidative effects of alpha-lipoic acid in experimentally induced acute otitis media. J Laryngol Otol. 2016;130:616–23.
47. Abdel-Razek O, Liu T, Chen X, Wang Q, Vanga G, Wang G. Role of surfactant protein D in experimental otitis media. J Innate Immun. 2021;8:1–14.
48. Abdel-Razek O, Ni L, Yang F, Wang G. Innate immunity of surfactant protein A in experimental otitis media. Innate Immun. 2019;25:391–400.
49. Gülmez Mİ, Okuyucu Ş, Dokuyucu R, Gökçe H. The effect of caffeic acid phenethyl ester and thymoquinone on otitis media with effusion in rats. Int J Pediatr Otorhinolaryngol. 2017;96:94–9.
50. Pang B, Swords WE. Haemophilus parainfluenzae strain ATCC 33392 forms biofilms *in vitro* and during experimental otitis media infections. Infect Immun. 2017;85(9):01070–16.
51. Bailey MT, Lauber CL, Novotny LA, Goodman SD, Bakaletz LO. Immunization with a biofilm-disrupting nontypeable Haemophilus influenzae vaccine antigen did not alter the gut microbiome in chinchillas, unlike oral delivery of a broad-spectrum antibiotic commonly used for otitis media. mSphere. 2020;5(2):e00296–20.
52. Novotny LA, Chiang T, Goodman SD, Elmaraghy CA, Bakaletz LO. Humanized anti- DNABII Fab fragments plus ofloxacin eradicated biofilms in experimental otitis media. Laryngoscope. 2021;131(10):E2698–704. https://doi.org/10.1002/lary.29497. Epub ahead of print.
53. Avci P, Karimi M, Sadasivam M, Antunes-Melo WC, Carrasco E, Hamblin MR. In-vivo monitoring of infectious diseases in living animals using bioluminescence imaging. Virulence. 2018;9:28–63.

Critical Appraisal of Published Research in Otitis Media or How to Sort the Wheat from the Chaff!

13

Joel Lavinsky, Vagner Antonio Rodrigues da Silva, and Luiz Lavinsky

Introduction

While we have witnessed considerable growth in the number of publications related to otitis media, this does not necessarily constitute a proportional step up in the quality of what is being published. Busy clinicians often lack the time required for interpretation and critical appraisal of publications and therefore rely on opinion formers in the area to publish guidelines or review articles. However, delegating interpretation to third parties exposes it to certain risks since such analyses may be biased by personal positions. It is therefore essential that clinicians are trained to be able to go directly to the original source and interpret results in a manner analogous to the approach they adopt when, starting with the clinical examination of a patient, they follow a process culminating in establishing the correct diagnosis. Clinicians should be capable of delving deeper into the data presented in a publication than can be achieved by merely reading the abstract.

One fundamental concept that clinicians must internalize is that not everything that is published is necessarily reliable, even if it has been peer-reviewed, published in a scientific journal of international renown, or has a high impact factor. This chapter is therefore intended to provide tools and strategies to enable clinicians to conduct their own critical analyses of publications on otitis media and select what they should actually incorporate into their clinical practice.

The first task is to select articles that merit reading in depth. On PubMed, a search using the terms "otitis" AND "media" returns a total of 31,347 publications. We must therefore be a little more specific with regard to the subject we are interested in, such as "acute otitis media", "chronic otitis media", or "otitis media with effusion". However, even these terms return lists of thousands of publications, so we need to apply filters based on the period of publication and type of study (meta-analysis, randomized clinical trial, literature review, etc.). This strategy can narrow our search and help us separate out those publications that are worth the effort of exploring in greater detail.

The subject of otitis media is undoubtedly the most advanced area within otorhinolaryngology in terms of incorporating the concepts of evidence-based medicine. For decades, management of acute otitis media and otitis media with effusion has been based on the results of large randomized clinical trials and meta-analyses. As a result, this is where we will find the studies considered to have the highest evidence levels, in particular because of the high prevalence of these diseases in the population. In contrast, in the area of chronic otitis media, it is more difficult to produce large-scale randomized clinical trials, both because of its lower prevalence and also because of the highly heterogeneous nature of clinical presentation and course in this population. The great majority of studies of surgical treatment for chronic otitis media are therefore retrospective observational studies. Even so, several randomized clinical trials have been conducted in the area over recent years, especially for the evaluation of surgical techniques.

Irrespective of the subject being studied, reading any article should always adhere to the principles of reading with

J. Lavinsky (✉)
Federal University of Rio Grande do Sul, Porto Alegre, RS, Brazil

Santa Casa de Porto Alegre, Porto Alegre, Brazil

V. A. R. da Silva
State University of Campinas (Unicamp), Campinas, Brazil

Faculty of Medical Sciences—UNICAMP, Campinas, Brazil

L. Lavinsky
Federal University of Rio Grande do Sul, School of Medicine, Porto Alegre, Brazil

Sul-Rio-Grandense Academy of Medicine, Porto Alegre, Brazil

M. V. Goycoolea et al. (eds.), *Textbook of Otitis Media*, https://doi.org/10.1007/978-3-031-40949-3_13

critical analysis that takes into account the size of the study, its clinical relevance, and the capacity for generalization of results. The act of reading a scientific article cannot be passive but must include a critical interpretation of the data presented. Furthermore, it is important to emphasize that a single study in isolation should not be enough to definitively change our practice. We need additional evidence that presents the results in a reproducible form and, when possible, in meta-analyses that support the findings.

Which Articles Should I Choose to Read?

Starting from a list of tens or hundreds of publications on otitis media, the initial selection will be based on the titles and abstracts. Providing that the author has been able to express it adequately, the relevance of what an article will present can be discerned from its title. An abstract that manages to clearly summarize the objectives and results increases the probability that the article is of interest for more in-depth reading.

As we select the articles, we can rapidly read through them to identify the basic elements that should be part of all scientific publications. The introduction should be clear, concise, and logical and should end by stating the primary objective of the research. The methods should be described in sufficient detail to enable the study to be reproduced. The results must be well organized and presented. The discussion section should integrate the results with those of the extant literature on the subject. The conclusions must follow the research objectives and be supported by the results.

Gehlbach [1] compares reading an article to eating a meal. The title is the menu, and the abstract is the taster for the dishes. However, this is not close enough to a meal to satisfy. The introduction to the article introduces the appetizers, which, when well served, increase the diner's appetite for the main course. The methods and results represent the main course and need to be well digested and analyzed. The discussion represents the dessert and can be rich in creativity and speculation. In some cases, it may be the part of the meal that is most appreciated, but it is not the most nutritious.

Once we have chosen which articles we will read in depth, we need to train ourselves to conduct a critical reading of a given publication. These considerations apply equally to articles on otitis media and to those on any other topic.

The impact factor of a given scientific journal may be indicative of an article's quality, but it is not a determinant factor. This can be exemplified by articles published on the subject of acute otitis media, which have wide coverage in many areas of medicine (otorhinolaryngology, pediatrics, family medicine, etc.), compared with the limited audience for articles on surgical treatment of chronic otitis media, which is restricted in interest to otological surgeons. As a result, it is easier to publish articles on acute otitis media in high-impact scientific journals compared with articles on surgical subjects. It is also important to take into account the credibility of the authors and the institution that promoted the research.

A study's evidence level may be related to the importance of a given publication. Figure 13.1 shows a diagram illustrating evidence levels, but these are not always a determinant factor in the quality of a publication. The fact is that a randomized clinical trial is not necessarily better than a cohort study. We could have a randomized clinical trial with several selection or measurement biases, for example. Conversely, we could have a large, well-delineated cohort with good follow-up.

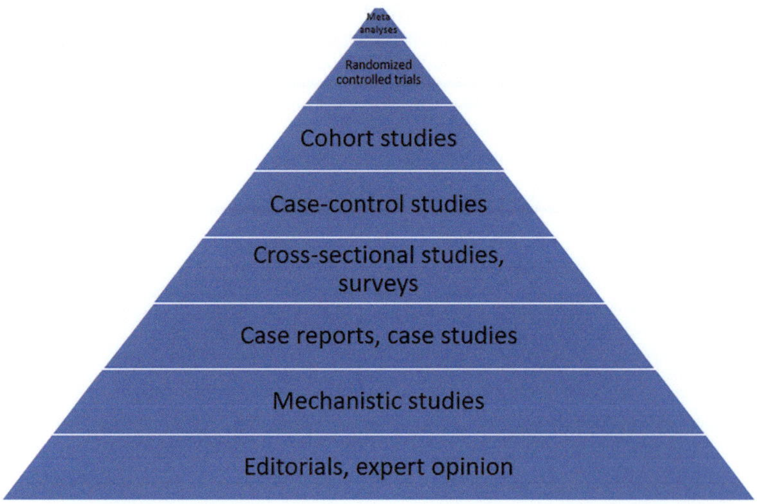

Fig. 13.1 Pyramid of scientific evidence with hierarchy of different types of publication in the literature

Methodology

The methodology is a crucial section of any scientific article, and so here we can already get a good preview of the quality of what will be presented further on. In this section, we will read how the research was conducted, and the proper critical analysis begins with the methods.

The first point is to check how the data were collected. As a general rule, prospective intervention studies yield higher-quality data because data collection is conducted under more carefully controlled conditions, as seen in randomized clinical trials. In contrast, the data used in retrospective studies generally come from medical records or are based on the research participants' recollections, thus increasing the probability of biases. For example, there will be less precision in a subjective assessment of the degree of otalgia during an episode of acute otitis media that occurred in the past or was recorded in medical records in an uncontrolled manner when compared with the collection of the same data as part of a prospective follow-up of the episode by a single evaluator trained for this purpose. This does not mean that data collected retrospectively is unreliable, but, in general, it is of lower quality when compared to intervention studies.

Articles on the treatment of otitis media should ideally include a group for comparison. If not, the study will simply be a description of a case series without the capacity to provide data on associations or efficacy. A comparison of different clinical and surgical treatments is essential to establishing reliable conclusions. When possible, a placebo control can amplify the assessment of the efficacy of the different treatments studied. Considering that untreated acute otitis media (adopting a "watchful waiting" approach) tends to have favorable outcomes, the inclusion of a control group is considered even more important. Along the same lines, it is to be expected that the number of recurrent infections reduces as children grow and their immune systems mature, and otitis media with effusion can also be expected to resolve as children grow and tube function improves. Therefore, a control group enables an adequate comparison with the natural history of otitis media.

Relationships of causality can be assessed to test hypotheses, either prospectively or retrospectively. Cross-sectional studies do not provide grounds for drawing conclusions of causality but only for the identification of associations, as in research investigating diagnostic tests or prevalence studies.

According to the CONSORT recommendations [2], randomization is generally an excellent strategy for achieving a better balance between potential factors of bias across different groups. This is why nonrandomized studies may need to adjust for confounding factors. However, this does not mean that just because a study is a randomized clinical trial, it is guaranteed to be of good quality; it just means that an observational study is not as reliable. Randomization is only one part of the methodology, and so it is also essential that the other methods are appropriate. In addition to randomization, blinding is also considered important and, preferably, should be conducted in such a manner that neither subjects nor investigators know which group participants are allocated to ("double blinding"). Finally, the analysis should ideally be on an "intention-to-treat" basis, that is, the analysis should include all subjects, even those who did not adhere to the treatment. This is considered very important in studies of acute otitis media because there are often failures to follow the treatment correctly.

As already mentioned, a randomized clinical trial is not always the best study design. For studies investigating treatments, such as the management of acute otitis media, a randomized clinical trial will certainly yield the best evidence. However, a cross-sectional design is more appropriate for studies conducted to evaluate diagnostic tests, such as the determination of the sensitivity and specificity of computed tomography for intracranial complications of acute mastoiditis, for example. In turn, cohort studies may be the most appropriate design if the objective is to assess prognosis, such as the risk of delayed speech acquisition among individuals with otitis media with effusion. As such, the level of evidence does not necessarily prove that a study has a better design. However, as a general rule, when discussing treatments, a randomized clinical trial is considered the most appropriate strategy for assessing the therapeutic effects of a given intervention.

The measurement method is considered an important part of the methodology, especially in relation to otitis media. Standardization of the method is a fundamental element in guaranteeing the reproducibility of the results in other studies. Instruments for documenting otoscopy findings, audiometers, the collection of samples from the middle ear, and imaging exams are some examples of methods frequently used in research into otitis media. Similarly, the methodology for measuring subjective data such as otalgia and other symptoms should also be standardized, whether collected prospectively or retrospectively. For example, it is unacceptable for a study investigating otitis media to assess the degree of otalgia in a haphazard manner. The preferred method is to use a visual analog scale. It is also recommended that a single model of audiometer be employed and that it be duly calibrated.

In surgical studies, such as those of chronic otitis media, standardization of the intervention is very often difficult because neither the surgeons nor the pathologies encountered intraoperatively are uniform. For example, when assessing the surgical treatment of individuals with uncomplicated chronic otitis media, perforations of the tympanum may have different shapes, positions, and sizes. Along the same lines, cholesteatoma is highly variable in terms of the route of formation, its extent, and its aggressiveness. In the case of tympanic membrane retraction, variations can be even greater. As a result, it is very difficult to generalize the conclusions drawn from a limited sample of surgical interventions.

It is important that the methods section present the provenance of the research participants and the inclusion and exclusion criteria. For randomized clinical trials, it is recommended that a flow diagram be constructed to illustrate how individuals were selected and the methods used for randomization. Additionally, the methods used to blind the membership of the intervention and control groups should be covered. When possible, the sample size calculation should be included in the methods because a sample that is too small can lead to type II error, which occurs if a null hypothesis is not rejected despite being false in the population. The statistical analysis methods must also be fully described in the methods section.

Results

It is very important for clinicians to be able to interpret the results through an understanding of the basic concepts of descriptive and analytical statistics.

One important concept is how to differentiate between a statistically significant difference and a clinically relevant difference. We may observe a p-value of <0.05 but find that the difference between groups is small in percentage terms, that is, a large number of individuals would have to be treated to benefit a small number of them. The larger the sample size, the easier it is to attain significant p values with relatively small percentage differences. This is why research into otitis media often employs the number necessary to treat (NNT). This value shows how many people would have to be given a certain intervention to achieve an outcome for one person. This is an important public health strategy. For example, it has been estimated that it is necessary to prescribe 2500 antibiotic courses for acute otitis media to prevent one episode of acute mastoiditis [3]. This is why cases of acute mastoiditis continue to occur during treatment with antibiotics despite the routine use of antibiotics for acute otitis media.

Effect sizes based on NNT are highly relative. These analyses are dependent on the severity of the disease and the side effects of the treatment. In the case of otitis media, and specifically in relation to antibiotic therapy, there is an intense debate about the effects on the community caused by increased bacterial resistance. Often, the NNT may not be available in publications on otitis media; only relative measures of effect size, such as relative risk or odds ratio, are available, which are no help in determining the impact oftreatment on the population level. In such cases, the NNT can be calculated as the inverse of the absolute risk reduction (ARR), that is, the absolute difference in the occurrence of events between the treatment group and the control group.

It is also important that the results are presented well in tables and figures to facilitate understanding of the study findings. Figure legends should be clear.

Internal Validity

Internal validity is related to the measurement methodology and the appropriate analysis of results. In the case of studies of otitis media, audiometric and otoscopic analysis, for example, are often used. These instruments must be valid, precise, and reproducible.

Along the same lines, an appropriate design is crucial for a study to have internal validity. It is also essential that the statistical tests employed are compatible with the analysis proposed. Consideration should be given to whether observations are interrelated or independent samples, whether the objective is to compare groups or associate an outcome with one or more predictive variables, and to the measurement of continuous variables.

External Validity

Assuming that the study has internal validity, the next step is to determine whether the results can be generalized to the universe beyond the study. This is closely related to the sampling process and especially to the use of representative and broad samples. A sample considered representative starts with careful selection on the basis of appropriate inclusion and exclusion criteria. One example of this would be to analyze the efficacy of a new antibiotic for the treatment of acute otitis media using a sample in which 90% of subjects are institutionalized and have Down syndrome. In such a case, the results of the study would not be generalizable to the population. External validity is greatly compromised if the investigators choose their sample based on convenience or subjective judgments. Additionally, highly restrictive exclusion criteria impede adequate generalization of the results.

Precision is a very important aspect and is based on the number of observations, that is, on the sample size. A larger sample size can be associated with reduced variability in observations through increased precision. The result is to narrow the 95% confidence interval and increase our confidence in the results.

The discussion gives the author an opportunity to evaluate the results and relate them to published data. This section may present speculations about the study, limitations, and future directions for a given investigation. It is important that the conclusions be based on the objectives and results of the study. The references should be presented in an up-to-date manner and, preferably, cover what is most relevant in the area.

Studies with In Vivo Experiments

Much important research into otitis media comes from animal experimentation studies. As is the case for clinical studies, guidelines containing recommendations for the publication of experimental research also exist. The ARRIVE 2.0 guidelines [4] deal with the format of scientific articles describing studies with animals. To a certain extent, they stipulate that studies should be reported with sufficient data to contribute to existing knowledge, enabling readers and reviewers to analyze the study in an appropriate manner and assess its methodological rigor while enabling the reproduction of the methods and results.

These guidelines are considered important for any study in the life sciences involving live animals, from mammals to fish. The guidelines are divided into two blocks, with no hierarchy. They are considered useful both when writing a manuscript to guarantee that it contains all of the relevant information and when reviewing a manuscript to check that all of the relevant information is available for assessment of the study.

There is a minimum set of 10 items considered essential to be included in the manuscript. If these data are not provided, readers and reviewers will not be able to assess the reliability of the results.

(a) Study design: When there are comparisons between groups, a control group should be included. If one is not used, this should be justified.
(b) Sample size: The exact number of experimental units in each group and the total number in each experiment should be specified, in addition to the total number of animals used. It should also be demonstrated how the sample size was established using the sample size calculation.
(c) Exclusion and inclusion criteria: It is recommended that any criteria used for including or excluding animals be described, especially if these criteria were defined a priori. For each experimental group, the reasons for exclusions and the exact value of n in each experimental group should be reported.
(d) Randomization: If randomization was used, the method employed to generate the randomization sequence should be described. The strategy used to minimize potential confounding variables, such as animals' locations in the animal house, should also be described.
(e) Blinding: It is recommended that who was aware of the allocation of experimental units at different stages of the experiment be stated.
(f) Outcomes: All outcomes assessed should be defined, and the primary outcome used to calculate the sample size should be specified.
(g) Statistical methods: It is recommended that details be provided on the statistical methods used for each analysis, especially the software employed.
(h) Experimental animals: Details should be provided of the species of animals used, including strain, substrain, age, and sex. Further information on the provenance of animals should be given and, if possible, health status and genotyping.
(i) Experimental procedures: All procedures should be described in enough detail to allow reproducibility, including materials used, frequency, locations, and reasons.
(j) Results: For each experiment, summary/descriptive statistics should be reported for each experimental group with a measure of variability where possible (mean, standard deviation, and median). The effect size and confidence interval should also be provided.

There is another list of items defined as the recommended set, including elements such as a precise abstract, a clear scientific background, a definition of objectives, an ethical statement, housing and husbandry conditions, care and monitoring of animals, interpretation and scientific implications, applicability and translation, protocol registration, free access to data, and a declaration of interests.

Randomized Clinical Trials

Treatment of otitis media has advanced greatly with the publication of large-scale randomized clinical trials over recent decades. We now have answers to the majority of questions about the treatment of acute otitis media and otitis media with effusion. For chronic otitis media, there is a growing effort to publish more clinical trials on which to base clinical and surgical decisions. However, we must be careful about the quality of randomized clinical trials that are being published. There is a checklist of the information that should be included in the publication that can be used to verify this, based on the CONSORT 2010 Statement [5]. As with ARRIVE 2.0, CONSORT considers that the results of a randomized clinical trial should enable readers to understand the study design, analysis, and interpretation. The checklist covers 25 items, the presentation of which is considered essential to the reliability of the results, especially in relation to the effects of a given treatment.

(a) Title and abstract: It is recommended that the study title identify it as a randomized clinical trial. The abstract should cover the trial design, methods, results, and conclusions.
(b) Introduction: This should include the scientific background and explanation of the rationale, specific objectives, and hypotheses.
(c) Study design: Description of trial design, such as parallel, including allocation ratio. Additionally, important changes to methods after the clinical study's outset, such as eligibility criteria, are explained.
(d) Participants: The methods section should clearly define the eligibility criteria for participants, with information on the locations where the data were collected.
(e) Interventions: The interventions for each group, with sufficient details to allow replication, including when they took place.
(f) Outcomes: Primary and secondary outcomes were defined in advance, including how they were assessed. Any changes to outcomes after the clinical trial has commenced should also be stated.
(g) Sample size: State how the sample size was determined and whether there were any trial-stopping guidelines.
(h) Randomization sequence generation: Show the method used to generate the allocation randomization sequence. Types of randomization, such as simple or blocking.
(i) Allocation: Mechanism employed to implement the random allocation sequence (such as sequentially numbered containers), describing the steps taken to conceal the sequence until interventions were assigned.
(j) Implementation of allocation: State who generated the random allocation sequence, who enrolled participants, and who assigned participants to interventions.
(k) Blinding: If done, who was blinded after the assignment to interventions, and how was this done?
(l) Statistical methods: Describe the statistical methods used to compare groups for primary and secondary outcomes, as well as for subgroup analyses and adjusted analyses.
(m) Participant flow: It is strongly recommended that a diagram be used. Show the numbers of participants who were randomly assigned, received the treatment assigned, and were analyzed for the primary outcome. For each group, show losses and exclusions after randomization with their respective reasons.
(n) Recruitment: Define when participants were recruited and follow-up times. State the reasons for ending or stopping the trial.
(o) Baseline data: Include a table showing baseline demographic and clinical characteristics for each group.
(p) Numbers analyzed: For each group, the number of participants in each analysis with the denominator.
(q) Outcomes and estimates: For each primary and secondary outcome, the results for each group and the estimated effect size and its respective precision (95% confidence interval). For binary outcomes, it is recommended that both absolute and relative effect sizes are presented.
(r) Ancillary analyses: Subgroup analyses and adjusted analyses, distinguishing prespecified from exploratory.
(s) Harms: All important harms or unintended effects in each group.
(t) Limitations: Indicate trial limitations, including sources of potential bias and imprecision.
(u) Generalization: Describe the external validity and applicability of the clinical trial findings.
(v) Interpretation: Interpretation consistent with the results, with a balance of benefits and harms.
(w) Registration: Registration number and name of the registered clinical trial.
(x) Protocol: State where the full clinical trial protocol can be accessed.
(y) Funding: State the sources of funding and other support, and the role of funders.

This CONSORT checklist enables the reader of a randomized clinical trial of otitis media to check that it meets all of the criteria recommended to consider it an appropriate publication to possibly influence clinical practice.

Systematic Reviews and Meta-Analyses

Systematic reviews and meta-analyses have been crucial in defining otitis media management practice. They are used as the starting point for developing instructions for clinical practices. Guidelines for the publication of systematic reviews and meta-analyses have been constructed based on the definitions used by the Cochrane Collaboration. A systematic review is a review of a clearly formulated question that employs systematic and explicit methods to identify, select, and critically evaluate relevant research and collect and analyze data from these studies, which are included in the review. Statistical methods (meta-analysis) may or may not be used to analyze and summarize the results of the studies included. Meta-analysis is the use of statistical techniques to integrate the results of the studies included in a systematic review.

An executive committee evaluated which items were crucial for systematic reviews and meta-analyses to be considered satisfactory, developing the PRISMA statement [6], which defines the following checklist:

(a) Title: The title should identify the report as a systematic review, meta-analysis, or both.

(b) Abstract: Should include a structured summary covering theoretical background, data sources, eligibility criteria, participants, interventions, study appraisal and synthesis methods, results, limitations, conclusions, and registration number.
(c) Rationale: Describe the rationale for the review in the context of what is already known.
(d) Objectives: Make an explicit statement of questions such as participants, interventions, comparisons, outcomes, and study design.
(e) Protocol and registration: Indicate whether a review protocol exists that can be accessed and provide information about the registration of the review.
(f) Eligibility criteria: Define characteristics of the study and the report, such as eligibility criteria with rationale.
(g) Information sources: Describe all information sources used in the search (database, contact with authors) and the date of the most recent search.
(h) Search: State the complete electronic search strategy, including limits, so it can be repeated.
(i) Study selection: State the process for selecting studies, that is, the search for eligible studies.
(j) Data collection process: Methods for extracting data from articles and processes for obtaining and confirming data from researchers.
(k) List of data items: List all variables collected, with references or simplifications.
(l) Risk of bias in each study: Describe the methods used to assess the risk of bias in each study and how this information was used in the analysis of the data.
(m) Summary measures: Should define the principal measures for summarizing results.
(n) Synthesis of results: Describe the methods for analyzing data and combining the results of studies with measures of consistency for each meta-analysis.
(o) Risk of bias across studies: It is recommended that any assessment of the risk of bias that may affect the cumulative evidence, such as publication bias, be specified.
(p) Additional analyses: All additional methods of analysis should be described, and those that were prespecified should be identified.
(q) Study selection: The results should state the number of studies screened, assessed for eligibility, and included in the review.
(r) Study characteristics: For each study, present characteristics for data extraction with their respective citations.
(s) Risk of bias for each study and between studies: It is recommended that data on risk of bias for each study and outcome be presented in the results.
(t) Results of individual studies: For each study and for all outcomes considered, present a simple summary of data for each intervention group and effect estimates and confidence intervals using forest plots.
(u) Synthesis of results: Present results for each meta-analysis conducted, including confidence intervals and measures of consistency.
(v) Additional analyses: Present additional analyses such as subgroup analyses and meta-regressions.
(w) Summary of evidence: It is recommended that the main findings be summarized, especially the strength of evidence for each outcome and its relevance to key groups.
(x) Limitations: Discuss limitations at the level of studies and outcomes and at the review level.
(y) Conclusions: Give a general interpretation of the results and their relationship to other evidence. Similarly, state the implications for future research.
(z) Funding: Declare sources of funding and the role of funders in the review.

Publications in the form of meta-analyses and systematic reviews are increasingly common in the area of otitis media. We therefore consider that it is important that readers are familiar with the PRISMA guidelines to enable them to use the checklist to critically appraise a meta-analysis or systematic review.

Observational Studies

The majority of studies of otitis media are observational, especially those conducted in the past. Such studies are essential to enable us to understand the many different clinical entities related to otitis media and enable developments in the area to be achieved through intervention studies. However, it is common for observational studies to be conducted inappropriately, making it less likely that correct extrapolation will be possible. An initiative known as Strengthening the Reporting of Observational Studies in Epidemiology (STROBE) published a 22-item checklist named the STROBE Statement, containing recommendations on what should be included in a more precise and complete description of such studies [7].

(a) Title and abstract: Indicate the study design in the title or abstract. Provide an informative and balanced summary in the abstract.
(b) Rationale: Include in the introduction the theoretical background and the reasons for the research.
(c) Objectives: State the specific objectives and hypotheses.
(d) Study design: The methods should describe the key elements of the study design.

(e) Setting: Describe the setting with locations and important dates, with periods of recruitment, exposure, follow-up, and data collection.
(f) Participants: For cohort studies, present the eligibility criteria, sources, and methods of selection of participants and follow-up. For case-control studies, present the eligibility criteria and the sources and diagnostic criteria for the separation of cases from controls. For cross-sectional studies, present the eligibility criteria and the sources and methods of selection of participants. In cohort studies and paired case-control studies, criteria for pairing and the number of exposed and non-exposed participants should be given.
(g) Variables: All outcomes should be clearly defined, with exposures, predictors, confounders, and effect modifiers. Diagnostic criteria likewise.
(h) Data sources and measurement: For each variable, the source of data and details of assessment methods are described.
(i) Bias: List all methods used to avoid potential sources of bias.
(j) Study size: The sample size should be clearly defined.
(k) Quantitative variables: It is recommended that the way that quantitative variables were treated and any categorizations used should be explained.
(l) Statistical methods: It is recommended that all statistical methods and the control of confounding factors be described. Likewise, describes subgroup and interaction analyses, how missing data were dealt with, losses to follow-up in cohort studies, pairing of cases and controls, sampling strategies, and sensitivity analyses.
(m) Participants: Number of participants in each stage and number who completed follow-up.
(n) Descriptive data: Demographic characteristics of participants and information on exposures and confounders. State the number of participants with missing data for each variable. For cohort studies, it is essential to state the follow-up time.
(o) Outcomes: Number of outcome events or summary measures over time for cohort studies. For case-control studies, the number of participants in each exposure category. For cross-sectional studies, the number of outcome events or summary measures.
(p) Main results: Estimates unadjusted and, if necessary, adjusted for confounding variables. If continuous variables were categorized, state the cut-offs used. If possible, transform relative risk estimates into absolute risk.
(q) Other analyses: Report on any analyses of subgroups that have been conducted.
(r) Key results: In the discussion, it is recommended that the main findings be related to the study objectives.
(s) Limitations: In the discussion, it is recommended that limitations be discussed, especially potential biases or imprecision.
(t) Interpretation: The interpretation of results should be cautious, taking into account objectives, limitations, multiplicity of analyses, and results of similar studies.
(u) Generalization: The external validity of the results should be discussed.
(v) Funding: State sources of study funding and the role of funders.

Conclusions

The objective of this chapter was to present an organized strategy for conducting a critical analysis of a scientific publication, specifically for the otitis media area, in which there have been significant increases in both the quantity and quality of publications over recent years. Researchers and clinicians thus have the tools to independently form their own opinions on the scientific content they analyze and incorporate this knowledge into their practice when they consider it truly relevant.

References

1. Gelbach SH. Interpreting the medical literature. 4th ed. Norwalk: Appleton & Lange; 2002.
2. Consolidated Standards of Reporting Trials, Altman DG, et al. The revised CONSORT statement for reporting randomized trials. Ann Intern Med. 2001;134:663–94.
3. Kassirer JP, Campion EW. Peer review: crude and understudied, but indispensable. JAMA. 1994;287:259–60.
4. Percie du Sert N, Ahluwalia A, Alam S, et al. Reporting animal research: explanation and elaboration for the ARRIVE guidelines 2.0. PLoS Biol. 2020;18(7):e3000411.
5. Schulz KF, Altman DG, Moher D, CONSORT Group. CONSORT 2010 statement: updated guidelines for reporting parallel group randomised trials. BMJ. 2010;340:c332.
6. Moher D, Liberati A, Tetzlaff J, Altman DG, The PRISMA Group. Preferred reporting items for systematic reviews and meta-analyses: the PRISMA statement. PLoS Med. 2009;6(7):e1000097.
7. von Elm E, Altman DG, Egger M, Pocock SJ, Gøtzsche PC, Vandenbroucke JP, STROBE Initiative. The strengthening the reporting of observational studies in epidemiology (STROBE) statement: guidelines for reporting observational studies. Prev Med. 2007;45(4):247–51.

Translational Histopathology in Otitis Media: The Real Evidence-Based Medicine!

14

Suanur M. Kayaalp, Sebahattin Cureoglu, and Michael M. Paparella

Pathology, the gold standard for discerning diseases in humans, is essential to every discipline in the medical field. Human ear structures are usually inaccessible during life, with the exception of surgical biopsies. However, such biopsies include only minuscule specimens of ear tissue and are often unrepresentative of the overall condition of the ear. Organs of the body, other than the ear, are routinely studied in hospital pathology laboratories. However, because of the difficulties and expense of ear tissue acquisition and preparation, human otopathology has evolved as a separate research discipline. The study of otitis media in human ear sections has been and continues to be the foundation for advancements in patient care (Fig. 14.1).

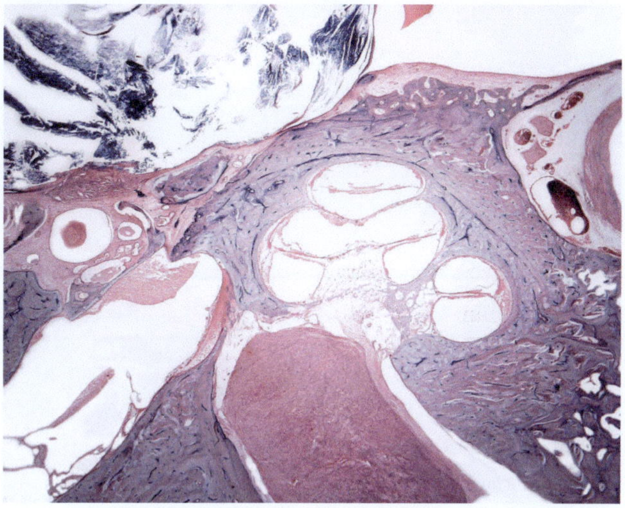

Fig. 14.1 An 86-year-old patient with diverticulitis and diabetes who was born deaf. Her ears showed multiple otopathologic problems, including cholesteatoma, cholesterol granuloma, tympanosclerosis, vestibular schwannoma, serous labyrinthitis, cochlear hydropic changes, and otosclerosis, all of which could be managed surgically

Although light microscopy of human temporal bones has profoundly influenced our knowledge of otitis media (Fig. 14.2a–c) and irreversible pathologies in the middle ear (Fig. 14.3), significant gaps remain in our understanding of their molecular mechanisms. The adaptation of new molecular and imaging techniques can provide researchers with the tools necessary to study normal function and pathology of the ear. However, the studies of underlying ear pathologies and disease mechanisms heavily depend on postmortem times, which affect middle and inner ear structures as well as the preservation of proteins, DNA/RNA, and other molecules (Fig. 14.4). Breakthrough human otologic studies will require high-quality human ear tissues, advanced techniques, and highly trained researchers. Human studies should be performed on human specimens with short postmortem periods that contain all the structures of the ear, including the entire Eustachian tube and mastoid, which is not possible in samples obtained at routine autopsies at this time.

The laboratory should have a multidisciplinary team in temporal bone procurement, clinical data collection, and methodologic analysis, such as pathology, histology, immunohistochemistry, proteomics, polymerase chain reaction, cDNA microarray, in situ hybridization, light and electron microscopy, and three-dimensional (3D) reconstruction from serial temporal bone sections, to understand the pathogenesis, pathophysiology, and etiology of middle ear infections through analysis of human ear tissues. The combined approach of ultrastructural and molecular analysis with temporal bone pathology will greatly enhance our understanding of the mechanisms involved in ear diseases.

We have previously shown that fresh dissected human ear tissues are suitable for studying mRNA and protein expression using techniques such as polymerase chain reaction (PCR), in situ hybridization, and immunohistochemistry (Fig. 14.5) [1, 2]. Current standard procedures have proven useful for many imaging and molecular studies of human temporal bones; however, because of long postmortem, fixation, and decalcification times, such procedures can

S. M. Kayaalp · S. Cureoglu (✉) · M. M. Paparella
Otopathology Laboratory, Department of Otolaryngology, University of Minnesota Physicians (UMP), University of Minnesota, Minneapolis, MN, USA
e-mail: cureo003@umn.edu

M. V. Goycoolea et al. (eds.), *Textbook of Otitis Media*, https://doi.org/10.1007/978-3-031-40949-3_14

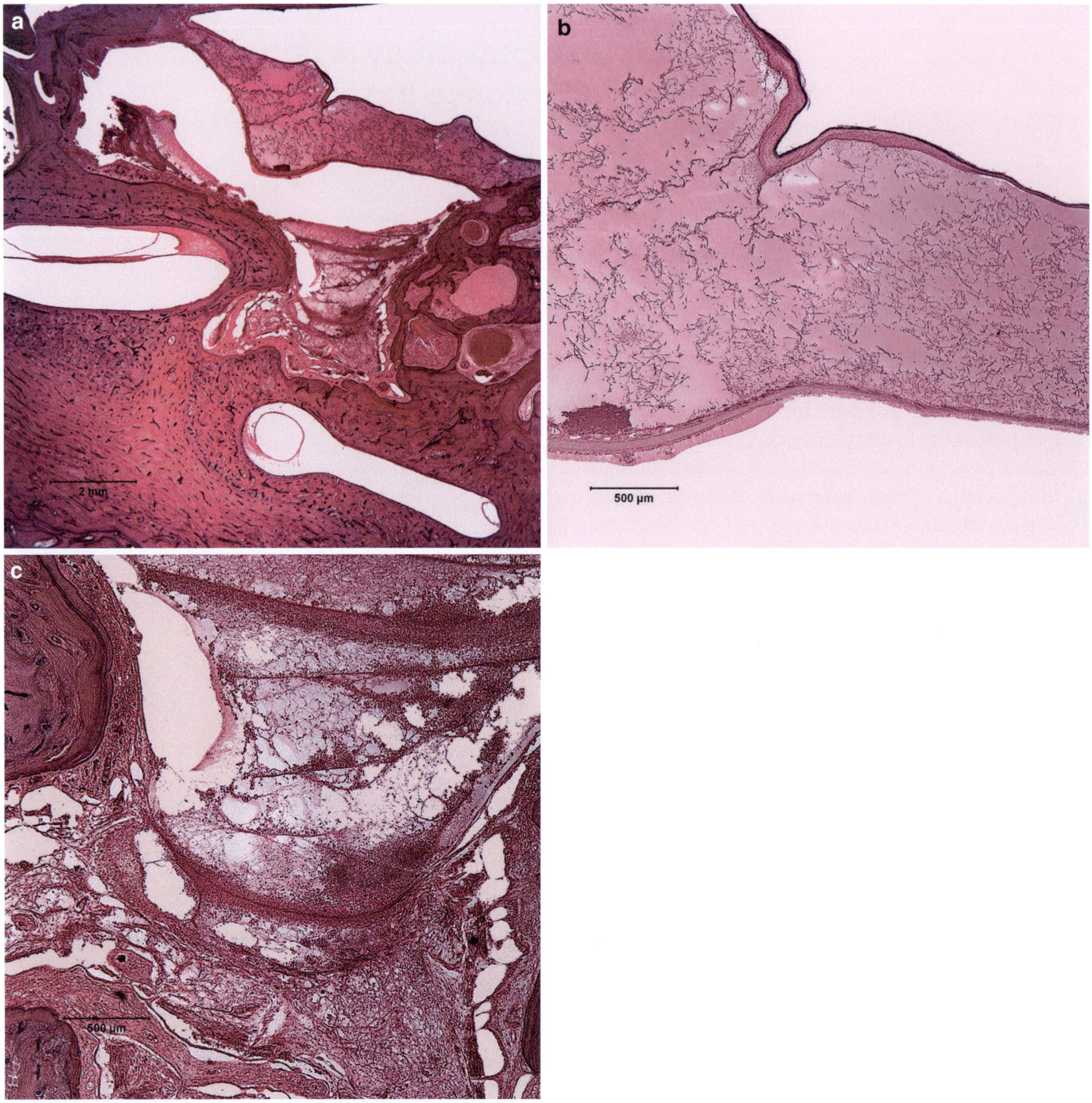

Fig. 14.2 This patient had a long-term history of ear pain, prolonged antibiotic treatment, and an immunocompromised status due to chronic myeloid leukemia. His histopathologic examination showed (**a**) an intact tympanic membrane, (**b**) otomycosis of the tympanic membrane, (**c**) in addition to bacterial communities such as biofilm like structures in the middle ear

fail to conserve the structure of specimens or preserve their nucleic acids and proteins. The limitations of DNA retrieval from archived temporal bones are as follows [3]: (1) the amount of DNA extracted from a single section (~500 ng) is low; (2) extracted DNA does not allow PCR amplification of fragments exceeding approximately 300–400 bp; (3) extracted DNA is labile and degrades rapidly; and (4) formalin fixation can induce alterations in template sequence that can inhibit alignment [4]. We found rapid degradation of RNA in bones when postmortem times exceeded 6 h [1]. Long preparation and storage times can also result in poor preservation of ear structures, degradation of DNA/RNA, and decreased antigenicity of proteins. Contamination of DNA/RNA is a significant problem [3]. Some reasons for

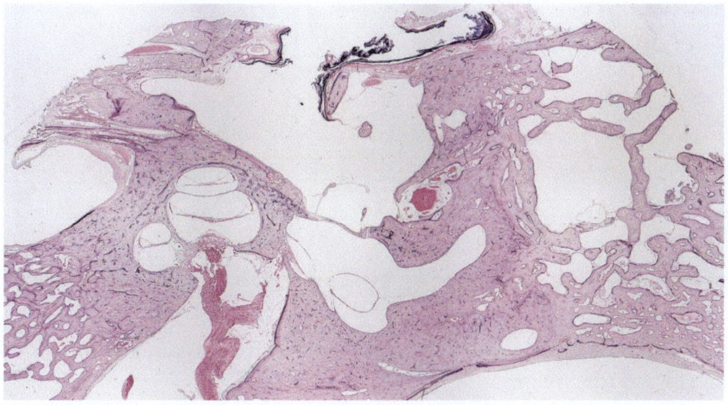

Fig. 14.3 An 88-year-old male with hx of chronic otitis media and dizzy spells showed mixed typed hearing loss and a perforated ear drum, Note that ear canal keratinized epithelium moves into the middle ear, creating acquired cholesteatoma

the contamination of archived specimens include: (1) before the development of molecular methods, there was no reason to follow the sterile technique; (2) temporal bones were processed in various concentrations of celloidin that were reused in multiple specimens; and (3) multiple specimens were stored in the same solutions. With newly acquired human temporal bones with specific requests regarding disease, fixative, or embedding media, as well as microdissected structures and modified fixative, avoiding the pitfalls of reusing embedding material and storing multiple specimens in the same solution, studies will use ear tissues with less contamination and better preservation of morphology and molecular footprints, enhancing immunohistochemical, electron microscopic, and proteomic analysis. However,

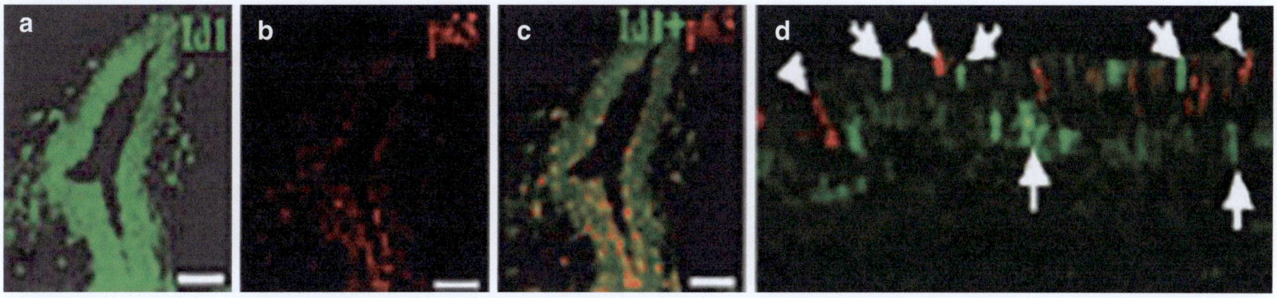

Fig. 14.4 Double immunolabeling of proteins co-expressed in cholesteatoma. (**a**) Id1 (green). (**b**) NF-kB p65 (red). (**c**) Yellow-orange dots = overlap of both Id1 and NF-kB p65. (**d**) In situ hybridization showing *MUC5AC* (arrowheads) and *MUC5B* (arrows)

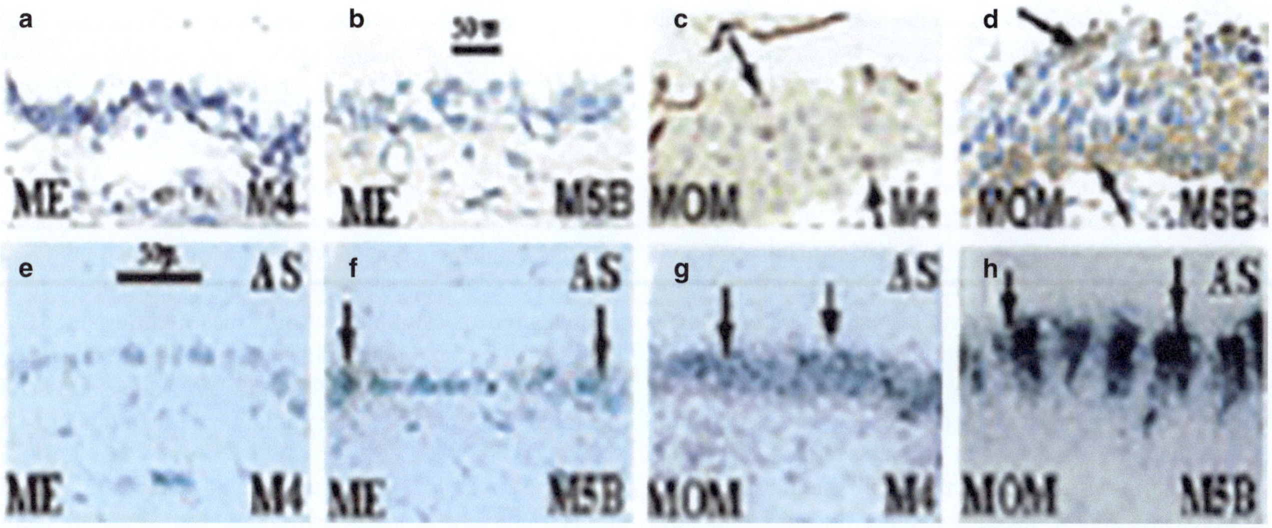

Fig. 14.5 (**a–d**) Immunohistochemical analysis. Noninflamed middle ear (ME) epithelia did not react with MUC4 (**a**) or MUC5B (**b**) antibodies but reacted positively with MUC4 (**c**, arrows) and MUC5B (**d**, arrows) antibodies in specimens with mucoid otitis media (MOM). (**e–h**) In situ hybridization. Control mucosa expressed no *MUC4* (**e**) or limited *MUC5B* (**f**), while ears with mucoid otitis media expressed abundant *MUC4* (**g**) and *MUC5B* (**h**) mRNA transcripts

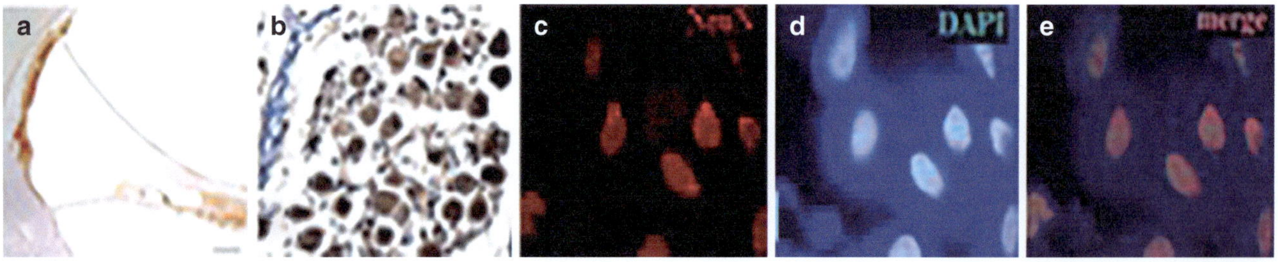

Fig. 14.6 (**a**) Immunolabeling of Na^+ and K^+-ATPase in the stria vascularis and spiral ligament Spiral ganglion cells immunostained with NE-14 (**b**) and NeuN (**c**) antibodies. (**d**) The nuclei, stained with DAPI. (**e**) Merge of (**c**) and (**d**) images

transmission electron microscopy can be applied to unstained celloidin sections; if those studies are performed in human specimens with minimal postmortem times, the morphologic analysis will demonstrate excellent structural detail. *Immunohistochemistry* of decelloidinized human temporal bones using the avidin–biotin–horseradish peroxidase method or immunofluorescent labeling is routinely performed (Fig. 14.6). We have applied several antigen retrieval methods (heat, chemical, and proteolytic-induced epitope retrieval). We observed mucin upregulation by immunohistochemistry (Fig. 14.5a–d) and mRNA by in situ hybridization (Fig. 14.5e–h) in mucoid otitis media using human temporal bones with postmortem times <6 h [2, 5].

A novel processing technique with a laser microtomeand automatic noncontact sectioning of human temporal bone without decalcification will be possible in the near future. As the laser microtome is automatic and requires minimal tissue manipulation, it *improves the quality of sectioning*, which is frequently affected by deficient decalcification and human-related issues. It *minimizes processing artifacts* related to the *presence of metallic implants* (such as cochlear implants), as contactless sectioning avoids the sheer stress artifacts that result from standard sectioning with rotary/sliding microtomes [6, 7]. Because of its built-in optical coherence tomography, it provides a means to *preview and section areas of interest in 3D*: This allows optimal quality of whole-mount sectioning, which yields tissue of uneven quality through standard manual dissection even for highly-skilled technicians. It allows the use of *different embedding media* such as Spurr epoxy and methyl-methacrylate, which can be *better for the preservation of proteins and nucleic acids* than celloidin but are impractical to use in standard processing because they are too dense for whole-specimen sectioning using the sliding microtome. This novel system can process the whole temporal bone, including the mastoid and Eustachian tubes.

Double labeling. Using immunohistochemistry to analyze temporal bones with cholesteatoma, we have found that Id1 (Fig. 14.4a) and nuclear factor-kappa B (NF-kB) p65 (Fig. 14.4b) proteins were coexpressed in the middle ear mucosa (Fig. 14.4c). We demonstrated NF-kB p65 (stained with MAB3026 antibody against "activated" p65) in the nuclei of cholesteatoma epithelium cells. Figure 14.4d shows double-labeled in situ hybridization of the Eustachian tube. Two genes, *MUC5AC* (TRITC) and *MUC5B* (FITC), were targeted in a specimen autopsied 3 h after death.

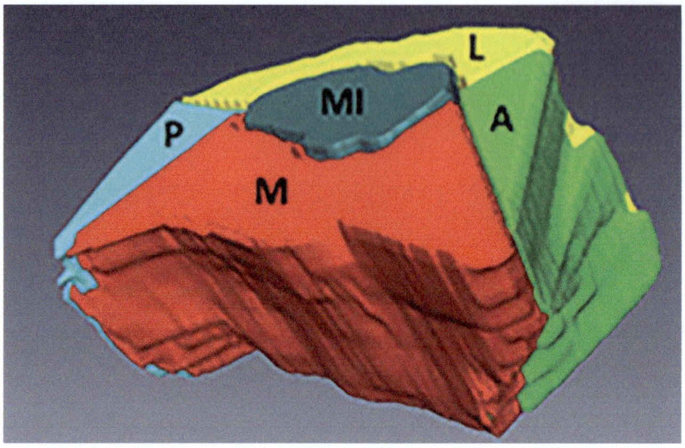

Fig. 14.7 Example of a 3D model generated for volume calculation for epitympanic compartments of the human temporal bone. A = anterior compartment; L = lateral compartment; M = medial compartment; MI = malleus/incus compartment; and P = posterior compartment of human temporal bone

Expression of toll-like receptors (TLRs) in chronic otitis media (COM). TLRs are membrane proteins that play a crucial role in the induction and activation of innate immunity in the course of infection [8]. Activation of TLRs leads to the mobilization of cytokines, chemokines, interferons, defensins, lysozyme, and other molecules in otitis media [9, 10]. We have found that both TLR2 and TLR4 were expressed in the middle ear mucosa and granulation tissue of donors with COM.

3D Reconstruction. Knowledge of many structures in human temporal bones is better achieved using 3D reconstruction (Fig. 14.7). We have applied 3D models generated from sections with 3D reconstruction software (Amira, Visualization Sciences Group, Bordeaux, France; and Zuse Institute, Berlin, Germany). The 3D reconstruction of the temporal bone is a validated mechanism to study the anatomical relationships between the structures within the ear [11–13]. We have studied the 3D model of epitympanic bony volume and tympanic isthmus area in temporal bones with COM [14]. It is also possible, with these reconstructions, to evaluate potential pathophysiological mechanisms leading to different diseases, such as otitis media, Meniere's disease, and hearing loss of all causes [11–13].

An air-containing middle ear is fundamental for normal hearing. The major aeration pathway of the epitympanum is the tympanic isthmus, which provides a major ventilation route to the upper epitympanum. The aeration pathway from the Eustachian tube leads directly to the mesotympanic and hypotympanic spaces, whereas the epitympanum is aside from the direct air stream and aerated [16]. The epitympanic diaphragm, which consisted of the incus, malleus, and their folds, was described as the floor of the epitympanum, dividing the structure from the mesotympanum. It is believed that the epitympanum and mastoid aeration occur through a tympanic isthmus (Palva 1991) [11, 15, 16]. Obstruction of the tympanic isthmus is a very common finding in various types of middle ear diseases, and that causes a disturbance in air diffusion within the temporal bone pneumatic system [15]. Dysventilation of the tympanic cavity due to blockage of or a narrowed ventilation/drainage route predisposes the middle ear to COM [16]. Swollen mucosa and tympanosclerotic deposits can obstruct the tympanic isthmus, resulting in the accumulation of exudates above the level of the epitympanic diaphragm [15]. A PE tube placement will only aerate the mesotympanum but not the epitympanic compartments if the tympanic isthmus is blocked.

On the other hand, it has been known that Eustachian tube dysfunction is one of the initial factors for chronic ear disease development and retraction pockets. The upper segment of the Eustachian tube, close to the tympanic cavity, is commonly exposed to the majority of childhood middle ear inflammatory diseases, making it a logical candidate for acquired inflammatory stenosis and irreversible damage to the temporo-mastoid system. Eustachian tube dysfunction, caused by a blockage or a narrow protympanic space, may be the main factor that triggers middle ear diseases [17]. A reduced volume of its bony segment, the protympanum, was observed in our temporal bones with middle ear diseases [13].

Proteomic analysis. Proteomic analysis in formalin-fixed, paraffin-embedded, and celloidin-embedded tissues has been described in the literature [18, 19]. However, the degradation of proteins can occur in celloidin-embedded tissues due to the methods used to embed and remove celloidin before performing the proteomic analysis. We continue to perform proteomic analysis of celloidin-embedded archived bones and plan to perform studies using our newly acquired temporal bones from patients with COM. We generally develop methodologic protocols using our archived chinchilla temporal bones before applying them to our valuable human specimens. We used tandem mass spectrometry at the Center for Mass Spectrometry and Proteomics at the University of Minnesota. Analysis of formalin-fixed, celloidin-embedded chinchilla temporal bones yielded more than 50 proteins, including collagen (alpha 1, 2, and 3), cytokeratins (CK-1, CK-10, and CK-2e), cochlin, vitronectin (isoform X1), and fibronectin (isoform X6). We believe those studies will provide intact protein identification combined with a protein database for human specimens from otitis media cases. As a result, the proteomic profile of the pathologic tissue can be compared to the normal protein distribution. In addition, abnormal proteins detected during proteomic analysis can be further evaluated by immunohistochemistry. Those analyses will provide insight into the underlying mechanisms of ear problems and propose potential treatment approaches.

Validation of Animal Models and Potential for Clinical Application. Many researchers have relied on experimental animal models; however, the application of such models to the human ear needs to be validated, given the genetic and anatomic differences between various animals and humans. Furthermore, no animal models currently exist for many otologic syndromes, irreversible ear pathologies such as cholesteatoma (Fig. 14.8a, b). Furthermore, experimental animal models do not always mimic the human condition; experimental otitis media has been induced by the inoculation of bacteria or obstruction of the Eustachian tube, whereas in humans, acute otitis media is often preceded by a viral upper respiratory tract infection [20, 21]. Knockout mice can develop spontaneous otitis media involving bacterial pathogens that are not common in human ear infections [22]. Finally, animal and human ears have significant anatomic differences. We have had many years of experience validating our experimental animal models against our human temporal bones, including their potential for translational applications. For example, in our animal model, we demonstrated the passage of bacterial toxins and inflammatory mediators through the round window membrane, thereby damaging the inner ear and causing hearing loss. However, our comparative studies of rodent models and the human round window membrane have shown differences in thickness (the human membrane is about 4–5 times thicker), despite structural similarity—possibly resulting in a slower rate of diffusion and decreased permeability in humans.

We have conducted many studies validating various aspects of the chinchilla model of otitis media (pioneered at the University of Minnesota) with respect to our human temporal bones from deceased donors with otitis media. We compared the ultrastructure of the normal human round window to that of various animal species [23, 24] (Fig. 14.9) and evaluated its permeability to different substances. Similar changes of inflammatory cell infiltration of the round window membrane and scala tympani due to otitis media in our chinchilla model [25–29] and our human temporal bones

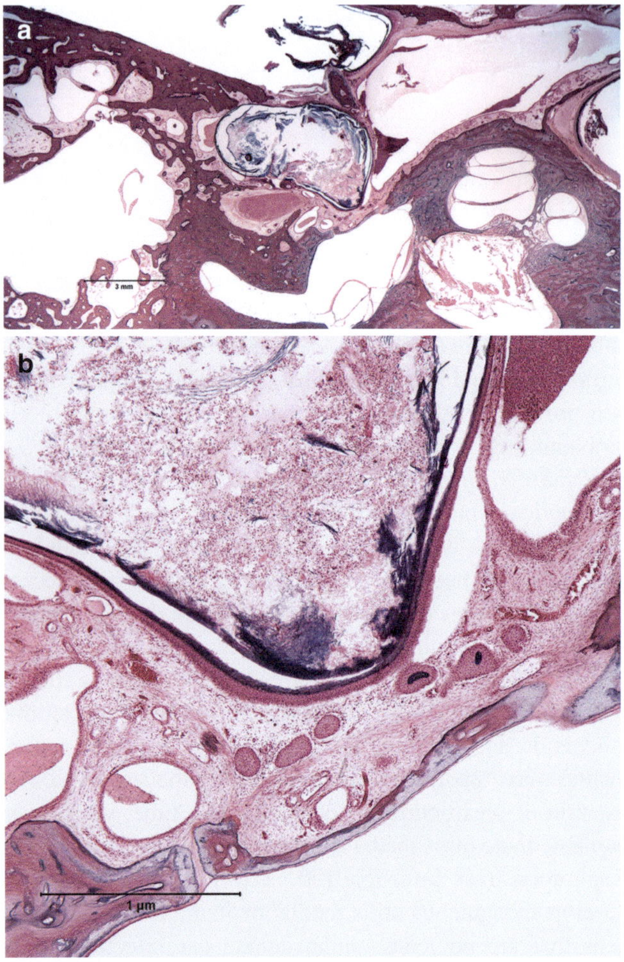

Fig. 14.8 A 64-year-old male patient had a history of otogenic meningitis. He had bilateral chronic otitis media and presence of cholesteatoma in the left ear. (**a**) Note the cholesteatoma destroyed ossicles and is located in between tympanic membrane and the stapedial footplate, creating a columellar effect in the sound conduction. (**b**) Higher magnification showed small cholesteatoma pearls under the mucosal surface of the stapedial footplate

with otitis media [30] have been shown. We also demonstrated sensorineural hearing loss secondary to otitis media in our chinchilla model [31], a sequela described in humans.

Our laboratory has made significant progress in *otitis media-related translational research* using our collection of human temporal bones and experimental animal models. The inner ear is intimately associated with the middle ear, both functionally and anatomically. Functional changes in the middle ear mechanics affect the transmission of sound to the inner ear, while areas of anatomical connections allow for the passage of microorganisms, cytokines, toxins, or drugs from the middle to the inner ear with potentially serious

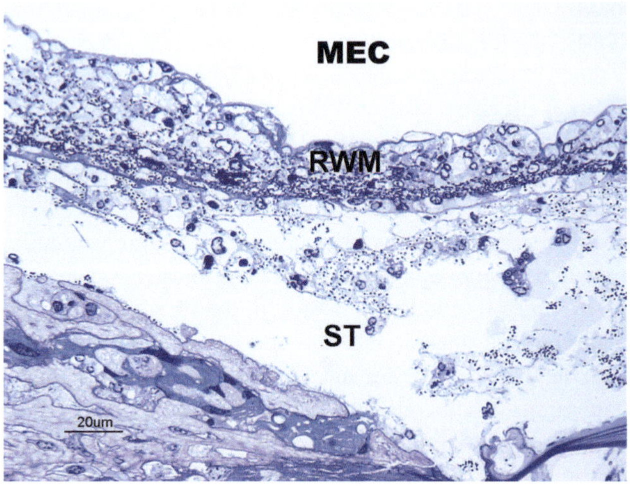

Fig. 14.9 In a chinchilla model, we have seen similar changes and mechanisms to those we sseen in human studies in terms of interaction in between the middle and inner ears. *MEC* middle ear cavity, *RWM* round window membrane; and *ST* scala tympani. Inflammatory cells, such as polymorphonuclear cells, mononuclear cells, bacteria in the membrane, and scala tympani. Note vacuolization and edema of the membrane (RWM). All specimens were processed in a similar manner to test the validity of the animal model in human patients

sequelae. The round window membrane, which is the only soft tissue barrier between the middle and inner ear and which lies within a niche and adjacent to the sinus tympani, facilitating the accumulation of pus, is vulnerable to toxic substances within the middle ear (Fig. 14.10a, b) [32]. This research transformed the treatment of patients with otitis media [33].

Dr. Paparella and his colleagues initiated the concept of the otitis media continuum [34, 35] (Fig. 14.11). It has been suggested that all types of otitis media represent different stages of a continuum of events. It can occur along a continuum, with the acute stage of otitis media leading to the chronic stage. One form of otitis media may resolve or lead to a more chronic stage of the disease. Although otitis media with effusion is characterized by the presence of a clear fluid in the middle ear cleft, there is no evidence of secretory cell proliferation at an earlier stage. Over time, subepithelial space is widened by edema, vascular dilation, and the infiltration of host defense cells. With the reabsorption of watery components of the fluid, the increased density of goblet cells, and the formation of secretory glands, the middle ear effusion becomes mucoid, in addition to the chronic inflammatory changes in the middle ear cleft.

COM has been clinically defined as a chronic discharge from the middle ear in the presence of a perforation of the tympanic membrane. It is defined when the inflammatory

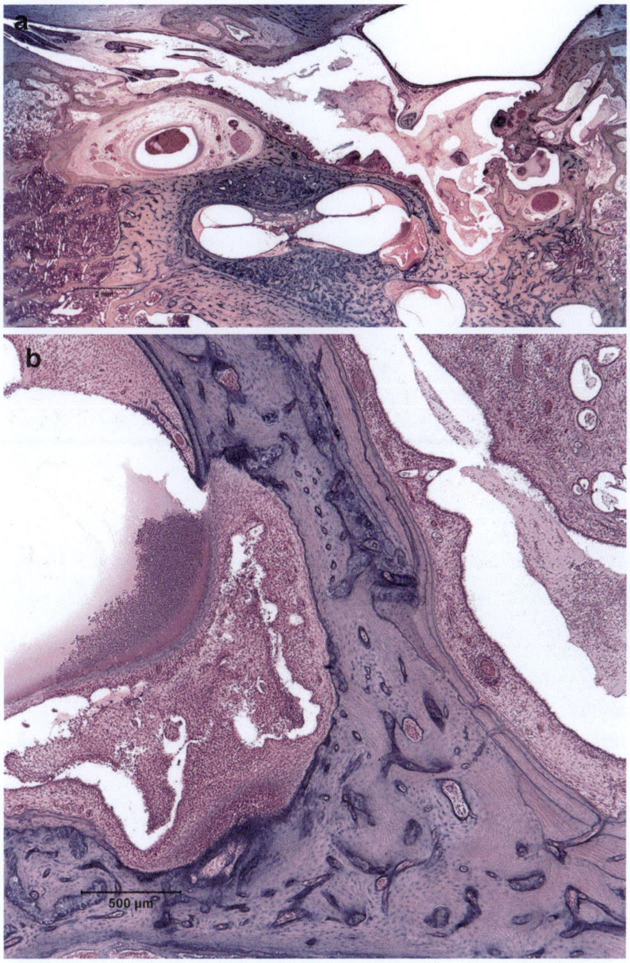

Fig. 14.10 A 1-year-old patient had a history of otogenic meningitis. (**a**) Horizontal sections of the right temporal bone showed irreversible pathologies such as granulation tissue and fibrous structures in the middle ear. (**b**) Higher magnification of round window membrane indicated purulent secretion around the niche in the middle ear has been crossing the membrane into the scala tympani as an example of middle ear/inner ear interaction

process has entered a chronic phase and permanent alteration of middle ear structures is seen [36]. The pathologic changes in the tympanic membrane due to COM include perforation, retractions, myringosclerosis, pseudocystic spaces, and hemorrhage [37]. Paparella et al. introduced the concept of chronic silent otitis media based on histopathologic evidence of chronic infection in the middle ear cleft in the absence of obvious ear-related symptoms and changes in the tympanic membrane or intractable tissue pathology behind an intact tympanic membrane [38, 39]. Because the chronic pathology is undetected, there is a lack of clinical treatment for otitis media, increasing the risk of complications due to the underlying problems [39]. As a result of the silent middle ear infection process, intratemporal problems such as endolymphatic hydrops, labyrinthitis, facial palsy, sensorineural hearing loss, and/or intracranial complications such as meningitis or brain abscess can be seen [39, 40]. The clinician should, therefore, be aware that an intact tympanic membrane does not necessarily preclude the presence of pathologic changes in the middle ear cleft (Fig. 14.12). In addition, ventilation tube placement does not guarantee the resolution of middle ear effusion if there are associated pathologies, such as granulation tissues in hidden areas, including the facial recess or sinus tympani (Fig. 14.13). As seen in the section, a dimeric membrane is observed due to several tube placements and residual effusion in addition to posterior fibrocystic granulation tissue around the sinus tympani and round window niche (Fig. 14.13).

As a result of human otopathologic studies, we will have a better understanding of the structural and molecular mechanisms, which will have a major impact on facilitating the development of new strategies to prevent and treat different types of otitis media and their complications.

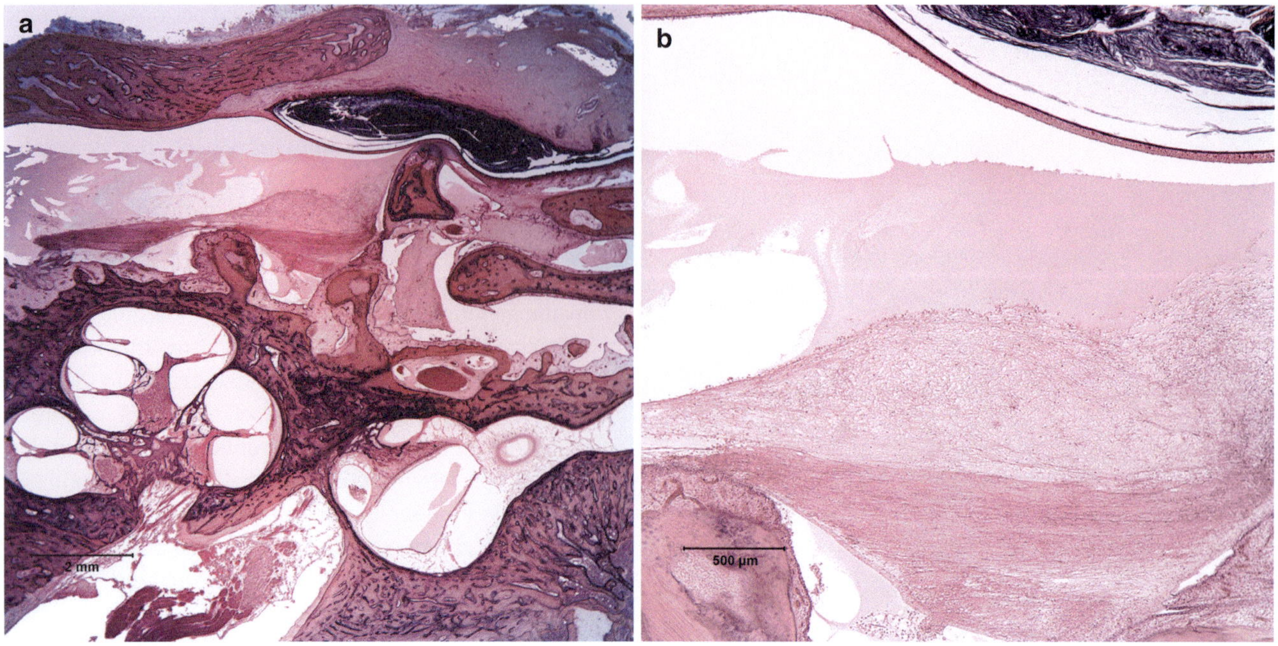

Fig. 14.11 (**a**) This was a 5-year-old male patient who had a history of immunodeficiency and bone marrow transplant. Histopathologic examination showed bilateral otitis media with effusion. (**b**) Higher magnification showed the continuation of effusion from serous to sero-mucoid and mucoid character in the middle ear

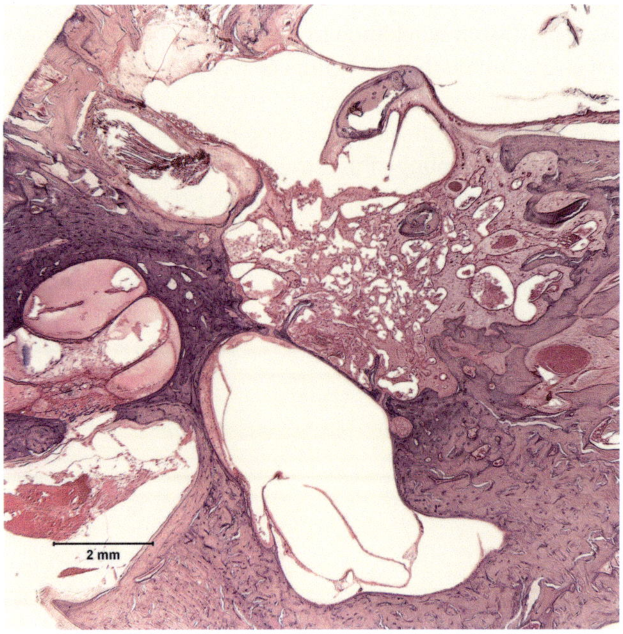

Fig. 14.12 This was an 18-month-old patient with bilateral chronic otitis media and meningitis. Fibrocystic granuloma, cholesterol granuloma, and residual mesenchyme can be seen behind the intact tympanic membrane. Purulent labyrinthitis showed biofilm structures in the inner ear. The concept of chronic silent (masked) otitis media depends on the basis of clinical and otopathological evidence of chronic infection in the middle ear cleft in the absence of obvious pathologic findings in the tympanic membrane

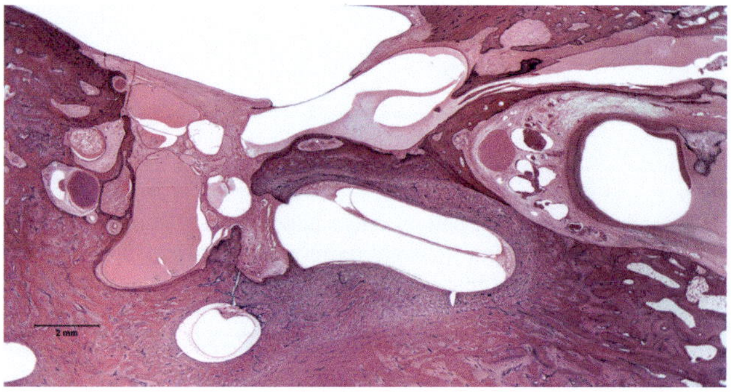

Fig. 14.13 This histopathologic section shows a dimeric membrane intact with serous effusion in the middle ear. A fibrocystic granulation tissue is seen around the round window niche and sinus tympani

References

1. Lin J, Kawano H, Paparella MM, Ho SB. Improved RNA analysis for immediate autopsy of temporal bone soft tissues. Acta Otolaryngol. 1999;119:787–95.
2. Lin J, Tsuprun V, Kawano H, Paparella MM, Zhang Z, Anway R, Ho SB. Characterization of mucins in human middle ear and Eustachian tube. Am J Physiol Lung Cell Mol Physiol. 2001;280:L1157–67.
3. McKenna M, Kristiansen AG, Author G, Tropitzsch AS, Trannelyzerg L, Merchant SN. Contamination in archival human temporal bones: a potential significant problem. Otol Neurotol. 2002;23:789–92.
4. Di Giorgi C, Sialer MF, Lamberti F. Formalin-induced infidelity in PCR-amplified DNA fragments. Mol Cell Probes. 1994;8:459–62.
5. Kawano H, Paparella MM, Ho SB, Schachern PA, Morizono N, Le CT, Lin J. Identification of MUC5B mucin gene in human middle ear with chronic otitis media. Laryngoscope. 2000;110:668–73.
6. Kunert-Keil C, Richter H, Zeidler-Rentzsch I, Bleeker I, Gredes T. Histological comparison between laser microtome sections and ground specimens of implant-containing tissues. Ann Anat. 2019;222:153–7. https://doi.org/10.1016/j.aanat.2018.12.001.
7. Richter H, Ratliff J. A non-contact method of sectioning cardiovascular arteries containing metallic stents using laser technology. J Histotechnol. 2012;35(4):205.
8. Kopp E, Medzhitov R. Recognition of microbial infection by Toll-like receptors. Curr Opin Immunol. 2003;15:396–401.
9. Lee YC, Kim C, Shim JS, Byun JY, Park MS, Cha CI, et al. Toll-like receptors 2 and 4 and their mutations in patients with otitis media and middle ear effusion. Clin Exp Otorhinolaryngol. 2008;1:189–95.
10. Leichtle A, Lai Y, Wollenberg B, Wasserman SI, Ryan AF. Innate signaling in otitis media: pathogenesis and recovery. Curr Allergy Asthma Rep. 2011;11:78–84.
11. da Costa Monsanto R, Pauna HF, Kaya S, et al. Epitympanum volume and tympanic isthmus area in temporal bones with retraction pockets. Laryngoscope. 2016;126(11):E369–74. https://doi.org/10.1002/lary.25937.
12. da Costa Monsanto R, Pauna HF, Kwon G, et al. A three-dimensional analysis of the endolymph drainage system in Ménière disease. Laryngoscope. 2017;127(5):E170–5. https://doi.org/10.1002/lary.26155.
13. Pauna HF, Monsanto RC, Schachern P, Paparella MM, Cureoglu S. A 3-D analysis of the protympanum in human temporal bones with chronic ear disease. Eur Arch Otorhinolaryngol. 2017;274(3):1357–64. https://doi.org/10.1007/s00405-016-4396-4.
14. Shirai K, Schachern PA, Schachern MG, Paparella MM, Cureoglu S. Volume of the epitympanum and blockage of the tympanic isthmus in chronic otitis media: a human temporal bone study. Otol Neurotol. 2015;36(2):254–9.
15. Aimi K. The tympanic isthmus: its anatomy and clinical significance. Laryngoscope. 1978;88(7 Pt 1):1067–81.
16. Marchioni D, Piccinini A, Ciufelli MA, Presutti L. Endoscopic anatomy and ventilation of the epitympanum. Otolaryngol Clin North Am. 2013;46(2):165–78.
17. Tarabichi M, Najmi M. Site of Eustachian tube obstruction in chronic ear disease. Laryngoscope. 2015;125:2572–5.
18. Aarnisalo AA, Green KM, O'Malley J, et al. A method for MS(E) differential proteomic analysis of archival formalin-fixed celloidin-embedded human inner ear tissue. Hear Res. 2010;270:15.
19. Palmer-Toy ED, Krastins B, Sarracino DA, Nadol JB Jr, Merchant SM. Efficient method for the proteomic analysis of fixed and embedded tissues. J Proteome Res. 2005;4(6):2404–11.
20. Heikkinen T. Role of viruses in the pathogenesis of acute otitis media. Pediatr Infect Dis J. 2006;19:S17–22.
21. Winther B, Doyle WJ, Alper CM. A high prevalence of new onset otitis media during parent diagnosed common colds. Int J Pediatr Otorhinolaryngol. 2006;70:1725–30.
22. MacArthur CJ, Pillers DA, Pang J, Degagne JM, Kempton JB, Trune DR. Gram-negative pathogen Klebsiella oxytoca is associated with spontaneous chronic otitis media in Toll-like receptor 4-deficient C3H/HeJ mice. Acta Otolaryngol. 2008;128(2):132–8.
23. Schachern PA, Paparella MM, Duvall AJ. The normal chinchilla round window membrane. Arch Otolaryngol. 1982;108:550–4.
24. Schachern PA, Paparella MM, Duvall AJ, Choo YB. The human round window membrane. An electron microscopic study. Arch Otolaryngol. 1984;110:15–21.
25. Schachern P, Tsuprun V, Cureoglu S, Ferrieri P, Briles D, Paparella M, Juhn S. The round window membrane in otitis media: effect of pneumococcal proteins. Arch Otolaryngol Head Neck Surg. 2008;134(6):658–62.
26. Schachern PA, Tsuprun V, Cureoglu S, Ferrieri P, Briles DE, Paparella MM, Juhn S. Virulence of pneumococcal proteins on the inner ear. Arch Otolaryngol Head Neck Surg. 2009a;135(7):657–61.
27. Schachern PA, Tsuprun V, Ferrieri P, Briles DE, Goetz S, Cureoglu S, Juhn S. Pneumococcal PspA and PspC proteins: potential vaccine candidates for experimental otitis media. Int J Pediatr Otorhinolaryngol. 2014;78(9):1517–21.
28. Schachern PA, Tsuprun V, Goetz S, Cureoglu S, Juhn SK, Briles DE, Ferrieri P. Viability and virulence of pneumolysin, pneumococcal surface protein A, and pneumolysin/pneumococcal surface protein A mutants in the ear. JAMA Otolaryngol Head Neck Surg. 2013;139(9):937–43.
29. Schachern PA, Tsuprun V, Wang B, Apicella MA, Cureoglu S, Paparella MM, Juhn SK. Effect of lipooligosaccharide mutations of Haemophilus influenzae on the middle and inner ears. Int J Pediatr Otorhinolaryngol. 2009b;73(12):1757–60.
30. Joglekar S, Morita N, Cureoglu S, Schachern PA, Deroe AF, Tsuprun V, Paparella MM, Juhn S. Cochlear pathology in human temporal bones with otitis media. Acta Otolaryngol. 2010;130(4):472–6.
31. Tsuprun V, Cureoglu S, Schachern PA, Ferrieri P, Briles DE, Paparella MM, Junh SK. Role of pneumococcal proteins in the sensorineural hearing loss due to otitis media. Otol Neurotol. 2008;29(8):1056–60.
32. Cureoglu S, Schachern PA, Rinaldo A, Tsuprun V, Ferlito A, Paparella MM. Round window membrane and labyrinthine pathological changes: an overview. Acta Otolaryngol. 2005;125(1):9–15.
33. deSouza C, Paparella MM, Sperling N, editors. Atlas of otitis media–clinicopathologic correlations and operative techniques. Mumbai: Bhalani Publishing House; 2005.
34. Paparella MM, Schachern PA, Yoon TH, Abdelhammid MM, Sahni R, da Costa SS. Otopathologic correlates of the continuum of otitis media. Ann Otol Rhinol Laryngol Suppl. 1990;148:17–22.
35. Yoon TH, Paparella MM, Schachern PA, Lindgren BR. Morphometric studies of the continuum of otitis media. Ann Otol Rhinol Laryngol Suppl. 1990;148:23–7.
36. Meyerhoff WL, Kim CS, Paparella MM. Pathology of chronic otitis media. Ann Otol Rhinol Laryngol. 1978;87:749–60.
37. Jaisinghani VJ, Paparella MM, Schachern PA, Le CT. Tympanic membrane/middle ear pathologic correlates in chronic otitis media. Laryngoscope. 1999;109:712–6.
38. Ferlito A, Paparella MM, Rinaldo A, Schachern PA, Cureoglu S. The entity known as chronic silent (subclinical) otitis media: a common lesion and a forgotten diagnosis. Acta Otolaryngol. 2003;123:751–3.
39. Paparella MM, Schachern PA, Cureoglu S. Chronic silent otitis media. ORL J Otorhinolaryngol Relat Spec. 2002;64(2):65–72.
40. Tovi F, Leiberman A. Silent mastoiditis and bilateral simultaneous facial palsy. Int J Pediatr Otorhinolaryngol. 1983;5:303–7.

15 Patulous Eustachian Tube and the Differential Diagnosis of Autophony

Bryan K. Ward, Carrie L. Nieman, and Dennis S. Poe

There are three primary functions of the Eustachian tube, including (1) ventilating and equalizing pressure in the middle ear; (2) draining secretions from the middle ear by gravity or by mucociliary clearance; and (3) protecting the middle ear from sounds and reflux of pathogens and contents from the nasopharynx [1]. This third function of the Eustachian tube is often overlooked. The Eustachian tube functions as a dynamic valve that is closed in its resting position and opens intermittently due to muscular action. Patulous Eustachian tube dysfunction can occur when the Eustachian tube is in a persistently opened state. The middle ear is no longer protected from the transmission of internal sounds and nasopharyngeal material. This chapter will review the diagnosis and management of patulous Eustachian tube dysfunction as well as consider the differential diagnosis of autophony for disorders that may overlap with the clinical presentation of patulous Eustachian tube dysfunction.

Introduction: Patulous Eustachian Tube Dysfunction

A patulous Eustachian tube was initially described by Hermann Schwartze in 1864 when he noticed that a patient's tympanic membrane was moving with breathing [2]. There have been numerous subsequent reports of patients in whom ipsilateral nasal breathing evoked excursions of the tympanic membrane, and this was associated with having patulous Eustachian tube dysfunction [3–7]. The common symptoms that patients report are a sense of aural fullness, hearing their nasal breathing loudly in their ears, and hearing that their own voice can be perceived as abnormally loud or distorted on the affected side. These two latter symptoms are called autophony. Some common descriptions that patients provide are that they feel that their voice sounds like it has an "echo" or that they sound like they are speaking "in a bucket or barrel." Sometimes patients will change their voice in response to this feedback, and it may be noticed by others. Patients with patulous Eustachian tube dysfunction can report hearing their heartbeat loudly in the affected ear when the other symptoms occur. Typically, the symptoms all occur together, and they are often intermittent. Commonly, there are triggers for the symptoms, such as public speaking, singing, yawning, or exercise. Anecdotally, symptoms can occur more frequently after drinking beverages containing caffeine or when taking diuretics or decongestant medications. There is also often a relief in symptoms when patients lie supine. An explanation for this is the dilation of the venous plexus around the Eustachian tube lumen [8]. Similar effects can occur if patients apply gentle pressure to their ipsilateral jugular vein or when lying supine with their head below the level of the heart.

The cause of patulous Eustachian tube dysfunction is a concave defect longitudinally through the valve within the cartilaginous portion of the Eustachian tube, usually located in the membranous (anterolateral) wall. Less commonly, there can be a deficiency in the cartilaginous (posteromedial) wall. In a normal situation, there is typically a convex bulge of the membranous wall, and this can be observed via nasopharyngoscopy (Fig. 15.1). Any deficiency in the valve region may prevent it from fully closing at rest, resulting in impairment of the usual function of preventing reflux of sound or secretions from entering the middle ear. A patulous Eustachian tube provides a new route for sound or nasopharyngeal secretions to access the inner ear.

B. K. Ward · C. L. Nieman
Department of Otolaryngology-Head and Neck Surgery, Johns Hopkins University School of Medicine, Baltimore, MD, USA
e-mail: bward15@jh.edu; cnieman1@jhmi.edu

D. S. Poe (✉)
Department of Otolaryngology-Head and Neck Surgery, Boston Children's Hospital, Boston, MA, USA
e-mail: dennis.poe@childrens.harvard.edu

M. V. Goycoolea et al. (eds.), *Textbook of Otitis Media*, https://doi.org/10.1007/978-3-031-40949-3_15

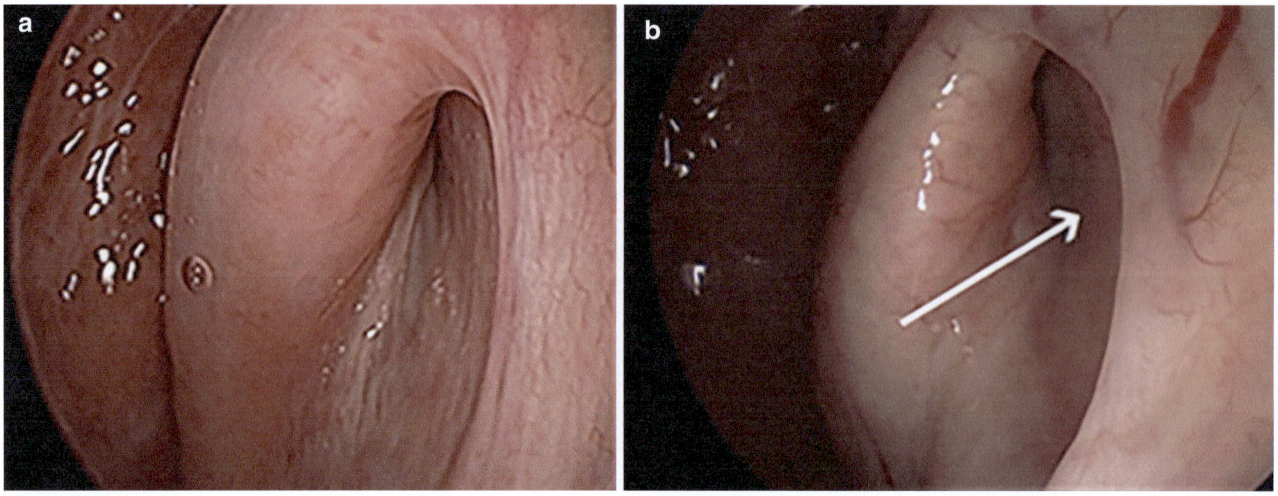

Fig. 15.1 An endoscopic examination of the left Eustachian tube. (**a**) A normal examination of an Eustachian tube in the closed position with a convex defect of the membranous wall. (**b**) Example of a patient with patulous Eustachian tube dysfunction with a hollowed-out concave deformity of the membranous wall at the mucosal valve (arrow)

Risk Factors for Patulous Eustachian Tube Dysfunction

In the healthy state, the usual bulge in the membranous wall of the Eustachian tube is caused by several factors that include mucosa, submucosa, muscle from the tensor veli palatini muscle, the lateral cartilaginous lamina, and fat. A depot of fat called Ostmann's fat pad is located in the region of the membranous wall. A deficiency in any or all of these structures can result in an increased likelihood that the valve will open and remain open, resulting in all of the classic symptoms of patulous Eustachian tube dysfunction. Several conditions may alter these structures, making patulous Eustachian tube dysfunction more likely. Allergic rhinitis is the most commonly associated condition with patulous Eustachian tube dysfunction [7]. Rapid weight loss is the next most common, and it is thought to cause atrophy of Ostmann's fat pad. An increased resting tension of the tensor veli palatini muscle and medial pterygoid muscle can flatten the membranous wall, increasing patency. Excessive tension can result from temporomandibular disorders (TMD), such as clenching of the muscles of mastication. Chronic inflammation in the nasopharynx, such as from environmental allergies or laryngopharyngeal reflux, may lead to atrophy of the secretory mucosa and submucosa. In clinical studies of patients with patulous Eustachian tube dysfunction, clinical diagnoses such as weight loss, chronic autoimmune or neuromuscular disorders, anxiety (possibly associated with TMD), and a history of environmental allergy are more prevalent than would be expected. Furthermore, findings on nasopharyngoscopy have correlated with the underlying diagnoses [7]. In any patient, the cause of a patulous Eustachian tube may be multifactorial, and in addition to the above-acquired issues, it could include congenital phenomena such as the shape of the medial cartilaginous lamina, the cartilage that supports the torus tubarius and cartilaginous wall, or the lateral cartilaginous lamina that contributes to the convex bulge in the membranous wall.

Diagnosis of Patulous Eustachian Tube Dysfunction

Clinicians can suspect patulous Eustachian tube dysfunction when they see a patient with aural fullness by asking about the classic symptoms of patulous eustachian tube dysfunction (autophony of voice and nasal breathing). The diagnosis is made by observation of pressure changes transmitted to the ear with ipsilateral nasal breathing. This pressure transmission can be observed by viewing the tympanic membrane with otoscopy or binocular microscopy. Observation is made for medial and lateral excursions of the tympanic membrane while the patient occludes the contralateral nostril and breathes through the nose, mildly deeper and faster than normal, similar to breathing while auscultating the lungs. Often, the movements of the tympanic membrane are best seen in the posterior-superior quadrant. These medial and lateral excursions of the tympanic membrane with nasal breathing are typically best seen when the patient is sitting upright. It is important to keep in mind that the movements will not be observed if symptoms are absent at the time of the examination. Sometimes patients can perform a maneuver to cause the symptoms, such as yawning or exercising, prior to the examination. On the other hand, patients may inadvertently perform frequent sniffing maneuvers to close the Eustachian tube when it opens [9]. To maximize the chances of seeing the tympanic membrane move with breathing, patients should be asked to avoid sniffing during the encounter.

Audiologists may be able to record these tympanic membrane excursions on tympanometry using the acoustic reflex decay setting on their audiometer. By performing tympanometry and asking the patient to perform ipsilateral nasal breathing, the movements of the tympanic membrane can be recorded as fluctuations in the immittance that are timed with nasal breathing [10]. Similar to examining the tympanic membrane in the clinic, however, fluctuations will not be observed if symptoms are absent at the time of the study. Finally, some patients may have a continuous column of air identifiable on computed tomography (CT) imaging, extending from the nasopharynx up to the middle ear. It can best be seen by cone beam CT in the sitting position. A continuous column of air is also diagnostic of a patulous Eustachian tube [11].

Since the sensation of ear fullness can be present in both patulous Eustachian tube dysfunction and obstructive Eustachian tube dysfunction, patients with ear fullness are often initially diagnosed with obstructive dysfunction. Furthermore, patients with patulous Eustachian tube dysfunction may have retractions of the tympanic membrane from repeated sniffing, generating negative pressure in the middle ear space to try to close the patulous Eustachian tube [12]. A strong sniff can generate a negative pressure in the nasopharynx, forcing air out of the middle ear space and closing the Eustachian tube by a Bernoulli effect. This can result in temporary relief of symptoms of the patulous Eustachian tube, but it can also result in retraction pockets, middle ear effusions, and cholesteatoma. Ordinarily, patients with negative middle ear pressure would be expected to try to improve their symptoms by performing a nasal Valsalva maneuver, forcing air from the nasopharynx to the middle ear (auto insufflation). Any patient with repeated sniffing despite evidence of negative pressure should be evaluated for patulous Eustachian tube dysfunction.

Finally, adding to the complexity of the diagnosis of patulous Eustachian tube dysfunction is that patients may fall along a spectrum of Eustachian tube dysfunction. As discussed above, the Eustachian tube is a valve that, for some of its functions, must open intermittently to ventilate the middle ear, while others stay closed to protect the middle ear from reflux of sound or nasopharyngeal secretions. In any person, there may be episodes in which the Eustachian tube is too frequently open, causing symptoms associated with patulous Eustachian tube dysfunction, and subsequently, episodes in which the Eustachian tube becomes closed too often (obstructive). The transition between obstructive and patulous dysfunction most commonly occurs in allergic rhinitis patients. Initially, they may have obstructive dysfunction, but over time, atrophy of the valve may occur, causing patulous dysfunction, even while there may still be evidence of inflammation elsewhere in the nose, nasopharynx, or torus tubarius. During exacerbations of allergic disease, obstructive dysfunction could recur, but during periods of quiescence or overmedicated for allergies, patulous symptoms may resume. Patients may alternate between these conditions, yet only report that they consistently have a "blocked ear." Therefore, the diagnosis of patulous Eustachian tube dysfunction requires a high index of suspicion.

Treatment of Patulous Eustachian Tube Dysfunction

When treating patients with patulous Eustachian tube dysfunction, the primary aim is to restore competence to the functional valve of the Eustachian tube to facilitate its closure more frequently. Patients should be made aware of behaviors that can make their symptoms less noticeable. Some will already have noticed that when they lie supine or put their head below the level of the heart, the symptoms are lessened. Similarly, gentle pressure on the neck ipsilateral to the symptoms can cause temporary venous congestion around the Eustachian tube, alleviating symptoms temporarily. Gentle sniffing can decrease symptoms in some patients, but strong sniffing as practiced by some patients should not be recommended due to the long-term effects on the tympanic membrane of inducing frequent negative pressure in the middle ear, such as tympanic membrane retractions and cholesteatoma.

The initial management of patulous Eustachian tube dysfunction is to discontinue any treatments with the potential to exacerbate symptoms. Dehydration makes symptoms more likely to occur. Therapies such as decongestants, diuretics, and caffeine should be discontinued if possible [13]. It may be helpful to increase oral water intake or to improve local hydration by delivering normal saline to the area with nasal saline drops. Topical estrogen drops (non-FDA approved) or irritants delivered to the surface of the Eustachian tube can help induce mucosal thickening and may be effective first-line agents [14, 15]. Patients need to be instructed on how to best apply the drops to the nose in order to deliver them to the surface of the Eustachian tube. We instruct patients to lie on their backs with their heads hanging 15°. After applying the drops, the head is turned approximately 45° to the side being treated to take on a nearly Hallpike position, except that the head is only hanging 15°. For example, when applying drops to the right nostril, the patient should lie supine. They then place the drops in the right nostril and rotate their head 45° to the right side to allow them to drain to the surface of the Eustachian tube. For irritants like hypertonic saline or ascorbic acid, patients often report feeling a twinge of irritation or pain that radiates toward the ear being treated when the drops contact the orifice of the Eustachian tube. This is often followed by relief of symptoms of variable duration. Patients are instructed to apply the drops as needed, generally three drops at a time. Hypertonic saline can be prepared at home with two teaspoons of table salt in a cup of water (~2.4 dL), varying the concentration if desired. Ascorbic acid preparations generally provide the maximal irritation that most patients would readily accept. They can be used three drops daily or, two to three times daily for 2 months in an attempt to obtain lasting benefits. Although weight loss has been associated with the onset of symptoms in some patients, it appears that weight gain is not an effective method for reducing symptoms and should only be recommended if the patient is medically underweight [7].

Surgical Management of Patulous Eustachian Tube Dysfunction

The majority of patients with patulous Eustachian tube dysfunction can be managed with behavioral changes and mucosal irritants, as described above [7]. Surgical treatments for patulous Eustachian tube dysfunction can be divided into two categories: (1) procedures that aim to modify the vibratory functions of the tympanic membrane (mass loading) to decrease symptoms such as autophony of voice and nasal breathing; and (2) procedures aimed at decreasing the diameter of the lumen of the valve of the Eustachian tube.

Procedures to Modify the Tympanic Membrane

Tympanostomy tubes have been reported as helping to alleviate symptoms in up to 54% of patients in one series [16]; however, symptoms of altered hearing and aural fullness may also be exacerbated by placing a tympanostomy tube [17]. Patients with frequent sniffing will be unable to alleviate their symptoms with a tympanostomy tube in place and should be counseled about this prior to placement. It may be that, when effective, tympanostomy tubes apply a mass load to the tympanic membrane or modify its vibratory features in a way that minimizes symptoms of autophony. Other groups have reported success with mass-loading the tympanic membrane using a variety of materials, such as tape, paper strips, eggshells, or putty-like adhesives [18–22]. We have observed that mass loading is more likely to be beneficial in patients in whom autophony of breathing or the sensation of tympanic membrane excursions are the dominant symptoms. We place one or more layers of adhesive skin closure strips, cut to about 4 mm in diameter, onto the posterior and superior tympanic membranes. These strips can stay in place for several weeks.

The above methods of addressing patulous Eustachian tube dysfunction are temporary, and symptoms are expected to recur once the materials migrate off the tympanic membrane with the normal epithelial migration of the ear canal skin. If patients report temporary relief, however, they may be more likely to benefit from a tympanostomy tube. Alternatively, mass loading by performing a tympanoplasty using auricular cartilage could provide enduring relief of symptoms [19, 21].

Procedures to Decrease the Diameter of the Lumen of the Valve of the Eustachian Tube

The other major category of procedures for patulous Eustachian tube dysfunction aims to address the Eustachian tube directly (Fig. 15.2). One approach includes inserting a shim to fill a gap in the valve of the Eustachian tube [13, 23–25]. Prior to the procedure, a CT scan is always performed to ensure there is no bony dehiscence of the internal carotid artery, as this would be contraindicated for this procedure. The shims may be inserted either via the nasopharynx or via the middle ear. For the nasopharynx insertion, a transnasal or combined transnasal and transoral approach is used to access the Eustachian tube. A non-FDA-approved shim is constructed using a 14-gauge or, less commonly, 16-gauge angiocatheter. Molten bone wax is aspirated into the angiocatheter, and this is trimmed to a size such that the full length of the Eustachian tube is included, plus an additional 5 mm. The final length is usually between 38 and 42 mm. After the wax hardens within the angiocatheter, it is trimmed to the appropriate size, placed within a piston-like insertion tool, and then inserted slowly into the nasopharyngeal end of the Eustachian tube via the oral or nasal cavity, using endoscopic guidance via the nasal passage. Although the shim is advanced into the Eustachian tube like the balloon catheter during balloon dilation of the Eustachian tube, the shim is advanced through the isthmus to hold it in place, while a balloon catheter does not pass the isthmus. Once the shim is inserted, the tympanic membrane is inspected to ensure the shim is not contacting the tympanic membrane. Following the nasopharyngeal placement of a shim, approximately 75% of patients can expect to have relief of symptoms at 1 year following the procedure; however, there is a risk that the shim can become dislodged in about 10% of cases and that about 50% of patients will develop a middle ear effusion that can be managed with tympanostomy tubes [26]. Shims have also been placed via a trans-tympanic approach, inserting the shim into the bony Eustachian tube. Using binocular microscopy, an otolaryngologist can place the shim by raising an anterior tympanomeatal flap, as initially described by Bluestone [23], or via a myringotomy.

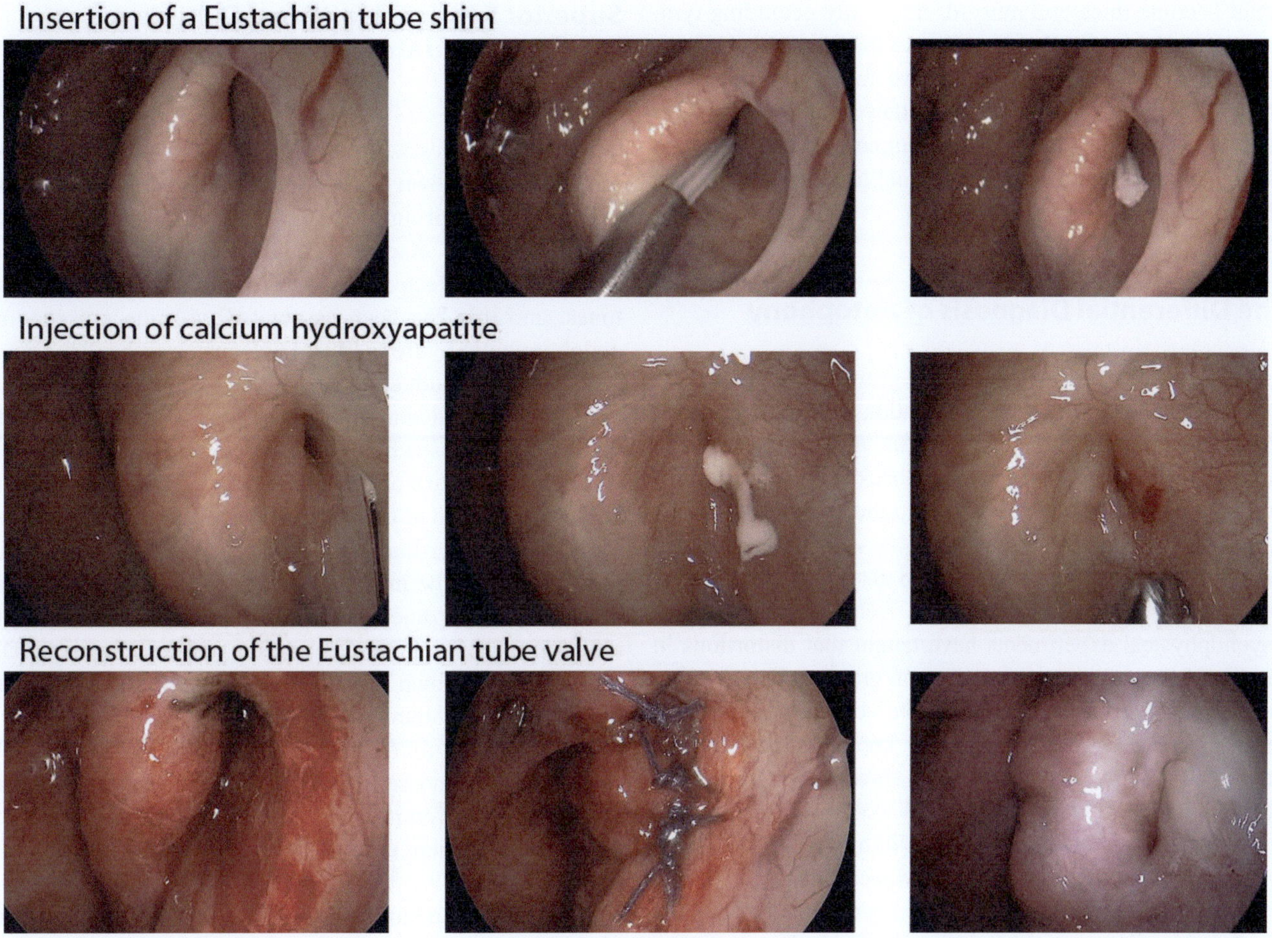

Fig. 15.2 Procedures to decrease the diameter of the Eustachian tube via the nasopharyngeal approach are shown, including insertion of a shim (upper panel), injection of calcium hydroxyapatite (middle panel), and reconstruction of the Eustachian tube valve by augmentation of the membranous wall (lower panel)

Materials used have included angiocatheters constructed similar to those described above [27, 28] and custom silicone plugs [29]. In either the nasopharyngeal approach or the transcanal approach, the procedure is reversible via a clinic visit, either by performing a myringotomy or nasopharyngoscopy and removal using sinus forceps.

Other attempts to narrow the lumen of the Eustachian tube have included injecting agents like calcium hydroxyapatite paste (non-FDA-approved) or performing procedures on the cartilaginous portion of the Eustachian tube to augment the soft tissue and facilitate closure of the valve. Calcium hydroxyapatite is a permanent filler material that can be injected beneath the surface of the mucosa. A needle is guided either transorally or transnasally and inserted just immediately beneath the mucosa, near the concave defect in the membranous wall of the Eustachian tube. Larger defects and those in which there is a defect at the 12 o'clock position (i.e., roof) in the Eustachian tube may not respond as well to the injection technique. Other injected materials have been reported, including morselized cartilage [30], fat [31], absorbable gelatin [32], Teflon paste [33], and polydimethylsiloxane elastomer [34]. Teflon has been abandoned following instances of cerebral embolus and death, potentially related to intravascular injection.

There have been additional methods described in which the Eustachian tube valve is reconstructed to narrow its lumen [26, 35, 36]. These procedures involve using combined transnasal and transoral approaches. The goal of the procedure is to narrow the diameter of the lumen without obliterating it entirely. Most commonly, incisions are made in the mucosa along the cartilaginous wall, beginning at the torus tubarius. Less commonly, the membranous wall may be augmented. Submucosal flaps are elevated, and materials are inserted into the pocket to reduce the diameter of the lumen [37]. The incisions are then closed. Still, other techniques have been developed, addressing the tensor veli palatini muscle or its tendon [38, 39]. Complete obliteration of the Eustachian tube can relieve symptoms [6, 26], but, chronic middle ear effusions are expected, at least initially. In instances of excessive closure of the valve, the effusion could become thick and mucoid, frequently occluding tympanostomy tubes. Total obliteration of the Eustachian tube is reserved only for patients who have failed multiple prior attempts to improve symptoms, as they would require permanent ventilation through the tympanic membrane and there is an increased risk of developing troublesome mucoid effusions.

The Differential Diagnosis of Autophony

From the time we begin to speak, we grow accustomed to the sound of our own voice, a combination of bone-conducted sounds transmitted directly from our vocal cords through bone to our ears combined with feedback from reflections of our self-generated acoustic sounds in the environment. This sensation is "normal." The lack of bone-conducted sound is the reason why our own voices sound distorted when we first hear recorded versions of them played back to us. Psychophysical experiments have taught that distortions in the perception of one's own voice can greatly affect the way one speaks. For instance, we raise the volume of our voices in the presence of background noise, known as the Lombard effect [40]. If one hears their own voice played back in a delayed manner, it begins to cause discomfort. Small delays (<10 ms) will distort the sound, medium delays (10–30 ms) will cause a hollow sound to the voice, and larger delays (>30 ms) are perceived as an "echo," with delays >200 ms resulting in difficulty communicating [41]. These studies support the idea that even a subtle variation in the way either bone- or air-conducted sounds reach our ear can significantly alter the comfort we experience when we perceive our own voice. Autophony is the term used to describe the enhanced, distorted perception of one's own voice.

Any method by which the sound of one's own voice becomes distorted can cause a sensation of autophony. Patients with patulous Eustachian tube dysfunction describe their own voice as sounding like they are speaking "in a bucket," and symptoms correlate temporally with the other symptoms of patulous Eustachian tube dysfunction, suggesting the opening in the Eustachian tube alters the transmission of sounds to the middle ear, resulting in a perceived distortion to one's voice. A loss in conductive hearing will cause distortion in the air-conducted component of one's own voice. This can be assessed by occluding the ear canal and speaking. Excessive cerumen, middle ear effusions, or ossicular chain abnormalities would cause a similar distortion. These alternative causes of autophony can be identified by pure tone audiometry, tympanometry, and a careful physical examination, including binocular microscopy. Patients with patulous Eustachian tube dysfunction typically do not have conductive hearing loss on pure tone audiometry, and conventional tympanometry is often normal.

Superior Semicircular Canal Dehiscence Syndrome and Other Third Mobile Window Syndromes

Altered mechanics within the inner ear can also cause distortion in one's own voice. For instance, diplacusis is the sensation of hearing two tones simultaneously. Patients with Meniere's disease occasionally report that some sounds in the affected ear can be perceived as having two tones, and this has been associated with the presence of endolymphatic hydrops [42]. Diplacusis can be disturbing, and similar to conductive hearing loss, the symptoms occur for both external and internal noises. However, patients with patulous Eustachian tube dysfunction often report that external sounds are often undisturbed, yet internal sounds, notably the sound of their own voice, are distorted. Another inner ear disorder that can alter the mechanics of acoustic transmission in the inner ear is superior semicircular canal dehiscence syndrome (SCDS) [43]. Like patients with patulous Eustachian tube dysfunction, patients with SCDS report that their own voice is disturbed but that their hearing for external sounds is minimally affected. Because of the overlap in symptoms of autophony, aural fullness, pulsatile tinnitus, and sensitivity to internal noises, SCDS is often in the differential when evaluating a patient with patulous Eustachian tube dysfunction and will be reviewed in greater detail.

SCDS has been modeled as a "third mobile window" syndrome. In a healthy state, there are two mobile windows in the inner ear: the oval and round windows. Vibrations of the tympanic membrane are transmitted through the ossicles to the inner ear at the oval window and are decompressed at the round window. In this way, acoustic energy is transmitted through the cochlea, facilitating normal hearing. There may be additional openings into the inner ear, caused either by surgeons or by disease processes. An extra opening or dehiscence in the superior semicircular canal is the best understood of these disorders. In some patients, an anatomic dehiscence in the superior semicircular canal can serve as a third mobile window and cause symptoms of superior semicircular canal dehiscence syndrome. The extra opening in the superior semicircular canal functions to shunt acoustic energy entering the oval window away from the round window and toward the dehiscence [44]. This causes an apparent increase in thresholds for low-frequency air-conducted sound on audiometry as this acoustic energy is shunted away from the cochlea. This alternate pathway traverses the sensory epithelium of the utricle and superior semicircular canal, causing the sound- and/or pressure-induced vertigo that patients report when exposed to loud low-frequency sounds. At the same time, the dehiscence creates a new low-impedance pathway into the inner ear for bone-conducted sounds. This allows patients with SCDS to hear bone-conducted sounds better than normal, leading to symptoms of autophony, pulsatile tinnitus, audible eyeball movements, footfalls, chewing, etc.

Risk Factors for Superior SCDS

The etiology of SCDS remains unknown, but there are two primary theories about its cause. The first is that SCDS is a congenital phenomenon, based on a large temporal bone study that found an anatomic dehiscence over the superior semicircular canal in approximately 0.5% of specimens without bony remodeling [45]. Furthermore, the otic capsule bone continues to develop several years after birth, with higher rates of anatomic dehiscence in young children [46]. Patients tend to present in their fourth and fifth decades of life; however, as many as a quarter of patients note an inciting traumatic event such as a head injury, noise exposure, or a strong Valsalva just prior to the onset of symptoms [47]. Others have suggested that SCDS may develop from progressive erosion of the bone over the superior semicircular canal and have pointed to the observation that patients with SCDS often have numerous defects in the tegmen [48]. The etiology may involve a combination of a congenital opening and progressive thinning of the bone or dura overlying the superior semicircular canal, eventually leading to the onset of symptoms.

Diagnosis of Superior SCDS

The International Classification for Vestibular Disorders recently published diagnostic criteria for SCDS [49]. For a diagnosis of SCDS, patients must have (1) at least one symptom consistent with a third mobile syndrome; (2) evidence of pressure transmission through the third mobile window on physiologic testing; and (3) the presence of dehiscence on high-resolution CT imaging. The symptoms that can be best attributed to a third mobile window include bone conduction hyperacusis (including autophony and abnormally loud internal noises like eye movements), sound or pressure-induced vertigo, and pulsatile tinnitus. There are several sensitive and specific diagnostic tests for SCDS. Classically, patients with SCDS have eye movements in the plane of the dehiscent semicircular canal when loud sounds or pressure are applied to the affected ear [43]. Additional diagnostic tests have become available, including the observation of negative or better-than-normal bone conduction thresholds on pure tone audiometry and enhanced responses on ocular or cervical vestibular-evoked myogenic potential (VEMP) testing. Patients with SCDS must also have anatomic dehiscence on high-resolution temporal bone CT imaging with multiplanar reconstruction in the plane of the affected semicircular canal (Fig. 15.3). Due to the frequent overlap of symptoms of SCDS with patulous Eustachian tube dysfunction and the observation that more patients with patulous Eustachian tube dysfunction than would be expected also have SCDS [7], any patient with symptoms consistent with SCDS should undergo a high-resolution temporal bone CT scan to evaluate for a possible third mobile window syndrome. Additional vestibular or VEMP testing can then be performed if an anatomic dehiscence is discovered. In patients with conductive hearing loss, stapedial reflex testing should be performed to distinguish SCDS from other diagnoses that cause conductive hearing loss, like otosclerosis. Stapedial reflexes should be present in patients with SCDS and absent in patients with other causes of conductive hearing loss.

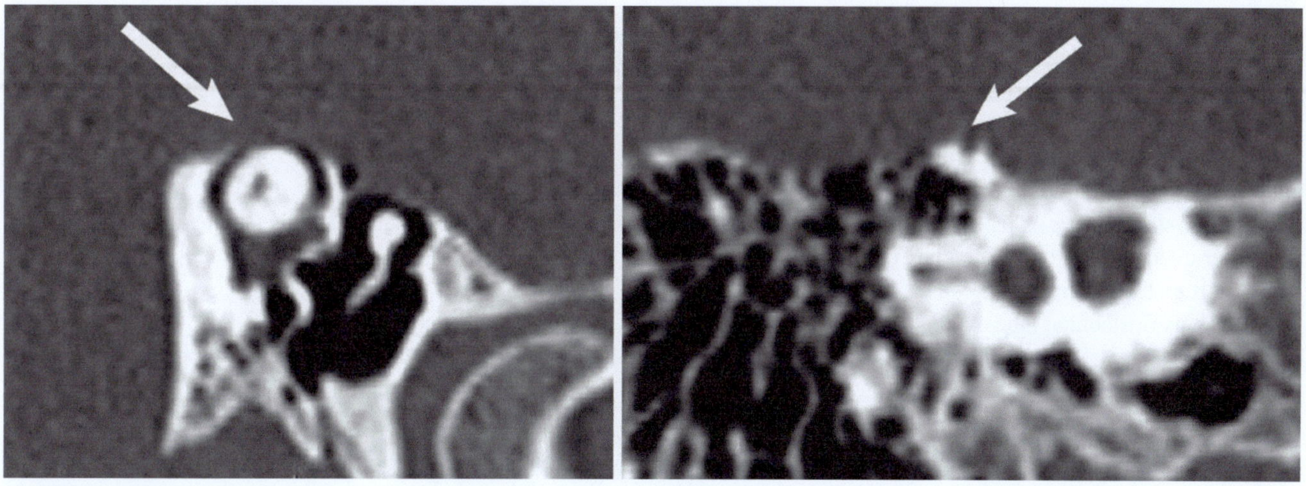

Fig. 15.3 Computed tomography imaging reconstructed in the plane of the superior semicircular canal and orthogonal to the canal, demonstrating a dehiscence (arrows)

Treatment of Superior SCDS

While there are no known medical treatments for SCDS, there are effective surgical interventions. Many patients (about half in our experience), however, are content to have an explanation for their symptoms and do not pursue surgical intervention. Surgery is offered when patients meet the diagnostic criteria for SCDS and find their symptoms debilitating. The original series by Minor et al. described plugging the superior semicircular canal via the middle cranial fossa approach [43]. The aim of surgery is to eliminate the pathophysiology of the third mobile window. Early attempts at resurfacing alone without plugging the affected canal led to recurrences of symptoms, and plugging was therefore preferred. Surgeons have used a variety of materials, including autologous tissues such as fascia, bone dust, bone chips, bone wax, or bone dust with fibrin glue. Often, the floor of the middle fossa is then resurfaced using calcium hydroxyapatite cement. Patients generally do well after surgery to plug the affected canal, with improvements in autophony [50], dizziness handicap [51], and overall health-related quality of life [52]. The transmastoid approach to plugging the canal has also been used with excellent results [53, 54]. Following surgery to plug the affected canal, patients have a reduction in the function of the affected superior canal, and about one-third of patients have a temporary reduction in the function of all three semicircular canals [55]. Profound hearing loss is a rare complication, occurring in fewer than 3% of cases, but approximately 25% of patients can have a high-frequency hearing loss [56]. The long-term recurrence rate following plugging is generally low, and most patients are content with the improvement in symptoms [57].

Conclusions

Autophony can be a debilitating symptom and seems to be particularly bothersome for patients with patulous Eustachian tube dysfunction and superior semicircular canal dehiscence syndrome. A careful history and physical examination can help differentiate the causes of autophony, but additional diagnostic testing may be needed. The workup typically begins with pure-tone audiometry and tympanometry. Additional evaluations such as nasopharyngoscopy, CT imaging, and vestibular-evoked myogenic potentials can help aid the diagnosis. Fortunately, there are excellent treatment options for both patulous Eustachian tube dysfunction and SCDS.

References

1. Schilder AGM, Bhutta MF, Butler CC, Holy C, Levine LH, Kvaerner KJ, et al. Eustachian tube dysfunction: consensus statement on definition, types, clinical presentation and diagnosis. Clin Otolaryngol. 2015;40:407–11.
2. Rumbold TF. A practical treatise on the medical, surgical and hygienic treatment of catarrhal diseases of the nose, throat, and ears. Medical Journal Publishing Company; 1888.
3. Shambaugh GE. Continuously open eustachian tube. Arch Otolaryngol. 1938;27:420–5.
4. Moore PM, Miller JB. Patulous, Eustachian tube. AMA Arch Otolaryngol. 1951;54:643–50.
5. Pulec JL, Simonton KM. Abnormal patency of the eustachian tube: report on 41 cases. Laryngoscope. 1964;74:267–71.
6. O'Connor AF, Shea JJ. Autophony and the patulous eustachian tube. Laryngoscope. 1981;91:1427–35.
7. Ward BK, Ashry Y, Poe DS. Patulous Eustachian tube dysfunction: patient demographics and comorbidities. Otol Neurotol. 2017;38:1362. https://doi.org/10.1097/MAO.0000000000001543.
8. Oshima T, Ogura M, Kikuchi T, Hori Y, Mugikura S, Higano S, et al. Involvement of pterygoid venous plexus in patulous eustachian tube symptoms. Acta Otolaryngol. 2007;127:693–9.
9. Yoshioka S, Naito K, Fujii N, Katada K. Movement of the Eustachian tube during sniffing in patients with patulous Eustachian tube: evaluation using a 320-row area detector CT scanner. Otol Neurotol. 2013;34:877–83.
10. Henry DF, DiBartolomeo JR. Patulous eustachian tube identification using tympanometry. J Am Acad Audiol. 1993;4:53–7.
11. Kikuchi T, Oshima T, Ogura M, Hori Y, Kawase T, Kobayashi T. Three-dimensional computed tomography imaging in the sitting position for the diagnosis of patulous eustachian tube. Otol Neurotol. 2007;28:199–203.
12. Ikeda R, Oshima T, Oshima H, Miyazaki M, Kikuchi T, Kawase T, et al. Management of patulous eustachian tube with habitual sniffing. Otol Neurotol. 2011;32:790–3.
13. Poe DS. Diagnosis and management of the patulous eustachian tube. Otol Neurotol. 2007;28:668–77.
14. DiBartolomeo JR, Henry DF. A new medication to control patulous eustachian tube disorders. Am J Otol. 1992;13:323–7.
15. Oshima T, Kikuchi T, Kawase T, Kobayashi T. Nasal instillation of physiological saline for patulous eustachian tube. Acta Otolaryngol. 2010;130:550–3.
16. Chen DA, Luxford WM. Myringotomy and tube for relief of patulous eustachian tube symptoms. Am J Otol. 1990;11:272–3.
17. Mackeith SAC, Bottrill ID. Polydimethylsiloxane elastomer injection in the management of the patulous eustachian tube. J Laryngol Otol. 2016;130:805–10.
18. Murakami S, Nakazawa M, Watanabe N, Takahashi M, Honda N, Goode RL. Role of tympanic membrane in symptoms of patulous eustachian tube syndrome: a new treatment with use of adhesive tape on the tympanic membrane. In: Middle ear mechanics in research and otology. World Scientific; 2004. p. 438–440.
19. Brace MD, Horwich P, Kirkpatrick D, Bance M. Tympanic membrane manipulation to treat symptoms of patulous eustachian tube. Otol Neurotol. 2014;35:1201–6.
20. Boedts M. Paper patching of the tympanic membrane as a symptomatic treatment for patulous eustachian tube syndrome. J Laryngol Otol. 2014;128:228–35.
21. Si Y, Chen Y, Li P, Jiang H, Xu G, Li Z, et al. Eardrum thickening approach for the treatment of patulous Eustachian tube. Eur Arch Otorhinolaryngol. 2016;273:3673–8.
22. Kim SJ, Shin SA, Lee HY, Park Y-H. Paper patching for patulous eustachian tube. Acta Otolaryngol. 2019;139:122–8.
23. Bluestone CD, Cantekin EI. "How I do it"—otology and neurotology. A specific issue and its solution. Management of the patulous Eustachian tube. Laryngoscope. 1981;91:149–52.
24. Dyer RK Jr, McElveen JT Jr. The patulous eustachian tube: management options. Otolaryngol Head Neck Surg. 1991;105:832–5.
25. Dean M, Lian T. Transnasal endoscopic Eustachian tube surgery. Otolaryngol Clin North Am. 2016;49:1163–71.
26. Ward BK, Chao W-C, Abiola G, Kawai K, Ashry Y, Rasooly T, et al. Twelve-month outcomes of Eustachian tube procedures for man-

agement of patulous Eustachian tube dysfunction. Laryngoscope. 2019;129:222–8.
27. Yu BJ, Kim HM, Jin SK, Park SN. Therapeutic efficacy of angiocatheter insertion surgery in the bony orifice of patulous Eustachian tube. Korean J Otorhinolaryngol Head Neck Surg. 2014;57:54–60.
28. Park JM, Han JS, Park SY, Park SN. Transtympanic tripod-shaped angiocatheter insertion for patients with intractable patulous Eustachian tube. Otol Neurotol. 2021;42:e1273–8.
29. Kikuchi T, Ikeda R, Oshima H, Takata I, Kawase T, Oshima T, et al. Effectiveness of Kobayashi plug for 252 ears with chronic patulous Eustachian tube. Acta Otolaryngol. 2017;137:253–8.
30. Oh S, Kong S-K. Endoscopic autologous cartilage injection for the patulous Eustachian tube: presenting author: Sejoon Oh. J Laryngol Otol. 2016;130:S215–6.
31. Doherty JK, Slattery WH 3rd. Autologous fat grafting for the refractory patulous eustachian tube. Otolaryngol Head Neck Surg. 2003;128:88–91.
32. Ogawa S, Satoh I, Tanaka H. Patulous Eustachian tube. A new treatment with infusion of absorbable gelatin sponge solution. Arch Otolaryngol. 1976;102:276–80.
33. Pulec JL. Abnormally patent eustachian tubes: treatment with injection of poly-tetrafluoroethylene (teflon) paste. Laryngoscope. 1967;77:1543.
34. Schröder S, Lehmann M, Sudhoff HH, Ebmeyer J. Treatment of the patulous Eustachian tube with soft-tissue bulking agent injections. Otol Neurotol. 2015;36:448–52.
35. Yañez C, Pirrón JA, Mora N. Curvature inversion technique: a novel tuboplastic technique for patulous Eustachian tube—a preliminary report. Otolaryngol Head Neck Surg. 2011;145:446–51.
36. Rotenberg BW, Busato G-M, Agrawal SK. Endoscopic ligation of the patulous eustachian tube as treatment for autophony. Laryngoscope. 2013;123:239–43.
37. Adil E, Poe D. What is the full range of medical and surgical treatments available for patients with Eustachian tube dysfunction? Curr Opin Otolaryngol Head Neck Surg. 2014;22:8–15.
38. Stroud MH, Spector GJ, Maisel RH. Patulous eustachian tube syndrome. Preliminary report of the use of the tensor veli palatini transposition procedure. Arch Otolaryngol. 1974;99:419–21.
39. Virtanen H, Palva T. Surgical treatment of patulous eustachian tube. Arch Otolaryngol. 1982;108:735–9.
40. Lombard E. Le signe de l'elevation de la voix. Ann Mal de L'Oreille et Du Larynx. 1911:101–119.
41. Appel R, Beerends JG. On the quality of hearing one's own voice. J Audio Eng Soc. 2002;50:237–48.
42. Tonndorf J. The mechanism of hearing loss in early cases of endolymphatic hydrops. Ann Otol Rhinol Laryngol. 1957;66:766–84.
43. Minor LB, Solomon D, Zinreich JS, Zee DS. Sound- and/or pressure-induced vertigo due to bone dehiscence of the superior semicircular canal. Arch Otolaryngol Head Neck Surg. 1998;124:249–58.
44. Rosowski JJ, Songer JE, Nakajima HH, Brinsko KM, Merchant SN. Clinical, experimental, and theoretical investigations of the effect of superior semicircular canal dehiscence on hearing mechanisms. Otol Neurotol. 2004;25:323–32.
45. Carey JP, Minor LB, Nager GT. Dehiscence or thinning of bone overlying the superior semicircular canal in a temporal bone survey. Arch Otolaryngol Head Neck Surg. 2000;126:137–47.
46. Meiklejohn DA, Corrales CE, Boldt BM, Sharon JD, Yeom KW, Carey JP, et al. Pediatric semicircular canal dehiscence: radiographic and histologic prevalence, with clinical correlation. Otol Neurotol. 2015;36:1383–9.
47. Minor LB. Clinical manifestations of superior semicircular canal dehiscence. Laryngoscope. 2005;115:1717–27.
48. Schutt CA, Neubauer P, Samy RN, Pensak ML, Kuhn JJ, Herschovitch M, et al. The correlation between obesity, obstructive sleep apnea, and superior semicircular canal dehiscence: a new explanation for an increasingly common problem. Otol Neurotol. 2015;36:551.
49. Ward BK, van de Berg R, van Rompaey V, Bisdorff A, Hullar TE, Welgampola MS, et al. Superior semicircular canal dehiscence syndrome: diagnostic criteria consensus document of the committee for the classification of vestibular disorders of the Bárány Society. J Vestib Res. 2021;31:131–41. https://doi.org/10.3233/ves-200004.
50. Crane BT, Lin FR, Minor LB, Carey JP. Improvement in autophony symptoms after superior canal dehiscence repair. Otol Neurotol. 2010;31:140–6.
51. Crane BT, Minor LB, Carey JP. Superior canal dehiscence plugging reduces dizziness handicap. Laryngoscope. 2008;118:1809–13.
52. Remenschneider AK, Owoc M, Kozin ED, McKenna MJ, Lee DJ, Jung DH. Health utility improves after surgery for superior canal dehiscence syndrome. Otol Neurotol. 2015;36:1695–701.
53. Crovetto M, Areitio E, Elexpuru J, Aguayo F. Transmastoid approach for resurfacing of superior semicircular canal dehiscence. Auris Nasus Larynx. 2008;35:247–9.
54. Agrawal SK, Parnes LS. Transmastoid superior semicircular canal occlusion. Otol Neurotol. 2008;29:363–7.
55. Agrawal Y, Migliaccio AA, Minor LB, Carey JP. Vestibular hypofunction in the initial postoperative period after surgical treatment of superior semicircular canal dehiscence. Otol Neurotol. 2009;30:502–6.
56. Ward BK, Agrawal Y, Nguyen E, Della Santina CC, Limb CJ, Francis HW, et al. Hearing outcomes after surgical plugging of the superior semicircular canal by a middle cranial fossa approach. Otol Neurotol. 2012;33:1386–91.
57. Alkhafaji MS, Varma S, Pross SE, Sharon JD, Nellis JC, Santina CCD, et al. Long-term patient-reported outcomes after surgery for superior canal dehiscence syndrome. Otol Neurotol. 2017;38:1319–26.

Office Examination in Otitis Media

16

Fábio André Selaimen, Alice Lang Silva,
Wiquinylson França de Oliveira,
and Sady Selaimen da Costa

Office Examination in Otitis Media

- How to collect and store high-quality images and data
- The challenge of examining the tympanic membrane: advantages and disadvantages of the otoscopes, microscopes, and endoscopes.
- Telemedicine otoscopy: Is it possible to make remote diagnostics?

Introduction

Otorhinolaryngology is a specialty that examines regions with difficult access. Evaluating structures such as the larynx, paranasal sinus, and ear has always been challenging since adequate angulation and lighting are simultaneously necessary. The technological improvements that occurred in the last decade brought a series of advances in the diagnosis process in otorhinolaryngology. Such progress led to a series of benefits, such as a greater understanding of the pathogenesis of diseases and the development of new therapeutic possibilities.

In otology, more specifically, it was not different. In the twentieth century, the otolaryngologist relied mainly on the otoscope, which has some limitations, such as limited amplification, angulation, and poor lighting. Although the otoscope has received several improvements over the years, such as the evolution of the halogen lamp to the LED lamp, today, it is just one more instrument among the many available in the office.

The microscopes, previously present only in operating rooms as large and heavy volumes, have evolved into much more compact and lightweight structures. In addition, there was a reduction in the cost of microscopes, a product of the dissemination of manufacturing techniques. As a result of these factors, today, the microscope can already be found in the office of most otologists.

The microscope is of foremost importance in manipulating the external and middle ear, allowing the removal of discharges, crusts, and granulations. It makes it possible to perform procedures with greater efficiency and less discomfort for the patient. Its significant difference is that it provides a three-dimensional and enlarged view, which allows better observation of the tympanic membrane and its relationship with structures of the external auditory canal and the middle ear. These features allow, for example, better identification and grading of tympanic retractions and better detailing of other aspects of the tympanic membrane and the external auditory canal.

Otoendoscopy, performed with the aid of 0°, 30°, and 45° rigid optics, emerged in the 1980s and was popularized in the twenty-first century. For otological examination in the office, perhaps the most evident benefit is the possibility of visualizing the anterior tympanic borders in patients whose external auditory canals are more tortuous. With the arrival of this technology, the tympanic membrane perforations previously classified as marginal can often be reclassified as central since the edges, hidden by the tortuosity of the external acoustic meatus, now become visible.

Otoendoscopy allows greater angulation in the external auditory canal, more efficient image amplification, and the possibility of more proximity with the tympanic membrane (often almost in direct contact). Also, it allows for the recording of the otoscopy, qualifying for reanalysis as often as required. New perspectives for studying chronic otitis media (COM) [1] emerged with the aid of those technologies.

F. A. Selaimen (✉)
Hospital de Clínicas de Porto Alegre, Porto Alegre, Brazil

Instituto Gaúcho de Otorrinolaringologia, Porto Alegre, Brazil

A. L. Silva
Instituto Gaúcho de Otorrinolaringologia, Porto Alegre, Brazil

W. F. de Oliveira
Universidade Federal do Rio Grande do Sul, Porto Alegre, Brazil

S. S. da Costa
Hospital de Clínicas de Porto Alegre, Porto Alegre, Brazil

Instituto Gaúcho de Otorrinolaringologia, Porto Alegre, Brazil

Universidade Federal do Rio Grande do Sul, Porto Alegre, Brazil

M. V. Goycoolea et al. (eds.), *Textbook of Otitis Media*, https://doi.org/10.1007/978-3-031-40949-3_16

Our research group has used otoendoscopy since 2002. Based on the serial analysis of cases of COM, we have already proposed a new classification for middle ear cholesteatomas [2], with the description of new growth patterns until then not observed. Furthermore, considering the tympanic membrane perforations, as previously mentioned, many were reclassified when we could see the tympanic borders with the otoendoscopy. Also, we were able to recognize essential factors related to perforation's pathogenesis. An example is the description of signs [3] that suggest tympanic membrane retraction before tympanic perforation, an association not previously portrayed in the literature, namely:

1. Medialization of the malleus handle,
2. Tympanic remnants in touch over the promontory,
3. Tympanic remnants in touch with the ossicular chain (incus and stapes),
4. Erosion of the ossicular chain.

These signs, analyzed adequately from the pathogenesis perspective, culminated in the proposal of a new classification for tympanic membranes.

This chapter aims to help the reader assemble their equipment for assistance or research purposes. It is important to emphasize that, at present, the availability of equipment on the market is endless, making it impossible to determine which system would be the best. The message to be conveyed in the chapter refers to the general lines of assembling a video otoscopy system, as well as some tricks and techniques that we have learned in the last 20 years of experience in our group. The reader should adapt the system to their possibilities and needs.

How to Collect and Store High-Quality Images and Data

The studies mentioned above, like countless others that aim to increase knowledge about pathogenesis and improve the treatment of COM, are possible only through proper compilation and storage of data. Therefore, routine use and the combination of good visualization with storage systems are essential for research. In addition, it ensures the replicability and reliability of data from many patients and different data from the same patient at different moments, which allows for a perspective on the progression of chronic disease.

Technology has added unanimous benefits to the daily care of patients in the otolaryngologist's clinic. High-resolution otoendoscopy and storage systems used initially for research purposes rapidly migrated to our clinics. Today, we can easily and quickly manipulate the middle ear with a microscope and, later, visualize and record the otoendoscopy. In addition, such storage allows for further reanalysis and case discussion with colleagues, which leads to overall improved care.

Table 16.1 Example of the information on the protocol used at the Chronic Otitis Media Outpatient Clinic at Hospital de Clínicas de Porto Alegre

Identification information	Individual record number Patient information (age, race, sex)
Subjective information	Subjective information about the case (chief complaint, chronology, associated symptoms) Standardized scoring tests for hearing loss and tinnitus Medical history (comorbidities, risk factors, past procedures, family history)
Objective information	Physical exam annotations Audiometry test results Detailed description of the tympanic membrane and middle ear

Therefore, in the following pages, we will present the protocol developed in our research group over the last 20 years. We remind you that it is necessary to obtain the Informed Consent Form from the patient (or their guardian) to store and use data from the anamnesis and physical examination.

Anamnesis Protocol

Mainly used for research purposes [1], we will show our group's anamnesis and otoscopy description protocols. Table 16.1 shows the protocol in its current version. In order to avoid mistakes in data transposition, our anamnesis and description protocols have been the same for the last 20 years. We strongly suggest avoiding frequent changes in protocols.

In recent years, the same protocol has been computerized and is currently applied through the RedCap tool. It is a secure web application for building and managing online surveys and databases.

Preparation of the Ears

The first step in recording an adequate otoscopy is, without a doubt, the proper preparation of the ears. The external auditory canal must be thoroughly cleaned, removing accumulated discharge, debris, epithelial desquamation, or any other obstacles to the tympanic membrane. Any crusts adhered to the tympanic membrane or in the attic region must be removed, as they may hide underlying retractions or cholesteatomas. Granulation tissue should also be treated with focal cauterization, antibiotics, and topical corticosteroids, whether it comes from the external auditory canal or the middle ear. Often, proper registration may not be performed on the patient's first visit to the clinic. Sometimes, it is only after proper otological care that a proper diagnosis can be made. Figure 16.1 shows the same ear at three different times.

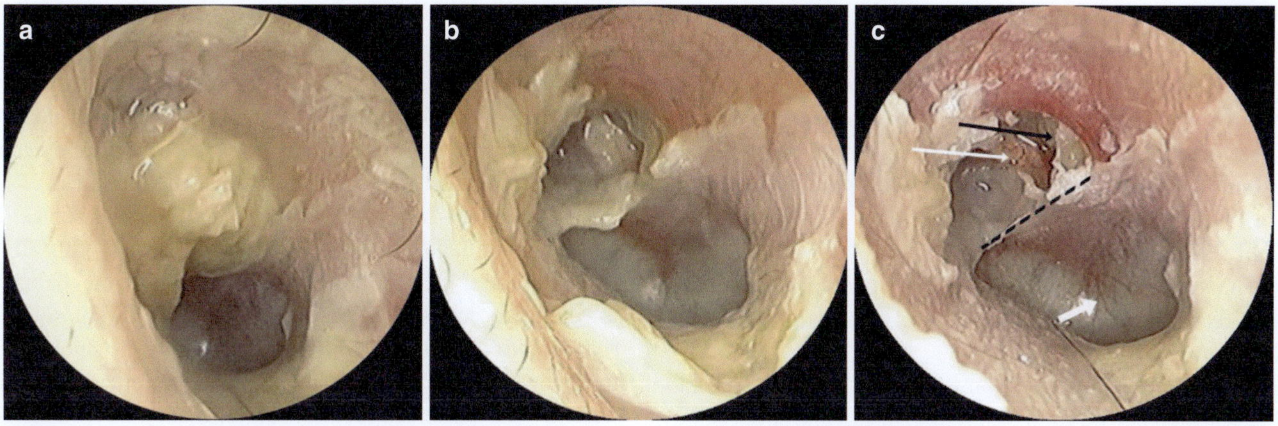

Fig. 16.1 Same ear at different moments. (**a**) At the patient's first visit, otorrhea, and epithelial debris make the diagnosis impossible. (**b**) After proper cleaning, reveal the infected attic cholesteatoma. (**c**) After the use of topical antibiotics and corticosteroids, with improvement in the infection and better definition of the attic cholesteatoma, with blockage of the tympanic diaphragm (dotted line), erosion of the malleus head (long white arrow), epithelial accumulation toward the aditus (long black arrow), and radial hypervascularization suggesting effusion in the mesotympanum (short white arrow)

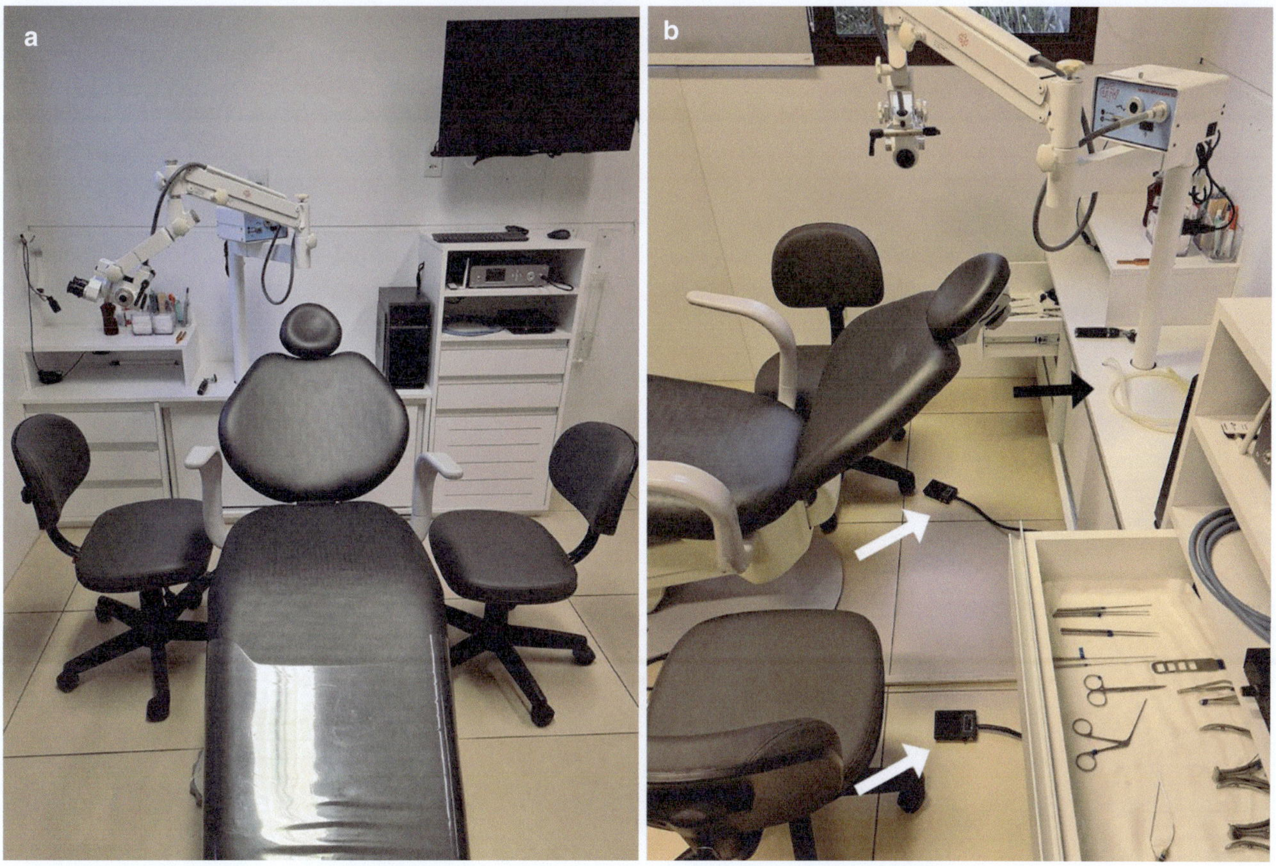

Fig. 16.2 Examination room with otomicroscopy and otoendoscopy with a recording system. (**a**) View of the dental chair, with a microscope at the top and chairs with backrests on both sides. (**b**) Detail of the aspiration system (black arrow) with pedal actuation on both sides (white arrows) and instruments for otological manipulation also available on both sides

These cleaning and preparative procedures should preferably be performed with a microscope. It is more comfortable for the patient because it allows for better control of instruments since binocular vision provides three-dimensional visualization of the ear. In these cases, an ENT chair or dental chair can be used.

Aspiration must be potent, and the room must allow the physician to perform the procedures with the proper posture without causing discomfort during a whole day of appointments. Figure 16.2 shows the ideal setting idealized by this chapter's authors.

Videoendoscopy System

Image-capturing systems are constantly improving with the technological innovations that are in unceasing development. Therefore, we reiterate that we will present the principles for different video endoscopy systems so that each professional can assemble their own complete system according to their reality, availability, and needs.

The systems are composed of three parts: image acquisition, recording, and storage/editing. A system overview is shown in Fig. 16.3.

The image acquisition components consist of an endoscope, which can be rigid (telescope) or flexible (fiber optic), a camera, a light source, and a monitor. While flexible fiber optics are used more in other areas of otolaryngology, telescopes are the choice for video otoscopy. In our routine, we have three telescope options:

- 0°, 4 mm, and 18 cm are preferred for use as they have a larger image area.
- 0°, 2.7 mm, and 11 cm are preferable for children or patients with a narrow external auditory canal.
- 30°, 2.7 mm, and 11 cm are used in specific situations, such as the analysis of attic retractions or others that require more angulation.

Cameras, previously found only with traditional suppliers and at very high costs, are now popularized and can even be found on traditional shopping websites (eBay and Amazon, among others). Therefore, we strongly recommend at least a full HD resolution. Nevertheless, 4K-resolution systems are more easily found nowadays and provide a great-quality image. Also, we believe that 3D visualization will be available soon at a feasible price for use at medical clinics.

Light sources have also gone through several stages of evolution. Initially, halogen lamps associated with fiber optics granted much better visualization than battery-powered otoscopes or Garcia's mirror with a light source. The evolution of light developed xenon lamps, which were more powerful and had less energy consumption, and LED is currently the preferred technology. The adaptation of LED lamps to medical equipment made much more powerful lighting possible and reduced the light sources' size. Alternatively, we can also find LED sources integrated with micro-camera devices in a single volume. In Fig. 16.4, we demonstrate an example of each of these devices.

The monitor can be specifically built for this purpose, or a regular television monitor with Full HD resolution can be used with good performance. The monitor can also be connected to the physician's computer to demonstrate endoscopy images or procedures.

We must remember that there is no "free lunch." In other words, we should remember that despite the wide variety of camera systems and LED sources, quality may vary a lot between them. The technical specifications provided can often lead us to misassessments in the assembly of the video

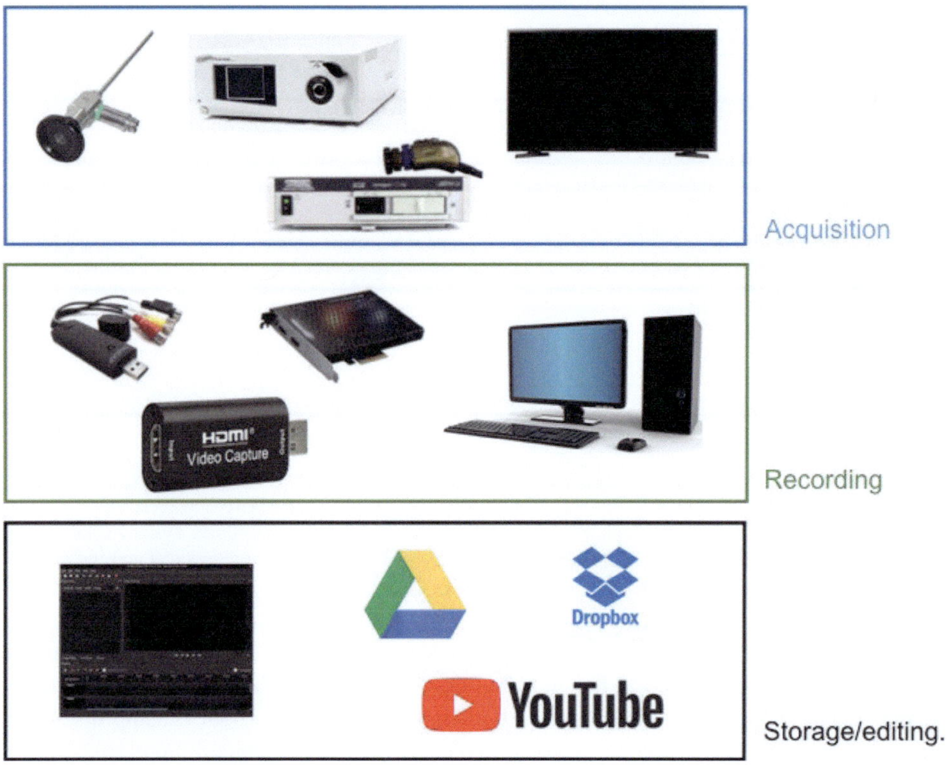

Fig. 16.3 Components of a complete video otoendoscopy system

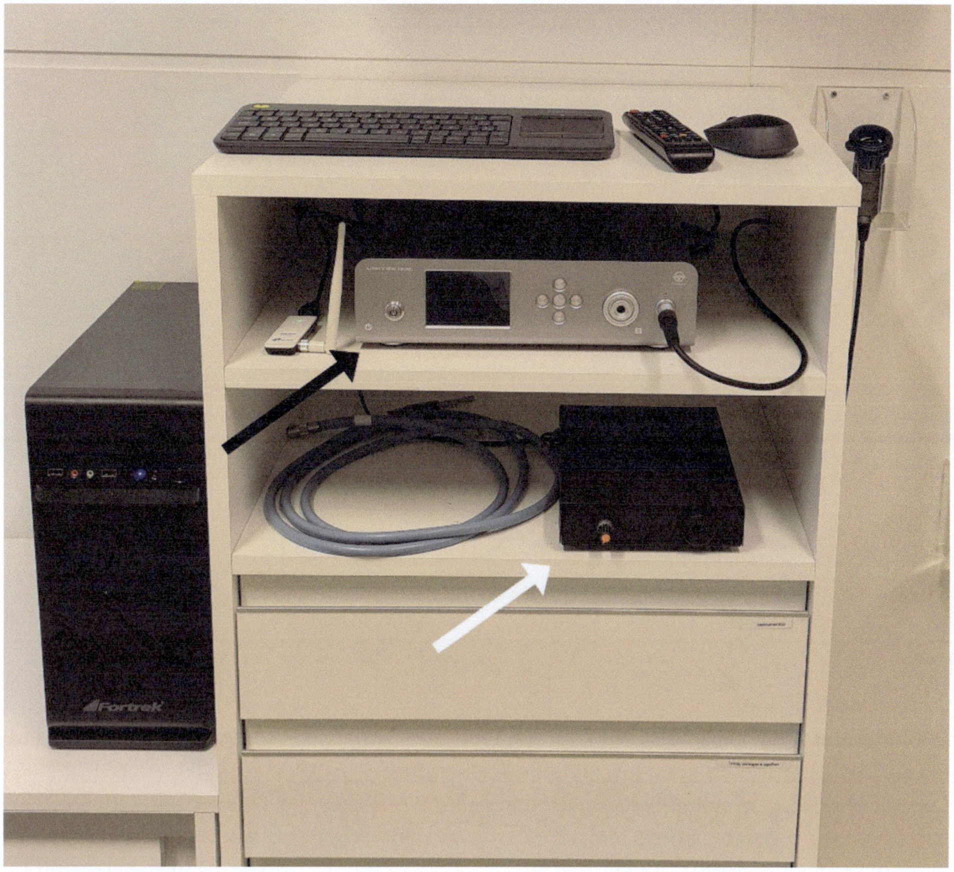

Fig. 16.4 Camera system with integrated LED source in the same volume (black arrow). LED light source (white arrow), with very reduced dimensions compared to those previously built with a halogen or xenon lamp

system. Just as an example, a camera with Full HD resolution (1920 × 1080 pixels) can provide an image with less quality than an HD (1280 × 720 pixels), which has a better-planned construction and higher-quality materials (lenses, conductors). At this point, it should be noted that traditional (and more expensive) brands tend to perform better than emerging brands and have surprisingly lower values, even if the technical specifications are the same. The professional should test the products whenever possible before making their final purchase.

Recording systems consist of image-capturing and recording devices. They are essential for teaching and research purposes but are optional for assistance. A video capture card and recording software are the items needed. The recording card must be compatible with the camera's output format (HDMI standard is the most modern and preferred standard nowadays). The HDMI interface is fully digital and capable of transmitting uncompressed audio and video data, representing an improved alternative to analog. It is still possible to use analogic technology (coax cable, S-Video, and composite video, among others), but these are in disuse and will probably disappear in a few years. The computer interface should preferably be USB to maximize compatibility and avoid data loss or delay.

As for the software used for capture, the options are extensive and very varied. The choice should be made according to the professional's choice and the sophistication required. Our clinic uses very simple and intuitive freeware, reducing the chances of wrong recordings or unintentional data loss.

Once the images are acquired and can be recorded, editing and storage systems are needed for future use of the images. Editing can be done with freeware too, which is usually very simple and intuitive. Most of the time, the physician is alone to record the otoendoscopy, generating unnecessary seconds of recording at the beginning and end of each video. Therefore, editing the video to cut the first and last seconds is necessary. Furthermore, it is also possible to perform cuts and add frames with structure names, captions, and other improvements that are currently available in programs for these purposes. Storage can be performed on physical media (computers, external hard drives, DVDs) or in clouds, the current preferred form. The best options are Google Drive, Dropbox, and YouTube.

Our Ideal System

The ideal system comprises all the requirements above and is shown in Fig. 16.5. A computer used exclusively to aid in video otoscopy seems perfect (regardless of whether it is a notebook, desktop, or all-in-one). Hardware used exclusively for this purpose has a lower chance of delays and crashes.

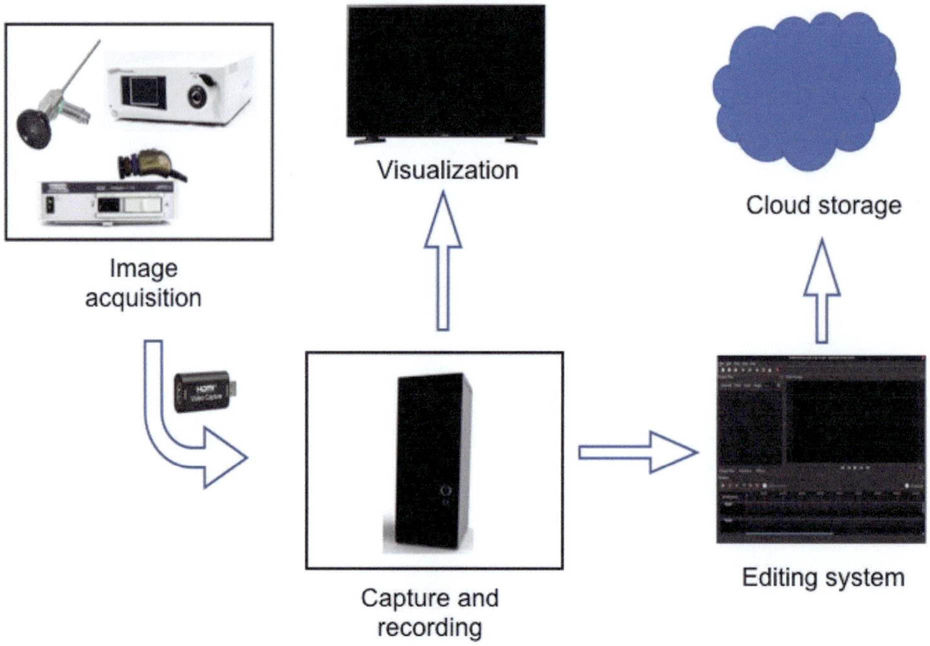

Fig. 16.5 Ideal video system composed of all previous requirements, with a computer used exclusively for this purpose. It consists of a camera for image acquisition, a video capture card, and a computer (with a monitor for visualization and software for editing) connected to cloud storage

Alternative System

Alternatively, the computer already used at the medical office can be the hardware for recording. Everything will depend on the positioning inside the room, and the possibility of using a wireless mouse and keyboard can help at the beginning and end of recordings. It is also possible to duplicate the image, favoring ergonomics in the service room. In this case, we suggest the use of image splitters so that the image does not suffer a delay with the capture before returning to the preview. The alternative system is shown in Fig. 16.6.

Software Tools for Analysis of the Tympanic Membrane

After recording and editing the video otoscopy, the assessment and quantification of tympanic membrane pathologies can either be performed manually by an expert or by specialized software.

Developed in 2006 in a partnership between the Federal Universities of Rio Grande do Sul and Santa Catarina and used for research at the Chronic Otitis Media Outpatient Clinic at Hospital de Clínicas de Porto Alegre, Cyclops Auris Wizard [4] (Fig. 16.7) is a tool used for quantitative analysis of the size and localization of tympanic membrane perforations. The software uses static frames from video otoscopy and provides accurate and reliable analysis using a semi-automated approach. The developers have published a validation study of the method using a subset of 39 cases randomly performed using images generated by experts [4]. Other researchers have used it to successfully correlate tympanic perforation characteristics to hearing loss patterns and to propose a new classification based on pathogenesis.

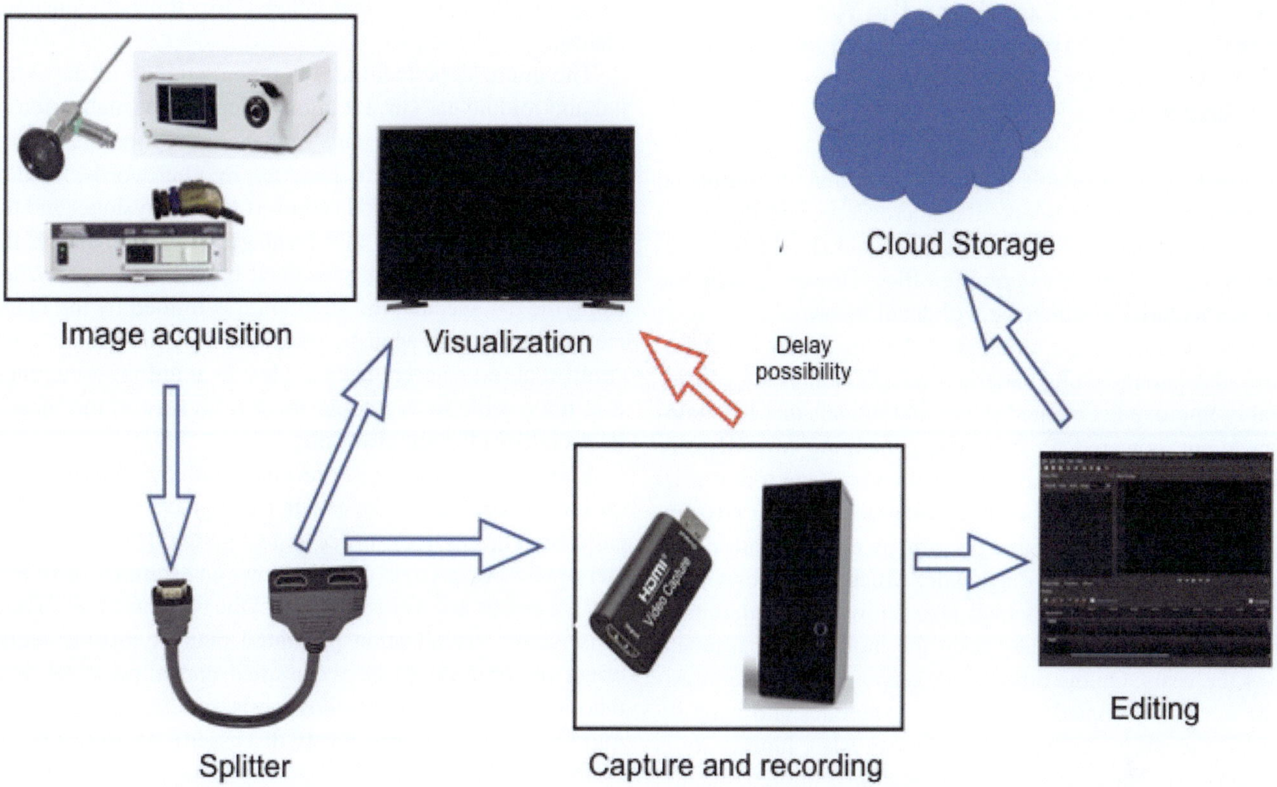

Fig. 16.6 Alternative video system

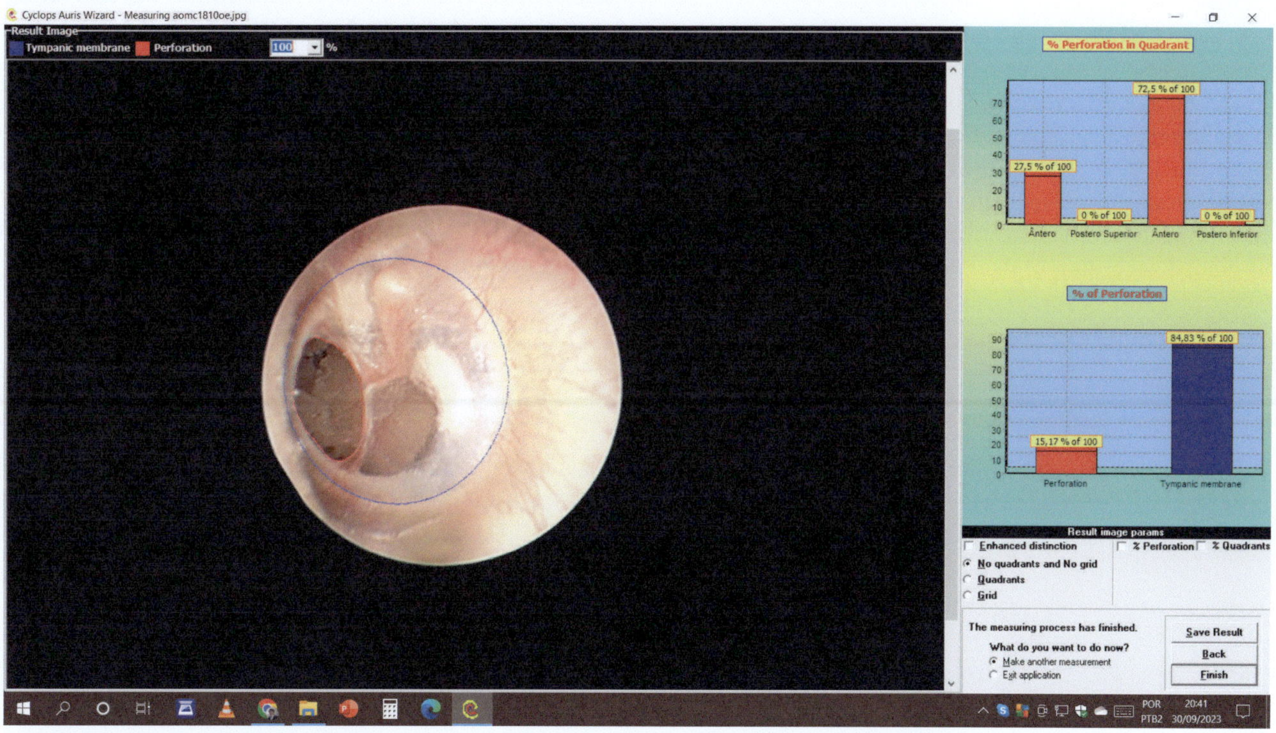

Fig. 16.7 Cyclops Auris Wizard interface

The Challenge of Examining the Tympanic Membrane: Advantages and Disadvantages of the Otoscopes, Microscopes, and Endoscopes

The instruments available today for examining the tympanic membrane are the otoscope, the microscope, and the endoscope. All three fulfill their objectives and should be available in the otologist's examining office. However, each one has particularities, which we will detail below.

The otoscope has evolved a lot in recent decades. Nowadays, long-lasting batteries and LED lamps are considerably improved compared to the first models that had halogen lamps powered by batteries, generating low-intensity lighting. However, perhaps, the main advantage today is its practicality and availability. In a case of less than 20 × 10 cm, we can take it anywhere and perform an excellent otoscopy.

The otoscope can be diagnostic, which only allows visualization, or operating, which also allows manipulation of the ear. It has undoubtedly been the most used instrument over the years. On the other hand, keeping one of the physician's hands occupied can reduce ergonomics and partially impair the ability to manipulate the ear. Also, luminosity is lower than in other devices, and angulation is limited. Finally, recording is impossible with most otoscopes, except for some clinical otoscopes that allow video equipment to be attached.

As described above, microscopes have suffered a significant reduction in size and cost in recent decades. That allowed many otolaryngologists to acquire this instrument for use in the office. Image magnification, with augmentation as much as 5, 10, 16, or 25 times, allows for a much more accurate diagnosis than the otoscope in many situations. Tympanic retractions, for example, can be identified and graded according to their severity with high precision since the binocular view allows for three-dimensional vision.

The microscope facilitates the manipulation of the external and middle ear since it allows amplified visualization of anatomical structures and enhances ergonomics, thus increasing the examiner's dexterity. In other words, in addition to better vision, it adds comfort to the physician and the patient. However, as a disadvantage, we can mention the same lack of angulation presented by the otoscope. When using the ear specula, the angulation is limited by the diameter of the external acoustic meatus and by the patient's discomfort at more accentuated angles. In addition, sometimes, it is impossible to overcome some tortuosity in the meatus (especially in the anterior wall).

Endoscopes are the most recent technology (compared to otoscopes and microscopes), but they have revolutionized ear examinations in the office and surgeries. The small diameter of telescopes (rigid optics) allows an examination of narrow ear canals and a closer vision of the tympanic membrane. This nearer visualization permitted many tympanic membrane perforations to be reclassified and allowed for new theories regarding the pathogenesis of different types of middle ear otitis (as previously discussed). An example can be found in Fig. 16.8.

However, as with any instrument, it also has its liabilities. As it occurs with the otoscope, it also provides two-dimensional vision, even if sometimes we can almost forget that given the quality of the image. Another disadvantage is the higher cost involved in having a complete set of endoscopic image acquisitions. As to manipulation, it has been argued by many experienced otologists that after some time of training, external and even middle ear procedures can be performed with good one-hand dexterity. Table 16.2 summarizes the advantages and disadvantages of each method.

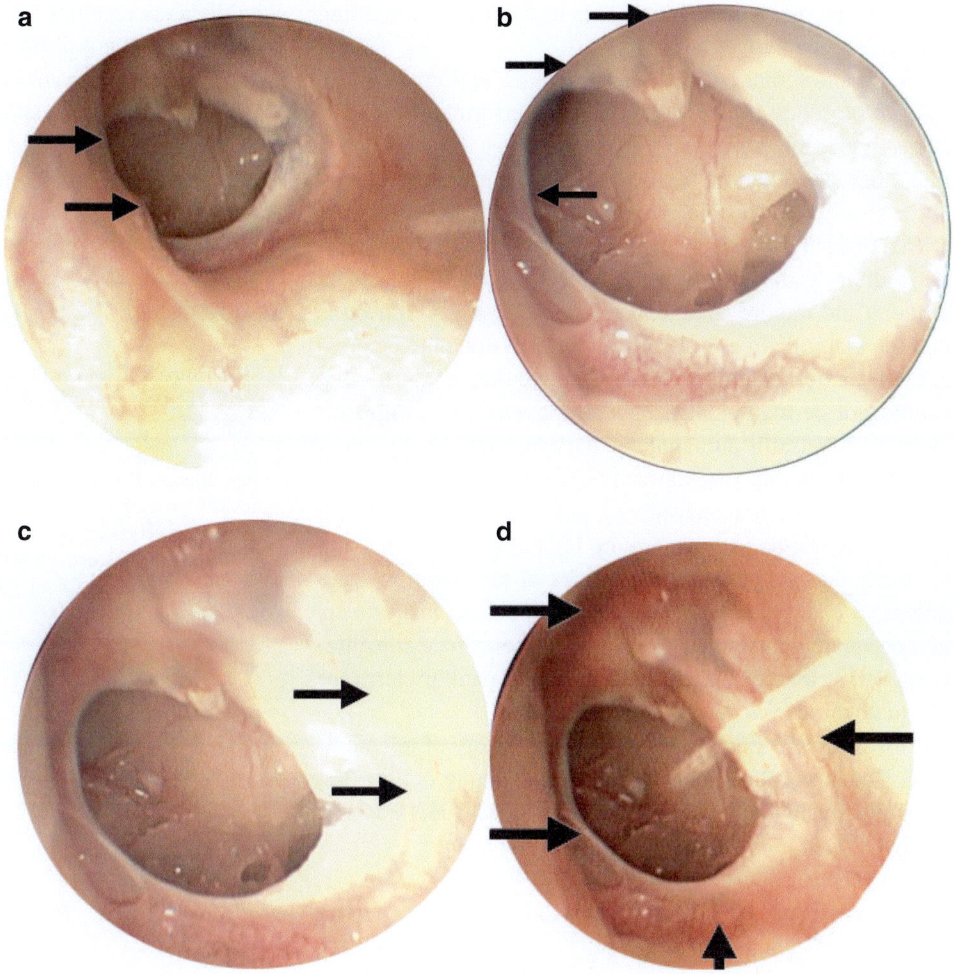

Fig. 16.8 Sequence of images from the same video otoscopy. (**a**) Tortuosity of the external auditory canal does not allow visualization of the anterior region (black arrows). (**b**) Proximity of the endoscope prevents visualization of the entire tympanic membrane on the same screen (black arrows). (**c**) Excessive light impairs the definition of the posterior edges (black arrows). (**d**) All criteria are met: visualization of the whole tympanic membrane and the perforation borders, good visualization of the attic, and adequate light power (black arrows)

Table 16.2 Advantages and disadvantages of each ear examining method

	Otoscope	Microscope	Endoscope
Advantages	• Availability • Quickness • Versatility	• Amplification • Three-dimensional vision • Ergonomics • Better manipulation	• Angulation • Ear canal tortuosity • Different diameters (for narrow ear canal)
Disadvantages	• Little amplification • Limited angulation • Allows for manipulation but with less precision	• More expensive • Limited angulation	• More expensive • Limited manipulation • Two-dimensional vision

Telemedicine Otoscopy: Is it Possible to Make the Diagnosis from a Distance?

Objectively answering the subtitle question: yes, it is possible. Currently, there is excellent availability and variability in image-recording devices, and the exchange of information between physicians is greatly facilitated. In addition to the devices and systems detailed previously in this chapter, we can also record ear examinations with smartphones using portable adapters.

Portable adapters can range from specific models for a particular smartphone to universal models. The adaptation and focus can be adjusted manually, and the device itself performs the recording, facilitating the sharing of images. We reiterate that the patient's consent is necessary for recording and storing the images.

We believe that, regardless of the technology used to acquire otoscopy images, it should be performed by physicians, preferably otolaryngologists, for two main reasons: first, the visualization of the tympanic membrane is not always easily accessible. Due to the presence of earwax, crusts, discharge, or even anatomical variations of the external auditory canal, access to the tympanic membrane can be arduous and require some experience. The second reason is that the manipulation of specific structures that may be present in the external auditory meatus may indicate injuries that should not be manipulated outside the surgical setting. An example is pulsatile aural polyps that can correspond to paragangliomas, highly vascularized lesions.

For now, we are unaware of portable devices that the patient can use to perform remote ENT appointments using telemedicine. Due to the singularities of the otorhinolaryngological examination, which requires specific instruments and adequate lighting, we believe that face-to-face consultations will still be essential in the short and medium term for adequate diagnoses.

However, teleconsultation is just one feature of telemedicine. The possibility of discussing cases among colleagues, remotely evaluating consultancies for other doctors, and even distance teaching has dramatically improved in recent years. All these possibilities for exchanging information and knowledge are of paramount importance for the evolution of otorhinolaryngology, especially because some diseases are more typical of specific populations. The possibility of exchanging knowledge with professionals from various parts of the world brings many benefits, especially for patients.

References

1. da Costa SS, Rosito LPS, Dornelles C, Sperling N. The contralateral ear in chronic otitis media. Arch Otolaryngol Head Neck Surg. 2008;134(3):290–3.
2. Rosito LPS, Silveira Netto LF, Teixeira AR, da Costa SS. Classification of cholesteatoma according to growth patterns. JAMA Otolaryngol Head Neck Surg. 2016;142(2):168–72. https://doi.org/10.1001/jamaoto.2015.3148.
3. Selaimen FA, Rosito LPS, da Silva MNL, de Souza Stanham V, Sperling N, da Costa SS. Tympanic membrane perforations: a critical analysis of 1003 ears and proposal of a new classification based on pathogenesis. Eur Arch Otorhinolaryngol. 2022;279:1277. https://doi.org/10.1007/s00405-021-06776-8.
4. Comunello E, Von Wangenheim A, Heck V Jr, Dornelles C, Costa SS. A computational method for the semi-automated quantitative analysis of tympanic membrane perforations and tympanosclerosis. Comput Biol Med. 2009;39(10):889–95. https://doi.org/10.1016/j.compbiomed.2009.07.002.

Non-surgical Strategies to Restore Middle Ear Aeration

17

Bernard Ars and Dominique Estève

The main function of the middle ear, provided by the tympano-ossicular system, is the initial phase of the mechanical-electrical transduction of sound energy of atmospheric origin. The quality of this function requires a perfect and permanent balance between the pressure of the endotympanic gas and the atmospheric pressure. This balance is ensured by a system called the isobaric system of the middle ear cleft [1–4]. (cfr. to the chapter "Regulated balance of pressure variations in the temporal pneumatic spaces").

The most important function of the middle ear cleft isobaric system is to prevent the development of a state of endotympanic gas depression. This is, moreover, the main pathogen responsible for the lytic and progressive lesions encountered in chronic otitis media.

Technique Necessary for the Diagnosis of Dysregulation of Pressure Variations in the Middle Ear Cleft: the Tubomanometry®

Tubomanometry allows the functional exploration of the isobaric system of the middle ear cleft by measuring the active gas transport of the rhinopharynx into the middle ear cleft (Fig. 17.1) after the tubal opening caused by a dysbaric event [5–8] (Table 17.1).

The measurements are taken at three intensities of the dysbaric event (30, 40, and 50 mbar); this makes it possible to determine the value of the opening latency index (R-value), which reflects the latency between the application of pressure in the rhinopharynx and the measurement of a pressure change in the external auditory canal in relation to the opening of the tube. This latency describes the function of the fibro-cartilaginous Eustachian tube. Three results are possible: early opening ($R \leq 1$), late opening ($R > 1$), or no opening (R not measurable).

In normal subjects, this opening latency, because it results from a reflex phenomenon [9–11], has a fixed value, whatever the intensity of the stimulation for a given middle ear cleft. This means that the variability between the three stimulation levels (30, 40, and 50 mbar), which is translated mathematically by the variance of the index R (VarR), is very small.

The results of the tubomanometry examination are presented on a so-called expert system, which combines two parameters: the average index R (MoyR) carried on the horizontal axis and the variance of its index (VarR) carried on the vertical axis. The expert system comprises seven ordered zones numbered from 1 to 7, making it possible to characterize the reactivity of the middle ear cleft isobaric system as a function of the position of this middle ear cleft on the expert system. This position in the expert system also makes it possible, depending on the normal or pathological state of the middle ear cleft examined, to determine rehabilitative or therapeutic behavior.

In the case of a normal middle ear cleft, tubomanometry tests the ability of the ear to respond to a dysbaric situation that may be the cause of the constitution of a middle ear barotrauma. In this context, the ear can only occupy four of the seven areas of the expert system (Fig. 17.2).

In the case of a middle ear cleft with chronic otitis media, the tubomanometry tests the same function as in the case of a normal middle ear cleft. This function can be more or less altered during chronic otitis media, and the degree of dysfunction depends on the intensity of the endotympanic gas depression and the time during which the middle ear cleft is subjected to this situation of endotympanic gas depression. The ear with chronic otitis media can occupy one of the seven zones of the expert system (Fig. 17.3), evolving over time (Fig. 17.3).

This reflects a progressive gradation of the pathology, from zone 1 (diseased ear but whose functionality of the isobaric system of the middle ear cleft is still considered normal)

B. Ars (✉)
University of Namur, Namur, Belgium

Temporal Bone Foundation, Brussels, Belgium

D. Estève
Manosque, France

M. V. Goycoolea et al. (eds.), *Textbook of Otitis Media*, https://doi.org/10.1007/978-3-031-40949-3_17

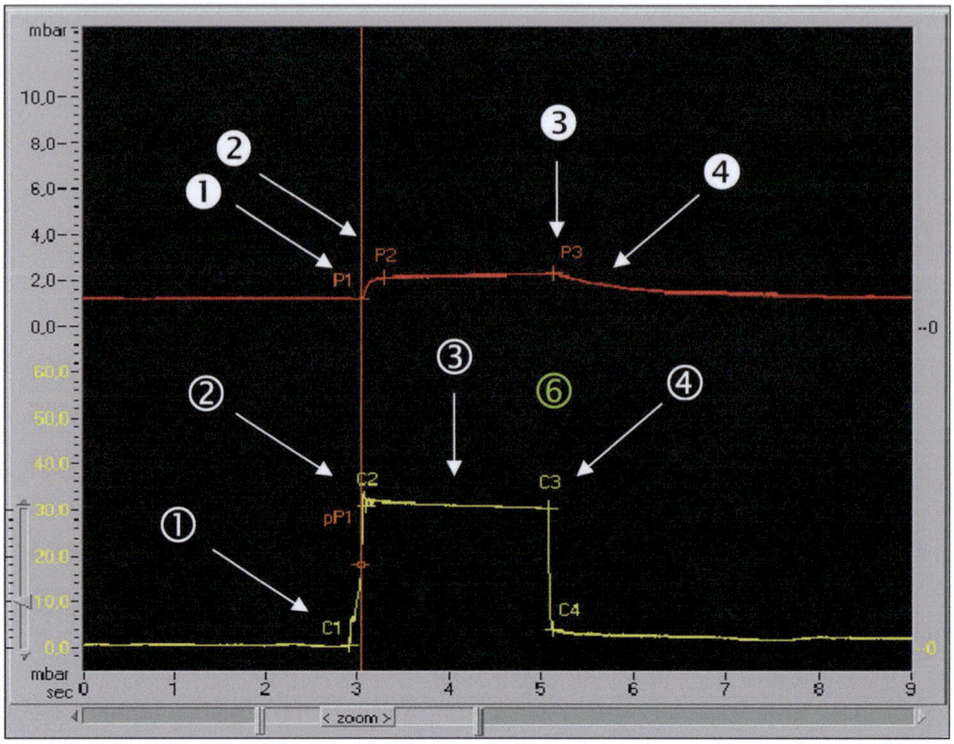

Fig. 17.1 Specimen tubomanometry curve for a normal subject (right ear with intact tympanic membrane, stimulus at 30 mbar, early eustachian tube opening). Lower curve (yellow) = change in rhinopharyngeal pressure over time: (1) C1: soft palate closed, start of reflex swallowing phase and of increasing pressure in rhinopharynx. (2) C2: rhinopharyngeal pressure reaches stimulus level (30 mbar). The C2–C1 phase lasts less than 0.30 s. (3) C2–C3: isometric contraction of soft palate muscle. This phase lasts 2 s and (4) relaxation of soft palate muscle and return to baseline rhinopharyngeal pressure. Upper curve (red) = changes in EAC pressure over time: (1) P1: opening of Eustachian tube. (2) P2: end of rising pressure phase in external auditory canal (P1–P2). P2–P3: pressure remains constant in the absence of change in tympanic membrane position. (3) P3: closure of Eustachian tube. (4) Middle ear emptying phase, beginning at P3. (5) Note that P3 is directly below C3, indicating that the tube remains open as long as a difference exists between nasopharyngeal pressure and atmospheric pressure, and demonstrating continual transmission of pressure status information to the integration center

Table 17.1 Value of MoyR and VarR depending on the area of the expert system and belonging to the group of normal ears or those with chronic otitis media

		Zone 1	Zone 2	Zone3	Zone 4
Normal ears	MoyR	0.68	1.53	1.86	No Ears
	VarR	0.02	0.09	0.66	No Ears
Ears + COM	MoyR	1.00	1.40	1.74	3.94
	VarR	003	0.07	1.15	6.65

VarR variance of the index R, *MoyR* average index R

up to zone 7 (total areflexia zone, acquired in chronic otitis media). The pathological evolution takes place over time and is marked by a joined increase in the two parameters retained (MoyR and VarR), in the case of chronic otitis media, with a very large increase in the VarR parameter, and this from the entry of the middle ear cleft into zone 3 of the expert system on (Table 17.1).

This stage (zone 3 of the expert system) is characterized by central neuronal damage, which reflects a loss of sensitivity to endotympanic gas depression, in relation to the physiological capacities of adaptation and accommodation of barosensitive neuronal structures. This sensory loss, if left unchecked, can increase over time, causing the middle ear cleft to shift to the right on the expert system. The entry of the middle ear cleft into zone 5 of the expert system results in an absence of response that initially concerns the lowest stimulation intensity, that is, 30 mbar (Fig. 17.4), responsible for the appearance of a grade I neurosensory scotoma (Fig. 17.4).

The ultimate evolution of this state is the absence of response to the three stimulation intensities (ear in zone 7 of the expert system), a stage corresponding to a grade III neurosensory scotoma.

In the event of chronic otitis media, we can schematize the therapeutic attitude according to the position of the middle ear cleft on the expert system:

- Zone 1: zone of absolute normality of the middle ear cleft isobaric system. The ear with chronic otitis media should be monitored (tubomanometry at 12 or 18 months). Treatments aimed at reducing inflammation of the middle

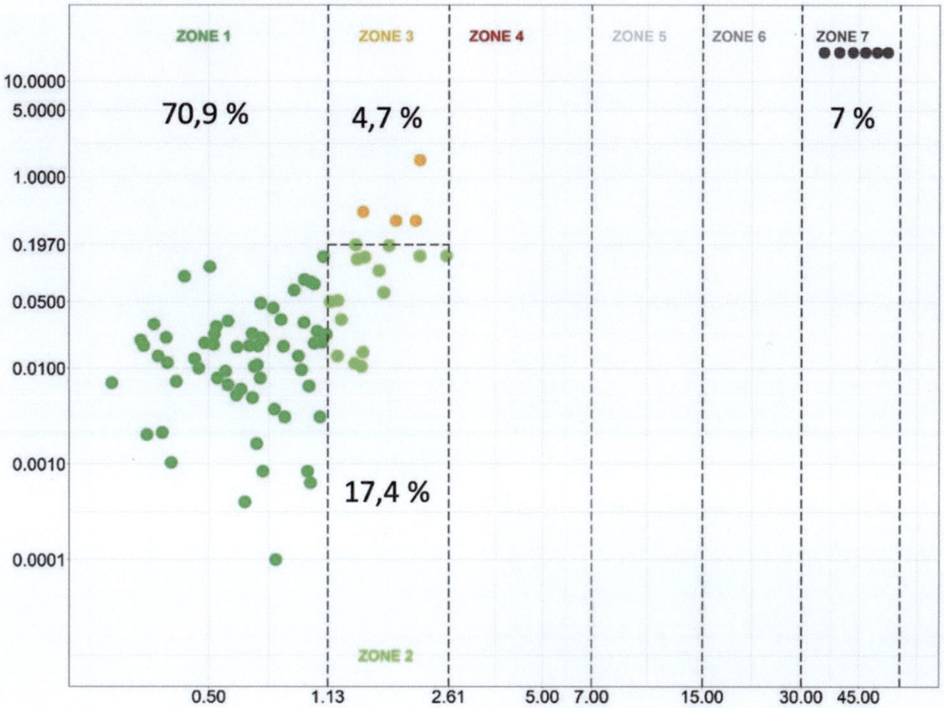

Fig. 17.2 Distribution of middle ears of a cohort of normal subjects on the tubomanometry expert system. Zone 1: zone of optimum efficiency of the isobaric system of the middle ear cleft. There is no risk of barotrauma for the middle ears located in this area. Zone 2: slight isolated increase in the MoyR parameter. Low risk of barotrauma for the middle ears located in this area. Zone 3: slight coupled increase in the parameters, MoyR and VarR. A significant risk of barotrauma for the middle ear is located in this area. Zone 7: strong increase in the MoyR parameters. Zone of so-called physiological areflexia, with a certain risk of barotrauma for the middle ears contained in this zone. The presence of a normal middle ear cleft in one of the above four areas of the expert system is a genetically determined trait, and this trait is fixed, that is, it is nonevolving over time in the absence of pathogenic elements. If necessary, it can be modified by the application of a specific rehabilitation

Fig. 17.3 Distribution of a cohort of middle ears with chronic otitis media on the tubomanometry expert system

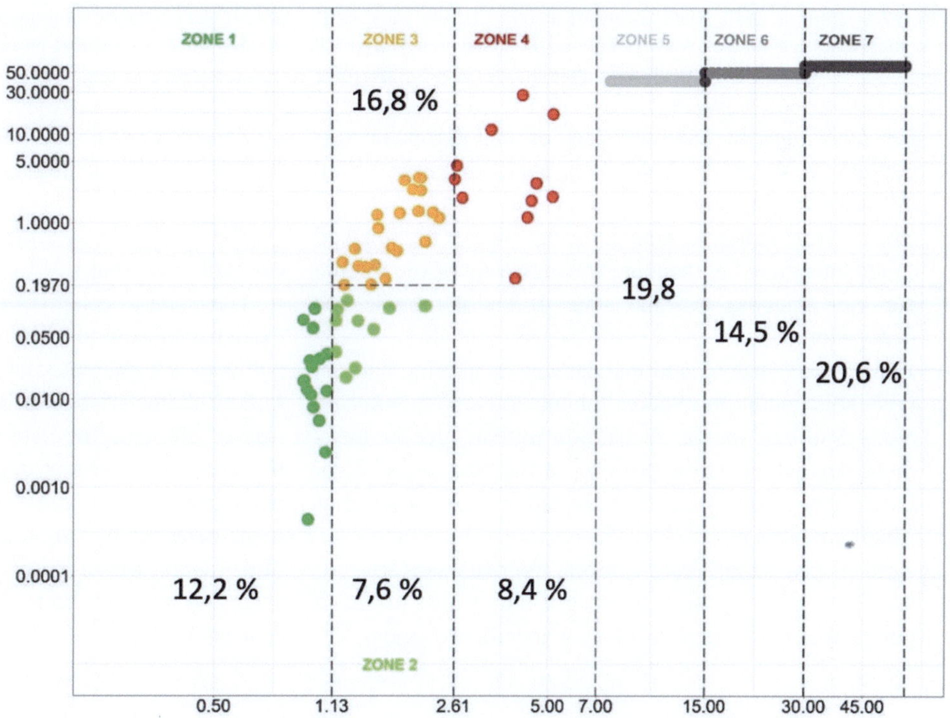

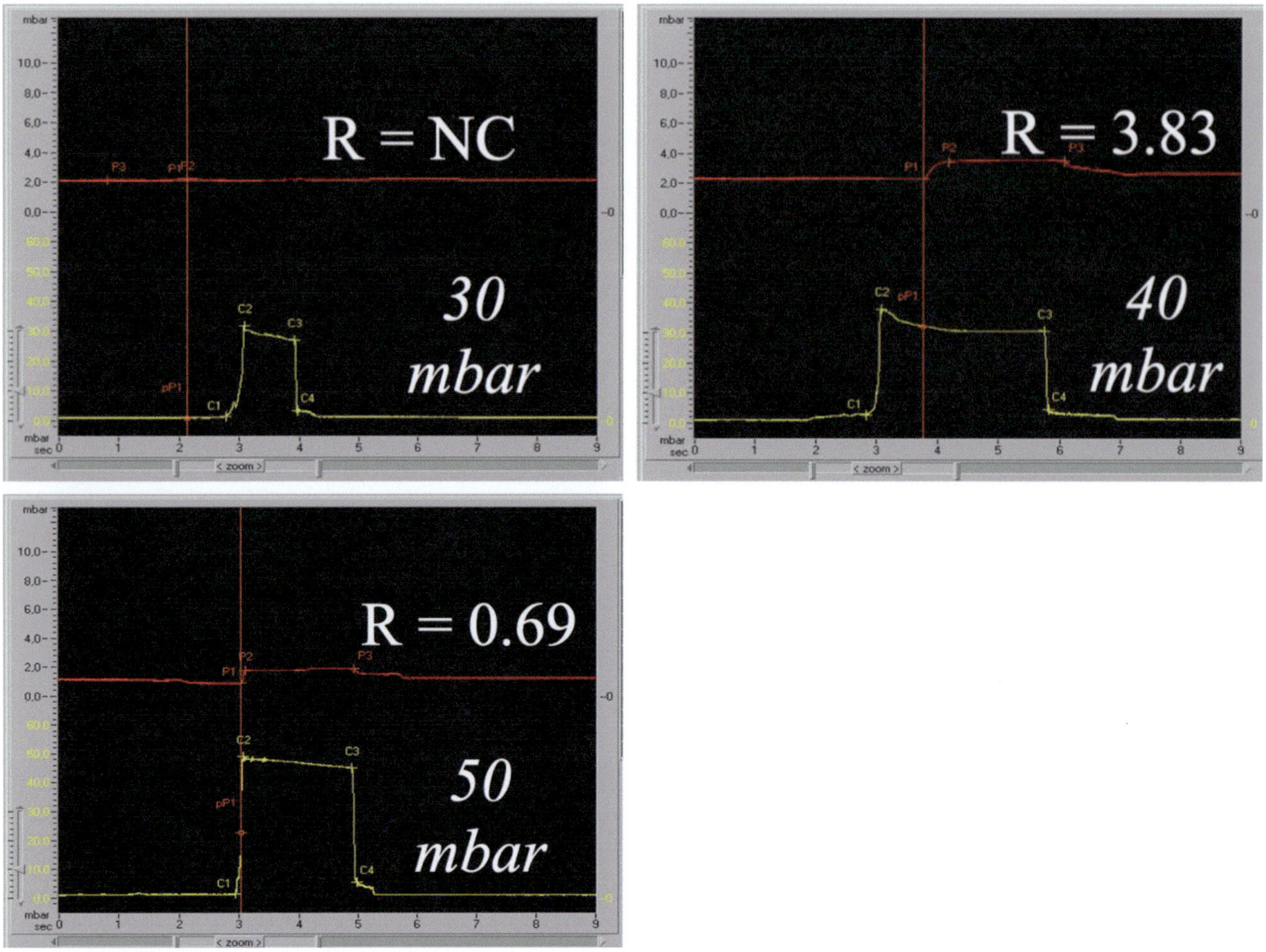

Fig. 17.4 Chronic oFFs media, result of a right ear: the value of R becomes dependent on the intensity of sFmulaFon, and there is a parFal anesthesia of the isobaric system of the middle ear, revealing the presence of neurosensory scotoma (here of grade I) and resulFng in an alteraFon of the tubal opening more marked for low sFmulaFon values

ear cleft mucosa and the state of endotympanic gas depression should be initiated to avoid or minimize an unfavorable outcome.

- Zone 2: tubomanometry monitoring every 6 months and treatments aimed at reducing inflammation of the middle ear cleft mucosa and the state of endotympanic gas depression.
- Zone 3: existence of neuronal damage, beginning but certain. This condition requires tubomanometry monitoring every 3 months or the decision to initiate specific treatment depending on the position in the area and clinical data. Entry into this state is irreversible in the absence of specific treatment.
- Zone 4: last stage before entering the neurosensory scotoma. Decision of a specific treatment to avoid crossing a course that would require a longer specific treatment.
- Zone 5, zone 6, and zone 7: zones of grade I, II, and III neurosensory scotoma. Specific treatment decision.

The aim of the specific treatment is to bring the affected ear back into zone 1.

The isobaric system of the middle ear cleft is based on the existence of a complex reflex neurosensory loop. If the reflex pathway is a guarantee of speed and efficiency, the physiological characteristics of its components have the disadvantage of allowing the deterioration of their performances in the event of persistent depressive stimulation by endotympanic gas. This explains the progressive neurological impairment detected by tubomanometry in the event of chronic otitis media, which is irreversible spontaneously at a certain stage and may worsen to the state of areflexia (neurosensory scotoma).

Technique Necessary for the Reeducational Management of Dysregulation of Pressure Variations in the Middle Ear Cleft: The Kinetube

This state of plasticity, which is based on the important neuronal contingent of the isobaric system of the middle ear cleft (neuroplasticity), is, however, not unambiguous: if a pejorative evolution is possible, an evolution toward improvement is also possible, based on the fact that every reflex of the organism is re-educable. This is the basis of a rehabilitative treatment of chronic otitis media whose tubomanometry shows that it has crossed the threshold of zone 3 of the expert system. This specific treatment is called Kinétube® [5, 12–14].

The Kinetube is a portable device similar to the calibrated pressure generator of the tubomanometer, that is, it delivers a succession of positive pressures in the rhinopharynx during swallowing, simulating high-amplitude dysbaric events (30, 40, and 50 mbar).

Indications for Treatment with Kinetube

- Normalization of dysfunctions of the isobaric system of the middle ear cleft observed by tubomanometry in the context of chronic otitis media. The prescription of Kinetube treatment will take place after the eradication of a cholesteatoma, but ideally before any tympanoplasty indicated outside of a cholesteatoma, in order to guarantee the best chance of success for this surgical procedure.
- Rehabilitation of an isobaric system of the middle ear cleft that is innately incapable (i.e., in normal subjects without an otological history) to prevent the occurrence of barotrauma.
- Rehabilitation of the velar musculature in the event of infantile swallowing with an operated or irradiated soft palate.

Contraindications to Treatment with Kinetube

- Children under the age of seven
- Subjects with chronic otitis media and for whom it is suspected that they will not be able to complete the treatment (due to its duration): lack of motivation, insufficient intellectual development, trisomy 21.
- An acute inflammatory episode in the ENT sphere (rhinitis, rhinopharyngitis, angina, otitis, etc.) is a temporary contraindication.

Methods of Treatment with Kinetube:

- The treatment is carried out at home, one session per day with 15 swallows at 30 mbar, 15 swallows at 40 mbar, 15 swallows at 50 mbar.
- Six days a week.
- By specifying never to exceed the prescribed doses, and to respect a period of at least 20 h between two sessions. Failure to comply with these instructions would generate the absence of results to treatment, due to the exhaustion and nonrenewal of the neurotransmitters at the origin of the meaningful message to the barostat of the middle ear cleft isobaric system.
- The duration of treatment will be at least 3 months, up to 6 months, rarely more.
- In France: rental of the device in pharmacies.

Criteria for Assessing the Result

Clinical, audiometric, and tubomanometric evolution (tubomanometry control at 1, then 3 months; possibly at 6 months). More rarely: middle ear cleft CT scan.

Visualization of the effects of treatment with Kinetube (Figs. 17.5 and 17.6).

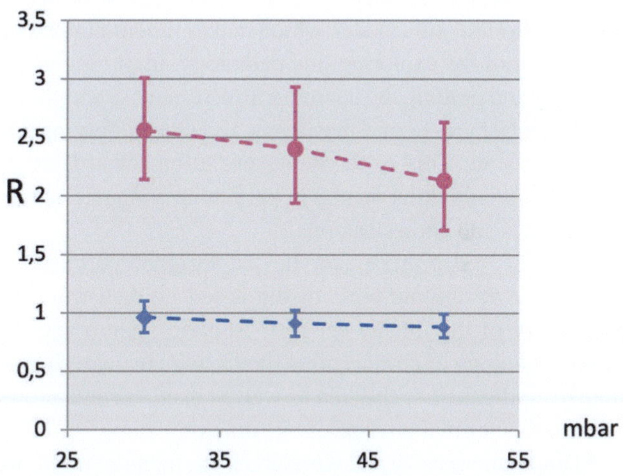

Fig. 17.5 109 ears with chronic oFFs media (in pink). In blue, 111 normal ears, which are the "model" to reach for ears with chronic oFFs media

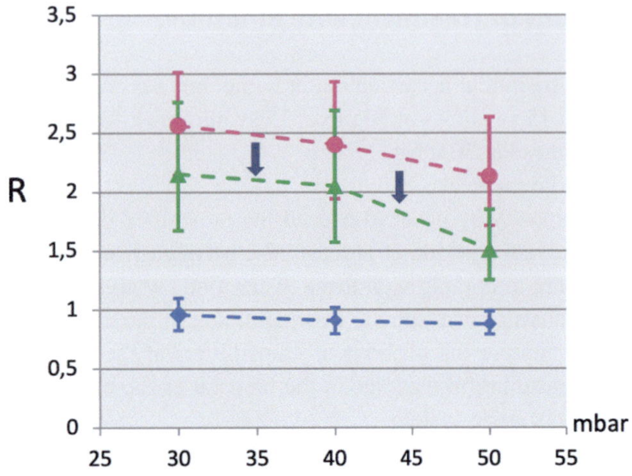

Fig. 17.6 109 ears with chronic oFFs media before (in pink) and the same (in green) aSer 21 days of treatment with Kinetube. In blue, 111 normal ears, which are the "model" to be reached for ears with chronic oFFs media

Conclusion

Tubomanometry®* is a means of exploring the capacity of the fibro-cartilaginous Eustachian tube to prevent (or not) barotrauma of the middle ear. It has been shown that this capacity is very frequently more or less strongly disturbed in cases of chronic otitis media, which makes tubomanometry a powerful tool for exploring this pathology, in particular for detecting and grading the neuronal involvement synonymous with sensory hypo or anesthesia, vis-à-vis the endotympanic gas depression. This explains the evolution toward severe forms of chronic otitis media, in particular tympanic retraction pockets and cholesteatoma.

Kinétube®* is a therapeutic device designed and used in the context of chronic otitis media based on data from the physiology of the middle ear cleft isobaric system and the pathophysiology of chronic otitis media, which makes it possible to eradicate it in children as well as in adults and allows a return to a normal physiological situation.

*Tubomanometer® and Kinétube® are manufactured by: DTF médical—Diffusion technique française. 13 rue de la Presse—CS 60132. F42003 SAINT-ETIENNE cedex 1—France. (dtf@dtf.fr).

Acknowledgments We wish to thank Professor Jean Lebacq for thoroughly reviewing the manuscript.

References

1. Estève D, Dubreuil C, Della Vedova C, Normand B, Lavieille JP, Martin C. Physiology and physiopathology of the Eustachian tube function: interest of tubomanometry. J Français d'ORL. 2001;50:233–42.
2. Estève D, Vecellio L, Lavieille JP. Middle ear cleft pressure regulation in health and disease. Sustained approach for a central regulating system: the middle ear isobaric system. In: Chronic otitis media. Pathogenesis-oriented therapeutic management. Amsterdam: Kugler Publications; 2008. p. 213–25.
3. Salburgo F, Garcia S, Lagier A, Estève D, Lavieille JP, Montava M. Histological identification of neuropharyngeal mechanoreceptors. Eur Arch Otorhinolaryngol. 2016;273:4127–33.
4. Alshukry A, Lagier C, Della Vedova C, Salburgo F, Lavieille JP, Montava M. The effects of hypoxia on middle ear pressure regulation. High Alt Med Biol. 2020;21(1):99–104.
5. Estève D, Dubreuil C, Della Vedova C, Normand B, Martin C. Évaluation par tubomanométrieâ de la fonction d'ouverture tubaire et de la réponse tympanique chez le sujet normal et chez le sujet porteur d'une otite séro-muqueuse chronique. Comparaison des résultats. J Français d'ORL. 2001;5(50):223–32.
6. Estève D. Tubomanometry and pathology. In: Fibrocartilaginous eustachian tube—middle ear cleft. Amsterdam: Kugler Publications; 2003. p. 159–75.
7. Ars B, Dirckx JJ. Tubomanometry. In: Fibrocartilaginous eustachian tube—middle ear cleft. Amsterdam: Kugler Publications; 2003. p. 151–8.
8. Collin M, Coulange M, Devèze A, Montava M, Estève D, Lavieille JP. Middle ear barotrauma due to thinopharyngeal scar tissue: tubomanometry diagnostic and therapeutic contribution. Rev Laryngol Otol Rhinol. 2012;133:157–61.
9. Eden A. Neural connections between the middle ear, eustachian tube and brain: implication for the reflex control of middle ear aeration. Ann Otol. 1981;90:566–9.
10. Eden A, Gannon P. Neural control of middle ear aeration. Arch Otolaryngol Head Neck Surg. 1987;113:133–7.
11. Martin C, Karkas A, Prades JM. Tubotympanic system functioning. Eur Ann Otorhinolaryngol Head Neck Dis. 2017;134:177–84.
12. Estève D. Re-adaptation of the baroreceptors of the fibrocartilaginous eustachian tube and middle ear cleft by the mean of the Kinétube®. In: Fibrocartilaginous eustachian tube—middle ear cleft. Amsterdam: Kugler Publications; 2003. p. 203–17.
13. Estève D. Rehabilitative management of the imbalance of pressure variations in the middle ear cleft. In: Chronic otitis media. Pathogenesis-oriented therapeutic management. Amsterdam: Kugler Publications; 2008. p. 341–9.
14. Barbut J. Place de la réhabilitation tubaire dans la prise en charge des otites moyennes chroniques. Thèse de Doctorat en médecine de l'Université Aix-Marseille. 2014. pp. 1–126.

Drug Delivery Across the Intact Tympanic Membrane: Methods, Mechanisms and Potential Impact

18

Arwa Kurabi, Molly Cooper, Emily Sereno, and Allen F. Ryan

Diseases of the Middle Ear

The middle ear (ME) is an air-filled cavity enclosed by the temporal bone. The impermeable tympanic membrane (TM) separates the outer ear from the ME, while the oval and round windows connect to the inner ear. The eustachian tube (ET) connects the nasopharynx to the ME and functions to equalize ME pressure to atmospheric changes. When there is ET dysfunction, symptoms such as earache, congestion, discomfort, and dizziness may occur [1].

ME infections (otitis media ([OM]), a serious disease of childhood, are the most common reason for physician visits and surgery in children [2, 3]. While most children recover quickly from acute OM, 10–15% of US children experience chronic or recurrent disease. Moreover, in many developing countries with limited access to medical care, undertreated OM progresses to chronic supurrative OM, the most serious form, which is estimated to cause 28,000 annual deaths and to be responsible for half of the world's burden of handicapped hearing loss [4, 5], making it the world's leading hearing loss cause.

Since acute OM typically resolves spontaneously, watchful waiting is recommended for children over 2 years of age. Systemic antibiotics are recommended for OM in children under two and for more complicated chronic or recurrent OM in older children [6]. However, systemic antibiotics can cause significant gastrointestinal side effects [7] and the exposure of off-target organisms throughout the body [8]. Moreover, in up to 15% of children, little or no systemically administered antibiotic reaches the ME [9]. Local antibiotic delivery to the ME can alleviate these issues, but it requires breaching the TM, which must be performed by a trained surgeon. Local ME delivery is typically performed when tympanostomy tubes are surgically inserted (considered invasive since the TM is breached). Ciprodex drops or other drug formulations are administered locally into the ME through tubes [10].

Cholesteatoma, in which keratinocytes invade the ME and often grow aggressively, can damage both the ME and inner ear and, in the worst case, progress intracranially [11]. Surgical removal of cholesteatoma tissue, the only treatment, often fails to remove all of the cholesteatoma. Remnants can continue to grow, leading to the need for further surgery [12]. Drugs to inhibit tissue growth, which have been proposed as potential treatments [13], have yet to be applied to this disease.

In both OM and cholesteatoma, local drug delivery could be beneficial. Noninvasive delivery would be especially useful, as it would not require surgery. Moreover, when access to ENT surgeons is limited, it would provide a practical means of local ME treatment. In this review, we describe our recent efforts to discover and validate peptides that can cross the intact TM into the ME while carrying large cargo. These peptides can be developed to deliver drugs and drug packages. As well, we provide a summary of other recent progress in the field of noninvasive intratympanic drug delivery and some of the available approaches.

Phage Display Reveals Rare Peptides that Can Cross the Intact TM

Many tissue barriers possess mechanisms by which select substances can be transported. We reasoned that the TM might harbor such a capacity. We also felt that transport would involve the recognition, by cellular receptors on the

A. Kurabi (✉) · M. Cooper · E. Sereno
Department of Surgery/Otolaryngology, UCSD School of Medicine, San Diego, CA, USA
e-mail: akurabi@ucsd.edu

A. F. Ryan
Department of Surgery/Otolaryngology, UCSD School of Medicine, San Diego, CA, USA

Department of Neurosciences, UCSD School of Medicine, San Diego, CA, USA

San Diego VA Healthcare System, La Jolla, CA, USA

M. V. Goycoolea et al. (eds.), *Textbook of Otitis Media*, https://doi.org/10.1007/978-3-031-40949-3_18

external surface of the TM, of biomolecules. Since many biologically relevant molecules are proteins, we used bacteriophage display to screen a library of peptides to identify amino acid sequences that could cross the TM [14]. Phage display is a high-throughput tool for the identification of molecules with specific characteristics [15].

Bacteriophages are bacterial viruses that, upon infecting their targets, replicate in large numbers, followed by release and continued bacterial infection. For phage display, each phage is engineered to express a different molecule, which is fused to the free end of a filamentous capsular protein [16, 17]. With a sufficiently large library of phages, each expressing a different molecule, this provides rapid combinatorial power to identify molecules of interest.

We initially screened a 7-mer peptide M13 phage library (PhD-C7C™, New England Biolabs, Cambridge, MA, USA), with 2.5×10^8 unique peptide sequences in the library. OM was induced in rats by ME injection with nontypeable *Haemophilus influenzae* (NTHi). After 48 h, when OM was well established, a library aliquot containing four copies on average of each peptide clone was applied to the TM in saline for 2 h. The external canal was rinsed and the ME contents harvested, after which bacteriophage were tittered. The resulting phages were amplified and screened for three additional rounds. However, there was no evidence of library "collapse" to a small number of peptides that would indicate selection for transport across the TM.

We felt it possible that the peptide length chosen was too short to interact with a possible transport mechanism. We therefore switched to a library expressing peptides that are 12 amino acids in length (Ph.D-12TM Phage Display Peptide Library; New England Biolabs), expressed on the free end of the M13 pIII protein. Five copies per phage of this filamentous, capsular protein mediate the recognition of and binding to the *Escherichia coli* hosts of the phage. The expressed peptides were thus well positioned to contact TM cells. Ten phages expressing one of 10^9 random peptides, thus totaling 10^{10} phages, were applied to the TMs of NTHI-infected rat MEs as above. Two screening strategies were employed.

First, sequential biopanning was used to screen for phage that first bound to, then internalized into, and finally crossed the TM. To accomplish this, the library was applied to TMs for 1 h, after which the external canal was extensively rinsed to remove any phage that had not bound to TMs. The TMs were harvested and homogenized. The homogenate was then applied to *E. coli*, the bacterial target of the M13 phage, and any phage present infected and multiplied within. These phages were harvested and used to repeat the binding screen two additional times. The resultant "TM-binding" library was then applied to rat TMs for 1 h. The TMs were again rinsed with saline, but then a low pH wash was applied to remove any phage bound to the TM surface. The TMs were then dissected from the M bulla, homogenized, applied to *E. coli,* and the phage was harvested. Repeated twice, this process yielded a "TM-penetrating" library, which was again applied to the TMs of NTHi-infected rats for 1 h. After extensive external canal rinsing with saline and low pH, the contents of the ME were harvested, used to infect *E. coli*, phage harvested, and the process repeated twice. From the resultant "TM-transiting" library, 30 colonies were selected for DNA sequencing to identify the peptide inserts. Each phage clone and corresponding peptide sequence were given a sequential name Binding-Penetrating-Transiting (BPT).

For the second strategy, the unselected 12-mer peptide library was applied to the TMs of NTHi-infected MEs for 1 h, and the external canal was rinsed with saline and low pH. The ME contents were then used to infect *E. coli*, and the process was repeated twice. From the resultant library, 30 phage clones were selected and sequenced. The phage clones were given names with a TMT (TM transmigrating) acronym.

For strategy 1, seven unique BPT peptide phages were present more than once among the 30 sequenced phages, suggesting efficient crossing of the TM, labeled BPT1–7. Strategy 2 yielded five unique peptides present multiple times in the sequence sample, labeled TMT1–5. These 12 sequences were aligned to determine sequence relationships (Fig. 18.1). Four peptides formed a group characterized by all or part of STKx consensus motif within the sequence. Five peptides formed a second group that exhibited all or part of a PxxP motif. Two peptides aligned separately but were more closely related to the STKx group than the PxxP group.

Analysis of the peptides using SAROTUP (Scanner and Reporter of Target Unrelated Peptides; [18]) found that the peptides are novel, not having been reported from earlier phage display studies. However, the MimoBlast tool [19] revealed that the BPT-1 sequence was identified in a biopanning study [20] as part of a human single-chain variable fragment (HuScFv) that targets the dengue virus envelope protein and blocks its infectivity.

To compare transport rates, 10^{10} of each trans-TM phage was applied to the TMs of NTHi-infected rat MEs for 1 h. Phage recovery was then used to assess trans-TM transport efficiency. A phage not expressing a peptide (wild type [WT]) was controlled for possible contamination. All the peptide-bearing phages were recovered in amounts significantly greater than those of the WT phage. While this validated the success of our biopanning strategies, it was clear that the different phages crossed the TM with different efficiencies.

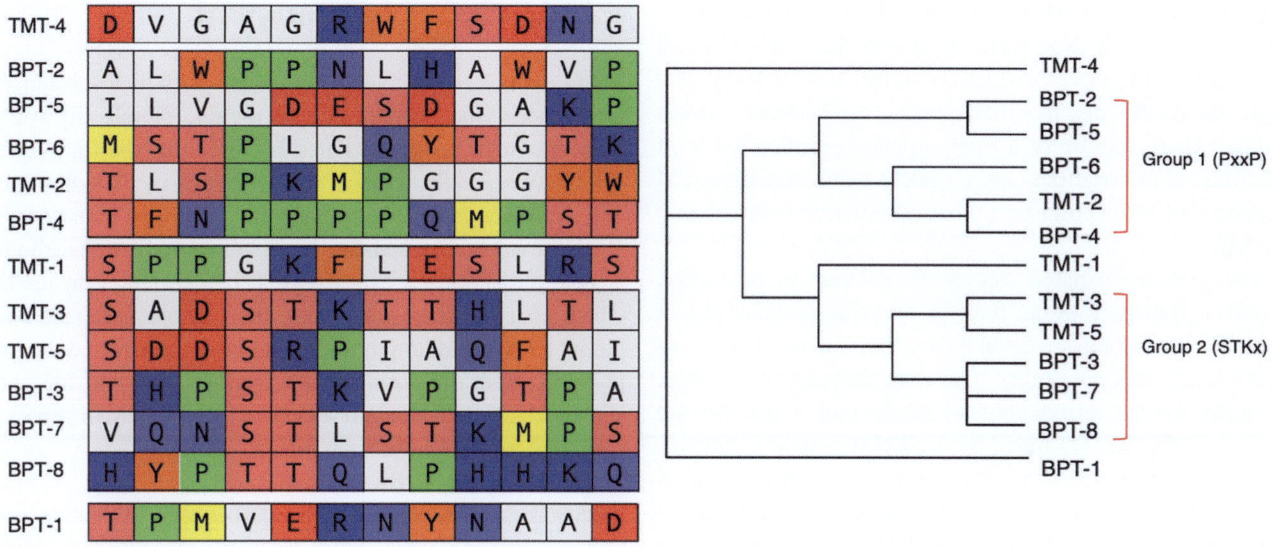

Fig. 18.1 Amino acid sequences of pIII extension peptides recovered from phage display biopanning against the tympanic membrane for transport into the middle ear. (Left) Amino acids (aa) are colored by side-chain functional characteristics and show a high degree of diversity. Blue is basic aa, red is acidic aa, orange is aromatic aa, yellow is sulfur-containing aa, polar hydroxylic aa are light red, polar amidic aa are light blue, and green is proline. (Right) The phylogenic tree sequence analysis reveals any potential homology between the peptides and divides them into two groups with shared common motifs: "ST(K/R)T" and "PxxP"

Trans-TM Phage Transport Is Active

To investigate the mechanism of phage transport, we varied the time of TM exposure, phage concentration, temperature, and oxygen level. When time on the TM was increased from 1–4 h, ME phage recovery increased exponentially [14]. Increasing phage concentration proportionally also increased recovery. The sensitivity of transport to oxygen deprivation and temperature was evaluated ex vivo using intact ME bullae. Transport was observed up to 6 h after death, but not at later times. At bulla temperature of 4 °C, transport was almost completely eliminated. These results strongly suggest that trans-TM transport occurs via an active, not passive, mechanism.

Additional Amino Acids Can Increase Transport

Given that 7-mer peptides were too short to mediate trans-TM transport, we reasoned that 12 amino acids might not be sufficient for optimal interaction with the TM transport mechanisms. We therefore used two 12-mer trans-TM phage with different transport rates, TMT-2 and TMT-3, as backbones for the construction of two new phage libraries. For each phage, we added six random amino acids to the free end of the peptide [21]. We exposed each library briefly (15 min) to the TMs of infected rat MEs. After three rounds of selection, we sequenced 30 phages recovered from the ME for each library and tested phages with multiple copies in the sample for transport rate. For TMT-2, which had a low transport rate, the best 6-mer extension doubled ME recovery. However, for TMT-3, a 12-mer with a high transport rate, the best 18-mer showed an eightfold increase.

Trans-TM Peptide Phage Do Not Damage the Middle or Inner Ear

Obviously, the usefulness of peptides for drug delivery depends on their safety. To evaluate trans-TM phage middle and inner ears, we applied 10^{10} WT, TMT1, TMT2, TMT3, or TMT4 phage in saline into normal rat MEs for 1, 2, or 3 days via transbullar injection. A saline injection was used as a control. ME morphology was evaluated on day 3. Auditory brainstem response (ABR) thresholds were measured before and at 1, 2, and 3 days after ME injection. ME morphology was comparable across all treatments. ABR thresholds were increased by approximately 20 dB in all groups at day 1, presumably due to the presence of fluid in the ME. Thresholds for all groups had recovered to normal by day 3 [22]. Titers of perilymph on day 3 indicated that transport of phage into the inner ear was minimal. The results indicate that trans-TM phages are safe as a potential drug delivery technique, at least in the short term.

Peptides Mediate Transport Across the Human TM

Since trans-TM peptides mediate the transport of bacteriophage, which are nearly 1 μm in length, they seem likely to support the noninvasive transport of other large cargo, including drugs or drug particles, across the intact TM and into the ME. Moreover, phages are in fact gene therapy vectors; the genetically modified phages used in our studies induce the expression of a foreign peptide in their hosts. It can thus be inferred that appropriately expressed trans-TM peptides could also transport other gene therapy vectors into the ME.

For peptide-mediated therapeutic delivery to be useful, however, transport would have to occur across the TM of patients. We therefore developed a two-chamber *in vitro* assay to test this possibility. The assay consists of an upper chamber for the introduction of phage plus a dye for the detection of leaks, separated by the TM from a lower chamber for phage recovery. A silicone rubber membrane is used to seal a TM fragment in between the upper and lower chambers. The device was first tested with WT phages, which we found were excluded by the TM from the lower chamber [23].

We then tested TM fragments from uninfected rat, guinea pig, and rabbit MEs. We found that TMs from uninfected rat MEs transported at a similar rate to TMs from infected MEs, indicating that the transport mechanism is not induced by infection but is a native property of the TM. We also found that transport for all three species occurred at similar rates. This mechanism of transport appears to be widespread in mammals separated by millions of years of evolution. We then tested TM fragments discarded as waste from human patients undergoing repair for TM perforations. Transport across the human TM also occurred at comparable levels [23], indicating the usefulness of transport for therapeutic purposes.

Trans-TM Peptides Cross the TM Independent of Phage

We next determined whether peptides could mediate transport across the TM independently or whether the ability to cross the TM was dependent on the phage particle. We linked a 130-bp DNA oligomer, which served as a polymerase chain reaction (PCR) template, to the trans-TM peptide TMT3. We used the *in vitro* model for this test since the *in vivo*-infected ME would likely contain DNases that could degrade the DNA tag. After the application of the peptide/DNA hybrid to the upper chamber for 1 h, recovery from the lower chamber was quantified by quantitative PCR. Unexpectedly, we found that transport of the much smaller peptide/DNA construct occurred at a comparable rate to that peptide phage, indicating that the transport mechanism is largely independent of cargo size [23].

Transport Occurs Via Transcytosis

There are several possible mechanisms by which substances can cross tissue barriers. These include simple diffusion, paracellular transport mediated by loosening the tight junctions between cells, transport through cells mediated by specific transmembrane molecular transporters, or transcytosis. Transcytosis involves endocytosis, followed by transcellular vesicle transport and exocytosis. It is a common means by which specific cargos are transported across polarized epithelial cells, including in the blood–brain barrier and the gut [24, 25]. Both diffusion and paracellular transport are passive mechanisms, which makes their involvement in peptide-mediated trans-TM transport unlikely.

To identify an active mechanism responsible for peptide-mediated trans-TM transport [26], we began by evaluating peptide structure. As noted above, we found that two amino acid motifs were shared by trans-TM peptides: ST(K/R)T or PxxP. To refine this identification, we used Multiple Em for Motif Elicitation (MEME; Bailey and Elkan [27]; web version 4.12.0). MEME analysis generated expanded versions of the motifs: MEME motif 1: S(T/P)K(Y/M)PG, and MEME motif 2: (T/P)(P/L)(S/P)P(Q/K)M. To identify the position of the MEME motif within the peptide, as expressed at the free end of the M13 pIII protein, we used PEPFOLD [28] software to predict the structure of each peptide plus the adjacent four amino acids of M13 pIII. We found that the position of a motif at the free end of a peptide was strongly associated with its rate of transport (Fig. 18.2). This result is consistent with motif interaction with surface proteins of TM cells to engage an active transport process. This could occur either by specific transmembrane transporters or by transcytosis. However, it seemed unlikely that a specific transporter could move cargo as large as a phage across cell membranes.

We then used the Motif Alignment and Search Tool (MAST) software to search the Ensembl Ab Initio Protein Sequence Database of all known proteins for relationships with the MEME motifs. We reasoned that the interacting partners of these proteins would be candidates for involvement in transport. The highest proteins identified by MAST for MEME motif 1 were Exocyst complex 1, Golgi-associated secretory pathway kinase, Sortilin 2, and Tetraspanin 5. The highest proteins identified by MAST for MEME motif 2 were importin subunit alpha, zinc finger homeobox protein 1, secretory carrier membrane protein 5, and GABA type alpha 4 subunit. The majority of these proteins are involved in transport across membranes and through cells and would almost certainly have interactions with other proteins involved in these processes. These results are consistent with transcytosis as the peptide-mediated trans-TM transport mechanism.

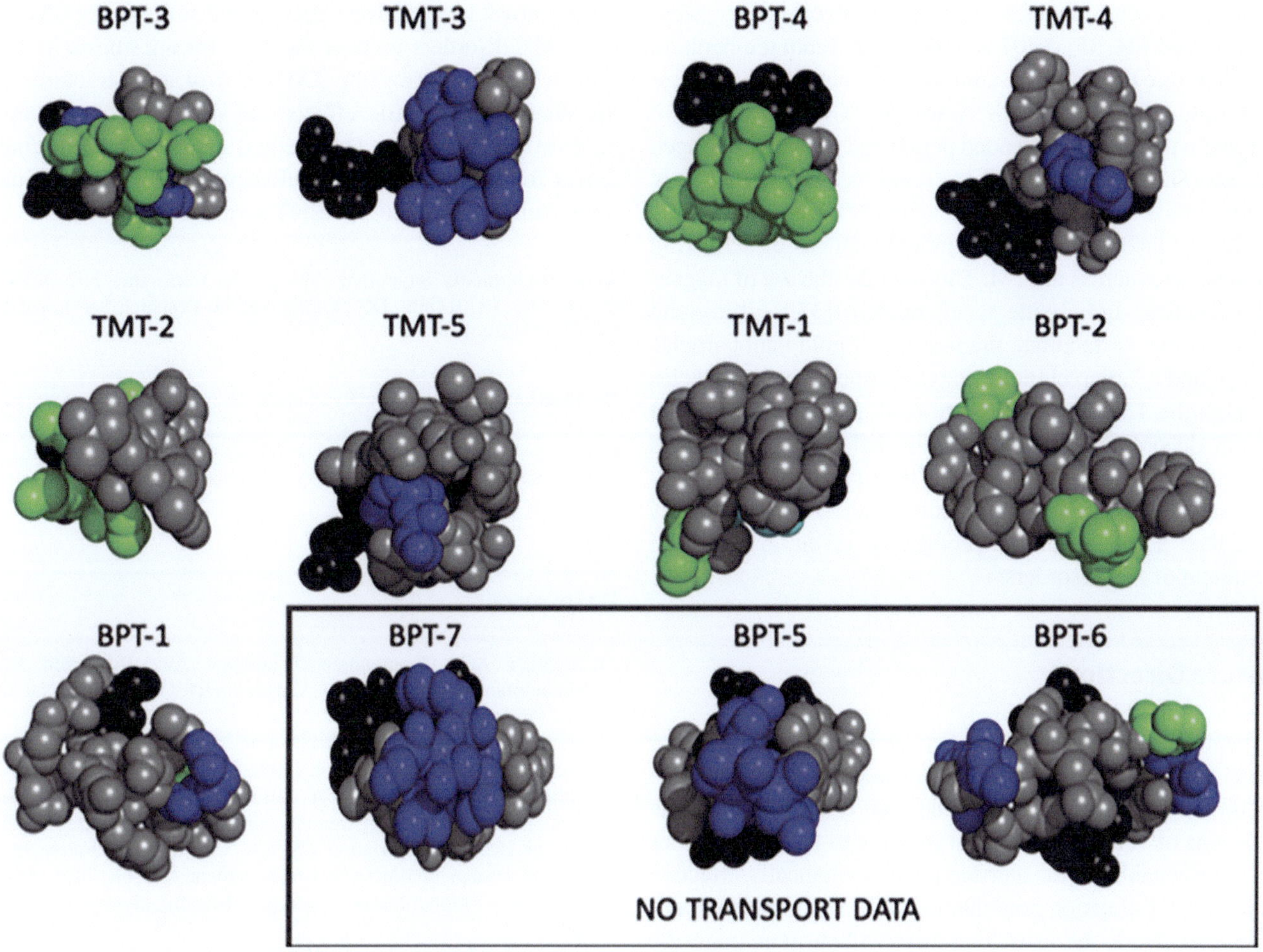

Fig. 18.2 Predicted 3D renderings of the 12-mer phage peptides, identified in Fig. 18.1, predicted by PEPFOLD. The conserved ST(K/R) and PxxP motifs are indicated in blue and green, respectively. The remaining amino acids of the expressed peptide are in gray, while the pIII chain is in black and positioned to the back to reveal a head-on view of the displayed peptide. The first nine structures are arranged in order of the amount recovered from the middle ear after 1 h of incubation (from top left to bottom right). A clear relationship is apparent between the display of motif aa's at the end of the peptide and transport rate. The last three peptides do not have transport data available

To test this possibility, we employed inhibitors of the various processes of transcytosis. We found that wortmannin, an inhibitor of the micropinocytosis mechanism of endocytosis, completely blocked trans-TM transport. Similarly, Retro2, an inhibitor of retrograde transport into the Golgi apparatus, dramatically reduced transport. Retrograde transport into the Golgi initiates one form of transcellular vesicle transport. Endosidin-2, an inhibitor of the EXO70 subunit of the exocyst complex involved in exocytosis, reduced transport by 80%. Taken together, the inhibitor data strongly support the conclusion that trans-TM transport occurs via transcytosis.

Potential for Noninvasive Therapeutic Delivery

Trans-TM peptides mediate the movement of large phage particles through the intact TM. This indicates the potential for noninvasive delivery of large therapeutic packages into the ME. The demonstrated ability of peptides to transit the TM at rates equivalent to peptide-phage suggests that they can be used to label and then transport large drug packages such as nanoparticles or liposomes. Moreover, the transport of a bacterial transduction vector through the TM suggests that peptides could also transport human gene therapy vectors, which are also modified viruses, to express therapeutic proteins or correct ME genetic disorders. Gene mutations that confer OM susceptibility have been discovered (e.g., [29, 30]). A number of these, especially those that affect innate immunity (e.g., [31]), could be appropriate targets for gene therapy to induce resistance to OM.

Other platforms for noninvasive delivery of drugs across the intact TM are also under development. Kohane and colleagues [32, 33] have used permeability enhancers to increase the movement of drugs across the TM in a thermo-reversible 407 hydrogel. They have successfully employed this method to treat NTHi OM in a chinchilla model [33]. This system was also shown to be effective against *Streptococcus pneumoniae* OM [34, 35]. P407 is a solution at room temperature and therefore can easily be administered, but it forms a depot (gelling) upon contacting the warm (37 °C) TM, allowing it to remain there for an extended period and provide prolonged release. The poloxamer 407 hydrogel has been extensively tested for safety in the external ear and ME [36].

Several laboratories have explored methods of delivering nanoparticles across the TM. This includes the use of magnetism to drive iron oxide nanoparticles ([37]), ultrasound microbubbles to facilitate the passage of gold nanoparticles ([38]), and a "microshotgun" device to power nanoparticles through the TM [39]. Abdelbary et al. [40] used propylene glycol decorations on antibiotic-loaded nanoliposomes to increase transit through the TM. These physical and chemical methods, plus peptide-mediated trans-TM transport as described above, offer the promise of revolutionizing the treatment of ME disorders.

Future Directions

If peptide-mediated ME delivery of therapeutics is to be developed for clinical use, significant additional work will be required. While trans-TM peptides can clearly mediate the transport of very large cargo, it remains to be seen whether they are capable of transporting pharmacologically effective quantities of drugs or gene therapy. Whether trans-TM peptides can clearly be used long-term without damaging the middle or inner ear needs to be established. Moreover, it is possible that peptides discovered in rats are not optimal for transport in humans. The *in vitro* assay that we developed to test transport in humans can be used to screen a phage library using the human TM. This would clarify whether even higher rates of transport can be achieved with human-specific peptides. These issues will need to be clarified to further assess the potential of peptide-mediated transport of therapies for treatment in patients.

Conclusions

Phage display of random peptides has identified rare peptides that mediate transport across the intact TM, from the external to the ME. This transport is active, mediated by transcytosis, does not negatively affect the middle or inner ears over the course of days, and occurs across the human TM. The peptides are able to mediate the transport of M13 bacteriophage, nearly 1 μm in length, across the two epithelia and stromal layers of the TM. It seems very likely that this cargo capacity can be harnessed for the noninvasive delivery of large drug packages and gene therapy vectors. This represents a novel local delivery therapeutic strategy for OM and other ME disorders without the need for anesthesia in children while preserving the TM integrity and structure and avoiding systemic side effects and exposure of off-target bacteria to antibiotics. The method could prove especially useful for noninvasive drug delivery to the ME in populations with limited access to ENT surgeons.

Acknowledgments Supported by grants from the NIH/NIDCD (DC012595, DC014801, DC000129) and the Research Service of the VA (BX001205).

Declaration of Interest Dr Ryan is the co-founder of Otonomy Inc., serves as a member of the Scientific Advisory Board, and holds an equity position in the company. The UCSD Committee on Conflict of Interest has approved this relationship. Otonomy, Inc. played no part in the research reported here.

References

1. Schilder AG, Chonmaitree T, Cripps AW, Rosenfeld RM, Casselbrant ML, Haggard MP, Venekamp RP. Otitis media. Nat Rev Dis Primers. 2016;2:16063.
2. Elden LM, Coyte PC. Socioeconomic impact of otitis media in North America. J Otolaryngol. 1998;27 Suppl 2:9–16.
3. Infante-Rivard C, Fernandez A. Otitis media in children: frequency, risk factors, and research avenues. Epidemiol Rev. 1993;15:444–65.
4. World Health Organization (WHO). Chronic suppurative otitis media: burden of illness and management options. 2004. http://www.who.int/pbd/deafness/activities/hearing_care/otitis_media.pdf.
5. World Health Organization (WHO). Deafness and hearing loss: key facts. 2020. https://www.who.int/en/news-room/fact-sheets/detail/deafness-and-hearing-loss.
6. Lieberthal AS, Carroll AE, Chonmaitree T, Ganiats TG, Hoberman A, Jackson MA, Joffe MD, Miller DT, Rosenfeld RM, Sevilla XD, Schwartz RH, Thomas PA, Tunkel DE. The diagnosis and management of acute otitis media. Pediatrics. 2013;131:e964–99.
7. Levy J. The effects of antibiotic use on gastrointestinal function. Am J Gastroenterol. 2000;95(Suppl 1):S8–S10.
8. Llor C, Bjerrum L. Antimicrobial resistance: risk associated with antibiotic overuse and initiatives to reduce the problem. Ther Adv Drug Saf. 2014;5:229–41.
9. Pichichero ME, Reed MD. Variations in amoxicillin pharmacokinetic/pharmacodynamic parameters may explain treatment failures in acute otitis media. Paediatr Drugs. 2009;11:243–9.
10. Zhang Z, Li X, Zhang W, Kohane DS. Drug delivery across barriers to the middle and inner ear. Adv Funct Mater. 2021;31(44):2008701.
11. Kuo CL, Shiao AS, Yung M, Sakagami M, Sudhoff H, Wang CH, Hsu CH, Lien CF. Updates and knowledge gaps in cholesteatoma research. Biomed Res Int. 2015;2015:854024.
12. Richter GT, Lee KH. Contemporary assessment and management of congenital cholesteatoma. Curr Opin Otolaryngol Head Neck Surg. 2009;17:339–45.
13. Hamed MA, Nakata S, Sayed RH, Ueda H, Badawy BS, Nishimura Y, Kojima T, Iwata N, Ahmed AR, Dahy K, Kondo N, Suzuki K. Pathogenesis and bone resorption in acquired cholesteatoma: current knowledge and future prospective. Clin Exp Otorhinolaryngol. 2016;9:298–308.

14. Kurabi A, Pak KK, Bernhardt M, Baird A, Ryan AF. Discovery of a biological mechanism of active transport through the tympanic membrane to the middle ear. Sci Rep. 2016;6:22663.
15. Pasqualini R, Ruoslahti E. Organ targeting *in-vivo* using phage display peptide libraries. Nature. 1996;380:364–6.
16. Barbas CF, Burton DR, Scott JK, Silverman GJ. Phage display: a laboratory manual. New York: CSHL Press; 2004.
17. Smith GP. Filamentous fusion phage: novel expression vectors that display cloned antigens on the virion surface. Science. 1985;228:1315–7.
18. Huang J, Ru B, Li S, Lin H, Guo FB. SAROTUP: scanner and reporter of target-unrelated peptides. J Biomed Biotechnol. 2010;2:1019–32.
19. Huang J. MimoDB 2.0: a mimotope database and beyond. Nucleic Acids Res. 2012;40(Database issue):D271–7.
20. Saokaew N, Poungpair O, Panya A, Tarasuk M, Sawasdee N, Limjindaporn T, Chaicumpa W, Yenchitsomanus P. Human monoclonal single-chain antibodies specific to dengue virus envelope protein. Lett Appl Microbiol. 2014;58:270–7.
21. Kurabi A, Schaerer D, Chang L, Pak K, Ryan AF. Optimisation of peptides that actively cross the tympanic membrane by random amino acid extension: a phage display study. J Drug Target. 2018a;26:127–34.
22. Kurabi A, Beasley KA, Chang L, McCann J, Pak K, Ryan AF. Peptides actively transported across the tympanic membrane: functional and structural properties. PLoS One. 2017;12:e0172158.
23. Kurabi A, Noack V, Schaerer D, Bernhardt M, Pak K, Alexander T, Husseman J, Nguyen Q, Harris JP, Ryan AF. Active transport of peptides across the intact human tympanic membrane. Sci Rep. 2018b;8(1):11815.
24. Pulgar VM. Transcytosis to cross the blood brain barrier, new advancements and challenges. Front Neurosci. 2019;12:1019.
25. Tuma P, Hubbard AL. Transcytosis: crossing cellular barriers. Physiol Rev. 2003;83(3):871–932.
26. Kurabi A, Pak K, Chavez E, Doan J, Ryan AF. A transcytotic transport mechanism across the tympanic membrane. Sci Rep. 2022;12(1):984.
27. Bailey TL, Elkan C. Fitting a mixture model by expectation maximization to discover motifs in biopolymers, In Proceedings of the Second International Conference on Intelligent Systems for Molecular Biology, AAAI Press. Menlo Park. 1994;pp 28–36.
28. Maupetit J, Derreumaux P, Tuffery P. PEP-FOLD: an online resource for *de novo* peptide structure prediction. Nucleic Acids Res. 2009;37(Web Server issue):W498–503.
29. Bhutta MF, Lambie J, Hobson L, Goel A, Hafrén L, Einarsdottir E, Mattila PS, Farrall M, Brown S, Burton MJ. A mouse-to-man candidate gene study identifies association of chronic otitis media with the loci TGIF1 and FBXO11. Sci Rep. 2017;7(1):12496.
30. Santos-Cortez RLP, Chiong C, Chonmaitree T, Frank DN, Ryan AF, Giese APJ, Roberts TB, Daly KA, Steritz MJ, Szeremeta W, Pedro M, Pine H, Yarza TKL, Scholes MA, Llanes EGDV, Yousaf S, Friedman N, Tantoco MLC, Wine TM, Labra PJ, Benoit J, Ruiz AG, de la Cruz RAR, Greenlee C, Yousaf A, Cardwell J, Nonato RMA, Ray D, Ong KMC, So E, Robertson CE, Dinwiddie J, Lagrana-Villagracia SM, University of Washington Center for Mendelian Genomics (UWCMG), Gubbels SP, Shaikh RS, Cass SP, Einarsdottir E, Lee NR, Schwartz DA, Gloria-Cruz TLI, Bamshad MJ, Yang IV, Kere J, Abes GT, Prager JD, Riazuddin S, Chan AL, Yoon PJ, Nickerson DA, Cutiongco-de la Paz EM, Streubel SO, Reyes-Quintos MRT, Jenkins HA, Mattila P, Chan KH, Mohlke KL, Leal SM, Hafrén L, Chonmaitree T, Sale MM, Ahmed ZM. *FUT2* variants confer susceptibility to familial otitis media. Am J Human Genet. 2018;103:679–90.
31. Hafrén L, Einarsdottir E, Kentala E, Hammarén-Malmi S, Bhutta MF, MacArthur CJ, Wilmot B, Casselbrant M, Conley YP, Weeks DE, Mandel EM, Vaarala O, Kallio A, Melin M, Nieminen JK, Leinonen E, Kere J, Mattila PS. Predisposition to childhood otitis media and genetic polymorphisms within the toll-like receptor 4 (TLR4) locus. PLoS One. 2015;10:e0132551.
32. Khoo X, Simons EJ, Chiang HH, Hickey JM, Sabharwal V, Pelton SI, Rosowski JJ, Langer R, Kohane DS. Formulations for trans-tympanic antibiotic delivery. Biomaterials. 2013;34(4):1281–8.
33. Yang R, et al. Treatment of otitis media by transtympanic delivery of antibiotics. Sci Transl Med. 2016;8(356):356ra120.
34. Yang R, Okonkwo OS, Zurakowski D, Kohane DS. Synergy between chemical permeation enhancers and drug permeation across the tympanic membrane. J Control Release. 2018a;289:94–101.
35. Yang R, Sabharwal V, Shlykova N, Okonkwo OS, Pelton SI, Kohane DS. Treatment of Streptococcus pneumoniae otitis media in a chinchilla model by transtympanic delivery of antibiotics. JCI Insight. 2018b;3(19):e123415.
36. Piu F, Wang X, Fernandez R, et al. OTO-104: a sustained-release dexamethasone hydrogel for the treatment of otic disorders. Otol Neurotol. 2011;32:171–9.
37. Huang PC, Chaney EJ, Shelton RL, Boppart SA. Magnetomotive displacement of the tympanic membrane using magnetic nanoparticles: toward enhancement of sound perception. IEEE Trans Biomed Eng. 2018;65(12):2837–46.
38. Lin YC, Shih CP, Chen HC, Chou YL, Sytwu HK, Fang MC, Lin YY, Kuo CY, Su HH, Hung CL, Chen HK, Wang CH. Ultrasound microbubble-facilitated inner ear delivery of gold nanoparticles involves transient disruption of the tight junction barrier in the round window membrane. Front Pharmacol. 2021;12:689032.
39. Liang Z, Yu H, Lai J, Wen L, Chen G. An easy-to-prepare microshotgun for efficient transmembrane delivery by powering nanoparticles. J Control Release. 2020;321:119–31.
40. Abdelbary AA, Abd-Elsalam WH, Al-Mahallawi AM. Fabrication of levofloxacin polyethylene glycol decorated nanoliposomes for enhanced management of acute otitis media: statistical optimization, trans-tympanic permeation and in vivo evaluation. Int J Pharm. 2019;559:201–9.

19 Viral Otitis Media and Acute Otitis Media and Recurrent Acute Otitis Media. An Evidence-Based Approach

José Faibes Lubianca Neto, João Pedro Neves Lubianca, and Marcelo Neves Lubianca

Introduction

The evidence-based approach is a modern, although not recent, way of supporting diagnostic and therapeutic decision-making in which the emphasis is removed from the pathophysiological mechanism, experimental work in animals, and nonsystematic clinical experience, placing it in the analysis of methodologically well-designed and properly conducted clinical studies [1]. Ideally, medical management should be aligned in light of the results of meta-analyses of large randomized, double-blind, placebo-controlled clinical trials with relevant clinical outcomes (decreased mortality, clinical cure, etc.). Most clinical approaches in otorhinolaryngology are still based on case series [2], and good level randomized clinical trials are insignificant in percentages [3]. The situation looks a little better in the diagnostic field than in the therapeutic one [4].

The clinical studies in acute/recurrent otitis media and otitis media with effusion, however, were the first to bring the evidence-based approach to otolaryngology, with clinical trials published in the 1980s and meta-analyses from the 1990s on. The pioneers in clinical trials of otitis media in children, such as the North Americans from Pittsburgh (Charles Bluestone, Sylvan Stool, and Jack Paradise) and the Europeans (Richard Maw and Louk van Buchem), deserve mention. Regarding meta-analyses, the North American Richard Rosenfeld and the Australians Christopher Del Mar and Paul Glasziou stand out.

J. F. Lubianca Neto (✉)
Graduate Program of Pediatrics of Federal University of Health Sciences of Porto Alegre, Porto Alegre, RS, Brazil

Otorhinolaryngology Service at Santa Casa de Misericórdia de Porto Alegre Hospital, Porto Alegre, RS, Brazil

Pediatric Otorhinolaryngology Service at Santo Antonio Children's Hospital, Porto Alegre, RS, Brazil
e-mail: lubianca@otorrinospoa.com.br

J. P. N. Lubianca
Federal University of Rio Grande do Sul, Hospital de Clínicas de Porto Alegre, Porto Alegre, RS, Brazil

M. N. Lubianca
Pontifical Catholic University of Rio Grande do Sul, São Lucas Hospital, Porto Alegre, RS, Brazil

Definitions

Acute otitis media (AOM) is defined as the prompt appearance of signs and symptoms of acute inflammation (fever, poor appetite, vomiting, otalgia, irritability, pulling the ear) associated with the presence of purulent exudate in the tympanic cavity. Recurrent AOM (RAOM) is defined as the occurrence of three or more episodes of AOM in a 6-month period or the occurrence of four or more episodes of AOM in a 12-month period that includes at least one episode in the preceding 6 months [5]. AOM peak incidence was between 6 and 11 months of age; until 3 years old, up to 85% of children will have had one or more episodes, of whom up to 20% had RAOM by 1 year of age and up to 40% will have six or more episodes during their lifetime [6]. A population-based birth cohort with more than 50,000 children born in southwestern British Columbia in 1999–2000 reported that almost half (48.6%) of children had 1 or more episodes of AOM by age 3 years, and 7.8% met the definition for recurrent AOM [7].

Risk Factors for Acute and Recurrent Acute Otitis Media

The risk factors for RAOM can be classified as host-associated and environmental. Usually, the factors most susceptible to intervention are environmental risk factors. There is scarce evidence, however, that intervention in these risk factors could decrease the incidence of RAOM. An exception to this was shown by studies that evaluated the effect of decreasing pacifier usage and frequency on daycare attendance, as well as the effect of adenoidectomy, on reducing RAOM.

M. V. Goycoolea et al. (eds.), *Textbook of Otitis Media*, https://doi.org/10.1007/978-3-031-40949-3_19

Host-Associated Risk Factors

Allergy

Even though there is epidemiologic, mechanical, and therapeutic evidence suggesting that allergic rhinitis contributes to the pathogenesis of otitis media, it is controversial that this entity is a risk factor in RAOM. In a cohort of 707 children with RAOM, Pukander and Karma [8] found more persistent middle-ear effusion (MEE) for 2 months or longer in children with atopic manifestations than in those that were nonallergic. Bernstein et al. [9] followed up on 77 children who had RAOM with chronic middle ear effusion and who had at least one ventilation tube placement performed. There was increased IgE in the MEE in 14 out of 32 children with allergic rhinitis, compared with two out of 45 children considered to be nonallergic. In an interesting German cohort study through the first 2 years of life, children diagnosed with otitis media during infancy were at greater risk for developing late-onset allergic eczema and asthma during school age, and associations were stronger for frequent otitis media [7].

On the other hand, there are two meta-analyses of risk factors for RAOM with conflicting results, preventing allergic rhinitis from becoming a well-established risk factor for RAOM. While Uhary et al. [10] did not find significance in the association between atopy and RAOM, Zhang et al. [11] have shown a significant pooled odds ratio (OR) of 1.36 (confidence interval [CI] 1.13–1.64).

Craniofacial Abnormalities

Children with an uncorrected cleft palate have a higher incidence of otitis media than normal children, especially when considering those aged up to 2 years old, as shown by Bluestone [12]. Since the cleft is corrected, RAOM reduces [13], possibly because Eustachian tube function improves in these cases [14]. The presence of craniofacial deformities increased the chance of the child requiring multiple interventions for ventilation tube placements, as shown in a retrospective cohort by Boston et al. [15].

Gastroesophageal Reflux (GER)

In a recent systematic review dealing only with the association between otitis media and GER, Miura et al. [16] concluded that "the prevalence of GER in children with RAOM may be higher than the overall prevalence for children. The presence of pepsin or pepsinogen in MEE could be related to physiologic reflux. A cause-and-effect relationship between pepsin and pepsinogen in MEE and otitis media is unclear". Antireflux therapy for otitis media cannot be endorsed based on existing research.

Adenoids

There are some articles that point out a great correlation (approximately 70%) between the rhinopharyngeal bacteria and those cultivated in the MEE in acute episodes [17]. Others demonstrate larger numbers of adenoid colony counts in patients operated on due to RAOM compared to those operated on due to obstruction [18]. Currently, the theory that suggests adenoids as a bacterial reservoir is more accepted than the one that their growth obstructs the Eustachian tube, a fact rarely proved in clinical practice [18], but that may exist [19]. A positive effect of adenoidectomy on reducing many endpoints related to otitis media has been demonstrated by randomized clinical trials [20–23]. Meantime, well-conducted randomized clinical trial results conflict with this, presenting that adenoidectomy alone or associated with ventilation tube placement has no solid role in the prophylaxis of RAOM in children less than 2 years old, at least at the first ventilation tube placement [23–25]. A meta-analysis analyzed the potential role of large adenoids as a risk factor for RAOM [11]. This study evaluated chronic nasal obstruction and snoring, two factors linked to large adenoids. Whereas results did not show any association between chronic nasal obstruction and RAOM, they showed that persistent snoring almost doubled its frequency (OR 1.96; CI 1.78–2.16). A more detailed analysis of the effect of adenoidectomy will be presented in the prophylactic treatment section of this chapter.

Genetic Susceptibility

Genetic factors and their influence on the genesis of otitis media are just beginning to be understood. We already have a few studies that can provide evidence for this. A positive parental story for RAOM remained a significant predictor for RAOM in children even after the logistic regression was performed, as shown by a huge prevalence study in Greenland [26]. The strongest evidence was demonstrated in research with twins and triplets. In a Norwegian retrospective study with 2750 twin pairs, 45% and 74% of heritability were found in boys and girls, respectively. Another retrospective study with a sample of 1373 twin pairs estimated heritability for RAOM in the ages of 2, 3, and 4 years, on average, close to 0.57 [27]. In the prospective twins and triplets Pittsburgh study, in which monthly monitoring of the middle ear was done, at the 2-year endpoint, the estimated heritability of otitis media was 0.79 in girls and 0.64 in boys. Of the original 140 pairs of twins and triplets with determined zygosity, 114 were followed up to the age of 3, and 83 were followed up for 5 years. The monozygotic twins had a significantly longer time with MEE (0.65–0.77) than the dizygotic twins (0.31–0.39) for each year until the third. After that, there was a decrease in these rates, probably explained by the lower incidence of otitis media in older children. The discordance estimates for three or more MEE episodes were 0.02 for monozygotic twins and 0.40 for dizygotic twins, both followed up until the fifth year ($p = 0.07$). The estimated heritability of the proportion of time spent with MEE in the first

5 years of life was 72% ($p < 0.001$). The boys' estimative was 0.66 and the girls' were 0.75. These results support the impact of genetics on otitis media [28]. There are linkage studies that search for genes that predispose to RAOM, and they have already pointed out some hotspots in the genome. Daly et al. found evidence of linkage in the 10q26.3 and 19q13.43 chromosomes. Another study was conducted at Pittsburgh on a population of full siblings (two or more) who had a history of tympanostomy tube insertion thanks to a significant history of otitis media; their parents and other full siblings had no history of tympanostomy tube insertion. Chromosome 17q12, which includes AP2B1, CCL5, and some other CCL genes, and chromosome 10q22.3 (STFPA2) were the most relevant linkage peaks [29].

Environmental Risk Factors

Upper Respiratory Tract Infections (URTI)

Both epidemiological and clinical evidence indicate that otitis media is a frequent URTI complication. The incidence of URTI increases during autumn and winter stations in both hemispheres, paralleling AOM incidence. In the summer, they both decrease [30–33]. A pooled analysis from a meta-analysis conducted by Zhang et al. showed an increase in the risk of otitis media in the presence or shortly after a URTI nearly sevenfold (OR 6.59; 95% CI 3.13–13.89). An AOM-associated incidence of 30% was found in 623 URTI episodes in 112 children aged between 6 and 35 months, as evaluated by Revai et al. [34]. In a 2010 study, recurrent URTI in the past 12 months was one of the variables in the multivariable model that significantly increased the risk of RAOM [35]. These studies provide enough evidence to support the idea of URTI as an important risk factor for otitis media (level of evidence II) and to speculate that preventing virus infections may decrease RAOM incidence. Both viral antigens and even live viruses have been isolated in the MEE of children [36–38]. Inflammation and harm to the mucociliary movement of the auditory tube epithelium are two of the mechanisms that can explain why URTI predisposes to RAOM, which has already been demonstrated experimentally [39] and clinically [40].

Daycare Center Attendance

Alho et al. examined questionnaires that were sent to 2512 randomly selected children's parents and reviewed their clinical record cards. The authors estimated a relative risk (RR) of 2.06 (95% CI 1.81–2.34) for the development of AOM in children who frequented daycare centers when compared to children who received home care [41]. In Uhari et al.'s meta-analyses, AOM risk increased with childcare outside the home too (RR 2.45; 95% CI 1.51–3.98) [10]. The same finding was shown by other studies, and this incidence increases with the number of companies [5, 6]. Large group childcare centers increase otitis media incidence and have been defined as those in which professional educators provide care for up to 10 groups of 8–12 children in the same setting [42]. Beyond that, children in daycare centers need more ventilation tubes than those who receive care at home [41]. The large prevalence of URTI in children exposed to other substances can be one mechanism related to this phenomenon [43]. Alho et al. [44], in a hypothetical cohort, estimated that if 825 children were transferred from daycare centers to home care and followed up for 2 years, approximately two out of five affected would have RAOM. Strong clinical evidence from the clinical practice of otolaryngologists confirms this presumption. During the COVID-19 pandemic, there was a significant reduction in cases of AOM in children in countries that adopted the strategy of closing daycare centers. In conclusion, daycare attendance is a risk factor for RAOM (evidence level II).

Family Size (Siblings)

A higher incidence of AOM is described in children belonging to large families (notably if many of them are under 5 years old) [12, 45]. Birth order was also associated with otitis media episode rate and time with middle ear effusion; the former children have lower rates in the first 2 years of life when compared to their younger siblings [46]. The risk of RAOM increases by 4.18 times (95% CI 2.74–6.36) in younger siblings [47]. However, these findings are not unanimous. Vinther et al. [48], in a population study, did not find that family size is a risk factor for otitis media, nor did Teele et al. in their classical cohort study [36]. The impact of genetics and the influence of daycare centers are two risk factors that make the exclusive analysis of sibling number as a risk factor a challenge. Finally, an increase of 92% in the incidence of otitis media if there is at least one sibling (RR 1.92; 95% CI 1.29–2.85) was shown by Uhari et al. in their meta-analysis, which pooled the results of two previous conflicting studies [36, 37].

Passive Smoking

It is one of the most studied risk factors for RAOM. However, the first studies were controversial, showing both positive [38, 49–51] and negative [48, 52–55] associations between otitis media and second-hand smoke exposure. Posterior studies, however, showed more conclusive results. Mother's heavy smoking (20 or more cigarettes per day) was a significant risk factor for RAOM, with an RR of 1.78 (95% CI 1.01–3.11) in a multivariate analysis, as demonstrated by Ey et al., who prospectively analyzed 1013 children from birth to 1 year [56]. In another prospective cohort with a sample of 918 children, the ones who had heavy-smoker mothers were at significantly increased risk of having four or more AOM episodes (RR 1.8; 95% CI 1.1–3.0) and made the first AOM episode earlier (RR 1.3; 95% CI 1.0–1.8). The more cigarettes smoked, the greater the risk of RAOM [57]. Maternal smoking enhanced the risk of RAOM (OR 4.15; CI 1.45–11.9) after ventilation tube insertion in another prospective cohort [58]. Some studies tried to measure objectively tobacco exposure through cotinine (a nicotine metabolite) concentrations in saliva and urine. One of these studies, using salivary cotinine, was a retrospective cohort of 9 years with 132 daycare children [59]. The incidence rate of MEE was 1.39 (95% CI 1.15–1.69) in the first year of life and 1.38 (95% CI 1.21–1.56) in the first 3 years. Nonetheless, when other variables were included in the logistic regression, the significance disappeared. Stratchan et al. did not find an association between salivary cotinine and otitis media. The association between early AOM onset and the rate of cotinine-creatinine in urine was also not able to be demonstrated by Daly et al. [60]. Stratchan and Cook's meta-analysis demonstrated estimated RRs, if at least one of the parents smoked, of 1.48 (95% CI 1.08–2.04) and 1.38 (95% CI 1.23–1.55) for RAOM and MEE, respectively [49]. Another meta-analysis calculated a risk of 1.92 (95% CI 1.29–2.85) for RAOM [11]. Finally, this association (passive smoking and otitis media) remains a controversial subject in otorhinolaryngology. However, regarding RAOM, passive smoking is a probable risk factor (level of evidence II).

Breastfeeding

Breastfeeding is considered a protective factor against otitis media by most authors. A prospective cohort demonstrated that children who were breastfed until 6 months of age did not have any episodes of AOM, whereas 10% of those who started with cow's milk before 2 months old presented AOM episodes during this period. The incidence of two or more otitis media episodes at the end of the first year was 6% and 19% for breastfed children and artificially fed children, respectively. From the end of the first year until the third, four or more episodes of otitis occurred in 6% of the former group and 26% of the latter. These results point out that prolonged breastfeeding (6 months or longer) protects against RAOM up to the third year of life, despite some individuals who were lost through follow-up [61]. An important lower number of otitis episodes in the first 2 years of breastfed children (0.3 episodes, 9/30) compared to cow's milk-fed children (2.9, 86/30) was shown by a case-control study [62]. Duncan et al. followed up on 1013 nursing infants for 1 year and showed that those who were exclusively breastfed for 4 months or longer had half of the AOM episodes when compared to non-breastfed infants and 50% less otitis than those breastfed up to 4 months [63]. In a cohort that followed up 306 children for their first 2 years, it was demonstrated that between 6 and 12 months of age, the cumulative incidence of first episodes increased from 25% to 51% and from 54% to 76% in exclusively breastfed infants and nursing infants fed with formula since birth, respectively. An inverse relation between the peak of AOM incidence (and MEE) and breastfeeding rates after 3 months of age was shown. During the same period of life, nursing infants exclusively breastfed for 6 months had half the risk of the first AOM episode compared to those exclusively fed formula [64]. In the Mandel et al. study, 148 children aged 1.0–8.6 years were followed up, and the results revealed that a lack of breastfeeding was a relevant predictor of otitis media with effusion (OME) and AOM incidences. Uhari et al.'s meta-analysis [10] demonstrated that children breastfed for at least 3 months reduced the risk of AOM by 13% (RR 0.87; 95% CI 0.79–0.95). The theory of "positional otitis media" says that children breastfed in an unsuitable position (lying down) are at greater risk for otitis media and finds support in some studies [63, 65].

In conclusion, most authors and the actual evidence point toward the protective effect of breastfeeding in the RAOM course (level of evidence II). At the same time, when it comes to the duration of breastfeeding required for protection, controversy remains. A study focused on this question demonstrated that AOM risk was significantly reduced for up to 4 months after breastfeeding ceased, but 12 months after the stop, the risk was virtually the same among the children who were still getting breastfed and the ones who were not [66].

Use of Pacifier

In a sample of 938 children, Niemela et al. [67] showed that those who used pacifiers had a higher risk of presenting RAOM than the ones who did not. In another study, Niemela et al. [68, 69], prospectively following 845 daycare children, demonstrated that pacifier use increased AOM annual incidence and was responsible for up to 25% of its cases. Pacifier sucking was significantly associated with otitis media from the sixth to the ninth month and presented a strong trend towards statistical significance in the period from 9 to 12 months ($p = 0.56$) [70]. Lastly, in the Uhari et al. [10] meta-analysis, pacifier use enhanced AOM risk by 25% (estimated RR 1.24; 95% CI 1.06–1.46) (level of evidence II). An open randomized clinical trial picked up 14 baby welfare clinics and paired them according to the number of students and their parents' social class. In each pair, one clinic was randomly allocated for intervention, while the other served as a control. The intervention consisted of a leaflet containing explanations about the deleterious effects of pacifier use and instructions for how to restrict it (essentially to use it only when going to sleep). Intervention clinics recruited 272 children under 18 months of age, while control clinics recruited 212. A decrease of 21% in continuous pacifier use from 7 to 18 months of age ($p = 0.0001$) and 30% less AOM occurrence were found among the intervention clinics. Children who did not use pacifiers continuously in any of the clinics had 33% fewer episodes of AOM when compared to those who did [68]. So, pacifiers have evidence of their deleterious effect, both in terms of association and in terms of intervention, and should be routinely discouraged.

Diagnosis of Acute Otitis Media

At least three papers have analyzed the value of different symptoms and otoscopic signs in the diagnosis of AOM. As early as 1968, Halsted et al. [71] aspirated fluid from the middle ears of 81 children who had moderate or marked bulging of the tympanic membrane, with or without erythema, stating that this sign is probably the most useful indicator of AOM. Karma et al. [72] have found that although a combination of otoscopic signs and symptoms is better than an isolated finding, bulging of the tympanic membrane is the best isolated sign, with a specificity of 96.8% and a positive predictive value of 96%. We found a similar result (97% and 94%, respectively) [73]. We question the appropriateness of performing tympanometry in cases of AOM in practice, as advocated by Saeed et al. [74]. It is an uncomfortable, painful procedure in acute cases and is not necessary for the great majority of children, even in uncertain cases. Pneumotoscopy and even otoscopy, in the hands of an otolaryngologist, are enough to diagnose at least the most severe cases, where bulging is almost always present.

Treatment of Recurrent Acute Otitis Media

The treatment of RAOM can be clinical and/or surgical. There are two main approaches: the treatment of repeated episodes and the prophylactic treatment to avoid or reduce the recurrence of acute episodes.

At least for the first and second days, the most important treatment is analgesia. The use of analgesics and antipyretics should be immediate since antibiotics take up to 48 h to relieve fever and otalgia. Among the most commonly used analgesics are dipyrone, acetaminophen (paracetamol), and ibuprofen [5].

Bacteriology and Antibiotics in RAOM

Antibiotic treatment should ideally be based on the bacterial profile and the resistance of bacteria in the place where we work. It is known that the bacterial resistance profile can vary between different countries and even in different cities within the same country [75], reinforcing the need to carry out microbiological studies in different regions [76]. This premise is not accepted, however, in different places like ours, where pediatric ethics committees do not approve such studies, as they consider tympanostomy an invasive procedure that usually, although there are exceptions [77, 78], is performed under general anesthesia.

Nowadays, antibiotic therapy options for RAOM are based on the results of sensitivity tests from large surveillance studies. However, these studies evaluate microorganisms from invasive infections (for instance, System of Surveillance Networks for Agents Responsible for Pneumonia and Bacterial Meningitis in Latin America and the Caribbean [SIREVA]). There is a lack of systematic studies seeking to identify the type of bacteria and its degree of resistance among upper airway infections. Traditionally, *Pneumococcus pneumoniae*, *Haemophilus influenzae*, and *Moraxella catharralis* (the hell trio), in that order, were the most common bacteria in AOM [79]. The order of frequency, however, changed with the implementation of the heptavalent pneumococcal vaccination, with *H. influenzae* appearing as the most common bacterium in place of *S. pneumoniae* [80], especially on RAOM [81]. Among the less commonly found bacteria are *S. aureus* and *S. pyogenes*, the latter being the second most frequent bacteria in acute mastoiditis [82, 83].

Evidence has modified some dogmas about the treatment of AOM. Children with AOM younger than 6 weeks, traditionally considered to be potentially contaminated with Gram-negative, demonstrated almost the same bacteriology as older children [84]. Another important observation with direct implications for the choice of antimicrobial is that relapses in less than 30 days of treatment are usually caused by bacteria different from those of the first episode and not by the same bacteria that would have become resistant [85].

Bacterial resistance became a public health problem secondary to the inappropriate use of antibiotics in the last few decades. It is estimated that in developed countries such as the USA and Canada, 30–50% of antibiotic prescriptions are inappropriate [86–88]. There is evidence showing that the greater the consumption of antibiotics in the community, the greater the bacterial resistance [89].

As for the cases that require treatment with antibiotics, these should cover the most commonly involved bacteria. The recommended treatment for uncomplicated cases is amoxicillin (45 mg/kg/day, divided into two or three doses), which may be associated with beta-lactamase inhibitors in patients with aggravating comorbidities or suspected or confirmed resistant infections (for instance, culture-proving resistance, previous poor outcome with the drug, recent antibiotic use) [5, 90, 91]. For patients with nonsevere allergies to penicillin, second- or third-generation cephalosporins, clindamycin, and macrolides, especially clarithromycin, may be used. Azithromycin and cefaclor should not be used due to their high resistance indexes. Sulfa drugs should be avoided due to their low therapeutic efficacy in children [5]. If resistant pneumococci are suspected, a double dose of amoxicillin (90 mg/kg/day) with or without clavulanate should be used [5]. In case of failure of this dose, intramuscular ceftriaxone is the next option, for 3 days [5]. In Brazil, we have no third-generation cephalosporins to be used orally.

Treatment of AOM Episode

The decision to use or not to use antibiotics in cases of AOM has been discussed in the literature over the last few decades. The natural history of nonsevere AOMs shows that the cure of this condition usually occurs regardless of the use of antibiotics. Although there is indeed an additional benefit to prescribing antibiotics to resolve the AOM picture, this benefit is modest, increasing the resolution rate by only 12–14% when compared to placebo (resolution of 92–94% with ATB use vs. 80% without ATB use) [92]. Antibiotics have a beneficial effect in reducing effusion up to 6 weeks after the end of treatment, preventing early recurrence of AOM and perforation onset, but they are all clinically modest. However, antibiotic use does not prevent more serious complications, such as mastoiditis, the presence of effusion, or late recurrences (after 3 months). On the other hand, adverse effects such as vomiting, diarrhea, and skin rashes are significantly more frequent in children who receive antibiotics [93]. In two studies that performed culture by tympanic membrane puncture before and after the treatment, 3–7% of patients who had negative cultures between days 3 and 7 failed to respond to the antibiotic. On the other hand, of those who maintained a positive culture, the failure rate was 37–38%. However, this result also means that 62–63% of the patients achieved clinical cure, even while maintaining a positive culture between days 3 and 7 [94, 95].

It is indisputable, however, that the use of antimicrobials should be reserved only for cases with bulging of the tympanic membrane [96, 97]. A meta-analysis of individual cases determined that the bilaterality of AOM and/or the presence of otorrhea would be the most important indicators for the prescription of antimicrobials [98] based on the reduction in the number of patients needed to treat (NNT) to benefit one. The overall NNT, which varies from 7 to 10, dropped to 5 and 3 in cases with bilateral AOM and with otorrhea, respectively. Other accepted criteria for routine antibiotic prescription, according to the last North American consensus on AOM, would be age younger than 6 months (there are no randomized clinical trials that include children of this age) and a severe course of AOM (severe otalgia and/or fever >39 °C) [5]. In this same consensus, due to the presence of AOM in cases older than 2 years, expectant treatment is an alternative even in bilateral cases without otorrhea. For children under 2 years, on the other hand, expectant treatment is only considered in unilateral cases [5].

Taking into account the indications for the optional use of antimicrobials, there are three approaches to the treatment of these acute episodes (do not forget that antibiotics do not treat pain acutely, so all approaches must be accompanied by analgesics): (1) immediate treatment of all cases of acute bulging; (2) expectant treatment (advise parents to only return for a new evaluation if the child still has fever or otalgia after 48 h) [99]; or (3) dispensing a delayed prescription, that is, prescribing the antimicrobial and asking that the prescription be used only if symptoms persist after 48 h [100].

A recent study showed that whereas some clinical characteristics were moderate determinants for watchful waiting, clinician antibiotic prescribing volume and specialty were strong determinants. Low-volume antibiotic prescribers (≥80% of AOM episodes managed with watchful waiting) had 11.61 (95% CI 10.66–12.64) higher odds of using watchful waiting for the index AOM episode than high-volume antibiotic prescribers (≥80% treated). Otolaryngologists were more likely to adopt watchful waiting (OR 5.45, 95% CI 5.21–5.70) than pediatricians, whereas other specialties deferred more commonly to antibiotics. Among 2,176,617 AOM episodes, 77.8% were treated within 3 days [101]. This result reinforces the need to invest in medical education, whether in medical schools or in the form of continuing medical education, in order to achieve more rational levels of antimicrobial prescribing, especially for pediatricians.

Prophylactic Treatment of Recurrent AOM

The prophylactic treatment of RAOM can be clinical and/or surgical. Clinical prophylactic treatment includes antibiotic prophylaxis, vaccines, and others. Surgical prophylactic treatment includes an adenoidectomy and ventilation tubes.

Antibiotic Prophylaxis

When compared to placebo [102–104] and even to tubes [102] and adenoidectomy [104], antibiotic prophylaxis had a variable but statistically significant greater protection against RAOM. A meta-analysis of studies using various antimicrobials indicated an overall reduction, with a rate difference of 0.11 episodes per patient-month during the period of prophylaxis [105]. The clinical significance, however, is less. This rate difference of 0.11 episodes per patient-month translated into NNT is nine, that is, I must treat one child for 9 months or nine children for 1 month with antibiotic prophylaxis to prevent one episode of AOM. Also, it should be highlighted that RAOM has a self-limiting natural history. The minority of children (17%) included in the randomized clinical trials in the placebo group will continue to have RAOM after 3 months to 2 years of their inclusion in the study (only one in eight children will continue to have RAOM if they are followed up for a while) [106]. Finally, the strongest argument not to use antibiotic prophylaxis nowadays is that antimicrobial use is a main contributor to bacterial resistance, so the risks of sustained prophylaxis now seem to generally outweigh the likely benefits.

Vaccines

There are two kinds of vaccines that play a role in the prophylaxis of RAOM: pneumococcal and influenza vaccines. The three licensed pneumococcal vaccines include a 7-valent PCV containing the polysaccharides of seven serotypes (4, 6B, 9V, 14, 18C, 19F, and 23F) conjugated to the diphtheria-derived carrier protein CRM197 (CRM197-PCV7), a 10-valent PCV containing the capsular polysaccharides of 10 serotypes (1, 4, 5, 6B, 7F, 9V, 14, 18C, 19F, and 23F) mostly conjugated to protein D, which is a surface lipoprotein of *H. influenzae* (PHiD-CV10), and a 13-valent PCV containing the capsular polysaccharides of 13 serotypes (1, 3, 4, 5, 6A, 6B, 7F, 9V, 14, 18C, 19A, 19F, and 23F) conjugated to CRM197 (CRM197–PCV13).

For AOM due to *S. pneumoniae*, the release of CRM197–PVC7 in 2000 resulted in a 69–91% decrease in invasive pneumococcal disease. However, despite also being associated with both a 56–57% decrease in AOM associated with the pneumococcal serotypes included in the vaccine [107–109] and a notable reduction in tympanostomy tube insertion [110], PCV7 yielded only a modest overall decrease in AOM (approximately 6–7%) [111]. The effects in the real world were more pronounced and appeared in both developed and developing countries. In the United States, for example, the incidence of RAOM decreased by 28%, there were 23% fewer grommet insertions, there was a 42% decrease in antibiotic prescriptions, and there was a 43% decrease in office visits related to otitis media in infants [110, 112, 113]. The same was seen in Australia, with a significant reduction in ventilation tube insertions seen in 23% of infants younger than 1 year, 16% of children aged 1–2 years, and 6% of children aged 2 years [114]. In Great Britain, the incidence rate of otitis media in children younger than 10 years decreased by 22% after the introduction of PV7, with an additional 19% reduction after the change from PVC7 to PVC13 [115]. In Goiânia, a Midwest city in Brazil, the equivalent reduction in office visits related to AOM was 44% in children between 2 and 23 months after the introduction of PVC10 [116].

It should be noted, however, that pneumococcal vaccines work mainly in early infants (children aged less than 1 year), with the first dose ideally at 2 months and two other booster shots during the first year [117].

Regarding the influenza vaccine, initial studies have shown a 35% reduction in the incidence of AOM in daycare centers during acute outbreaks of influenza [118, 119]. A recent meta-analysis confirmed the protection but found a small but still significant protective effect of the vaccine against RAOM if applied before the influenza season began [120]. Topical intranasal vaccines have been studied with welcome results. At least one nonlicensed intranasal inactivated influenza vaccine prevented AOM in 43.7% of children with RAOM (95% CI 18.6–61.1%; $p = 0.002$) [121].

Other Medical Treatments

Xylitol is a pentitol (i.e., a five-carbon polyol sugar alcohol). Studies have shown that 1 and 5% xylitol could markedly reduce the *in vitro* growth [122] and respiratory-cell adhesion [123] of several otopathogens. A double-blind randomized clinical trial with 306 daycare children with RAOM was conducted in Finland. It showed that at least one episode of AOM was experienced by 31/149 (20.8%) children who received a placebo compared with 19/157 (12.1%) of those receiving chewing gum containing xylitol (five times per day) during a 2-month period (difference 8.7%; 95% CI 0.4–17.0%; $p = 0.04$). Significantly fewer antibiotics were prescribed to children who were using xylitol [124]. However, those results are not unanimous. Another trial that tried to make xylitol dosage more accessible was not able to confirm previous positive results. They have used a dose of 5 g three times a day, administered in the form of a syrup. In this study, 326 subjects were enrolled, and the hazard ratio for time to first clinically diagnosed AOM episode for xylitol versus placebo recipients was 0.88 (95% CI 0.61–1.3). In secondary analyses, the incidence of AOM was 0.53 episodes per 90 days in the xylitol group versus 0.59 in the placebo group (difference 0.06; 95% CI −0.25 to 0.13) [125]. A 2011 meta-analysis concluded that there is fair evidence that the prophylactic administration of xylitol among healthy children attending daycare centers reduces the occurrence of AOM by 25%. The author emphasized the inclusion of only four randomized clinical trials, and almost all were from the same study group [126]. We agree with the statement to not use xylitol for RAOM prophylaxis in the Guidelines of the Italian Society of Pediatrics on Prevention of RAOM [127] because the available evidence comes from studies with different xylitol dosages, administrations, and preparations, which makes the results difficult to compare.

Probiotics are live microorganisms that offer health benefits by modulating an individual's microbial community and enhancing host immunity (mainly *Lactobacillus* and *Streptococcus* species). Despite a few exceptions for oral probiotic studies [128], AOM data are scarce and often controversial. In general, any reduction in respiratory infection incidence observed in children receiving probiotics was marginal at best [128–130]. The nasal route for probiotic administration was also tried as a prophylactic treatment for RAOM in children. The most studied microorganism is alpha-hemolytic Streptococcus (AHS), an infectious agent with low infectivity that could interfere with the survival and multiplication of pathogens carried in the nasopharynx and is more frequently associated with AOM [131]. However, despite initially positive results [132], RAOM prophylaxis via nasal AHS administration has been rapidly abandoned due to the fear that AHS could cause infection as well as findings from a well-conducted study [132]. More recently, attention has focused on *Streptococcus salivarius*, an AHS isolated from healthy individuals that has never been demonstrated to cause infection.

A recent meta-analysis analyzed 16 Randomized Clinical Trials, of which 11 evaluated Lactobacillus-containing probiotics and six evaluated Streptococcus-containing probiotics [133]. The proportion of children (i.e., the number of children in each group) experiencing one or more episodes of AOM during the treatment was lower for those taking probiotics (RR 0.77, 95% CI 0.63–0.93; 16 trials; 2961 participants; NNT = 10; moderate-certainty evidence). However, this effect was restricted to children not prone to RAOM. *Post hoc* subgroup analysis found that among children not prone to otitis media, a lower proportion of children receiving probiotics experienced AOM (RR 0.64, 95% CI 0.49–0.84; 11 trials; 2227 participants; NNT = 9; moderate-certainty evidence). Unfortunately, among children who were otitis prone, there was no difference between probiotic and comparator groups (RR 0.97, 95% CI 0.85–1.11; five trials; 734 participants; high-certainty evidence). Probiotics decreased the proportion of children taking antibiotics for any infection (RR 0.66, 95% CI 0.51–0.86; eight trials; 1768 participants; NNT = 8; moderate-certainty evidence). The test for subgroup differences (use of antibiotics specifically for AOM and use of antibiotics for infections other than AOM) was not significant. Probiotic strains studied and their dose, frequency, and duration of administration varied considerably across studies, which likely contributed to the substantial levels of heterogeneity and the difficulty of extrapolating the results. The inconsistency of the subgroup analyses suggests caution in interpreting the results. The optimal strain, duration, frequency, and timing of probiotic administration still need to be established. We can conclude that the available evidence does not recommend the use of probiotics to prevent RAOM.

Vitamin D (VD) has been found to play a crucial role in immune system regulation by governing macrophage and dendritic cell activities and various Toll-like receptor-mediated events in neutrophils [134, 135]. VD also induces the expression of antimicrobial peptides such as cathelicidin and b-defensins. Finally, VD shifts cytokine expression from Th1 to Th2. Children with RAOM have significantly lower serum 25 (OH)D levels (<30 ng/mL) than healthy controls, and administering VD can significantly reduce the incidence of new AOM episodes [136]. In a double-blind, placebo-controlled trial, the number of children with RAOM who experienced more than one AOM episode was significantly lower among the group who received 1000 IU of VD than among untreated controls (26 vs. 38; $p = 0.03$). We should conclude that perhaps (the evidence is too scarce) for children with hypovitaminosis D, supplementation could decrease the incidence of RAOM. However, for children with normal serum levels of VD, there is no evidence that VD can reduce RAOM. So, for the moment, the use of vitamin D is not recommended for RAOM prophylaxis.

Surgical Prophylactic Treatment of RAOM

Ventilation Tubes

Myringotomy with the insertion of a ventilation tube is the most frequently performed ambulatory pediatric surgery in North America after the newborn period [137]. Almost 700,000 such procedures are performed every year in the United States, and 6.8% of the population had TTs placed before the age of 3 [137]. One of the main indications is RAOM. The indication of surgery is a balance between the risks of myringotomy and tubes (general anesthesia, tube recurrent otorrhea, blockage, extrusion, or retraction of the tube into the middle ear, tympanosclerosis and associated potential mild conductive hearing loss, residual perforation, and contradictory necessity of water precautions) and benefits (change from oral antibiotics to topical antibiotics to treat acute otorrhea, hearing improvement, decrease in pain, and a debatable reduction in the frequency of AOM episodes).

Many classic trials supporting the efficacy of tympanostomy tubes [102] were conducted before the introduction of conjugate pneumococcal vaccines, which decreased the incidence and changed other epidemiologic and bacteriologic features of AOM. Besides presenting mixed results, they have some limitations: they include children with questionable diagnoses of AOM, have short follow-up periods, and have small study samples. A 2018 meta-analysis including five randomized clinical trials, all of the pre-pneumococcal vaccine era, concluded that low- to very-low-quality evidence suggests that children receiving grommets are less likely to have AOM recurrences compared to those managed by active monitoring and placebo medication, but the magnitude of the effect is modest, with around one fewer episode at 6 months and a less noticeable effect by 12 months, and claimed for new and high-quality randomized clinical trials of grommet insertion in children with RAOM. These trials should not only focus on the frequency of AOM recurrences but also collect data on the severity of AOM episodes, antibiotic consumption, and adverse effects of both surgery and antibiotics [138].

Since the introduction of PCV7 and PCV13, there have been at least two main randomized clinical trials comparing the efficacy of tympanostomy tube insertion versus observation with episodic antimicrobial therapy among children with recurrent AOM [139, 140]. The European randomized clinical trial among 300 children 10–24 months of age with RAOM showed intervention failure (defined as two or more episodes of AOM in 2 months, three or more episodes in

6 months, or persistent effusion for 2 months) was lower in the tympanostomy tube group than in the observation group (21% vs. 34%, respectively; 95% CI −25 to −1%; $p = 0.04$). The tympanostomy group also had a lower 1-year incidence rate of AOM (1.15 vs. 1.70; difference of −0.55, 95% CI −0.93 to −0.17) [139]. A 2021 United States randomized clinical trial among 250 children 6–35 months of age with recurrent AOM found no significant difference in the rate of episodes of AOM during a 2-year period in the intention-to-treat analysis (mean of 1.5 episodes, risk ratio 0.97; 95% CI 0.84–1.12; $p = 0.66$). However, a substantial number of patients (54 of 121 patients; 44.6%) who were initially assigned to medical management crossed over to the tympanostomy tube group, prompting a per-protocol analysis that slightly favored tympanostomy tubes, with rates (±SD) of 1.47 ± 0.08 and 1.72 ± 0.11 episodes of AOM per year over a 2-year period in the tympanostomy tube and medical-management groups, respectively (a rate that was modestly lower, by 0.25 episodes per year, in the tympanostomy tube group). The time to first occurrence of AOM was longer in the tympanostomy tube group than in the observation group (4.34 months vs. 2.33 months; hazard ratio = 0.68, 95% CI 0.52–0.90; $p = 0.01$). Children in the surgical group had higher mean days per year with tube otorrhea (7.96 [1.10] vs. 2.83 [0.78] days), but had fewer mean days per year with other otitis-related symptoms (2.00 [0.29] vs. 8.33 [0.59] days), and had fewer children with treatment failure (45% vs. 62%; $p = 0.006$). The tympanostomy tube group also received shorter mean oral antibiotic treatment (8.76 [0.94] vs 12.92 [0.90] days) [140]. The results of both studies are generally consistent in that the benefit of tympanostomy tube surgery is seen in the first year after the procedure, but this benefit disappears by the end of the second year.

The American Academy of Otolaryngology-Head and Neck Surgery recommended in the original 2013 Clinical Practice Guideline on tympanostomy tubes in children that tubes be offered for RAOM if a middle-ear effusion (MEE) is present on an otolaryngologist's examination [141]. Patients with no MEE between intervals are not good candidates. The natural history of RAOM without persistent effusion is favorable, with more than 40% of children in randomized clinical trial control groups having no additional AOM episodes in the next 6 months and only about 15% continuing to have RAOM [106]. The only RCT of tubes for recurrent AOM that specifically excluded children with baseline MEE found no benefit of tube insertion for reducing subsequent AOM incidence [102]. Likewise, a 2019 retrospective chart review followed children with RAOM aged 6 months to 12 years without MEE on presentation who were assigned to watchful waiting treatment. Treatment failure was defined as any continued AOM or MEE on follow-up leading to tube placement and occurred in 42 out of 123 patients (34% failure rate). Tubes were prevented in the majority of patients—in 81 out of 123 patients (66% success rate) [142]. So, this recommendation was sustained in the 2022 updated guideline, which recommends that clinicians offer bilateral tympanostomy tube insertion to children with RAOM who have unilateral or bilateral MEE at the time of assessment for tube candidacy [143].

There is a role for shared decision-making with caregivers in almost all indications for tympanostomies to insert tubes [144]. Recent interest in office-based tympanostomy tube placement without general anesthesia has been welcomed by caregivers but currently lacks the support of most otolaryngologists [78].

Adenoidectomy

Several randomized clinical trials analyzed the efficacy of adenoidectomy in RAOM, with diverging results [23, 104, 139, 145, 146]. The first was published in 1999 and involved 461 children less than 3 years old. A significant reduction in the mean rate of occurrence of AOM episodes per patient was seen in the adenotonsillectomy group compared to the control group, but only in the first year of follow-up (1.4 episodes vs. 2.1 episodes, in the adenoidectomy and control groups, respectively, $p < 0.001$). The same result also occurred in the first year of follow-up, with the mean of total days per year classified as otitis present at 18.6% vs. 29.9%, a difference of 11.3% fewer days with MEE in the adenotonsillectomy group, $p < 0.002$ [23]. In another trial that involved 217 RAOM children >12 months and <48 months of age, the risk of more than three AOM episodes in the next year of follow-up was not reduced in the group randomized to adenoidectomy plus tympanostomy, compared to the group of isolated tympanostomy [145]. At least three randomized trials evaluated the effect of adenoidectomy on the RAOM course, specifically in children younger than 2 years. Mattila et al., comparing isolated tympanostomy to tympanostomy plus adenoidectomy in 137 children, did not find any significant difference between groups (cumulative hazard of all otitis media episodes = 19%, 95% CI −14 to 43%) [146]. Koivunen et al. compared the failure proportion (defined as two episodes of AOM in 2 months or three episodes in 6 months, or middle ear effusion persistent for >2 months) among three groups: adenoidectomy, sulfafurazole, and placebo, and found similar treatment failure among the adenoidectomy and placebo groups (0% at 24 months, 95% CI −17 to 17%) [104]. Kujala et al. randomly assigned and followed for 1 year 300 children who had RAOM to receive tympanostomy tubes ($n = 100$), tympanostomy tubes with adenoidectomy ($n = 100$), or neither ($n = 100$). The intervention failed (two AOM episodes in 2 months, three in 6 months, or persistent effusion lasting for 2 months) in 21% of cases in the tympanotomy group, in 16% in the tympanostomy plus adenoidectomy group, and 34% in the control group. The absolute differences were −13% (95% CI −25 to −1%,

$p = 0.04$] between the tympanostomy and control groups and −18% (95% CI −30 to −6%, $p = 0.004$) between the tympanostomy plus adenoidectomy and control groups [139].

Two systematic reviews and meta-analyses published in 2014 analyzed the effect of adenoidectomy on RAOM, the need for repeated tympanostomy tube insertion, OME, and otorrhea. Mikals and Brigger compared tympanostomy tube insertion alone with combined surgery (tympanostomy plus adenoidectomy). Fifteen studies were included, and the main outcome measure was repeated surgery with a tympanostomy tube. Ten studies ($n = 71,353$) reported that primary adenoidectomy plus tympanotomy decreased the risk of reoperation or risk of RAOM, OME, or otorrhea compared with tympanostomy alone. The estimated rate of reoperation for children undergoing primary adenoidectomy was 17.2% (95% CI 12.2–22.2%) versus 31.8% (95% CI 23.9–39.8%) for children undergoing primary tympanostomy only. The protective effect was restricted to children greater than 4 years of age [147].

The last one, an individual patient data meta-analysis, investigated adenoidectomy with or without grommets with nonsurgical treatment or grommets only. The primary outcome was failure at 12 months after surgery, defined as four or more episodes of AOM, the presence of effusion for >6 months, the need for additional surgery, or hearing improvement of <10 dB. There were fewer failures at 12 months in the adenoidectomy group. In terms of reducing the occurrence of RAOM, there was a rate difference favoring the adenoidectomy group of −10% (95%CI −0.18 to −0.02). This translates into a modest NNT of 10. The RR for RAOM was 0.58 (95% CI 0.36–0.94), which corresponds to a protection for RAOM of 42%. Further analysis showed that two groups specifically had a favorable effect of adenoidectomy: children <2 years old with RAOM (16% failure rate vs. 27% with or without adenoidectomy, respectively) and children ≥4 years with persistent OME [148]. The last 2022 recommendation of the American Academy of Otolaryngology-Head & Neck Surgery is that "clinicians may perform adenoidectomy as an adjunct to tympanostomy tube insertion for children with symptoms directly related to the adenoids (adenoid infection or nasal obstruction) or in children aged 4 years or older to potentially reduce future incidence of RAOM or the need for repeat tube insertion" [143].

Conclusion

RAOM represents a public health problem, either because of its importance in the global prescription of antibiotics for children and its association with an increase in microbial resistance to antibiotics or because of its frequent association with surgery. The last decades have seen many etiological and epidemiological transformations in the RAOM. There are several viable and effective forms of treatment for the acute episode itself and prophylaxis. An alternative for the treatment of the crisis is watchful waiting, which has its indications and the potential to reduce the prescription of antimicrobials. Prophylactic measures include intervention in modifiable risk factors (daycare attendance, passive smoking, pacifiers, breastfeeding), influenza and pneumococcal vaccination, and tympanotomy with ventilation tubes with or without adenoidectomy.

References

1. Evidence-Based Medicine Working Group. Evidence-based medicine. A new approach to teaching the practice of medicine. JAMA. 1992;268(17):2420–5.
2. Bentsianov BL, Boruk M, Rosenfeld RM. Evidence-based medicine in otolaryngology journals. Otolaryngol Head Neck Surg. 2002;126(4):371–6.
3. Yao F, Singer M, Rosenfeld RM. Randomized controlled trials in otolaryngology journals. Otolaryngol Head Neck Surg. 2007;137(4):539–44.
4. Wasserman JM, Wynn R, Bash TS, Rosenfeld RM. Levels of evidence in otolaryngology journals. Otolaryngol Head Neck Surg. 2006;134(5):717–23.
5. Lieberthal AS, Carroll AE, Chonmaitree T, Ganiats TG, Hoberman A, Jackson MA, et al. The diagnosis and management of acute otitis media. Pediatrics. 2013;131:964–99.
6. Rovers MM, Schilder AG, Zielhuis GA, Rosenfeld RM. Otitis media. Lancet. 2004;363:465–73.
7. Macintyre EA, Karr CJ, Koehoorn M, Demers P, Tamburic L, Lencar C, et al. Otitis media incidence and risk factors in a population-based birth cohort. Paediatr Child Health. 2010;15:437–42.
8. Pukander J, Karma P. Persistence of middle-ear effusion and its risk factors after an acute attack of otitis media with effusion. In: Lim DJ, Bluestone CD, Klein JO, Nelson JD, editors. Recent advances in otitis media. Proceedings of the fourth international symposium. Toronto: BC Decker; 1988. p. 8–11.
9. Bernstein JM, Lee J, Conboy K, Ellis E, Li P. The role of IgE mediated hypersensitivity in recurrent otitis media with effusion. Am J Otol. 1983;5:66–9.
10. Uhari M, Matsyaari K, Niemela M. A meta-analytic review of the risk factor for acute otitis media. Clin Infect Dis. 1996;22:1079–83.
11. Zhang Y, Xu M, Zhang J, Zeng L, Wang Y, Zheng KY. Risk factors for chronic and recurrent otitis media. A meta-analysis. PLoS One. 2014;9:e86397.
12. Bluestone CD. Studies in otitis media: Children's Hospital of Pittsburgh—University of Pittsburgh Progress Report—2004. Laryngoscope. 2004;114(suppl 105):1–26.
13. Frable MA, Brandon GT, Theogaraj SD. Velar closure and ear tubings as a primary procedure in the repair of cleft palates. Laryngoscope. 1985;95:1044–6.
14. Doyle WJ, Reilly JS, Jardini L, Rovnak S. Effect of palatoplsty on the function of the Eustachian tube in children with cleft palate. Cleft Palate J. 1986;23:63–8.
15. Boston M, McCook J, Burke B, Derkay C. Incidence of and risk factors for additional tympanostomy tube insertion in children. Arch Otolaryngol Head Neck Surg. 2003;129:293–6.

16. Miura MS, Mascaro M, Rosenfeld RM. Association between otitis media and gastroesophageal reflux: a systematic review. Otolaryngol Head Neck Surg. 2012;146:354–2.
17. Howie VM, Plousard JH. Bacterial etiology and antimicrobial treatment of exudative otitis media: relation of antibiotic therapy to relapses. South Med J. 1971;64:233–9.
18. Pillsbury HC 3rd, Kveton JF, Sasaki CT, Frazier W. Quantitative bacteriology in adenoid tissue. Otolaryngol Head Neck Surg. 1981;89:355–63.
19. Kindermann CA, Roithmann R, Lubianca Neto JF. Obstruction of the eustachian tube orifice and pressure changes in the middle ear: are they correlated? Ann Otol Rhinol Laryngol. 2008;117:425–9.
20. Gates GA, Avery CA, Prihoda TJ, Cooper JC Jr. Effectiveness of adenoidectomy and tympanostomy tubes in the treatment of chronic otitis media with effusion. N Engl J Med. 1987;317:1444–51.
21. Maw R, Bawden R. Spontaneous resolution of severe chronic glue ear in children and the effect of adenoidectomy, tonsillectomy and insertion of ventilation tubes (grommets). BMJ. 1993;306:756–60.
22. Paradise JL, Bluestone CD, Rogers KD, Taylor FH, Colborn DK, Bochman RZ, et al. Efficacy of adenoidectomy for recurrent otitis media in children previously treated with tympanostomy tube placement. Results of parallel randomized and nonrandomized trials. JAMA. 1990;263:2066–73.
23. Paradise JL, Bluestone CD, Colborn DK, Bernard BS, Smith CG, Rockette HE, et al. Adenoidectomy and adenotonsillectomy for recurrent acute otitis media: parallel randomized clinical trial in children not previously treated with tympanostomy tubes. JAMA. 1999;282:945–53.
24. Kouvunem P, Uhari M, Luotonen J, Kristo A, Rask R, Pokka T, et al. Adenoidectomy versus chemoprophylaxis and placebo for recurrent acute otitis media in children aged under 2 years: randomised controlled trial. BMJ. 2004;328:487–91.
25. Mattilla OS, Joki-Erkkila VP, Kilpi T, Jokinen J, Herva E, Phakka H. Prevention of otitis media by adenoidectomy in children younger than 2 years. Arch Otolaryngol Head Neck Surg. 2003;129:163–8.
26. Homoe P, Christensen RB, Bretlau P. Acute otitis media and sociomedical risk factors among unselected children in Greenland. Int J Pediatr Otorhinolaryngol. 1999;49:37–52.
27. Rovers M, Haggard M, Gannon M, et al. Heritability of symptom domains in otitis media: a longitudinal study of 1373 twin pairs. Am J Epidemiol. 2002;155:958–64.
28. Casselbrant ML, Mandel EM, Rockette HE, et al. The genetic component of middle ear disease in the first 5years of life. Arch Otolaryngol Head Neck Surg. 2004;130:273–8.
29. Casselbrant ML, Mandel EM, Jung J, Ferrel RE, Tekely K, Szatkiewicz JP, Ray A, Weeks DE. Otitis media: a genome-wide linkage scan with evidence of susceptibility loci within the 17q12 and 10q22.3 regions. BMC Med Genet. 2009;10:85–94.
30. Castagno LA, Lavinsky L. Otitis media in children: seasonal changes and socioeconomic level. Int J Pediatr Otorhinolaryngol. 2002;62:129–34.
31. Casselbrant ML, Brostoff LM, Cantekin EI, Flaherty MR, Doyle WJ, Bluestone CD, et al. Otitis media with effusion in preschool children. Laryngoscope. 1985;95:428–36.
32. Van Cauwenberge PB. Relevant and irrelevant predisposing factors in secretory otitis media. Acta Otolaryngol Suppl. 1984;414:147–53.
33. Alho OP, Oja H, Koivu M, Sorri M. Risk factor for chronic otitis media with effusion in infancy. Each acute otitis media episode induces a high but transient risk. Arch Otolaryngol Head Neck Surg. 1995;121:839–43.
34. Revai K, Dobbs LA, Nair S, Patel JA, Grady JJ, Chonmaitree T. Incidence of acute otitis media and sinusitis complicating upper respiratory tract infection: the effect of age. Pediatrics. 2007;119:1408–12.
35. Chonmaitreee T, Revai K, Grady JJ, Clos A, Janak AP, Nair S, Fan J, Henrickson KJ. Viral upper respiratory tract infection and otitis media complication in young children. Clin Infect Dis. 2008;46:815–23.
36. Teele DW, Klein JO, Rosner B, Greater Boston Otitis Media Study Group. Epidemiology of otitis media during the first seven years of life in children in greater Boston: a prospective cohort study. J Infect Dis. 1989;160:83–94.
37. Pukander J, Luotonem J, Timonen M, Karma P. Risk factors affecting the occurrence of acute otitis media among 2-3 year-old urban children. Acta Otolaryngol. 1985;100:260–5.
38. Kraemer JK, Richardson MA, Weis NS, Furukawa CT, Shapiro GG, Pierson WE, et al. Risk factors for persistent middle-ear effusions. JAMA. 1983;249:1022–5.
39. Buchman CA, Doyle WJ, Skoner D, Fireman P, Gwaltney JM. Otologic manifestations of experimental rhinovirus infection. Laryngoscope. 1994;104:1295–9.
40. Bylander A. Upper respiratory tract infection and Eustachian tube dysfunction in children. Acta Otolaryngol. 1984;97:343–9.
41. Alho OP, Koivu M, Sorri M, Rantakallio P. Risk factor for recurrent acute otitis media and respiratory infection in infancy. Int J Pediatr Otorhinolaryngol. 1990;19:151–61.
42. Côté SM, Peticlerc A, Rynault MF, et al. Short- and long-term risk of infections as a function of group child care attendance: a 8-year population-based study. Arch Pediatr Adolesc Med. 2010;164:1132–7.
43. Wald ER, Dashefsky B, Byers C, Guerra N, Taylor F. Frequency and severity of infections in day care. J Pediatr. 1988;112:540–6.
44. Alho OP, Läärä E, Oja H. Public health impact of various risk factors for acute otitis media in northern Finland. Am J Epidemiol. 1996;143:1149–56.
45. Ladomenou F, Kafatos A, Tselentis Y, Galanakis E. Predisposing factor for acute otitis media in infancy. J Infect. 2010;61:49–53.
46. Lim DJ. Recent advances in otitis media with effusion. Report of the fourth research conference. Ann Otol Rhinol Laryngol. 1989;98(suppl 139):10–55.
47. Daly KA, Rich SS, Levine S, Margolis RH, Le CT, Lidgren B, et al. The family study of otitis media: design and disease and risk factor profiles. Genet Epidemiol. 1996;13:451–68.
48. Vinther B, Elbrond O, Pedersen B. A population study of otitis media in childhood. Acta Otolaryngol Suppl. 1979;360:135–7.
49. Stratchan DP, Cook DG. Health effects of passive smoking. 4. Parental smoking, middle ear disease and adenotonsillectomy in children. Thorax. 1998;53:50–6.
50. Strenstrom R, Bernard PA, Bem-Simhon H. Exposure to environmental tobacco smoke as a risk factor for recurrent acute otitis media in children under the age of five years. Int J Pediatr Otorhinolaryngol. 1993;27:127–36.
51. Kitchens GG. Relationship of environmental tobacco smoke to otitis media in young children. Laryngoscope. 1995;105:1–13.
52. Blakley BW, Blakley JE. Smoking and middle ear disease: are they related? A review article. Otolaryngol Head Neck Surg. 1995;112:441–6.
53. Birch L, Elbrond O. A prospective epidemiological study of secretory otitis media in young children related to the indoor environment. ORL J Otorhinolaryngol Relat Spec. 1987;49:253–8.
54. Hinton AE, Buckley G. Parental smoking and middle ear effusion in children. J Laryngol Otol. 1988;102:992–6.
55. Lubianca Neto JF, Burns AG, Lu L, Mombach R, Saffer M. Passive smoking and non-recurrent acute otitis media in children. Otolaryngol Head Neck Surg. 1999;121:805–8.
56. Ey JL, Holberg CJ, Aldous MB, Wright AL, Martinez FD, Taussig LM. Passive smoke exposure and otitis media in the first year of life. Pediatrics. 1995;95:670–7.

57. Collet JP, Larson CP, Boivin JF, Suissa S, Pless IB. Parental smoking and risk of otitis media in pre-school children. Can J Public Health. 1995;86:269–73.
58. Hammaren-Malmi S, Saxen H, Tarkkanen J, Mattila PS. Passive smoking after tympanostomy and risk of recurrent acute otitis media. Int J Pediatr Otorhinolaryngol. 2007;71:1305–10.
59. Etzel RA. Smoke and ear effusions. Pediatrics. 1987;79:309–11.
60. Daly KA, Brown JE, Lindgren BR, Meland MH, Le CT, Giebink GS. Epidemiology of otitis media onset by six months of age. Pediatrics. 1999;103:1158–66.
61. Saarinen UM. Prolonged breast feeding as prophylaxis for recurrent otitis media. Acta Pediatr Scand. 1982;71:567–71.
62. Chandra RK. Prospective studies of the effect of breast feeding on incidence of infection and allergy. Acta Pediatr Scand. 1982;71:567–71.
63. Duncan RB. Positional otitis media. Arch Otolaryngol. 1960;72:454–63.
64. Duffy LC, Faden H, Wasielewski R, Wolf J, Krystofik D. Exclusive breastfeeding protects against bacterial colonization and day care exposure to otitis media. Pediatrics. 1997;100:E7.
65. Beauregard RB. Positional otitis media. J Pediatr. 1971;79:294–6.
66. Sassen ML, Brand R, Grote JJ. Breast-feeding and acute otitis media. Am J Otolaryngol. 1994;15:351–7.
67. Niemela M, Uhari M, Hannuksela A. Pacifiers and dental structure as risk factors for otitis media. Int J Pediatr Otorhinolaryngol. 1994;29:121–7.
68. Niemela M, Uhari M, Mötönen M. A pacifier increases the risk of recurrent acute otitis media in children in day-care centers. Pediatrics. 1995;96:884–8.
69. Niemela M, Phakari O, Pokka T, Uhari M. Pacifier as a risk factor for acute otitis media: a randomized controlled trial of parental counseling. Pediatrics. 2000;106:483–8.
70. Warren JJ, Levy SM, Kirchner HL, Nowak AJ, Bergus GR. Pacifier use and the occurrence of otitis media in the first year of life. Pediatr Dent. 2001;23:103–7.
71. Halsted C, Lepow ML, Balassanian N, Emmercih J, Wolinsky E. Otitis media: clinical observations, microbiology, and evaluation of therapy. Am J Dis Child. 1968;115:542–6.
72. Karma PH, Sipilä MM, Kataja MJ, Penttilä MA. Pneumatic otoscopy and otitis media, II: value of different tympanic membrane findings and their combinations. In: Lim DJ, Bluestone CD, Klein JO, Nelson JD, Ogra PL, editors. Recent advances in otitis media: proceedings of the fifth international symposium. Burlington: Decker; 1993. p. 41–45.
73. Saffer M, Lubianca Neto JF. Avaliação do poder diagnostico dos sintomas e sinais otomicroscópicos na otite média aguda em crianças. Rev Bras Otorrinolaringol. 1994;60:246–50.
74. Saeed K, Coglianese CL, McCormick DP, Chonmaitree T. Otoscopic and tympanometric findings in acute otitis media yielding dry tap at tympanocentesis. Pediatr Infect Dis J. 2004;23:1030–4.
75. Garbutt J, Rosenbloom WJ, Storch GA. Empiric first-line antibiotic treatment of acute otitis in the era of the heptavalent pneumococcal conjugate vaccine. Pediatrics. 2006;117:1087–94.
76. Piltcher OB, Lubianca Neto JF. Bacterial upper respiratory tract infections in Brazil: bacterial resistance, human resistance, scientific darkness. Braz J Otorhinolaryngol. 2021;87:123–4.
77. Rosenfeld RM, Sury K, Mascarinas C. Office insertion of tympanostomy tubes without anesthesia in young children. Otolaryngol Head Neck Surg. 2015;153:1067–70.
78. Schild SD, Rosenfeld RM. Otolaryngologist's attitudes toward in-office pediatric tympanostomy tube placement without general anesthesia. Ann Otol Rhinol Laryngol. 2022;131:101–7.
79. Bluestone CD, Stephenson JS, Martin LM. Ten-year review of otitis media pathogens. Pediatr Infect Dis J. 1992;11:S7–S11.
80. Kaur R, Morris M, Pichichero ME. Epidemiology of acute otitis media in the postpneuococcal conjungate vaccine era. Pediatrics. 2017;140:e20170181.
81. Ngo CC, Massa HM, Thornton RB, Cripps AW. Predominant bacteria detected from the middle ear fluid of children experiencing otitis media: a systematic review. PLoS One. 2016;11:e0150949.
82. Kordeluk S, Orgad R, Kraus M, Puterman M, Kaplan DM, Novak L, Dagan R, Leibovitz E. Acute mastoiditis in children under 15 years of age in southern Israel following the introduction of pneumococcal conjugate vaccines: a 4-year retrospective study (2009-2012). Int J Pediatr Otorhinolaryngol. 2014;78:1599–604.
83. Mansour T, Yehudai N, Tobia A, Shihada R, Brodsky A, Khnifies R, et al. Acute mastoiditis: 20 years of experience with a uniform management protocol. Int J Pediatr Otorhinolaryngol. 2019;125:187–91.
84. Karma PH, Pukander JS, Sipilä MM, Vesikari TH, Grönroos PW. Middle ear fluid bacteriology of acute otitis media in neonates and very young infants. Int J Pediatr Otorhinolaryngol. 1987;14(2–3):141–50.
85. Kaur R, Casey JR, Pichichero ME. Relationship with original pathogen in recurrence of acute otitis media after completion of amoxicillin/clavulanate: bacterial relapse or new pathogen. Pediatr Infect Dis J. 2013;32:1159–62.
86. McCullough AR, Pollack AJ, Plejdrup Hansen M, Glasziou PP, Looke DF, Britt HC, et al. Antibiotics for acute respiratory infections in general practice: comparison of prescribing rates with guideline recommendations. Med J Aust. 2017;207:65–9.
87. Fleming-Dutra KE, Hersh AL, Shapiro DJ, Bartoces M, Enns EA, File TM Jr, et al. Prevalence of inappropriate antibiotic prescriptions among US ambulatory care visits, 2010-2011. JAMA. 2016;315:1864–73.
88. Bjornsdottir I, Kristinsson KG, Hansen EH. Diagnosing infections: a qualitative view on prescription decisions in general practice over time. Pharm World Sci. 2010;32:805–14.
89. van de Sande-Bruinsma N, Grundmann H, Verloo D, Tiemersma E, Monen J, Goossens H, Ferech M, European Antimicrobial Resistance Surveillance System Group; European Surveillance of Antimicrobial Consumption Project Group. Antimicrobial drug use and resistance in Europe. Emerg Infect Dis. 2008;14:1722–30.
90. Ovnat Tamir S, Shemesh S, Oron Y, Marom T. Acute otitis media guidelines in selected developed and developing countries: uniformity and diversity. Arch Dis Child. 2017;102:450–7.
91. Kitamura K, Iino Y, Kamide Y, Kudo F, Nakayama T, Suzuki K, et al. Clinical practice guidelines for the diagnosis and management of acute otitis media (AOM) in children in Japan—2013 update. Auris Nasus Larynx. 2015;42:99–106.
92. Rosenfeld RM, Vertrees JE, Carr J, Cipolle RJ, Uden DL, Giebink GS, et al. Clinical efficacy of antimicrobial drugs for acute otitis media: metaanalysis of 5400 children from thirty-three randomized trials. J Pediatr. 1994;124:355–67.
93. Venekamp RP, Sanders SL, Glasziou PP, Del Mar CB, Rovers MM. Antibiotics for acute otitis media in children. Cochrane Database Syst Rev. 2015;2015:CD000219.
94. Carlin SA, Marchant CD, Shurin PA, Johnson CE, Super DM, Rehmus JM. Host factors and early therapeutic response in acute otitis media. J Pediatr. 1991;118:178–83.
95. Dagan R, Leibovitz E, Greenberg D, Yagupsky P, Fliss DM, Leiberman A. Early eradication of pathogens from middle ear fluid during antibiotic treatment of acute otitis media is associated with improved clinical outcome. Pediatr Infect Dis J. 1998;17:776–82.
96. Hoberman A, Paradise JL, Rockette HE, Shaikh N, Wald ER, Kearney DH, Colborn DK, Kurs-Lasky M, Bhatnagar S, Haralam MA, Zoffel LM, Jenkins C, Pope MA, Balentine TL, Barbadora KA. Treatment of acute otitis media in children under 2 years of age. N Engl J Med. 2011;364(2):105–15.

97. Tähtinen PA, Laine MK, Huovinen P, Jalava J, Ruuskanen O, Ruohola A. A placebo-controlled trial of antimicrobial treatment for acute otitis media. N Engl J Med. 2011;364(2):116–26.
98. Rovers MM, Glasziou P, Appelman CL, Burke P, McCormick DP, Damoiseaux RA, Little P, Le Saux N, Hoes AW. Predictors of pain and/or fever at 3 to 7 days for children with acute otitis media not treated initially with antibiotics: a meta-analysis of individual patient data. Pediatrics. 2007;119:579–85.
99. Little P, Gould C, Williamson I, Moore M, Warner G, Dunleavey J. Pragmatic randomized controlled trial of two prescribing strategies for childhood acute otitis media. BMJ. 2001;322(3):36–42.
100. Spiro DM, Tay KY, Arnold DH, Dziura JD, Baker MD, Shapiro ED. Wait-and-see prescription for the treatment of acute otitis media: a randomized controlled trial. JAMA. 2006;296:1235–41.
101. Smolinski NE, Antonelli PJ, Winterstein AG. Watchful waiting for acute otitis media. Pediatrics. 2022;150:e2021055613.
102. Casselbrant ML, Kaleida PH, Rockette HE, Paradise JL, Bluestone CD, Kurs-Lasky M, et al. Efficacy of antimicrobial prophylaxis and of tympanostomy tube insertion for prevention of recurrent acute otitis media: results of a randomized clinical trial. Pediatr Infect Dis J. 1992;11:278–86.
103. Sih T, Moura R, Caldas S, Schwartz B. Prophylaxis for recurrent acute otitis media: a Brazilian study. Int J Pediatr Otorhinolaryngol. 1993;25:19–24.
104. Koivunen P, Uhari M, Luotonen J, Kristo A, Raski R, Pokka T, Alho OP. Adenoidectomy versus chemoprophylaxis and placebo for recurrent acute otitis media in children aged under 2 years: randomised controlled trial. BMJ. 2004;328:487–92.
105. Williams RL, Chalmers TC, Stange KC, Chalmers FT, Bowlin SJ. Use of antibiotics in preventing recurrent acute otitis and in treating otitis media with effusion: a meta-analytic attempt to resolve the brouhaha. JAMA. 1993;270:1344–51.
106. Rosenfeld RM, Kay DJ. Natural history of untreated otitis media. Laryngoscope. 2003;113:1654–7.
107. Block SL, Hedrick J, Harrison CJ, Tyler R, Smith A, Findlay R, et al. Community-wide vaccination with the heptavalent pneumococcal conjugate significantly alters the microbiology of acute otitis media. Pediatr Infect Dis J. 2004;23(9):829–33. PMID: 15361721.
108. Eskola J, Kilpi T, Palmu A, Jokinen J, Haapakoski J, Herva E, et al. Efficacy of a pneumococcal conjugate vaccine against acute otitis media. N Engl J Med. 2001;344(6):403–9. PMID: 11172176.
109. Kilpi T, Ahman H, Jokinen J, Lankinen KS, Palmu A, Savolainen H, et al. Protective efficacy of a second pneumococcal conjugate vaccine against pneumococcal acute otitis media in infants and children: randomized, controlled trial of a 7-valent pneumococcal polysaccharide-meningococcal outer membrane protein complex conjugate vaccine in 1666 children. Clin Infect Dis. 2003;37(9):1155–64. PMID: 14557958.
110. Poehling KA, Szilagyi PG, Grijalva CG, Martin SW, LaFleur B, Mitchel E, et al. Reduction of frequent otitis media and pressure-equalizing tube insertions in children after introduction of pneumococcal conjugate vaccine. Pediatrics. 2007;119(4):707–15. PMID: 17403841.
111. Fletcher MA, Fritzell B. Brief review of the clinical effectiveness of PREVENAR against otitis media. Vaccine. 2007;25(13):2507–12. PMID: 17011085.
112. Grijalva CG, Poehling KA, Nuorti JP, et al. National impact of universal childhood immunization with pneumococcal conjugate vaccine on outpatient medical care visits in the United States. Pediatrics. 2006;118:865–73.
113. Zhou F, Shefer A, Kong Y, Nuorti JP. Trends in acute otitis media-related health care utilization by privately insured young children in the United States, 1997–2004. Pediatrics. 2008;121:253–60.
114. Jardine A, Menzies RI, Deeks SL, Patel MS, McIntyre PB. The impact of pneumococcal conjugate vaccine on rates of myringotomy with ventilation tube insertion in Australia. Pediatr Infect Dis J. 2009;28:761–5.
115. Lau WC, Murray M, El-Turki A, et al. Impact of pneumococcal conjugate vaccines on childhood otitis media in the United Kingdom. Vaccine. 2015;33:5072–9.
116. Sartori AL, Minamisava R, Bierrenbach AL, Toscano CM, Afonso ET, Morais-Neto OL, Antunes JLF, Cristo EB, Andrade AL. Reduction in all-cause otitis media-related outpatient visits in children after PCV10 introduction in Brazil. PLoS One. 2017;12(6):e0179222.
117. de Sévaux JL, Venekamp RP, Lutje V, Hak E, Schilder AG, Sanders EA, Damoiseaux RA. Pneumococcal conjugate vaccines for preventing acute otitis media in children. Cochrane Database Syst Rev. 2020;11:CD001480.
118. Heikkinen T, Ruuskanen O, Waris M, Zieger T, Arola M, Halonen P. Influenza vaccination in the prevention of acute otitis media in children. Am J Dis Child. 1991;145:445–8.
119. Clements DA, Langdon L, Bland C, Emmanuel W. Influenza A vaccine decreases incidence of otitis media in 6- to 30 month-old-children in day care. Arch Pediatr Adolesc Med. 1995;149:1113–7.
120. Norhayati MN, Ho JJ, Azman MY. Influenza vaccines for preventing acute otitis media in infants and children. Cochrane Database Syst Rev. 2017;10(10):CD010089.
121. Marchisio P, Cavagna R, Maspes B, et al. Efficacy of intranasal virosomal influenza vaccine in the prevention of recurrent acute otitis media in children. A randomized single-blind clinical trial. Clin Infect Dis. 2002;35:168–74.
122. Kontiokari T, Uhari M, Koskela M. Effect of xylitol on growth of nasopharyngeal bacteria in vitro. Antimicrob Agents Chemother. 1995;39:1820–3.
123. Kontiokari T, Uhari M, Koskela M. Antiadhesive effects of xylitol on otopathogenic bacteria. Antimicrob Agents Chemother. 1998;41:563–5.
124. Uhari M, Kontiokari T, Koskela M, et al. Xylitol chewing gum in prevention of acute otitis media: double blind randomized trial. BMJ. 1996;313:1180–4.
125. Vernacchio L, Corwin MJ, Vezina R, et al. Xylitol syrup for the prevention of acute otitis media. Pediatrics. 2013;133:289–95.
126. Azarpazhooh A, Limeback H, Lawrence HP, Shah PS. Xylitol for preventing acute otitis media in children up to 12 years of age. Cochrane Database Syst Rev. 2011;11:CD007095.
127. Marchisio P, Bortone B, Ciarcià M, Motisi MA, Torretta S, Castelli Gattinara G, et al. Updated guidelines for the management of acute otitis media in children by the Italian Society of Pediatrics: prevention. Pediatr Infect Dis J. 2019;38:S22–36.
128. Niittynen L, Pitkäranta A, Korpela R. Probiotics and otitis media in children. Int J Pediatr Otorhinolaryngol. 2012;76:465–7052.
129. Cohen R, Martin E, de La Rocque F, et al. Probiotics and prebiotics in preventing episodes of acute otitis media in high-risk children: a randomized, double-blind, placebo-controlled study. Pediatr Infect Dis J. 2013;32:810–4.
130. Principi N, Tagliabue C, Tenconi R, Esposito S. Probiotics and prevention of pediatric upper respiratory tract infections. Eur J Inflamm. 2013;11:581–9.
131. Santagati M, Scillato M, Patanè F, et al. Bacteriocin-producing oral streptococci and inhibition of respiratory pathogens. FEMS Immunol Med Microbiol. 2012;65:23–31.
132. Roos K, Hakansson EG, Holm S. Effect of recolonization with "interfering" alpha streptococci on recurrences of acute and secretory otitis media in children: randomized placebo-controlled trial. BMJ. 2001;322:210–1259.
133. Scott AM, Clark J, Julien B, Islam F, Roos K, Grimwood K, Little P, Del Mar CB. Probiotics for preventing acute otitis media in children. Cochrane Database Syst Rev. 2019;6:CD01294.

134. Shaw NJ, Mughal Z. Vitamin D and child health (skeletal aspects). Arch Dis Child. 2013;98:363–7.
135. Shaw NJ, Mughal Z. Vitamin D and child health (extra skeletal aspects). Arch Dis Child. 2013;98(3):68–7270.
136. Marchisio P, Consonni D, Zampiero A, et al. Vitamin D supplementation reduces the risk of acute otitis media in otitis-prone children. Pediatr Infect Dis J. 2013;32:1055–60.
137. Cullen KA, Hall MJ, Golosinskiy A. Ambulatory surgery in the United States, 2006. Natl Health Stat Rep. 2009;11:1–25.
138. Venekamp RP, Mick P, Schilder AG, Nunez DA. Grommets (ventilation tubes) for recurrent acute otitis media in children. Cochrane Database Syst Rev. 2018;5(5):CD012017.
139. Kujala T, Alho OP, Luotonen J, Kristo A, Uhari M, Renko M, et al. Tympanostomy with and without adenoidectomy for the prevention of recurrences of acute otitis media: a randomized controlled trial. Pediatr Infect Dis J. 2012;31:565–9.
140. Hoberman A, Preciado D, Paradise JL, Chi DH, Haralam M, Block SL, et al. Tympanostomy tubes or medical management for recurrent acute otitis media. N Engl J Med. 2021;384(1):789–99.
141. Rosenfeld RM, Schwartz SR, Pynnonen MA, et al. Clinical practice guideline: tympanostomy tubes in children. Otolaryngol Head Neck Surg. 2013;149(Suppl 1):S1–S35.
142. Lavere PF, Ohlstein JF, Smith SP, Szeremeta W, Pine HS. Preventing unnecessary tympanostomy tube placement in children. Int J Pediatr Otorhinolaryngol. 2019;122:40–3.
143. Rosenfeld RM, Tunkel DE, Schwartz SR, Anne S, Bishop CE, Chelius DC, Hackell J, Hunter LL, Keppel KL, Kim AH, Kim TW, Levine JM, Maksimoski MT, Moore DJ, Preciado DA, Raol NP, Vaughan WK, Walker EA, Monjur TM. Clinical practice guideline: tympanostomy tubes in children (update). Otolaryngol Head Neck Surg. 2022;166(1 suppl):S1–S55.
144. Rosenfeld RM. Shared decision making and office insertion of tympanostomy tubes. Otolaryngol Head Neck Surg. 2016;154:807–9.
145. Hammarén-Malmi S, Saxen H, Tarkkanen J, Mattila PS. Adenoidectomy does not significantly reduce the incidence of otitis media in conjunction with the insertion of tympanostomy tubes in children who are younger than 4 years: a randomized trial. Pediatrics. 2005;116:185–9.
146. Mattila PS, Joki-Erkkilä VP, Kilpi T, Jokinen J, Herva E, Puhakka H. Prevention of otitis media by adenoidectomy in children younger than 2 years. Arch Otolaryngol Head Neck Surg. 2003;129:163–8.
147. Mikals SJ, Brigger MT. Adenoidectomy as an adjuvant to primary tympanostomy tube placement: a systematic review and meta-analysis. JAMA Otolaryngol Head Neck Surg. 2014;140(2):95–101.
148. Boonacker CW, Rovers MM, Browning GG, Hoes AW, Schilder AG, Burton MJ. Adenoidectomy with or without grommets for children with otitis media: an individual patient data meta-analysis. Health Technol Assess. 2014;18(5):1–118.

The Microbiology of Otitis Media, Biofilms and Its Implication in the Clinical Treatment

20

Maria Beatriz Rotta Pereira, Manuel Ruttkay Pereira, Denise Rotta Ruttkay Pereira, and Vlademir Cantarelli

Acute otitis media (AOM) is one of the most prevalent childhood diseases, with a peak incidence between 6 and 24 months of age. Viral infections of the upper respiratory tract almost always precede and predispose to an episode of AOM [1, 2]. The etiology of infectious diseases is constantly changing due to a series of factors, including the identification of previously unknown, potentially pathogenic microorganisms; increased virulence of long-known pathogens; changing incidence patterns; the introduction of vaccines; and changes in susceptibility to antimicrobial agents [2, 3]. Knowledge regarding the etiology of otitis media has evolved in recent years, mainly with the introduction of molecular diagnostic methods such as polymerase chain reaction (PCR) and next-generation sequencing (NGS), which have allowed the detection and identification of microorganisms previously unrecognized, either because of difficulty in their isolation or due to low representativeness in relation to other pathogens classically implicated in these infections [4]. Nevertheless, the bacteria most commonly involved in the etiology of otitis media (OM)—*Streptococcus pneumoniae, Haemophilus influenzae*, and *Moraxella catarrhalis*, also known as otopathogens—have remained the same in recent decades, in children and adults alike [3, 5, 6].

The microbiology of otitis media has been recorded both by bacterial cultures and molecular techniques, usually on middle ear effusion collected by needle aspiration [7, 8]. The application of molecular amplification techniques for the detection of otopathogens has contributed to a better understanding of the etiology of OM, especially in cases in which culture fails to reveal the presence of bacteria in a sample obtained from the middle ear. The use of PCR panels targeting key otopathogens has revealed an average threefold to fourfold increase in the detection of these pathogens when compared to traditional culture methods [9, 10]. Since the 2000s, the introduction of the quantitative real-time PCR (qPCR) technique, in which all reaction cycles can be monitored as they occur, has made this method even more sensitive and specific for the detection of otopathogens, and it is now often used in parallel with culture methods for the microbiological analysis of middle ear effusions. In addition to enhanced sensitivity, continuous improvement of primers and probes allows more accurate detection of pathogens, especially *S. pneumoniae*, avoiding cross-reactivity with similar species present in the upper respiratory tract. The development of qPCR techniques for serotyping *S. pneumoniae* directly from clinical specimens without previous isolation in culture has been particularly useful. This method even allows the study of the evolution of pneumococcal serotypes in response to the introduction of new pneumococcal vaccines [11].

When molecular methods were employed, bacteria were identified in up to 92%, viruses in 70%, and bacteria and viruses simultaneously in up to 66% of middle ear effusion specimens [12]. The most common otopathogens are isolated in more than two-thirds of effusions aspirated from the ears of children with AOM and, with the advent of the aforementioned molecular techniques, in an equally high proportion of specimens from ears with recurrent acute otitis media (rAOM) and chronic otitis media with effusion (COME) [10]. Thus, *Streptococcus pneumoniae* and *Haemophilus*

M. B. R. Pereira
Department of Otolaryngology and Head and Neck Surgery, Hospital Sao Lucas, Pontificia Universidade Católica do Rio Grande do Sul (PUCRS), Porto Alegre, RS, Brazil

M. R. Pereira
Department of Pediatrics, School of Medicine, Pontificia Universidade Católica do Rio Grande do Sul (PUCRS), Porto Alegre, RS, Brazil

Department of Pediatrics, School of Medicine, Universidade Federal do Rio Grande do Sul (UFRGS), Porto Alegre, RS, Brazil

D. R. R. Pereira (✉)
Department of Otolaryngology and Head and Neck Surgery, Hospital de Clinicas de Porto Alegre, Universidade Federal do Rio Grande do Sul (UFRGS), Porto Alegre, RS, Brazil

V. Cantarelli
Department of Basic Health Sciences, Universidade Federal de Ciencias da Saude de Porto Alegre (UFCSPA), Porto Alegre, RS, Brazil

M. V. Goycoolea et al. (eds.), *Textbook of Otitis Media*, https://doi.org/10.1007/978-3-031-40949-3_20

influenzae predominate in the various presentations of otitis media, alternating as the most prevalent species across different countries and geographic regions. Other bacterial pathogens, including anaerobic species, may, to a lesser extent, be found in middle ear effusions from ears with otitis media [9, 13].

The Role of Viruses in the Etiopathogenesis of AOM

Several animal experiments and clinical studies in humans have shown that respiratory viruses play an important role in the etiopathogenesis of otitis media. Viruses are detected in the nasopharyngeal aspirate of up to 45% of children with AOM [12].

Provided that viral replication takes place, along with associated symptoms, several viruses can cause AOM or facilitate bacterial infection of the middle ear. Viral infections of the upper respiratory tract trigger a cascade of events that precede bacterial otitis media. Respiratory viruses induce the release of inflammatory mediators in the nasopharynx, increase bacterial colonization and adhesion, and exert a suppressive effect on host defense mechanisms. Bacteria that colonize the nasopharynx and exhibit middle ear tropism apparently do not become pathogenic before a virus initiates an inflammatory process in the ear [14]. Rhinoviruses were detected in nearly half of the 800 nasopharyngeal specimens from a sample of children with AOM, and, using PCR techniques, respiratory syncytial virus (RSV) was identified in more than half of the ears of children with AOM during an outbreak of RSV infection [15, 16]. Studies have shown a higher rate of treatment failure when bacteria and viruses coexist in the middle ear compared to ears in which only bacteria were detected, suggesting that the presence of a viral component in AOM may interfere with the clinical and bacteriological response to antimicrobial agents. In addition to RSV, rhinoviruses, adenoviruses, influenza and parainfluenza viruses, coronaviruses, and enteroviruses are often found in the nasopharynx of children with AOM [17–19].

Bacteria in AOM and rAOM

Analyses of AOM effusions carried out in the last four decades confirm the presence of *S. pneumoniae, H. influenzae,* and *M. catarrhalis* as the most prevalent pathogens. They are often found alone or in combination in specimens from the upper respiratory tract, where they colonize mucous membranes and from which they can travel upwards through the Eustachian tube to the middle ear. Group A streptococci, *Staphylococcus aureus, Pseudomonas aeruginosa, Staphylococcus epidermidis, Alloiococcus otitidis, Klebsiella pneumoniae*, and *Escherichia coli* are also found, albeit with a lower prevalence [20].

There is some age-related variation, with *S. pneumoniae* and *H. influenzae* being the most common pathogens found in neonates and infants, while other bacteria usually associated with systemic infections are identified in more than 20% of cases in this age group [21].

The isolated bacteria also change according to the techniques, objectives, methodologies, and geographic area of the study, but the three species mentioned above are still inarguably the most relevant otopathogens [9].

Importantly, several studies based on cultures of middle ear fluid identified other species whose pathogenic role in AOM is debatable. *Alloiococcus otitidis* and *Turicella otitidis* are two species of gram-positive microorganisms frequently isolated from the middle ear fluid of children in several parts of the world, and their role in AOM has been debated in recent decades without, however, any definitive conclusions being reached regarding their pathogenicity [22]. Despite their abundance in the middle ear fluid of children with OM, two main factors hinder their definitive acceptance as pathogens causing or associated with OM: both can be isolated from the external auditory meatus in patients with OM and likewise in individuals without this condition. Unlike other pathogens, *A. otitidis* and *T. otitidis* are rarely detected in nasopharyngeal samples; therefore, their presence in middle ear effusions is not easily explained by their ascent through the Eustachian tube. [22, 23] Conversely, evidence in favor of a pathogenic role of these organisms in OM includes the detection of a specific immune response with antibodies and proinflammatory cytokines in the middle ear fluid of children with OM, from which *A. otitidis* was isolated in the absence of other classic otopathogens. It is possible that the pathogenic role of *A. otitidis* in OM is more complex and involves its co-occurrence with other microorganisms. Consistent with this hypothesis, there is evidence that *A. otitidis* is not only capable of producing biofilms but also polymicrobial biofilms, particularly stimulating the growth of *H. influenzae* without the need for the presence of any specific growth factors [24]. Studies involving the pathogenic potential of *T. otitidis* are much scarcer, and the mechanism of its pathogenicity in OM, if any, remains unknown.

It bears stressing that colonization of the nasopharynx with bacteria potentially pathogenic to the middle ear is considered a condition that precedes an episode of AOM, which in turn is often preceded by or associated with a viral infection [18]. Research has already confirmed, through DNA sequencing, the striking similarity between otopathogenic strains isolated from the nasopharynx and middle ear of children with AOM [25].

Role of Pneumococcal Conjugate Vaccines

The prevalence and resistance profiles of microorganisms have changed in recent years due to the advent of pneumococcal conjugate vaccines and the frequent use of antibiotics. A relative increase in beta-lactamase-producing strains of *H. influenzae* and *M. catarrhalis* has been observed, as has variation in rates of penicillin resistance across different strains of *S. pneumoniae*. [26]

The introduction of universal pneumococcal vaccination through conjugate vaccines has changed the microbiology of OM, interfering with the proportions of the most commonly implicated bacteria and changing the profile of pneumococcal strains isolated from the middle ear. Before the advent of the first (7-valent) pneumococcal conjugate vaccine, serotypes covered by this vaccine were detected in approximately 65% of cases [27]. Prospective studies performed after its introduction have documented reductions of up to 45% in pneumococci identified in the middle ear and a concomitant increase in the isolation of non-typeable *H. influenzae*. The advent of vaccination with the 7-valent pneumococcal vaccine was also followed by a change in serotype profile; serotypes not present in the vaccine, mainly 19A, became predominant among pneumococci isolated from the middle ear and nasopharynx [28–30]. The prevalence of pneumococci has become even lower after the introduction of the 13-valent conjugate vaccine, while the detection of *H. influenzae* and *M. catarrhalis* continues to rise [3]. Some studies conducted after the introduction of the 13-valent vaccine documented a decrease both in the general incidence of AOM and in the incidence of episodes caused by the serotypes covered by the vaccine. Unfortunately, more recent studies have already identified a higher prevalence of pneumococcal serotypes not present in the 13-valent vaccine in the middle ear of children with AOM [31].

The Role of Bacteria in COME

For many years, the effusion present in the middle ear of patients with COME was presumed to be sterile. The relative failure to grow bacteria from these effusions, combined with the ineffectiveness of antibiotic therapy, appeared to corroborate the "sterile effusion" theory and suggest a minor or absent role of bacteria in the etiopathogenesis of this condition.

During the second half of the twentieth century, the first studies that confirmed the presence of bacteria in the middle ear of children with AOM and COME were published. These first authors found a 30% culture positivity rate as well as a significant number of white blood cells [32]. Subsequently, several authors documented culture positivity rates ranging from 18 to 45% in effusion specimens from patients with protracted courses of OM. The advent of PCR finally allowed significant advances and clearly demonstrated that the degree of bacterial and viral involvement in the various presentations of otitis media had been grossly underestimated, especially in COME. Early studies using the PCR technique detected bacteria in up to 80% of effusions from ears with COME [10, 33, 34].

The concept of a continuum of disease states linking the various forms of otitis media with increasingly competent detection of pathogenic microorganisms in the middle ear helps to understand the existence of a causative role for bacteria in AOM and COME. As noted above, the key otopathogens remain the same, but with a clear predominance of *H. influenzae*, followed by *S. pneumoniae* and *M. catarrhalis*. It is now known that most cases of AOM are self-limited and thus resolve spontaneously, but patients sometimes present with recurrent forms (rAOM) or progress to chronic conditions such as COME [35, 36]. Several studies carried out in the last 25 years have confirmed the presence of bacterial communities—in the form of biofilms—living in the nasopharynx, middle ear, and even in tympanostomy tubes. These findings are consistent with the low efficacy of systemic antibiotics, prescribed at conventional doses, in the management of rAOM and COME [37, 38].

The Role of Bacteria in Chronic Otitis Media

Significant microbiological differences can be observed in the chronic forms of OM, especially in chronic suppurative otitis media (CSOM) and when there is cholesteatoma. *P. aeruginosa* and *S. aureus* represent the two most commonly isolated aerobic species from samples of patients with CSOM and chronic otitis media with cholesteatoma, followed by Enterobacteriaceae such as *E. coli*, *K. pneumoniae*, and *Proteus* sp. Unlike the classic otopathogens that colonize the mucous membranes of the upper respiratory tract, *P. aeruginosa* and *S. aureus* are found mainly in the external auditory meatus, from where they can reach the middle ear. *P. aeruginosa* is intrinsically resistant to several antibiotics and can evade immune defenses by producing several virulence factors [39]. The role of other species, including fungi, is difficult to assess because they are also present in the external auditory meatus as part of its normal microbiota [40].

Several studies carried out from the 1970s through the 2000s assessed the presence of anaerobic microorganisms in middle ear fluids. In general, these studies reported more frequent isolation of anaerobic species in CSOM and chronic OM with cholesteatoma; however, in approximately half of the cases, the isolates were found in combination with other aerobic and anaerobic species. Several genera of gram-positive and gram-negative anaerobic bacteria have been isolated from middle ear effusions, especially *Peptostreptococcus* sp., *Prevotella, Porphyromonas, Bacteroides*, and *Fusobacterium*. Interestingly, many of these species are beta-lactamase producers, and their hydrolytic activity on penicillins and cephalosporins can be measured directly in the middle ear effusions of these patients. The use of antibiotics with adequate coverage against anaerobes and combinations of penicillins and beta-lactamase inhibitors may be useful for the treatment of these polymicrobial infections [41].

The Role and Relevance of Biofilms

The term "biofilm" was first used in 1975 in reference to mixed colonies of bacteria detected in an aquatic environment. Bacteria have the ability to avoid destruction and extinction by existing in two modes in nature: planktonic (free-living) and sessile (grouped into biofilms). Currently, both modes are believed to form part of the life cycle of a bacterium. When in planktonic form, bacteria are able to reproduce rapidly and are associated with acute infections. In the form of biofilms, they tend to be less aggressive but are able to survive in adverse conditions [42]. A biofilm represents a complex organization of bacteria that attach themselves to a surface (biological or nonbiological) in order to live in the form of organized structures in which they can share nutrients and communicate cooperatively. Biofilms are produced by the bacteria themselves as a means of protection, nutrition, and growth [43]. The bacteria are contained within a structure composed of polysaccharides, proteins, and nucleic acids called the *glycocalyx*, or, more appropriately, *exopolysaccharides* or *extracellular polymeric substances* (EPS). The vast majority of bacteria live in biofilms, and all otopathogens have this ability [44].

To form a biofilm, bacteria must first adhere firmly to a surface, and then enter a maturation stage in which they organize themselves into microcolonies within an EPS matrix. In this state, they are able to communicate with one another (via so-called *quorum sensing*), share nutrients and oxygen, and eliminate waste products of their metabolism through open channels that play the role of a primitive circulatory system. In addition, biofilms protect bacteria from changes in pH, temperature, humidity, and exposure to ultraviolet light. Biofilms found on mucosal surfaces are physiologically different from those formed on inert surfaces and are modulated by the host's immune responses. Host cells may even be incorporated into the composition of the polysaccharide matrix [45].

Specifically in the field of otolaryngology, several acute, recurrent, and chronic infections affect the pharyngeal and palatine tonsils, paranasal sinuses, and ears. Biofilms cause the majority of recurrent and chronic infections and their importance in rAOM and COME is well documented. Bacterial communities in biofilms have the ability to disperse bacteria in planktonic form into their surroundings (dispersion), which explains the pathogenesis of recurrent acute infections [42, 45].

The presence of otopathogens in biofilm form in the nasopharynx has been proven, and some authors suggest that episodes of AOM and rAOM occur when bacteria leave the biofilm in the region of the pharyngeal tonsils and, in the presence of Eustachian tube dysfunction, migrate to the middle ear [46]. In support of this theory is the fact that children with rAOM have more biofilms on their pharyngeal tonsils than those with AOM (97.6% versus 27.7%) [47].

The identification of bacteria in biofilms by conventional culture methods is difficult, but the evolution of PCR techniques, with an increase in both sensitivity and specificity, has allowed the detection of *S. pneumoniae*, *H. influenzae*, and *M. catarrhalis* in metabolically active forms in effusion specimens from patients with COME. Subsequently, biofilms were identified in the middle ear of children with COME, with effusions being 100% positive on PCR testing, even though only 22% of specimens were culture-positive [34, 48]. These findings confirmed the role of bacteria in biofilms in the development and maintenance of chronic infectious processes in the middle ear, contributing decisively to the near extinction of the early concern that molecular techniques were mostly detecting the genetic remains of nonviable bacteria ("fossilized remains").

Biofilms are also present in cholesteatomas, and recurrent episodes of otorrhea are probably attributable to their presence. Strains of *Pseudomonas aeruginosa* present in cholesteatomas have been demonstrated to form biofilms [49].

The emergence of new antibiotic-resistant strains of otopathogens, especially *S. pneumoniae,* can be explained at least in part by the existence of biofilms, insofar as they function as a "reservoir" of microorganisms capable of interrupting complete healing and causing reinfections. Although some antibiotics are able to penetrate biofilms, phenotypic changes in bacteria, which decrease their metabolic rates and their ability to divide, make these organisms particularly drug-resistant [45, 50]. On the other hand, resistance to host defense mechanisms occurs due to bacterial aggregation within polysaccharide structures that make them too large to undergo phagocytosis and reduce their accessibility to the humoral immune system. It is important to bear in mind that a strain of a bacterium can be very susceptible to a particular antibiotic when it is in its planktonic (free-living) form and highly resistant when within a biofilm [51]. In addition to these mechanisms, cooperation among the bacteria that constitute the biofilm can also interfere with the action of antibiotics. One example is the production of beta-lactamases by

M. catarrhalis, which protects pneumococci and *Haemophilus* from the action of amoxicillin by inactivating the drug [52].

Implications of Biofilms for the Treatment of Otitis

Current management strategies for rAOM and COME involve antibiotic therapy (with only relative success) and removal of the effusion through a tympanostomy, along with the placement of a tympanostomy tube. In addition to other benefits, evacuation of the effusion performs biofilm removal. Adenoidectomy is also effective in the treatment of rAOM and COME, as the pharyngeal tonsils are well known to be rich in biofilms containing one or more otopathogens [53]. In episodes of chronic otitis with cholesteatoma, topical antibiotics (when there is discharge) and surgical removal of the cholesteatoma are the cornerstones of treatment.

In some ear infections, flares occur due to the formation of granulation tissue, which, in turn, surrounds the tympanostomy tube and causes persistent discharge. In these cases, the scar tissue and the tube must both be removed and a new tube placed if necessary [54, 55]. Tympanostomy tubes coated with silver oxide or antibiotics decreased the incidence of otorrhea, possibly due to an anti-biofilm effect [56].

The Upper Respiratory Tract Microbiome and Its Relationship with Otitis Media

Microbiological and molecular techniques have always correlated otitis media with the presence of classic otopathogens, as well as with some other species associated with this condition, but without definitive proof of their pathogenic role. More recently, the possibility of detecting microorganisms has expanded considerably with the evolution of DNA sequencing techniques, especially the use of 16S rRNA gene sequencing for bacterial detection and identification, which can be applied directly to clinical specimens [57].

With about 1500 base pairs, the 16S rRNA gene is an integral part of the ribosome and is present in all bacteria, being composed of highly conserved regions (i.e., with the same nucleotide sequence present in all species) interspersed with variable regions, which, once characterized, allow identification of the species. The evolution of sequencing techniques, especially with the advent of NGS, now allows for the complete and simultaneous sequencing of all species present in a given clinical sample, thus providing crucial data on its constituent microbiome. The relative abundance of each species in the analyzed sample can also be assessed. Use of these methods has also made it possible to follow the evolution over time of one's normal and pathogenic microbiota since the initial colonization after birth, to compare their variations throughout the life course or even during the emergence of disease states, and, in the latter case, to assess whether the normal microbiota is being replaced by new, potentially pathogenic species [58].

Studies have tried to correlate the microbiota of the upper respiratory tract, especially the nasopharynx and pharyngeal tonsils, with that found in the middle ear. The results suggest the presence of certain bacterial genera, such as *Dolosigranulum, Corynebacterium, Lactococcus, Cutibacterium (Propionibacterium),* and *Staphylococcus*, in an amount inversely proportional to that of classic otopathogens, such as pneumococci, *Haemophilus*, and *Moraxella*. The inverse also seems to hold true; that is, the presence of increased colonization by classic otopathogens, especially in the pharyngeal tonsils, seems to be associated with a smaller number and reduced variety of the species mentioned above. Furthermore, in children with otitis media, there seems to be a significantly reduced diversity of other bacterial species in nasopharyngeal and pharyngeal tonsil samples when compared to healthy controls. Interestingly, molecular techniques point to the existence of a normal microbiota in the middle ear, which is no longer considered a sterile site [4, 59]. Unfortunately, studies based on traditional bacteriological techniques fail to disclose bacteria in middle ear samples from healthy individuals, casting doubt on the results of molecular methods, whose identified bacterial sequences could have been the result of inevitable contamination of the reagents used in the process rather than the actual presence of the detected organisms in the clinical sample [60, 61].

At any rate, it now seems undeniable that some bacterial species may play a protective role when present in the upper respiratory tract. Two of these genera, *Dolosigranulum* and *Corynebacterium*, are found in significantly increased proportions in the nasopharynx of children without OM, suggesting that they are part of a normal and protective microbiota [62].

In summary, new molecular methods have confirmed the importance of the so-called otopathogens as causative agents of OM. These same studies also provide evidence of the abundant presence of certain bacterial genera, such as *Alloiococcus* and *Turicella,* in middle ear fluid samples from children with AOM or rAOM; these are also present in significant amounts in the outer ear but are practically absent in the nasopharynx. These potential pathogens act as adjuvants within biofilms formed by classic otopathogens, facilitating the persistence of these species in the middle ear and hindering their elimination either by the immune system or by antimicrobial therapy, a hypothesis that warrants further investigation [22, 63].

Conclusions and Recommendations

Ongoing, global monitoring of the bacteria involved in the pathogenesis of OM is essential for the development of vaccines and the establishment of new therapeutic strategies. Improvement of vaccines against the organisms that cause middle ear infections is essential for the prevention of otitis media in its acute, recurrent, and chronic forms [10].

Finally, it is beyond question that greater knowledge regarding biofilm function is essential for the development of new therapeutic options [43, 64]. These options can target different stages of biofilm formation (adhesion, maturation, *quorum sensing*, and dispersion), bearing in mind that different bacterial species and strains can employ different methods in the development of their biofilms and that the genetic exchange that occurs between communities within biofilms can increase and modify existing resistance mechanisms [42].

References

1. Coker T, Chan L, Newberry S, et al. Diagnosis, microbial epidemiology, and antibiotic treatment of acute otitis media in children? A systematic review. JAMA. 2010;304:2161.
2. Marom T, Tan A, Wilkinson G, et al. Trends in otitis media-related health care use in the United States, 2001-2011. JAMA Pediatr. 2014;168:68.
3. Kaur R, Morris M, Pichichero M. Epidemiology of acute otitis media in the postpneumococcal conjugate vaccine era. Pediatrics. 2017;140:e20170181.
4. Folino F, Ruggiero L, Capaccio P, et al. Upper respiratory tract microbiome and otitis media intertalk: lessons from the literature. J Clin Med. 2020;9(9):2845.
5. Teele D, Klein J, Rosner B. Epidemiology of otitis media during the first seven years of life in children in greater Boston: a prospective cohort study. J Infect Dis. 1989;160:83.
6. Bluestone C, Stephenson J, Martin L. Ten-year review of otitis media pathogens. Pediatr Infect Dis J. 1992;11:7–11.
7. Bluestone C, Klein J. Epidemiology. In: Otitis media in infants and children. 4th ed. Hamilton: BC Decker; 2007. p. 73.
8. Van Dyke M, Pirçon J, Cohen R, et al. Etiology of acute otitis media in children less than 5 years of age: a pooled analysis of 10 similarly designed observational studies. Pediatr Infect Dis J. 2017;36:274.
9. Ngo C, Massa H, Thornton R, Cripps A. Predominant bacteria detected from the middle ear fluid of children experiencing otitis media: a systematic review. PLoS One. 2016;11(3):e0150949.
10. Rotta Pereira MB, Pereira MR, Cantarelli V, Costa SS. Prevalence of bacteria in children with otitis media with effusion. J Pediatr (Rio J). 2004;80(1):41–8.
11. Slinger R, Duval M, Langill J, et al. Direct molecular detection of a broad range of bacterial and viral organisms and Streptococcus pneumoniae vaccine serotypes in children with otitis media with effusion. BMC Res Notes. 2016;9:247.
12. Ruohola A, Meurman O, Nikkari S, Skottman T, Salmi A, Waris M, Osterback R, Eerola E, Allander T, Niesters H, Heikkinen T, Ruuskanen O. Microbiology of acute otitis media in children with tympanostomy tubes: prevalences of bacteria and viruses. Clin Infect Dis. 2006;43(11):1417.
13. Brook I. Anaerobic bacteria in upper respiratory tract and head and neck infections: microbiology and treatment. Anaerobe. 2012;18(2):214–20.
14. Schilder A, Chonmaitree T, Cripps A, Rosenfeld R, Casselbrandt M, Haggard M, Venekamp R. Otitis media. Nat Rev Dev Primers. 2016;2:16063.
15. Chonmaitree T, Alvarez-Fernandez P, Jennings K, et al. Symptomatic and asymptomatic respiratory viral infections in the first year of life: association with acute otitis media development. Clin Infect Dis. 2015;60:1–9.
16. Pitkaranta A, Virolainen A, Jero J, et al. Detection of rhinovirus, respiratory syncytial virus, and coronavirus infections in acute otitis media by reverse transcriptase polymerase chain reaction. Pediatrics. 1998;102:291.
17. Ruuskanen O, Arola M, Heikkinen T, Ziegler T. Viruses in acute otitis media: increasing evidence for clinical significance. Pediatr Infect Dis J. 1991;10:425.
18. Stockman C, Ampofo K, Hersh A, et al. Seasonality of acute otitis media and the role of respiratory viral activity in children. Pediatr Infect Dis J. 2013;32:314.
19. Chonmaitree T, Trujillo R, Jennings K, Alvarez-Fernandez P, Patel J, Loeffelholz M, et al. Acute otitis media and other complications of viral respiratory infection. Pediatrics. 2016;137(4):e20153555.
20. Revai K, Mamidi D, Chonmaitreee T. Association of nasopharyngeal bacterial colonization during upper respiratory tract infection and the development of acute otitis media. Clin Infect Dis. 2008;46(4):e34–7.
21. Ziv O, Kraus M, Holcberg R, et al. Acute otitis media in infants younger than two months of age: epidemiologic and microbiologic characteristics in the era of pneumococcal conjugate vaccines. Int J Pediatr Otorhinolaryngol. 2019;119:123.
22. Pereira MBR, Cantarelli V, Pereira DRR, Costa SS. High incidence of Alloiococcus otitidis in otitis media with effusion measured by multiplex PCR. Braz J Otorhinolaryngol. 2004;70(2):217–24.
23. Lappan R, Jamieson SE, Peacock CS. Reviewing the pathogenic potential of the otitis-associated bacteria *Alloiococcus otitidis* and *Turicella otitidis*. Front Cell Infect Microbiol. 2020;10:51.
24. Chan CL, Richter K, Wormald PJ, Psaltis AJ, Vreugde S. *Alloiococcus otitidis* forms multispecies biofilm with *Haemophilus influenzae*: effects on antibiotic susceptibility and growth in adverse conditions. Front Cell Infect Microbiol. 2017;7:344.
25. Kaur R, Chang A, Xu Q, et al. Phylogenetic relatedness and diversity of non-typable Haemophilus influenzae in the nasopharynx and middle ear fluid of children with acute otitis media. J Med Microbiol. 2011;60:1841–8.
26. Nagai K, Kimura O, Domon H, et al. Antimicrobial susceptibility of Streptococcus pneumoniae, Haemophilus influenzae, and Moraxella catarrhalis clinical isolates from children with acute otitis media in Japan from 2014 to 2017. J Infect Chemother. 2019;25(3):229–32.
27. Hausdorff WP, Yothers G, Dagan R, et al. Multinational study of pneumococcal serotypes causing acute otitis media in children. Pediatr Infect Dis J. 2002;21:1008.
28. Pichichero ME, Casey JR. Emergence of a multiresistant serotype 19A pneumococcal strain not included in the 7-valent conjugate vaccine as an otopathogen in children. JAMA. 2007;298:1772.
29. McEllistrem MC, Adams JM, Patel K, et al. Acute otitis media due to penicillin-nonsusceptible Streptococcus pneumoniae before and after the introduction of the pneumococcal conjugate vaccine. Clin Infect Dis. 2005;40:1738.
30. Couloigner V, Levy C, François M, et al. Pathogens implicated in acute otitis media failures after 7-valent pneumococcal conjugate vaccine implementation in France: distribution, serotypes, and resistance levels. Pediatr Infect Dis J. 2012;31:154.
31. Marchisio P, Esposito S, Picca M, et al. Serotypes not included in 13-valent pneumococcal vaccine as causes of acute otitis media

with spontaneous tympanic membrane perforation in a geographic area with high vaccination coverage. Pediatr Infect Dis. 2017;36:521.
32. Senturia BH, Gessert CF, Carr CD, et al. Studies concerned with tubotympanitis. Ann Otol Rhinol Laryngol. 1958;67:440–67.
33. Gok U, Bulut Y, Keles E, et al. Bacteriological and PCR analysis of clinical material aspirated from otitis media with effusions. Int J Pediatr Otorhinolaryngol. 2001;60:49.
34. Hall-Stoodley L, Hu FZ, Gieseke A, et al. Direct detection of bacterial biofilms on the middle-ear mucosa of children with chronic otitis media. JAMA. 2006;296:202.
35. Juhn S, Paparella M, Kim C, Goycoolea M, Giebink G. Pathogenesis of otitis media. Ann Otol Rhinol Laryngol. 1977;86:481–92.
36. Giebink GS. Progress in understanding the pathophysiology of otitis media. Pediatr Rev. 1989;11:133–8.
37. Habashi N, Marom T, Steinberg D, et al. Biofilm distribution on tympanostomy tubes: an ex vivo descriptive study. Int J Pediatr Otorhinolaryngol. 2020;138:110350.
38. Monroy GL, Hong W, Khampang P, et al. Direct analysis of pathogenic structures affixed to the tympanic membrane during chronic otitis media. Otolaryngol Head Neck Surg. 2018;159:117.
39. Mittal R, Lisi CV, Gerring R, et al. Current concepts in the pathogenesis and treatment of chronic suppurative otitis media. J Med Microbiol. 2015;64(10):1103–16.
40. Singh G, Solo M, Kaur R, et al. Mycology of chronic suppurative otitis media-cholesteatoma disease: an evaluative study. Am J Otolaryngol. 2018;39(2):157–61.
41. Brook I. The role of anaerobic bacteria in chronic suppurative otitis media in children: implications for medical therapy. Anaerobe. 2008;14(6):297–300.
42. Kao W, Chole R. Biofilms disease and otitis. In: Kania R, Ars B, editors. Biofilms and otitis. Amsterdam: Kugler; 2015. p. 21.
43. Urquiza R, Pérez-Lázaro J. The non-natural history of otitis media and biofilms. In: Kania R, Ars B, editors. Biofilms in otitis. Amsterdam: Kugler; 2015. p. 13.
44. Post C, Hiller N, Nistico L, et al. The role of biofilms in otolaryngologic infections: update 2007. Curr Opin Otolaryngol Head Neck Surg. 2007;15:347–51.
45. Post J, Stoodley P, Hall-Stoodley L, et al. The role of biofilms in otolaryngologic infections. Curr Opin Otolaryngol Head Neck Surg. 2004;12:185–90.
46. Vermee Q, Cohen R, Hays C, et al. Biofilm production by Haemophilus influenzae and Streptococcus pneumoniae isolated from the nasopharynx of children with acute otitis media. BMC Infect Dis. 2019;19:44.
47. Hoa M, Tomovic S, Nistico L, et al. Identification of adenoid biofilms with middle ear pathogens in otitis-prone children utilizing SEM and FISH. Int J Pediatr Otorhinolaryngol. 2009;73:1242–8.
48. Post J, Preston R, Aul J, et al. Molecular analysis of bacterial pathogens in otitis media with effusion. JAMA. 1995;273(20):1598–604.
49. Wang E, Jung J, Pashia M, et al. Otopathogenic Pseudomonas aeruginosa strains as competent biofilm formers. Arch Otolaryngol Head Neck Surg. 2005;131(11):983–9.
50. Stewart P, Costerton J. Antibiotic resistance of bacteria in biofilms. Lancet. 2001;358(9276):135–8.
51. Whiteley M, Bangera M, Bumgarner R, et al. Gene expression in Pseudomonas aeruginosa biofilms. Nature. 2001;413(6858):860–4.
52. Schaar V, Nordström T, Mörgelin M, et al. Moraxella catarrhalis outer membrane vesicles carry β-lactamase and promote survival of Streptococcus pneumoniae and Haemophilus influenzae by inactivating amoxicillin. Antimicrob Agents Chemother. 2011;55:3845.
53. Hoa M, Syamal M, Schaeffer M, et al. Biofilms and chronic otitis media: an initial exploration into the role of biofilms in the pathogenesis of chronic otitis media. Am J Otolaryngol. 2010;31(4):241–5.
54. Costerton W, Veeh R, Shirtliff M, et al. The application of biofilm science to the study and control of chronic bacterial infections. J Clin Invest. 2003;112:1466–77.
55. Pereira MBR, Pereira DRR, Costa SS. Tympanostomy tube sequelae in children with otitis media with effusion: a three-year follow-up study. Braz J Otorhinolaryngol. 2005;71(4):415–20.
56. Chole R, Hubbell R. Antimicrobial activity of silastic tympanostomy tubes impregnated with silver oxide. A double-blind randomized multicenter trial. Arch Otolaryngol Head Neck Surg. 1995;121(5):562–5.
57. Liu C, Cosetti M, Aziz M, et al. The otologic microbiome? A study of the bacterial microbiota in a pediatric patient with chronic serous otitis media using 16SrRNA gene-based pyrosequencing. Arch Otolaryngol Head Neck Surg. 2011;137(7):664–8.
58. Xu Q, Gill S, Xu L, et al. Comparative analysis of microbiome in nasopharynx and middle ear in young children with acute otitis media. Front Genet. 2019;10:1176.
59. Minami SB, Mutai H, Suzuki T, et al. Microbiomes of the normal middle ear and ears with chronic otitis media. Laryngoscope. 2017;127(10):e371–7.
60. Laufer A, Metlay J, Gent J, et al. Microbial communities of the upper respiratory tract and otitis media in children. mBio. 2011;2(1):e00245–10.
61. Jervis-Bardy J, Leong LE, Papanicolas LE, et al. Examining the evidence for an adult healthy middle ear microbiome. mSphere. 2019;4(5):e00456–19.
62. Lappan R, Imbrogno K, Sikazwe C, et al. A microbiome case-control study of recurrent acute otitis media identified potentially protective bacterial genera. BMC Microbiol. 2018;18(1):13.
63. Chan C, Richter K, Wormald P, et al. Alloiococcus otitidis forms multispecies biofilm with Haemophilus influenzae: effects on antibiotic susceptibility and growth in adverse conditions. Front Cell Infect Microbiol. 2017;7:344.
64. Thornton R, Wiertsema S, Kirkham L, et al. Neutrophil extracellular traps and bacterial biofilms in middle ear effusion of children with recurrent otitis media—a potential treatment target. PLoS One. 2013;8(2):e53837.

21 Otitis Media with Effusion: Pathophysiology, Clinical Picture and Management

María José Herrera J and José Alzerreca

Overview

One of the most frequently diagnosed middle ear diseases is otitis media with effusion (OME), which is defined as the presence of fluid behind an intact tympanic membrane, without any acute signs or symptoms [1].

First described by Mawson in 1976, it was originally referred as seromucous otitis media, a condition that have received multiples synonyms over the past such as nonsuppurative otitis media or ear fluid [1].

It occurs mostly in children and about 90% of them have had at least one episode of OME before school age, being the most frequent cause of acquired hearing loss in preschool children [2].

The vast majority of OME cases resolve spontaneously in less than 3 months from its onset without producing any hearing impairment. However, at least 25% of OME episodes can last longer and may be associated with hearing loss, balance difficulties, ear discomfort, and behavioral and sometimes social concerns [1, 2].

Incidence and Prevalence

OME is a disease predominantly seen in children, with an incidence of 0.6% between the adult population. Almost 50–90% of children will have at least one episode of OME by the age of 5 years, with a peak in the first year of life and a per year prevalence of 15–30% [1, 2].

Having an early age first OME episode may be the primary event that predisposes a child to recurrent and chronic otitis media by setting up an inflammatory process in the middle ear and eustachian tube.

There is no difference in prevalence between gender, but there are studies that determine a higher prevalence in Native American and Inuit population. Also, some American Indian and Eskimo communities have reported a low prevalence of OME [1].

About 4 episodes of new onset OME occur annually in young children with a mean duration of 17–20 days per episode, with 13–21% having bilateral involvement. Recurrence in OME is also common, with an estimated rate of 50% within 24 months [1, 2].

At least 40% of ear fluid episodes can last longer than 30 days, and sometimes becoming a reason for outpatient visits to pediatricians, accounting for almost 11% of office consultations in primary care practices [2].

Etiology

It has been suggested that the etiology of OME is multifactorial and that different conditions can contribute to the appearance and persistence of OME.

There are several theories and determined risk factors for the development of OME. These conditions can be categorized as:

Eustachian Tube Dysfunction

The eustachian tube connects the middle ear to the nasopharynx via a 24-mm length bony cartilaginous tube which main function is to allow adequate ventilation of the middle ear. In children, the eustachian tube is wider and more horizontal-oriented. This difference with the eustachian tube of and adult increases the possibility of an upper respiratory tract infection to rise to the middle ear [1, 3].

Apart from the anatomical differences of the eustachian tube in children, there are other causes of dysfunction such as obstruction for hypertrophied adenoids or inflammation secondary to upper respiratory infections [1, 2].

M. J. Herrera J (✉) · J. Alzerreca
Department of Otolaryngology, Clínica Universidad de Los Andes, Santiago, Chile

M. V. Goycoolea et al. (eds.), *Textbook of Otitis Media*, https://doi.org/10.1007/978-3-031-40949-3_21

Craniofacial Abnormalities

Any condition or syndrome that affects the anatomy of the middle third of the face or the skull base can be a risk factor for OME. Most common examples of this condition are Down's syndrome and cleft palate abnormalities, since this kind of syndromes can present with abnormal muscle insertion of the soft palate leading to an inadequate opening of the eustachian tube during swallowing [2].

Acute Otitis Media Sequelae

Up to 45% of children diagnosed with acute otitis media were found to have a middle ear effusion at 1 month and 10% at 3 months after the initial diagnosis [3, 4].

Gastroesophageal Reflux Disease (GERD)

Pepsin-related association with middle ear effusion is well studied. Pepsin found in middle ear effusion is thought to arise as a result of reflux; however since not all effusion have pepsin, it is unlikely a factor for all cases of OME [5, 6].

Allergies

Allergies may predispose to OME by generating edema around the eustachian tube or as a primary mucosal disease of the middle ear. Some studies have found up to 63% of positive skin test on children with OME [7].

Pathogenesis

The pathogenesis of OME is mainly considered to be initiated by an inflammatory reaction against a rhinopharyngeal infection. This inflammatory process leads the production of cytokines and the secretion of a protein and inflammatory mediators' rich exudate. Also, there is a vasodilatation process that is responsible for an increased gaseous exchange with an endotympanic pressure drop consequently. This pressure changes in the middle ear affects the tympanic membrane mostly in its pars flaccida which is the most fragile area, sometime developing a retraction at this site [1, 8].

If the middle ear pressure drops continues without correction, tympanic atelectasis progresses to the pars tensa and may lead to a complete atelectasis of the tympanic membrane.

Also, when a prolonged inflammation of the middle ear mucosa is present, it is common to observe cell differentiation with an increased number of mucus cells. This factor contributes to a higher exudate production that fills the middle ear space.

Some researchers have studied the presence of biofilms in the middle ear cavity estimating that almost 65% of chronic infections involve biofilms. This structure of bacterial and fungal origin is formed from polysaccharides, proteins, and nucleic acids, that give protection against antibodies, phagocytosis, and antibiotics, perpetuating the presence of effusion or infection in time [9].

Many other factors are considered to play a role in the pathogenesis of OME, and they include GERD, pollution, allergies, which in theory alter the middle ear mucosa in the same way as previously exposed.

Clinical Presentation

Children with OME may present as an asymptomatic patient and be detected on routine screening, since children rarely complain about hearing loss, making diagnosis of OME more difficult.

OME can produce a variety of clinical scenarios, but physicians should always be aware of a hearing disorder, a delayed language acquisition, difficulties at school, and behavioral and/or sleep disorders [1].

Other symptoms that may indicate the presence of OME include clumsiness, bumping into things, or balance issues, and it is very common that these patients are assessed for a neurological disorder initially [2].

Also, any children with nasal obstruction, snoring, or mouth breathing should be assessed for OME, since adenoid hypertrophy is related with middle ear effusion.

Diagnosis

The diagnosis is essentially clinical. The probability of OME is defined by the balance between symptoms and signs and the review of the medical history and possible risk factors. Due to the multiple factors that must be considered in the diagnosis, there is considerable interobserver variation. Another consideration is the significant difference in diagnosis between pediatricians and otolaryngologists [1, 2, 8].

Otoscopy is diagnostic in around 78% of cases, with 95% specificity, when performed by an otolaryngologist [1, 2, 8].

The medical history should consider epidemiological factors such as age, gender, race, and seasonality. Risk factors considered are the age of the first AOM, bilaterality, history of allergic rhinitis and family history of OME, childcare assistance, and parental smoking. In adults, the risk factors are the history of allergy and radiation therapy of the head and neck [1, 8].

Most cases are asymptomatic, with hearing loss being the most frequent symptom. Because children do not usually report hearing loss, the diagnosis is usually late, resulting in language delay or deterioration of school performance. Screening at school entrance can trigger a referral to the otolaryngologist who ends up diagnosing an OME [2].

The head and neck examination should be complete because it may reveal predisposing anatomical factors or airway inflammation. The examiner should determine the presence of craniofacial dysmorphias, upper respiratory infections, complications, or other ear pathologies [1, 8]. In the examination of the tympanic membrane in recent OME, a translucent membrane and middle ear with aqueous liquid, sometimes with air bubbles or an airfluid level, are usually observed. In chronic OME mucosal effusion is observed, the membrane is thickened, opaque, and without inflammation [1]. Microscopic examination helps to increase accuracy and should be used when the diagnosis is unclear. The use of the fingerboard can also contribute to the diagnosis of driving hearing loss [1].

The accuracy of diagnosed OME by otoscopy is difficult to measure because the gold standard—the true condition of the middle ear—can only be documented by myringotomy or tympanocentesis. There is consensus that the diagnosis can be challenging, and even experienced otolaryngologists require the use of adjuvant diagnostic methods such as the microscope or tympanometry to better discern the presence of middle ear fluid in difficult cases [10, 11].

Determining membrane mobility is important, and pneumatic otoscopy is recommended but there is great interobserver variability. Actually, visible light pneumatic otoscopy is considered as the best currently available diagnostic tool for otitis media. A systematic review for diagnosing OME showed a sensitivity of 94% and specificity of 80% [12]. The Clinical Practice Guideline of the American Academy of Otolaryngology 2016 strongly recommends the use of pneumatic otoscope to document the presence of middle ear effusion to diagnose otitis media with effusion in a child and to assess for OME in a child with otalgia, hearing loss, or both with the pneumatic otoscope [2].

However, pneumatic otoscopy has various limitations. The speculum must create an adequate seal against the external auditory canal to obtain tympanic membrane movement, which is seldom possible with the standard disposable speculum. Also, sufficient training is required for effective pneumatic otoscopy, but there is frequently a gap in training for most clinicians. The implementation of pneumatic otoscopy by primary care physicians in their practice has not been optimal, leading to a lack of resident training and a perception that pneumatic otoscopy is difficult [11].

Recently, an otoscope sensitive to shortwave infrared (SWIR, 1–2 μm) wavelengths of light with the objective of improving middle ear disease diagnoses has been described. SWIR otoscopy provides two fundamental advantages over conventional visible light-based pneumatic otoscopy. First, a SWIR otoscope could help identify middle ear effusions based on the strong light absorption by middle ear fluid in the SWIR spectral region. Second, due to a longer wavelength, SWIR light can penetrate deeper through tissue, enabling a better view of middle ear anatomy behind the tympanic membrane [11].

The differentiation of OME versus OMA is the determining factor in the therapeutic decision. For this, it is important to determine the presence of tympanic effusion and signs of acute inflammation. Paradise suggested a useful algorithm to differentiate OME from OMA based on the presence of otalgia, otorrhea, and the degree of erythema and gloom of the tympanic membrane, classifying them as suppurative and nonsuppurative. Kempthorne created a clinical severity scale for each entity based on the presence of signs found in otoscopy [1].

The tympanometer provides more objective information. The presence of a smaller amplitude or a wider or absent pick are associated with a greater probability of effusion. An OME will show a B-curve and absence of stapedial reflection [1]. Clinicians should obtain tympanometry in children with suspected OME for whom the diagnosis is uncertain after performing pneumatic otoscopy [2]. The acoustic reflectometer is another instrument used to determine the probability of effusion, but its pressure is questioned.

Pure tonal audiometry will show mild to moderate driving hearing loss. It is essential to evaluate the impact of OME on the child's hearing, given the disorder's frequent occurrence during the language acquisition period. Around 50% of children with OME have a loss of more than 20 dB, 20% have a loss of more than 35 dB, and 5–10% have a loss of more than 50 dB. A hearing loss greater than 50 dB must be considered as a possible inner ear damage [11, 13–15]. Ideally, the hearing assessment should include tonal audiometry with air and bone conduction and age-appropriate vocal audiometry. If an audiometric examination is impossible, auditory evoked potentials or the auditory steady state response is recommended [3, 8].

It is important to obtain a hearing test prior to surgery when a child becomes a candidate for tympanostomy tube insertion. To confirm the indication of surgery and to discard sensorineural hearing loss [1, 3], reevaluation at 3–6 months intervals, until the effusion is no longer present, significant hearing loss is identified, or structural abnormalities of the eardrum or middle ear are suspected, is recommended [2].

Children who are at risk for developmental difficulties would likely be disproportionately affected by hearing problems from OME. Clinicians should determine if a child with OME is at increased risk for speech, language, or learning problems from middle ear effusion because of baseline sensory, physical, cognitive, or behavioral factors and should evaluate at-risk children for OME.

At-risk patients are patients with permanent hearing loss, speech and language delay or disorder, autism spectrum disorder and other developmental disorders, syndromes or craniofacial disorders that include cognitive, speech, or language delays, and visual impairment or cleft palate [2].

The use of nasal endoscopy should be used in cases of associated nasal obstruction or prolonged or unilateral OME to confirm adenoid hypertrophy. Flexible nasal endoscopy also enables the differential diagnosis of a rhino pharyngeal tumor, and it should be used more routinely in areas with high HIV prevalence due to the increased risk of nasopharyngeal anomalies such as lymphoma [3]. It is important to screen for an associated palatal disorder or craniofacial dysmorphism that are risk factors for the onset, persistence, and recurrence of OME [1, 8]. The cavum radiography may help only when you cannot do a nasal endoscopy.

Among the predisposing factors of OME, allergy plays a crucial role in the etiology of OME. Many publications show that OME is associated with allergy. Allergies may predispose to OME by causing edema around the eustachian tube or primary mucosal disease in the middle ear. Allergy can induce an inflammatory reaction in the middle ear cavity and increase the susceptibility to infection by microbes. Skin tests of children with OME were found to be negative in 37.1% and positive in 62.9% of cases [16, 17]. The presence of atopy or allergic rhinitis represents an important risk factor for OME, so it seems important to diagnose and treat it [13, 14, 18]. Studies on interventional strategies to reduce these risk factor and the impact on OME and evaluate the impact of treatment of allergic rhinitis and rhinosinusitis on OME are needed [19].

GERD has been associated with OME, and pepsin and H. Pylori have been found in middle ear fluid [3]. In a recent study, at long-term follow-up, the prevalence of OME in adults was higher in the GERD group. The same study found that allergic rhinitis, asthma, or chronic rhinosinusitis showed increase in the risk of developing OME than those without these conditions [6].

In the case of a persistent OME, it is recommended to explore the most frequent risk factors such as GERD and all causes of nasopharyngeal obstruction.

Treatment

Treatment should be individualized and aimed at managing predisposing factors. The goal is to reverse hearing loss and prevent an OMC with permanent sequelae and complications by eliminating the effusion in the middle ear [1].

Treatment will depend on the patient's history and age, the type of OME, the presence and degree of hearing loss, bilaterality, and duration of the effusion.

An OME secondary to an IRA can last 1–2 months and resolve spontaneously without the need for treatment. When secondary to an AOM, the effusion slowly disappears after the treatment of the AOM. Fifty percent have effusion after 2 weeks, 20% after 4 weeks, and 10% after 8 weeks. These cases also do not require additional treatment [8]. So, OME generally resolves spontaneously with watchful waiting.

Clinician decisions for the correct interventional treatment of OME for a specific patient include a variety of factors such as comorbidities, severity of hearing loss, unilaterally or bilaterally, effusion duration, age, social factors, costs, adherence to treatment, and familial assistance with treatment. A patient-focused approach should be adopted when assessing hearing disability. How the child is coping socially and at school is more important than the results of audiometry investigations. Although most OME patients will warrant a conservative management approach, all physical and social factors should be examined to provide a patient-centered treatment plan that optimizes outcomes for the patient [20].The recommendation is to watchful waiting for 3 months from the date of effusion onset(if known) or the date of diagnosis [2, 8, 15].

Medical Therapy

Antibiotics

Venecamps and cols review randomized controlled trials comparing oral antibiotics with placebo, no treatment, or therapy of unproven effectiveness in children with OME. They present evidence of both benefits and harms associated with the use of oral antibiotics to treat children up to 16 years with OME. Although evidence indicates that oral antibiotics are associated with an increased chance of complete resolution of OME, they found evidence that these children are more likely to experience diarrhea, vomiting, or skin rash. The impact of antibiotics on short-term hearing was uncertain, and low-quality evidence did not show that oral antibiotics were associated with fewer ventilation tube insertions. They found no data on the impact of antibiotics on speech, language, and cognitive development or quality of life [13]. The recommendation is against the use of antibiotics for OME [2].

A study investigated the therapeutic effect of erythromycin, clarithromycin, azithromycin, and roxithromycin on a histamine-induced animal model of OME. They recommended the use of macrolide antibiotics, as they show antibacterial and anti-inflammatory efficacy on OME [21]. The international recommendation guidelines do not recommend the use of macrolides in the treatment of OME [3].

Decongestants and Antihistamines

Its use is based on reducing the congestion of the eustachian tube. A systematic review of 2010 found no benefit on hearing, but some benefits in improvement of nasal and ocular allergic symptomatology. They found more adverse effects (11%) in treated versus untreated subjects. They recommended against using antihistamines, decongestants, or both for treating OME [22].

Mucolytics might relieve the symptoms of OME but do not have proven for long-term efficacy [8]. Mucolytics can be used as support in the watchful waiting period because these agents have low cost and are safe [3].

Corticoids

Local inflammation that causes eustachian tube dysfunction in OME could be treated with systemic and/or intranasal corticoids.

In the Cochrane Review of 2011, the analyses of 12 studies shows that there was no evidence of benefit for systemic steroid treatment for OME or hearing loss associated with OME in the longer term [23]. Furthermore, systemic corticoids are associated with a range of adverse reactions, such as diarrhea, nausea, hyperactivity, and epistaxis [8].

Compared with systemically administered steroids, intranasal steroids have limited side effects. Patients with OME and allergic rhinitis may benefit for topical intranasal steroids, targeting the inflammatory component of allergic rhinitis. More prolonged treatment protocols and long-term clinical outcomes will require critical assessment (7). There may be a short-term benefit of topical intranasal steroids in children with adenoidal hypertrophy, although the magnitude of the effect is small, and dosing in one report was higher than recommended [22].

In the 2011 review, no evidence of benefit from treatment of OME with topical intranasal steroids, alone or in combination with an antibiotic, was found [23].

The recommendation is against the use of these medications for OME [2, 8].

Autoinflation

The use of autoinflation balloons is also an option. Autoinflation (Politzer maneuver) is a technique consists in the eustachian tube which is partially reopened by raising pressure in the nose. This can be achieved by forced exhalation with closed mouth and nose, blowing up a balloon through each nostril or using an anesthetic mask. The aim is to introduce air into the middle ear, via the eustachian tube, equalizing the pressures and allowing better drainage of the fluid. Studies of this technique are small of limited treatment duration and had short follow-up, and no double-blind trials have been performed [8, 24].

Table 21.1 Medical treatment of OME [3, 4]

Treatment	Recommended
Oral or nasal steroids	No
Oral antihistamines	No
Antibiotics	No
Mucolytics	No
Decongestants	No
Autoinflation	Yes (limited evidence)

A literature review found a trend toward rapid improvement of the symptoms. The audiometry and tympanometry results were not statistically significant. But, because of the low cost and absence of adverse effects it is reasonable to consider autoinflation while awaiting natural resolution of OME [25] (Table 21.1).

In children, the EarPopper® shows to be a safe and effective treatment option for hearing loss from persistent OME, and reduces the rate of ventilation tube insertion [26]. Another study of 320 children with OME (unilateral and bilateral) showed tympanometric resolution at 3 months in a nasal balloon autoinflation (Otovent®) group versus no nasal balloon autoinflation group. The study concludes that the treatment shows to be feasible, safe, and effective in clearing effusions and in improving important ear symptoms [27]. The use of Otovent® in cleft palate children accelerates the improvement of middle ear status and hearing thresholds at 6 months [28].

In adults, the combined treatments including medication and the use of a modified Politzer device (Streamsys) show to be more effective than medical treatment alone. Younger age, smaller air bone gap, and higher tubomanometry value are good predictors for treatment success too [29].

PPIs

Although the link between gastroesophageal reflux disease and OME is increasingly well documented, there is no evidence regarding the treatment of reflux and OME. It is not recommended to use anti-reflux medication for OME at this time [6].

Immunization

Medical therapy should be attempted before a surgical solution, but there is nothing proven for it. Active observation is considered an appropriate strategy for most children because the effusion resolves spontaneously in most of them [10].

Hearing Aids

Other alternative is the use of hearing aids and osseous conduction hearing aids in children with craniofacial abnormalities, Down's syndrome, and cleft palate. They have been found to overcome the hearing loss associated with this condition. Childhood hearing loss can affect language development. Therefore, hearing aids may be considered as a noninvasive option to treat OME [20].

Surgical Treatment

Ventilation Tubes (VT)

The use of ventilation tubes is widespread, with different indication schemes. VT helps to ventilate the cavities of the middle ear and balance the pressures on each side of the tympanic membrane, preventing re-accumulation of fluid. After this procedure, many patients do not need additional therapy due to the growth and development of the eustachian tube angle, which will allow for drainage [14].

Short-term VTs are used for first-line treatment and fall out after between 6 and 18 months. Thus, the risk of complications is correspondingly lower. Long-term VTs stay in place for 2 years or more. Even though the complication rate increases with the VTs' duration of use, these devices are still indicated when OME recurs in a child who has already had short-term VTs. They are also recommended in children with chronic eustachian tube dysfunction [14].

The current clinical practice guidelines for OME recommend surgical management for children with 3 or more months of OME with persistent hearing loss or symptoms that are likely attributable to OME, for recurrent or persistent OME in children with developmental risks regardless of hearing status or for OME with structural damage to the middle ear or tympanic membrane [15]. Also, the individual difficulties related to the hearing loss, which vary from one child to another and are not always correlated with the hearing threshold, need to be considered [6]. In children at risk of language or learning disorders, rapid treatment is recommended to limit the impact of additional deafness. This concerns children with autistic spectrum disorders, perception deafness unrelated to OME, a speech delay, a craniofacial syndrome or malformation, blindness (or other visual disorders), a cleft palate, or a global development delay [15].

When OME is detected in an at-risk child, tympanostomy tubes should be offered when the likelihood of spontaneous resolution is low (type B tympanogram or persistence for 3 months) [2].

In 2010, Browning et al. review of 10 randomized studies show the effectiveness of ventilation tubes versus myringotomy or nonsurgical treatment in children with OME. Randomized controlled studies are included. Tubes installed after 12 weeks of effusion with documented hearing loss show benefit in the first 6 months in hearing as does nonsurgical treatment. The studies showed a small difference in relation to the decibels gained between those treated with tubes and controls. At 12–18 months, no differences were found. There are no differences in language, behavior, cognitive development, or quality of life. Tympanosclerosis was observed in one-third of the ears receiving tubes. Otorrhea is common in infants but in children over 3 years of age it occurs in <2% of the ears in 2 years of follow-up. No studies evaluate benefits in children with developmental or language delays. Therefore, the tubes would be beneficial only in the short term in the hearing of healthy children [10].

Consequences for tympanic retractions and cholesteatoma are difficult to interpret from available evidence as the ears with the most severe disease are usually those which require ventilation tubes, so it is difficult to dissociate disease from treatment as cause of complications [3].

The tympanic membrane generally benefits from tympanostomy tubes, avoiding posterosuperior retraction pockets, ossicular erosion, adhesive atelectasis, and retraction pockets that accumulate keratin debris [15]. A prospective study shows that early tympanostomy tubes do not prevent the progression of OME toward tympanic retraction [30]. Concerning cholesteatomatous chronic otitis media, tubes prevent the appearance of cholesteatoma on a population level, but individually the absolute risk reduction is very small [31]. There is insufficient literature to assess the possible benefit of tubes on cholesteatoma prevention [3].

The use of tympanostomy with tubes decreased OME for 2 years compared with watch and wait or myringocentesis and improved hearing for 6 months compared with watch and wait [32].

Adenoidectomy

Adenoidectomy is currently utilized in cases of OME that involve enlarged adenoids and is an important addition to management in patients with OME.

The increase of adenoid hypertrophy cells can enhance local inflammation, resulting in abnormal physiological function of eustachian tube and middle ear effusion. It is found that many pathogenic microorganisms in the middle ear effusion are like the bacteria in adenoid tissues [33].

Biofilms contribute to the pathogenesis of OME [9]. Many therapeutic strategies have been attempted, and the role of topical therapies is still being investigated. A review of 30 articles shows that antibiotics were ineffective for eradicating biofilm. Mupirocin irrigation, gentian violet, and thiamphenicol glycinate acetylcysteine effectively eradicated biofilms. Physical disruption, surfactants, and probiotics were also shown to be beneficial [34].

An animal experiment found that middle ear biofilms can be treated safely and effectively reducing the surface area of biofilm by washing the middle ear with saline solution or children's shampoo. An hydrodebrider demonstrated to be more effective at eradicating biofilm than manual irrigation [35].

Adenoidectomy removes the physical obstruction of the eustachian tube, restores the drainage of mucus, and equilibrates the pressure in the middle ear [8]. Adenoidectomy was significantly more effective in the treatment of OME when large adenoids were in contact with the torus tubarius. The viscosity of the middle ear effusion does not influence the effectiveness of adenoidectomy [36]. Adenoidectomy may enhance the clinical effectiveness of TTs in OME, for at least 2 years. Adenoidectomy is most beneficial in children with persistent OME aged ≥4 years [18].

In 2010, Van den Aardweg et al. review shows that the 22% and 29% risk differences at 6 months and 12 months, respectively, for children with persistent otitis media with effusion in the trials that compared adenoidectomy with unilateral tympanostomy tubes versus a unilateral tympanostomy tube alone, in which the non-operated ears were used as the control, that shows a significant benefit of adenoidectomy as far as the resolution of middle ear effusion in children with OME is concerned. The results of studies of adenoidectomy with or without myringotomy versus nonsurgical treatment or myringotomy only, and those of adenoidectomy in combination with bilateral tympanostomy tubes versus bilateral tympanostomy tubes only, showed a small beneficial of adenoidectomy on the resolution of the effusion. The benefit to hearing is small, and the effects on changes in the tympanic membrane are unknown. The risks operating should be weighed against these potential benefits [37].

Adenoidectomy used as an adjunct to grommet insertion reducing hearing loss by a further 4 dB. As well as improving thresholds, there is a prolongation in the duration of improvement in hearing of up to 18 months. This extended period creates a reduction in reinsertion rate of 21% [38].

Compared with simple tube insertion, tympanostomy tubes combined with adenoidectomy can effectively shorten the duration of middle ear effusion, reduce the recurrence rate, and improve the curative effect. But it has no obvious advantage in improving the postoperative hearing level [33].

The American guidelines recommend adenoidectomy for the treatment of OME as a function of the child's age. For children under the age of 4 years, adenoidectomy must only be performed in cases of nasal obstruction or recurrent infections. In children over the age of 4 years, it can be combined with TT placement [2, 8].

Balloon Dilatation on Eustachian Tube

The aim of this procedure is to improve the ventilatory and pressure-equalizing function of the eustachian tube to treat OME by widening the medial cartilaginous part of the eustachian tube.

A recent study shows that patients treated with dilatation and grommet insertion had good outcomes, improving subjective symptoms and objective evaluations and achieved good results in eustachian tube function and structure (enlarged and effectively improves the active and passive opening) [39].

Eustachian tube balloon dilatation combined with grommet insertion could be a treatment for refractory otitis media with effusion [39].

References

1. Goycoolea MV, Hueb MM, Ruan C. Otitis media. The pathogenesis approach. Otolaryngol Clin North Am. 1991;24(4):757–61.
2. Rosenfeld RM, Shin JJ, Schwartz SR, et al. Clinical practice guideline: otitis media with effusion (update). Otolaryngol Head Neck Surg. 2016;154:S1–S41. https://doi.org/10.1177/0194599815623467.
3. Simon F, Haggard M, Rosenfeld RM, Jia H, Peer S. International consensus (ICON) on management of otitis media with effusion in children. Eur Ann Otorhinolaryngol Head Neck Dis. 2018;1:S33–9. https://doi.org/10.1016/j.anorl.2017.11.009.
4. Atkinson H, Wallis S, Coatesworth AP. Otitis media with effusion. Postgrad Med. 2015;127:381–5. https://doi.org/10.1080/00325481.2015.1028317.
5. Miura MS, Mascaro M, Rosenfeld RM. Association between otitis media and gastroesophageal reflux: a systematic review. Otolaryngol Head Neck Surg. 2012;146:345–52.
6. Yeo CD, Kim JS, Lee EJ. Association of gastroesophageal reflux disease with increased risk of chronic otitis media with effusion in adults: a nationwide population-based cohort study. Medicine. 2021;100:33–9.
7. Lack G, Caulfield H, Penagos M. The link between otitis media with effusion and allergy: a potential role for intranasal corticosteroids. Pediatr Allergy Immunol. 2011;22(3):258–66. https://doi.org/10.1111/j.1399-3038.2010.01130.x.
8. Vanneste P, Page C. Otitis media with effusion in children: pathophysiology, diagnosis, and treatment. A review. J Otol. 2019;14:33–9. https://doi.org/10.1016/j.joto.2019.01.005.
9. Bakaletz LO. Bacterial biofilms in the upper airway—evidence for role in pathology and implications for treatment of otitis media. Paediatr Respir Rev. 2012;13(3):154–9. https://doi.org/10.1016/j.prrv.2012.03.001.
10. Browning GG, Rovers MM, Williamson I. Grommets (ventilation tubes) for hearing loss associated with otitis media with effusion in children. Cochrane Database Syst Rev. 2010;(10):CD001801. https://doi.org/10.1002/14651858.CD001801.pub3.
11. Valdez TA, Carr JA. Initial findings of shortwave infrared otoscopy in a pediatric population. Int J Pediatr Otorhinolaryngol. 2018;114:15–9. https://doi.org/10.1016/j.ijporl.2018.08.024.
12. Shekelle P, Takata G, Chan LS, Mangione-Smith R, Corley PM, Morphew T, Morton S. Diagnosis, natural history, and late effects of otitis media with effusion. Evid Rep Technol Assess (Summ). 2002;(55):1–5. https://doi.org/10.1037/e439822005-001. PMID: 12945555; PMCID: PMC4781261.

13. Venekamp RP, Burton MJ, van Dongen TMA, van der Heijden GJ. Antibiotics for otitis media with effusion in children. Cochrane Database Syst Rev. 2016;2016:CD009163. https://doi.org/10.1002/14651858.CD009163.pub3.
14. Isaacson G. Tympanostomy tubes—a visual guide for the young otolaryngologist. Ear Nose Throat J. 2020;99(1_suppl):8S–14S. https://doi.org/10.1177/0145561320929885.
15. Rosenfeld RM, Schwartz SR, Pynnonen MA, et al. Clinical practice guideline: tympanostomy tubes in children. Otolaryngol Head Neck Surg. 2013;149(1_suppl):S1–S35. https://doi.org/10.1177/0194599813487302.
16. Songu M, Islek A, Imre A, et al. Risk factors for otitis media with effusion in children with adenoid hypertrophy. Acta Otorhinolaryngol Ital. 2020;40:133–7. https://doi.org/10.14639/0392-100X-245.
17. Martinez F, Bentivegna D, Di Piazza F, et al. The point prevalence of otitis media with effusion among primary school children in Western Sicily. Eur Arch Otorhinolaryngol. 2010;267:709–14. https://doi.org/10.1007/s00405-009-1131-4.
18. Boonacker CW, Rovers MM, Browning GG, Hoes AW, Schilder AG, Burton MJ. Adenoidectomy with or without grommets for children with otitis media: an individual patient data meta-analysis. Health Technol Assess. 2014;18(5):1–118. https://doi.org/10.3310/hta18050.
19. Zernotti ME, Pawankar R, Ansotegui I, Badellino H. Otitis media with effusion and atopy: is there a causal relationship? World Allergy Organ J. 2017;10(1):37–41.
20. Searight FT, Singh R, Peterson DC. Otitis media with effusion. In: StatPearls [Internet]. Treasure Island: StatPearls Publishing; 2022. PMID: 30855877.
21. Ersoy B, Aktan B, Kilic K, Sakat M, Sipal S. The anti-inflammatory effects of erythromycin, clarithromycin, azithromycin and roxithromycin on histamine-induced otitis media with effusion in Guinea pigs. J Laryngol Otol. 2018;132(7):579–83. https://doi.org/10.1017/S0022215118000610.
22. Bhargava R, Chakravarti A. A double-blind randomized placebo-controlled trial of topical intranasal mometasone furoate nasal spray in children of adenoidal hypertrophy with otitis media with effusion. Am J Otolaryngol. 2014;35(6):766–70. https://doi.org/10.1016/j.amjoto.2014.06.006. Epub 2014 Jun 20. PMID: 25151658.
23. Simpson SA, Lewis R, van der Voort J, Butler CC. Oral or topical nasal steroids for hearing loss associated with otitis media with effusion in children. Cochrane Database Syst Rev. 2011;2011(5):CD001935. https://doi.org/10.1002/14651858.CD001935.pub3.
24. Griffin G, Flynn CA. Antihistamines and/or decongestants for otitis media with effusion (OME) in children. Cochrane Database Syst Rev. 2011;2011(9):CD003423. https://doi.org/10.1002/14651858.CD003423.pub3. PMID: 21901683; PMCID: PMC7170417.
25. Perera R, Glasziou PP, Heneghan CJ, McLellan J, Williamson I. Autoinflation for hearing loss associated with otitis media with effusion. Cochrane Database Syst Rev. 2013;(5):CD006285. https://doi.org/10.1002/14651858.CD006285.pub2. PMID: 23728660.
26. Banigo A, Hunt A, Rourke T, Whiteside O, Aldren C. Does the EarPopper® device improve hearing outcomes in children with persistent otitis media with effusion? A randomised single-blinded controlled trial. Clin Otolaryngol. 2016;41(1):59–65.
27. Williamson I, Vennik J, Harnden A, Voysey M, Perera R, Kelly S, Yao G, Raftery J, Mant D, Little P. Effect of nasal balloon autoinflation in children with otitis media with effusion in primary care: an open randomized controlled trial. CMAJ. 2015;187(13):961–9. https://doi.org/10.1503/cmaj.141608. Epub 2015 Jul 27. PMID: 26216608; PMCID: PMC4577342.
28. Rosso C, Pisani A, Stefanoni E, et al. Nasal autoinflation devices for middle ear disease in cleft palate children: are they effective? Acta Otorhinolaryngol Ital. 2021;41:364–70. https://doi.org/10.14639/0392-100X-N1277.
29. Zhong Z, Zhang J, Ren L, Liu Y, Zhen Z, Xiao S. Predictors of conservative treatment outcomes for adult otitis media with effusion. J Int Adv Otol. 2020;16(2):248–52. https://doi.org/10.5152/iao.2020.8091. PMID: 32784164; PMCID: PMC7419099.
30. Johnston LC, Feldman HM, Paradise JL, Bernard BS, Colborn DK, Casselbrant ML, Janosky JE. Tympanic membrane abnormalities and hearing levels at the ages of 5 and 6 years in relation to persistent otitis media and tympanostomy tube insertion in the first 3 years of life: a prospective study incorporating a randomized clinical trial. Pediatrics. 2004;114(1):e58–67. https://doi.org/10.1542/peds.114.1.e58. PMID: 15231974.
31. Djurhuus BD, Christensen K, Skytthe A, Faber CE. The impact of ventilation tubes in otitis media on the risk of cholesteatoma on a national level. Int J Pediatr Otorhinolaryngol. 2015;79(4):605–9. https://doi.org/10.1016/j.ijporl.2015.02.005. Epub 2015 Feb 11. PMID: 25724629.
32. Berkman ND, Wallace IF, Steiner MJ, Harrison M, Greenblatt AM, Lohr KN, Kimple A, Yuen A. Otitis media with effusion: comparative effectiveness of treatments [internet]. Rockville: Agency for Healthcare Research and Quality (US); 2013. Report No.: 13-EHC091-EF. PMID: 23762917.
33. Hao J, Chen M, Liu B, et al. Compare two surgical interventions for otitis media with effusion in young children. Eur Arch Otorhinolaryngol. 2019;276:2125–31. https://doi.org/10.1007/s00405-019-05421-9.
34. Smith A, Buchinsky FJ, Post JC. Eradicating chronic ear, nose, and throat infections: a systematically conducted literature review of advances in biofilm treatment. Otolaryngol Head Neck Surg. 2011;144(3):338–47. https://doi.org/10.1177/0194599810391620. Epub 2011 Jan 24. PMID: 21493193.
35. Abi Hachem R, Goncalves S, Walker T, Angeli S. Middle ear irrigation using a hydrodebrider decreases biofilm surface area in an animal model of otitis media. Laryngoscope Investig Otolaryngol. 2018;3(3):231–7. https://doi.org/10.1002/lio2.164. PMID: 30062140; PMCID: PMC6057225.
36. Skoloudik L, Kalfert D, Valenta T, Chrobok V. Relation between adenoid size and otitis media with effusion. Eur Ann Otorhinolaryngol Head Neck Dis. 2018;135(6):399–402. issn:1879-7296. https://doi.org/10.1016/j.anorl.2017.11.011.
37. Van den Aardweg MT, Schilder AG, Herkert E, Boonacker CW, Rovers MM. Adenoidectomy for otitis media in children. Cochrane Database Syst Rev. 2010;(1):CD007810. https://doi.org/10.1002/14651858.CD007810.pub2.
38. MRC Multicentre Otitis Media Study Group. Adjuvant adenoidectomy in persistent bilateral otitis media with effusion: hearing and revision surgery outcomes through 2 years in the TARGET randomised trial. Clin Otolaryngol. 2012;37(2):107–16. https://doi.org/10.1111/j.1749-4486.2012.02469.x. PMID: 22443163.
39. Li L, Mao Y, Hu N, Yan W, Lu Y, Fan Z, Wang H, Han Y. The effect of balloon dilatation eustachian tuboplasty combined with grommet insertion on the structure and function of the eustachian tube in patients with refractory otitis media with effusion. Ann Palliat Med. 2021;10(7):7662–70. https://doi.org/10.21037/apm-21-1280. PMID: 34353054.

Inflammatory Mediators in the Pathogenesis of Otitis Media: A Brief Review

22

Timothy T. K. Jung

Otitis media (OM) is a common childhood disease. OM can be defined as an inflammation or infection of the middle ear cavity. Among many causative factors of OM, infection and eustachian tube (ET) dysfunction are most important. These causative factors stimulate middle ear epithelia and inflammatory cells to secrete inflammatory mediators (IMs) such as cytokines, eicosanoids, platelet-activating factor (PAF), tumor necrosis factor (TNF)-a, and nitric oxide. These IMs increase vascular permeability and secretory activity resulting in middle ear effusion (MEE) [1]. Thus, IMs play a central role in the pathogenesis of OM.

Pathogenesis of OM has been studied in humans and various animal models. Various forms of OM have been studied in longitudinal and parallel studies including acute purulent otitis media (POM), serous otitis media (SOM), mucoid or secretory otitis media (MOM), and chronic suppurative otitis media (COM). When these forms of OMs are followed longitudinally, they seem to change in continuum and interrelated [2].

The purpose of this study was to better understand the role of IMs in the pathogenesis of OM by finding levels of IMs in samples of human middle ear effusion (MEE) and in animal models of OMs and by studying the effect of the therapeutic use of inhibitors of IMs.

Methods

The topic of IMs in the pathogenesis of OM was searched in the National Center for Biotechnology Information (NCBI) and at the U.S. National Library of Medicine (NLM).The articles were reviewed, organized, and discussed. Only common IMs studied in OM were included. Most of the studies start with assaying samples of MEE in humans obtained at the time of myringotomy and tympanostomy tube (TT) insertions or in different types of animal models at different time intervals. Many of the animal studies also examined corresponding temporal bone histopathology.

Results

Lysozyme and Lactic Dehydrogenase (LDH)

Both lysozyme and LDH have been used as an index of inflammation.

Human MEE

Levels of lysozyme and LDH were higher in mucoid MEE than serous MEE [2].

Animal MEE

In POM model using chinchilla infected with pneumococcus, concentration of lysozyme and LDH were highest on day 7 and decrease over time. In SOM model induced by blocking eustachian tube in chinchilla and cat, levels of these IMs were lower than POM [2].

Histopathology of the temporal bones showed inflammations in mucoperiosteum corresponding to levels of IMs [2].

Eicosanoids, Prostaglandins (PGs), and Leukotrienes (LTs)

Among the various IMs of OM, arachidonic acid (AA) metabolites (eicosanoids) such as PGs and LTs appear to play an important role in the pathogenesis of OM. To investigate the role of AA metabolites on the pathogenesis of OM, concentrations of AA metabolites were measured in the MEE from human and paralleling animal models of OM and effects of inhibiters of AA metabolism, antibiotics, and tympanostomy tube (TT) on the outcome of animal models of

T. T. K. Jung (✉)
Department of Otolaryngology-Head & Neck Surgery, Loma Linda University School of Medicine, Jerry L. Pettis Veterans Medical Center, Loma Linda, CA, USA

Inland Ear Head & Neck Clinic, Riverside, CA, USA

M. V. Goycoolea et al. (eds.), *Textbook of Otitis Media*, https://doi.org/10.1007/978-3-031-40949-3_22

OM were studied [3]. AA is released from membrane phospholipids by the action of phospholipase. This step is inhibited by corticosteroids. Once released, AA can be converted to two metabolic pathways, one through cyclo-oxygenase into PGs and the other through lipoxygenase into LTs. Most of nonsteroidal anti-inflammatory drugs (NSAIDS) like aspirin or ibuprofen inhibit the activity of cyclo-oxygenase.

Human and Animal MEE

PGE2 and PGF2a in human pooled MEE were measured by radioimmunoassay (RIA) and found that mucoid effusions had higher concentrations of PGs than serous effusion [4]. In more extensive studies concentrations of major AA metabolites, both PGs and LTs were assayed and analyzed according to type of fluids, age groups, and bacterial culture results. It was found that AA metabolites were higher in younger age group than from older age groups. Levels of LTs were generally higher in mucoid MEEs than in serous MEEs. LTB4 was the only AA metabolite with higher levels in bacterial culture-positive human MEE.

Effect of Inhibitors of AA Metabolism

From the study of the therapeutic use of inhibitors of AA metabolism, combination of penicillin and corticosteroid was the best mode of therapy, followed by penicillin alone and penicillin plus NSAID. Therapy with ibuprofen alone induces more inflammation and increased effusion probably because of increased LTs due to inhibition of cyclo-oxygenase [3].

Effect of LT and Its Inhibitor on the Clearance of the Eustachian Tube

Using guinea pigs, this study demonstrated that LTC4 impaired mucociliary clearance function of the eustachian tube in dose-dependent manner. This inhibition of mucociliary clearance function was prevented by pretreatment with LT inhibitor. The findings of this study suggest that LT plays an important role in the pathogenesis of OME by impairing eustachian tube clearance function. LT inhibitors may have future prophylactic or therapeutic implications for OME [5].

Platelet-Activating Factor (PAF)

A biologically active phospholipid PAF is known to have wide-ranging effects on acute inflammation and allergy. It is released from human neutrophils, platelets, eosinophils, macrophages, mast cells, and vascular endothelial cells [6]. It has been identified in human MEE and has been suggested to participate in developing OME and maintaining MEE by stimulating vascular permeability and chemotaxis [7].

To test hypothesis that PAF can induce OME, PAF was injected into the chinchilla bullae which induced dose-dependent OME. PAF antagonist, WEB 2170, prevented the development of OME. The findings of this study suggest that PAF plays an important role in the pathogenesis of OME [8].

Tumor Necrosis Factor-a (TNF-a)

TNF is produced by activated macrophages and has various activities. It activates neutrophils, induces production of intercellular adhesion molecules from lymphocyte, directs tumoricidal action on certain tumor cell line, enhances production of interleukins such as interferon, interleukin (IL)-1, IL-2, IL-6, and IL-8, and stimulates production of collagenase, prostaglandin, and pyrogen [9].

To clarify the role of TNF in experimental OME, OME was induced by transtympanic injection of TNF in rats. MEE was developed in 70% of specimens, and histopathological changes such as subepithelial edema and marked infiltration of neutrophils were present in 100% at 24 h after injection. MEE was prevented by pretreatment with TNF antagonist, TNF-soluble receptor type I (TNFsolRI) [10]. Another study performed by same group showed that treatment with TNF antagonist prevents MEE induced by pseudomonas lipopolysaccharide (LPS) in rats[11].

Nitric Oxide Metabolites

Free radicals such as nitric oxide (NO) seem to be important in the pathogenesis of OME. This study measured concentrations of NO in human MEE. Type of MEE was determined at the time of collection as SOM, MOM, and POM. Concentrations of NO metabolites were highest in MOM followed by SOM and POM. This study suggests that NO is present in human MEE and may play an important role in the pathogenesis of OME [12].

Review of IMS, OM, and Connection to Inner Ear Function

Here is a review article dealing with the characteristics of various inflammatory mediators identified in the middle ear during otitis media and in cholesteatoma. The role of each inflammatory mediator in the pathogenesis of otitis media and cholesteatoma has been discussed. Further, the relation of each inflammatory mediator to the pathophysiology of the middle and inner ear along with its mechanisms of histopathological change has been described. The mechanisms of hearing loss including sensorineural hearing loss (SNHL) as a sequela of otitis media are also discussed. The passage of inflammatory mediators through the round window membrane into the scala tympani is discussed. In an experimental animal model, an application of cytokines and lipopolysaccharide (LPS), a bacterial toxin, on the round window membrane induced sensorineural hearing loss as identified through auditory brainstem response threshold shifts. An increase in permeability of the blood–labyrinth barrier (BLB) was observed following the application of these inflammatory mediators and LPS[13].

Inflammasome and OME

The nucleotide-binding oligomerization domain-like receptor protein 3 (NLRP3) inflammasome is a critical molecule mediating interleukin-1β (IL-1β) responses. However, the role of the NLRP3 inflammasome in otitis media has not been fully examined. The purpose of this study was to assess the expression of NLRP3, ASC (apoptosis-associated speck-like protein containing a caspase recruitment domain and a pyrin domain), and caspase-1 in lipopolysaccharide-induced otitis media. BALB/c mice received a transtympanic injection of either lipopolysaccharide or phosphate-buffered saline. The mice were sacrificed 24 h after injection. Concentrations of IL-1β, NLRP3, ASC, and caspase-1 in the middle ear effusions were measured by enzyme-linked immunosorbent assay. Temporal bones were processed for histologic examination and immunohistochemistry.

The transtympanic injection of lipopolysaccharide significantly upregulated levels of IL-1β, NLRP3, ASC, and caspase-1 in the middle ear as compared with the control mice. The proteins of NLRP3, ASC, and caspase-1 were observed in infiltrating inflammatory cells induced by lipopolysaccharide in the middle ear cavity. Lipopolysaccharide induces NLRP3 inflammasome components in the middle ear. The NLRP3 inflammasome may play an important role in the pathogenesis of otitis media. Modulation of inflammasome-mediated inflammation may be a novel therapeutic strategy for otitis media [14].

Viral and Bacterial Pathogens and IMs in MEE

Secretory *otitis media* (SOM) is characterized by persistence of fluid in the middle ear, often following an episode of acute *otitis media*. The hypothesis is that failure to eliminate bacterial or viral pathogens may result in persistent low-grade inflammation. In this study, inflammatory mediators in middle ear fluids from 67 children with SOM were analyzed. This was combined with determinations of viable bacteria by culture along with detection of bacterial and viral genetic material by real-time polymerase chain reaction (PCR). The inflammatory mediators found at the highest concentrations (>30 ng/mL) were stem cell growth factor-β (median 110 ng/mL), CXCL1, IL-16, IL-8, migration inhibitory factor, CXCL10, and CXCL9. Among bacterial pathogens, *Moraxella catarrhalis* and *Haemophilus influenzae* dominated, regardless of detection methods, while rhinovirus dominated among viral pathogens. Middle ear fluid levels of interleukin (IL)-1α, IL-17, IL-1β, fibroblast growth factor basic, and tumor necrosis factor correlated strongly with the presence of bacteria detected either by culture or PCR, while IL-1RA, IL-3, IL-6, IL-8, CCL3, CCL4, and granulocyte colony-stimulating factor correlated significantly with real-time PCR values. CXCL10, CXCL9, CCL2, and TRAIL correlated significantly with viral nucleic acid levels. To conclude, persistence of viral and bacterial pathogens may fuel persistent inflammation in SOM. Bacteria caused a broad inflammatory response, while viruses chiefly elicited the interferon-induced chemokines CXCL9 and CXCL10 [15].

Discussion

The goal of this review is to find the role of IMs on the pathogenesis of OM. Typical OM starts with viral upper respiratory infection followed by bacterial infection. It may start with eustachian tube (ET) dysfunction creating negative pressure in the middle ear. Frequently, OM may start with the combination of both bacterial infection and ET dysfunction. Either bacterial infection or ET or both stimulate middle ear epithelia and inflammatory cells to secrete inflammatory mediators (IMs) such as cytokines, eicosanoids, platelet-activating factor (PAF), tumor necrosis factor (TNF)-a, and nitric oxide. These IMs increase vascular permeability and secretory activity resulting in middle ear effusion (MEE) [1]. IMs can start, perpetuate MEE, and cause sequelae such as sensorineural hearing loss.

Most of the studies of IMs in OM start with assaying samples of MEE from human or animal model of OM. Usually, samples are divided by the type of fluids such as SOM, MOM, or POM either from human or experimental animal models.

Next step is injecting IMs either transtympanic membrane or through the top of the bullae and checking whether MEE is produced or not. This step is followed by treating with blockers of IMs being tested and checking whether formation of MEE is blocked or not. As much as possible histopathology of middle ear mucosa is examined.

The IMs that have been gone through these tests include cytokines, prostaglandins, leukotrienes, platelet-activating factor (PAF), tumor necrosis factor (TNF)-a, and nitric oxide. No doubt there are more IMs involved in the pathogenesis of OM, and more will be discovered and added to the list.

Goal of these studies is to find better treatment of OM. Finding how IMs induce OMs and inhibitors of IMs may reduce or block OM can be used clinically to treat patients with OM. One example of this is the judicious use of glucocorticoid with antibiotics to treat POM. This practice came from extensive animal and human studies using glucocorticoid which blocks the formation of both LTs and PGs from AA. It will be possible that more inhibitors of IMs could be used to treat OM in the future.

Conclusion

This brief review demonstrates that various IMs such as lysozyme, LDH, PGs, LTs, PAF, TNF, ILs, and NO are involved in the pathogenesis of OM. These IMs were measured in the samples of MEE in human and animal models of OME and histopathological effect studied. Effects of blockers of these IMs on the outcome of animal models of OM were studied to discover better treatment for OM. One example of such finding was better outcome when OM was treated with antibiotic in combination with glucocorticoids.

Goal of these studies is to find therapeutic use of inhibitors of IMs. Further study is needed to determine if more of these IM blockers can be implemented into the clinical setting.

References

1. Jung TT, Park SK, Rhee CK. Effect of inhibitors of leukotriene and/or platelet activating factor on killed H. influenzae induced experimental otitis media with effusion. Int J Pediatr Otorhinolaryngol. 2004;68:57–63.
2. Juhn SK, Paparella MM, Kim CS, Goycoolea MV, Giebink S. Pathogenesis of otitis media. Ann Otol Rhino Laryngo. 1977;86:481–93.
3. Jung TTK. Prostaglandins, leukotrienes, and other arachidonic acid metabolites in the pathogenesis of otitis media. Laryngoscope. 1988;98:980–93.
4. Jakson RT. Autonomic stimulation, osmolarity and prostaglandin effects in the Eustachian tube. Ann Otol Rhino Laryungol. 1976;85(Suppl 25):187–93.
5. Rhee CK, Jang YJ, Jeong PS, Hyun MH, Kim YH, Ju CY, Jung TTK. The effect of leukotriene and its inhibitor on the mucociliary clearance of the eustacyhian tube in Guinea pigs. In: Tos M, Thomsen J, Balle V, editors. Otitis media today. Hague, The Netherlands: Kugler Publications; 1999. p. 199–203.
6. Barnes P, Chung K, Page C. Platelet-activating factor as a mediator of allergic disease. J Allergy Clin Immunol. 1988;81:919–34.
7. Cauwenberge P, Bernstein J. Inflammatory mediators inmiddle ear disease. In: Bernstein J, Ogra P, editors. Immunology of the ear. New York, NY: Raven Press; 1987. p. 338–9.
8. Rhee CK, Jung TTK, Miller S, Weeks D. Experimental otitis media with effusion induced by platelet activating factor. Ann Otol Rhinolo Laryngol. 1993;102:600–5.
9. Ophir D, Hahn T, Schattner A, Wallach D, Aviel A. Tumor necrosis factor in middle ear effusions. Arch Otolaryngol Head Neck Surg. 1988;114:1256–8.
10. Lee DH, Park YS, Jung TTK, Yeo SW, Choi YC, Jeon EJ. Effect of tumor necrosis factor—a on experimental otitis media with effusion. Laryngoscope. 2001;111:728–33.
11. Jeon EJ, Park YS, Choi YC, Yeo SW, Jung TTK. Effect of inhibitor of tumor necrosis factor—a on experimental otitis media with effusion. Ann Otol Rhinol Lryngol. 2001;110:917–21.
12. John EO, Russell PT, Nam BH, Jinn TH, Jung TTK. Concentration of nitric oxide metabolites in middle ear effusion. Int J Pediatr Otorhinolaryngol. 2001;60:55–8.
13. Juhn SK, Jung MK, Hoffman MD, Drew BR, Preciado DA, Sausen NJ, Jung TTK, Kim BH, Park SY, Lin J, Ondrey FG, Mains DR, Huang T. The role of inflammatory mediators in the pathogenesis of otitis media and sequelae. Clin Exp Otorhinoaryngol. 2008;3:117–38. https://doi.org/10.3342/ceo.2008.1.3.117.Epub2008.
14. Kariya S, Okano M, Zhao P, Maeda Y, Kataoka Y, Hiaki T, Noda Y, Makihara S, Nishizaki K. NLRP3 inflammasome expression in lipopolysaccharide-induced otitis media. Acta Otolaryngol. 2018;138:1061–5. https://doi.org/10.1080/00016489.2018.1515499.
15. Skovbjerg S, Roos K, Andersson M, Rabe H, Nilsson S, Lindh M, Wold A. Inflammatory mediator profiles in secretory otitis media in relation to viable bacterial pathogens and bacterial and viral nucleic acids. J Interf Cytokine Res. 2020;40:555–69. https://doi.org/10.1089/jir.2020.0075.

Retraction Pockets and Adhesive Otitis Media

23

María José Herrera J and Javiera Pardo

Definition

A retraction of the tympanic membrane occurs when a portion or the entirety of the membrane collapses within the middle ear cavity, as a result of negative pressure from impaired airflow in this space.

The importance of retraction pockets lies in the loss of the original histological and anatomical structure, which is associated with the development of ossicular chain erosion, cholesteatoma formation, and potentially life-threatening complications from cholesteatoma. The development of retraction pocket presumes a change in the histological structure of the tympanic membrane, typically the loosening of the elastic fibers in the middle layer and reductions in thickness and tensile strength and in the layer's abilities to maintain the shape and position of the tympanic membrane and to return to its original thickness and strength. Retraction pockets are considered sequels of abnormal pressure regulation in the middle ear; however, inflammation or earlier perforations may also contribute to the development of retraction pockets [1].

Prevalence

Retractions are much more common in children than in adults. The incidence of atrophy increases from 4% at age 4 years to 11% at age 16 years [2]. In a study of 294 healthy children between 5 and 16 years old, the prevalence of atelectasis of the eardrum was estimated at 14%–26% in the pars flaccida and only 0.3%–3.7% in the pars tensa [3]. Re-examinations of children who had secretory otitis media noticed that 34% of the ears had developed different degrees of attic retractions after 3–8 years [4].

In 2011, Maw et al. used video-otoscopy to perform an important longitudinal cohort study with 6908 healthy children, whose ages ranged from birth to 10 years. They found pars flaccida retractions in 9.6% of cases and pars tensa retractions in 7.9%. Most of these retractions were mild, and a few cases were severe [5]. The prevalence of retractions in adults has been reported in a population sample as 9.6% for pars flaccida and 7% for pars tensa [5].

Bilateral retraction pockets are often present. The association between pars tensa and pars flaccida abnormalities in the same ear shows that pars flaccida retractions are frequently associated with pars tensa abnormalities, but when abnormalities have been found in the pars tensa, the pars flaccida has been completely normal [5].

Many studies have reached a similar conclusion: When otitis media is present, the frequency of tympanic membrane pathology is significantly higher. Abnormalities in the tympanic membrane in ears without histories of otitis have been present in 11% of cases. In children with a history of otitis, the rates of abnormalities have been 46% and 92% (as found with the use of a ventilation tube, or VT) for 8-year-olds. In the same study, a high number of mild retractions that were present during the initial examination at this age had substantially diminished at 10-year follow-ups [6].

Pathogenesis

Tympanic retraction is a sequel secondary to an inflammatory process of the tympanic membrane, such as otitis media with effusion or recurrent acute otitis media, and it is associated with the poor ventilation of the middle ear. Anatomically, the tympanic membrane is formed by three layers of skin, connective tissue, and mucosa. At the level of the pars tensa, the lamina propria, corresponding to the middle layer, has two layers: the stratum radiatum and the stratum circulare. On one hand, in the posterosuperior part of the pars tensa, the

M. J. Herrera J (✉)
Otolaryngologist Department of Otolaryngology, Clínica Universidad de Los Andes,, Santiago, Chile

J. Pardo
Otolaryngologist Department of Otolaryngology, Clínica Universidad de Los Andes, Santiago, Chile
e-mail: jpardo@clinicauandes.cl

M. V. Goycoolea et al. (eds.), *Textbook of Otitis Media*, https://doi.org/10.1007/978-3-031-40949-3_23

stratum circulare is poorly developed and more vascularized, which makes it a weaker zone. On the other hand, at the level of the pars flaccida, this zone has no annulus (Rivinus segment), and its lamina propria has few elastic and collagen fibers, which are also disorganized. This exacerbates the weakness of this zone and increases the risk of retraction [7].

From a ventilation point of view, the middle ear is divided into two compartments by the tympanic diaphragm: a posterosuperior compartment, which includes the superior epitympanum and mastoid, and an anteroinferior compartment, which includes the mesotympanum, protympanum, hypotympanum, inferior retrotympanum, and inferior epitympanum (Prusak's space). The ventilation of the posterosuperior compartment depends on the tympanic diaphragm and its isthmus, whereas the anteroinferior compartment is ventilated directly by the Eustachian tube. In addition, the inferior epitympanum, which lies below the diaphragm and is independent of the superior epitympanum, is ventilated through the posterior pocket of the Von Tröltsch fascia into the mesotympanum.

Mastoid cells exhibit pneumatization, which occurs progressively from birth, from which age it eventually reaches only the antrum and is completed in adolescence. The mucosa of the mastoid is cuboidal, and its main function is gas exchange. In contrast, the mucosa of the middle ear is secretory, and its main function is mucociliary clearance.

When the middle ear mucosa becomes inflamed, it tends to reabsorb more gas, thus generating more negative pressure [8]. In addition, the inflamed mucosa tends to obstruct the airways, both at the level of the isthmus and at the level of the Eustachian tube. Obstruction at the level of the Eustachian tube generates poor diffuse ventilation, which predisposes the membrane to the generation of otitis media with effusion and to the global retraction of the tympanic membrane. On the other hand, altering segmental ventilation at the level of the isthmus predisposes the membrane to focal retractions and the formation of attic cholesteatomas.

At the cellular level, the infiltration of the eardrum by inflammatory cells in cases of otitis media with effusion destroys the lamina propria of the tympanic membrane, through the secretion of collagenase and elastase, which also generates atrophy [9, 10]. Atrophy is what predisposes the membrane to the formation of retraction pockets.

Formation of Retraction Pockets in the Pars Tensa

During otitis media with effusion, the chronic inflammatory process around the ossicular chain is more severe than in other areas of the middle ear. Draining this area around the ossicular chain is difficult, so the effusion tends to remain there, and granulation tissue could form [11]. This tissue can obstruct the superior retrotympanic airway, resulting in the poor ventilation of the posterior retrotympanum. The anatomical passage through which this area drains into the inferior mesotympanum is easily blocked by mucosal folds and by the infrastructure of the tympanic isthmus.

The inflame area around the ossicular chain irritates the eardrum and triggers the infiltration of inflammatory cells in the squamous layer of the pars flaccida and the posterosuperior quadrant of the pars tensa of the tympanic membrane. The inflammatory process's invasion into the tympanic membrane plays an important role in the development of retraction pockets and subsequent cholesteatoma formation, through the destruction of the lamina propria and the stimulation of keratinocyte growth and proliferation [12–14].

Formation of Retraction Pockets in the Pars Flaccida

Ventilation routes to the attic compartments are secured by the tympanic isthmus and by the anterior route through the incomplete tensor tympani fold in an anterior epitympanic recess of normal size.

Selective epitympanic dysventilation syndrome occurs when the tympanic isthmus of a complete tensor tympani fold has been blocked, resulting in the complete isolation of the epitympanum from the mesotympanum. This event induces a gas deficit and could be the basis for the selective decrease of gas pressure in the attic, which leads to the development of an attic retraction pocket and its possibly evolving into a cholesteatoma, even in subjects with normal Eustachian tube function [14].

An incomplete tensor tympani fold prevents the development of extensive pathology around the malleus and the attic, even in the presence of chronic otitis media [14]. In one study, the blockage of the isthmus and a complete tensor tympani fold were present in more than 96% of patients with attical disease, whereas only present in 19% in the control group [15].

The anterior epitympanic recess is important in the recurrence of otitis media with effusion. Complete control of the retraction pocket was not achieved even with a tympanoplasty with cartilage or the reconstruction of the lateral wall of the attic if there the surgery on the aeration of the anterior epitympanic recess was insufficient [14, 16].

Clinic

Clinical evaluations of a retraction pocket allow for differentiation between a stable retraction pocket and an unsafe retraction pocket, which progresses and is at risk of evolving into a cholesteatoma. Retraction pockets can remain silent for a long time. Their clinical symptoms depend on their extent and severity. Mild retractions are usually asymptomatic, and they may be associated middle ear effusion.

Retractions of the tympanum are incidentally diagnosed during examinations. Their symptoms, such as otorrhea and conductive hearing loss, as a result of a middle ear effusion, splinting of the tympanic membrane, or ossicular chain erosion, are recurrent. Otalgia may be present because of changes in middle ear pressure or infection [17]. Dizziness is a very rare symptom [14].

Otorrhea is mostly intermittent and can be spontaneous or can follow exposure to water. Hearing loss is mostly of the mild conductive type but can reach up to 45–55 dB in some cases. No correlation has been established between hearing threshold and retraction stages [14, 18]. But improvement in audiometry exams has been found over time in mild retraction pockets [19].

Diagnosis

Diagnosis is clinical and requires a visual examination of the tympanic membrane using an otoscope or microscope. A retraction is defined as an intact tympanic membrane that has been transformed into a very thin epidermal membrane retracted toward the medial wall of the tympanic cavity [14]. It is important to describe the severity of a retraction. The description should include its position, its depth, whether it is fixed or mobile, the presence of discharge, the accumulation of keratin, and the presence of bony erosion. This could be carried out by using one of the published staging methods or by describing it with text, drawings, or photographs [20].

Descriptions of Retractions

Retractions are localized to the pars flaccida and pars tensa; they are marginal, nonmarginal, or bilateral [14]. The location can be made more specific by describing the involved quadrant [1]. For adherence, the mobility of a retraction can be tested via the Valsalva maneuver; via delicate suctioning, which requires exercising caution so as not to disrupt the pocket membrane [14]; or by using a pneumatic otoscope [20].

In the pars tensa, descriptions should include the adhesion to the ossicular structures, the facial recess, the sinus tympani, the promontory, and the area deep into the retrotympanum. In the pars flaccida, descriptions should include the adhesion to the malleus.

For the external auditory canal's status, descriptions should include the presence of keratin accumulation at the retraction pocket and granulations; any bone erosion in the scutum and the posterosuperior quadrant; and the presence of otorrhea.

Ossicular status includes the focal lysis of the incus, any interruption of the incudostapedial joint, myringostapediopexy, and the lysis of the stapes.

Descriptions of the bottom of the retraction pocket should include whether it is visible, any crusting, and the presence of debris accumulation. If all the frontiers of the retraction pocket can be seen, it is called a controllable retraction pocket. This could be assessed by using an endoscope.

Descriptions of the neck of the retraction pocket should include whether it stays large and wide enough and whether it is capable of self-cleaning. A constricted neck results in debris accumulation inside the pocket and runs the risk of cholesteatoma formation [14].

In addition to their clinical uses, classification systems for retractions are useful for research, where the behavior of retractions can be studied. Also, any system must be validated and reproducible. All the currently used systems suffer from a high degree of interobserver variability by an individual and between individuals [17, 21]. Grading a retraction is considered a good protocol for the evaluation of its risk factors, especially those for developing a cholesteatoma, and helpful for making comparative assessments over time, once the retraction has progressed. However, studies have lacked a universally accepted or adopted staging system for retraction pockets. In addition, the functional deficit has not been included in any staging system [14], and none of these systems has a specific treatment method [1].

Retraction of the Pars Tensa

When the retraction compromises the pars tensa, it could be seen as retraction pocket, atelectasis, or adhesive otitis media. A retraction pocket is defined by a retraction of a fragile portion of the tympanic membrane, such as the pars tensa or the pars flaccida. Also, retraction pockets in both portions can occur in the same ear. The collapse of the whole membrane is called atelectasis. When the atelectatic membrane adheres to the middle ear floor, it is called adhesive otitis media [14]. An instance of general retraction or atelectasis is not called a retraction pocket until specific sections have been more retracted [1].

Retraction Pockets

A retraction pocket is a dynamic pathology with variable outcomes, and it's important to describe the stage of the retraction. For pars tensa retractions, the Sadé classification is the most popular [10], although others have been reported, such as Charachon [22]. Dornhoffer's staging is like the Sadé classification except that stage 4 is assigned to retraction pockets with invisible depths [1].

The Sadé classification is divided as follows:

Sadé I—retracted tympanic membrane
Sadé II—retraction with contact on the incus
Sadé III—middle ear atelectasis (tympanic membrane on the promontory, but mobile)
Sadé IV—adhesive otitis media (tympanic membrane on the promontory, but fixed) [17]

The Charachon classification is divided as follows:

Stage 1—mobile retraction pocket
Stage 2—fixed and controllable retraction pocket
Stage 3—fixed and uncontrollable retraction pocket [17]

Atelectasis or Adhesive Otitis Media

Mansour et al. described atelectatic ears as follows: when the middle ear space has been partially or completely obliterated but the tympanic membrane has not adhered to the medial wall of the middle ear and the mucosal lining of the middle ear is intact. They also described adhesive otitis media: when the tympanic membrane has been partially or totally bound to the medial wall of the middle ear by fibrous adhesions with no possibility of reversing the retraction. In cases of partial adhesions, there may be effusion in the middle ear. In mild cases, only a few adhesions may be present, while in more severely affected ears, the space area of the middle ear cavity has vanished and the ossicular system is no longer functional. Fibroadhesive otitis media is characterized by the presence of fibrosis in the middle ear cavity [14]. Finally, a cholesteatoma is defined as a non-self-cleaning retraction pocket with keratin accumulation inside the pocket even if the ear is free of discharge [20].

It is not possible to predict the course of a retraction. Those that will remain stable and safe might form a cholesteatoma or might even resolve. Cholesteatoma development occurs in 1%–5% of patients [19]. For this, the timing and the nature of any intervention remain unclear [17].

Retraction of the Pars Flaccida

The most used staging system is the Tos classification for pars flaccida retractions [2]. The Tos classification is divided as follows:

Tos I—the pars flaccida not in contact with the malleus head
Tos II—the pars flaccida in contact with the malleus head
Tos III—limited outer attic wall erosion
Tos IV—severe outer attic wall erosion

Evaluation

As part of an assessment of a patient with a tympanic membrane retraction, an audiometric evaluation with a pure-tone audiogram and tympanometry is usually performed [17]. CT or magnetic resonance imaging (MRI) scans could also be invaluable in assessing deep retraction pockets where the bottom cannot be seen on otoscopy [20]. CT imaging of retraction pockets is an important diagnostic tool when assessing the localization, the extension and the status of the ossicular chain, and the involvement of the middle ear compartments. Finding an associated evolving inflammatory process (via condensation images) of the middle ear on the CT scan may indicate an active disease and consequently point to an unfavorable prognosis [14].

Investigations into a retraction should include assessments of the upper respiratory tract. This is particularly important for patients with nasal or sinal symptoms [20]. Formal Eustachian tube function (ETF) tests are not standard investigations for retraction pockets. They are performed mainly for research purposes or considered on an individual basis [20]. Any patient that has a retraction pocket should be evaluated for ETF, though [1].

A scoring system (ETS-7) that assigns a score for ETF after combining physical exams, the ability to perform the Valsalva maneuver, and normal tubomanometry results has been developed, but tubomanometers are used at some clinical research centers. There are other ETF testing methods, but they are also less available. Many tympanometer brands feature software to test the ETF. Another option is to decrease the ear canal pressure to −200 daPa, which increases the middle ear pressure (MEP) to +200 daPa, and then to ask the patient to swallow, in order to determine how much can be corrected after one swallow and after five swallows. Then this process is repeated with the ear canal pressure increased to +200 daPa, increasing the MEP to −200 daPa. If a patient is able to correct the positive and negative MEPs with swallows, this indicates that their ETF is normal. Another method is to measure the baseline MEP and then ask the patient to perform a Valsalva maneuver; after this, measure the MEP to determine whether it has increased. If the patient can generate significant pressure, the Eustachian tube (ET) should open. If the ET does not open after the patient has performed the Valsalva maneuver, there may be ET dysfunction (ETD). If successful, the patient is then asked to swallow and correct the MEP difference. Achieving a similar degree of correction with one swallow and/or five swallows should indicate normal ETF. Abnormal test results are not always accurate in showing ETD, but ETD is easy to interpret when normal. Also, the ETD may be intermittent and not show up on exams [1].

Evolution

The progression should be monitored, especially in children. Regular observation is important to assess disease progression and monitor for complications, such as cholesteatoma formation. The untreated retraction pocket may stay unchanged in many cases, may show spontaneous resolution (which has been observed in about 40% of mild retraction cases), or may continuously progress to a precholesteatomatous stage or into a cholesteatoma [14]. A deep retraction pocket that cannot be completely visualized should be considered as carrying a significant risk of developing a cholesteatoma [23].

Kokko found that in 1%–4% of patients with otitis media with effusion who underwent ventilation tube insertions with or without adenoidectomy developed an attic cholesteatoma. The determinant factor in the evolution of a retraction pocket is the presence of the active and persistent inflammatory process inside the middle ear spaces and its effect on the neighboring segment of the tympanic membrane [24].

Treatment

There is no consensus among otologists on the indications, timing, or options for the adequate management of tympanic membrane retraction pockets. The literature does not offer enough studies with high levels of evidence to support any surgical intervention over watchful waiting in the management of mild to moderate degrees of tympanic membrane retraction pockets. There is also no good evidence to favor one treatment over other [14, 17, 20].

A systematic review by Nankivell et al. found two randomized controlled trials with small numbers of patients to analyze. Another randomized controlled trial was excluded because it lacked an appropriate control group. One aspect that affects the risk of bias in the included and excluded studies is the reliability of grading retraction pockets by using a staging system. This makes the interpretation of any studies performed using these systems difficult. No good evidence for the role of any individual surgical intervention for the management of atelectasis of the tympanic membrane was found. Nankivell et al.'s review does not show any statistical benefit of surgical intervention over taking a watch-and-wait approach [17]. Bayoumy et al.'s systematic review concluded that the evidence is heterogenous and depends on the patient population, location, and severity of the retractions [19].

In general, a clean, asymptomatic retraction pocket with normal hearing does not require surgery, even if it is in contact with the intact ossicular chain. The indications for surgery for retraction pockets are generally the same for children and adults. However, in children, assessing the upper respiratory tract is an important part of the management, and any retraction pockets should be more closely monitored in children than in adults [20].

If there is evidence that the patient has ETD, this should be assessed and managed if possible. Decisions for management may be made on the assumption that the dysfunction may continue. Other risk factors include exposure to viral respiratory tract infections, allergies, recurrent acute otitis media, recurrent sinusitis, and acid reflux, which should be evaluated and treated. Nasopharyngeal or parapharyngeal tumors can also manifest with ETD, and if the masses grow slowly, retraction pockets may develop [1].

Surgical Procedures

Indications for surgery on a retraction pocket include the following:

1. Otorrhea
2. Hearing impairment
3. Keratin accumulation within the retraction pocket
4. An inability to see the bottom of the retraction pocket or the polyp formation suggestive of cholesteatoma

However, the decision for surgery also depends on factors such as the degree of hearing loss, hearing in the opposite ear, patient compliance with follow-up monitoring, and the efficiency of the local treatment. A functional deficit of more than 30 dB could be an indication for surgery to improve hearing. The surgical indication for repairing a functional deficit is relative and must be formally studied and counseled. In children, asymptomatic but fixed retraction pockets may need to be monitored more frequently and for a longer period. In cases where compliance with the follow-up monitoring is in doubt, surgical intervention should be considered early, especially if the bottom of the retraction pocket cannot be seen. Surgical intervention is undoubtedly proposed in all cases featuring skin suffering and otorrhea with scutum erosion. A preoperative CT scan is recommended as part of an adequate workup [14, 20].

Ventilation Tubes

Myringotomy with a ventilation tube is indicated for the early stages to promote the ventilation of the middle ear. The indication for a grommet or T-tube is based on the progression of the retraction.

Using subannular ventilation tubes aims to avoid the early extrusion of the tube and recurrences and to avoid the risk of persistent tympanic membrane perforation [14]. Such a tube is placed beneath the annulus in the posteroinferior quadrant. A small skin flap is elevated with the annulus. A small burr is used to drill a canal in the posterior bony wall, then the tube is placed with the inner flange medial to the annulus of the middle ear [23]. This procedure confers good and lasting control over retraction pockets, but complications such as occluding the tube with debris or cerumen, chorda tympani injury and persisting otorrhea, may occur [14, 23].

Treatment of Eustachian Tube Dysfunction

Many medical and surgical treatments for Eustachian tube dysfunction (ETD) have been investigated, but none has been proven effective in high-quality randomized controlled trials. Medical treatments primarily include decongestants, antihistamines, and nasal steroids [17]. Several devices can equilibrate the middle ear pressure to the environment, such as the Otovent nasal balloon device and the EarPopper [1]. Preventive treatment must be taken as early as possible to stop the process before it reaches the end stage: severe adhesive otitis media [14].

Several surgical treatments are available when medical therapy fails. Surgical treatments aim to enlarge the narrowed Eustachian tube. The most common procedures are laser tuboplasty and balloon tuboplasty [25]. Laser tuboplasty with the ablation of some pathological findings at the posterior half of the tube in cases of tubal tonsils, a narrow orifice of the tubal ending, or an adenoid has been reported in 70% of cases, and patients who had these were offered an improvement to their ET function [14]. Balloon tuboplasty has been shown to significantly improve ETD and, compared with laser tuboplasty, has shown a greater tympanometry improvement rate [25]. A systematic review by Huisman et al. found that this procedure reduced the symptoms associated with ETD [26]. Huhnd et al. showed that 31% patients with tympanic membrane retraction experienced an improvement in middle ear ventilation and that 54% of the patients perceived an improvement in their clinical symptoms after a Eustachian tube dilatation [27].

There are no randomized clinical trials showing the efficacy of balloon dilation, but in experienced hands, this procedure is considered safe. Therefore, if this procedure were to be tried on some patients, the recommendation is in the group of patients with ongoing ETD [1].

Adenoidectomy improves tubal function. The effect of cleft palate repair on improving tubal function has been variously reported in literature. The impact of septal deviations on the middle ear has been demonstrated; it has reflected tubal dysfunction caused by turbulence from inspiratory air at the nasopharynx. The beneficial effect of septoplasty on tubal function has been demonstrated by several studies [14].

Tympanectomy

Tympanectomy is a surgical procedure that resects the retracted portion of the ear, leaving a perforation. A ventilation tube is placed in the tympanic remnant. In a 2-year study, tympanectomy was performed on 50 ears, and the indication of this technique was retraction Sadé II or larger. After an average of 12 months of follow-up, 34 cases (68%) showed a normal eardrum. In nine cases, the eardrum retracted again, and six showed a perforation. On average, spontaneous closure occurred in 4–7 weeks [28]. Other authors have considered not excising too-large areas because large perforations may result. Such an excision should be performed only if retraction has been limited to one quadrant. Cases must be followed long enough after the extrusion of the tube to look for recurrence [14]. A systematic review showed that created perforations persist in 3%–13% and showed recurrences in 11%–25% of the patients [19].

Tympanoplasty

This intervention involves the excision of the retraction and then reconstruction [19]. A cartilage graft is considered to provide good reinforcement for the tympanic membrane and resists middle ear pressure variations, even in the case of severe Eustachian tube dysfunction. But the cartilage is less compliant, has a negative impact during higher sudden pressure variations, may hide possible future cholesteatoma formation, and does not relieve the middle ear from its causal pathology. The reported recurrence rate of retraction with this procedure is between 5% and 45% [14]. Different techniques for cartilage tympanoplasty have been described [23]. Finally, at 10-year follow-ups examining the retraction pockets reconstructed with perichondrium or temporalis fascia, the recurrence rates were as follows: 80% of the ears were repaired with fascia and 40% with perichondrium [14].

In the Cochrane revision of 2010, the findings from one study [29] suggest that surgical intervention with the tragal cartilage reconstruction of the lateral attic wall reduces the risk of the progression of the retraction pocket, but the study design had a high potential risk of bias. The findings of another study [30] suggest no additional benefit would come from also inserting ventilation tubes into patients undergoing cartilage tympanoplasty [17].

If an ear exhibits reasonably normal ETF, a VT may not be placed, and the retraction pocket should be surgically managed with a tympanoplasty. If ETD is suspected, the recommendation is to insert a VT at the time of tympanoplasty. With evidence or suspicion of ongoing ETD, medial grafts can be used, but they carry higher risks of failure. It's important to prevent the graft from medializing. In general, using a lateral graft is better but more difficult to perform for ongoing ETD, and it carries a higher risk of blunting, lateralization, and cholesteatoma formation if not carried out by experienced hands. If the lateral graft technique is used, it is better to completely remove the retraction pocket [1].

Tympanoplasty and ossiculoplasty should be considered to treat hearing loss caused by middle ear atelectasis and ossicular chain interruption. Mastoidectomy does not add a favorable prognostic factor to the management of retraction in terms of hearing recovery or recurrence rate [31].

Patients who have undergone a successful cartilage tympanoplasty for either pars tensa retraction pockets or pars flaccida retraction pockets should be followed up with for at least 3–5 years. The patients should be informed of the symptoms of otorrhea and hearing loss and inform of the need to return for review [20].

Endoscopic Ear Surgery

Using an endoscope allows surgeons to explore the hidden areas of the middle ear, such the retrotympanum and its surrounding structures, the epitympanum, and the protympanum. This surgical technique preserves the healthy mucosa of the middle ear and the mastoid. The Eustachian tube plays an important role in the aeration of the middle ear, but other anatomic factors are likewise important, such are the epitympanic diaphragm and the tympanic isthmus. The tympanic isthmus is crucial in the ventilation of the attic, and the blockage of it is defined as selective epitympanic dysventilation syndrome. To treat this condition, a surgery of the isthmus must be performed to restore the ventilation pathway. Thanks to the endoscope, new concepts have been developed in the surgical treatment of middle ear pathologies [32]. Endoscopic tympanoplasty for retractions is a promising surgical technique, but further studies are needed to confirm previous results [19].

Atticotomy

Limited pars flaccid retraction may be approached by performing an endaural atticotomy. The amount of bone removed depends on the degree of exposure required to investigate the presence of squamous epithelium and explore the tympanic isthmus. Any surgical defects can be reconstructed by using cortical bone, bone wax, or cartilage [23]. The epitympanum needs open ventilation routes, so the physiological pathways of aeration for the diseased compartments must be restored and the adequate gas exchange of the middle ear must be ensured to avoid the recurrence of the retraction [14].

Resection of the Retraction and Mastoid Obliteration

Mastoid obliteration reduces the degree of transmucosal gas exchange in the middle ear and the need for ventilation to be compensated for by using a Eustachian tube. The indication for this procedure relies on the grade of aeration of the tympanum, as shown on CT scan images of the temporal bone. This procedure decreases the incidence of cholesteatoma development but cannot eliminate the recurrence of a retraction pocket [14].

Treatment of Middle Ear Atelectasis

Atelectasis may be reversible with the use of ventilating tubes. Atelectatic tympanic membranes can be restored to their normal position via the administration of nitrous oxide to a patient under general anesthesia and via the insertion of a ventilating tube. Ventilating the middle ear may bring back the tympanic membrane to its normal position and restore its consistency, thus preventing its progressing to adhesive otitis media [14].

Tympanoplasty consists of carefully elevating the thin tympanic membrane from the medial wall of the middle ear, reconstructing the ossicular chain and inspecting the antrum, and then reinforcing the eardrum with cartilage to maintain an air-filled tympanic cavity [1, 23]. This procedure carries a high risk of inducing an iatrogenic cholesteatoma and hearing loss and has a high rate of failure. The surgery is not indicated in asymptomatic adhesive otitis media with normal hearing, because hearing function is not easy to improve. Recurrent otorrhea, cholesteatoma, and conductive hearing loss are indications for intervention. The risks and benefits of surgery must be discussed with the patient [14].

The European Academy of Otology and Neurotology (EAONO) wrote a consensus-based practical guide featuring several recommendations for retractions [20].

For an adult with a pars tensa retraction pocket requiring surgery, the EAONO recommends cartilage reinforcement for the retraction pocket or cartilage tympanoplasty. The added benefit of using a ventilation tube remains uncertain, except in cases with concomitant middle ear effusion.

It is prudent to monitor these pockets for at least 12 months, to check that they remain stable. Upon discharge from outpatient follow-up, patients should be informed of the symptoms of otorrhea and hearing loss and informed of the need to return for review.

For a child with a pars tensa retraction pocket requiring surgery, the EAONO recommends inserting a ventilation tube as the first line of treatment. Cartilage tympanoplasty should be reserved for retractions that persist following the failure of ventilation tube insertion. The combination of ventilation tube insertion and a simple excision of the retraction pocket is a simple technique used by some surgeons, but it may cause a residual perforation or iatrogenic cholesteatoma.

For an adult or a child with a pars flaccida retraction pocket requiring surgery, atticotomy and cartilage reconstruction for the outer attic wall is generally the surgery of choice. In less-severe cases, it may be possible to clear the debris and observe.

For patients with complete atelectasis who present with hearing loss, the EAONO recommends that they be monitored for at least 12 months with hearing rehabilitation using a hearing aid if necessary. Children may need to be monitored more frequently and for a longer period. However, the long-term results from hearing restoration surgery have been disappointing overall.

References

1. Alpert C, Olszewska E. Assessment and management of retraction pockets. Otolaryngol Pol. 2017;71(1):1–21.
2. Tos M. Anatomy and histology of the middle ear. Clin Rev Allergy. 1984;2:267–84.
3. Stangerup SE, Tos M, Arnesen R, Larsen P. A cohort study of point prevalence of eardrum pathology in children and teenagers from age 5 to age 16. Eur Arch Otorhinolaryngol. 1994;251(7):399–401.
4. Tos M, Poulsen G. Attic retractions following secretory otitis. Acta Otolaryngol. 1980;89(5–6):479–86.
5. Maw AR, Hall AJ, Pothier DD, Gregory SP, Steer CD. The prevalence of tympanic membrane and related middle ear pathology in children: a large longitudinal cohort study followed from birth to age ten. Otol Neurotol. 2011;32(8):1256–61.
6. De Beer BA, Schilder AG, Zielhuis GA, Graamans K. Natural course of tympanic membrane pathology related to otitis media and ventilation tubes between ages 8 and 18 years. Otol Neurotol. 2005;26(5):1016–21.
7. Mansour S, et al. Comprehensive and clinical anatomy of the middle ear. Berlin/Heidelberg: Springer; 2013.
8. Ruah CB, Schachern PA, Paparella MM, Zelterman D. Mechanisms of retraction pocket formation in the pediatric tympanic membrane. Arch Otolaryngol Head Neck Surg. 1992;118(12):1298–305.
9. Ars BM, Dirckx JJ, Decraemer WF, Ars-Piret NM. Faulty aeration of the middle ear: repercussion on the tympanic membrane lamina propria. In: Sadé J, editor. The Eustachian tube, basic aspects. Amsterdam: Kugler and Ghedini Publications; 1991. p. 365–71.
10. Sadé J, Berco E. Atelectasis and secretory otitis media. Ann Otol Rhinol Laryngol. 1976;85(Suppl 25 Pt 2):66–72.
11. Zhang Q, Liang J. Transformation of effusion and formation of granulation tissue in the pathologic process of otitis media with effusion. Lin Chuang Er Bi Yan Hou Ke Za Zhi. 1999;13(1):8–11.
12. Hueb MM, Goycoolea MV, Muchow D, Duvall AJ, Paparella MM, Sheridan C. In search of missing links in otology, III: development of a new animal model for cholesteatoma. Laryngoscope. 1993;103(7):774–84.
13. Massuda ET, Oliveira JA. A new experimental model of acquired cholesteatoma. Laryngoscope. 2005;115(3):481–5.
14. Mansour S et al. Tympanic membrane retraction pocket: overview and advances in diagnosis and management. doi: https://doi.org/10.1007/978-3-319-13996-8_8.
15. Marchioni D, Mattioli F, Alicandri-Ciufelli M, Presutti L. Prevalence of ventilation blockages in patients affected by attic pathology: a case-control study. Laryngoscope. 2013;123(11):2845–53.
16. Mansour S, Nicolas K, Naim A, Yamine F, Moukarzel N, Nehme A. Inflammatory chronic otitis media and the anterior epitympanic recess. J Otolaryngol. 2005;34(3):149–59.
17. Nankivell PC, Pothier DD. Surgery for tympanic membrane retraction pockets. Cochrane Database Syst Rev. 2010;(7):CD007943. https://doi.org/10.1002/14651858.CD007943.pub2.
18. Amioni, et al. Tympanic atelectasis in children and early surgical approach. Int Adv Otol. 2011;7:293–8.
19. Bayoumy AB, Veugen CCAFM, van der Veen EL, Bok JM, de Ru JA, Thomeer HGXM. Management of tympanic membrane retractions: a systematic review. Eur Arch Otorhinolaryngol. 2022;279(2):723–37. https://doi.org/10.1007/s00405-021-06719-3. Epub 2021 Mar 10.
20. Yung M, Neumann C. A consensus-based practical guide on the management of retraction pockets of pars tensa and pars flaccida. J Int Adv Otol. 2013;9:12–5.
21. Pothier D. Sade and Tos classifications of the tympanic membrane: Ot reliable? Clin Otolaryngol. 2006;31(3):249.
22. Charachon R, Barthez M, Lejeune JM. Spontaneous retraction pockets in chronic otitis media medical and surgical therapy. Ear Nose Throat J. 1992;71(11):578–83.
23. Goycoolea MV, de Souza C. Atlas of otologic surgery and magic otology, vol. 1. 2nd ed. p. 739–54.
24. Kokko E. Chronic secretory otitis media in children. A clinical study. Acta Otolaryngol Suppl. 1974;327:1–44.
25. Wang TC, Lin CD, Shih TC, Chung HK, Wang CY, Tsou YA, Huang CH, Tsai MH. Comparison of balloon dilation and laser eustachian tuboplasty in patients with eustachian tube dysfunction: a meta-analysis. Otolaryngol Head Neck Surg. 2018;158(4):617–26. https://doi.org/10.1177/0194599817753609. Epub 2018 Mar 20.
26. Huisman JML, Verdam FJ, Stegeman I, de Ru JA. Treatment of Eustachian tube dysfunction with balloon dilation: a systematic review. Laryngoscope. 2018;128(1):237–47. https://doi.org/10.1002/lary.26800. Epub 2017 Aug 11.
27. Huhnd LE, Wirtz SP, Schrom T. Stellenwert der Tubendilatation bei Mittelohradhäsivprozess [Balloon dilation oft the Eustachian tube in tympanic membrane retraction]. Laryngorhinootologie. 2018;97(10):688–93. https://doi.org/10.1055/a-0640-9270. German. Epub 2018 Jun 28.
28. Bonilla G. Timpanectomy for eardrum retractions. Rev otorrinolaringol cir cabeza cuello. 1998;58(3):135–9.
29. Barbara M. Lateral attic reconstruction technique: preventive surgery for epitympanic retraction pockets. Otol Neurotol. 2008;29(4):522–5.
30. Elsheikh MN, Elsherief HS, Elsherief SG. Cartilage tympanoplasty for management of tympanic membrane atelectasis: is ventilatory tube necessary? Otol Neurotol. 2006;27(6):859–64.
31. Dispenza F, Mistretta A, Gullo F, Riggio F, Martines F. Surgical management of retraction pockets: does mastoidectomy have a role? Int Arch Otorhinolaryngol. 2021;25(1):e12–7. https://doi.org/10.1055/s-0040-1709196. Epub 2020 Apr 24.
32. Marchioni D, Rubini A, Soloperto D. Endoscopic ear surgery: redefining middle ear anatomy and physiology. Otolaryngol Clin North Am. 2021;54(1):25–43. https://doi.org/10.1016/j.otc.2020.09.003. Epub 2020 Nov 2.

Ventilation Tubes

24

Ann Hermansson

Background

Acute otitis media (AOM) and secretory otitis media (SOM) or otitis media with effusion (OME) [1] is fairly well defined in international recommendations. The difference basically is that while AOM is an infectious disease with acute onset, SOM is the presence of effusion in the middle ear without any associated signs of acute ear infection. It is thus different from AOM, which causes pain and symptoms of acute illness, in having much less obvious symptoms and not having an acute onset. SOM might cause a substantial hearing loss which if present for longer periods can affect both speech development and behavior [2].

Most children experience a few episodes of AOM, while almost all will suffer SOM for shorter periods during and after upper airway infections [3]. Also, most episodes of AOM are followed by an episode of SOM. In most countries, the recommended treatment for both uncomplicated sporadic AOM and SOM is watchful waiting. This is since they tend to be self-limiting, healing well in most cases without treatment or sequele.

In some instances, however, the child will experience recurrent episodes of AOM. The definition of recurrent AOM (rAOM) is agreed to be when there is three or more episodes in 6 months, or four in 1 year with the most recent in the last 6 months [4]. These children and their families experience a substantial impact on quality of life that actually has been shown to be comparable to childhood asthma [5]. Repeated episodes of AOM are also related to frequent antibiotic use, since most guidelines recommend antibiotic treatment of these children. Children with rAOM will also suffer frequent, perhaps prolonged, periods of SOM.

SOM might also have a more complicated course with repeated or perhaps long-standing periods of hearing loss. It has been suggested that these episodes could affect not only hearing but also speech development, general behavior, and perhaps vestibular function [6, 7]. No long-term effect of antibiotics has been shown in the treatment of SOM [8], and no other medical treatments are recommended [9].

History of Ventilation Tubes

Already in 400 BC, the Hippocratic school described middle ear effusion that could be relieved by incising the eardrum [10]. Myringotomy was practiced to relieve "deafness" with various success during the centuries thereafter. A more scientific approach to myringotomy was begun in the late eighteenth century, and in 1801 Astley Cooper presented two papers to the Royal Society showing that myringotomy indeed could improve hearing. He was aware that bone conduction must be present and to ensure this he placed a watch on the patients' incisors or mastoid and made sure they could hear it better than when it was held near the outer ear [11]. Later in the nineteenth century, Adam Politzer is credited with the first use of suction to remove fluid [12]. He is also thought to have designed the first ventilation tube, in an attempt to overcome the problem of keeping the perforation open for a longer period. Several other attempts were done to keep the perforation open. They however met with very little success, and the attempts were abandoned. It was not until 1954 that a vinyl tube that was successful in airing the middle ear was introduced by Beverly Armstrong [13], and the use of ventilation tubes was introduced worldwide.

Effect of Ventilation Tubes

Ventilation tubes have now been used in the treatment of middle ear problems for many years. The tubes are not supposed to drain the ear but to overcome the pressure differences and ventilate the ear. In this way, they fulfill the double purpose of preventing collection of fluid in the middle ear and create a better environment for the middle ear mucosa.

A. Hermansson (✉)
Department of ENT, Lund University Hospital, Lund, Sweden
e-mail: ann.hermansson@med.lu.se

M. V. Goycoolea et al. (eds.), *Textbook of Otitis Media*, https://doi.org/10.1007/978-3-031-40949-3_24

Ventilation tubes are used in both rAOM and SOM, and indeed many of the children treated with ventilation tubes will suffer from a combination of both. When used in rAOM, the main indication is reducing the numbers of AOM episodes while in SOM the main indication is to better the hearing [9].

In a Cochrane review [14] published in 2018, it is concluded that children receiving grommets are less likely to have AOM recurrences compared to those managed by active monitoring or placebo medication. However, the effect is modest already during the first six months and even lower after 12 months.

Another Cochrane review [15] states that no effect was seen on speech development in otherwise healthy children after ventilation tube placement.

Some studies have however shown a positive effect on quality of life (QoL) of children with OM after insertion of ventilating tube [16], especially in those suffering from both rAOM and severe SOM. There are also indications in all studies that ventilation tubes should be considered earlier in otherwise impaired children. In several studies, it has been stated that ventilation tubes for rAOM should only be considered if there are persistent SOM in one or both ears [17–20]. There is also an ongoing discussion on the additive effect of ventilation tubes and adenoidectomy in the treatment of rAOM. There seems indeed to be a modest effect on the number of recurrences, especially in children under the age of two years, if adenoidectomy is done when placing tubes [21, 22].

Since keeping antibiotic use low in children is strongly suggested to reduce the risk of antibiotic resistance in upper airway pathogens, prolonged antibiotic treatment is not recommended as first-line treatment in rAOM. It has also been suggested that ventilation tubes may reduce the severity of AOM recurrences and allow for topical rather than oral antibiotic treatment of AOM episodes which would make the impact on antibiotic use greater than the reduction in numbers of episodes would suggest.

SOM mostly resolves spontaneously; thus, all current guidelines recommend a three-month period of watchful waiting in children with SOM who are not at particular risk for speech, language, or learning problems. Medical treatments such as decongestants, antihistamines, and oral/intranasal corticosteroids are either ineffective or may cause adverse effects [23–25]. Ventilation tubes are thus the main option in children with SOM and hearing impairment lasting more than 3 months [26, 27].

The most common problem in children treated with ventilation tubes is ear discharge. It has been shown that in small children, it is often caused by an AOM while in older children it is more often caused by contamination through the ear canal. It has also been shown that topical treatment with ear drops is sufficient in most cases and oral antibiotics seldom are needed [28, 29]. Probably due to biofilm formation, some patients will experience prolonged periods of otorrhea, sometimes resulting in the need for removal of the tube [30].

The other major risk is that of persistent perforation of the tympanic membrane. When using modern tubes, it has been shown to be low. The long-term results after ventilation tube treatment are good, although more tympanosclerosis are seen in patients treated with ventilation tubes [31, 32]. Some have claimed that the use of ventilation tubes might cause more cholesteatomas to develop, while others have claimed that tubes could prevent the formation of cholesteatomas. No conclusive evidence has been found of either theory [33, 34].

Different types of ventilation tubes have been tried both concerning design, material, and coating. Tubes designed to stay longer have a greater risk of causing persistent perforations and tympanosclerosis [35]. On the other hand, early extrusion is a problem in some patients causing re-operations. This risk seems to differ with different kinds of tubes [36].

It is interesting to note that there are great regional differences in the use of ventilation tubes, indicating that indications vary not only over time but also regionally. Denmark is probably the country where most tubes are used with a prevalence as high as almost 30% during the first three years of life [37], while neighboring Sweden have much lower rates. It is also interesting to note that although some countries have shown a declining rate of ventilation tube use after the introduction of vaccine against pneumococci, this has not been the case in Denmark.

References

1. Rosenfeld RM, Shin JJ, Schwartz SR, Coggins R, Gagnon L, Hackell JM, et al. Clinical practice guideline: otitis media with effusion (update). Otolaryngol Head Neck Surg. 2016;154:S1–S41.
2. Roberts J, Hunter L, Gravel J, Rosenfeld R, Berman S, Haggard M, Hall J, Lannon C, Moore D, Vernon-Feagans L, Wallace I, Carey WB. Otitis media, hearing loss, and language learning: controversies and current research. J Dev Behav Pediatr. 2004;25:122.
3. Todberg T, Koch A, Andersson M, Olsen SF, Lous J, Homøe P. Incidence of otitis media in a contemporary Danish National Birth Cohort. PLoS One. 2014; https://doi.org/10.1371/journal.pone.0111732.
4. Goycoolea MV, Hueb MM, Ruah C. Otitis media: the pathogenesis approach. Definitions and terminology. Otolaryngol Clin N Am. 1991;24:757–61.
5. Brouwer CN, Rovers MM, Maillé AR, Veenhoven RH, Grobbee DE, Sanders EA, et al. The impact of recurrent acute otitis media on the quality of life of children and their children and caregivers. Clin Otolaryngol. 2005;30(3):258–65.
6. Cohen MS, Mandel EM, Furman JM, Sparto PJ, Casselbrant ML. Tympanostomy tube placement and vestibular function in children. Otolaryngol Head Neck Surg. 2011;145(4):666–72.
7. Herzog C, Homøe P, Koch A, Niclasen J, Dammeyer J, Lous J, Kørvel-Hanquist A. Effects of early childhood otitis media and ventilation tubes on psychosocial wellbeing—a prospective cohort study within the Danish National Birth Cohort. Int J Pediatr Otorhinolaryngol. 2020;133:109961.

8. Venekamp RP, Burton MJ, van Dongen TMA, van der Heijden GJ, van Zon A, Schilder AGM. Antibiotics for otitis media with effusion in children. Cochrane Database Syst Rev. 2016;2016(6):CD009163.
9. Simon M, Haggard RM, Rosenfeld H, Jia S, Peer M-N, Calmels V, Couloigner N, Teissier. International consensus (ICON) on management of otitis media with effusion in children. Eur Ann Otorhinolaryngol Head Neck Dis. 135(1):S33–9.
10. Black NA. Is glue ear a modern phenomenon?—a historical review of the medical literature. Clin Otolaryngol. 1984;9(3):155–63.
11. McGovern FH. Sir Astley Cooper and his otological papers. Ann Otol Rhinol Laryngol. 1984;93(6 pt 1):531–3.
12. Mudry A. The role of Adam Politzer (1835-1920) in the history of otology. Am J Otol. 2000;21(1):753–63.
13. Armstrong BW. A new treatment for chronic secretory otitis media. Arch Otolaryngol. 1954;59(4):653–65.
14. Venekamp PM, Schilder AGM, Nunez DA. Grommets(ventilation tubes) for recurrent acute otitis media in children. Cochrane Database Syst Rev. 2018;2018(5):CD012017.
15. Browning G, Rovers M, Williamson I, Lous J, Burton M. Grommets (ventilation tubes) for hearing loss associated with otitis media with effusion in children. Cochrane Database Syst Rev. Review—Intervention Version published: 06 October 2010 Version history.
16. Heidemann, Lauridsen HH, Kjeldsen AD, Faber CE, Johansen ECJ, Godballe C. Quality-of-life differences among diagnostic subgroups of children receiving ventilating tubes for otitis media. Otolaryngol Head Neck Surg. 2015;153(4):636–43.
17. McDonald S, Langton Hewer CD, Nunez DA. Grommets (ventilation tubes) for recurrent acute otitis media in children. Cochrane Database Syst Rev. 2008;4:CD004741.
18. Rosenfeld RM, et al. Clinical practice guideline: tympanostomy tubes in children. Otolaryngol Head Neck Surg. 2013;149:S1–35. 179. Boonacker, C. W. et al.
19. Hellström S, et al. Ventilation tube treatment: a systematic review of the literature. Otolaryngol Head Neck Surg. 2011;145:383–95.
20. Lous J, Ryborg CT, Thomsen JL. A systematic review of the effect of tympanostomy tubes in children with recurrent acute otitis media. Int J Pediatr Otorhinolaryngol. 2011;75:1058–61.
21. Boonacker CW, et al. Adenoidectomy with or without grommets for children with otitis media: an individual patient data meta-analysis. Health Technol Assess. 2014;18:1–118.
22. Kujala T, Alho OP, Loutonen J, Kristo A, Uhari M, Renko M, et al. Tympanostomy with and without adenoidectomy for the prevention of recurrences of acute otitis media: a randomized controlled trial. Pediatr Infect Dis J. 2012;31(6):565–9.
23. Griffin G, Flynn CA. Antihistamines and/or decongestants for otitis media with effusion (OME) in children. Cochrane Database Syst Rev. 2011;9:CD003423. 181.
24. Simpson SA, Lewis R, van der Voort J, Butler CC. Oral or topical nasal steroids for hearing loss associated with otitis media with effusion in children. Cochrane Database Syst Rev. 2011;5:CD001935.
25. Venekamp RP, et al. Antibiotics for otitis media with effusion in children. Cochrane Database Syst Rev. 2016;6:CD009163.
26. National Institute for Health and Clinical Excellence. Surgical management of otitis media with effusion in children. NICE Clinical Guideline 60. Developed by the National Collaborating Centre for Women's and Children's Health. NICE; 2008. http://www.nice.org.uk/nicemedia/pdf/CG60NICEguideline.pdf.
27. Rovers MM, et al. Grommets in otitis media with effusion: an individual patient data meta-analysis. Arch Dis Child. 2005;90:480–5.
28. van Dongen TM, van der Heijden GJ, Venekamp RP, Rovers MM, Schilder AG. A trial of treatment for acute otorrhea in children with tympanostomy tubes. N Engl J Med. 2014;370:723–33.
29. Granath A, Rynnel-Dagöö B, Backheden M, Lindberg K. Tube associated otorrhea in children with recurrent acute otitis media: results of a prospective randomized study on bacteriology and topical treatment with or without systemic antibodies. Int J Pediatr Otorhinolaryngol. 2008;72(8):1225–33.
30. Wang JC, Hamood AN, Saadeh C, Cunningham MJ, Yim MT. Cordero strategies to prevent biofilm-based tympanostomy tube infections. J Int J Pediatr Otorhinolaryngol. 2014;78(9):1433–8.
31. Cayé-Thomasen P, Stangerup SE, Jørgensen G, Drozdziewic D, Bonding P, Tos M. Myringotomy versus ventilation tubes in secretory otitis media: eardrum pathology, hearing, and eustachian tube function 25 years after treatment. Otol Neurotol. 2008;29(5):649–57.
32. Alenezi EMA, Robinson M, Choi RSM, Veselinovic T, Richmond PC, Eikelboom RH, Brennan-Jones CG. Long-term follow-up after recurrent otitis media and ventilation tube insertion: hearing outcomes and middle-ear health at six years of age. Int J Pediatr Otorhinolaryngol. 2022;163:111379.
33. Roland NJ, Phillips DE, Rogers JH, Singh SD. The use of ventilation tubes and the incidence of cholesteatoma surgery in the paediatric population of Liverpool. Clin Otolaryngol Allied Sci. 1992;17(5):437–9.
34. Djurhuus BD, Christensen K, Skytthe A, Faber CE. The impact of ventilation tubes in otitis media on the risk of cholesteatoma on a national level. Int J Pediatr Otorhinolaryngol. 2015;79(4):605–9.
35. Van Heerbeek N, De Saar GMAC, Mulder JJS. Long-term ventilation tubes: results of 726 insertions. Clin Otolaryngol Allied Sci. 2002;27(5):378–83.
36. Knutsson J, Priwin C, Hessén-Söderman AC, Rosenblad A, von Unge M. A randomized study of four different types of tympanostomy ventilation tubes—full-term follow-up. Int J Pediatr Otorhinolaryngol. 2018;107:140–4.
37. Pedersen TM, Mora-Jensen AC, Waage J, Bisgaard H, Stokholm J. Incidence and determinants of ventilation tubes in Denmark. PLoS One. 2016;11:e0165657–11.

Post-Tympanostomy Tube Otorrhea and Other Complications

25

Henrique Furlan Pauna, Rafael C. Monsanto,
Letícia A. Oyama, Ana Paula Chornobay, Karina Salvi,
Livia Tamie T. Sassaki, and Michael M. Paparella\

Introduction

Otitis media with effusion is one of the most common diseases of childhood [1]. It is estimated that 35–70% of prescholars experience at least one episode of otitis media with effusion (OME), and 17%–41% of children between 2 and 3 years old have chronic OME [2]. Ventilation tube surgery is frequently top ranked among the most performed surgery in the United States yearly. The American Academy of Otolaryngology—Head and Neck Surgery (AAO-HNS) clinical practice guideline recommends that tympanostomy tube insertion should be offered to children with bilateral OME exceeding 3 months and have documented hearing difficulties or symptoms that are likely attributable to OME (such as vestibular problems, poor school performance, behavioral problems, ear discomfort, or reduced quality of life) [3]. The ventilation tube provides middle ear pressure equalization and drainage of effusion; additionally, it allows topical administration of antibiotic therapy [4].

Untreated otitis media may result in clinically intractable middle-ear changes (such as chronic tympanic membrane perforations, fibrosis, cholesterol granuloma, ossicular chain erosion, and even cholesteatoma), in a process termed by Paparella as "otitis media continuum" [5–7]. Tympanostomy tubes are considered a safe, cost-effective treatment of chronic OME, potentially preventing the development of these tissue abnormalities [6]. The surgical procedure is simple, requiring only a small myringotomy and the use of adequate instruments to position the tube (Fig. 25.1). Regarding the optimal position of the ventilation tube, most protocols recommend the tube to be inserted in the anterior–inferior quadrant of the tympanic membrane. It is not recommended to position the tubes in the posterior–superior quadrant due to the risk of inadvertently damaging the ossicular chain. Although a few surgeons find the posterior–inferior quadrant ideal in cases presenting with stenotic external auditory canals, there is a risk of damaging the round window membrane and the jugular bulb (in cases it is high and dehiscent). Paparella [8] described that the anterior–superior quadrant would be ideal for the tube placement, adjacent to the handle of the malleus and halfway between the umbo, which often contacts the promontory and short process of the malleus (Fig. 25.2). The author hypothesized that the anterior quadrant would facilitate ventilation through the eustachian tube as it would be in a "valley" at the level of the protympanum. When placed inferiorly, the tube could be obstructed by the promontory in cases of retracted membranes (Fig. 25.2).

There are several types of ventilation tubes available for clinical use, and those can be classified in short-term (Shepard, Sheehy, Shah, Reuter-Bobbin, Paparella type 1, Donaldson, Armstrong) or long-term (butterfly, Paparella types 2 and 3, Per-Lee, Triune, Goode T-Tube) tubes. The short-term tubes are indicated for children who have a presumably temporary eustachian tube dysfunction (eustachian tube immaturity or blockage due to a hyperplastic adenoid), while long-term tubes are mostly indicated for cases where a prolonged or permanent eustachian tube dysfunction is expected, or after a short-term tube has failed to provide efficient ventilation [9]. Short-term tubes tend to extrude spontaneously at 6–18 months, but some may remain in the tympanic membrane years after insertion [9]. In comparison to short-term tubes, long-term tubes typically have a larger luminal diameter and medial flange [9].

H. F. Pauna
Hospital Universitário Cajuru, Curitiba, PR, Brazil

Hospital IPO, Curitiba, PR, Brazil

R. C. Monsanto (✉) · M. M. Paparella
Department of Otolaryngology, Head & Neck Surgery, University of Minnesota, Minnesota, MN, USA
e-mail: rdacosta@umn.edu

L. A. Oyama · A. P. Chornobay
Hospital Universitário Cajuru, Curitiba, PR, Brazil

K. Salvi · L. T. T. Sassaki
Department of Otolaryngology, Banco de Olhos de Sorocaba Hospital, Sorocaba, SP, Brazil
e-mail: rdacosta@umn.edu

M. V. Goycoolea et al. (eds.), *Textbook of Otitis Media*, https://doi.org/10.1007/978-3-031-40949-3_25

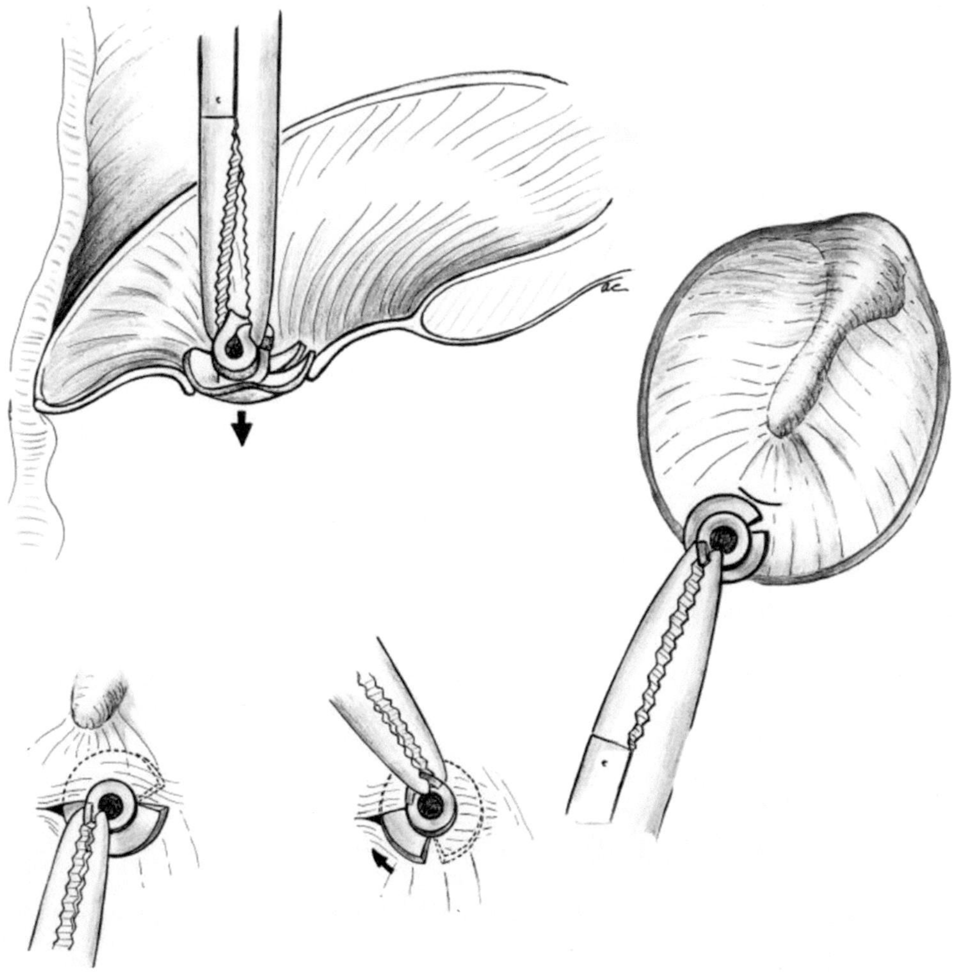

Fig. 25.1 A schematic drawing showing the placement of a Paparella tympanostomy tube. The top figure shows the inner flange of type 2 or 3 tube folding as the tube is pushed through a small myringotomy. The figure in the right, a type 2 tube, is placed close to the myringotomy incision. The figure in the bottom left represents the placement of part of the inner flange using an alligator forceps. The bottom right shows the tube being twisted until the remainder of the inner flange slides to the middle ear through the tympanic membrane

Paparella et al. [10] developed a series of ventilation tubes (Paparella type 1, type 2, and type 3) (Fig. 25.3) that are advantageous to other options of tubes for several reasons. They are made of soft, pliable rubber that is inert; they have been developed to be used for both routine and complicated cases; and they have a notch in the inner flange that allows insertion through a smaller incision, which works best for atrophic or atelectatic tympanic membranes [10, 11]. From tube 1 to 3, there is an increase in the diameter of the lumen and size of the inner flange (Fig. 25.3). The larger the lumen and inner flange, the longer the tube remains placed in the tympanic membrane. In all tubes, there is an outer flange to aid introduction (and removal, when necessary). Paparella's type 1 tube is used in routine cases whenever a tube is indicated, and it usually remains in location for four to eight months. The type 2 tube is indicated for chronic, difficult cases, as it remains functional and in place for periods ranging from 6 months to two years or more. The type 2 tubes are usually indicated for patients who had required numerous insertions of standard middle ear ventilation tubes. The type 3 tube was designed for the rare case in which the disease is so obstinate that a permanent tube with a large lumen is warranted. While the tubes type 1 are used in virtually all ventilation tube surgeries, the type 2 is used less frequently, and type 3 tubes are very rarely needed.

The most frequent complication of tympanostomy tubes is postoperative otorrhea (PTTO), which is defined as drainage of secretion through a ventilation tube caused by an infectious or inflammatory process [4]. The estimated incidence of PTTO ranges between 3.4 and 74% [12]. PTTO may be associated with fever, pain, and reduced quality of life [13]. PTTOs may be classified according to their evolution in Kay et al. [14] and Myer 3rd [15]: (1) early PTTO, otorrhea within the first two weeks of tube placement; (2) late PTTO, otorrhea after two weeks of tube placement; (3) chronic or persistent PTTO, otorrhea lasting above 6 or 8 weeks; and (4) recurrent PTTO, distinct episodes of otorrhea, with intervals of dry ears between them.

In this chapter, we further discuss the factors and characteristics of the PTTO in short- and long-term tubes and other potential complications.

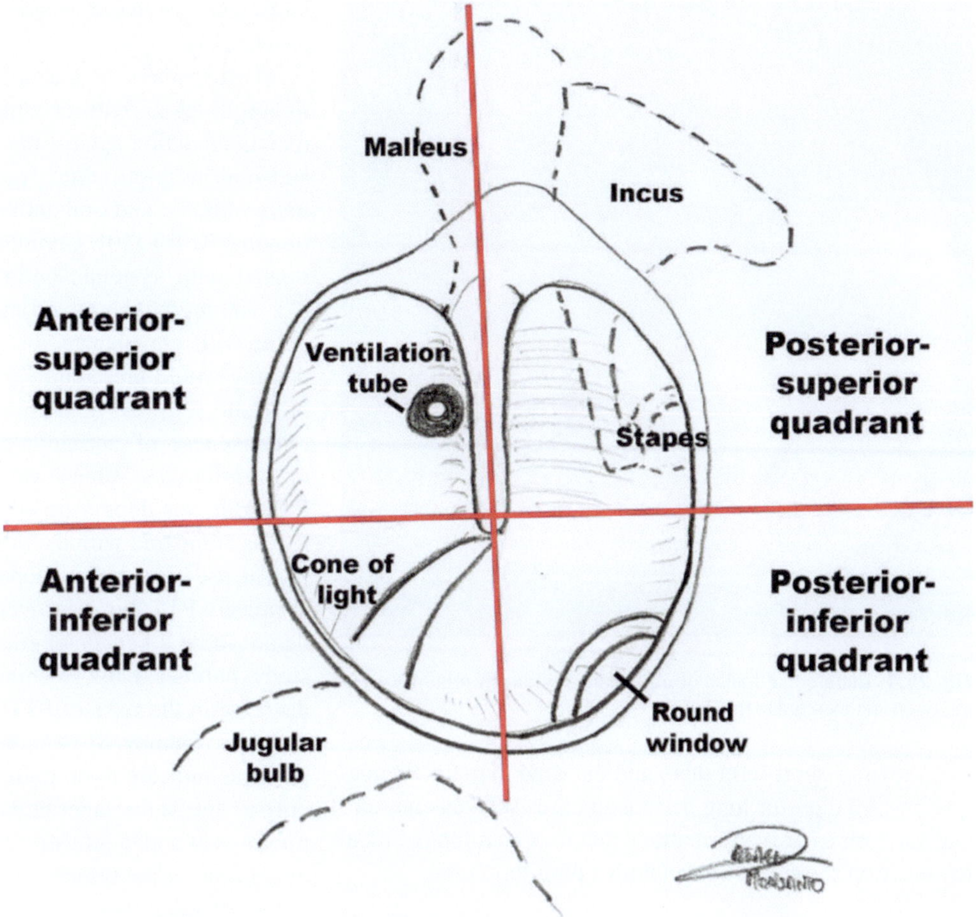

Fig. 25.2 Schematic drawing of the optimal placement of the ventilation tube [8]

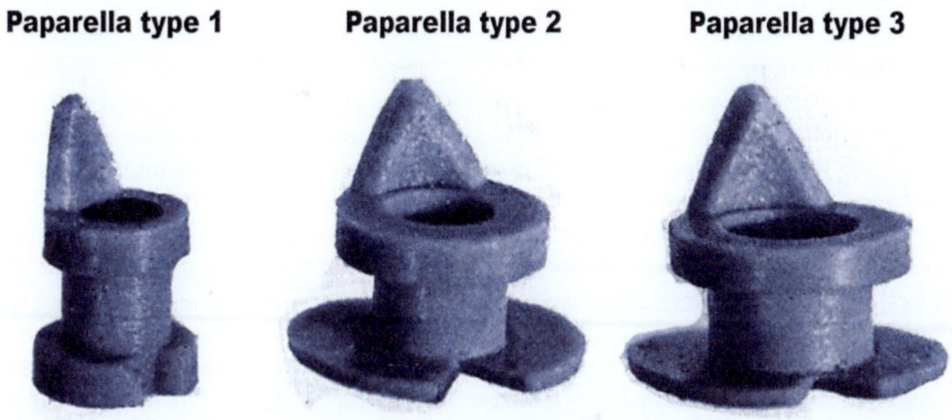

Fig. 25.3 Paparella's ventilation tubes

Short-Term Ventilation Tubes

Indications

Short-term ventilation tubes are indicated to the majority of OME cases (Fig. 25.4). The preference for short-term tubes is based on clinical data showing that only 15–30% of patients who underwent tympanostomy tube surgery needed an additional surgery over time [16]. There is no consensus on which type of tube should be used in each case, as studies dedicated to compare the results of these tubes failed to demonstrate significant differences in outcomes [17]. The tubes usually stay in place from 6 to 18 months and then extrude spontaneously. Although there is no consensus regarding which cases would not benefit from a short-term tube, it seems that cases with atelectatic tympanic membrane, failure

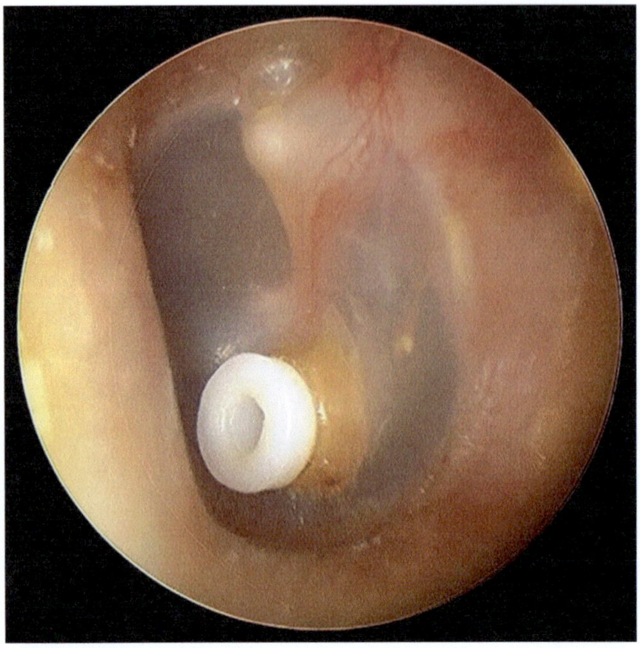

Fig. 25.4 Endoscopic image of a Shepard ventilation tube placed in the tympanic membrane in a left ear

of a previous short-term tube, and the need to maintain adequate ventilation for long periods in cases such as craniofacial syndromes or malformations that imply prolonged tubal dysfunction should be treated with a long-term tube.

Short-Term Tube Complications

Otorrhea (PTTO)

PTTO is the most frequent postsurgical complication of tympanostomy tubes. Several risk factors have been cited for PTTO, and these could be intrinsic or extrinsic. Extrinsic risk factors are the type of ventilation tube (short- versus long-term), location of the tympanotomy, perioperative antibiotic therapy, and environmental exposure to predisposing factors to upper respiratory infections (i.e., children who attend daycare centers). Intrinsic factors include age of the patient, bacteriology of middle ear effusion, previous diseases of nose, adenoids and paranasal sinuses, prior treatment for acute otitis media, and nasopharyngeal and gastroesophageal reflux [18]. However, it seems that the most important factor resulting in PTTO is the presence of intractable tissue pathology in the middle ear, including granulation tissue, hyperplasia and metaplasia of the mucosal lining, and cholesteatoma.

In younger children (<2 years old), the otorrhea is commonly caused by *Streptococcus pneumoniae, Moraxella catarrhalis,* and *Haemophilus influenza.* In younger children with persistent otorrhea and older children, the most prevalent agents are *Pseudomonas aeruginosa* and *Staphylococcus aureus* [19].

The treatment of uncomplicated acute PTTO is topical fluoroquinolone with or without steroids. There is a strong recommendation against the use of topical aminoglycosides and oral antibiotic therapy, as aminoglycosides are potentially ototoxic and oral antibiotics are largely ineffective for treating PTTO [20]. Complicated acute otorrhea should be treated with systemic antibiotic therapy with amoxicillin (75–100 mg/kg/day) two times a day for ten days or amoxicillin with clavulanate. In refractory cases, the antibiotic therapy would preferentially be guided by culture and antibiogram [20]. A randomized, controlled trial compared effectiveness of antibiotic-glucocorticoid eardrops versus oral antibiotics versus watchful waiting in treating mild PTTO: it was demonstrated that eardrops were more effective as compared with the other two treatment options [13].

The use of routine postoperative topical antibiotic therapy to prevent PTTO is controversial, as several studies failed to demonstrate a beneficial effect. However, the meta-analysis study published by Hochman et al. [12] showed a 48% decrease in the risks of PTTO by using prophylactic topical antibiotic therapy. Most studies that recommend topical prophylaxis indicate fluoroquinolones (ofloxacin or ciprofloxacin) as the safest alternative. The dosage depends on the presence of active infection at the time of the procedure (i.e., at the time of the tympanotomy). If signs of active infection are observed, it was suggested that a therapeutic dose of four drops should be used twice daily for five to seven days. In the absence of active infection, a prophylactic dose of three drops should be used twice daily for three days [20].

Considering the potential ototoxic effects of topical antibiotics in patients with ventilation tubes, two randomized, controlled studies revealed that ciprofloxacin did not associate with significant risks of hearing loss [21]. Other alternatives for the prevention of otorrhea with proven efficacy by randomized clinical studies and meta-analyses are intraoperative washing of the middle ear with saline solution after the tympanostomy [19, 21, 22].

Tympanostomy Tube Blockage

Mucus, blood, earwax, and granulation tissue can obstruct the lumen of the ventilation tubes. The tube blockage may occur immediately after surgery or after varying periods of time [14]. Eardrops can be used to clear the clogging, but none of the otic drops available for commercial use are currently approved by the FDA for this purpose.

One study compared the outcomes of children with tube blockage treated with 5% sodium bicarbonate otological solution, 3% hydrogen peroxide, or watchful waiting. Clearance of the tube block was observed in 56 and 71% of the patients treated with hydrogen peroxide and sodium bicarbonate, respectively, compared to 0% on the observation group [23]. An alternative therapeutic option proposed by some authors is to insert a 3-French metal suction catheter into the lumen of the tube to clear the obstruction. However, the risks of inserting a suctioning device into the tube should be carefully weighed against the potential benefits, as it may lead to pain, bleeding, dizziness, and tube medialization or extrusion.

Chronic Tympanic Membrane Perforation

The prevalence of chronic tympanic membrane perforation following short-term tubes is low (0%–2.2%), being lower than in long-term tubes [14, 24].

The factors contributing to a chronic tympanic membrane perforation are size of the myringotomy and the presence of tympanosclerosis [24]. The presence of a perforation may be seen in cases of early extrusion – in these cases, most heal spontaneously and no not demand additional treatment. However, persistent, chronic perforations may require myringoplasty [14].

Granulation Tissue

The formation of granulation tissue in the external auditory canal and tympanostomy site is uncommon in both short- and long-term tubes, with an estimated prevalence of 5% [14] (Fig. 25.5). The development of granulation tissue over the tube seems to associate with the presence of chronic inflammation and otorrhea. It can be treated with the use of eardrops containing antibiotics and corticosteroids, associated with oral antibiotic therapy and local cauterization with silver nitrate solution. In cases where the granulation tissue does not heal by clinical treatment, surgical removal may be necessary [19].

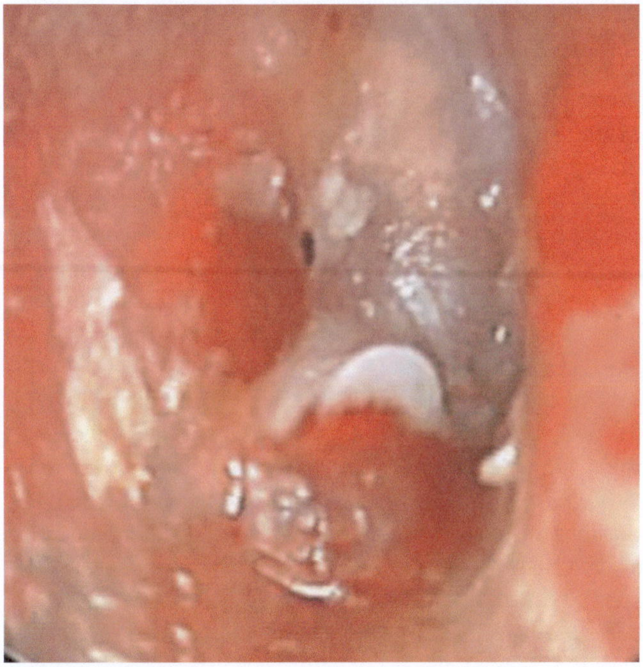

Fig. 25.5 Granulation tissue obstructing the lumen of a Shepard tympanostomy tube in the right ear

Tympanosclerosis

It occurs due to the accumulation of collagen fibers in the lamina propria, associated with hyaline degeneration and calcification. Most frequently, it is caused by inflammatory tissue changes secondary to otitis media. However, authors have hypothesized that it might occur because of foreign body reaction, fibrous hyperplasia, local hemorrhage, and free hemoglobin release after the myringotomy. It is a common consequence of the tympanostomy tubes (34.6%), and it usually locates in the lower quadrants. Hearing loss associated with tympanosclerosis secondary to ventilation tubes is rare [25]. The diagnosis is made through otoscopy, showing whitish plaques on the tympanic membrane. Pneumatic otoscopy can demonstrate reduced or absent tympanic membrane mobility [20].

Focal Atrophy of the Tympanic Membrane

The presence of a focal atrophy of the tympanic membrane is frequent after tympanostomy tube insertions, especially in cases where a large tympanostomy is performed. The atrophy can occur from several mechanisms, including middle ear dysventilation caused by otitis media, and as direct consequence of the lack of regeneration of the medial fibrous layer of the tympanic membrane, as only the epithelial and mucous layers regenerate. It affects approximately 25% of the ears that underwent tympanostomy tube insertions [20], and it can lead to areas of tympanic membrane fragility, with greater susceptibility to retraction and perforation over time.

Other Complications

Early extrusion (4%) and medial tube displacement (0.5%) [20].

Long-Term Ventilation Tubes

Indications

Long-term ventilation tubes (Fig. 25.6) are mostly indicated for patients with chronic eustachian tube dysfunction who have low perspective of improvements in the short term [9]. Although the exact indications of long-term tubes are controversial, it has been proposed that long-term tubes should preferred in the following situations: (1) anatomical obstructions such as malignant tumors (nasopharyngeal carcinoma, lymphoma, and chondrosarcoma), fibrosis, and adhesions caused by adenoidectomy or other surgical procedures [26]; (2) patulous eustachian tube [26]; (3) cranial malformations

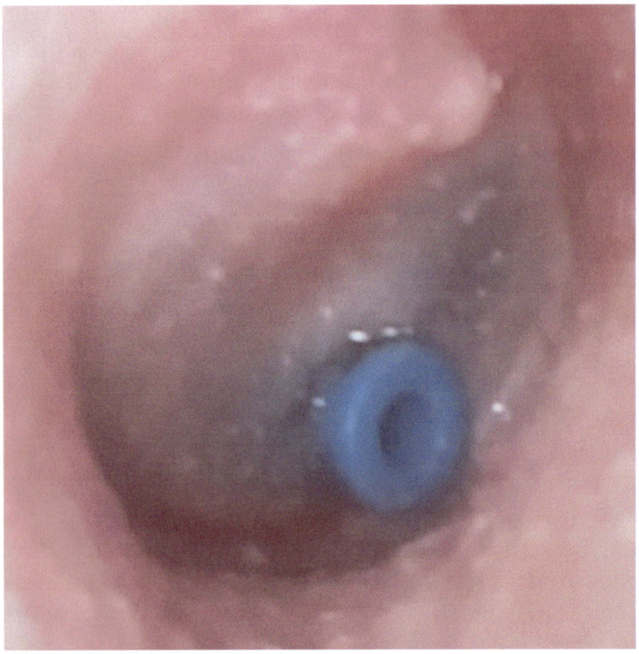

Fig. 25.6 A Paparella type 2 ventilation tube placed in posterior–inferior quadrant of the right ear tympanic membrane

associated or not with genetic syndromes (such as Treacher Collins syndrome, Robin sequence, Crouzon syndrome, and DiGeorge syndrome) [27]; (4) genetic disorders leading to poor clearance of mucus, such as Kartagener's, CHARGE, Young, mucopolysaccharidosis, primary ciliary dyskinesia [28]; (5) immunodeficiencies (acquired immunodeficiency syndrome, selective IgA immunodeficiency, and common variable immunodeficiency agammaglobulinemia) [29–31]; (6) hereditary factors and a family history of chronic ear disease [32]; (7) chronic inflammation of the nasal mucosa resulting in tubal obstruction (e.g., allergies and laryngopharyngeal reflux) [27]; (8) failure to treat OME using eustachian tube dilation [33]; (9) muscular problems causing dilatory dynamic dysfunction [26]; (10) adhesive otitis stage III or IV with or without conductive hearing loss [34]; and (11) deep retractions pockets and/or atrophic scars with tympanograms type C, Cs, or B [34].

The cost versus benefit should be weighed in the decision-making process for indicating long-term tubes. Eliachar et al. [34] described that the long-term tubes can prevent the development and formation of retraction pockets, reduce the frequency of middle ear infections, improve hearing, and provide a well-ventilated middle ear cavity. On the other hand, as compared with short-term tubes, they associate with an increased relative risk of chronic tympanic membrane perforations and cholesteatoma, and also with an increased cost of treatment, as patients will have longer follow-ups and might require additional procedures for removing the tube or treating a residual perforation [35].

Complications

Otorrhea (PTTO)

PTTO is the most frequent complication of ventilation tubes. The prevalence of PTTO following long-term tympanostomy tube surgery varies greatly among studies, ranging from 0.8% to 50%. There is a great debate on whether a long-term tube leads to increased risks of developing a PTTO as compared with short-term ones, with most studies showing that the incidence is higher in long-term tubes [35]. Kay et al. [14] hypothesized that long-term tubes are generally indicated for patients who have a chronic eustachian tube dysfunction or a more advanced underlying middle ear disease, and it seems that the increased risk of PTTO may correlate with the severity of the middle ear disease rather than being a direct consequence of the ventilation tube.

As in short-term tubes, there are many intrinsic and extrinsic factors that increase the risks of developing PTTO. The extrinsic factors include type of tympanostomy tube placed, environmental exposure to upper respiratory infections, tube type, ear canal sterilization, pacifier use, and perioperative antibiotic use. The intrinsic factors are the presence of eustachian tube dysfunction, nasopharyngeal reflux, status of the middle ear effusion at the time of the tympanostomy tube placement, swelling of the peritubal mucosa caused by allergic rhinitis or chronic rhinosinusitis, direct eustachian tube blockage by an enlarged adenoid, age of patient, and colonization of the middle ear by pathogenic bacteria [12].

Simon et al. [35] showed insufficient evidence to support that the PTTO could be prevented by precautions over water exposure. It seems that most PTTOs develop either from an upper respiratory tract infection or through penetration of bacteria from the external auditory canal to the middle ear. Most frequently, the otorrhea following eustachian tube insertion is caused by a bacterial infection—in younger children, the most common pathogens identified are *Streptococcus pneumoniae*, *Haemophilus influenzae*, and *Moraxella catarrhalis*. In older children, the otorrhea is frequently caused by pathogens arising from the external auditory canal, which include *Pseudomonas aeruginosa* and *Staphylococcus aureus*.

There is consensus that PTTO should be treated with topical antibiotic solutions, either with or without topical steroids [35]. As most PTTOs are caused by *Pseudomonas aeruginosa*, quinolone eardrops are sufficient to treat the otorrhea in most cases. There is a strong recommendation against treating PTTOs with oral antibiotics for several reasons [3]: first, the most common pathogen (*Pseudomonas aeruginosa*) is resistant to most oral antibiotics prescribed to children. Second, the use of antibiotics to treat otitis media is considered as one of the most critical vectors leading to bacterial resistance. Moreover, quinolone eardrops, which are safe and effective, can achieve local drug levels up to 1000 times higher than oral antibiotics [18]. Steele et al. [36] also demonstrated that treatment of PTTO with topical quinolones is more efficient than watchful waiting. Regarding the recommendation for removing the tube in cases of PTTO, there is no high-grade evidence in the literature supporting that it should be routinely performed, as (1) chronic PTTO could associate with the presence of a chronic suppurative otitis media, which—in turn—require specific treatment; and (2) removing the tube may lead back to OME. Thus, it is paramount that the pros and cons of keeping or removing the tubes are carefully discussed with the parents.

Chronic Tympanic Membrane Perforation

Some patients who receive tympanostomy tubes develop a chronic eardrum perforation. The prevalence of chronic perforation of the tympanic membrane following spontaneous extrusion of the tube is higher in patients who receive a long-term tympanostomy tube (16%) as compared with patients receiving short-term tubes (2%) [14]. In patients who have their grommets removed surgically, the prevalence seems to be much higher, ranging from 10% to 47% among studies [37].

There higher prevalence of persistent tympanic membrane perforation seen in patients with long-term tubes is most likely multifactorial. The larger mass and diameter of the long-term tubes, the need for a larger tympanostomy incision, and the longer permanence of the tube in the eardrum seem to play a pivotal role in the development of such complication. Patients who are predisposed to have recurrent or chronic ear infections (such as Down syndrome or with craniofacial malformations) also seem to have an increasing risk of developing a chronic perforation following tube extrusion. A persistent tympanic membrane perforation may result in a number of detrimental outcomes, including conductive hearing loss, increased risks of otorrhea and middle ear infections, and higher risks of developing a cholesteatoma over time. Furthermore, patients may need to undergo further surgical procedures to close the perforation (Brown and Behar 2019).

Cholesteatoma

Several studies showed that tympanostomy tubes could result in cholesteatoma formation (Fig. 25.7). The incidence of such complication is very low, being estimated at 0.03–1.1%, and it seems that there is a higher incidence in long-term than short-term tubes [38]. Kay et al. [14] showed that T-tubes (in relation to short-term tubes) associate with a 2.6 increase in the risk of developing cholesteatoma.

Many pathophysiological mechanisms were proposed. The cholesteatoma could be the result of (1) the accumulation of debri in cases where a tube is placed in a retraction pocket or an atrophic, flaccid area; (2) shedding and implantation of epithelial cells into the middle ear in cases of an improper tympanostomy; (3) ingrowth of epithelial cells through the margins of the perforation to the middle ear mucosa, a process that could be further facilitated by the flanges of the tube; and (4) progression of the tissue abnormalities that are inherent to chronic otitis media. It is possible that several of these pathological processes occur in association, and the tympanostomy tube is a facilitator. Although the hypothesis that the tympanostomy tube could create a pathway for the epithelium to migrate to the middle ear is compelling and corroborated by clinical evidence [38], this theory is still considered controversial. Kokko and Palva [39], Padgham et al. [40] and Kinsella [41] did not find a significant increase in the incidence of cholesteatoma in their patients despite a considerable increase in the number of ventilation tubes performed by their groups.

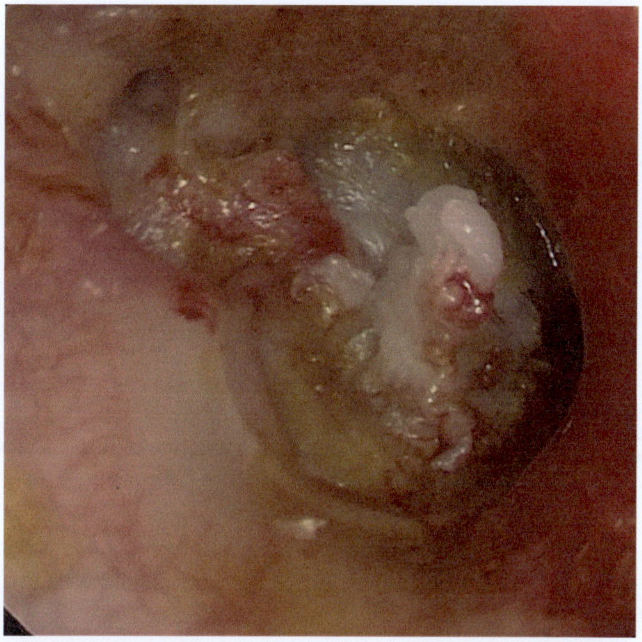

Fig. 25.7 Otoendoscopic image of the right tympanic membrane of a 28-year-old woman with adhesive otitis media who had underwent placement of a Sheppard ventilation tube 2 years before. The image shows global retraction of the tympanic membrane, and keratin debri located at the site where the tube had been previously placed. Exploratory tympanotomy later revealed the presence of mesotympanum cholesteatoma, located in the area adjacent to the residual perforation left after extrusion of the tympanostomy tube

Golz et al. [38] investigated a total of 2829 children who underwent a total of 6701 tympanostomy tube placements and observed that the incidence of cholesteatoma directly attributable to the tubes (behind an intact drum or next to a perforation at or near the site of the tube insertion, in the mesotympanum or hypotympanum) was 1.1%. The authors found that the most critical risk factors associated with this complication were (1) younger children (<5 years old); (2)

use of Goode T-tubes; (3) repeated tube insertions; (4) the tube exceeds 12 months placed in the tympanic membrane; and (5) patients with recurrent or intractable PTTO.

In conclusion, although cholesteatoma formation following tympanostomy tubes is a rare complication, it is important that the risks are discussed with the patients or parents, and that periodic examinations are performed to detect this complication as early as possible [38].

Indications for Tube Removal

There is no consensus as to when long-term tubes should be removed, or even whether they should be removed at all. As these tubes are indicated for patients with a worse prognosis of having adequate middle ear ventilation, authors may have proposed that the tubes should not be removed if there is no evidence of associated complications. Other authors proposed some potential indications for the removal of the tympanostomy tubes [42], which include (a) chronic otorrhea; b) granulation tissue that do not resolve with clinical treatment; (c) long-standing tube in patients who would be expected to have a functional eustachian tube; and (d) tubes that remain placed for over 2 years [42, 43].

Conclusion

It is established that the insertion of ventilation tube improves hearing and consequently the social and language development and reduces the risk of progression to chronic otitis media and its consequences. The indication of tube type must be individualized for each patient weighing the risk and benefits of the procedure.

References

1. Vlastos IM, Houlakis M, Kandiloros D, et al. Adenoidectomy plus tympanostomy tube insertion versus adenoidectomy plus myringotomy in children with obstructive sleep apnoea syndrome. J Laryngol Otol. 2011;125(3):274–8.
2. Allen J, Morton RP, Ahmad Z. Early post-operative morbidity after tympanostomy tube insertion. J Laryngol Otol. 2005;119(9):699–703.
3. Rosenfeld RM, Shin JJ, Schwartz SR, et al. Clinical practice guideline: otitis media with effusion (update). Otolaryngol Head Neck Surg. 2016;154:S1–S41.
4. Isaacson GC (2021a) Tympanostomy tube otorrhea in children: causes, prevention and management. In: essner AH, Kaplan SL, Armsby C, editor. UpToDate, Waltham, MA.
5. Paparella MM, Hiraide F, Juhn SK, Kaneko Y. Cellular events involved in middle ear fluid production. Ann Otol Rhinol Laryngol. 1970;79(4):766–79.
6. Paparella MM, Abdelhammid MM, Schachern PA, et al. Otopathologic correlates of the continuum of otitis media. Ann Otol Rhinol Laryngol. 1990;99:17–22.
7. Yoon TH, Paparella MM, Schachern PA, Lindgren BR. Morphometric studies of the continuum of otitis media. Ann Otol Rhinol Laryngol. 1990;148:23–7.
8. Paparella MM. Location of the ventilation tube. ENT. 2009;88:963.
9. Goode RL. Long-term middle ear ventilation with T-tubes: the perforation problem. Otolaryngol Head Neck Surg. 1996;115(6):500–1.
10. Jurgens GL, Paparella MM. Three new middle ear ventilation tubes. Trans Am Acad Opht Otolaryngol. 1972;76:P1017–9.
11. Paparella MM, Sugiura S. Silicones in middle ear reconstructive surgery. J Laryngol Otol. 1968;82:29–40.
12. Hochman J, Blakley B, Abdoh A, et al. Post-tympanostomy tube otorrhea: a meta-analysis. Otolaryngol Head Neck Surg. 2006;135:8–11.
13. van Dongen TMA, van der Heijden GJMG, Venekamp RP, et al. A trial of treatment for acute otorrhea in children with tympanostomy tubes. N Engl J Med. 2014;370:723–33.
14. Kay DJ, Nelson M, Rosenfeld RM. Meta-analysis of tympanostomy tube sequelae. Otolaryngol Head Neck Surg. 2001;124(4):374–80.
15. Myer CM 3rd. Post-tympanostomy tube otorrhea. Ear Nose Throat J. 2001;80:4.
16. Huyett P, Sturm JJ, Shaffer AD, et al. Second tympanostomy tube placement in children with recurrent acute otitis media. Laryngoscope. 2018;128:1476–9.
17. Tavin ME, Gordon M, Ruben RJ. Hearing results with the use of different tympanostomy tubes: a prospective study. Int J Ped Otorhinolaryngol. 1988;15(1):39–50.
18. Oberman JP, Derkay CS. Posttympanostomy tube Otorrhea. Am J Otolaryngol. 2004;25(2):110–7.
19. Syed MI, Suller S, Broning GG, et al. Interventions for the prevention of postoperative ear discharge after insertion of ventilation tubes (grommets) in children. Cochrane Database Syst Rev. 2013;30(4):CD008512.
20. Isaacson GC (2021b). Overview of tympanostomy tube placement, postoperative care and complications in children. In: Messner AH, Armsby C, editor. UpToDate, Waltham, Mass.
21. Mair EA, Park AH, Don D, et al. Safety and efficacy of intratympanic ciprofloxacin otic suspension in children with middle ear effusion undergoing tympanostomy tube placement: two randomized clinical trials. JAMA Otolaryngol Head Neck Surg. 2016;142(5):444–51.
22. Gabarain G, Baird R, Morisada M, et al. Early otorrhea rates: a randomized trial of ciprofloxacin versus saline drops after tympanostomy tubes. Ann Otol Rhinol Laryngol. 2019;128:760.
23. Spraggs PD, Robinson PJ, Ryan R, et al. A prospective randomized trial of the use of sodium bicarbonate and hydrogen peroxide ear drops to clear a blocked tympanostomy tube. Int J Ped Otorhynolaryngol. 1995;31:207–14.
24. Brown C, Behar P. Factors affecting persistent tympanic membrane perforation after tympanostomy tube removal in children. Int J Otorhinolaryngol. 2020;130:109779. https://doi.org/10.1016/j.iiporl.2019.109779.
25. Yaman H, Yalmaz S, Alkan N, et al. Shepard grommet tympanostomy tube complications in children with chronic otitis media with effusion. Eur Arch Otorhinolaryngol. 2010;267:1221–4.
26. Schilder AG, Bhutta MF, Butler CC, et al. Eustachian tube dysfunction: consensus statement on definition, types, clinical presentation and diagnosis. Clin Otolaryngol. 2015;40(5):407–11.
27. Sánchez-Borges M, Filho NR. Fatores de risco para otite média secretora. Arq Asma Alerg Imunol. 2017;1(1):55–8.
28. Santos JWAD, Waldow A, Figueiredo CWCD, et al. Discinesia ciliar primária. J Pneumol. 2001;27(5):262–8.

29. Araujo KM, Velloso LA, Mansour E, et al. Imunodeficiência comum variável: dificuldades no diagnóstico. Braz J Allergy Immunol. 2015;3(2):61–7.
30. Freitas EB, Lessa HA, Torres SS, et al. Imunodeficiência primária seletiva de IgA em crianças: Relato de 4 casos. Int Arch of Otorhinolaryngol. 1999;3(3):116–8.
31. Oliveira FTLB (2020) Alterações otológicas e audiológicas em pacientes com deficiência comum variável variável e agamaglobulinemia. Dissertação de Mestrado, Faculdade de Medicina de Ribeirão Preto, USP Ribeirão Preto.
32. Alshehri KA, Saggaf OM, Alshamrani HM, et al. Prevalence of and factors associated with Eustachian tube dysfunction among the public in Jeddah, Saudi Arabia: cross-sectional survey-based study. Interact J Med Res. 2020;9(4):e14640. https://doi.org/10.2196/14640.
33. Giunta AA, Liberati L, Pellegrino C, et al. Eustachian tube balloon dilation in treatment of equalization problems of freediving spearfishermen. Diving Hyperb Med. 2019;49(1):9–15.
34. Eliachar I, Joachims HZ, Goldsher Met al (1983) Assessment of long-term middle ear ventilation, Acta Otolaryngol 96(1–2): 105–112.
35. Simon F, Haggard M, Rosenfeld RM, et al. International consensus (ICON) on management of otitis media with effusion in children. Eur Ann Otorhnolaryngol Head Neck Dis. 2018;135: S33–9.
36. Steele DW, Adam GP, Di M. Prevention and treatment of Tympanostomy tube Otorrhea: ameta-analysis. Pediatrics. 2017;189(6):e20170667.
37. Brown C, Behar P. Factors affecting persistent tympanic membrane perforation after tympanostomyr tube removal in children. Int J Pediatr Otorhinolaryngol. 2020;130:109779. https://doi.org/10.1016/j.ijporl.2019.109779. Epub 2019 Nov 15.
38. Golz A, Netzer A, Goldenberg D, et al. Ventilation tubes and cholesteatoma: what is the association? Otolaryngol Head Neck Surg. 1999;121(2):148.
39. Kokko E, Palva T. Clinical results and complications of tympanostomy. Ann Otol Rhinol Laryngol. 1976;85:277–9.
40. Padgham N, Mills R, Christmas H. Has the increasing use of grommets influenced the frequency of surgery for cholesteatoma? J Laryngol Otol. 1989;103:1034–5.
41. Kinsella JB. Ventilation tubes and cholesteatoma. Ir Med J. 1996;89(6):223.
42. Saito T, Iwaki E, Kohno Y, et al. Prevention of persistent ear drum perforation after long-term ventilation tube treatment for otitis media with effusion in children. Int J Pediatr Otorhinolaryngol. 1996;38(1):31–9.
43. El-Bitar MA, Pena MT, Choi SS, et al. Retained ventilation tubes: should they be removed at 2 years? Arch Otolaryngol Head Neck Surg. 2002;128(12):1357–60. https://doi.org/10.1001/archotol.128.12.1357.

Vaccination Policies in Otitis Media

26

Ann Hermansson

Prevention of infectious diseases with vaccination is an effective way to avoid both the risk of serious disease, complications, and the drawbacks of antibiotic treatment in children. Vaccinations have been very effective in preventing, for instance, serious pediatric infections such as meningitis and epiglottitis caused by *Hemophilus influenzae* type b [1]. Conjugate *H. influenzae* type b (Hib) vaccine was introduced in the beginning of the 1990s and is since then administered as part of a routine childhood vaccination program in most countries.

Acute otitis media (AOM) is one of the main causes of antibiotic prescriptions to children worldwide, and a reduced number of infections should be important in the global fight against antibiotic resistance. It has therefore been a priority to try to find vaccination against otitis media. The obvious problem is, however, that "otitis media" is not one disease caused by one microbe but a multifaceted problem caused by a multitude of bacteria and viruses. In most studies, *Streptococcus pneumonia*, *Hemophilus influenzae* (Hi), *Moraxella catarrhalis* (Mc), and *Streptococcus pyogenes* are the four most important bacteria causing acute otitis media. The role for viruses in AOM has been debated, but it is agreed that viruses cause AOM and that they also play an important role in facilitating bacterial infections [2, 3].

Current Vaccines

The introduction of the conjugated Hib vaccine did not affect the number of AOM episodes significantly which probably is since the vaccine only confers protection against Hib and not to other types of capsulated H.infl. or non-typeable Hi (NTHi). It has been shown in several studies that *H. influenzae* AOM in most cases is caused by NTHi and that the relative number of *H. influenzae*–positive AOM probably have increased after the introduction of pneumococcal vaccines [4]. There has been a marked reduction in Hib meningitis though, and it might be argued that this could be related to a decrease in Hib AOM.

Polysaccharide vaccine against *Streptococcus pneumoniae* has been available for many years (23-valent vaccine was introduced in 1983) and confers a good protection in adults and older children against the included types. After the successful introduction of conjugated Hib vaccination in children, a conjugate 7-valent vaccine against pneumococci was introduced with the same protein as in the Hib vaccine, CRM_{197} derived from *Corynebacterium diphteriae*, as a carrier. These seven serotypes were responsible for eighty percent of invasive disease caused by *S. pneumoniae* in young children prior to the introduction of pneumococcal vaccination in the United States. It provided a good protection against invasive disease in the parts of the world where these strains were dominating. The reduction in AOM episodes was more moderate. The two large early studies of the 7-valent vaccine [5, 6] both showed only a modest reduction, around six percent, in the total number of AOM episodes in vaccinated children. This has also been shown in later studies [7]. However, there was a greater reduction of episodes caused by the included pneumococcal strains (57%), and a better protection was also later shown in otitis prone children if vaccinated early [8].

A 10-valent vaccine conjugated to a surface protein from Hi has also been introduced. This vaccine is designed to confer not only protection against pneumococcal disease but also to infections caused by NTHi [9]. Most of the antigens of this vaccine are carried by protein D a surface protein isolated from NTHi [10]. Thus, there are two slightly different pneumococcal vaccines on the market today: pneumococcal protein D-conjugate vaccine and CRM_{197}-conjugated vaccines.

Many viruses (e.g. influenza, rhinovirus, and coronavirus) have been found in conjunction with episodes of AOM and SOM. In many instances, bacterial and viral co-infections are seen in AOM and it seems as though the presence of

A. Hermansson (✉)
Department of ENT, Lund University Hospital, Lund, Sweden
e-mail: ann.hermansson@med.lu.se

M. V. Goycoolea et al. (eds.), *Textbook of Otitis Media*, https://doi.org/10.1007/978-3-031-40949-3_26

viruses are associated with prolonged clinical illness [3, 11–13]. The effect of viral vaccines on AOM has been studied in several settings with very different results depending on the settings. In Finland, influenzae A vaccination during season gave a better protection than pneumococcal vaccination [12, 13], but looking at long term the results are less impressive.

Effect

The impact of pneumococcal vaccines on OM is not easy to determine. The immediate reduction in episodes of AOM after vaccination has been modest in all controlled clinical trial settings, while most observational studies have shown a greater impact [14]. There are several confounding factors that could contribute to this discrepancy. The main problem in interpreting the observational studies is the introduction of "watchful waiting" policies in most countries during the same period as the introduction of pneumococcal vaccination [15]. In Sweden for instance where a reduction of over 30% in antibiotic prescriptions in children was seen between 1987 and 2004 after the introduction of a "watchful waiting" regime for AOM, it is hard to decide the effect of vaccination per se [16]. The same tendencies with a sharp decline in the numbers of uncomplicated episodes of AOM seen in primary care have been observed in other countries after the introduction of "watchful waiting" policies.

In the United States, a downward trend in OM visits was seen from 2004 to 2011, coinciding with both the introduction of pneumococcal vaccines and guidelines advocating watchful waiting in 2004.The incidence of tympanic membrane perforations and otorrhea cases remained unchanged throughout the study period, indicating that the reduction in visits mostly was in uncomplicated cases [17]. To study the reduction in more complicated AOM, several evaluations of the impact on mastoiditis have been made without consistent results. In most studies, there is no change in the number of serious complications. There is generally a reduction in mastoiditis caused by serotypes included in the vaccines, but the total number of complications seems not to have been affected, with other serotypes of pneumococci or other bacteria seen more frequently [18–20].

The effect of vaccination on secretory otitis media and chronic otitis media has been less studied. Potentially, an effect could be seen, and some studies have shown an effect while others have failed to prove a measurable impact [21–23].

Future

In some areas, a significant shift has taken place in AOM bacteriology after routine pneumococcal vaccinations. Strains not included in the vaccines have been taking over, and a need for more serotypes included is obvious. Vaccines containing more serotypes are currently introduced, but there are also attempts to develop a vaccine that will retain its efficacy for most pneumococcal serotypes [24, 25]. It has also been shown that other bacteria might be more frequently isolated in AOM after pneumococcal vaccination why vaccines with an effect also against H.infl and viruses are of interest.

Conclusion

Vaccines against Hib and pneumococci have reduced the burden of invasive diseases in children, but the effect on AOM has been modest in controlled clinical studies. The effect in observational studies has been much better, but these results might be affected by the introduction of regimes of "watchful waiting." These regimes as well as a known protection against serious disease could reduce the numbers of uncomplicated AOM being seen in primary care. Vaccination thus have definitively helped in reducing the need for antibiotic treatment for AOM, and further development of both bacterial and viral vaccines is of great importance.

References

1. Centers for Disease Control and Prevention. Progress toward elimination of Haemophilus influenza type b invasive disease among infants and children—United States, 1998–2000. MMWR Morb Mortal Wkly Rep. 2002;51:234–7.
2. Marom T, Nokso-Koivisto J, Chonmaitree T. Viral-bacterial interactions in acute otitis media. Curr Allergy Asthma Rep. 2012;12(6):551–8. https://doi.org/10.1007/s11882-012-0303-2.
3. Giebink GS, Berzins IK, Marker SC, Schiffman G. Experimental otitis media after nasal inoculation of Streptococcus pneumoniae and influenza A virus in chinchillas. Infect Immun. 1980;30(2):445–50.
4. Murphy T. Vaccines for Nontypeable Haemophilus influenzae: the future is now. Clin Vaccine Immunol. 2015;22(5):459–66.
5. Eskola J, Kilpi T, Palm A, Jokinen J, Haapakoski J, Herva E, Takala A, Käyhty H, Karma P, Kohberger R, Siber G, Mäkelä PH, Finnish Otitis Media Study Group. Efficacy of a pneumococcal conjugate vaccine against acute otitis media. N Engl J Med. 2001;344(6):403–9.
6. Black S, Shinefield H, Fireman B, et al. Efficacy, safety and immunogenicity of heptavalent pneumococcal conjugate vaccine in children. Pediatr Infect Dis. 2000;19:187–95.
7. Straetemans M, Sanders EA, Veenhoven RH, Schilder AG, Damoiseaux RA, Zielhuis GA. Pneumococcal vaccines for preventing otitis media. Cochrane Database Syst Rev. 2002;(2):CD001480.
8. Gisselsson-Solén M, Melhus A, Hermansson A. Pneumococcal vaccination in children at risk of developing recurrent acute otitis media - a randomized study. Acta Paediatr. 2011;100(10):1354–8.
9. Prymula R, Peeters P, Chrobok V, Kriz P, Novakova E, Kaliskova E, Kohl I, Lommel P, Poolman J, Prieels JP, Schuerman L. Pneumococcal capsular polysaccharides conjugated to protein D for prevention of acute otitis media caused by both Streptococcus pneumoniae and non-typeable Haemophilus influenzae: a randomised double-blind efficacy study. Lancet. 2006;367:740–74.

10. Janson H, Melhus A, Hermansson A, Forsgren A. Protein D the glycerophospodiester phosphodiesterase from Haemophilus influenzae with affinity for human immunoglobulin D, influences virulence in a rat otitis model. Infect Immun. 1994;62(11):4848–54.
11. Chonmaitree T, Revai K, Grady JJ, Clos A, Patel JA, Nair S, Fan J, Henrickson KJ. Viral upper respiratory tract infection and otitis media complication in young children. Clin Infect Dis. 2008;46:815–23.
12. Heikkinen T, Ruuskanen O, Waris M, Ziegler T, Arola M, Halonen P. Influenza vaccination in the prevention of acute otitis media in children. Am J Dis Child. 1991;145(4):445–8.
13. Heikkinen T, Block SL, Toback SL, Wu X, Ambrose CS. Effectiveness of intranasal live attenuated influenza vaccine against all-cause acute otitis media in children. Pediatr Infect Dis J. 2013;32(6):669–74.
14. Vojtek I, Nordgren M, Hoet B. Impact of pneumococcal conjugate vaccines on otitis media: a review of measurement and interpretation challenges. Int J Pediatr Otorhinolaryngol. 2017;100:174–82.
15. Venekamp R, Sanders S, Glasziou P, Del Mar C, Rovers M. Antibiotics for acute otitis media in children. Cochrane Database Syst Rev. 2015;23(6):CD000219.
16. Molstad S, Erntell M, Hanberger H, Melander E, Norman C, Skoog G, et al. Sustained reduction of antibiotic use and low bacterial resistance: 10-year follow-up of the Swedish Strama programme. Lancet Infect Dis. 2008;8(2):125–32.
17. Marom T, Tan A, Wilkinson GS, Pierson KS, Freeman JL, Chonmaitree T. Trends in otitis media-related health care use in the United States, 2001–2011. JAMA Pediatr. 2014;168:68–75.
18. Kaplan S, Center KJ, Barson WJ, Ling-Lin P, Romero JR, Bradley JS, Tan TQ, Hoffman JA, Peters TR, Gurtman A, Scott DA, Trammel J, Gruber WC, Hulten KG, Mason EO. Multicentre surveillance of Streptococcus pneumoniae isolates from middle ear and mastoid cultures in the 13-valent pneumococcal conjugate vaccine era. Clin Infect Dis. 2015;60:1339–45.
19. Groth A, Enoksson F, Hermansson A, Hultcrantz M, Stalfors J, Stenfeldt K. Acute mastoiditis in children in Sweden 1993–2007—no increase after new guidelines. Int J Pediatr Otorhinolaryngol. 2011;75(12):1496–501.
20. Balsamo C, Biagi C, Mancini M, Corsini I, Bergamaschi R, Lanari M. Acute mastoiditis in an Italian pediatric tertiary medical center: a 15—year retrospective study. Ital J Pediatr. 2018;44(1):71.
21. Leach AJ, Wigger C, Hare K, Hampton V, Beissbarth J, Andrews R, Chatfield M, Smith-Vaughan H, Morris PS. Reduced middle ear infection with non-typeable Haemophilus influenzae, but not Streptococcus pneumoniae, after transition to 10-valent pneumococcal non-typeable H. influenzae protein D conjugate vaccine. BMC Pediatr. 2015;15:162.
22. Toizumi M, et al. Effect of pneumococcal conjugate vaccine on prevalence of otitis media with effusion among children in Vietnam. Vaccine. 2022;40(36):5366–75.
23. Jespersen SI, Demant MN, Pedersen ML, Homøe P. Acute otitis media and pneumococcal vaccination—an observational cross-sectional study of otitis media among vaccinated and unvaccinated children in Greenland. Int J Circumpolar Health. 2021;80(1):1858615.
24. Briles DE, Paton JC, Mukerji R, Swiatlo E, Crain MJ. Pneumococcal vaccines. Microbiol Spectr. 2019;7(6)
25. Musher DM, Anderson R, Feldman C. The remarkable history of pneumococcal vaccination: an ongoing challenge Pneumonia (Nathan). 2022;14(1):5.

Managing Risk Factors in Otitis Media

27

Joshua A. Stramielo and Daniela Carvalho

Introduction

The cumulative incidence of at least one episode of otitis media (OM) by the age of 7 years is reported to be 61–99%, depending on the population [1–3]. Risk factors for otitis media include a spectrum of nonmodifiable and modifiable qualities specific to the patient. They can be described as patient characteristics, genetic influences, opportunistic morbidities, and socioeconomic practices (Table 27.1). A complete birth and medical history is the first step to identifying some of these risk factors. Frequent recurrence and co-morbidities may prompt referral for other testing and in some cases genetic testing. Regardless, educating parents and patients of their risk factors and how to minimize them is crucial to decrease the incidence of otitis media in children.

Table 27.1 Risk factors in otitis media: nonmodifiable, potentially modifiable, and modifiable

Risk factors in otitis media		
Nonmodifiable	Potentially modifiable	Modifiable
Patient characteristics	*Genetic influences*	*Socioeconomic behaviors*
Young age (2 yo, 4–5 yo)	Monozygotic twins	Second- and third-hand smoke
Male sex	Family history, sibling with history of OM	Obesity
Older sibling(s)	Aerodigestive tract mucociliary disorders (primary ciliary dyskinesia and cystic fibrosis)	Daycare
Ethnicity (Native American, Canadian Eskimo, and Australian Aborigine)	Immunodeficiency (hypogammaglobulinemia and leukocyte adhesion deficiency)	Short-term breastfeeding
Cesarean section delivery	Specific genotypes (ISL1 polymorph, A2LM1, SAMD9—MIRAGE syndrome)	Pesticide exposure in utero
Lo	*Opportunistic morbidities*	
	Upper respiratory infection	
	Winter season	
	Cleft palate	
	Trisomy 21 (Down's syndrome)	
	Craniofacial deformity	
	Adenoid hypertrophy	
	Environmental/food allergies	
	Gastroesophageal reflux	

J. A. Stramielo
Division of Otolaryngology Head and Neck Surgery, University of California, San Diego, La Jolla, CA, USA

D. Carvalho (✉)
Division of Otolaryngology Head and Neck Surgery, University of California, San Diego, La Jolla, CA, USA

Rady Children's Hospital, San Diego, San Diego, CA, USA
e-mail: dcarvalho@rchsd.org

M. V. Goycoolea et al. (eds.), *Textbook of Otitis Media*, https://doi.org/10.1007/978-3-031-40949-3_27

Nonmodifiable Risk Factors

Patient Characteristics

Risk factors for otitis media related to a patient's characteristics are inherently nonmodifiable. However, parent and patient education is helpful in offering reassurance and explaining why it does not necessarily portend serious underlying disorders. The first of these risk factors include male sex, which account for 51–55% of pediatric otitis media cases, as well as young age, with a bimodal increased incidence at 6–18 months old and 4–5 years old [1, 3–7]. While the slight male preponderance has been fairly consistent, no explanations have been proven as to why otitis media is more prevalent in males. Alternatively, it is widely accepted that the risk of young age is related to short, relatively horizontal eustachian tubes, which elongate and eventually develop a 30–40° upward angle toward the middle ear with increasing age [8]. Having an older sibling at home is also a risk factor, presumably due to earlier exposure to upper respiratory tract infections, which is supported by further increased risk if a room is shared with them [7].

Native American, Canadian Eskimo, and Australian Aborigine ethnicities have an increased risk for otitis media, compared to Caucasians [3, 7]. This is likely due to anatomical characteristics of the eustachian tube of these ethnicities. Children with Black ethnic backgrounds have a decreased risk [3, 5], though causality is unknown in all cases. Lastly, children delivered via cesarean section have a slightly increased risk of otitis media, as compared to nonoperative vaginal delivery [9, 10]. The hypothesis is that there are differences in the gut biome of children born by cesarian section and via vaginal delivery [10]. Interestingly, patients born via an operative vaginal delivery (defined as instruments placed in the birth canal) have the same increased risk as cesarean section [9]. Low birth preterm children are also at an increased risk for otitis.

Potentially Modifiable Risk Factors

Genetic Influences

It is clear that genetics play a strong role in the risk for otitis media as epidemiology studies have identified family history of a sibling with prior otitis media as a risk factor [4, 7, 11]. Even more telling, this association is stronger between monozygotic twins and triplets compared to dizygotic twins and triplets, though this difference no longer remains significant after 4 years of age [11]. While genetic counseling is not necessary for the majority of patients with otitis media, advances in genomics and genetic therapies may prompt genetic testing for patients with recurrent or severe disease. Arguably, the otolaryngologist's role in minimizing genetically influenced risk factors for otitis media is identification of the underlying cause, or more realistically, timely referral for work-up. The presence of these risk factors may also sharpen clinical acumen for the need of more aggressive preventive measures and more frequent follow-up to ensure hearing is protected.

Ciliary Motility Disorders

Genetic diseases that lead to aerodigestive motility disorders are important considerations for recurrent otitis media. Primary ciliary dyskinesia is a rare (1:10,000–20,000 live births) genetic disorder affecting the cilia of the upper respiratory tract which can lead to chronic rhinosinusitis, bronchiectasis, and otitis media. Clinical screening questionnaires and expired nasal nitric oxide concentrations are potentially cost-effective methods for identifying patients who warrant formal genetic testing [12]. Historically, cystic fibrosis was considered protective against otitis media due to well-aerated temporal bones and overly tenacious nasal secretions making translocation to the middle ear more difficulty [13]. However, recent review has noted increased incidence of otitis media coinciding with increased identification of subclinical genotypes [14]. Interestingly, cystic fibrosis patients without otitis media were found to have a lower density of goblet cells on postmortem analysis as compared to cystic fibrosis patients with otitis media, yet most have inner ear damage due to ototoxic drugs [13].

Immunodeficiency

Immunodeficiency is another important consideration. Leukocyte adhesion deficiency leads to a defect in transporting leukocytes to regions of tissue injury. A recent cohort analysis identified an otitis media prevalence of 10–21% in these patients. Suspicion is worked up with cytometric analysis of CD18 and CD11 expression of leukocytes, and diagnosis can be confirmed by the identification of a defect in the ITGβ2 gene [15]. Similarly, a cross-sectional study of pediatric patients with hypogammaglobulinemia identified an otitis media prevalence of 49%, which led to conductive hearing loss in 73% of patients. This includes X-linked agammaglobulinemia, common variable immunodeficiency, IgA deficiency, and hyper-IgM syndrome [16].

Specific Genotypes

The ubiquity of genomics has also led to the identification of specific genotypes with higher risk for otitis media with unclear etiology, which includes ISL1 and A2LM1 polymorphisms and SAMD9 mutations [17–19]. ISL1 is part of the insulin gene enhancer protein 1 homeodomain that regulates the insulin gene. Specific polymorphisms of this gene relating to different exons have been found to increase the risk of otitis media [19]. The A2LM1 encodes the α-2 macroglobulin-like-1 protein. A variant of which was identified in a Filipino community to have a significant odds ratio of 3.7 for OM [18]. SAMD9, or sterile alpha motif domain containing 9, encodes a protein of unknown significance; however, mutations in this gene are responsible for MIRAGE (myelodysplasia, infection, restriction of growth, adrenal hypoplasia, genital problems, and enteropathy) syndrome. MIRAGE syndrome has been associated with increased risk of otitis media. This may be related to cytopenias but has not been investigated [17]. Of note, other mutations of SAMD9 can also lead to normophosphatemic familial tumoral calcinosis but has not been linked to otitis media [20].

Alternatively, some genotypes may be protective, such as IFI44L minor homozygotes, who have a significate incidence rate ratio of 0.77 compared to other allele combinations [21]. IFI44L is a protein-encoding gene for the interferon-induced protein 44-like which has viral antiproliferative activity; however, the mechanism of this property is unknown [22].

The prevalence of otitis media in children with Down's syndrome has been reported to be 81–83% [23, 24]. Temporal bone studies have identified that Down's syndrome patients have smaller middle ear compartments and more collapsible eustachian tubes due to immature development of eustachian tube cartilage and the tensor veli palatini muscle [25]. These patients can also have immunodeficiencies that contribute to their increase risk of otitis media [26]. Otitis media in Down's syndrome patients has been shown to commonly cause significant physical symptoms and hearing loss [27]. While tympanostomy tubes significantly improve these symptoms, it is common for their otitis media to stay unresolved requiring subsequent tubes for a majority of young age [24, 27].

Opportunistic Morbidities

Several morphological morbidities have been identified as risk factors for otitis media, which offers an opportunity for potential medical or surgical intervention. Identifying these risk factors and educating parents and patients offers better informed perspectives of preventing OM. It may also obviate the need for further testing and offer reassurance regarding the overall health of the patient.

Upper Respiratory Infections

Likely the most common risk factor for otitis media is current or recent upper respiratory infection. In a prospective cohort study of 294 children aged 1–3 years, otitis media was found to complicate upper respiratory infection 61% of the time. While there were no associations with sex or ethnicity, age was significant with each increasing month of life after 1 year reducing the risk of otitis media by 4%. Interestingly, there was also a significant difference in the incidence of otitis media by virus type with adenovirus and coronavirus being the most associated with otitis media. The proposed pathophysiology of this association is nasopharyngeal edema leading to eustachian tube dysfunction, as well as increased production of mucus in the middle ear [28]. Similarly, as viral upper respiratory infections are most common in the fall and winter seasons [29], so is otitis media [30]. Intranasal steroids, antihistamines, and decongestants are not helpful as treatment for otitis media [31], and this likely holds true for prevention as well during an upper respiratory infection. However, symptomatic care with oral hydration and nasal saline irrigation are safe adjuncts [32]. Furthermore, yearly influenza vaccines have been linked to significant reductions in otitis media, and similarly, the pneumococcal conjugate vaccine [33, 34].

Craniofacial Abnormalities

Extra vigilance should be practiced in patients with craniofacial abnormalities that can predispose to otitis media. Patients with cleft palate ultimately have poor middle ear ventilation due to poor function of the palatine muscles and frequent velopharyngeal reflux [35, 36]. Greater than 95% of children with cleft palate have otitis media prior to palatal closure [37, 38], which can improve somehow along with hearing status at about 6–12 months after surgery [39]. However, pediatric patients with cleft palate have similar long-term chronicity and audiological outcomes when treated with tympanostomy tubes as compared to pediatric patients without cleft palate [40]. Patients with other forms of craniofacial deformity should also be considered to be at an increased risk for otitis media. Specifically, changes in the relative positions of the mandible, skull base, middle ear, sphenoid, and palate can increase the risk of otitis media [41].

Adenoids

The adenoid tissue can act as a reservoir for otitis media pathogens and can also cause eustachian tube dysfunction if enlarged and encroaching onto the tori tubarius [42, 43]. Inflammatory changes to the adenoids can also cause increased inflammation of the middle ear [44]. Interestingly, Streptococcus pneumoniae is the most common adenoidal pathogen in patients 7 years of age or younger and Staphylococcus aureus is the most common in those older than 7 years of age. However, there is no association between the risk of otitis media and the pathogen(s) colonizing adenoid tissue [45]. Adenoidectomy in the setting of hypertrophy has been shown to improve middle ear ventilation [46]. It may also decrease the number of repeated tympanostomy tube in children older than 4 years of age [47].

Allergies

While the relationship between environmental allergies and otitis media is complicated and controversial, immunological studies have identified IgE-mediated middle ear disease. Furthermore, the middle ear mucosa is an extension or the upper airway mucosa and has similar physiologic and immune mechanisms, including inflammation due to allergies. The prevalence of atopy, including allergic rhinitis in patients with recurrent otitis, ranges from 24% to 89% [48].

Because of the multifactorial nature of OM, it is difficult to measure the impact of allergy-related middle ear disease in the setting of other known risk factors. However, allergy testing can be considered for children with signs of atopia [49]. Similarly, the impact of food allergies and the need for avoidance practices remains controversial. Nonrandomized, prospective studies have researched food allergy associations and impact of dietary avoidance among children with OM with positive results [50, 51]. However, there remains a dearth of definitive studies and subsequent consensus statements. While food allergy is a consideration and can be tested, the risks and benefits of dietary avoidance therapy should be critically appraised specific to the patient and other risk factors should be minimized.

GERD

Gastroesophageal reflux in early childhood is another important concern, as it significantly increases the risk for otitis media [52, 53]. In fact, increasing the severity of reflux symptoms increases the risk of eustachian tube dysfunction, hearing loss, and tympanostomy tube placement [52]. Part of this may be related to pepsin or pepsinogen identified in middle ear aspirates, putting even laryngopharyngeal reflux patients at risk. However, this connection has not been confirmed [54].

Modifiable Risk Factors

Socioeconomic Practices

Lifestyle and access to healthy and clean food has important implications beyond the incidence of otitis media but may offer a tangible and evidence-based opportunity to educate parents and improve social and environmental factors affecting the patient. One of the most important in this category is exposure to second- and third-hand smoking. Passive smoke exposure is a clear, reproducible risk factor across ethnicities [4, 5, 18, 55–57]. The pathophysiology for this association has not been established; however, second- and third-hand smoke have been linked to significant alterations in the respiratory microbiome, with exposed children more likely to have inflamed upper airways with pathogenic and polymicrobial flora [58, 59].

Obesity has a significant role in increasing the risk of otitis media, though it is likely multifactorial. Obesity leads to poor eustachian tube dysfunction secondary to an increase in the Ostmann fat pad of the nasopharynx. There is also an increased risk of acid reflux, which is an independent risk factor for otitis media. Most importantly, obesity also leads to a local immune dysfunction of the middle ear with reduction in toll-like receptor-mediated expression of mRNA for multiple cytokines [60].

Daycare

Daycare attendance has an odds ratio of 1.3–1.5 for otitis media [61, 62]. However, an increasing number of caregivers is not significant [62], highlighting the increased microbial transmission rates among young children, inherent to their behavior. The risk is even higher when daycare attendance is started prior to age 12 months [63, 64], which emphasizes the multifactorial nature of risk factors for otitis media. While recommending removal from daycare may lead to significant concerns, such as the effects on social development, suggesting delaying admission and ensuring hygienic practices of the facilities, especially for patients with multiple risk factors, may be better received.

Breastfeeding

Breastfeeding has repeatedly been shown to reduce the risk of otitis media in infancy by 40–50% [65]. This risk reduction is most robust in infants who are breastfed ≥12 months as compared to those breastfed <6 months [66, 67]. This benefit may be derived from milk fat globule membranes, or fat globules, which transport high concentrations of phospholipids, gangliosides, and proteins [68]. Milk fat globule membrane-supplemented formula significantly reduces the incidence of otitis media compared to nonsupplemented, formula-fed infants [69]. Similarly, prospective research has correlated pesticide exposure in utero to increased risk of otitis media in childhood, as compared to mothers who consumed an organic, pesticide-free diet [70]. Breastfeeding position seems to cause different changes in negative pressure in the middle ear, and breastfeeding a child in the "flat" position might be related to increased risk of otitis media [71, 72].

Common Misconceptions

Pacifier use has had a long history of reported association with increased risk for otitis media. However, significant correlations fail to remain significant after multivariate logistic regression analysis [73]. Furthermore, other studies contradict this association, linking increased otitis media prevalence with decreased pacifier use [74]. This represents sampling errors. Likely more important, otitis media within the first month of life increases the risk of recurrent otitis media fourfold [75]. Given the clear reduction in sudden infant death syndrome [76] and the paucity of definitive relationships to otitis media, pacifier use should not be discouraged.

Swimming can often be a confusing topic for parents and caregivers of children with otitis media. While swimming can increase the risk of otitis externa [77], it does not increase nor decrease the risk of otitis media [78]. Similarly, there is no increased risk for otitis media in patients with tympanostomy tubes 1 month after placement and current tympanostomy tube guidelines do not recommend avoiding water exposure [79, 80].

Effects of Social Distancing During the COVID-19 Pandemic

SARS-CoV2 (server acute respiratory syndrome coronavirus 2) and the subsequent COVID-19 (2019 novel corona virus disease) pandemic has led to a radical change in daily life for most people around the world. Social distancing, social isolation, and increased frequency of hygienic practices have clearly mitigated the risk of contracting SARS-CoV2 and developing COVID-19 [81]. As such, these practices have simultaneously mitigated the risk of contact with other viruses, subsequentially leading to a significant 5–10 fold reduction in the incidence of otitis media in children [82, 83]. Interestingly, this has also led to a significant increase in resolution of chronic otitis media with effusion [83]. Though social distancing and isolation are likely not an appropriate measure for most children given the need for social development, it does highlight the importance of ensuring hygienic practices and a possible short-term adjunct for children severely affected by otitis media.

References

1. Todberg T, Koch A, Andersson M, Olsen SF, Lous J, Homoe P. Incidence of otitis media in a contemporary Danish National Birth Cohort. PLoS One. 2014;9(12):e111732.
2. Paradise JL, Rockette HE, Colborn DK, et al. Otitis media in 2253 Pittsburgh-area infants: prevalence and risk factors during the first two years of life. Pediatrics. 1997;99(3):318–33.
3. Infante-Rivard C, Fernandez A. Otitis media in children: frequency, risk factors, and research avenues. Epidemiol Rev. 1993;15(2):444–65.
4. Froom J, Culpepper L, Green LA, et al. A cross-national study of acute otitis media: risk factors, severity, and treatment at initial visit. Report from the International Primary Care Network (IPCN) and the Ambulatory Sentinel Practice Network (ASPN). J Am Board Fam Pract. 2001;14(6):406–17.
5. Qureishi A, Lee Y, Belfield K, Birchall JP, Daniel M. Update on otitis media—prevention and treatment. Infect Drug Resist. 2014;7:15–24.
6. Chen CH, Lin CJ, Hwang YH, Ku CJ. Epidemiology of otitis media in Chinese children. Clin Otolaryngol Allied Sci. 2003;28(5):442–5.
7. Baraibar R. Incidence and risk factors of acute otitis media in children. Clin Microbiol Infect. 1997;3(Suppl 3):S13–22.
8. Bluestone CD, Doyle WJ. Anatomy and physiology of eustachian tube and middle ear related to otitis media. J Allergy Clin Immunol. 1988;81(5 Pt 2):997–1003.
9. Auger N, Soullane S, Luu TM, Lee GE, Wei SQ, Quach C. Association of cesarean delivery with childhood hospitalization for infections before 13 years of age. J Pediatr. 2021;231:178.
10. Hartley M, Woolcott CG, Langley JM, Brown MM, Ashley-Martin J, Kuhle S. Birth by caesarean section and otitis media in childhood: a retrospective cohort study. Sci Rep. 2020;10(1):5219.
11. Casselbrant ML, Mandel EM, Rockette HE, et al. The genetic component of middle ear disease in the first 5 years of life. Arch Otolaryngol Head Neck Surg. 2004;130(3):273–8.
12. Brennan SK, Molter D, Menezes M, et al. Implementation of a screening tool for primary ciliary dyskinesia (PCD) in a pediatric otolaryngology clinic. Int J Pediatr Otorhinolaryngol. 2020;142:110586.
13. Yildirim N, Sone M, Mutlu C, Schachern PA, Paparella MM, Le CT. Histopathologic features of the temporal bone in patients with cystic fibrosis. Arch Otolaryngol Head Neck Surg. 2000;126(1):75–8.
14. McCoy JL, Kaffenberger TM, Yang TS, Shaffer AD, Dohar JE. Middle ear disease in CF? It's not just about the sinuses anymore! Int J Pediatr Otorhinolaryngol. 2020;134:110032.
15. Kambli PM, Bargir UA, Yadav RM, et al. Clinical and genetic spectrum of a large cohort of patients with leukocyte adhesion deficiency type 1 and 3: amulticentric study from India. Front Immunol. 2020;11:612703.
16. Tavakol M, Kouhi A, Abolhassani H, et al. Otological findings in pediatric patients with hypogammaglobulinemia. Iran J Allergy Asthma Immunol. 2014;13(3):166–73.
17. Tanase-Nakao K, Olson TS, Narumi S. MIRAGE syndrome. In: Adam MP, Ardinger HH, Pagon RA, et al., editors. GeneReviews((R)). Seattle, WA: University of Washington; 1993.
18. Santos-Cortez RL, Reyes-Quintos MR, Tantoco ML, et al. Genetic and environmental determinants of otitis media in an indigenous Filipino population. Otolaryngol Head Neck Surg. 2016;155(5):856–62.
19. Kondyarpu A, Ray CS, Panda KC, Biswal NC, Ramchander PV. Association of ISL1 polymorphisms and eosinophilic levels among otitis media patients. J Clin Lab Anal. 2021;35:e23702.
20. Jiang Q, Quaynor B, Sun A, et al. The Samd9L gene: transcriptional regulation and tissue-specific expression in mouse development. J Invest Dermatol. 2011;131(7):1428–34.
21. Lempainen J, Korhonen LS, Kantojarvi K, et al. Associations between IFI44L gene variants and rates of respiratory tract infections during early childhood. J Infect Dis. 2021;223(1):157–65.
22. Busse DC, Habgood-Coote D, Clare S, et al. Interferon-induced protein 44 and interferon-induced protein 44-like restrict replication of respiratory syncytial virus. J Virol. 2020;94(18):e00297-20.
23. Roizen NJ, Wolters C, Nicol T, Blondis TA. Hearing loss in children with Down syndrome. J Pediatr. 1993;123(1):S9–12.
24. Shott SR, Joseph A, Heithaus D. Hearing loss in children with Down syndrome. Int J Pediatr Otorhinolaryngol. 2001;61(3):199–205.
25. Nogaki T, Paparella MM, Cureoglu S. A structural analysis of tympanic compartments of the middle ear in patients with Down's syndrome: atemporal bone study. Otol Neurotol. 2020;41(8):1149–57.

26. Verstegen RHJ, Kusters MAA. Inborn errors of adaptive immunity in Down syndrome. J Clin Immunol. 2020;40(6):791–806.
27. Labby A, Mace JC, Buncke M, MacArthur CJ. Quality of life improvement after pressure equalization tube placement in Down syndrome: a prospective study. Int J Pediatr Otorhinolaryngol. 2016;88:168–72.
28. Chonmaitree T, Revai K, Grady JJ, et al. Viral upper respiratory tract infection and otitis media complication in young children. Clin Infect Dis. 2008;46(6):815–23.
29. Dasaraju PV, Liu C. Infections of the respiratory system. In: Baron S, editor. Medical microbiology. Galveston, TX: University of Texas Medical Branch; 1996.
30. Kim TH, Jeon JM, Choi J, Im GJ, Song JJ, Chae SW. The change of prevalence and recurrence of acute otitis media in Korea. Int J Pediatr Otorhinolaryngol. 2020;134:110002.
31. Rosenfeld RM, Shin JJ, Schwartz SR, et al. Clinical practice guideline: otitis media with effusion executive summary (update). Otolaryngol Head Neck Surg. 2016;154(2):201–14.
32. Marchisio P, Bortone B, Ciarcia M, et al. Updated guidelines for the management of acute otitis media in children by the Italian Society of Pediatrics: Prevention. Pediatr Infect Dis J. 2019;38(12S Suppl):S22–36.
33. Lieberthal AS, Carroll AE, Chonmaitree T, et al. The diagnosis and management of acute otitis media. Pediatrics. 2013;131(3):e964–99.
34. de Sevaux JL, Venekamp RP, Lutje V, et al. Pneumococcal conjugate vaccines for preventing acute otitis media in children. Cochrane Database Syst Rev. 2020;11:CD001480.
35. Azman A, Manuel AM. Otological outcome in cleft lip and palate children with middle ear effusion. Int J Pediatr Otorhinolaryngol. 2020;138:110274.
36. Hocevar-Boltezar I, Jarc A, Kozelj V. Ear, nose and voice problems in children with orofacial clefts. J Laryngol Otol. 2006;120(4):276–81.
37. Dhillon RS. The middle ear in cleft palate children pre and post palatal closure. J R Soc Med. 1988;81(12):710–3.
38. Paradise JL, Bluestone CD, Felder H. The universality of otitis media in 50 infants with cleft palate. Pediatrics. 1969;44(1):35–42.
39. Acharya P, Sahana BA, Desai A, Jalisatgi RR, Kumar N. Pre-operative and post-operative audiological assessment in cleft lip and palate patients-a prospective study. J Oral Biol Craniofac Res. 2021;11(2):321–9.
40. Inoue M, Hirama M, Kobayashi S, Ogahara N, Takahashi M, Oridate N. Long-term outcomes in children with and without cleft palate treated with tympanostomy for otitis media with effusion before the age of 2 years. Acta Otolaryngol. 2020;140(12):982–9.
41. Gremba AP, Weinberg SM, Swarts JD, Casselbrant ML. Craniofacial shape in children with and without a positive otitis media history. Int J Pediatr Otorhinolaryngol. 2016;84:110–5.
42. Musher DM. Pneumococcal vaccine-direct and indirect ("herd") effects. N Engl J Med. 2006;354:1522–4.
43. Wright ED, Alden JP, Manoukian JJ. Laterally hypertrophic adenoids as a contributing factor in otitis media. Int J Pediatr Otorhinolaryngol. 1998;45:207–14.
44. Abdullah B, Hassan S, Sidek D, Jaafar H. Adenoid mast cell and their role in the pathogenesis of otitis media with effusion. J Laryngol Otol. 2006;120:556–60.
45. Ungkanont K, Jootakarn S, Leelaporn A, et al. Association between adenoid bacteriology and clinical characteristics of adenoid-related diseases in children. SAGE Open Med. 2021;9:20503121211006005.
46. Manno A, Iannella G, Savastano V, et al. Eustachian tube dysfunction in children with adenoid hypertrophy: the role of adenoidectomy for improving ear ventilation. Ear Nose Throat J. 2021; https://doi.org/10.1177/0145561321989455.
47. Wang MC, Wang YP, Chu CH, Tu TY, Shiao AS, Chou P. The protective effect of adenoidectomy on pediatric tympanostomy tube re-insertions: a population-based birth cohort study. PLoS One. 2014;9(7):e101175. https://doi.org/10.1371/journal.pone.0101175.
48. Lack G, Caulfield H, Penagos M. The link between otitis media with effusion and allergy: a potential role for intranasal corticosteroids. Pediatr Allergy Immunol. 2011;22:258–66.
49. Hurst DS. The role of allergy in otitis media with effusion. Otolaryngol Clin N Am. 2011;44(3):637–54, viii–ix.
50. Aydogan B, Kiroglu M, Altintas D, Yilmaz M, Yorgancilar E, Tuncer U. The role of food allergy in otitis media with effusion. Otolaryngol Head Neck Surg. 2004;130(6):747–50.
51. Nsouli TM, Nsouli SM, Linde RE, O'Mara F, Scanlon RT, Bellanti JA. Role of food allergy in serous otitis media. Ann Allergy. 1994;73(3):215–9.
52. Lee JA, Schaffer CE, Mehta CH, Close MF, Nguyen SA, Meyer TA. Impact of early gastroesophageal reflux disease on childhood otologic outcomes. Int J Pediatr Otorhinolaryngol. 2020;134:110069.
53. Wu ZH, Tang Y, Niu X, Sun HY, Chen X. The relationship between otitis media with effusion and gastroesophageal reflux disease: ameta-analysis. Otol Neurotol. 2021;42(3):e245–53.
54. Lechien JR, Hans S, Simon F, et al. Association between laryngopharyngeal reflux and media otitis: asystematic review. Otol Neurotol. 2021;42:e801.
55. Tarhun YM. The effect of passive smoking on the etiology of serous otitis media in children. Am J Otolaryngol. 2020;41(3):102398.
56. Kalcioglu MT, Sallavaci S, Hrncic N, et al. Prevalence of and factors affecting otitis media with effusion in children in the region from Balkans to Caspian basin; a multicentric cross-sectional study. Int J Pediatr Otorhinolaryngol. 2021;143:110647.
57. van Ingen G, le Clercq CMP, Touw CE, et al. Environmental determinants associated with acute otitis media in children: a longitudinal study. Pediatr Res. 2020;87(1):163–8.
58. Kelley ST, Liu W, Quintana PJE, et al. Altered microbiomes in thirdhand smoke-exposed children and their home environments. Pediatr Res. 2021;90:1153.
59. Bugova G, Janickova M, Uhliarova B, Babela R, Jesenak M. The effect of passive smoking on bacterial colonisation of the upper airways and selected laboratory parameters in children. Acta Otorhinolaryngol Ital. 2018;38(5):431–8.
60. Ahmed S, Arjmand E, Sidell D. Role of obesity in otitis media in children. Curr Allergy Asthma Rep. 2014;14(11):469.
61. van Ingen G, le Clercq CMP, Jaddoe VWV, et al. Identifying distinct trajectories of acute otitis media in children: a prospective cohort study. Clin Otolaryngol. 2021;46:788.
62. Chen KK, Huang DT, Chou LT, Nieh HP, Fu RH, Chang CJ. Childhood otitis media: relationship with daycare attendance, harsh parenting, and maternal mental health. PLoS One. 2019;14(7):e0219684.
63. Lee JY, Kim SH, Song CI, Kim YR, Kim YJ, Choi JH. Risk factors for persistent otitis media with effusion in children: a case-control study. Yeungnam Univ J Med. 2018;35(1):70–5.
64. Korvel-Hanquist A, Koch A, Lous J, Olsen SF, Homoe P. Risk of childhood otitis media with focus on potentially modifiable factors: a Danish follow-up cohort study. Int J Pediatr Otorhinolaryngol. 2018;106:1–9.
65. Lodge CJ, Bowatte G, Matheson MC, Dharmage SC. The role of breastfeeding in childhood otitis media. Curr Allergy Asthma Rep. 2016;16(9):68.
66. Ardic C, Yavuz E. Effect of breastfeeding on common pediatric infections: a 5-year prospective cohort study. Arch Argent Pediatr. 2018;116(2):126–32.

67. Stordal K, Lundeby KM, Brantsaeter AL, et al. Breast-feeding and infant hospitalization for infections: large cohort and sibling analysis. J Pediatr Gastroenterol Nutr. 2017;65(2):225–31.
68. Raza GS, Herzig KH, Leppaluoto J. Invited review: milk fat globule membrane-a possible panacea for neurodevelopment, infections, cardiometabolic diseases, and frailty. J Dairy Sci. 2021;104:7345.
69. Ambrozej D, Dumycz K, Dziechciarz P, Ruszczynski M. Milk fat globule membrane supplementation in children: systematic review with meta-analysis. Nutrients. 2021;13(3):714.
70. Vigar V, Myers S, Oliver C, Arellano J, Robinson S, Leifert C. A systematic review of organic versus conventional food consumption: is there a measurable benefit on human health? Nutrients. 2019;12(1):7.
71. Narayanan I, Singh S, Mathur R, Jain BK. Ear infection and infant feeding practices. Indian J Pediatr. 1989;56(3):399–402. https://doi.org/10.1007/BF02722311.
72. Tully SB, Bar-Haim Y, Bradley RL. Abnormal tympanography after supine bottle feeding. J Pediatr. 1995;126(6):S105–11. https://doi.org/10.1016/s0022-3476(95)90249-x.
73. Salah M, Abdel-Aziz M, Al-Farok A, Jebrini A. Recurrent acute otitis media in infants: analysis of risk factors. Int J Pediatr Otorhinolaryngol. 2013;77(10):1665–9.
74. Ilia S, Galanakis E. Clinical features and outcome of acute otitis media in early infancy. Int J Infect Dis. 2013;17(5):e317–20.
75. Megged O, Abdulgany S, Bar-Meir M. Does acute otitis media in the first month of life increase the risk for recurrent otitis? Clin Pediatr (Phila). 2018;57(1):89–92.
76. Hauck FR, Omojokun OO, Siadaty MS. Do pacifiers reduce the risk of sudden infant death syndrome?A meta-analysis. Pediatrics. 2005;116(5):e716–23.
77. Caramia G, Serafini V, Loggi A. [The swimmer's otitis. An up to date and prevention options]. Pediatr Med Chir. 2013;35(4):177–82.
78. Sanchez L, Carney AS, Esterman A, Sparrow K, Turner D. Does access to saltwater swimming pools reduce ear pathology and hearing loss in school children of remote arid zone aboriginal communities? A prospective 3-year cohort study. Clin Otolaryngol. 2019;44(5):736–42.
79. Miyake MM, Tateno DA, Cancado NA, Miyake MM, Tincani S, Sousa Neto OM. Water protection in patients with tympanostomy tubes in tympanic membrane: a randomized clinical trial. Einstein (Sao Paulo). 2019;17(2):eAO4423.
80. Rosenfeld RM, Schwartz SR, Pynnonen MA, et al. Clinical practice guideline: tympanostomy tubes in children. Otolaryngol Head Neck Surg. 2013;149(1 Suppl):S1–35.
81. Lio CF, Cheong HH, Lei CI, et al. Effectiveness of personal protective health behaviour against COVID-19. BMC Public Health. 2021;29(1):827.
82. Torretta S, Capaccio P, Coro I, et al. Incidental lowering of otitis-media complaints in otitis-prone children during COVID-19 pandemic: not all evil comes to hurt. Eur J Pediatr. 2021;180(2):649–52.
83. Alde M, Di Berardino F, Marchisio P, et al. Effects of COVID-19 lockdown on otitis media with effusion in children: future therapeutic implications. Otolaryngol Head Neck Surg. 2021;165:710.

Otitis Media in Special Populations

28

Stephanie J. Wong and Daniela Carvalho

The rate of otitis media and other otologic problems is significantly higher in children with developmental anatomic issues such as Down syndrome or cleft palate, and physiologic issues such as primary ciliary dyskinesia or cystic fibrosis (CF). Furthermore, other predisposing conditions such as patients with sensorineural hearing loss or those prone to febrile seizures must also be considered in their overall clinical picture and otologic management.

Primary Ciliary Dyskinesia

Primary ciliary dyskinesia (PCD) is characterized by abnormal ciliary function impairing mucociliary clearance in the airway and middle ear, causing respiratory tract infections and otologic complications.

Pathophysiology

PCD is a genetically heterogenous disorder, which is predominantly inherited as an autosomal recessive trait [1]."Primary" was adopted for the term PCD, to distinguish it from secondary or acquired ciliary defects associated with infection and inflammation [2]. Ciliated epithelium covers most areas of the upper respiratory tract, including nasal mucosa, paranasal sinuses, middle ear, eustachian tube, and pharynx, and the lower respiratory tract from the trachea to the respiratory bronchioles. The normal ciliary axoneme is structurally made of nine peripheral doublet microtubules with attached dynein arms and radial spokes and two central single microtubules. Cilia propel overlying mucus via a ciliary beat cycle is mediated by dynein arms. Patients with primary ciliary dyskinesia can encompass a wide range and severity of axonemal defects [3–5], which ultimately impairs ciliary beating and mucociliary clearance. In approximately 30% of cases, there still may be abnormalities in function, despite normal ciliary structure [2].

Of note, Kartagener syndrome is part of the larger group of disorders referred to as primary ciliary dyskinesias and is characterized by the clinical trial of chronic rhinosinusitis, bronchiectasis, and *situs inversus*, which randomly occurs in approximately 50% of PCD cases.

Epidemiology

The estimated incidence of PCD is 1 in 10,000–40,000 births [6]. However, the prevalence of PCD in the United States is difficult to determine, largely due to inadequacies of diagnostic methods [7].

Clinical Presentation

The diagnosis of PCD is based on a combination of clinical phenotype, diagnostic tests such as nasal nitrous oxide measurement, inspection of mucosal cilia, and genetic testing. It is manifested clinically by neonatal respiratory distress in >80% of cases, evidence of chronic upper airway symptoms (daily nasal congestion, episodic facial pain, and anosmia), daily year-round wet cough starting soon after birth (nearly 100% of PCD patients), and early development of recurrent/chronic middle-ear and sinus disease [1, 2, 8].

In children with PCD, the ciliary function of the eustachian tube and the middle ear mucosa is impaired leading to mucous stasis and eustachian tube dysfunction. Recurrent otitis media with effusion (OME) seems to affect at least 80% of children with PCD, particularly in the first year of life [1, 9–11].

S. J. Wong
Pediatric Otolaryngology, Mount Sinai, NY, USA

D. Carvalho (✉)
Rady Children's Hospital, San Diego, San Diego, CA, USA

Division of Otolaryngology Head and Neck Surgery, University of California, San Diego, La Jolla, CA, USA
e-mail: dcarvalho@rchsd.org

M. V. Goycoolea et al. (eds.), *Textbook of Otitis Media*, https://doi.org/10.1007/978-3-031-40949-3_28

Otologic Management

The utility of tympanostomy tubes in this patient population is under some debate.

While OME in PCD patients can persist into adulthood, the hearing loss generally thought to resolve by the age of 12 years regardless of intervention [9, 12, 13]. Furthermore, several studies have found that tympanostomy tubes in PCD often results in prolonged and offensive otorrhea, multiple insertions, and permanent perforation [9, 13, 14]. Therefore, the 2009 European Respiratory Society Consensus Statement recommends managing OME in patients with PCD conservatively, with regular audiological assessment, hearing aids, and hearing therapy, since treatment with tympanostomy tubes can lead to significant morbidity without a long-term benefit to hearing.

On the other hand, more recent systematic reviews have shown benefit of tympanostomy tubes for patients with PCD. One 2009 literature review of eight studies found that ventilation tube insertion improves hearing in primary ciliary dyskinesia but may lead to higher rate of otorrhea (33%) when compared to the general population (3.8–13.2%) [15]. The 2016 PCD Foundation Consensus Recommendations advocate for tympanostomy tubes for children with PCD who have hearing deficits or speech delay and middle ear effusions based on literature review findings of significant hearing improvements post-tympanostomy tube placement in children with PCD compared to those managed with medical therapy alone [8]. Overall, it should be noted that the highest level of evidence found for the management of OME in children with PCD was level IV [15].

Regardless, all PCD patients considering tympanostomy tube placement should be counseled on the likelihood of multiple insertions, postoperative otorrhea, and possibility of permanent tympanic membrane perforation (up to 50% in one study) [16]. Furthermore, otolaryngologists should closely monitor these patients and always consider acquired cholesteatoma as a potential cause of persistent otorrhea in PCD given the poor eustachian tube function and multiple tympanostomy tube insertions. Pediatric PCD patients should visit a pediatric otolaryngologist at least once to twice annually, while adult patients should have otolaryngology care, as needed. An initial audiology assessment in all PCD patients is suggested at diagnosis, with subsequent evaluations coordinated through their otolaryngologist [8].

Cleft Palate

Orofacial clefts are the most common congenital malformations of the head and neck region, and approximately three-quarters of these patients have some form of cleft palate deformity [17]. Both cleft lip and cleft palate (CP) occur when tissues in the face and mouth do not fuse properly by the second or third month of pregnancy. Presentation can be varied, including with or without associated cleft lip, or be syndromic or nonsyndromic. Several subtypes of CP can be distinguished according to severity. At minimum, there can be cleaving of the uvula. A more severe form is a cleft of the soft palate. A submucous CP occurs when the cleft of the hard palate is covered by mucosa and continues through the soft palate. A complete CP is cleft of the hard palate, soft palate, and uvula. Meanwhile, a cleft anterior to the incisive foramen is also defined as a cleft of the primary palate. In all cases, CP can be associated with anatomic abnormalities that contribute to eustachian tube dysfunction [18].

Pathophysiology

Cleft palate results from the failure of the lateral palatine processes to meet and fuse with each other. This can be the result of (1) defective growth of the palatal shelves, (2) failure of the shelves to rise above the tongue, (3) lack of contact between shelves (such as in an excessively wide head), (4) failure to fuse, or (5) rupture after fusion of the shelves [18].

OME occurs in nearly all infants with an unrepaired cleft palate under the age of 2 years because of abnormal insertions of the tensor veli palatini, which causes limited ability of the eustachian tube to open actively. Failure of the eustachian tube opening and equalization of the pressure within the middle ear to that of the atmosphere leads to the accumulation of negative pressure and fluid stasis within the middle ear [19].

Epidemiology

The prevalence of CP alone is 0.5 per 1000 live births. The overall incidence of cleft lip with cleft palate is 1 per 700 live births. Sex differentiation (male:female ratio) for cleft lip and palate is about 2:1, and 1:2 for CP alone [18].

Clinical Presentation

At the time of cleft palate repair, more than 90% of the middle ears contain mucoid material ("glue ear") [20]. Approximately 75% of children with CP will have a history of nontrivial OME. In these patients, middle ear disease persists longer and leads to an increased incidence of conductive hearing loss, language delays, and cholesteatoma over that of their peers [21]. Furthermore, most children with CP have greater rates of acute otitis media (AOM). The incidence of AOM in these children is not comparable to that of the general population until adolescence [22].

In general, earlier age to cleft palate repair seems to correlate with a corresponding decrease in prevalence of middle ear dysfunction and hearing loss [23]. However, although its prevalence is reduced after surgical cleft palate repair, a significant number (13–36%) of these children continue to suffer from middle ear disease and sequelae into adolescence and adulthood [19, 24–27]. Severity or type of cleft palate does not seem to correlate with otologic or audiologic outcomes [25].

Otologic Management

The inability to establish adequate eustachian function leads to the near-universal recommendation that these children receive early tympanostomy tubes to prevent otologic complications related to the conductive hearing loss [28].

In the short term, patients treated early with ear tubes exhibit better audiometric results as well as better articulation and speech development compared with patients treated conservatively, whereas no significant differences have been observed regarding mid- or long-term outcomes [29, 30]. However, patients who received tympanostomy tube placement prior to time of palate repair (typically 9–12 months) was associated with increased repeat tympanostomy tube placement [31]. Thus, many doctors prefer to perform the repair of cleft palate and ventilation tube surgery simultaneously when the child is near 1 year old [31, 32].

The 2013 Clinical Practice Guidelines for tympanostomy tube codeveloped by the American Academy of Otolaryngology-Head and Neck Surgery Foundation (AAO-HNSF), the American Academy of Pediatrics (AAP), and the American Academy of Family Physicians (AAFP) advocate for a more individualized approach [33]. Specifically, that it may be appropriate to offer tympanostomy tubes on an individualized basis for cleft palate infants with OME that persists after failing hearing tests [33] because resolving the issue of middle ear effusion could facilitate the assessment of hearing status. Hearing aids are an alternative to tympanostomy tubes when hearing loss is present. Regardless, it is also recommended that clinicians evaluate children with cleft palate for OME and hearing loss at the time at which cleft palate is first diagnosed. It is recommended that middle ear status be assessed at 12–18 months of age, considering that this is a critical period in the development of language skills, speech, balance, and coordination. By 18 months of age, delays in language and speech development are easily identified. For children who do not receive tympanostomy tubes, the follow-up schedule to monitor OME and hearing loss until OME resolves should be more frequent than the 3–6-month intervals recommended for children without cleft palate.

Meanwhile, palatoplasty is observed to decrease the frequency of middle ear disease and improve hearing compared with untreated cleft palate [21]. The recovery rate of eustachian tube function after palatal surgery ranges from 40% to 86% [34, 35]. However, continued monitoring for OME and hearing loss should continue throughout childhood, including after palate repair, because of a continued high prevalence of effusion and hearing loss [33].

Down Syndrome

Down syndrome is characterized by dysmorphic facies, flat nasal bridge, epicanthal folds, brachycephaly with anterior–posterior flattening of the skull, a simian crease, learning disabilities, and generalized hypotonia [36]. Children with Down syndrome also experience an increased rate of recurrent AOM, OME, poor eustachian tube function, and stenotic ear canals that can impede the assessment of the tympanic membrane and middle ear status.

Pathophysiology

Down syndrome is genetically defined by a nondisjunction mutation resulting in trisomy of chromosome 21.

Patients with Down syndrome have a range of otologic problems including stenotic ear canals, increased incidence of otitis media, chronic ear disease, secondary hearing loss, as well as hearing loss caused by ossicular abnormalities and inner ear dysplasia.

Specifically, the high prevalence of serous otitis media in these patients is thought to be due to several factors. The major predisposing factors to otitis media in these children are thought to be the result of defective eustachian tube cartilage and musculature. In addition to histologically abnormal cartilage, the diameter of the eustachian tube is significantly smaller compared to the general population. Hypotonicity and muscular defects of the tensor palatini and dilator tubae have also been described. These produce stasis within the eustachian tube and allows easier ascent of bacteria from the nasopharynx [36].

Patients with Down syndrome also have midface and nasopharyngeal anatomy that predisposes them to chronic ear disease. Midface hypoplasia seen in many of these patients involves the nasopharynx and the eustachian tube openings. The bony confines of the nasopharynx are smaller in children with Down syndrome, and therefore even small- to medium-sized adenoids may give rise to eustachian tube dysfunction in these patients [37].

Finally, children with Down syndrome suffer from increased number of upper respiratory infections, thought to be related from both impaired immune function and nonimmunological factors. These episodes, in turn, can lead to more frequent middle ear effusions in the setting of increased nasal secretions and inflammation [37].

Epidemiology

The incidence of Down syndrome is approximately 1 in 700 [38]. This incidence increases proportionately with increasing maternal age, particularly after 35 years of age.

Clinical Presentation

As previously discussed, congenital and acquired otologic problems contribute to the relatively high incidence of hearing loss (conductive, sensorineural, and mixed) in patients with Down syndrome.

Patients with Down syndrome will often have their first encounter with an otolaryngologist for otologic issues. Narrowed ear canals predispose patients with Down syndrome to cerumen impaction, which adds to the difficulty to adequately examine the ear. Furthermore, prevalence of OME in this population is as high as 67–93% by age 1. Though, fortunately, this rate falls to 18–38% by the age of 8 years [39–41]. These patients are at significant risk for mixed or sensorineural hearing loss (up to 75%), which may persist throughout childhood and may require multiple tympanostomy tube placements [33, 42].

Otologic Management

Because of their increased risk of otologic complications, infants with Down syndrome should undergo complete audiologic evaluation, including behavioral sound field testing and auditory brainstem response by 1 month of age, and no later than 3 months. Thereafter, hearing assessments are recommended every 6 months, and evaluation by an otolaryngologist is recommended if middle ear status is uncertain or when hearing loss is found. Children with stenotic ear canals are best assessed with an otologic microscope every 3–6 months to remove cerumen and detect OME [33, 42, 43]. The presence or duration of MEE may be difficult to establish in some of these children because of limited ability to communicate, stenotic ear canals, and lack of cooperation for cerumen removal or tympanometry. These children are candidates for examination under anesthesia with the option of placing tympanostomy tubes if MEE is confirmed [33].

While the impact of tympanostomy tubes in this population has been variably reported in the literature regarding hearing outcomes and surgical complications (perforated tympanic membrane, recurrent or chronic otorrhea, and need for reoperation), there is a general consensus that children with Down syndrome may derive greater benefit from more timely tympanostomy insertion since they are at increased risk for speech, language, or learning problems from otitis media [33]. Some advocate tympanostomy tube placement earlier than in normal developing children without Down syndrome. However, the benefits of tympanostomy tube insertion are modest, though significant, and are offset by procedural risks. Ultimately, clinicians should offer tympanostomy tubes to children with Down syndrome with recurrent AOM or MEE that is unlikely to resolve quickly, but the final decision should incorporate provider experience, family values, and realistic expectations about the effect of reduced MEE and improved hearing on the child's developmental progress. If surgery is pursued, caregivers should also be counseled on the possible need for multiple sets of tympanostomy tubes and corresponding risk of long-term complications throughout the child's life [33, 37, 43].

Meanwhile, during surgery in patients with Down syndrome, the surgeon should always be aware of the possibility of atlantoaxial instability, and no dramatic head movement should be made.

Mucopolysaacharidoses

Mucopolysaacharidoses (MPS) represent a spectrum of disorders characterized by the genetic deficiency of specific lysosomal enzymes leading to glycosaminoglycan (GAGs) accumulation in tissues leading to progressive damage and a variety of multi-organ clinical manifestations.

Pathophysiology

There are currently seven recognized subtypes of MPS caused by a deficiency of 1 of 11 enzymes involved in the degradation of GAGs [44], but all forms ultimately result in cellular dysfunction from the progressive accumulation of partially degraded GAGs within the cells of various body tissues. These disorders are inherited primarily in an autosomal recessive pattern (except for MPS II, which is X-linked) [45]. Because of the ubiquitous presence of GAGs throughout the body, clinical manifestations are variable and often multisystemic. Clinical features are often absent at birth, appearing gradually as the disease progresses, and commonly ends with death before adulthood.

Epidemiology

MPS disorders are rare and have an overall incidence reported between 1 in 150,000 and 1 in 10,000 live births.

Clinical Presentation

Children have highly variable, multisystemic involvement, and the full comprehensive descriptions of each subtype are beyond the scope of this chapter. However, some unifying features include characteristic coarse facial features, developmental delay, mental retardation, and skeletal or joint dysplasia. Moreover, ENT disorders affect more than 90% of MPS patients and appear relatively early on (median age 2.8 years), including recurrent AOM, persistent OME, hearing loss, macroglossia, adenotonsillar hypertrophy, nasal obstruction, and progressive respiratory disorders [45–47]. Patients will often present with symptoms of sleep apnea, frequent respiratory and ear infections, chronic nasal discharge, and enlargement of the tongue, tonsils, and adenoids. Therefore, otolaryngologists are commonly the first clinicians to whom these patients present, with median age of a first ENT visit around 4 years of age [46–48]. This is often prior to definitive MPS diagnosis, so otolaryngologists are in optimal position to establish diagnosis by initiating workup and referral for definitive testing.

Patients with MPS are prone to AOM and OME due to the accumulation of GAGs in the postnasal space and middle ear, with reported prevalence ranging between 72% and 91% depending on subtype [44, 46, 49, 50]. They often have a number of ventilation tube insertions prior to the diagnosis of MPS being made. Furthermore, 53–100% patients with MPS will also frequently experience progressive hearing loss, which has both conductive and sensorineural components [47, 50]. While the conductive loss is generally attributed to chronic effusions and eustachian tube dysfunction, the etiology of the sensorineural component is less clear [45].

Traditionally, MPS disorders were regarded as incurable, progressing until causing death often before adulthood due to cardiac or respiratory failure. However, more recently enzyme replacement therapy and bone marrow transplantation have had some limited success in select cases [49].

Otologic Management

Given their predisposition for AOM and OME, patients with MPS will frequently require symptomatic treatment to improve the quality of life. The conductive hearing loss and recurrent AOM these patients frequently experience can be improved with insertion of tympanostomy tubes and adenoidectomy [50, 51]. When possible, it is generally recommended to opt for inserting long-term tympanostomy tubes, as opposed to short-term ones, once diagnosis of MPS has been made to decrease the number of anesthetic procedures these patients have to undergo. Despite this, patients may still require multiple sets of tubes in their lifetime [44, 52, 53]. Furthermore, as patients often present with mixed hearing loss, parents should be counseled that amplification is often still required to overcome what is generally permanent sensorineural hearing loss [45, 48].

The progressive nature of hearing loss means that continuous monitoring of hearing thresholds is necessary to optimize amplification [46, 48]. Some international guidelines have been published focusing on specific subtypes of MPS, which generally recommend age-adjusted audiology assessments to be done at diagnosis and on an annual basis thereafter [52, 54–57]. One guideline focusing on MPS IVa recommended ENT examination, including tympanometry, to be conducted every 3–6 months during childhood, and every 6–12 months thereafter [56].

Of note, children with MPS may also present with difficult intubations due to trismus, macroglossia, and short stiff neck. Furthermore, these patients potentially have neck instability (universal in MPS IV, but also may manifest in other MPS types) [49]. Both features should be taken into account when arranging for surgery in these patients.

Other Considerations

Immunodeficiency

Primary immunodeficiencies, also known as inborn errors of immunity, are rare congenital defects of the immune system with an estimated prevalence of 1 in 10,000 to 1 in 12,000 in the general population [58]. These conditions can manifest in a broad-spectrum of clinical presentations. However, in the pediatric population, recurrent otitis (4 or more ear infections in 1 year) should raise suspicion for possible underlying immunodeficiency or at least prompt further questioning for relevant personal or family history [59]. Similarly, for the adult population, the European Society of Immunodeficiencies identified clinical manifestations which would be significant for identifying primary immunodeficiency. These include four or more infections treated with antibiotics in 1 year (otitis, bronchitis, sinusitis, and pneumonia) and recurrent infections needing prolonged therapy with antibiotics [59]. Overall, clinicians should have a low threshold for investigating for immune defects in patients presenting with otitis evolving with mastoiditis, abscesses, or systemic infections; no response to appropriate antibiotic therapy; otitis media associated with other infections; recurrent otitis leading to failure to thrive and general developmental delay; and family history of primary immunodeficiency [59, 60].

Infectious complications can present a significant cause of mortality and morbidity among patients with immunodeficiencies. While exact guidelines do not exist, these patients should be treated more aggressively as they are more prone to severe complications from otologic problems. In the case of otitis media, this includes having a lower threshold for empirically treating with antibiotics and/or considering tympanocentesis, followed by aspiration and culture of middle ear fluid samples [61].

Sensorineural Hearing Loss

Otitis media with effusion (OME) is an important cause of transient moderate hearing loss in newborns that can result in a failed newborn hearing screen. However, it is critically important to remember that although many infants who fail screening because of transient middle ear effusion will normalize within several months of effusion resolution, some also have an underlying sensorineural hearing loss. The AAO-HNSF clinical practice guidelines on otitis media with effusion and the American Academy of Audiology guidelines for the diagnosis and treatment of otitis media in children both emphasize the importance of patient follow-up after a failed newborn screening, even if the cause is presumed to be secondary to OME [43, 62]. Insertion of tympanostomy tubes to resolve effusion and facilitate better assessment of hearing status may also be appropriate on an individualized basis for children with severe hearing loss (which cannot be attributed completely to OME), a history of congenital sensorineural hearing loss (SNHL) in the immediate family, or an at-risk status for developmental difficulties [43].

Similarly, patients with known SNHL should be considered at-risk patients who could be disproportionately affected by the conductive hearing loss associated with otitis media. These are patients who might benefit from an earlier intervention for acute otitis media or otitis media with effusion including more active and accurate surveillance of middle ear status [33, 43].

Meanwhile, recent studies have found chronic otitis media to also be associated with some degree of sensorineural hearing loss in addition to conductive hearing loss, suggestive of inner ear damage [63–71]. Reported prevalence of SNHL in these patients vary widely, ranging between <1% and 52% [65, 68, 72]. The exact etiology is unclear; however, patients with longer duration of disease seems to have greater susceptibility to develop SNHL [67]. Higher frequencies also appear to be more affected [63, 65]. Other potential risk factors include age, presence of cholesteatoma, and tympanic membrane perforation size [64, 67, 69–71]. There is also some evidence for an association between sudden sensorineural hearing loss and chronic otitis media [66, 73]. Ultimately, while the clinical significance requires more study, these findings suggest that the inner ear is vulnerable to otitis media and should be taken to account when considering treatment of otitis media.

Cystic Fibrosis

Cystic fibrosis (CF) is an autosomal recessive genetic disease caused by mutations in the gene that encodes the regulatory protein for transmembrane conductance (CFTR), resulting in a range of clinical phenotypes affecting the pulmonary, pancreatic, and sino-nasal systems. Historically, CF was once considered to be protective against otitis media, based on significantly lower reported rates of otitis media in age-matched CF and non-CF children [74]. More recent studies, however, have demonstrated that OM in CF children appears to be similar to OM in non-CF children [75]. This may be due to expanding diagnostic capabilities and refinements in the diagnostic criteria by the CF Foundation International Committee in 2017 [76]. As such, CF should no longer be considered protective against otitis media, as this seems to not hold true.

References

1. Barbato A, Frischer T, Kuehni CE, et al. Primary ciliary dyskinesia: a consensus statement on diagnostic and treatment approaches in children. Eur Respir J. 2009;34(6):1264–76. https://doi.org/10.1183/09031936.00176608.
2. Knowles MR, Daniels LA, Davis SD, Zariwala MA, Leigh MW. Primary ciliary dyskinesia. Recent advances in diagnostics, genetics, and characterization of clinical disease. Am J Respir Crit Care Med. 2013;188(8):913–22. https://doi.org/10.1164/rccm.201301-0059CI.
3. Rutland J, Cox T, Dewar A, Cole P. Screening for ciliary dyskinesia—a spectrum of defects of motility and structure. Eur J Respir Dis Suppl. 1983;127:71–7.
4. Sturgess JM, Chao J, Wong J, Aspin N, Turner JA. Cilia with defective radial spokes: a cause of human respiratory disease. N Engl J Med. 1979;300(2):53–6. https://doi.org/10.1056/NEJM197901113000201.
5. Sturgess JM, Chao J, Turner JA. Transposition of ciliary microtubules: another cause of impaired ciliary motility. N Engl J Med. 1980;303(6):318–22. https://doi.org/10.1056/NEJM198008073030606.
6. Kuehni CE, Frischer T, Strippoli M-PF, et al. Factors influencing age at diagnosis of primary ciliary dyskinesia in European children. Eur Respir J. 2010;36(6):1248–58. https://doi.org/10.1183/09031936.00001010.
7. Leigh MW, O'Callaghan C, Knowles MR. The challenges of diagnosing primary ciliary dyskinesia. Proc Am Thorac Soc. 2011;8(5):434–7. https://doi.org/10.1513/pats.201103-028SD.
8. Shapiro AJ, Zariwala MA, Ferkol T, et al. Diagnosis, monitoring, and treatment of primary ciliary dyskinesia: PCD foundation consensus recommendations based on state of the art review. Pediatr Pulmonol. 2016;51(2):115–32. https://doi.org/10.1002/ppul.23304.
9. Majithia A, Fong J, Hariri M, Harcourt J. Hearing outcomes in children with primary ciliary dyskinesia—a longitudinal study.

Int J Pediatr Otorhinolaryngol. 2005;69(8):1061–4. https://doi.org/10.1016/j.ijporl.2005.02.013.
10. Pederson M. Nose-, sinus- and ear-symptoms in 27 patients with primary ciliary dyskinesia. Eur J Respir Dis Suppl. 1983;127:96–101. Published 31 Dec 1982. Accessed 31 Mar 2021. https://europepmc.org/article/med/6604651.
11. Sommer JU, Schäfer K, Omran H, et al. ENT manifestations in patients with primary ciliary dyskinesia: prevalence and significance of otorhinolaryngologic co-morbidities. Eur Arch Otorhinolaryngol. 2011;268(3):383–8. https://doi.org/10.1007/s00405-010-1341-9.
12. Ghedia R, Ahmed J, Navaratnam A, Harcourt J. No evidence of cholesteatoma in untreated otitis media with effusion in children with primary ciliary dyskinesia. Int J Pediatr Otorhinolaryngol. 2018;105:176–80. https://doi.org/10.1016/j.ijporl.2017.12.015.
13. Hadfield PJ, Rowe-Jones JM, Bush A, Mackay IS. Treatment of otitis media with effusion in children with primary ciliary dyskinesia. Clin Otolaryngol Allied Sci. 1997;22(4):302–6. https://doi.org/10.1046/j.1365-2273.1997.00020.x.
14. el-Sayed Y, al-Sarhani A, al-Essa AR. Otological manifestations of primary ciliary dyskinesia. Clin Otolaryngol Allied Sci. 1997;22(3):266–70. https://doi.org/10.1046/j.1365-2273.1997.00895.x.
15. Campbell RG, Birman CS, Morgan L. Management of otitis media with effusion in children with primary ciliary dyskinesia: a literature review. Int J Pediatr Otorhinolaryngol. 2009;73(12):1630–8. https://doi.org/10.1016/j.ijporl.2009.08.024.
16. Prulière-Escabasse V, Coste A, Chauvin P, et al. Otologic features in children with primary ciliary dyskinesia. Arch Otolaryngol Head Neck Surg. 2010;136(11):1121–6. https://doi.org/10.1001/archoto.2010.183.
17. Woo AS. Evidence-based medicine: cleft palate. Plast Reconstr Surg. 2017;139(1):191e–203e. https://doi.org/10.1097/PRS.0000000000002854.
18. Bernheim N, Georges M, Malevez C, De Mey A, Mansbach A. Embryology and epidemiology of cleft lip and palate. B-ENT. 2006;2(Suppl 4):11–9.
19. Heidsieck DSP, Smarius BJA, Oomen KPQ, Breugem CC. The role of the tensor veli palatini muscle in the development of cleft palate-associated middle ear problems. Clin Oral Invest. 2016;20(7):1389–401. https://doi.org/10.1007/s00784-016-1828-x.
20. Muntz HR. An overview of middle ear disease in cleft palate children. Facial Plast Surg. 1993;9(3):177–80. https://doi.org/10.1055/s-2008-1064609.
21. Smith LK, Gubbels SP, MacArthur CJ, Milczuk HA. The effect of the palatoplasty method on the frequency of ear tube placement. Arch Otolaryngol Head Neck Surg. 2008;134(10):1085. https://doi.org/10.1001/archotol.134.10.1085.
22. Harman NL, Bruce IA, Kirkham JJ, et al. The importance of integration of stakeholder views in core outcome set development: otitis media with effusion in children with cleft palate. PLoS One. 2015;10(6):e0129514. https://doi.org/10.1371/journal.pone.0129514.
23. Lou Q, Zhu H, Luo Y, et al. The effects of age at cleft palate repair on middle ear function and hearing level. Cleft Palate Craniofac J. 2018;55(5):753–7. https://doi.org/10.1177/1055665618754632.
24. Dochy F, Vanheule E, Leenheer ED, et al. Middle ear problems in children with cleft palate: a cross-sectional study. Arch Otolaryngol Rhinol. 2019;5(3):078–82.
25. Funamura JL, Lee JW, McKinney S, Bayoumi AG, Senders CW, Tollefson TT. Children with cleft palate: predictors of otologic issues in the first 10 years. Otolaryngol Head Neck Surg. 2019;160(5):902–10. https://doi.org/10.1177/0194599818825461.
26. Sehhati-Chafai-Leuwer S, Wenzel S, Bschorer R, et al. Pathophysiology of the Eustachian tube—relevant new aspects for the head and neck surgeon. J Craniomaxillofac Surg. 2006;34(6):351–4. https://doi.org/10.1016/j.jcms.2006.03.006.
27. Sheahan P, Miller I, Sheahan JN, Earley MJ, Blayney AW. Incidence and outcome of middle ear disease in cleft lip and/or cleft palate. Int J Pediatr Otorhinolaryngol. 2003;67(7):785–93. https://doi.org/10.1016/s0165-5876(03)00098-3.
28. Berryhill W. Otologic concerns for cleft lip and palate patient. Oral Maxillofac Surg Clin North Am. 2016;28(2):177–9. https://doi.org/10.1016/j.coms.2015.12.001.
29. Azman A, Manuel AM. Otological outcome in cleft lip and palate children with middle ear effusion. Int J Pediatr Otorhinolaryngol. 2020;138:110274. https://doi.org/10.1016/j.ijporl.2020.110274.
30. Imbery TE, Sobin LB, Commesso E, et al. Long-term Otologic and audiometric outcomes in patients with cleft palate. Otolaryngol Head Neck Surg. 2017;157(4):676–82. https://doi.org/10.1177/0194599817707514.
31. Shaffer AD, Ford MD, Choi SS, Jabbour N. The impact of timing of Tympanostomy tube placement on sequelae in children with cleft palate. Cleft Palate Craniofac J. 2019;56(6):720–8. https://doi.org/10.1177/1055665618809228.
32. Kuo C-L, Shiao A-S. Tympanostomy tube placement for otitis media with effusion in children with cleft lip and palate. In: Designing strategies for cleft lip and palate care. IntechOpen. Published online 22 Mar 2017. https://doi.org/10.5772/67122.
33. Rosenfeld RM, Schwartz SR, Pynnonen MA, et al. Clinical practice guideline: tympanostomy tubes in children. Otolaryngol Head Neck Surg. 2013;149(1_Suppl):S1–S35. https://doi.org/10.1177/0194599813487302.
34. Alper CM, Losee JE, Mandel EM, Seroky JT, Swarts JD, Doyle WJ. Pre- and post-palatoplasty Eustachian tube function in infants with cleft palate. Int J Pediatr Otorhinolaryngol. 2012;76(3):388–91. https://doi.org/10.1016/j.ijporl.2011.12.017.
35. Alper CM, Losee JE, Mandel EM, Seroky JT, Swarts JD, Doyle WJ. Postpalatoplasty Eustachian tube function in young children with cleft palate. Cleft Palate Craniofac J. 2012;49(4):504–7. https://doi.org/10.1597/11-065.
36. Kanamori G, Witter M, Brown J, Williams-Smith L. Otolaryngologic manifestations of Down syndrome. Otolaryngol Clin N Am. 2000;33(6):1285–92. https://doi.org/10.1016/s0030-6665(05)70281-4.
37. Rodman R, Pine HS. The otolaryngologist's approach to the patient with down syndrome. Otolaryngol Clin N Am. 2012;45(3):599–629. https://doi.org/10.1016/j.otc.2012.03.010.
38. Mai CT, Isenburg JL, Canfield MA, et al. National population-based estimates for major birth defects, 2010–2014. Birth Defects Res. 2019;111(18):1420–35. https://doi.org/10.1002/bdr2.1589.
39. Barr E, Dungworth J, Hunter K, McFarlane M, Kubba H. The prevalence of ear, nose and throat disorders in preschool children with Down's syndrome in Glasgow. Scott Med J. 2011;56(2):98–103. https://doi.org/10.1258/smj.2011.011036.
40. Austeng ME, Akre H, Øverland B, Abdelnoor M, Falkenberg E-S, Kværner KJ. Otitis media with effusion in children with in Down syndrome. Int J Pediatr Otorhinolaryngol. 2013;77(8):1329–32. https://doi.org/10.1016/j.ijporl.2013.05.027.
41. Maris M, Wojciechowski M, Van de Heyning P, Boudewyns A. A cross-sectional analysis of otitis media with effusion in children with Down syndrome. Eur J Pediatr. 2014;173(10):1319–25. https://doi.org/10.1007/s00431-014-2323-5.
42. Bull MJ, Committee on Genetics. Healthsupervision for children with down syndrome. Pediatrics. 2011;128(2):393–406. https://doi.org/10.1542/peds.2011-1605.
43. Rosenfeld RM, Shin JJ, Schwartz SR, et al. Clinical practice guideline: otitis media with effusion (update). Otolaryngol Head Neck Surg. 2016;154:S1.Published online 1 Feb 2016. https://doi.org/10.1177/0194599815623467.

44. Wolfberg J, Chintalapati K, Tomatsu S, Nagao K. Hearing loss in mucopolysaccharidoses: current knowledge and future directions. Diagnostics (Basel). 2020;10(8) https://doi.org/10.3390/diagnostics10080554.
45. Wold SM, Derkay CS, Darrow DH, Proud V. Role of the pediatric otolaryngologist in diagnosis and management of children with mucopolysaccharidoses. Int J Pediatr Otorhinolaryngol. 2010;74(1):27–31. https://doi.org/10.1016/j.ijporl.2009.09.042.
46. Bianchi PM, Gaini R, Vitale S. ENT and mucopolysaccharidoses. Ital J Pediatr. 2018;44(Suppl 2) https://doi.org/10.1186/s13052-018-0555-0.
47. Murgasova L, Jurovcik M, Jesina P, et al. Otorhinolaryngological manifestations in 61 patients with mucopolysaccharidosis. Int J Pediatr Otorhinolaryngol. 2020;135:110137. https://doi.org/10.1016/j.ijporl.2020.110137.
48. Motamed M, Thorne S, Narula A. Treatment of otitis media with effusion in children with mucopolysaccharidoses. Int J Pediatr Otorhinolaryngol. 2000;53(2):121–4. https://doi.org/10.1016/s0165-5876(00)00320-7.
49. Simmons MA, Bruce IA, Penney S, Wraith E, Rothera MP. Otorhinolaryngological manifestations of the mucopolysaccharidoses. Int J Pediatr Otorhinolaryngol. 2005;69(5):589–95. https://doi.org/10.1016/j.ijporl.2005.01.017.
50. Mesolella M, Cimmino M, Cantone E, et al. Management of otolaryngological manifestations in mucopolysaccharidoses: our experience. Acta Otorhinolaryngol Ital. 2013;33(4):267–72.
51. Oghan F, Harputluoglu U, Guclu E, Guvey A, Turan N, Ozturk O. Permanent t-tube insertion in two patients with Hurler's syndrome. Int J Audiol. 2007;46(2):94–6. https://doi.org/10.1080/14992020600975287.
52. Hendriksz CJ, Berger KI, Giugliani R, et al. International guidelines for the management and treatment of Morquio A syndrome. Am J Med Genet A. 2015;167(1):11–25. https://doi.org/10.1002/ajmg.a.36833.
53. Nan H, Park C, Maeng S. Mucopolysaccharidoses I and II: brief review of therapeutic options and supportive/palliative therapies. Biomed Res Int. 2020;2020:1. https://doi.org/10.1155/2020/2408402.
54. Stapleton M, Hoshina H, Sawamoto K, et al. Critical review of current MPS guidelines and management. Mol Genet Metab. 2019;126(3):238–45. https://doi.org/10.1016/j.ymgme.2018.07.001.
55. Martins AM, Dualibi AP, Norato D, et al. Guidelines for the management of mucopolysaccharidosis type I. J Pediatr. 2009;155(4 Suppl):S32–46. https://doi.org/10.1016/j.jpeds.2009.07.005.
56. Akyol MU, Alden TD, Amartino H, et al. Recommendations for the management of MPS IVA: systematic evidence- and consensus-based guidance. Orphanet J Rare Dis. 2019;14:137. https://doi.org/10.1186/s13023-019-1074-9.
57. Scarpa M, Almássy Z, Beck M, et al. Mucopolysaccharidosis type II: European recommendations for the diagnosis and multidisciplinary management of a rare disease. Orphanet J Rare Dis. 2011;6:72. https://doi.org/10.1186/1750-1172-6-72.
58. Bucciol G, Moens L, Bosch B, et al. Lessons learned from the study of human inborn errors of innate immunity. J Allergy Clin Immunol. 2019;143(2):507–27. https://doi.org/10.1016/j.jaci.2018.07.013.
59. Bardou MLD, Pontarolli D, Grumach AS. Otitis media and inborn errors of immunity. Curr Allergy Asthma Rep. 2020;20(10):59. https://doi.org/10.1007/s11882-020-00957-x.
60. Urschel S. Otitis media in children with congenital immunodeficiencies. Curr Allergy Asthma Rep. 2010;10(6):425–33. https://doi.org/10.1007/s11882-010-0143-x.
61. Ramakrishnan K, Sparks RA, Berryhill WE. Diagnosis and treatment of otitis media. AFP. 2007;76(11):1650–8.
62. Audiologic guidelines for the diagnosis and treatment of otitis media in children. The American Academy of Audiology. Accessed 26 Jul 2021. https://www.audiology.org/practice-resources/practice-guidelines-and-standards/audiologic-guidelines-for-the-diagnosis-and-treatment-of-otitis-media-in-children/.
63. Amali A, Hosseinzadeh N, Samadi S, Nasiri S, Zebardast J. Sensorineural hearing loss in patients with chronic suppurative otitis media: is there a significant correlation? Electron Physician. 2017;9(2):3823–7. https://doi.org/10.19082/3823.
64. Kasemodel ALP, Costa LEM, da Costa Monsanto R, Tomaz A, de Oliveira Penido N. Sensorineural hearing loss in the acute phase of a single episode of acute otitis media. Braz J Otorhinolaryngol. 2020;86(6):767–73. https://doi.org/10.1016/j.bjorl.2019.06.001.
65. Lee D, Kim Y, Kim D-K. Sensorineural hearing loss after surgery to treat chronic otitis media. Ear Nose Throat J. 2021;100(3_Suppl):220S–4S. https://doi.org/10.1177/0145561320968929.
66. Choi HG, Min C, Lee CH, Kim SY. The relation of sudden sensorineural hearing loss in pediatric patients with recurrent otitis media: anested case-control study using a national sample cohort. Otol Neurotol. 2020;41(7):e836–41. https://doi.org/10.1097/MAO.0000000000002655.
67. Subramaniam V, Ashkar A, Rai S. Cochlear dysfunction in chronic otitis media and its determinants. Iran J Otorhinolaryngol. 2020;32(109):79–84. https://doi.org/10.22038/ijorl.2019.35045.2158.
68. Ali Zaidi SS, Pasha HA, Suhail A, Qureshi TA. Frequency of sensorineural hearing loss in chronic suppurative otitis media. J Pak Med Assoc. 2016;66(Suppl 3(10)):S42–4.
69. da Costa SS, Rosito LPS, Dornelles C. Sensorineural hearing loss in patients with chronic otitis media. Eur Arch Otorhinolaryngol. 2009;266(2):221–4. https://doi.org/10.1007/s00405-008-0739-0.
70. Papp Z, Rezes S, Jókay I, Sziklai I. Sensorineural hearing loss in chronic otitis media. OtolNeurotol. 2003;24(2):141–4. https://doi.org/10.1097/00129492-200303000-00003.
71. Singer AEA, Abdel-Naby Awad OG, El-Kader RMA, Mohamed AR. Risk factors of sensorineural hearing loss in patients with unilateral safe chronic suppurative otitis media. Am J Otolaryngol. 2018;39(2):88–93. https://doi.org/10.1016/j.amjoto.2018.01.002.
72. Rajput MS-E-A, Rajput MSA, Arain AA, Zaidi SS, Hatem A, Akram S. Mucosal type of chronic suppurative otitis media and the long-term impact on hearing loss. Cureus. 2020;12(9):e10176. https://doi.org/10.7759/cureus.10176.
73. Yen Y-C, Lin C, Weng S-F, Lin Y-S. Higher risk of developing sudden sensorineural hearing loss in patients with chronic otitis media. JAMA Otolaryngol Head Neck Surg. 2015;141(5):429–35. https://doi.org/10.1001/jamaoto.2015.102.
74. Haddad J Jr, Gonzalez C, Kurland G, Orenstein DM, Casselbrant ML. Ear disease in children with cystic fibrosis. Arch Otolaryngol Head Neck Surg. 1994;120(5):491–3. https://doi.org/10.1001/archotol.1994.01880290009002.
75. McCoy JL, Kaffenberger TM, Yang TS, Shaffer AD, Dohar JE. Middle ear disease in CF? It's not just about the sinuses anymore! Int J Pediatr Otorhinolaryngol. 2020;134:110032. https://doi.org/10.1016/j.ijporl.2020.110032.
76. Farrell PM, White TB, Ren CL, et al. Diagnosis of cystic fibrosis: consensus guidelines from the cystic fibrosis foundation. J Pediatr. 2017;181S:S4–S15.e1. https://doi.org/10.1016/j.jpeds.2016.09.064.

Early in Life Otitis Media and Its Impact in Hearing, Speech Development, and Central Auditory Processing

29

Berenice Dias Ramos

The strong interest in the neurobiological sequelae of human auditory deprivation in the form of otitis media (OM) is attributable to the high prevalence of OM in children [1]. At least 80% of the children have otitis media with effusion (OME) on at least one occasion before the age of 4 years [2]. The condition is common enough to be called an "occupational hazard" of early childhood [3] because about 90% of children have OME before school age [4] and they develop, on average, four episodes of OME every year [5]. It is postulated that middle ear effusion (MEE) is a "physiological" phenomenon at pre-school age with some pathological exceptions [2]. To understand the impact of OM on hearing, speech development, and central auditory processing (CAP), it is important to know that:

- Middle ear infection is the most common cause of pediatric temporary hearing loss [6].
- The ability to process two or more rapidly presented, successive, auditory stimuli is believed to underlie successful language acquisition [7]. MEE can delay sound transmission [1], interfering with the speed of auditory processing, which could impair language development.
- The auditory system is assumed to have its most sensitive period for speech perception between 0 and 2 years [8, 9], which is at the same time the period when OM occurrence has its highest incidence [10].
- The baby makes a brain map of all the phonemes of the native language until the end of the first year of life [8]. To make a good phonetic map, it is necessary to prevent OM before the first year of life.
- The primary risk factor for abnormalities in brain physiology, auditory perception, and speech receptivity that can accompany OM in childhood is not the presence of the disease state itself but the degradation of the afferent signal that can arise from OM [1].
- Degraded afferent signaling does not always accompany OM [11]. Sixty-seven percent of children with OM have average hearing levels (HLs) of 16 dB (decibel) or greater, 15% demonstrated hearing thresholds greater than 25 dB HL, while just 6% had threshold shifts that exceeded 35 dB HL [11].
- Early onset, degree of hearing loss, more frequent infections, and infections of longer duration have all been shown to act as risk factors for long-term consequences [1].

B. D. Ramos (✉)
Phoniatrics, Otorhinolaryngology Head and Neck Surgery Service, Hospital de Clínicas de Porto Alegre, UFRGS, Porto Alegre, RS, Brazil

Otitis media and hearing

Conductive Hearing Loss (CHL)

OM has both acute and persistent effects on hearing [1]. The middle ear pathology and accumulation of excess, viscous mucin that typically accompany OM can disrupt the acoustic-mechanical properties of the middle ear system, producing a conductive hearing loss (CHL) [1]. Although OM is physically restricted to the middle ear space, it can interfere with the transmission of acoustic signals to the inner ear and, by extension, the entire auditory system [1].

The conventional cutoff for normal-range hearing in children is 15 dB HL [6]. In a large sample of prospectively followed young children (years 1, 2, and 3) diagnosed with OM, 67% had average hearing levels of 16 dB HL or greater, 15% demonstrated hearing thresholds greater than 25 dB HL, while just 6% had threshold shifts that exceeded 35 dB HL [11]. During year 2, 68% of children OME positive had average hearing levels greater than 15 dB HL. In year 3, half of the children considered OME positive had average hearing levels greater than 15 dB HL [11]. The resilience of hearing sensitivity in the presence of MEE can be attributed to the

M. V. Goycoolea et al. (eds.), *Textbook of Otitis Media*, https://doi.org/10.1007/978-3-031-40949-3_29

transmission properties of the middle ear, which are relatively unaffected by large, yet incomplete, reductions in tympanum volume [1]. Even small bubbles in the fluid introduce a sufficient volume in the middle ear space to improve mechanical transmission [1]. Therefore, while the presence of MEE will likely produce an abnormal tympanogram, a middle ear transmission metric often used to diagnose OM, the quality of the afferent signal transmitted to the brain may be unaffected [1].

The characteristics of the CHL associated with OME differ from those of permanent CHL or cochlear hearing impairments [11]. Rather than a stable auditory deficit, the amount and viscosity of the fluid in both ears during any given episode influences the degree and configuration of the CHL [11]. The CHL associated with OME is temporary, but sometimes persistent or recurrent, and variable (fluctuating) in degree and symmetry [11].

During early childhood, especially in the first 3 years, active OME reduces the level of sound entering the ear by up to 38 dB [11] and delays the sound by up to 300 μs [12]. The impact of OME on hearing ranges from normal hearing to moderate CHL (0–55 dB) [13, 14]. The average CHL associated with OME in children is 28 dB HL (hearing level), while a lesser proportion (approximately 20%) exceed 35 dB HL [13, 15]. The air conduction configuration is roughly flat with a slight elevation at 2000 Hz and a nadir at 8000 Hz [16].

OME fluctuates between unilateral and bilateral, with individual episodes lasting from a few days to many weeks [17, 18]. In general, hearing threshold levels were highest in the youngest children tested with visual reinforcement audiometry and lowest in the oldest children tested with conventional audiometry [14]. On average, the presence of bilateral MEE was associated with hearing threshold levels 10–15 dB higher than the normative values for the corresponding age group [14]. Chronic OME prevents complete access to auditory language, which may limit the development of mature speech weighting strategies. Several investigators have reported that OME is often associated with an audiogram where sensitivity at 2000 Hz is better (by 7–10 dB) than at lower and higher frequencies [19, 20]. Dobie and Berlin (1979) speculated that the peak in sensitivity at 2000 Hz may be a result of intrinsic properties of the middle ear system, i.e., a crossover point between separate mass and stiffness components of the hearing loss [21]. They noted that even mild alterations in the speech spectrum could result in changes in speech perception in children with OME, particularly at poor signal-to-noise ratios [21]. The spectral region around 2000 Hz, where sensitivity is usually best and least variable over time in children with recurrent episodes of OME, is given more weight than lower and higher spectral regions [22]. This hypothesis is based on the idea that the abnormal spectral input experienced by children with chronic OME may result in adaptation of the neural structures that underlie the processing of speech [22]. Listeners with OME may compensate for degraded auditory input by placing high weight upon spectral information that is relatively reliable and by learning to accommodate the range of spectral configurations that they encounter because of chronic, intermittent CHL [22].

Extended High-Frequency Hearing Loss

The CHL that accompanies OM is reversible and hearing sensitivity returns to normal following resolution of OM [11]. Studies have found that frequencies above 4 kHz and up to as high as 20 kHz have poorer thresholds that persist after the recovery of middle ear function, including tympanometry, high frequency middle ear reflectance, and bone conduction [23–25]. The difference in thresholds increases with greater frequency, suggesting basal cochlear involvement [26]. Better hearing thresholds in the region from 6 to 12.5 kHz have been associated with better reception of speech in background noise [26]. Because OME is a common childhood condition, poorer extended high-frequency hearing could be a basis for poorer speech perception, especially in noise, for children with histories of recurrent or chronic OME [26].

Hunter et al. (2021) studying children with idiopathic listening difficulties found that extended high-frequency hearing thresholds, wideband tympanometry, contralateral middle ear muscle reflexes, distortion product, and transient evoked otoacoustic emissions were related to a history of pressure equalization tube surgery [26]. The physiologic measures were also associated with extended high-frequency hearing loss, secondary to pressure equalization tube history [26].

Decreased sensitivity in the extended high frequency (>8 kHz) could result from pathology in the basal cochlea, as has been reported in association with chronic childhood OME and treated with tubes [23–25]. Animal studies of experimentally induced OME have shown that the mechanism for extended high-frequency hearing loss is round window transmission of bacterial endotoxins with basilar cochlear damage [27–29]. Inner ear morphology shows pathologic changes in the stria vascularis, suggesting it is a target of OM-induced damage, which may lead to sensorineural hearing loss [29].

Electrophysiological Tests

Auditory development is a broadly defined term, which refers to the fact that perception is influenced by a combination of innate, genetically programmed changes in anatomy and physiology, combined with auditory experience [30]. Adequate sensory experience is critical to the developing nervous system for the expression as well as maintenance of sensory functions even when such functions are innately determined [31]. Development and maintenance of auditory sense is no exception [32]. In other words, reduced auditory input, early in life, may affect auditory processing later in life [32].

Years after the resolution of CHL and OM, absolute and interpeak wave latencies of the auditory brainstem response (ABR) are abnormally delayed, potentially suggesting immaturity in neural conduction [25, 32, 33]. OM in the first year of life leads to negative effects on brainstem signal processing even if it has occurred only for a short duration [32]. The mean central conduction time was significantly increased, and the mean amplitude of wave I and III of ABR was significantly reduced in children with early-onset OM compared to normal children [32].

Children with a history of OM and subsequent bilateral tubes placement surgery present significant latency delays and reduced amplitude ($p < 0.05$) of waves III and V for ABR, significant latency delay of potentials P2, N2, and P300 for Long Latency Auditory Evoked Potential (LLAEP), and significant latency delays and reduced amplitude ($p < 0.05$) for frequency following response (FFR) [33].

In addition, elevation of the brainstem-mediated contralateral acoustic stapedial reflex threshold is also observed in children with a history of OM and CHL, further suggesting persistent dysfunction of the neuronal circuitry within the auditory brainstem [25].

Otitis Media and the Critical Period for Language Acquisition

It is assumed that the auditory system has its most sensitive period for speech perception between 0 and 3.5 years (best in the first 2 years of life) [34], which is at the same time the period when OM occurrence has its highest incidence [10]. Middle ear status should therefore be observed at least in these years [10], as normal hearing is essential for the correct learning of an oral language [8].

An infant's auditory brain map is completely formed by 12 months of age [8]. The best known auditory examples of critical periods (CPs) were observed in language development [35]. Young children are able to discriminate phonetic contrasts of all languages; however, they specialize in mother language with increasing age and lose the ability to discriminate phonetic contrasts that do not exist in their mother language at around 8th–10th month after birth [8, 36]. There is a strong pattern of correlation between early speech perception skills and later language abilities [8].

Although phonetic learning can be affected by experience past childhood, phonetic learning exhibits the two principles for a CP [37]. A lack of exposure early in development to natural language, speech, or sign results in the lack of normal language and early experience with a particular language has indelible effects on speech perception [37]. Although lifelong learning is possible, neural plasticity during the CP is extreme, facilitating the adaptation of the developing brain to its environment and providing it with a stable long-lasting experiential foundation [37]. During a CP, appropriate experience must occur to produce the neural connections necessary for normal function, and the resulting patterns are irreversible [37].

The newborn can learn any language in the universe, and it is the contact with the native language that will make him/her form specific brain maps of the language of the environment in which he/she lives [8]. To facilitate decoding, the developing brain constructs acoustic maps of the sounds of its native language, thus allowing the child to respond in a fast automatic way to incoming language [8, 9]. Formation of this memory trace or "sensory map" is critical as it allows efficient discrimination of subsequent deviant stimuli [9]. Both the precision of biological encoding of sound and the "stability" of the neural representation throughout the auditory system are important contributors to accurate acoustic mapping [9].

Neural and behavioral research studies show that exposure to language in the first year of life influences the brain's neural circuitry even before infants speak their first words [8]. Studies indicate that the CP for phonetic learning occurs prior to the end of the first year, vocabulary development explodes at 18 months of age, whereas syntactic learning flourishes between 18 and 36 months of age [8].

Failure to receive proper excitatory input from the cochlea is known to cause the functional impairment in the central auditory system and various sound processing deficits [38].

Otitis Media and Speech Development

Otitis media may be related to difficulties in speech and reading, delayed response to auditory input, limited vocabulary, and disturbances in attention [39]. The effect of OME-related hearing loss on communication development is greatest when repeated or persistent episodes occur during early childhood and presumably depends on several factors, including severity, laterality, duration, and age of identification [3].

Too many variables are present in the learning process of children: amount of parental stimulation, quality of parental stimulation, innate intelligence, age of onset of hearing loss, personality factors, health conditions, and socioeconomic status [6]. These variables may so affect the learning abilities of children that a 15-dB HL loss may be a significant hindrance in hearing for one child, whereas a 20-dB HL loss will not be much of a problem for another child [6].

The world's languages contain approximately 600 consonants and 200 vowels [8]. Each language uses a unique set of about 40 distinct elements, *phonemes*, which change the meaning of a word (e.g., from *bat* to *pat* in English) [8]. The baby's task in the first year of life, therefore, is to make some progress in figuring out the composition of the 40-odd phonemic categories in their language(s) before trying to acquire words that depend on these elementary units [8].

During the first year of life, infants tune to the consonant and vowel categories of the native language [8]. By the middle of the second year of life, infants use their native phonetic categories to represent words and guide word learning [8]. Infants begin to use their native phonetic categories to direct word learning by 17–20 months of age [8]. The utilization of phonetic categories to direct word learning results in lexical (word-level) representations that are based on the phonetic categories established in infancy [8]. These become self-perpetuating as they direct uptake of phonetic detail in new word learning situations and simultaneously serve as the basis for later emerging rhyming and alliteration which in turn serve as the foundation for literacy acquisition [8]. Although the literature is by no means consistent, numerous studies indicate that children who had recurrent middle ear infections in infancy may have less sharp phonetic categories than expected even in childhood [40]. Infants, toddlers, and young children who are just learning and building speech and language relationships need to hear all the sounds clearly to implant the perceptions solidly in their developing brains [6]. Children are unable to "fill in the blanks" when speech is not heard clearly [6]. In hearing children, perceptual filling-in can be demonstrated only after the second year of life has been reached [41]. It is therefore tempting to assume that these phenomena are dependent on experience and consequently affected by hearing impairment [36].

Vowel sounds carry the most vocal energy (intensity) in speech, whereas the higher frequency consonant sounds contribute to the intelligibility of speech [6]. The voiceless consonants /s, p, t, k, th, f, sh/ often fall below normal hearing thresholds in average rapid conversation and may be missed [6]. Voiceless stops and voiced fricatives are 30 dB less intense than vowels and other consonants [6]. However, it is important to note that frequencies above 3000 Hz contribute approximately 25% to audibility of speech [6]. The frequency of the fricative /s/ sound may be between 6300 and 8300 Hz depending on the speaker's voice fundamentals [6]. The phoneme /s/ is one of the most frequently occurring sounds in the English language and carries significant linguistic and grammatical cues such as passive voice, plurality, possession, and verb tense [6].

There is no agreement between studies that evaluated the effect of OM on speech development [3]. More studies are needed that include hearing level, age at onset, laterality, and duration of hearing loss, as well as quantity and quality of parental stimulation, and socioeconomic status [3].

Otitis Media and Auditory Processing

Central Auditory Processing Definition

Central auditory processing (CAP) refers to the efficiency and effectiveness by which the central nervous system (CNS) utilizes auditory information [42]. In other words, CAP is a set of specific skills on which the individual depends to understand what he/she hears [42]. Sounds, after being detected by the inner ear, undergo numerous physiological and cognitive processes to be decoded and understood [42]. CAP is an umbrella term for all of the operations executed on peripheral auditory inputs, and which are required for the successful and timely generation of auditory percepts, their resolution, differentiation, and identification [43].

Whenever listening to a song, attending a class, or talking to someone, countless processes are triggered so that we can enjoy the melody, understand what is being explained by the speaker, or listen to a conversation and elaborate a response [44]. During the 24 h of the day, we are exposed to several auditory information, many of them simultaneous [44]. It is up to our auditory system to identify the messages that matter and ignore unimportant auditory information [44].

CAP includes the auditory mechanisms that underlie the following abilities or skills: sound localization and lateralization; auditory discrimination (ability to differentiate similar acoustic stimuli that differ in frequency, intensity, and/or temporal parameters); auditory pattern recognition; temporal aspects of audition, including temporal integration, temporal discrimination (e.g., temporal gap detection), temporal ordering, and temporal masking; auditory performance in competing acoustic signals (including dichotic listening); and auditory performance with degraded acoustic signals [42].

CAP is extremely important in a classroom, for example, where the student should focus attention on what the teacher says and ignore any other stimulus that might negatively interfere in the listening: classmate talks, chair-dragging, footsteps in the hallway, fan noise, street honking, or screaming in the schoolyard [45]. However, due to the slow maturation of the various mechanisms that support binaural hearing, even a child with normal development may have more difficulty than adults to understand speech if there is complex background noise [45].

To understand the effects of OM on auditory processing, it is important to know how the central auditory nervous system processes sounds [46].

Our sense of hearing depends on precisely organized circuits that allow us to sense, perceive, and respond to complex sounds in our environment, from music and language to simple warning signals [47].

Neuroscientists often consider the sensory systems with respect to their representational feature maps; in other words, they investigate how physical features of stimuli are represented in the brain [36]. In the auditory system, such features are sound frequency and intensity, binaural time and intensity differences, frequency modulation, amplitude modulation, etc. [36]. In recent times, considerable interest has shifted also to the way how the brain generalizes and abstracts from individual physical features to generate auditory objects or events [36]. The auditory object can be defined as a neuronal representation of a delimited acoustic pattern that is subject to figure–background separation [36].

Two of the primary goals of auditory neuroscience are to determine how acoustic information is progressively transformed along the auditory pathway and to understand the functional consequences of those transformations [48]. These goals have been difficult to achieve, in large part owing to the complexity of the auditory system [48].

The auditory system engages in an analysis of the auditory world so that the listener can accomplish the goal of communication and learning [30]. Auditory processing occurs in a series of analysis stages, beginning with peripheral auditory mechanisms devoted to encoding sound, and proceeding to more complex stages at which sound processing leads to perception and object recognition [30]. An important feature of the staging is the combination of inputs from the right and left ears, which takes place several synapses after the initial impact of sound on the auditory sensory organ, the cochlea [30].

Cochlea, Auditory Nerve, and Cochlear Nucleus

The cochlear transduction process confers on each afferent fiber narrow frequency tuning, and it is the role of each fiber to encode the presence, amplitude, and timing of stimulus energy within its frequency passband [43]. The cochlea has a tonotopic organization, with the basal region of the basilar membrane responding to high-frequency sound stimuli and the apical region responding to low-frequency sound stimuli [43]. Auditory processing begins in the cochlea of the inner ear, where sounds are detected by sensory hair cells and then transmitted to the central nervous system by spiral ganglion neurons, which faithfully preserve the frequency, intensity, and timing of each stimulus [47]. During the assembly of auditory circuits, spiral ganglion neurons establish precise connections that link hair cells in the cochlea to target neurons in the auditory brainstem, develop specific firing properties, and elaborate unusual synapses both in the periphery and in the CNS [47]. The ascending auditory system is composed of many nuclei connected through a series of parallel pathways [48]. The pathways begin with the auditory nerve, which branches to distribute information to the various cell groups in the cochlear nucleus [48](Fig. 29.1). Each cell group in the cochlear nucleus transforms the incoming spike trains uniquely and then distributes that information along a series of parallel pathways to a myriad of auditory nuclei in the medulla and pons [48]. Some of these nuclei are binaural, receiving innervation from the cochlear nuclei on both sides, whereas others are innervated from the cochlear nucleus on only one side and are monaural [48]. The outputs from all these binaural and monaural nuclei then converge on the inferior colliculus (IC) in the midbrain [48].

Superior Olivary Complex

It is a bilateral structure that contains two important groups of cells, involved in the neural encoding of binaural cues for the spatial location of sounds, organized tonotopically, and receiving inputs from both ears. Interaural time (ITD) and level (ILD) differences are the principal binaural cues used in sound localization [46]. Differences in the timing (ITD) and amplitudes (ILD) of acoustic signals arriving at the two ears play an essential role in spatial hearing, particularly in the horizontal plane [1]. The viscous fluid in the middle ear space can decrease the intensity and delay the transmission of the transduced sound waveform [1].

Inferior Colliculus (IC)

The central nucleus of the IC is a mandatory synaptic station for auditory sensory information ascending beyond the auditory midbrain [46]. It receives significant projections from the lateral superior olivary (LSO) nucleus bilaterally, from the ipsilateral medial superior olivary (MSO) nucleus, and from the dorsal nucleus of the lateral lemniscus (DNLL) bilaterally. The crossed projection from LSO is excitatory; projection from the ipsilateral LSO is inhibitory probably mediated by glycine [49]. Preserving the contra laterality of spatial representation, the DNLL contralateral projection is

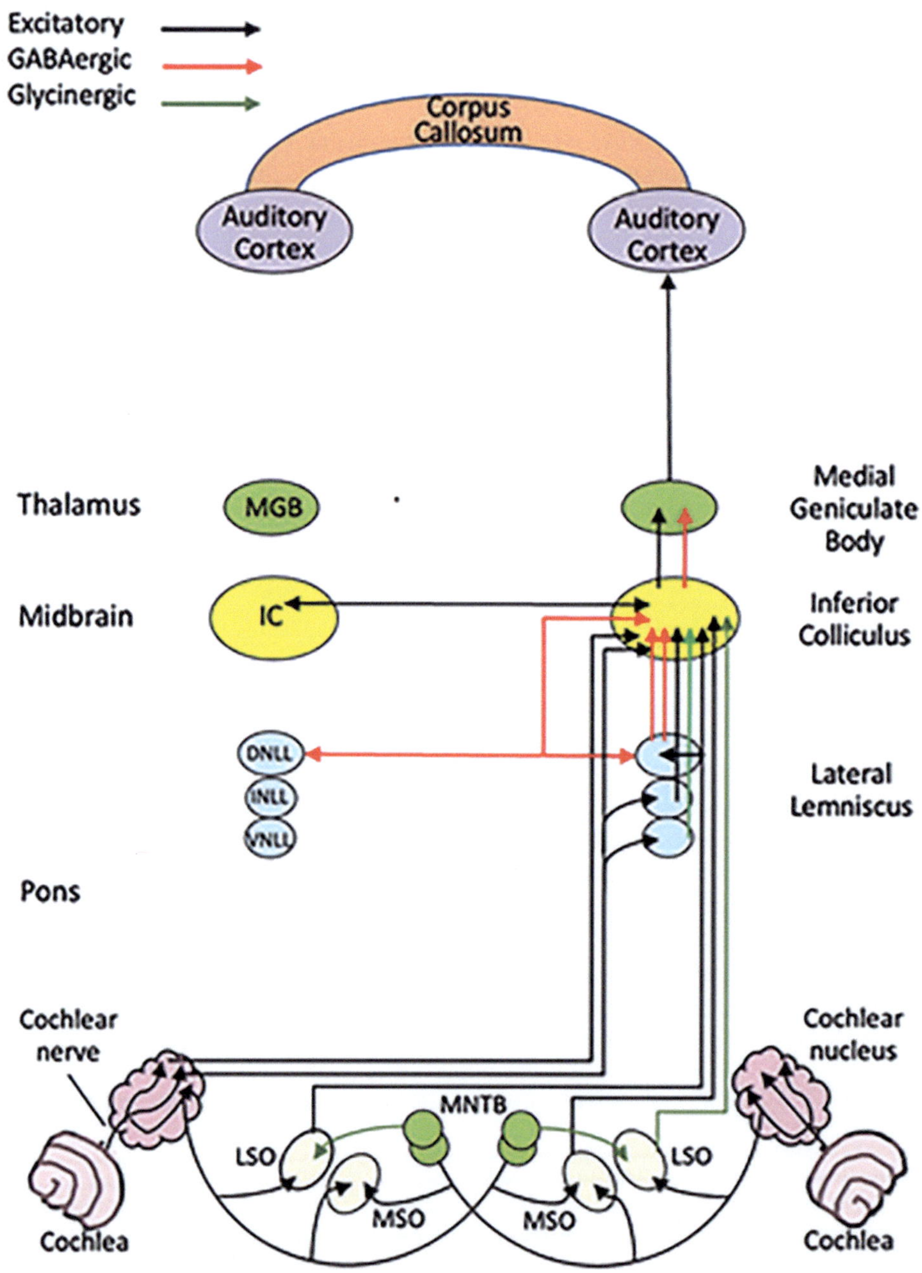

Fig. 29.1 Schematic representation of the main brainstem nuclei of the auditory pathway, their main connections, and neurotransmitters. *MSO* medial superior olivary nucleus, *LSO* lateral superior olivary nucleus, *MNTB* medial nucleus of the trapezoid body, *IC* inferior colliculus, and the three nuclei of the lateral lemniscus: *DNLL* dorsal nucleus of the lateral lemniscus, *INLL* intermediate nucleus of the lateral lemniscus, *VNLL* ventral nucleus of the lateral lemniscus [48]

inhibitory, likely mediated by gamma-amino-butyric acid (GABA) [50].

The IC provides the principal source of innervation to the medial geniculate body (MGB) and, thus, indirectly to the auditory cortex [48]. Therefore, the IC is the nexus of the auditory system because it processes and integrates almost all ascending acoustic information from lower centers and determines the form in which information is conveyed to higher regions in the forebrain [48]. The central auditory system has both parallel and hierarchical afferent architectures [43]. In the frequency domain, it is tonotopically constrained, and in the spatial domain, it is dominated by a representation of the contralateral acoustic hemifield [43]. The CHL at early age can disrupt the binaural integration of interaural level differences in the IC [38].

Medial Geniculate Body (MGB)

Neurons are arranged tonotopically, in sheet-like layers, each receiving its input from a single cochlear place [46]. They are narrowly tuned to tone frequency, have short response latencies, and show the familiar patterns of binaural input and interactions [46].

Auditory Cortex

Some of the fields are tonotopically organized, and these typically receive thalamic input from MGB, with the densest such projection serving the primary auditory cortex [46]. Tonotopic maps describe the spatial arrangement of neurons according to their frequencies [46]. The thalamocortical connections in the auditory system are largely reciprocal [46]. The cortical representation of a stimulus resides in the distribution of responses in space (and time) across the cortex [46].

The combined effect of CHL paired with a loss of temporal fidelity and disorganized binaural cues can substantially degrade the quality of afferent signals transmitted to brain areas that represent and shape our perceptions of the auditory world [1]. This hypothesis is supported by thousands of studies that characterize the development of higher (i.e., midbrain, thalamic, and cortical) sensory brain areas and describe significant alterations in the response properties of individual neurons, as well as their coordinated arrangement into functional circuits and topographic maps, based on the presence and quality of sensory-evoked afferent input [1].

Neurotransmitters

All aspects of audition, from pure tone hearing to complex spoken language processing, rely on the transmission of neural information across synapses [42]. Information about sound representation at the cochlea must be transmitted to the brain through a complex network of neural synapses [42]. Synaptic transmission, from neurotransmitter (NT) synthesis, through binding and activation of receptors, to reuptake and degradation of NT, is dependent on chemical processes [42].

NT is a molecule that is synthesized in neurons, which can modify the functioning of another cell. This chemical communication depends on the NT passing from one neuron to another through spaces known as synapses. The most important excitatory NTs in the auditory system are acetylcholine, dopamine, noradrenalin, and glutamate, and the most important inhibitory NTs are GABA and glycine [48] .

Moderate hearing loss during development can alter the temporal properties of synapses and spikes and prevent the synaptic inhibitory plasticity development which was regulated by the GABA-B receptors [38]. Hearing loss can impair sound tolerance by reducing GABA inhibition in the IC, which may be related to hyperacusis seen in children with OM [38]. Failure to receive proper excitatory input from the cochlea is known to cause the functional impairment in the central auditory system and various sound processing deficits [48]. Early age sound deprivation caused by CHL may cause an irreversible impairment in the central auditory system and increases the risk of developing hyperacusis [38].

Central Auditory Processing Disorder (CAPD)

Behaviors which are most indicative of auditory processing difficulties include difficulty hearing in background noise, difficulty following instructions, poor listening skills, academic difficulties, poor auditory association skills, distractibility, and inattention [51].

Recurrent acute OM and chronic OME, especially when they occur in the first 3 years of life, may be causes of central auditory processing disorder (CAPD), even after the resolution of middle ear disease and return of auditory thresholds to normal [45]. The degree of CHL (rather than the presence of OM per se) is decisive for the occurrence of central auditory deficits [1]. CHL attenuates and delays sound passing through the middle ear [1, 52].

A central auditory test battery should include measures that examine four different central processes: auditory pattern/temporal ordering; monoaural separation/closures; binaural integration/binaural separation; and binaural interaction (BI) [42]. Tests generally should include both nonverbal (e.g., tones, clicks, and complex waveforms) and verbal stimuli to examine different aspects of auditory processing and different levels of the auditory nervous system [42]. Unless tests incorporating verbal stimuli are available in the individual's native language, evaluation may require reliance on nonverbal stimuli [42]. We will discuss below the most performed tests in children with suspected CAPD secondary to OM.

Binaural Interaction (BI)

The 2005 American Speech-Language-Hearing Association technical report on CAPD identified BI as one of the main central processes that may need to be assessed as part of the evaluation for a CAPD, particularly if the referring complaint or clinical information indicates that there may be a deficit in this domain, e.g., difficulty with sound localization or hearing in a background noise [42]. There are several tests that have been designed to assess BI, and they are thought to be sensitive to brainstem pathology [45].

The neural connections subserving binaural processing are present at birth, but they are immature [53, 54]. The neural circuitry that underpins binaural hearing undergoes a structural reorganization after hearing onset [53, 54]. Postnatal maturation is experience-dependent, and reduced or altered cochlear output during the early postnatal period may change the normal development of the central auditory system [53, 54].

Several studies have investigated the effects of CHL caused by OM during early childhood on binaural processing abilities [1, 25, 55–57]. Studies have consistently shown disrupted binaural processing for years following reinstatement of hearing through either spontaneous resolution of effusion or placement of tympanostomy tubes [1, 55, 56]. This impairs binaural hearing and other central auditory functions dependent on high fidelity sound transmission [52]. For example, children who have had multiple episodes of OME in the first few years of life may have poor detection of sounds in noisy environments, evidenced by reduced binaural unmasking (BU) [52]. Recent research shows that a "threshold" level of OME is required to produce impaired BU [52]. Children who had OME in one or both ears for more than about 50% of the first 5 years had reduced BU [52]. Animal research, using long-term ear plugging, suggests that total OME duration, rather than age at the time of having the disease, determines its effect on BU [52]. Animals reared with bilateral (but not unilateral) ear plugs also have poor auditory temporal resolution, and reduced sensitivity to short tones in the presence of background noise, after plug removal [52]. However, given time (6–24 months) and training, all animals regained normal temporal resolution [52].

Impaired spatial processing and BI could underpin symptoms of listening difficulties, for example, impaired temporal processing, increased auditory filter width, or enhanced masking may lead to poor speech perception [58–60]. Children with BI deficit are at greater risk of difficulty in hearing and processing the teacher's speech when there is environmental noise, which may affect negatively in the learning process [1, 45].

Binaural Interaction Test: Masking Level Difference (MLD) Test

The binaural masking level difference (MLD) test is a measure of the ability to take advantage of interaural phase differences between the target and masker when detecting a tone in background noise [45]. Measures of BI are sensitive to low brainstem dysfunctions/lesions [42, 45]. BI tests involve the dichotic stimulation, i.e., the concurrent delivery of separate and different acoustic stimuli to the two ears [45]. The behavioral MLD may provide a measure of our ability to segregate sounds based on their location in space and is underpinned by early processing of spatial cues in the brainstem and subsequent gating of this information in the thalamus, although contributions by later processing stages are also involved [45]. The localization and the lateralization of auditory stimuli, the detection of acoustic signals in noisy environments, and the binaural fusion depend on this ability [45]. It is a perceptual test that affords researchers with an objective and parametric assessment of perceptual acuity that also relates to the real-world experience of hearing in noisy environments, such as classrooms or gymnasiums, by measuring a participant's sensitivity to interaural time and amplitude cues [1].

Pillsbury et al.(1991) found reduced binaural MLDs in children with OM (and associated CHL) during the disease as well as 1 and 3 months after ventilation tube surgery compared to normal hearing controls [61]. Furthermore, they reported a (nonsignificant) trend for the binaural MLDs of the OM children to increase over time [61]. Moore et al. (1991) observed significantly smaller binaural MLDs in children with more than five OM episodes (as assessed using parental reports) compared to normal hearing controls [62]. Hall et al. (1995) measured binaural MLDs in OM children 3 months, 1, 2, 3, and 4 years after the CHL had disappeared [58]. They observed reduced MLDs that persisted for up to 2 years, leading them to propose that binaural function in OM children recovers slowly [58]. Hogan and Moore (2003) studied the effects of OM history on the binaural MLD in 6-year-old children [56]. The middle ear status and the degree of CHL associated with OM of the children were prospectively documented from birth to the time of testing [56]. They found long-term negative effects of OM-related CHL on the binaural MLD, which was related to the number of experienced OM episodes [56]. Using a prospective study design, Gravel et al. (2006) investigated the long-term effects of CHL associated with OM in the first 3 years of life on the binaural MLD [25]. In contrast to the aforementioned studies, these authors did not find a significant effect on the binaural MLD at school age [25]. A possible explanation for the contrary outcomes of these studies might be the age at which these children were tested [25]. The auditory system may have recovered by the age of 8 years [25].

Monaural Low-Redundancy Speech Test: Speech-in-Noise Test

The main complaint of the patient with auditory processing disorder is the difficulty in understanding speech with background noise. The type of noise used in speech-in-noise tests can vary considerably [63]. White noise, multitalker babble, and even competing discourse have been used in various speech-in-noise tests [63]. These tests have moderate sensitivity for brainstem and cortical dysfunction [63].

Since performance on monoaural low-redundancy speech tests is not affected by interhemispheric involvement (i.e., corpus callosum), they are especially useful when used alongside dichotic tests or pattern tests that are sensitive to hemispheric as well as interhemispheric involvement [63]. The tests used are the Synthetic Sentence Identification (SSI) and the Pediatric Speech Intelligibility (PSI) [63]. The SSI test consists of the presentation of synthetic sentences (signal) in the presence of competitive noise, in the same ear [63]. The task is to listen to the sentence and point it in the frame [63]. The ability analyzed in this test is figure-ground [63]. The PSI test, for children who are not yet reading, consists of figures description (signal) in the presence of competitive noise, in the same ear [63]. The child is asked to point to the picture that is heard [63]. Patients with low to mid-brainstem involvement, as well as cortical lesions typically perform poorly on speech-in-noise tests [63].

Children with a history of OM and subsequent bilateral tubes placement surgery presented a lower performance than children with no history of OM in the mean responses for the SSI test of approximately 8% [33]. There is a causality between OM in early life and its accompanied hearing loss and lower performance on higher-order auditory skills, such as speech perception in noise, even up to the age of 7 years [10]. Poor speech perception in noise can have negative consequences in daily situations and impair communicative situations with background noise [10]. Especially in educational settings with background noise in the classroom, important information can be missed which consequently also affects other academic skills [10].

Gravel and Wallace (1992) demonstrated in a prospective study that 4-year-olds with a history of OM needed a significantly higher signal/noise ratio than children with a negative OM history [64]. Gravel et al. (2006) have used the PSI test to test 8-year-old children with a prospectively followed history of OM [25]. The authors found that functional auditory processes, evaluated by psychoacoustic measures, were not associated with early conductive hearing loss or experience with OM [25]. Also, the PSI test was not correlated to earlier OM, in contrast to the study by Gravel and Wallace (1992) [25, 64]. A possible explanation for the contrary outcomes of these two studies might be the age at which these children were tested [25, 64]. Consequences of OM on speech recognition in noise might still be present at the age of 4 years, while the auditory system may have recovered by the age of 8 years [25, 64].

Dichotic Digits (DD) Test

The dichotic digits (DD) test analyzes the ability of binaural integration performed by the corpus callosum [65]. Dichotic listening means simultaneous stimulation of both ears, but with different stimulus in each ear [65]. When asking patients to make a verbal response in a dichotic test, the primary auditory cortex and related areas are recruited [65]. In a majority of patients, this neural center is located in the left hemisphere [65]. As such, both left and right ear signals must reach the left hemisphere in order to be repeated back verbally. The right ear signal has a direct route to this region, as it ascends contralaterally to the left hemisphere [65]. The left ear signal, however, ascends to the right hemisphere and then must be transmitted across the corpus callosum to reach the left hemisphere [65]. The corpus callosum is a heavily myelinated structure, and rapid transmission of interhemispheric signals is dependent on the integrity of this myelin [65]. Neuroanatomic studies have shown that children do not have adultlike levels of myelin at birth, and the normal time course of myelin development is approximately 10–12 years of age [65]. Because right ear performance typically matures before left ear performance, most children will show normal interaural asymmetries on dichotic tests throughout the development process, with better results in the right ear [65].

The DD test consists of a list of digits, in which four different digits are presented simultaneously, two in each ear [65]. The participants are instructed to repeat all the numbers they have heard [65]. The order did not matter [65].

Children with a history of OM did not show as much improve in left ear performance as normal hearing controls when attending to the left ear on binaural separation tasks [65]. Children with a history of OM and subsequent bilateral tubes placement surgery presented a lower performance than children with no history of OM in the mean responses for the DD test of approximately 5% in both ears [33].

This suggests that a persistence of deprivation induced dichotic deficits [65].

Auditory Temporal Processing and Patterning Tests: Frequency Pattern Test (FPT)

Temporal ordering, or sequencing, refers to the processing of two or more auditory stimuli in their order of occurrence in time [66]. Accurate temporal ordering requires that both the left and the right hemispheres be anatomically and physiologically intact. It also requires integration of information from both hemispheres across the corpus callosum [66]. Pattern tests are sensitive to hemispheric lesions, as well as interhemispheric dysfunction [66].

The frequency pattern test (FPT) verifies temporal ordering ability [66]. The ability of the brain to decode incoming speech is dependent on the accurate perception of rapid acoustic changes [9].

It is composed of three tones that are either high frequency (H—1122 Hz) or low frequency (L—880 Hz) [66]. Each tone is 150 ms in duration and an intertone interval of 200 ms [66]. There are six possible combinations of the three-tone sequence (LLH, LHL, LHH, HLH, HLL, and HHL) [66]. The subjects were instructed that they would hear sets of three consecutive tones that varied in pitch [66].

The task of the subject was to repeat by humming and verbalizing the tonal pattern with the frequency patterns (e.g., high-low-high, low-low-high) [66].

Children with a history of OM and subsequent bilateral tubes placement surgery presented a lower performance than children with no history of OM in the mean responses for the FPT of 9.6% for humming and 30% for naming [33].

Auditory Temporal Processing and Patterning Tests: Gaps-in-Noise Test (GIN)

The gaps-in-noise (GIN) test measures temporal resolution ability [66]. The temporal processing is primarily mediated in the cerebrum [66]. Children aged 7 years demonstrate the same performance as adults, and no ear asymmetry is observed [66].

It consists of a series of six segments of broadband noise [66]. Each segment contains zero to three silent intervals or gaps per noise segment [66]. The gap durations presented 2, 3, 4, 5, 6, 8, 10, 12, 15, and 20 ms [66]. The approximate gap detection threshold is defined as the shortest gap duration which is correctly identified at least four out of six times [66]. The participants were instructed to indicate each time they perceived a gap [66].

Children with a history of OM and subsequent bilateral tubes placement surgery showed significantly poorer performance ($p < 0.001$) than children with no history of OM in the GIN test [33].

The ability of the brain to decode incoming speech is dependent on the accurate perception of rapid acoustic changes [9]. The higher the threshold obtained, the worse the test performance [66].

Note that no time gaps or explicit boundaries segment the ongoing speech stream into distinct phonemes or syllables [7]. For example, in the syllables /ba/ and /da/, the only differentiating cues occur within the initial 40-ms formant transition [7].

Recruitment Bias

Overall, recruitment bias in retrospective studies cannot be ruled out completely, and therefore a prospective study design is preferable. During an episode of upper respiratory infection (URI), at least a quarter of young children would have asymptomatic OM, without their parents realizing it [67]. Furthermore, retrospective studies can generally not provide information about the hearing threshold during an OM episode. The possibility of missing information regarding OM episodes in retrospective studies cannot be completely ruled out [67].

Several studies correlate mild peripheral hearing loss in early childhood with speech-in-noise hearing and various aspects of cognition [68], including speech and language development [69], selective attention [70], social use of language [71], and literacy [72].

Prospective studies with documented OM episodes and hearing thresholds are recommended for future research.

Prevention of CAPD

Delay the Start of Daycare at Least Until 12 Months

The common cold or upper respiratory infection (URI), a disease caused by a variety of viruses, is a universal illness. Particularly susceptible to URI are young children, especially those who attend day care centers. More than 60% of episodes of symptomatic URI among young children were complicated by acute OM (37%) and/or OME (24%) [67]. The strategy to prevent OM should involve prevention of viral URI, by delaying school starting age [67].

Insert Tympanostomy Tubes

For children with chronic OME, tube insertion reduces the prevalence of MEE by 32% in the first year and improves average hearing levels by 5–12 dB [73–75].

Motherese

The linguistically simplified and acoustically exaggerated speech that adults universally use when speaking to infants makes phonetic units more distinct from one another [8]. Talk slightly louder, slightly slower, clearly, and looking at the child's eyes [8].

Decrease Environment Noise

Children may have mild to moderate hearing loss for several weeks or months, during and possibly for some time after the middle ear effusion resolves. These children may experience considerable difficulties in perceiving the speech of teachers and peers in noisy classrooms, which can lead to increased listening effort, fatigue, and suboptimal quality of life [76]. It is important to assess this type of difficulty, improve the management of OME-related CHL, and advise educators on ways to improve disadvantageous classroom acoustic conditions and optimize the listening and learning environment for children with OME-related hearing loss [16]. Avoiding permanent background noise should also occur at home, as hearing sound stimuli clearly with interaction is necessary for the child to develop cortical auditory maps responsible for the perception of auditory-verbal language [8]. If the television, radio, or stereo system are always on, these maps will not develop properly [77].

Intervention

Listening Strategies

The simplest way to improve speech perception is to teach the child to look directly at the speaker and ask the speaker to direct speech toward the listener and ensure that their face is uncovered [42, 78].

Modifying the Listening Environment

More evidence-based than other strategies [78]. Increasing the signal (speech) level relative to that of the background noise will usually result in enhanced perception [42, 78]. This may be achieved by sitting or standing closer to a speaker (preferential seating) [42, 78]. Reducing the noise level of a listening environment may also be feasible and has been shown to be helpful [42, 78]. FM and Bluetooth wireless listening devices are becoming simpler to use, more affordable, and smaller [78]. Such systems can improve learning outcomes, auditory perception, and the fidelity with which the auditory brainstem encodes speech signals [42, 78].

Auditory Training

Mixed results [78]. Current software auditory training provides robust "on-task" learning of the exact skill trained, but little or no transfer of learning to untrained tasks or skills [78].

Compensatory Strategies

Not well validated [78]. Training in metacognitive and metalinguistic strategies can also be considered [78]. These strategies include self-regulation and problem-solving, by identifying individual listening strengths and weaknesses and listening situations that are more challenging [78].

Long-Term Benefit: Music and Exercise

To the extent that good listening strategies and acoustic enhancement may be lifelong changes in behavior, we can assume that the benefits of those interventions will persist [78]. After 1 year of music training, the children who actively engaged with sound through instrumental music training had faster and more robust neural processing of speech than the children who stayed in the music appreciation class, observed in neural responses to a speech sound /d/ [79]. The neurophysiological measures found to be enhanced in the instrumentally trained children have been previously linked to reading ability, suggesting a gain in neural processes important for literacy stemming from active auditory learning [79].

Aerobic exercise is the activity for which there is the best evidence of retention and enhancement of cognitive function, underpinning all aspects of hearing and listening [80].

Conclusions

Often, when caring for a child with OM, we do not know if this is the first episode, if there was already a MEE before the onset of symptoms, or if there is hearing loss. Therefore, we must monitor OM episodes and auditory thresholds.

The baby makes a brain map of all the phonemes of the native language until the end of the first year of life, but for this map to be perfect, it is necessary to ensure perfect hearing. The guidelines for talking while looking into the eyes, slower, a little louder, with higher intonation, and avoiding permanent background noise are very important at this age.

When we know that the child has had OM for a long time, there is no need to wait for the child to present complaints such as hyperacusis, difficulty understanding speech in noisy environment, or learning difficulties. We must recommend musical training, to strengthen the auditory system, the attention, and the memory.

References

1. Whitton JP, Polley DB. Evaluating the perceptual and pathophysiological consequences of auditory deprivation in early postnatal life: a comparison of basic and clinical studies. JARO. 2011;12(5):535–47.
2. Zielhuis GA, Rach GH, van den Broek P. The occurrence of otitis media with effusion in Dutch pre-school children. Clin Otolaryngol Allied Sci. 1990;15:147–53.
3. Rosenfeld RM, Shin JJ, Schwartz SR, Coggins R, Gagnon L, Hackell JM, Hoelting D, Hunter LL, Kummer AW, Payne SC, Poe DS, Veling M, Vila PM, Walsh SA, Corrigan MD. Clinical practice guideline: otitis media with effusion (update). Otolaryngol Head Neck Surg. 2016;154:S1–S41.
4. Tos M. Epidemiology and natural history of secretory otitis. Am J Otol. 1984;5:459–62.
5. Mandel EM, Doyle WJ, Winther B, Alper CM. The incidence, prevalence, and burden of OM in unselected children aged 1-8 years followed by weekly otoscopy through the "common cold" season. Int J Pediatr Otorhinolaryngol. 2008;72:491–9.
6. Northern JL, Downs MP. Hearing in children. 6th ed. San Diego: Plural Publishing; 2014, 720p.

7. Tallal P. Improving language and literacy is a matter of time. Nat Rev Neurosci. 2004;5:721–8.
8. Kuhl PK. Brain mechanisms in early language acquisition. Neuron. 2010;67(5):713–27.
9. Benasich AA, Choudhury NA, Realpe-Bonilla T, Roesler CP. Plasticity in developing brain: active auditory exposure impacts prelinguistic acoustic mapping. J Neurosci. 2014;34(40):13349–63.
10. Zumach A, Gerrits E, Chenault MN, Anteunis LJC. Otitis media and speech-in-noise recognition in school-aged children. Audiol Neurotol. 2009;14:121–9.
11. Gravel JS, Wallace IF. Effects of otitis media with effusion on hearing in the first 3 years of life. J Speech Lang Hear Res. 2000;43:631–44.
12. Hartley DEH, Moore DR. Effects of conductive hearing loss on temporal aspects of sound transmission through the ear. Hear Res. 2003;177(1–2):53–60.
13. Gravel JS. Hearing and auditory function. In: Rosenfeld RM, Bluestone CD, editors. Evidence-based otitis media. 2nd ed. Hamilton: BC Decker Inc.; 2003. p. 342–59.
14. Sabo DL, Paradise JL, Kurs-Lasky M, Smith CG. Hearing levels in infants and young children in relation to testing technique, age group, and the presence or absence of middle-ear effusion. Ear Hear. 2003;24(1):38–47.
15. Hunter LL, Margolis RH, Giebink GS. Identification of hearing loss in otitis media. Ann Otol Rhinol Laryngol. 1994;103:S59–61.
16. Cai T, McPherson B. Hearing loss in children with otitis media with effusion: a systematic review. Int J Audiol. 2017;56:1–11. Early Online.
17. Hogan SC, Stratford KJ, Moore DR. Duration and recurrence of otitis media with effusion in children from birth to 3 years: prospective study using monthly otoscopy and tympanometry. BMJ. 1997;314:350–5.
18. Paradise JL, Rockette HE, Colborn DK, Bernard BS, Smith CG, Kurs-Lasky M, Janosky JE. Otitis media in 2253 Pittsburgh-area infants: prevalence and risk factors during the first two years of life. Pediatrics. 1997;99(3):318–33.
19. Fria TJ, Cantekin EI, Eichler JA. Hearing acuity of children with otitis media with effusion. Arch Otolaryngol. 1985;111(1):10–6.
20. Hunter LL, Margolis RH, Giebink GS. Identification of hearing loss in children with otitis media. Ann Otol Rhinol Laryngol Suppl. 1994;163:59–61.
21. Dobie RA, Berlin CI. Influence of otitis media on hearing and development. Ann Otol Rhinol Laryngol. 1979;88(5):S48–53.
22. Eapen RJ, Buss E, Grose JH, Drake AF, Dev M, Hall JW. The development of frequency weighting for speech in children with a history of otitis media with effusion. Ear Hear. 2008;29(5):718–24.
23. Laitila P, Karma P, Sipilä M, Manninen M, Rakho T. Extended high frequency hearing and history of acute otitis media in 14-year-old children in Finland. Acta Otolaryngol. 1997;529:S27–S9.
24. Margolis RH, Saly GL, Hunter LL. High-frequency hearing loss and wideband middle ear impedance in children with otitis media histories. Ear Hear. 2000;21(3):206–11.
25. Gravel JS, Roberts JE, Roush J, Grose J, Besing J, Burchinal M, Neebe E, Wallace IF, Zeisel S. Early otitis media with effusion, hearing loss, and auditory processes at school age. Ear Hear. 2006;27(4):353–68.
26. Hunter LL, Chelsea M, Blankenship CM, Lin L, Sloat NT, Perdew A, Stewart H, Moore DR. Peripheral auditory involvement in childhood listening difficulty. Ear Hear. 2021;42(1):29–41.
27. Morizono T, Paparella MM, Juhn SK. Ototoxicity of propylene glycol in experimental animals. Am J Otolaryngol. 1980;1(5):393–9.
28. Schachern PA, Paparella MM, Goycoolea MV, Duvall AJ III, Choo YB. The permeability of the round window membrane during otitis media. Arch Otolaryngol Head Neck Surg. 1987;113(6):625–9.
29. Tsuprun V, Sebahattin C, Schachern PA, Ferrieri P, Briles DE, Paparella MM, Juhn SK. Role of pneumococcal proteins in sensorineural hearing loss due to otitis media. Otol Neurotol. 2008;29(8):1056–60.
30. Litovsky R. Development of the auditory system. Handb Clin Neurol. 2015;129:55–72.
31. Knudsen EI. Experiences alters the spatial tuning of auditory units in the optic tectum during a sensitive period in the barn owl. J Neurosci. 1985;5:3094–109.
32. Maruthy S, Mannarukrishnaiah J. Effect of early onset otitis media on brainstem and cortical auditory processing. Behav Brain Funct. 2008;4:1–17.
33. Colella-Santos MF, Donadon C, Sanfins MD, Borges LR. Otitis media: long-term effect on central auditory nervous system. Biomed Res Int. 2019;2019:8930904.
34. Sharma A, Campbell J. A sensitive period for cochlear implantation in deaf children. J Matern Fetal Neonatal Med. 2011;24(1):151–3.
35. Kuhl PK. Early language acquisition: cracking the speech code. Nat Rev Neurosci. 2004;5:831–43.
36. Kral A. Auditory critical periods: a review from system's perspective. Neuroscience. 2013;247:117–33.
37. Kuhl PK, Conboy BT, Padden D, Nelson T, Pruitt J. Early speech perception and later language development: implications for the "critical period". Lang Learn Dev. 2005;1(3–4):237–64.
38. Sun W, Manohar S, Jayaram A, Kumaraguru A, Fu Q, Li J, Allman B. Early age conductive hearing loss causes audiogenic seizure and hyperacusis behavior. Hear Res. 2011;282(1–2):178–83.
39. Bellussi L, Mandala M, Passali FM, Passali GC, Lauriello M, Passali D. Quality of life and psycho-social development in children with otitis media with effusion. Acta Otorhinolaryngol Ital. 2005;25:359–64.
40. Clarkson RL, Eimas PD, Marean GC. Speech perception in children with histories of recurrent otitis media. J Acoust Soc Am. 1989;85(2):926–33.
41. Newman RS. 2-Year-olds' speech understanding in multitalker environments. Infancy. 2011;16(5):447–70.
42. American Speech-Language-Hearing Association. (Central) auditory processing disorders (technical report). Working group on auditory processing disorders. 2005. Available at: http://www.akaw.de/sites/default/files/2016-12/ASHA_CAPD_2005.pdf.
43. Phillips DP. Central auditory system and central auditory processing disorders: some conceptual issues. In: Palmer CV, Chermak GD, editors. Management of auditory processing disorders. Semin Hear. 2002;23:251–61.
44. Ramos BD, Costa-Ferreira MID, Guedes MC, Alvarez AM. Auditory processing and language. In: Sih T, Chinski A, Eavey R, Godinho R, editors. XVII IAPO manual of pediatric otorhinolaryngology. IAPO—Interamerican Association of Pediatric Otorhinolaryngology. Guarulhos: Lis Gráfica e EditoraLtda; 2020. p. 265–82.
45. Mc Cullagh J, Bamiou DE. Measures of binaural interaction. In: Musiek FE, Chermak GD, editors. Handbook of central auditory processing disorder, Auditory neuroscience and diagnosis, vol. 1. San Diego: Plural Publishing; 2014. p. 435–69.
46. Phillips DP. An introduction to central auditory neuroscience. In: Musiek FE, Chermak GD, editors. Handbook of central auditory processing disorder, Auditory neuroscience and diagnosis, vol. 1. San Diego: Plural Publishing; 2014. p. 113–52.
47. Appler JM, Lisa V, Goodrich LV. Connecting the ear to the brain: molecular mechanisms of auditory circuit assembly. Prog Neurobiol. 2011;93(4):488–508.
48. Pollak GD, Burger RM, Klug A. Dissecting the circuitry of the auditory system. Trends Neurosci. 2003;26(1):33–9.
49. Glendenning KK, Baker BN, Hutson KA, Masterton RB. Acoustic chiasm V: inhibition and excitation in the ipsilateral and contralateral projections of LSO. J Comp Neurol. 1992;319(1):100–22.

50. Shneiderman A, Oliver DL, Henkel CK. Connections of the dorsal nucleus of the lateral lemniscus: an inhibitory parallel pathway in the ascending auditory system? J Comp Neurol. 1988;276(2):188–208.
51. Chermak G, Somers EK, Seikel J. Behavioral signs of central auditory processing disorder and attention deficit hyperactivity disorder. J Am Acad Audiol. 1998;9(1):78–84.
52. Moore DR, Hartley DEH, Hogan SCM. Effects of otitis media with effusion on central auditory function. Int J Pediatr Otorhinolaryngol. 2003;67:S63–6.
53. Kapfer C, Seidl AH, Schweizer H, Grothe B. Experience-dependent refinement of inhibitory inputs to auditory coincidence-detector neurons. Nat Neurosci. 2002;5(3):247–53.
54. Moore DR. Auditory development and the role of experience. Br Med Bull. 2002;63:171–81.
55. Hall JW, Grose JH. The effect of otitis media with effusion on the masking-level difference and the auditory brainstem response. J Speech Lang Hear Res. 1993;36(1):210–7.
56. Hogan SCM, Moore DR. Impaired binaural hearing in children produced by a threshold level of middle ear disease. JARO. 2003;4:123–9.
57. Koiek S, Brandt C, Schmidt JH, Neher T. Monaural and binaural phase sensitivity in school-age children with early-childhood otitis media. Int J Audiol. 2022;61:1054–61.
58. Hall JW III, Grose JA, Pillsbury HC. Long-term effects of chronic otitis media on binaural hearing in children. Arch Otolaryngol Head Neck Surg. 1995;121(8):847–52.
59. Cameron S, Dillon H, Glyde H, Kanthan S, Kania A. Prevalence and remediation of spatial processing disorder in indigenous children in regional Australia. J Audiol. 2014;53(5):326–35.
60. Hogan SC, Meyer SE, Moore DR. Binaural unmasking returns to normal in teenagers who had otitis media in infancy. Audiol Neurootol. 1996;1(2):104–11.
61. Pillsbury HC, Grose JH, Hall JW III. Otitis media with effusion in children binaural hearing before and after corrective surgery. Arch Otolaryngol Head Neck Surg. 1991;117(7):718–23.
62. Moore DR, Hutchings ME, Meyer SE. Binaural masking level differences in children with a history of otitis media. Audiology. 1991;30:91–101.
63. Krishnamurti S. Monaural low-redundancy speech tests. In: Musiek FE, Chermak GD, editors. Handbook of central auditory processing disorder, Auditory neuroscience and diagnosis, vol. 1. San Diego: Plural Publishing; 2014. p. 349–67.
64. Gravel JS, Wallace IF. Listening and language at 4 years of age: effects of early otitis media. Speech Hear Res. 1992;35(3):588–95.
65. Weihing J, Atcherson SR. Dichotic listening tests. In: Musiek FE, Chermak GD, editors. Handbook of central auditory processing disorder, Auditory neuroscience and diagnosis, vol. 1. San Diego: Plural Publishing; 2014. p. 369–404.
66. Shin JB. Temporal processing tests. In: Musiek FE, Chermak GD, editors. Handbook of central auditory processing disorder, Auditory neuroscience and diagnosis, vol. 1. San Diego: Plural Publishing; 2014. p. 405–34.
67. Chonmaitree T, Revai K, Grady JJ, Clos A, Patel JA, Nair S, Fan J, Henrickson KJ. Viral upper respiratory tract infection and otitis media complication in young children. Clin Infect Dis. 2008;46:815–23.
68. Moore DR, Zobay O, Ferguson MA. Minimal and mild hearing loss in children: association with auditory perception, cognition, and communication problems. Ear Hear. 2020;41(4):720–32.
69. Tomblin JB, Harrison M, Ambrose SE, Walker EA, Oleson JJ, Moeller MP. Language outcomes in young children with mild to severe hearing loss. Ear Hear. 2015;36:76S–91S.
70. Holmes E, Kitterick PT, Summerfield AQ. Peripheral hearing loss reduces the ability of children to direct selective attention during multi-talker listening. Hear Res. 2017;350:160–72.
71. Meinzen-Derr J, Wiley S, Grether S, Phillips J, Choo D, Hibner J, Barnard H. Functional communication of children who are deaf or hard-of-hearing. J Dev BehavPediatr. 2014;35(3):197–206.
72. Harris M, Terlektsi E, Kyle FE. Literacy outcomes for primary school children who are deaf and hard of hearing: a cohort comparison study. J Speech Lang Hear Res. 2017;60(3):701–11.
73. Rosenfeld RM, Tunkel DE, Schwartz SR, Anne S, Bishop CE, Chelius DC, Hackell J, Hunter LL, Keppel KL, Kim AH, Kim TW, Levine JM, Maksimoski MT, Moore DJ, Preciado DA, Raol NP, Vaughan WK, Walker EA, Monjur TM. Clinical practice guideline: tympanostomy tubes in children (update). Otolaryngol Head Neck Surg. 2022;166(1S):S1–S55.
74. Browning GG, Rovers MM, Williamson I, Lous J, Burton MJ. Grommets (ventilation tubes) for hearing loss associated with otitis media with effusion in children. Cochrane Database Syst Rev. 2010;10:CD001801.
75. Rovers MM, Black N, Browning GG, Maw R, Zielhuis GA, Haggard MP. Grommets in otitis media with effusion: an individual patient data meta-analysis. Arch Dis Child. 2005;90(5):480–5.
76. Rosenfeld RM, Goldsmith AJ, Lynne TL. Quality of life for children with otitis media. Arch Otolaryngol Head Neck Surg. 1997;123(10):1049–54.
77. Chang EF, Merzenich MM. Environmental noise retards auditory cortical development. Science. 2003;300:498–502.
78. Aksoy S, Zehnhoff-Dinnesen A, Atas A, Bamiou DE, Bartel-Friedrich S, Benton C, Brockmeir SJ, Campbell NG, Carr G, Caversaccio M, et al. Rehabilitation and prognosis of disorders of hearing development. In: Zehnhoff-Dinnesen A, Wiskirska-Woznica B, Neumann K, Nawka T, editors. European Manual of Medicine. Phoniatrics I: fundamentals—voice disorders—disorders of language and hearing development. Berlin: Spring-Verlag GmbH; 2020.
79. Kraus N, Slater J, Thompson EC, Hornickel J, Strait DL, Nicol T, White-Schwoch T. Auditory learning through active engagement with sound: biological impact of community music lessons in at-risk children. Front Neurosci. 2014;8:1–12.
80. Hillman C, Erickson K, Kramer A. Be smart, exercise your heart: exercise effects on brain and cognition. Nat Rev Neurosci. 2008;9:58–65.

Balance and Otitis Media

30

Rafael da Costa Monsanto, José Carlos Convento Júnior, José Vicente Boleli Scardini Alves, and Norma de Oliveira Penido

Introduction

The term "otitis media" (OM) refers to a group of inflammatory and infectious diseases that affect the middle ear [1]. Many different types of otitis media have been described in the past, most of which are variations of the three following groups: (1) otitis media with effusion (OME), characterized by the presence of chronic middle ear effusion (>3 months) [2]; (2) acute otitis media (AOM), defined as an acute onset of symptoms of middle ear inflammation [3]; and (3) chronic otitis media (COM), defined as the presence of a chronic inflammation inf the middle ear cleft associated with clinically intractable tissue changes (such as tympanic membrane perforation, cholesterol granuloma, fibrosis, and ossicular erosion) [1].

Otitis media is considered by the World Health Organization (WHO) a public health problem for several reasons [4]. The lofty burden of disease caused by otitis media has been recently described by Monasta et al. [5]. In their study, the authors showed that the different types of otitis media associate with high worldwide incidence rates, which reflects in the fact that it one the most frequent causes for antibiotic prescription yearly. Furthermore, otitis media associates with excessive healthcare costs and can cause a severe impact on the quality of life of patients. Concerning the incidence of acute otitis media (AOM), it has been demonstrated that 80% of children worldwide will have one episode of AOM before the age of 3 years [6], and over 40% will have six or more recurrences before the age of 7 years [7, 8]. The yearly global incidence of AOM is 10.85%, accounting for more than 700 million new cases [5]. Otitis media with effusion (OME) is even more common: it was estimated that virtually 100% of children will experience at least one episode of transitory effusion in the middle ear—these observations led authors to define OME as an "occupational hazard of the childhood" [2]. Finally, the yearly incidence of new cases of chronic otitis media (COM) is 4.76 per thousand people, resulting in ~31 million cases. Otitis media may also culminate in intracranial and extracranial complications in 8–12% of all cases, and these are associated with high mortality rates (5–26%) [9].

The association of otitis media and inner ear deficits (such as hearing loss, tinnitus, and vestibular impairment) has been demonstrated in the past [10]. Data from the WHO demonstrated that otitis media is the third leading cause of hearing impairment among all causes, ranking behind genetic hearing loss and presbycusis [4]. The estimated prevalence of permanent hearing loss (>25 dB in the best-hearing ear) was 30.82 per 10,000 cases [5]. Although otitis media leads to conductive hearing loss in most cases, studies demonstrated that it can also result in sensorineural hearing loss. The pioneer study in this regard was published by Paparella et al. [11]—in this translational study, the authors demonstrated the presence of high-frequency sensorineural hearing loss in patients with COM. The authors later demonstrated otopathological correlates of these findings, showing a significant decrease in number of inner and outer cochlear hair cells in temporal bone specimens with COM. These studies were later corroborated by several of experimental and clinical studies.

More recently, it has been hypothesized that otitis media may also cause vestibular damage in addition to the cochlear/auditory impairment [12]. Studies dedicated to evaluating vestibular dysfunction secondary to otitis media are scarce in the literature. The hypothesis of a direct vestibular damage

R. da Costa Monsanto (✉)
Department of Otolaryngology, Head and Neck Surgery, University of Minnesota, Minneapolis, MN, USA

Department of Otolaryngology, Head and Neck Surgery, Universidade Federal de São Paulo/Escola Paulista de Medicina (UNIFESP/EPM), São Paulo, Brazil
e-mail: rdacosta@umn.edu

J. C. C. Júnior · J. V. B. S. Alves
Department of Otolaryngology, Banco de Olhos de Sorocaba Hospital, Sorocaba, Brazil

N. de Oliveira Penido
Department of Otolaryngology, Head and Neck Surgery, Universidade Federal de São Paulo/Escola Paulista de Medicina (UNIFESP/EPM), São Paulo, Brazil

M. V. Goycoolea et al. (eds.), *Textbook of Otitis Media*, https://doi.org/10.1007/978-3-031-40949-3_30

caused by otitis media in the absence of perilymphatic fistula has been subject of an intense debate [13]. Although no study has yet peremptorily demonstrated that AOM and OME cause vestibular impairment, recent evidence showed that COM associates with a high prevalence of vestibular symptoms (40–60%) and abnormalities in several vestibular function tests (including caloric tests and cervical vestibular myogenic potentials). A meta-analysis [10] revealed that most of these studies have several potential biases and methodological problems that undermine the validity of their data. However, recent histological and clinical evidence have shed additional light in the subject, revealing that otitis media (more specifically COM) may result in direct vestibular impairment.

In this chapter, we explore the clinical and experimental evidence available in the literature showing the association between otitis media and vestibular impairment.

Pathophysiology

The first description of an inner ear sequelae of otitis media was published by Adam Politzer, in 1894 [14]. In this study, the author investigated the hearing of patients with chronic OME—although there was no objective way to test the hearing at the time, it was observed that these patients had worse hearing than controls. The hypothesis was later explored in the decade of 1920: Mackenzie [15], Turner and Fraser [16], and Druss [17] described potential pathways from which otitis media could progress to the inner ear, including through the oval and round windows, or through and hematogenic route.

It was only in the 1960s and 1970s that these theories were evaluated in an experimental setting: first, Arslan [18], in a study evaluating a potential osmotic mechanism leading to Meniere's disease, observed an outflow of perilymph through the round window membrane after placement of NaCl over this structure. This observation was later explored in a series of studies by Schachern and Goycoolea [19–22]: these studies revealed that the round window membrane is permeable to albumin, inflammatory mediators and genes, bacterial toxins, and even whole bacteria. The translational study published by Paparella et al. [11] observed that the most critical inner ear lesions in patients with COM occurred in the cochlear hair cells in the basal turn of the cochlea (Fig. 30.1). The lesion site in the inner ear in these patients with otitis media, together with the observation that the round window membrane is semi-permeable, has corroborated that the inner ear is susceptible to lesion in cases of otitis media, in a process called by Paparella as "middle ear/inner ear interactive disease" [13].

Recently, the group at the University of Pittsburgh evaluated the inner ear environment in otitis media models [23–26]. In these studies, it was shown that both acute and chronic otitis media impact on the expression of hundreds of middle and inner ear genes. It was demonstrated that otitis media associated with an upregulation in the concentration of pro-inflammatory cytokines and mediators (such as tumor necrosis factor TNF-alpha and interleukins) and downregulation of anti-inflammatory mediators in the middle and inner ears. Moreover, the elevation of these inflammatory mediators in the inner ear seemed to occur by two distinct mechanisms: (1) direct passage through the round window membrane; and (2) through an active immunological mechanism mediated by the spiral ligament, which amplify the inflammatory response in the inner ear following otitis media. Although such amplification would—hypothetically—aim to suppress an inflammatory issue in the inner ear, it could increase the risks of cochlear damage.

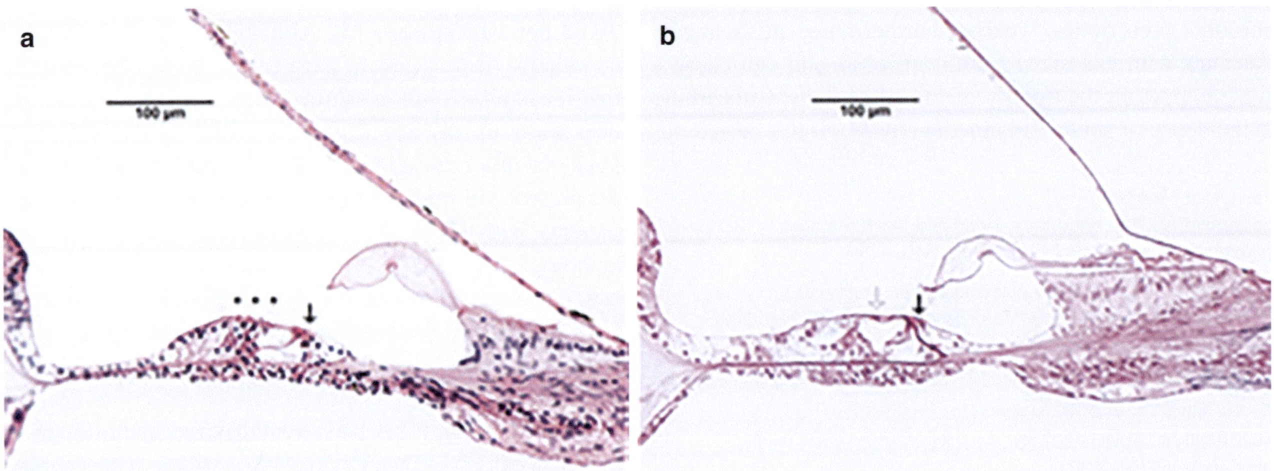

Fig. 30.1 Two representative human temporal bone sections, one from a healthy donor (**a**) and other from a donor with chronic otitis media (**b**) seen in optic microscopy (hematoxylin & eosin). In (**a**), the organ of Corti is normal, with normal number of inner (black arrow) and outer (*) hair cells. In (**b**), the inner hair cell (black arrow) is present, but there is a complete loss of outer hair cells (white arrow)

Studies evaluating peripheral vestibular damage secondary to otitis media are very scarce. In fact, the presence of a potential vestibular lesion secondary to otitis media has been a matter of great controversy for several reasons. First, the presence of vestibular symptoms and signs of vestibular dysfunction are much less frequent than auditory symptoms in otitis media [27, 28]. Second, in most cases, vestibular symptoms in patients with otitis media are frequently associated with a perilymphatic fistula or other causes of dizziness, such as metabolic diseases or benign paroxysmal vertigo (Monsanto et al. 2018). Also, Juhn et al. [29] demonstrated the presence of a blood–labyrinthine barrier, which is a protective mechanism to maintain the ionic balance and homeostasis in the inner ear fluids. Several substances and clinical conditions have been shown to alter the permeability of the blood–labyrinthine barrier, leading to loss of homeostasis and cochlear (and possibly vestibular) changes [30, 31]. Although otitis media could be one of these problems affecting the blood–labyrinthine barrier, this has not yet been explored in experimental studies yet. Nonetheless, growing evidence indicates a potential vestibular dysfunction secondary to COM: the prevalence of vestibular symptoms in patients with COM was estimated at 40–60%, and these symptoms frequently associate with abnormal results in vestibular function tests (caloric tests, cervical vestibular evoked myogenic potentials (cVEMPs), and rotatory chair) (Monsanto et al. 2018).

Paparella et al. [32] hypothesized, based on the clinical observation that many patients with otitis media have fluctuating sensorineural hearing loss, tinnitus, and episodic dizziness or vertigo, that otitis media could be a cause of secondary endolymphatic hydrops. Based on these observations, the authors performed an otopathologic study in 194 temporal bones specimens with otitis media. In these temporal bones, 75 (38.6%) had signs of endolymphatic hydrops. Later, Saito et al. [33] showed similar findings: in their temporal bones, there was a 44.8% prevalence of endolymphatic hydrops. These histopathological data have been later supported by clinical studies, observing that some patients with chronic otitis media tend to develop Meniere's disease over time [34, 35]. Additionally, Zou and Pyykkö [36] demonstrated the presence of obvious endolymphatic hydrops in a magnetic resonance imaging of a patient with chronic otitis media. Thus, it is possible that endolymphatic hydrops is one of the potential causes of vestibular impairment in patients with otitis media.

The first study to perform an otopathologic evaluation of the vestibular system in human temporal bones with COM was Kodama et al. [27]. In this study, the authors demonstrated eosinophilic deposits (suggestive of inflammatory response) in the endolymphatic and perilymphatic compartments, being more concentrated in the saccule. It was also observed the presence of saccular edema and an abnormal neuroepithelium, while no significant abnormalities were seen in the utricle and semicircular canals. Kodama et al. [27] also showed that the abnormalities affecting the cochlea (loss of cochlear hair cells and stria vascularis abnormalities) were much more frequent than the vestibular changes. After Kodama's study, there is a 30-year gap before the subject was revisited by Monsanto et al. [12], who studied the vestibular neuroepithelium (saccule, utricle, and semicircular canals) and dark and transitional cells in the crista ampullaris of the lateral and posterior semicircular canals in temporal bones with COM. The authors found a significant loss of vestibular hair cells type I and II in the saccular and utricular macula (more intense) and loss of type I cells in the anterior and posterior semicircular canals (less intense) (Fig. 30.2). Also, the authors found a significant loss of dark cells in the COM group as compared with controls. Kaya et al. [37] later studied vestibular abnormalities in temporal bones of patients with labyrinthitis (serous, suppurative, and ossificans). The authors showed that the presence of labyrinthitis caused by otitis media associated with a high prevalence of endolymphatic hydrops, and a significant loss of transitional and dark cells in the semicircular canals, and loss of vestibular hair cells type I and II in both otolithic organs and semicircular canals.

In 2017, following the theory of the continuum of otitis media as described by Paparella et al. [38], investigators at the University of Minnesota aimed to evaluate potential routes of progression of the inner ear lesions secondary to otitis media [10]. In this study, the authors analyzed losses of cochlear hair cells, stria vascularis, vestibular hair cells, and vestibular dark and transitional cells in temporal bones with different types of otitis media and controls. The results showed that early stages of otitis media associated with cochlear lesions limited to the basal turn of the cochlea (loss of outer hair cells and atrophy of the stria vascularis). As the disease progresses, structures from the middle turn of the cochlea are affected, and—in more advanced cases of COM—there is a significant loss of vestibular hair cells in the otolithic organs. The authors conclude that the cochlear damage precedes the vestibular damage secondary to otitis media, and that the severe and chronicity of the middle ear inflammation seem to directly associate with the degree of inner ear losses. These findings are supported by clinical evidence. Chang et al. [39] demonstrated that the inner ear deficits in patients with COM initiate at the cochlea, affecting the saccule/utricle and semicircular canals in a later stage of the disease. Monsanto et al. [28] also showed a similar pattern, revealing that the hearing loss in patients with COM initiates at an earlier stage and affects a significant higher portion of patients as compared with vestibular symptoms and abnormalities in the vestibular function tests.

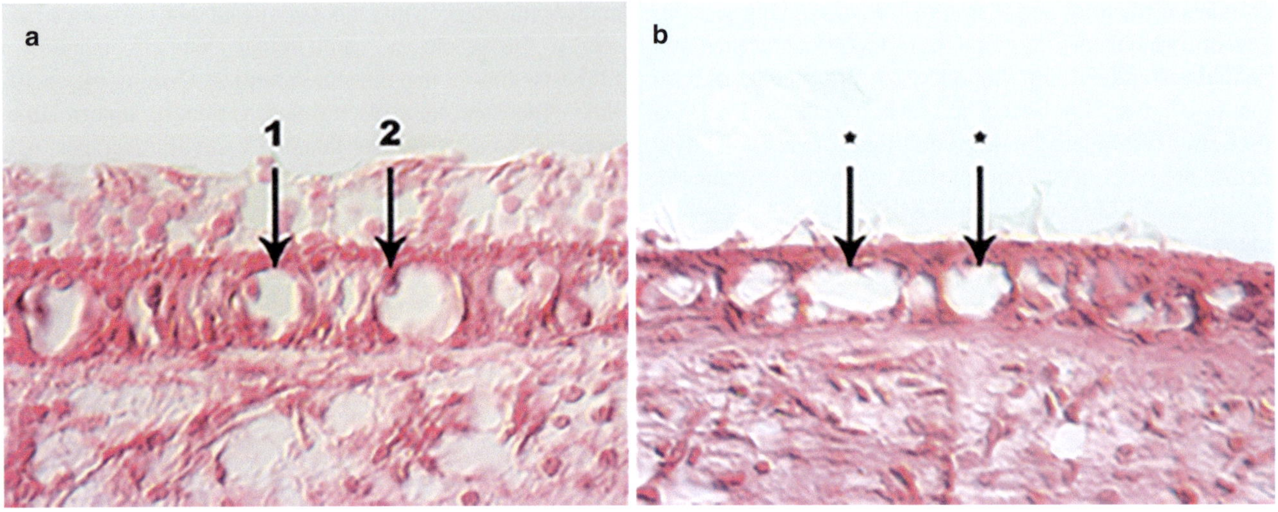

Fig. 30.2 Two representative human temporal bone sections, one from a healthy donor (**a**) and other from a donor with chronic otitis media (**b**) seen under Nomarsky microscopy (hematoxylin and eosin). In (**a**), the utricular macula seems normal, with normal number of type I (1) and type II (2) vestibular hair cells. In (**b**), the arrows (*) point to areas of loss of vestibular hair cells in the utricular macula

Vestibular Symptoms in Patients with Otitis Media

The association between otitis media and vestibular symptoms has been described in recent studies [40–42]. It is unclear what exact pathophysiologic mechanisms are involved with the development of these vestibular symptoms; in fact, no previous study has strongly determined the presence of a peripheral vestibular lesion secondary to otitis media. However, growing evidence support the hypothesis that otitis media does associate with vestibular dysfunction. A recent systematic review demonstrated that over 30% of patients with different types of otitis media experience some sort of symptom attributable to vestibular dysfunction (Monsanto et al. 2018) (Fig. 30.3). In patients with AOM, studies estimated that 30–48% of patients complain of dizziness or vertigo in the initial phase of the disease [43–46]. In OME cases, children were described as "clumsy" and had a higher tendency to fall as compared with children who did not have OME [47]. Also, OME associated with worse posturography results as compared with those of healthy children [48]. COM also associates with a high prevalence of vestibular symptoms, as a meta-analysis estimated the prevalence of dizziness or vertigo in this population at 40–60% (Monsanto et al. 2018). Despite these evidence, many authors have disputed the assumption that otitis media leads to a direct vestibular lesion, hypothesizing that the worse balance in these patients would be rather due to the active inflammation, through a difference in the pressure of the middle ear caused by the effusion, a direct effect of the hearing loss, or even due to other diseases or associated issues that could lead to vestibular dysfunction (such as metabolic diseases, benign paroxysmal positional vertigo (BPPV), and perilymphatic fistula) (Monsanto et al. 2018). However, a 30-year cohort has demonstrated that the prevalence of self-reported dizziness in adulthood was significantly higher among people who had a history of chronic otitis media in the past as compared with people who did not, showing that otitis media do lead to permanent (although potentially subclinical) peripheral vestibular damage [49].

The first study associating middle ear effusion with disequilibrium was published in 1977 [50]. Nowadays, OME is acknowledged as the most common cause of dizziness in childhood—however, the real incidence may be even higher than reported, as children rarely complain of balanced-related symptoms. Instead, vestibular symptoms are reported by caregivers as frequent falls, clumsiness, or bumping into things [47, 48, 51, 52]. Most studies demonstrated that children with OME have worse results in balance tests, delayed gross/fine skills acquisition, and abnormal posturography results. These abnormalities seem to subside after adequate treatment of the middle ear effusion: the symptoms and signs of balance disturbances resolved in 96% of the children after ventilation tube insertion [53]. However, even after the improvements, these children have lower scores than controls in balance tests as compared with controls [53–55]. A possible explanation for this is that chronic or repeated inflammation may cause permanent damage to the vestibular sensory epithelium [56]. Furthermore, adults who had OME or recurrent AOM during childhood may experience dizziness during their life [49]. Although speculative, it is possible that inflammatory mediators or toxins arising from the

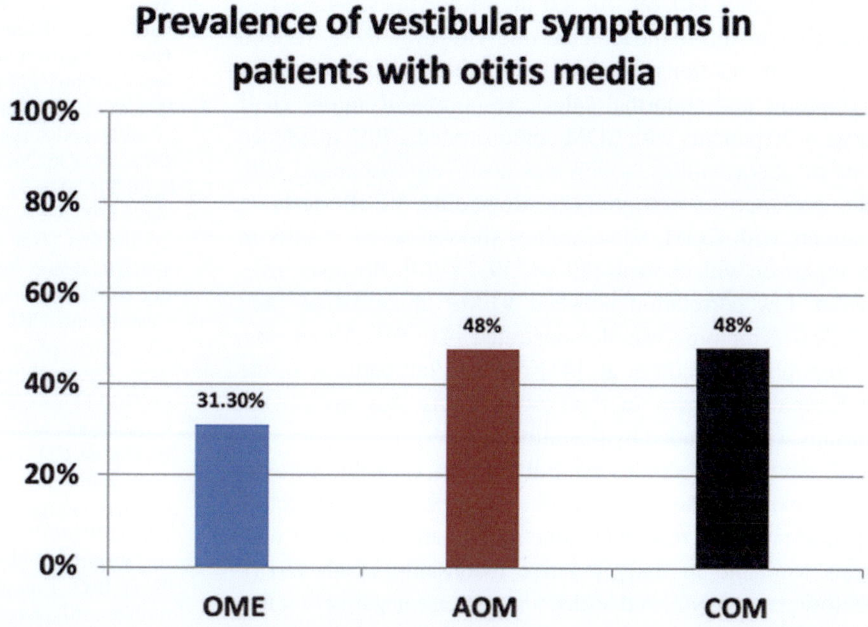

Fig. 30.3 Prevalence of vestibular symptoms in patients with different types of otitis media

middle ear inflammation may lead to a permanent effect on the vestibular system [10, 24, 25].

The long-term sequelae due to AOM have been sparsely studied. Several authors described the presence of vestibular deficits after ear infection, which resolved completely after treatment [57]. It seems that only patients who develop suppurative labyrinthitis as a consequence of AOM seem to be at an increased risk of developing a permanent vestibular sequela [37, 58]. It is possible that future studies in this regard will shed additional light in this yet pending aspect of AOM.

The prevalence of vestibular symptoms in patients who have COM was estimated at 40–60% [41, 59]. It was reported that the most critical factors associating with the vestibular symptoms in COM patients are the presence of perilymphatic fistulae or exacerbations of the middle ear inflammation. The vestibular symptoms in patients with COM are much less frequent than the auditory [28, 39]. In fact, it was observed that less than 20% include the vestibular symptoms as their chief complaints [39]. A possible explanation to that fact is that the chronic progression of the vestibular impairment caused by COM would allow central compensation for daily situations [60], or that the vestibular system is more resistant to inflammatory damage as compared with the cochlea [10].

Vestibular Function Tests

The matter of vestibular testing in patients with otitis media will be discussed in detail in a different chapter. The different types of otitis media (OME, AOM, and COM) were evaluated in relation to vestibular impairment with vestibular function tests (Monsanto et al. 2018), which included electronystagmography (ENG), caloric tests, vestibular evoked myogenic potentials (VEMP), dynamic and static posturography, sway magnetometry, craniocorpography, and the subjective vertical visual (SVV). Furthermore, scales and clinical tests were used to evaluate coordination, balance, and motor skills: Peabody Developmental Motor Scales (PDMS), Bruininks-Oseretsky Test of Motor Proficiency (BOTMP), Stott Test of Motor Impairment (STMI), and the Motor Accuracy Test-Revised (MAT-R).

All studies consistently demonstrated that children with OME had worse performance compared with controls, regarding the PDMS and BOTMP tests [53, 54, 61–64]. However, the association between low scores in these tests and presence of vestibular symptoms was inconsistent among studies. No significant differences existed in the results of STMI and MAT-R tests of OME and control groups [65]. Of ENG tests, rates of abnormalities were significantly higher compared with controls in all studies except in the study of Engel-Yeger et al. [62]. Regarding VEMP testing, no consistent results were found between OME patients and controls [64, 66, 67]. VEMP tests using air-conducted stimuli and bone-conducted stimuli varied greatly among studies (2–30% of absence of responses). The patients subjected to dynamic or static posturography demonstrated abnormal results compared with controls in some studies [47, 51, 52, 68]. In contrast, Ben-David et al. did not find differences in posturography between OME patients and controls [50].

The studies regarding AOM patients, 93% with AOM had abnormalities on the ENG and/or caloric tests. Also, caloric tests demonstrated decreased function in the affected ear in 30.7% of the subjects (Monsanto et al. 2018). Of patients with COM, ENG tests demonstrated that 56% had spontaneous nystagmus [40, 69, 70]. Of the caloric tests, 34.3% had abnormal results in the affected side. However, there were no significant relations between the presence of vestibular symptoms and abnormal caloric responses. Rotatory chair tests in 60 patients with COM demonstrated a 70% incidence rate of abnormalities, which was positively associated with the presence of vertigo [41]. Regarding VEMP tests in patients with COM, some studies showed worse results in comparison with controls [39, 41, 59, 71–74]. However, over again, low correlation between VEMP abnormalities and clinical symptoms was demonstrated [41, 59]. About posturography, Mostafa et al. [41] did not find patterns in the abnormal responses in their 60 subjects, but no control groups were included by the authors.

Despite many studies using these tests to evaluate possible damage in the inner ear due to otitis media, objective quantification of vestibular function is hard to achieve with tests available in daily practice (Monsanto et al. 2018). Caloric tests, ENG, and VEMPs results are negatively influenced by the status of the middle ear, and their results should be interpreted with caution. Further, children's cooperation for those tests is often limited [61, 62]. Some vestibular tests that are not affected by the presence of conductive hearing loss are viable alternatives to estimate whether the vestibular system was affected by otitis media or not. Those tests include clinical bedside tests (gait, static and dynamic postural tests, tests of the vestibule-ocular reflexes, cerebellar function tests, and neurologic evaluation), the video head impulse test (vHIT), static and dynamic posturography, and the SVV test [40, 41, 48].

Conclusions

Currently, there is consistent histopathologic and clinical evidence associating otitis media with peripheral vestibular system injury, which makes the search for vestibular symptoms and vestibular tests important in the evaluation of patients with otitis media. However, some aspects regarding the pathophysiological mechanisms leading to the vestibular lesion still need further clarification.

References

1. Bluestone CD, Gates GA, Klein JO, Lim DJ, Moji J, Ogra PL, et al. 1. Definitions, terminology and classification of otitis media. Ann Otol Rhinol Laryngol. 2002;111:8–18.
2. Rosenfeld RM, Shin J, Schwartz SR, Coggins R, Cagnon L, Hackell JM, et al. Clinical practice guideline: otitis media with effusion (update). Otolaryngol Head Neck Surg. 2016;154:S1–S41.
3. Lieberthal AS, Carrol AE, Chonmaitree T, Ganiats TG, Hoberman A, Jackson MA, et al. Clinical practice guideline: the diagnosis and management of acute otitis media. Pediatrics. 2013;131:e964–99.
4. World Health Organization. Chronic suppurative otitis media: burden of illness and management options. Geneva: World Health Organization; 2004. Available at: https://apps.who.int/iris/handle/10665/42941.
5. Monasta L, Ronfani L, Marchetti F, et al. Burden of disease caused by otitis media: systematic review and global estimates. PLoS One. 2012;7(4):e36226. https://doi.org/10.1371/journal.pone.0036226. Epub 2012 Apr 30.
6. Teele DW, Klein JO, Rosner B. Epidemiology of otitis media during the first seven years of life in children in greater Boston: aprospective, cohort study. J Infect Dis. 1989;160(1):83–94. https://doi.org/10.1093/infdis/160.1.83.
7. Casselbrant ML, Rubenstein E, Furman JM, Mandel EM. Effect of otitis media on the vestibular system in children. Ann Otol Rhinol Laryngol. 1995;104(8):620–4. https://doi.org/10.1177/000348949510400806.
8. Casselbrant ML, Mandel EM, Kurs-Lasky M, Rockette HE, Bluestone CD. Otitis media in a population of black American and white American infants, 0–2 years of age. Int J Pediatr Otorhinolaryngol. 1995;33(1):1–16. ISSN: 0165-5876. https://doi.org/10.1016/0165-5876(95)01184-D.
9. de Oliveira Penido N, Chandrasekhar SS, Borin A, Maranhão AS, Testa JRG. Complications of otitis media e a potentially lethal problem still present. Braz J Otorhinolaryngol. 2016;82(3):253–62. https://doi.org/10.1016/j.bjorl.2015.04.007.
10. Monsanto RDC, Schachern P, Paparella MM, Cureoglu S, de Oliveira Penido N. Progression of changes in the sensorial elements of the cochlear and peripheral vestibular systems: the otitis media continuum. Hear Res. 2017;351:2–10. ISSN: 0378-5955. https://doi.org/10.1016/j.heares.2017.05.003.
11. Paparella MM, Oda M, Hiraide F, et al. Pathology of sensorineural hearing loss in otitis media. Ann Otol Rhinol Laryngol. 1972;81:632–47. https://doi.org/10.1177/000348947208100503.
12. Monsanto RDC, Erdil M, Pauna HF, et al. Pathologic changes of the peripheral vestibular system secondary to chronic otitis media. Otolaryngol Head Neck Surg. 2016;155:494–500. https://doi.org/10.1177/0194599816646359.
13. Paparella MM. Interactive inner-ear/middle-ear disease,including perilymphatic fistula. Acta OtolaryngolSuppl. 1991;485:36–45.
14. Anon. Politzer's text-book of the diseases of the ear for students and practitioners. Indian Med Gaz. 1927;62:410–1.
15. Mackenzie GW. LXXXIX. Suppurative labyrinthitis with report of cases. Ann Otol Rhinol Laryngol. 1927;36:1019–77. https://doi.org/10.1177/000348942703600412.
16. Turner AL, Fraser JS. Labyrinthitis, a complication of middle-ear suppuration: aclinical and pathological study. J Laryngol Otol. 1928;43:609–44. https://doi.org/10.1017/S0022215100032485.
17. Druss JG. Pathways of infection in labyrinthitis: report of three different types. Arch Otolaryngol. 1929;9:392–403. https://doi.org/10.1001/archotol.1929.00620030414004.
18. Arslan M. Modifications of the osmotic pressure of perilymph and endolymph. An hypothesis on the pathogenesis of Menière's disease. Acta Otolaryngol (Stockh). 1969;67:360–77. https://doi.org/10.3109/00016486909125463.
19. Cureoglu S, Schachern PA, Rinaldo A, et al. Round window membrane and labyrinthine pathological changes: an overview. Acta Otolaryngol (Stockh). 2005;125:9–15. https://doi.org/10.1080/00016480410022534.
20. Goycoolea MV, Paparella MM, Goldberg B, et al. Permeability of the middle ear to staphylococcal pyrogenic exotoxin in otitis media. Int J Pediatr Otorhinolaryngol. 1980;1:301–8.
21. Goycoolea MV, Lundman L. Round window membrane. Structure function and permeability: a review. Microsc Res Tech. 1997;36:201–11. https://doi.org/10.1002/(SICI)1097-0029(19970201)36:3<201::AID-JEMT8>3.0.CO;2-R.

22. Schachern PA, Paparella MM, Goycoolea MV, et al. The permeability of the round window membrane during otitis media. Arch Otolaryngol Head Neck Surg. 1987;113:625–9.
23. Ghaheri BA, Kempton JB, Pillers D-AM, et al. Cochlear cytokine gene expression in murine chronic otitis media. Otolaryngol Head Neck Surg. 2007;137:332–7. https://doi.org/10.1016/j.otohns.2007.03.020.
24. MacArthur CJ, Pillers D-AM, Pang J, et al. Altered expression of middle and inner ear cytokines in mouse otitis media. Laryngoscope. 2011;121:365–71. https://doi.org/10.1002/lary.21349.
25. MacArthur CJ, Hausman F, Kempton JB, et al. Otitis media impacts hundreds of mouse middle and inner ear genes. PLoS One. 2013;8:e75213. https://doi.org/10.1371/journal.pone.0075213.
26. Trune DR, Kempton B, Hausman FA, et al. Correlative mRNA and protein expression of middle and inner ear inflammatory cytokines during mouse acute otitis media. Hear Res. 2015;326:49–58. https://doi.org/10.1016/j.heares.2015.04.006.
27. Kodama A, Ishii T, Oka Y, et al. Histopathology of the inner ear in chronic otitis media. Equilib Res. 1988;47:94–100.
28. Monsanto RDC, Kasemodel ALP, Tomaz A, Elias TGA, Paparella MM, Penido NO. Evaluation of vestibular symptoms and postural balance control in patients with chronic otitis media. J Vestib Res. 2020;30(1):35–45. https://doi.org/10.3233/VES-200691.
29. Juhn SK, Meyerhoff WL, Paparella MM. Clinical application of middle ear effusion analyses. Laryngoscope. 1981 Jun;91(6):1012-1015. https://doi.org/10.1288/00005537-198106000-00023.
30. Ishiyama G, Lopez IA, Ishiyama P, et al. The blood labyrinthine barrier in the human normal and Meniere's disease macula utricle. Sci Rep. 2017;7:253. https://doi.org/10.1038/s41598-017-00330-5.
31. Ishiyama G, Wester J, Lopez IA, Beltran-Parrazal L, Ishiyama A. Oxidative stress in the blood labyrinthine barrier in the macula utricle of Meniere's disease patients. Front Physiol. 2018;9:1068. https://doi.org/10.3389/fphys.2018.01068.
32. Paparella MM. Middle ear effusions: definitions and terminology Ann. Otol. Rhinol. Laryngol., 85 (2 Suppl. 25 Pt 2) (1976 Mar-Apr), pp. 8–11.
33. Saito H, Kitahara M, Kitajima K, Takeda T, Yazawa D, Matsubara H, Kitano J. Distended Reissner's membrane and otitis media (in Japanese). Pract Otol (Kyoto). 1981;74(Suppl 5):2413–8.
34. Paparella MM, Morizono T, Le CT, et al. Sensorineural hearing loss in otitis media. Ann Otol Rhinol Laryngol. 1984;93(6):623–9. https://doi.org/10.1177/000348948409300616.
35. Yamamoto E, Mizukami C. Endolymphatic hydrops induced by chronic otitis media. In: Kitahara M, editor. Ménière's disease. Tokyo: Springer; 1990. https://doi.org/10.1007/978-4-431-68111-3_25.
36. Zou J, Pyykkö I. Endolymphatic hydrops in Meniere's disease secondary to otitis media and visualized by gadolinium-enhanced magnetic resonance imaging. World J Otorhinolaryngol. 2013;3(1):22–5.
37. Kaya S, Schachern PA, Tsuprun V, et al. Deterioration of vestibular cells in labyrinthitis. Ann Otol Rhinol Laryngol. 2017;126:89–95.
38. Paparella MM, Abdelhammid MM, Schachern PA, Sahni R, Yoon TH, da Costa SS. Otopathologiccorrelates of the continuum of otitis media. Ann Otol Rhinol Laryngol. 1990;99(6_Suppl):17–22. https://doi.org/10.1177/00034894900990S606.
39. Chang C-W, Cheng P-W, Young Y-H. Inner ear deficits after chronic otitis media. Eur Arch Otorhinolaryngol. 2014;271:2165–70. https://doi.org/10.1007/s00405-013-2714-7.
40. Lee JS, Lee SK, Shin IH, et al. Vestibular evoked myogenic potential according to middle ear condition in chronic otitis media with tympanic membrane perforation. Acta Otolaryngol. 2014;134: 34–40.
41. Mostafa BE, Shafik AG, El Makhzangy AMN, et al. Evaluation of vestibular function in patients with chronic suppurative otitis media. ORL J Otorhinolaryngol Relat Spec. 2013;75:357–60.
42. Paparella MM. Interactive inner-ear/middle-ear disease, including perilymphatic fistula. Acta Otolaryngol. 1991;485:36–45.
43. Eliashar R, Gross M, Saah D, et al. Vestibular involvement in myringitis bullosa. Acta Otolaryngol. 2004;124:249–52.
44. Kim CH, Yang YS, Im D, et al. Nystagmus in patients with unilateral acute otitis media complicated by serous labyrinthitis. Acta Otolaryngol. 2016;136:559–63.
45. Nishimura M, Doi K, Kubo T, et al. Inner ear damage in acute otitis media. Pract Otorhinolaryngol. 2000;93:455–9.
46. Yamaguchi J, Yagi T, Baba S, et al. Inner ear damage in acute otitis media. OtolJpn. 1992;2:259–63.
47. Casselbrant ML, Furman JM, Rubenstein E, et al. Effect of otitis media on the vestibular system in chil-dren. Ann Otol Rhinol Laryngol. 1995;104:620–4.
48. Casselbrant ML, Furman JM, Mandel EM, et al. Past history of otitis media and balance in four-year-old children. Laryngoscope. 2000;110:773–8.
49. Aarhus L, Tambs K, Hoffman HJ, et al. Childhood otitis media is associated with dizziness in adulthood: the HUNT cohort study. Eur Arch Otorhinolaryngol. 2016;273:2047–54.
50. Ben-David J, Podoshin L, Fradis M, et al. Is the vestibular system affected by middle ear effusion? Otolaryngol Head Neck Surg. 1993;109:421–6.
51. Casselbrant ML, Redfern MS, Furman JM, et al. Visualinduced postural sway in children with and without otitis media. Ann Otol Rhinol Laryngol. 1998;107:401–5.
52. Gawron W, Pospiech L, Orendorz-Fraczkowska K. An evaluation of postural stability and the effects of middle-ear drainage on vestibulo-spinal reflexes of children with chronic otitis media with effusion. Int J Pediatr Otorhinolaryngol. 2004;68:1175–9.
53. Golz A, Netzer A, Angel-Yeger B, et al. Effects of middle ear effusion on the vestibular system in children. Otolaryngol Head Neck Surg. 1998;119:695–9.
54. Orlin MN, Effgen SK, Handler SD. Effect of otitis media with effusion on gross motor ability in preschool-aged children: preliminary findings. Pediatrics. 1997;99:334–7.
55. Wang M-C, Lee G-S. Vestibular evoked myogenic potentials in middle ear effusion. Acta Otolaryngol. 2007;127:700–4.
56. Joglekar S, Morita N, Cureoglu S, et al. Cochlear pathology in human temporal bones with otitis media. Acta Otolaryngol. 2010;130:472–6.
57. Balatsouras DG, Kaberos A, Assimakopoulos D, et al. Etiology of vertigo in children. Int J Pediatr Otorhinolaryngol. 2007;71:487–94.
58. Igarashi M, O-Uchi T, Isago H, et al. Utricular and saccular volumetry in human temporal bones. Acta Otolaryngol. 1983;95:75–80.
59. Ho K-Y, Chien C-Y, Tsai S-M, et al. Clinical significance of vestibular function with caloric and vestibular evoked myogenic potential testing for patients with simple chronic otitis media. J Int Adv Otol. 2012;8:447–52.
60. Lacour M, Helmchen C, Vidal P-P. Vestibular compensation: the neuro-otologist's best friend. J Neurol. 2016;263:54–64.
61. Cohen H, Friedman EM, Lai D, et al. Balance in children with otitis media with effusion. Int J Pediatr Otorhinolaryngol. 1997;42:10107–15.
62. Engel-Yeger B, Golz A, Parush S. Impact of middle ear effusion on balance performance in children. Disabil Rehabil. 2004;26:97–102.
63. Hart MC, Nichols DS, Butler EM, et al. Childhood imbalance and chronic otitis media with effusion: effect of tympanostomy tube insertion on standardized tests of balance and locomotion. Laryngoscope. 1998;108:665–70.
64. Said EA, Ahmed MK, Mohamed ES. Role of vestibular testing in deciding treatment strategies for children with otitis media with effusion. Egypt J Ear Nose Throat Allied Sci. 2015;16:151–9.
65. Von T, Deitz JC, McLaughlin J, et al. The effects ofchronic otitis media on motor performance in 5- and 6-year-old children. Am J Occup Ther. 1988; 42:421–426.400R.

66. Wang M-C, Lee G-S. Vestibular evoked myogenicpotentials in middle ear effusion. Acta Otolaryngol. 2007;127:700–4.
67. Kolkaila EA, Emara AA, Gabr TA. Vestibular evaluation in children with otitis media with effusion. J Laryngol Otol. 2015;129: 326–36.
68. Jones NS, Prichard AJN, Radomskij P, et al. Imbalance and chronic secretory otitis media in children: effect of myringotomy and insertion of ventilation tubes on body sway. Ann Otol Rhinol Laryngol. 1990;99:477–81.
69. Kanaya T, Shirato M, Unno T. Equilibrium findings of chronic otitis media. Pract Otorhinolaryngol. 1982;75:2392–8.
70. Kanoh Y, Yagi T, Yoshimoto Y, et al. A study on preoperative electronystagmography in chronic otitis media. Equilib Res. 1980;39:43–8.
71. Seo T, Miyamoto A, Saka N, et al. Vestibular evoked myogenic potential induced by bone-conducted stimuli in patients with conductive hearing loss. Acta Otolaryngol. 2008;128:639–43.
72. Wang M-C, Liu C-Y, Yu EC-H, et al. Vestibular evoked myogenic potentials in chronic otitis media before and after surgery. Acta Otolaryngol. 2009;129:1206–11.
73. Yang T-L, Young Y-H. Comparison of tone burst and tapping evocation of myogenic potentials in patients with chronic otitis media. Ear Hear. 2003;24:191–4.
74. Zhou G, Poe D, Gopen Q. Clinical use of vestibular evoked myogenic potentials in the evaluation of patients with air-bone gaps. Otol Neurotol. 2012;33:1368–74.

The Use of Topical Treatment and Middle–Inner Ear Interaction

31

Marcos V. Goycoolea, Leandro Rodríguez, and Pilar Epprecht

Introduction

The use of otologic drops as topical treatment for external otitis, for some forms of otitis media, in otologic surgery and for mastoid cavities is well established. Potential ototoxicity involves the concept that under specific circumstances, some of the components of these preparations (ototoxic components) can reach the inner ear and cause sensory damage.

Until 1995 [1], there were at least nine reports totaling 165 documented patients who developed sensorineural hearing loss owing to the use of ear drops for otitis media. In a survey composed of 2235 otolaryngologists, 3.4% reported having seen cochlear damage owing to otologic drops [2, 3]. If each of these otolaryngologists would have seen at least one case, this would represent 76 additional cases. Moreover, if 3.4% of otolaryngologists worldwide (ear drops are used universally) would see, at the very least, one case (a very conservative estimate), ototoxicity to otologic drops would constitute a significant problem. To our knowledge, no new reviews documenting groups of publications describing patients who developed sensorineural hearing loss owing to the use of ear drops have been available. However, isolated case reports keep appearing in the literature. Moreover, in our daily otologic practice, we occasionally receive patients who are referred because they developed sensorineural hearing loss after using ear drops with ototoxic components. In brief, ototoxicity due to components of ear drops is a reality to be addressed and with awareness it can be significantly diminished. Therefore, to avoid this complication while benefiting from the use of these preparations, it is important to review the potential routes of passage of these components to the inner ear, the pathogenesis of these events, and the experimental and clinical evidence available. With this information in hand, safer means of using drops can be developed.

Potential Routes from Middle to Inner Ear

Potential routes include round and oval windows, bony fistulae, micro-fissures, and blood and/or lymph vessels. Bony fistulae, micro-fissures, and the oval window do not seem to play a significant role, and lymphatics which are abundant in the round window membrane seem to participate in a peripheral rather than in a central direction. This is because the inner ear is of neurectodermal origin; therefore, it should not have lymphatics [3]. Blood vessels are an important route to consider because of the abundant vascular connections between the middle and inner ear in the round window [3–5].

The predominant pathway—and the most evaluated—seems to be the round window membrane. This membrane is the only soft tissue barrier between the middle and the inner ear. It is located inferiorly in the medial wall of the middle ear and lies in a niche, being therefore susceptible to exposure to fluids in the middle ear cavity.

Ultrastructural studies of the round window membrane of humans, monkeys, felines, and rodents have disclosed three basic layers: an outer epithelium, a middle core of connective tissue, and an inner ear epithelium. Despite being formed by three layers, experimental evidence has suggested that it behaves like a semipermeable membrane. Such evidence suggests that the layers of the round window participate in resorption and secretion of substances to and from the inner ear. Different substances, including antibiotics and tracers, when placed in the middle ear, traverse the membrane. Permeability is selective. Factors affecting permeability include size, concentration, electrical charge, thickness of the membrane, and facilitating agents [6, 7].

M. V. Goycoolea (✉)
Department of Otolaryngology, Clínica Universidad de Los Andes, Santiago, Chile

L. Rodríguez
Department of Otolaryngology, Clínica Universidad de Los Andes, and Hospital del Salvador, Santiago, Chile

P. Epprecht
Department of Otolaryngology, Clínica Universidad de Los Andes and Exequiel González Cortés Hospital, Santiago, Chile

M. V. Goycoolea et al. (eds.), *Textbook of Otitis Media*, https://doi.org/10.1007/978-3-031-40949-3_31

Available evidence of ototoxicity and/or passage of the components of commonly used ear drops that can be detected directly or indirectly in the inner ear after placing them in experimental animals in the round window niche are described in Table 31.1. Those detected when placed in the middle ear of humans are described in Table 31.2.

Table 31.1 Components of commonly used ear drops that can be detected directly or indirectly in the inner ear after placing them in experimental animals in the round window niche

Antibiotics
Chloramphenicol
Gentamicin
Neomycin
Polymyxin B
Antiseptics
Acetic acid
Ethanol
Local anesthetics
Lidocaine
Solvents
Propylene glycol
Corticosteroids (beneficial)
Hydrocortisone
Betamethasone

Table 31.2 Components of commonly used ear drops that can be detected directly or indirectly in the inner ear after placing them in the middle ear of humans

Antibiotics
Chloramphenicol
Gentamicin
Neomycin
Polymyxin B
Local anesthetics
Lidocaine
Corticosteroids (beneficial)
Dexamethasone

Inner Ear Effects of Ear Drop Components

Chloramphenicol, neomycin, polymyxin B, and gentamicin have been shown to cause hair cell damage [3, 8, 9]. Propylen gycol is ototoxic and in addition causes inflammatory reactions in the middle ear mucosa[10]. On the other hand, ciprofloxacin [11], dexamethasone, and methyl prednisolone [12, 13] traverse the round window membrane and are safe to use.

Permeability of the Round Window Membrane in Otitis Media

The question that comes up is what happens to the permeability of otologic drop components in middle ears with otitis media. The round window membrane in otitis media undergoes the same histopathologic changes that the mucoperiosteum of the middle ear does (it is part of it). These changes suggest that in early stages (the first 3–5 days of active inflammation), there may be an increase in permeability but that, as the inflammatory process develops (1 week of inflammation and thereafter), the membrane becomes thicker and develops protective mechanisms in terms of decreased permeability. As the active inflammatory process decreases (and the membrane regains its normality), so does the thickness and the protective mechanisms of the membrane decrease. Experimental evidence in cats, chinchillas, and guinea pigs using tracers and neomycin has confirmed this suggestion [6, 8].

There is an apparent discrepancy between experimental studies and clinical impressions in terms of ototoxicity of ear drops. As mentioned, animal studies have shown that during an established active inflammatory process (draining ears), round window membrane permeability drastically decreases owing to an increase in the thickness of the membrane to defensive mechanisms in the membrane [14] and dilution effects by the middle effusion. In my opinion, this is what happens in clinical cases because the physician uses otologic drops once the inflammatory process is already established. Therefore, in light of the available experimental evidence, it comes as no surprise that in these cases, ototoxic drugs traverse the membrane less readily and are less likely to cause inner ear damage, leading to an "apparent discrepancy." However, once the active inflammatory process decreases or subsides, the defensive mechanisms decrease, and the membrane becomes more permeable. Moreover, if one reviews the documented cases of patients who have developed sensorineural hearing loss owing to the use of otologic drops for otitis media [1], these tend to coincide with this explanation. Most of the reported cases are related to prolonged use of drops and/or in patients who continued their use once the drainage had subsided. That is to say, ototoxicity occurred once the active inflammatory process had subsided, the defensive mechanisms had decreased, and the membrane had become more permeable.

Although the subject of discussion of this chapter is ototoxicity, there are two aspects to be mentioned as complications in the use of ear drops. The relatively high incidence of allergic reactions to the neomycin contained in ototopical drops, and the significant vertigo that develops when drops containing lidocaine enter the middle ear cavity.

Which Drops Are Safe to Use?

Based on the available evidence, our indications and rationale for the use of otologic drops are as follows:

In chronic otitis media (chronic draining ears), topical treatment is our main modality. In our Clinical Department, we consider it safe to use quinolones as a first line of treatment, based on their safety profile. It is also possible that shorter courses of other drops could be safe and reasonable, should quinolones be either unavailable or contraindicated (e.g., allergy) or that the bacteria are resistant to them, assuming that the round window membrane has an established inflammatory process, and its permeability is drastically reduced.

In recently draining ears, we consider it safe to use quinolones and, if needed, other types of otologic drops while drainage persists, assuming that the round window membrane has an inflammatory process and that patients are closely monitored, and as soon as the drainage decreases, if needed, we switch to quinolone drops (e.g., ciprofloxacin), assuming that the membrane becomes more permeable.

In ears without drainage (e.g., placement of ventilation tubes in patients with "cloudy" effusion), we use only quinolone drops.

Future Trends

In terms of future trends or alternatives, some of our experimental approaches include the following:

Developing slow-release biodegradable membranes that could release substances over time in the middle ear [15], because otologic drops achieve adequate local levels but only for very short periods of time. Another experimental approach that has been described is the use of a sustained-release ciprofloxacin hydrogel that could be used as a single administration [16].

Developing spheres of a size that would not traverse the round window membrane or be absorbed by the middle ear mucosa, to which ototoxic drugs could be attached (provided that they would stay attached and remain effective) [3].

Developing means of defining the stage of reactivity of the middle ear mucosa and of permeability of the round window to use ototoxic drugs safely. The stage of reactivity should eventually be determined by evaluating middle ear effusions, since they are a reflection of the stage of reactivity of the middle ear mucosa [17].

Better defining the "defense" mechanisms of the round window membrane (round window membrane defense system) [3].

Developing research protocols that would evaluate not only passage but also mechanisms, routes, and distribution in the inner ear. This would also allow the eventual development of therapeutic approaches.

References

1. Linder TE, Zwuky S, Brandle P. Ototoxicity of ear drops: a clinical perspective. Am J Otol. 1995;16:653–7.
2. Lundy LB, Graham MD. Ototoxicity and ototopical medications: a survey of otolaryngologists. Am J Otol. 1993;14:141–6.
3. Goycoolea MV, Jung TK. Complications of suppurative otitis media. In: Paparella MM, Shumrick DA, Gluckman JL, Meyerhoff WI, editors. Otolaryngology, vol. 2. Philadelphia: W.B. Saunders; 1991. p. 1381–403.
4. Axelsson A. The vascular anatomy of the cochlea in the guinea pig and man. Acta Otolaryngol (Stockh). 1968;243:1–30.
5. Nakashima T, Ito A. Blood flow of the round window. Arch Otorhinolaryngol. 1981;230:57–9.
6. Goycoolea MV. Clinical aspects of round window membrane permeability under normal and pathological conditions. Acta Otolaryngol (Stockh). 2001;121:437–47.
7. Goycoolea MV, Muchow D, Schachern PA. Experimental studies on round window membrane structure function and permeability. Laryngoscope. 1988;98(Suppl 44):1–20.
8. Palomar GV, Palomar AV. Are some ear drops ototoxic or potentially ototoxic? Acta Otolaryngol (Stockh). 2001;121:565–8.
9. Smith BM, Myers MG. The penetration of gentamicin and neomycin into perilymph across the round window membrane. Otolaryngol Head Neck Surg. 1979;87:888–91.
10. Wright CG, Meyerhoff WL. Ototoxicity of otic drops applied to the middle ear in the chinchilla. Am J Otolaryngol. 1984;5:166–76.
11. Bagger-Sjoback D, Lundman L, Nilsson-Ehle I. Ciprofloxacin and the inner ear: a morphological and round window membrane permeability study. ORL J Otorhinolaryngol Relat Spec. 1992;54:5–9.
12. Itoh A, Sakata E. Treatment of vestibular disorders. Acta Otolaryngol Suppl (Stockh). 1991;481:617–23.
13. Parnes LS, Sun AH, Freeman DJ. Corticosteroid pharmokinetics in the inner ear fluids: an animal study followed by clinical application. Laryngoscope. 1999;109(Suppl 91):1–17.
14. Goycoolea MV, Lundman L. Round window membrane. A review. Microsc Res Tech. 1997;36:201–11.
15. Goycoolea MV, Muchow D, Sirvio L, Winandy RM. In search of missing links in otology. Part II. Development of an implantable middle ear drug delivery system: initial studies of sustained ampicillin release for the treatment of otitis media. Laryngoscope. 1991;101:727–32.
16. Wang X, Fernández R, Tsivkovskaia N, Harrop-Jones A, et al. Nonclinical assessment of a sustained-release ciprofloxacin hydrogel for the treatment of otitis media. Otol Neurotol. 2014;35(3):459–69.
17. Goycoolea MV, Paparella MM, Juhn SK, Carpenter AM. A longitudinal study of cellular changes in otitis media. Otolaryngol Head Neck Surg. 1979;87:685–700.

Silent Otitis Media and Subtle Complications

32

Rafael da Costa Monsanto and Michael M. Paparella

Introduction

Otitis media (OM) is a ubiquitous health problem in the United States that is associated with significant morbidity [1]. OM is increasingly impacting upon public health: it is the primary reason for visits to the Emergency Room, the second ranking reason for visits to a physician's office, the number one reason for antibiotic prescriptions in childhood (accounting for greater than 40% of all outpatient use of oral antibiotics), the primary reason for hearing loss in children and the third leading cause of hearing impairment in people of all ages, the primary reason for the use of general anesthesia in the pediatric population (for the purpose of inserting tympanostomy tubes) and is a significant cause of vestibular impairment [2–6]. The direct and indirect cost of medical, surgical, and rehabilitation management of OM is approximately 5 billion dollars in the United States alone [6, 7]. The chronic form of otitis media (COM) has an extremely high disease burden: it results in over 3 million disability-adjusted life years lost and results in 28,000 deaths yearly, mostly associated with intracranial complications [8, 9]. Over 60% of patients with COM have significant hearing impairment, accounting for a prevalence of up to 200 million people worldwide [1, 10]. More recently, a systematic review demonstrated that COM associates with a 40–60% prevalence of vestibular impairment, resulting in delayed acquisition of developmental milestones, abnormalities in several vestibular function tests, and increased risk of falls as compared with controls [11, 12].

Throughout the decades, many authors have described that chronic otitis media required the presence of a perforation of the tympanic membrane in association with persistent middle ear inflammation and otorrhea [13]. However, in a groundbreaking study published in 1979, Paparella et al. [5] introduced the concept of silent otitis media, demonstrating that even patients with an intact tympanic membrane could present "undetected or undetectable" clinically intractable chronic tissue (Fig. 32.1). Such hypothesis was later consistently corroborated by human temporal bone and clinical studies demonstrating similar findings [5, 14, 15]. As the diagnosis of this condition may be delayed because of the mild symptomatology and absence of a tympanic membrane perforation, the disease can progress through significant time periods without adequate diagnosis or treatment, which—in turn—could result in severe complications and sequelae.

Numerous studies have described the presence of intractable tissue pathology behind an intact eardrum. Meyerhoff et al. [3] studied 123 temporal bones with chronic otitis media. Only 24 of these patients (36 ears) had symptoms of otological disease recorded on their charts, and—of these—only 19.5% had an associated tympanic membrane perforation. In another study [16], 144 temporal bones with chronic

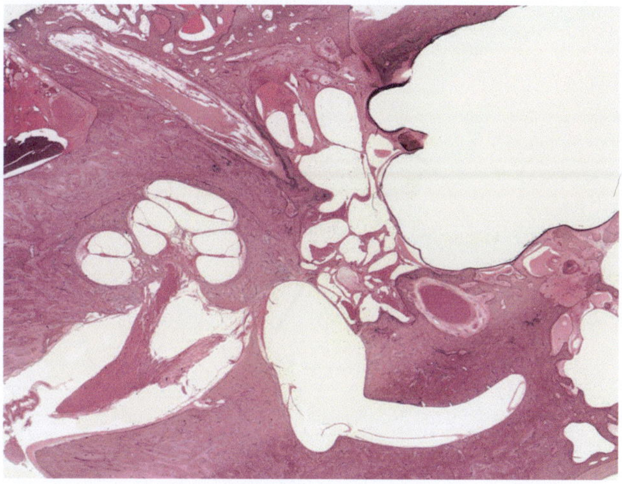

Fig. 32.1 A representative human temporal bone horizontal section showing signs of silent otitis media: the tympanic membrane is intact, although a retraction pocket is seen in the posterior aspect of the drum. In the middle ear, mucoid-purulent effusion permeated by fibrosis is seen

R. da Costa Monsanto (✉) · M. M. Paparella
Department of Otolaryngology, Head and Neck Surgery, University of Minnesota, Minneapolis, MN, USA
e-mail: rdacosta@umn.edu

M. V. Goycoolea et al. (eds.), *Textbook of Otitis Media*, https://doi.org/10.1007/978-3-031-40949-3_32

otitis media were divided into two groups: 28 with perforated and 116 with nonperforated tympanic membranes. The authors observed that the prevalence of granulation tissue, ossicular erosion, middle ear effusion, cholesterol granuloma, and tympanosclerosis were not significantly different between ears with and without tympanic membrane perforation.

Silent otitis media is a common finding in children. Paparella et al. [5] studied 111 infant ears; 54 of these showed histological evidence of otitis media. Of these, 20 cases presented with clinical manifestations, while 34 did not and were identified as silent otitis media. Mehta [17] examined 60 temporal bones of stillborns and neonates who died of causes other than septicemia for evidence of otitis media. He found 23.3% had silent otitis media.

Pathophysiological Mechanisms: The "Otitis Media Continuum"

Paparella et al. [18], in 1970, were the first authors to hypothesize and demonstrate that otitis media occurs in a continuum of mucoperiosteal changes that finally result in chronic inflammatory disease and clinically intractable tissue changes in the middle ear cleft (such as fibrosis, bony erosion, cholesterol granuloma, and cholesteatoma) (Fig. 32.2). In their study, the authors demonstrated progressive tissue changes that followed obstruction of the eustachian tubes of squirrel monkeys. These patterns have been also observed in clinical studies over the years. Collectively, the data suggest that the "acute" forms of otitis media (such as purulent, serous, and mucoid otitis media), when unresolved, may progress over time to more advanced degrees of pathological middle and inner ear changes [19]. As the disease advances

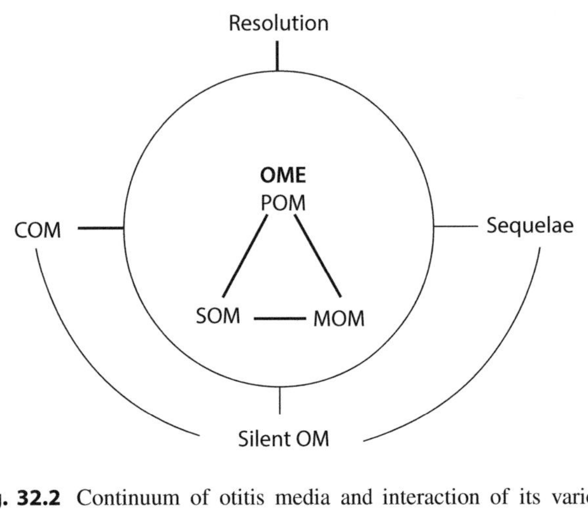

Fig. 32.2 Continuum of otitis media and interaction of its various forms. *OME* otitis media with effusion, *POM* purulent otitis media, *SOM* serous otitis media, *MOM* mucoid otitis media, *COM* chronic otitis media, *OM* otitis media

to the chronic, end stages of the continuum, the risks of inner ear sequelae also increase, resulting in sensorineural hearing loss and peripheral vestibular impairment [20]. The continuum of otitis media pathologic tissue changes was consistently seen in the otitis media temporal bone collection at the University of Minnesota, even in specimens with an intact tympanic membrane. Meyerhoff et al. [14] reproduced the series of events leading to silent otitis media in animals: using 38 chinchillas who received intratympanic bacterial inoculation, the authors later found the presence of effusion, mucosal edema, granulation tissue, hyperemia of the subepithelial space, hemorrhage in the middle ear space, and abundant polymorphonuclear leukocytes in the middle ear cleft despite the presence of a normal or subnormal tympanic membrane.

Paparella et al. [4] performed a longitudinal morphometric study of the middle ears of cats with otitis media in different time points (ranging from 1 week to 6 months). The authors showed the series of events following obstruction of the eustachian tube: at 1 week, a thin effusion could be observed in the middle ear cleft, possibly resulting from the negative middle ear pressure causing vascular transudate [21]. In the following weeks, a distinct metaplasia of the middle ear mucosal lining could be seen: the epithelium became cuboid, with enlargement of the blood vessels; also, goblet cells (who are not seen in a healthy middle ear mucosa) were seen in the epithelium. The middle ear effusion became increasingly thicker, being intensely stained by hematoxylin and eosin possibly due to a high protein content secondary to active secretion of the goblet cells. There is also an increasing concentration of inflammatory cells in the middle ear, polymorphonuclear leukocytes being the most frequent cell type. Months after the eustachian tube blockage, progressive development of intractable tissue changes occurred, including granulation tissue and fibrosis. These series of events, which are highly consistent with the concept of "otitis media continuum," were also demonstrated by following studies. Yoon et al. [22] observed a significant trend toward the development of these clinically intractable tissue changes in the later stages of the continuum (mucoid and chronic otitis media), further corroborating that time and the severity of the middle ear inflammation are pivotal factors in the development of these changes.

Although the pathophysiological mechanism resulting in otitis media and its subtypes are multifactorial, it has been demonstrated that obstruction of the middle ear ventilation in isolation can both initiate and perpetuate the cellular abnormalities that result in otitis media. This obstruction to the ventilation pathways may occur in different locations of the temporal bone, including the bony and cartilaginous eustachian tube, *protympanum*, *mesotympanum*, *isthmus*, attic, *aditus ad antrum*, and/or isolated groups of mastoid air cells [15]. In a study that included a total of 229 temporal bones with otitis media, obstruction of the epitympanum and mastoid antrum by pathological tissue (granulation tissue, residual mesenchyme, cholesterol granuloma, or cholesteatoma) was seen in 44 (19.2%) [23]. Palva and Johnsson [24] also demonstrated the patterns of ventilation within the *mesotympanum* and *epitympanum*, showing that the presence of fibrosis and granulation tissue secondary to otitis media can result in selective dysventilation. The decreased ventilation to specific parts of the middle ear can also result in the continuum of changes described by Paparella and colleagues [3]. Monsanto et al. [25] showed that the volume of the *epitympanum* and the area of the posterior tympanic *isthmus* are significantly decreased in human temporal bones with chronic otitis media. The authors hypothesized that the ventilation blockage caused by the tissue changes can result in negative pressure and hypodevelopment of the *epitympanum* and mastoid, being one potential pathophysiological mechanism involved with retraction pockets and cholesteatoma formation. Similar findings were later described in computed tomography studies [26].

In children, questions have been raised regarding the role residual mesenchyme in the pathogenesis of otitis media. Guggenheim et al. [27] commented on whether the residual mesenchyme would provide a predisposition toward or if it would act as a protective immunologic mechanism against development of otitis media. Kasemsuwan et al. [28] evaluated the temporal bone specimens of children who were younger than 5 years old and observed that the peak incidence of unresolved mesenchyme occurred between the ages of 4 months and 1 year. Furthermore, they observed that bones who had residual mesenchymal had a much higher prevalence of histological signs of otitis media. Considering the high association between mesenchyme and otitis media, as well as the observation that the highest prevalence of mesenchymal tissue was within the ages of peak incidence of otitis media, the authors argued that the presence of mesenchymal tissue in the middle ear would most likely contribute with the development of otitis media.

Subtle Complications of Otitis Media

The clinical symptoms of silent otitis media are frequently mild, and some patients may present only with intermittent aural fullness or tinnitus. As the disease might progress over significant periods of time (even decades) without adequate diagnosis or treatment, the risks of silent otitis media resulting in acute complications or sequelae might be even higher than in normal cases of acute or chronic otitis media presenting with tympanic membrane perforation [29]. Among the most frequent subtle complications are sensorineural hearing loss, labyrinthitis, vestibular impairment, and endolymphatic hydrops [5, 20, 30]. Although the exact pathophysiological mechanisms leading to these inner ear changes are still unknown, they most likely result from the passage of inflammatory mediators and bacterial products to the middle ear through the semipermeable round window membrane [31, 32]. This hypothesis was raised following observations that proteins, toxins, pharmaceutical substances, and even whole bacteria can penetrate the round window membrane during episodes of otitis media [33].

Endolymphatic Hydrops

Endolymphatic hydrops is a histopathological finding that has been associated as a causative mechanism of Meniere's disease. Paparella et al. were the first authors to describe a potential association between otitis media and secondary endolymphatic hydrops [34]. In their studies, the authors described the presence of significant cochlear hydrops in 20 temporal bones with chronic otitis media. The authors also hypothesized that the presence of an intact tympanic membrane would favor the development of inner ear sequelae, including endolymphatic *hydrops*, as the inflammatory mediators would be concentrated in the hypoventilated middle ear environment. However, studies dedicated to evaluating the pathophysiological mechanisms involved with the development of endolymphatic *hydrops* secondary to otitis media are very scarce in the literature.

Labyrinthitis

Although labyrinthitis can occur through meningogenic, hematogenic, or tympanogenic origins, otitis media has been described as one of the most frequent causative agents [29, 30]. The association between otitis media, labyrinthitis, and meningitis has been receiving a renewed interest after a study revealed an unexpected positive relationship between abnormal tympanometry and mortality rates in children with nontraumatic coma [35].

Three different types of labyrinthitis have been described: serous, suppurative, and ossificans. Serous labyrinthitis refers to the presence of "serous," proteinic material in the labyrinth, with fibrous or granular precipitate in the inner ear in the absence of bacteria, viruses, or inflammatory cells [30]. The serous labyrinthitis is most likely secondary to a change in the concentration of protein in the endolymphatic and perilymphatic fluids due to an inflammatory process. Kaya et al. [30] showed in a human temporal bone study involving patients with silent otitis media that serous labyrinthitis resulted in significant loss of outer hair cells in the basal and middle cochlear turns and increased degrees of cochlear *hydrops*. However, authors showed that serous labyrinthitis did not result in loss of cochlear inner hair cells, spiral ligament fibrocytes, and spiral ganglion neurons.

Suppurative labyrinthitis, on the other hand, refers to the presence of an active bacterial infection of the inner ear, resulting in conspicuous inner ear changes [36]. Studies from the otopathology laboratory at the University of Minnesota recently showed some of these cochlear changes secondary to suppurative labyrinthitis [36]. In their studies, the authors found not only loss of outer hair cells but also significant damage to the inner and outer hair cells, spiral ganglion cells, stria vascularis, and signs of severe endolymphatic hydrops in bones with suppurative labyrinthitis.

Labyrinthitis ossificans refers to the process of deposition of new bone in the cochlea following suppurative labyrinthitis or meningitis. Labyrinthitis ossificans is a critical problem that may affect patients with inner ear complications of otitis media, as it frequently results in complete deafness and could result in impossibility to perform a cochlear implant. Therefore, patients with labyrinthitis and meningitis must be carefully evaluated for the presence of progressive hearing loss, as delays in the diagnosis might result in irreversible deafness. The group at the University of Minnesota studied temporal bone specimens with labyrinthitis ossificans (Fig. 32.3), demonstrating significant abnormalities of the cochlear architecture, with critical damages to all cellular and neural structures of the cochlea and signs of severe endolymphatic hydrops [37]. Paparella et al. [38] reported that silent otitis media can also result in tympanogenic labyrinthitis and complete cochlear deafness. The authors also hypothesized that the absence of a tympanic membrane perforation can increase the chances of inner ear complications secondary to otitis media, as the infection is confined to a cavity with minimum or no drainage. Kaya et al. [39] also evaluated the sensorial epithelium of the peripheral vestibular system secondary to labyrinthitis: while all three types of labyrinthitis showed losses of vestibular hair cells (Fig. 32.4), loss of transitional and dark cells were seen only in the suppurative and ossificans group. The authors finally argue that labyrinthitis secondary to otitis media can significantly affect vestibular function.

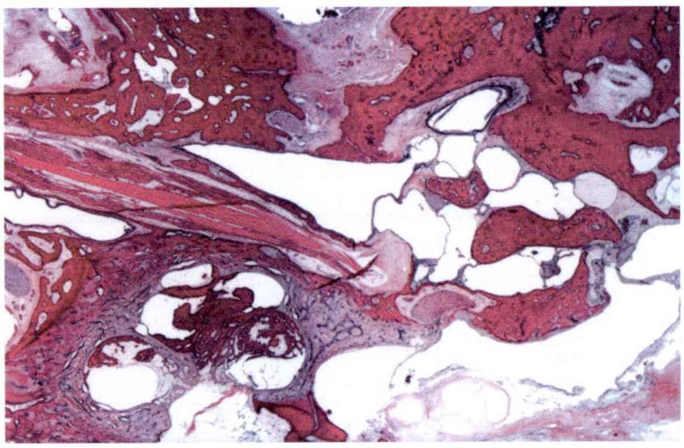

Fig. 32.3 A representative human temporal bone from a donor with signs of chronic otitis media behind an intact tympanic membrane. The cochlea is seen at the midmodiolar level, showing intense fibrosis and cochlear ossification within the cochlear turns

Sensorineural Hearing Loss

In 1972, Paparella et al. [38] were the first authors to demonstrate a concrete association between chronic otitis media and sensorineural hearing loss. The authors studied 279 cases of chronic otitis media and revealed that the otopathologic findings (loss of cochlear hair cells in the basal turn of the cochlea) were tonotopically consistent with the high-frequency hearing loss seen in most patients with the disease [38, 40]. Furthermore, they hypothesized that the round window membrane was the portal of entry from the middle to inner ear, which was later corroborated by experimental studies (Fig. 32.5) [41–43]. The passage of inflammatory mediators and bacterial toxins through the round window membrane results in serofibrinous precipitates and inflammatory cells in the perilymph of the scala tympani of the basal turn [40]. In a study of sensorineural hearing loss in chronic otitis media involving six centers from five countries, all centers showed significant levels of sensorineural hearing losses in patients with chronic otitis media. Through the following decades, studies continued to support these early observations [44, 45]. More recently, clinical studies showed that even a single episode of uncomplicated acute otitis media can result in permanent sensorineural hearing loss affecting the extended high frequencies, as demonstrated in long follow-up studies [46, 47].

Vestibular Impairment

The association between otitis media and vestibular symptoms has been a matter of great controversy [12]. Frequently, the presence of vestibular symptoms in patients with otitis media are immediately associated with a perilymphatic fistula or other causes of dizziness, such as metabolic diseases or benign paroxysmal vertigo [12]. Nonetheless, growing evidence indicate that otitis media, most frequently chronic and silent otitis media, can cause vestibular impairment even in the absence of perilymphatic fistula: studies revealed that the prevalence of vestibular symptoms in patients with COM ranged from 40% to 60%, and these symptoms frequently associate with abnormal results in vestibular function tests (caloric tests, cervical vestibular evoked myogenic potential (cVEMPs), and rotatory chair) [12].

The first author to evaluate potential causes for vertigo and vestibular symptoms in patients with silent otitis media

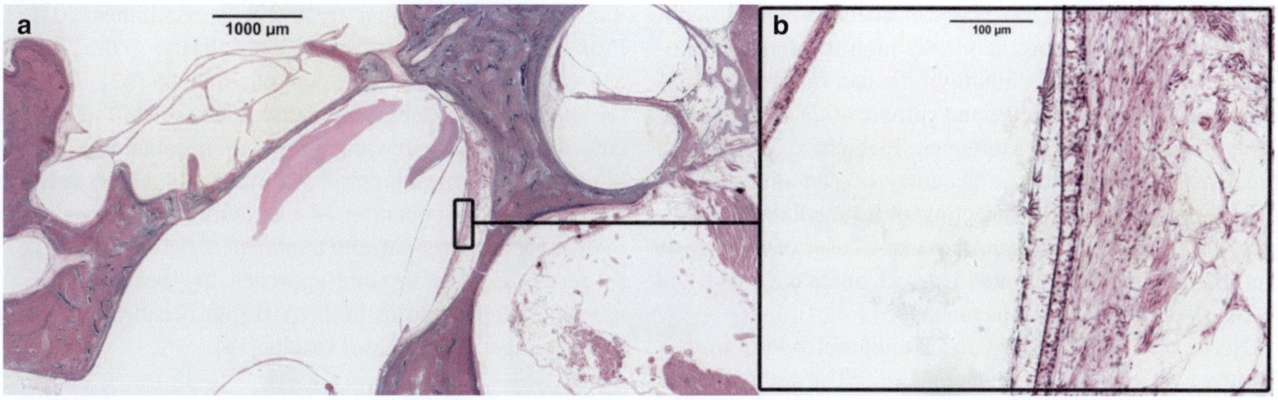

Fig. 32.4 (**a**) A representative human temporal bone specimen showing signs of serous labyrinthitis in the vestibule. (**b**) Squared area of the sensorial epithelium of the saccule from the top image seen under a higher magnification. The sensorial epithelium shows cellular disorganization, with areas of loss of vestibular hair cells (*)

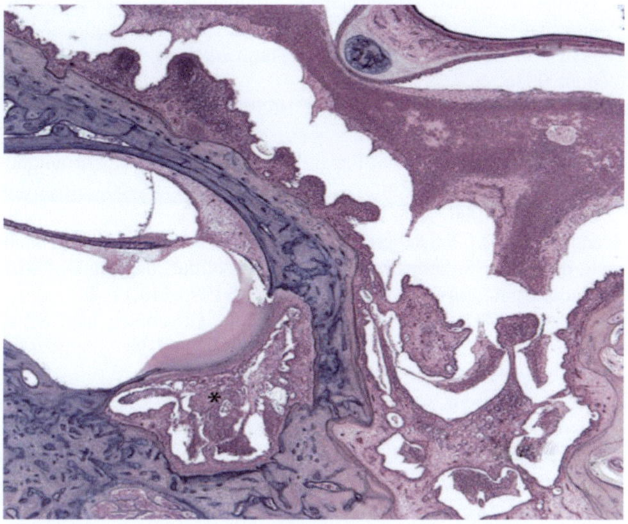

Fig. 32.5 A human temporal bone specimen with purulent otitis media, sectioned horizontally at the level of the round window membrane. Several inflammatory cells are seen in the round window niche (*), with an adjacent inflammatory infiltrate in the basal turn of the cochlea

was Paparella et al. [34] In their observations, the authors noted that some patients with otitis media have fluctuating sensorineural hearing loss, tinnitus, and episodic dizziness or vertigo, which were consistent with symptoms caused by *endolymphatic hydrops*. Based on these observations, the authors performed an otopathologic study in 194 temporal bones specimens with otitis media, revealing a 40% prevalence of endolymphatic hydrops. Later, clinical studies showed that some patients with chronic otitis media tend to develop Meniere's disease over time [48–50].

Histopathological examinations of the vestibular structures in bones with otitis media are very scarce. Kodama et al., in 1988 [51], demonstrated eosinophilic deposits in the endolymphatic and perilymphatic compartments, being more concentrated in the saccule. The authors also showed the presence of saccular edema and an abnormal neuroepithelium, while no significant abnormalities were seen in the utricle and semicircular canals. Monsanto et al. [52], in 2016, were the first authors to reveal a significant loss of vestibular hair cells type I and II in the saccular and utricular macula (more intense) and loss of type I cells in the anterior and posterior semicircular canals (less intense). Also, the authors found a significant loss of dark cells in the COM group as compared with controls. A later follow-up study from the same authors revealed that the cochlear changes secondary to otitis media initiated at an earlier stage and seemed to be more severe as compared with the vestibular losses [20]. Clinical studies showed similar findings: a systematic review demonstrated that over 30% of patients with different types of otitis media experience some sort of symptom attributable to vestibular dysfunction [12]. In children with otitis media with effusion and chronic silent otitis media, children were described as "clumsy" and had a higher tendency to fall as compared with children who did not have otitis media [53]. Additionally, a 30-year cohort has demonstrated that the prevalence of self-reported dizziness in adulthood was significantly higher among people who had a history of otitis media in the past as compared with people who did not, showing that otitis media do lead to permanent (although potentially subclinical) peripheral vestibular damage [54].

Severe Complications

Although in most cases silent otitis media result in subtle changes and mild symptoms, they might also result in severe complications. In this regard, meningitis is considered the most typical intracranial complication of otitis media [9, 29, 55, 56]. Although several otolaryngological societies dedicated to proposing diagnostic guidelines and the widespread use of antibiotics, intracranial complications of otitis media are still very common, especially in underdeveloped countries [9]. Among the reasons for the high incidence of otogenic meningitis, we can highlight the fact that in children, the symptomatology of acute and chronic otitis media can be highly unspecific [57]. Moreover, Pichichero et al. [58] revealed that the diagnostic accuracy of pediatricians and general practitioners for detecting otitis media was lower than 50%. Therefore, it seems that many cases of meningitis in children could be prevented if an adequate diagnosis and treatment of otitis media was made [35].

Djeric et al. [59] evaluated 16 temporal bones from 8 children who died of otogenic meningitis. The authors found signs of chronic inflammation of the round window membrane, with inflammatory cell infiltration within the membrane and the adjacent scala tympani. All cases had suppurative labyrinthitis, with a significant number of bacteria and inflammatory cells in all cochlear turns and the vestibule. Most interestingly, the tympanic membrane was intact in all 16 specimens. Yildirim-Baylan et al. [56] also found an 82% prevalence of bacteria embedded within a fibrous matrix in the middle ear of infants with tympanogenic meningitis who had silent otitis media. The authors also comment that clinicians must be aware that an intact tympanic membrane does not necessarily preclude the presence of pathologic changes in the middle ear cleft that could result in severe intracranial complications. The authors discussed on potential pathways for the spread of these bacteria to the central nervous system, of which the most likely would be through the round window membrane. In this regard, Schachern et al. [60] revealed findings that corroborate this hypothesis: in an animal study, they compared chinchillas with and without grafted round window membranes that were inoculated with Streptococcus pneumoniae. The authors demonstrated that none of the animals who received round window membrane grafts had signs of active labyrinthitis. Non-grafted animals, however, frequently showed bacteria in the cerebrospinal fluid, suggesting meningitis of tympanogenic origin. Thus, the authors further corroborate the round window membrane as the most likely route for spread of infection from the middle to the inner ear and central nervous system.

Treatment of Silent Otitis Media

Considering the risks of hearing loss, vestibular impairment, and intratemporal and intracranial complications, patients with a suspected silent otitis media must be adequately followed and diagnosed for optimal prevention and treatment strategies [56]. In children at the initial stages of the otitis media continuum, patients can be adequately treated by tympanostomy tubes [5]. In patients with a suspected chronic silent otitis media with the presence of intractable tissue in the middle ear, surgical treatment is recommended [61]. Prof. Michael Paparella has proposed the use of the "flexible approach" to treat chronic silent otitis media [62]. Although the surgical procedure will be discussed in detail in a different chapter, this approach proposes an endaural approach aimed to perform an exploratory tympanotomy, removal of tissue pathology, opening of the ventilation spaces in the middle ear and mastoid, and treatment of ossicular pathology as necessary. The flexible approach has been extensively used by many surgeons in the past four decade, with excellent hearing and functional results [15].

References

1. Monasta L, Ronfani L, Marchetti F, Montico M, Brumatti LV, Bavcar A, Grasso D, Barbiero C, Tamburlini G. Burden of disease caused by otitis media: systematic review and global estimates. PLoS One. 2012;7:e36226. https://doi.org/10.1371/journal.pone.0036226.
2. Acuin J. Chronic suppurative otitis media. BMJ Clin Evid. 2007;2007:0507.
3. Meyerhoff WL, Kim CS, Paparella MM. Pathology of chronic otitis media. Ann Otol Rhinol Laryngol. 1978;87:749–60. https://doi.org/10.1177/000348947808700602.
4. Paparella MM, Schachern PA, Yoon TH, Abdelhammid MM, Sahni R, da Costa SS. Otopathologic correlates of the continuum of otitis media. Ann Otol Rhinol Laryngol Suppl. 1990;148:17–22.
5. Paparella MM, Shea D, Meyerhoff WL, Goycoolea MV. Silent otitis media. Laryngoscope. 1980;90:1089–98. https://doi.org/10.1288/00005537-198007000-00003.
6. Teele DW, Klein JO, Chase C, Menyuk P, Rosner BA. Otitis media in infancy and intellectual ability, school achievement, speech, and language at age 7 years. Greater Boston Otitis Media Study Group. J Infect Dis. 1990;162:685–94. https://doi.org/10.1093/infdis/162.3.685.
7. Klein JO. The burden of otitis media. Vaccine. 2000;19:S2–8. https://doi.org/10.1016/S0264-410X(00)00271-1.
8. Hay SI, Abajobir AA, Abate KH, Abbafati C, Abbas KM, Abd-Allah F, et al. Global, regional, and national disability-adjusted life-years (DALYs) for 333 diseases and injuries and healthy life expectancy (HALE) for 195 countries and territories, 1990–2016: a systematic analysis for the Global Burden of Disease Study 2016. Lancet. 2017;390:1260–344. https://doi.org/10.1016/S0140-6736(17)32130-X.
9. de Oliveira Penido N, Chandrasekhar SS, de Albuquerque Maranhão AB AS, Testa JRG. Complications of otitis media—a potentially lethal problem still present. Braz J Otorhinolaryngol. 2016;82:253–62. https://doi.org/10.1016/j.bjorl.2015.04.007.
10. World Health Organization. Addressing the rising prevalence of hearing loss. 2018.
11. da Costa Monsanto R, Kasemodel ALP, Tomaz A, Abrahão Elias TG, Paparella MM, de Oliveira Penido N. Evaluation of vestibular symptoms and postural balance control in patients with chronic otitis media. J Vestib Res. 2020;30:35. https://doi.org/10.3233/VES-200691.
12. da Costa Monsanto R, Kasemodel ALP, Tomaz A, Paparella MM, de Oliveira Penido N. Current evidence of peripheral vestibular symptoms secondary to otitis media. Ann Med. 2018;50:391–401. https://doi.org/10.1080/07853890.2018.1470665.
13. Bluestone CD, Gates GA, Klein JO, Lim DJ, Mogi G, Ogra PL, Paparella MM, Paradise JL, Tos M. 1. Definitions, terminology,

and classification of otitis media. Ann Otol Rhinol Laryngol. 2002;111:8–18. https://doi.org/10.1177/00034894021110S304.
14. Meyerhoff WL, Giebink GS, Shea DA. Silent otitis media: an animal study. Ann Otol Rhinol Laryngol. 1984;93:136–9. https://doi.org/10.1177/000348948409300207.
15. Paparella MM, Schachern PA, Cureoglu S. Chronic silent otitis media. ORL J Otorhinolaryngol Relat Spec. 2002;64:65–72. https://doi.org/10.1159/000057783.
16. da Costa SS, Paparella MM, Schachern PA, Yoon TH, Kimberley BP. Temporal bone histopathology in chronically infected ears with intact and perforated tympanic membranes. Laryngoscope. 1992;102:1229–36. https://doi.org/10.1288/00005537-199211000-00005.
17. Mehta S. Silent otitis media: an autopsy study in stillborns and neonates. Ear Nose Throat J. 1990;69:296, 299–300, 311–317.
18. Paparella MM, Brady DR, Hoel R. Sensori-neural hearing loss in chronic otitis media and mastoiditis. Trans Am Acad Ophthalmol Otolaryngol. 1970;74:108–15.
19. Juhn SK, Paparella MM, Goycoolea MV, Kim CS, Giebink S. Pathogenesis of otitis media. Ann Otol Rhinol Laryngol. 1977;86:481–92. https://doi.org/10.1177/000348947708600407.
20. da Costa Monsanto R, Schachern P, Paparella MM, Cureoglu S, de Oliveira Penido N. Progression of changes in the sensorial elements of the cochlear and peripheral vestibular systems: the otitis media continuum. Hear Res. 2017;351:2–10. https://doi.org/10.1016/j.heares.2017.05.003.
21. Hiraide F, Paparella MM. Vascular changes in middle ear effusions. Arch Otolaryngol. 1972;96:45–51. https://doi.org/10.1001/archotol.1972.00770090083010.
22. Yoon TH, Paparella MM, Schachern PA, Lindgren BR. Morphometric studies of the continuum of otitis media. Ann Otol Rhinol Laryngol Suppl. 1990;148:23–7. https://doi.org/10.1177/00034894900990s607.
23. Schachern P, Paparella MM, Sano S, Lamey S, Guo YH. A histopathological study of the relationship between otitis media and mastoiditis. Laryngoscope. 1991;101:1050–5. https://doi.org/10.1288/00005537-199110000-00004.
24. Palva T, Johnsson L-G. Epitympanic compartment surgical considerations: reevaluation. Otol Neurotol. 1995;16:505–13.
25. da Costa Monsanto R, Pauna HF, Kaya S, Hızlı Ö, Kwon G, Paparella MM, Cureoglu S. Epitympanum volume and tympanic isthmus area in temporal bones with retraction pockets. Laryngoscope. 2016;126:E369–74. https://doi.org/10.1002/lary.25937.
26. Marchioni D, Piccinini A, Alicandri-Ciufelli M, Presutti L. Endoscopic anatomy and ventilation of the epitympanum. Otolaryngol Clin N Am. 2013;46:165–78. https://doi.org/10.1016/j.otc.2012.10.002.
27. Clements L, Guggenheim P, Schlesinger A. The significance and fate of the mesenchyme of the middle ear. Laryngoscope. 1956;66:1303–26. https://doi.org/10.1288/00005537-195610000-00004.
28. Kasemsuwan L, Schachern P, Paparella MM, Le CT. Residual mesenchyme in temporal bones of children. Laryngoscope. 1996;106:1040–3. https://doi.org/10.1097/00005537-199608000-00025.
29. Schachern PA, Paparella MM, Hybertson R, Sano S, Duvall AJ. Bacterial tympanogenic labyrinthitis, meningitis, and sensorineural damage. Arch Otolaryngol Head Neck Surg. 1992;118:53–7.
30. Kaya S, Tsuprun V, Hızlı Ö, Schachern PA, Paparella MM, Cureoglu S. Cochlear changes in serous labyrinthitis associated with silent otitis media: a human temporal bone study. Am J Otolaryngol. 2016;37:83–8. https://doi.org/10.1016/j.amjoto.2015.10.002.
31. Goycoolea MV. Clinical aspects of round window membrane permeability under normal and pathological conditions. Acta Otolaryngol. 2001;121:437–47.
32. Schachern PA, Paparella MM, Goycoolea MV, Duvall AJ, Choo Y-B. The permeability of the round window membrane during otitis media. Arch Otolaryngol Head Neck Surg. 1987;113:625–9. https://doi.org/10.1001/archotol.1987.01860060051014.
33. Cureoglu S, Schachern PA, Paparella MM, Lindgren BR. Cochlear changes in chronic otitis media. Laryngoscope. 2004;114:622–6. https://doi.org/10.1097/00005537-200404000-00006.
34. Paparella MM, Goycoolea MV, Meyerhoff WL, Shea D. Endolymphatic hydrops and otitis media. Laryngoscope. 1979;89:43–58.
35. Gwer S, Chengo E, Newton CRJC, Kirkham FJ. Unexpected relationship between tympanometry and mortality in children with nontraumatic coma. Pediatrics. 2013;132:e713–7. https://doi.org/10.1542/peds.2012-3264.
36. Kaya S, Tsuprun V, Hizli Ö, Paparella MM, Cureoglu S. Quantitative assessment of cochlear histopathologic findings in patients with suppurative labyrinthitis. JAMA Otolaryngol Head Neck Surg. 2016;142:364–9. https://doi.org/10.1001/jamaoto.2015.3803.
37. Kaya S, Paparella MM, Cureoglu S. Pathologic findings of the cochlea in labyrinthitis ossificans associated with the round window membrane. Otolaryngol Head Neck Surg. 2016;155:635–40. https://doi.org/10.1177/0194599816651245.
38. Paparella MM, Oda M, Hiraide F, Brady D. Pathology of sensorineural hearing loss in otitis media. Ann Otol Rhinol Laryngol. 1972;81:632–47. https://doi.org/10.1177/000348947208100503.
39. Kaya S, Schachern PA, Tsuprun V, Paparella MM, Cureoglu S. Deterioration of vestibular cells in labyrinthitis. Ann Otol Rhinol Laryngol. 2017;126:89–95. https://doi.org/10.1177/0003489416675356.
40. Paparella MM, Morizono T, Le CT, Mancini F, Sipilä P, Choo YB, Lidén G, Kim CS. Sensorineural hearing loss in otitis media. Ann Otol Rhinol Laryngol. 1984;93:623–9. https://doi.org/10.1177/000348948409300616.
41. Goycoolea MV, Lundman L. Round window membrane. Structure function and permeability: a review. Microsc Res Tech. 1997;36:201–11. https://doi.org/10.1002/(SICI)1097-0029(19970201)36:3<201::AID-JEMT8>3.0.CO;2-R.
42. Goycoolea MV, Paparella MM, Carpenter AM, Juhn SK. A longitudinal study of cellular changes in experimental otitis media. Otolaryngol Head Neck Surg. 1979;87:685–700. https://doi.org/10.1177/019459987908700524.
43. Goycoolea MV, Paparella MM, Goldberg B, Schlievert PM, Carpenter AM. Permeability of the middle ear to staphylococcal pyrogenic exotoxin in otitis media. Int J Pediatr Otorhinolaryngol. 1980;1:301–8.
44. Hunter LL, Margolis RH, Rykken JR, Le CT, Daly KA, Giebink GS. High frequency hearing loss associated with otitis media. Ear Hear. 1996;17:1–11. https://doi.org/10.1097/00003446-199602000-00001.
45. Margolis RH, Nelson DA. Acute otitis media with transient sensorineural hearing loss: acase study. Arch Otolaryngol Head Neck Surg. 1993;119:682–6. https://doi.org/10.1001/archotol.1993.01880180102020.
46. Cordeiro FP, da Costa MR, Kasemodel ALP, de Almeida GL, de Oliveira PN. Extended high-frequency hearing loss following the first episode of otitis media. Laryngoscope. 2018;128:2879–84. https://doi.org/10.1002/lary.27309.
47. Kasemodel ALP, Costa LEM, da Costa Monsanto R, Tomaz A, de Oliveira Penido N. Sensorineural hearing loss in the acute phase of a single episode of acute otitis media. Braz J Otorhinolaryngol. 2019;86:767. https://doi.org/10.1016/j.bjorl.2019.06.001.
48. Paparella MM. Interactive inner-ear/middle-ear disease, including perilymphatic fistula. Acta Otolaryngol Suppl. 1991;485:36–45.
49. Paparella MM, de Sousa LC, Mancini F. Meniere's syndrome and otitis media. Laryngoscope. 1983;93:1408–15.
50. Yamamoto E, Mizukami C. Endolymphatic hydrops induced by chronic otitis media. In: Kitahara M, editor. Ménière's disease. Tokyo: Springer; 1990. p. 191–8.

51. Kodama A, Ishii T, Oka Y, Uebo K. Inner ear histopathology of human temporal bone with chronic otitis media. 1988.
52. da Costa MR, Erdil M, Pauna HF, Kwon G, Schachern PA, Tsuprun V, Paparella MM, Cureoglu S. Pathologic changes of the peripheral vestibular system secondary to chronic otitis media. Otolaryngol Head Neck Surg. 2016;155:494–500. https://doi.org/10.1177/0194599816646359.
53. Casselbrant ML, Furman JM, Rubenstein E, Mandel EM. Effect of otitis media on the vestibular system in children. Ann Otol Rhinol Laryngol. 1995;104:620–4. https://doi.org/10.1177/000348949510400806.
54. Aarhus L, Tambs K, Hoffman HJ, Engdahl B. Childhood otitis media is associated with dizziness in adulthood: the HUNT cohort study. Eur Arch Otorhinolaryngol. 2016;273:2047–54. https://doi.org/10.1007/s00405-015-3764-9.
55. Penido ND, Borin A, Iha LCN, Suguri VM, Onishi E, Fukuda Y, Cruz OLM. Intracranial complications of otitis media; 15 years of experience in 33 patients. Otolaryngol Head Neck Surg. 2005;132:37–42. https://doi.org/10.1016/j.otohns.2004.08.007.
56. Yildirim-Baylan M, Schachern P, Tsuprun V, Shiabata D, Paparella MM, Cureoglu S. The pathology of silent otitis media: a predecessor to tympanogenic meningitis in infants. Int J Pediatr Otorhinolaryngol. 2014;78:451–4. https://doi.org/10.1016/j.ijporl.2013.12.015.
57. Niemela M, Uhari M, Jounio-Ervasti K, Luotonen J, Alho OP, Vierimaa E. Lack of specific symptomatology in children with acute otitis media. Pediatr Infect Dis J. 1994;13:765–8. https://doi.org/10.1097/00006454-199409000-00002.
58. Pichichero ME, Poole MD. Assessing diagnostic accuracy and tympanocentesis skills in the management of otitis media. Arch Pediatr Adolesc Med. 2001;155:1137–42. https://doi.org/10.1001/archpedi.155.10.1137.
59. Djerić DR, Schachern PA, Paparella MM, Jaramillo M, Haruna S, Bassioni M. Otitis media (silent): a potential cause of childhood meningitis. Laryngoscope. 1994;104:1453–60. https://doi.org/10.1288/00005537-7990632.
60. Schachern PA, Paparella MM, Goycoolea MV. Experimental grafting of the round window membrane: part I. Laryngoscope. 1987;97:790–6. https://doi.org/10.1288/00005537-198707000-00002.
61. Patterson MH, Paparella MM. Otitis media with effusion and early sequelae—flexible approach. Otolaryngol Clin N Am. 1999;32:391. https://doi.org/10.1016/S0030-6665(05)70141-9.
62. da Costa SS, de Souza LCA, Piza MRD. The flexible endaural tympanoplasty—pathology-guided, pathogenesis-oriented surgery for the middle ear. Otolaryngol Clin N Am. 1999;32:413. https://doi.org/10.1016/S0030-6665(05)70143-2.

Complications of Otitis Media Limited to Within the Temporal Bone

33

Diane Biju, Aishan Patil, Shaila Sidam, Aditi Govil, Kanchan Gupta, Vishal Tyagi, Rosemarie de Souza, and Chris de Souza

Intratemporal Bone Complications

Complications are different from sequelae. Sequalae are limited to the mucoperiosteum, while complications extend beyond it. An example of a sequelae is tympanosclerosis. An example of a complication is a perforation of the tympanic membrane or a brain abscess. Acute otitis media can exist behind an intact tympanic membrane. The inflammation may involve the entire middle ear cleft or rarely the middle ear cavity alone. In the era that was before the widespread availability and use of antibiotics, infections of the middle ear cavity rapidly spread to involve the entre middle ear cleft and thus were able to cause complications. Chronic otitis media presents in two forms: (a) cholesteatoma and (b) perforations of the tympanic membrane. In the era of the understanding of otologic diseases, the surgical management of cholesteatomas was evolving. While cholesteatomas themselves are not infectious, they harbor infections which allowed infections to spread through the channels created by cholesteatomas. Chronic otitis media also presented in the form of perforations. These perforations rarely healed and allowed egress of infection into the middle ear cavity and middle ear cleft through frequent attacks of otitis media. In general, it was chronic otitis media (with cholesteatoma or with perforations) that was primarily associated with complications. Acute otitis media could and did cause complications, especially if the infection was a particularly virulent one.

D. Biju
Holy Spirit Hospital, Mumbai, India

A. Patil
Vascular Surgery, Borders General Hospital, Melrose, Scotland, UK

S. Sidam
All India Institute of Medical Sciences, Bhopal, Madhya Pradesh, India

A. Govil
Lilavati Hospital and Research Centre, Mumbai, India

BJ Medical College, Ahmedabad, India

K. Gupta
Lilavati Hospital and Research Centre, Mumbai, India

V. Tyagi
Holy Family Hospital, Holy Spirit Hospital, Mumbai, India

Department of ENT, VN Desai Hospital, Mumbai, India

R. de Souza
Internal Medicine, BYL Nair Hospital and TNM College, Mumbai, India

C. de Souza (✉)
Faculty SUNY, Brooklyn, NY, USA

LSUHSC, Shreveport, LA, USA

Lilavati Hospital, Holy Family Hospital, Holy Spirit Hospital, Mumbai, India

Tympanic Membrane Perforation

Tympanic membrane perforations of the tympanic membrane are the single most common complication of otitis media. Perforations develop in the presence of either acute or chronic ear disease. The pathogenic pathway that causes perforations are excessive pressure on the TM, resulting either from pressurized purulent matter in the middle ear or from long-standing eustachian tube dysfunction which in turn causes atelectasis. The resulting perforation usually occurs in the pars tensa and can vary considerably in size.

Most perforations heal spontaneously. There are a few patients who present with chronic perforation. A patient with a chronic perforation classically presents with a conductive hearing loss. Hearing loss will depend on the type and location of the perforation and the status of the ossicular chain. Diagnosis of a perforation can be confirmed by direct visualization with otomicroscopy or otoendoscopy. The treatment of perforations is through surgery. The results of tympanoplasty for chronic TM perforations are excellent.

M. V. Goycoolea et al. (eds.), *Textbook of Otitis Media*, https://doi.org/10.1007/978-3-031-40949-3_33

Acute Mastoiditis

Mastoiditis is the acute inflammation of mastoid air cells which are epithelium-lined bone septations that are continuous with the middle ear cavity.

Coalescent Mastoiditis [1–3]

Coalescent mastoiditis with presence of a subperiosteal abscess occurs when the air cells in the mastoid that are separated from each other by multiple septa break down and form a single pus-filled cavity. This in turn causes the infection to spread to the periosteum resulting in a subperiosteal abscess. Although this much dreaded complication has declined considerably, the mortality of mastoiditis sequela in children remains 10% [4].

Acute mastoditis is a clinical diagnosis. The pathognomonic triad of symptoms of acute mastoiditis are (1) severe unrelenting otalgia, (2) postauricular swelling indictive of a subperiosteal abscess, and (3) fever. Otorrhea and hearing loss are also present. The most common presenting sign, postauricular tenderness, is seen in a majority of cases. In addition, protrusion of the pinna and postauricular erythema and swelling are classic findings. On otoscopy, bulging of the posterosuperior wall of the external auditory canal and a bulging erythematous tympanic membrane can be seen.

Induration over the mastoid is often a sign of an impending sub-periosteal abscess.

Temporal bone computed tomographic (CT) scanning is the imaging modality of choice, and a loss of bony trabeculae in a single inflamed pus filled cavity is the commonest finding (Fig. 33.1). CT scans of the temporal bone can also pick up other conditions like Bezold's abscess and venous thrombosis.

The natural progression of acute otitis media to coalescent mastoiditis follows a well-described sequence of stages [5].

Stage 1. At first, there is hyperemia and edema of the mucoperiosteal lining of the pneumatized mastoid air cells. This results in obstruction of the narrow aditus which in turn disrupts aeration (ventilation and drainage).

Stage 2. The thickened mucous membrane and impaired ciliary function prevent drainage of secretions of the middle ear through the eustachian tube. The exudates in the early stages of the infection are serous.

Stage 3. They become purulent once inflammatory cells invade. These series of events result in venous stasis, local acidosis, and dissolution of calcium from the bony septae. Osteoclastic activity in the inflamed periosteum softens and dissolves the bony partitions, causing the small air cells to coalesce into larger cavity that results in.

Stage 4. Coalescent mastoiditis

Histological examination shows that areas of coalescent bone erosion are combined with adjacent areas of bone deposition. The healing processes cause the normal mucoperiosteum to be replaced with maturing granulation tissue. Osteitis occurs in the areas of bone destruction which results in the production of dense, compact bone resulting in a sclerotic contracted mastoid bone.

Masked Mastoiditis

Acute mastoiditis has frequently been reported in patients with a well-aerated tympanic cavity and normal appearing tympaniç membrane and present with minimal symptoms. This has been termed masked mastoiditis and is attributed to

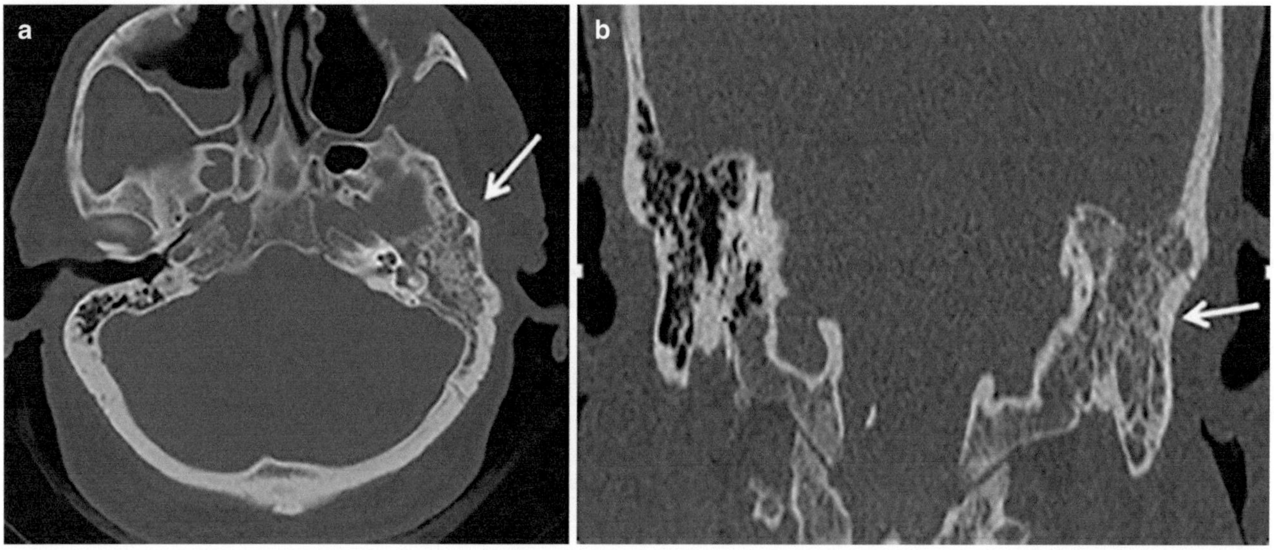

Fig. 33.1 CT scan demonstrating coalescent mastoiditis (white arrow). This can be easily compared to the opposite mastoid which is clearly uninvolved. **a** CT scan coronal view of the temporal bone. **b** CT scan coronal sections of the te with coalescent mastoiditismporal bone. white arrow points towards the affected side

inadequate antibiotic management of acute otitis media which suppress but not completely eliminate infection within the middle ear cleft. Although the incidence of surgical mastoiditis appears to be decreasing, there is still a high index of suspicion required in children with otitis media that could be masked by antibiotic therapy. The clinical course is more insidious than that of classical coalescent mastoiditis. In a recent review, 72% of 18 patients with acute mastoiditis had no history of ear disease, and 67% had middle ear symptoms for less than 7 days before developing a clinically significant mastoiditis that required surgical intervention.

This condition necessitates that the appropriate antibiotic be given for the appropriate period of time in the appropriate dosage for it to be effective. Mastoidectomy is required to remove necrotic bone and infected material, provide drainage for pus, and prevent intracranial extension of infection. This needs to be carried out in conjunction with antibiotic treatment.

Facial Nerve Paralysis

With the advent of antibiotics, facial nerve paralysis has become very rare. The frequency of facial nerve paralysis has reduced drastically [6, 7].

High-resolution temporal bone CT scanning is necessary, especially when facial nerve palsy occurs in the presence of otitis media. HR CT scans of the temporal bone help accurately identify the location and possible cause of the facial nerve lesion.

Antibiotic treatment and surgery are directed at the removal of the cause of facial nerve edema which should result in the restoration of facial nerve function.

Some authors advocate the use of corticosteroids when facial paralysis occurs in the presence of OM. The tympanic segment is the most common area of involvement.

Facial nerve decompression is usually not indicated. However, should a complete facial paralysis occur that does not respond to conservative treatment, then decompression of the nerve should be performed. When decompressing the facial nerve, the sheath of the nerve should not be opened, and this could lead to neuritis which could damage the nerve permanently.

Labyrinthitis

Labyrinthitis usually occurs when infections in the middle ear/mastoid enter the labyrinth via the round and/or oval windows. It can also enter the inner ear through fistulae in the semicircular canals. Labyrinthitis presents as either a circumscribed or serous labyrinthitis without total and permanent loss of function or as adiffuse, purulent, or suppurative labyrinthitis with permanent total destruction of the sensory elements within the labyrinth [8, 9].

Serous Labyrinthitis

The symptoms of serous labyrinthitis are vertigo, nausea, and vomiting. Spontaneous nystagmus toward the unaffected ear and some degree of ataxia with past-pointing is present. The cochlear symptoms of serous labyrinthitis are high-frequency sensorineural hearing loss with distortion of hearing and diplacusis.

Treatment of the serous labyrinthitis is the aggressive use of the appropriate antibiotic. If the cause is acute otitis media, then the treatment consists of myringotomy and the appropriate antibiotic. On occasion, corticosteroids may also need to be simultaneously administered. This is needed to halt the sequelae of inflammation which is usually ossification of the inner ear. If the cause is cholesteatoma, then mastoidectomy with removal of diseased bone along with antibiotic coverage should be proven to be sufficient.

Suppurative Labyrinthitis

The exact same etiologic factors and pathways of invasion of the inner ear that result in serous labyrinthitis can also result in suppurative labyrinthitis.

The most feared result of suppurative labyrinthitis is intracranial extension of infection. Antibiotics will need to be given at high doses until it becomes apparent that the infection is coming under control. Any evidence of intracranial spread indicates the need for a labyrinthectomy.

Labyrinthine Fistula

Fistulae are a consequence of bone erosion usually caused by cholesteatoma. Common findings associated with labyrinthine fistulae include granulation tissue and cholesteatoma debris.

Patients with labyrinthine fistulae present with episodic vertigo. The "fistula test" can be easily performed by the bedside. It is easily performed using either pneumatic insufflation or manual tragal pressure to apply positive or negative pressure to the ear. A positive test consists of a quick component of nystagmus toward the affected ear with the application of positive pressure. As the vast majority of fistulae occur in the lateral semicircular canal, the nystagmus is most frequently horizontal. Conversely, when the nystagmus is vertical, then the fistula is likely located in the superior (vertical) semicircular canal. With a large (>2 mm), far-anterior fistula, which exposes simultaneously the ampullae of the horizontal and superior canals, the nystagmus is rotary.

The fistula test can be elicited only when vestibular function is present. Therefore, a negative fistula test does not rule out fistula. It has been found that the fistula test is positive in less than half of all patients with confirmed fistulae. A false-negative fistula test occurs when the fistula is accompanied by a localized loss of function of the ampulla of the involved canal or by a generalized loss of labyrinthine response. A false-positive fistula test can be seen if the stapes is hypermobile. Occasionally, patients with a labyrinthine fistula will experience momentary vertigo when exposed to loud noise. This is known as the Tullio phenomenon.

Computed tomographic scanning of the temporal bone is imaging modality of choice to determine if a labyrinthine fistula is present. Labyrinthine fistulae can be readily identified on CT scan.

Management of a fistula depends on their location, size, and the status of hearing. Even in experienced hands, there is the real risk of damage to the inner ear in patients with labyrinthine fistula [10–13], with rates of total hearing loss between 8% and 56%. Even attempted removal of the matrix overlying a large fistula involving a single semicircular canal can result in profound irreversible sensorineural hearing loss. On the other hand, the matrix can generally be removed from fistulae measuring less than 2 mm in size, i.e., "small" fistulae. Small fistula involving the semicircular canals can be managed more aggressively by removing cholesteatoma matrix from the fistula. The defect (fistula) is repaired with bonepaté.

Acute Petrositis

Inflammation of the petrous portion (the apex of the temporal bone) is referred to as petrositis. It is seen in temporal bones with pneumatic cells in the petrous pyramid [14, 15]. As less than one-third of petrous bones are pneumatized right up to the apex, petrositis is not seen frequently. Natural drainage pathways are absent in petrous bone, with the bottleneck to drainage by bony labyrinth further blocking the base of the pyramid. The petrous bone proximity to the base of skull combined with virulent bacterial organisms makes it a very threatening site of infection because of its proximity to the midbrain.

Petrositis most commonly presents with complaints of otorrhea, deep-boring pain, and diplopia. Air cells extend into the petrous pyramid in two main groups: a posterior group of air cells from the epitympanum and antrum that finds its way around the semicircular canals into the base of the pyramid, frequently extending to the apex, and an anterior group of cells from the tympanum, hypotympanum, and eustachian tube that finds its way around the cochlea into the apex of the pyramid. The posterior group of cells are most commonly present, in about 30% of temporal bones. The diagnosis can be made by the location of the pain. In the case of posterior petrositis, the pain is occipital, parietal, or temporal, and the discharge is from the mastoid. In the case of anterior petrositis, the pain is frontal or behind the eye, and the discharge is from the tympanum.

Gradenigo's syndrome: triad of diplopia (from ipsilateral abducens nerve palsy), retrobulbar pain, and persistent otorrhea are pathognomonic to making a diagnosis of petrositis.

Diplopia is caused by sixth cranial nerve paralysis, since the abducens nerve (the sixth cranial nerve) passes near the petrous apex. Inflammation caused by petrositis causes the nerve to get compressed by surrounding edema when it passes through Dorello's canal beneath the petroclinoid (Gruber's) ligament at the tip of the petrous apex.

Petrositis can present without the full triad of symptoms. Less common symptoms of petrositis are transient facial nerve paresis, mild recurrent vertigo, and low grade and intermittent fever.

Persistent, purulent discharge and pain, despite a well-done mastoidectomy should raise the suspicion of petrositis. It should be confirmed by a high-resolution temporal bone CT scan (Fig. 33.2).

Gallium 67 and technetium 99m bone scans show increased radioactive uptake on the affected side.

Management of acute petrositis consists of intravenous antibiotics and surgical drainage of the suppurative focus in the petrous apex. This is a procedure that requires significant expertise, since it should be carried out without damage to the facial nerve or labyrinth.

Several viable surgical approaches to the petrous apex are available, all of which include a preliminary complete simple mastoidectomy with skeletonization of the semicircular canals. Even if symptoms and imaging studies point toward one particular group of cells as the site of disease, a systematic surgical routine should be employed.

Petrous apicitis drainage route selection depends on three primary factors (1) the location of the infection, (2) the pneu-

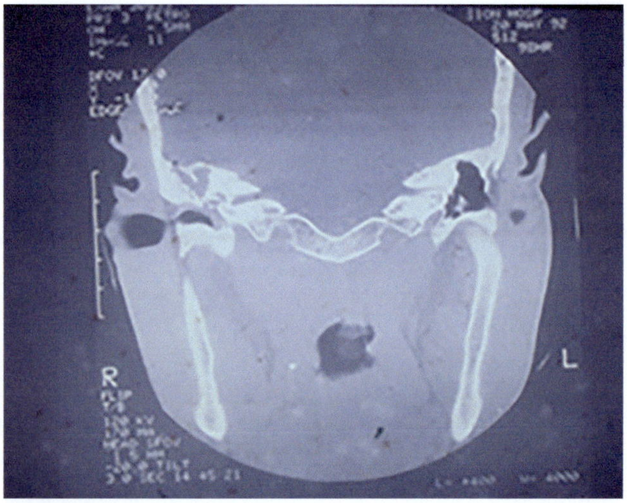

Fig. 33.2 Axial CT scan demonstrating coalescent mastoiditis. The tegmen tympani is eroded

matization of the temporal bone, and (3) the status of the hearing.

The translabyrinthine approach: In the absence of hearing, it provides excellent exposure of the entire posterior portion of the petrous apex.
The transcochlear approach: If more anterior exposure is required, this approach can usually be accomplished without rerouting the facial nerve.
The subtemporal or infracochlear approach: If anterior drainage is necessary in a patient with hearing. The infracochlear approach provides a very narrow window of access as compared with the subtemporal but does provide a sustained route of gravity-dependent drainage.
The retrolabyrinthine or subarcuate route: It can be used in posterior petrous apicitis. In a well-pneumatized bone, both approaches provide adequate access as well as allow both hearing preservation and drainage.

Extratemporal Complications

Subperiosteal Abscess (Figs. 33.3, 33.4, and 33.5)

Subperiosteal abscesses frequently occur as a complication of acute otitis media, and the incidence rate has decreased in the antibiotic era. However, in the past few years, it is on the rise again probably due to the increase in the incidence of antibiotic-resistant bacteria. Direct destruction of cortical bone or hematogenous spread through small vascular channels are the mechanisms that lead to the creation of a subperisosteal abscess [16]. Subperiosteal abscesses are seen in situations of very well pneumatised mastoid bone in comparisoon with ssclerotic mastoids. Macewens' triangle with its thin trabecular bone is the most common site of cortex break down. This pushes the pinna forward and outward, and a fluctuant mass can be palpated behind the ear. On rare occasions, frequent drainage of subperiosteal access can result in a mastoid fistula (Fig. 33.5).

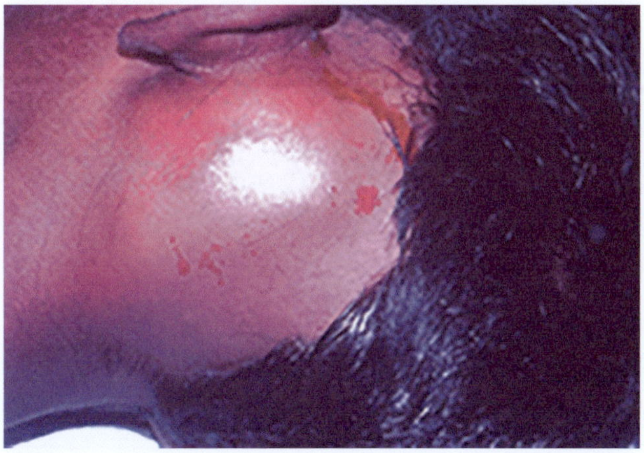

Fig. 33.3 A significant subperiosteal abscess as a result of coalescent mastoiditis

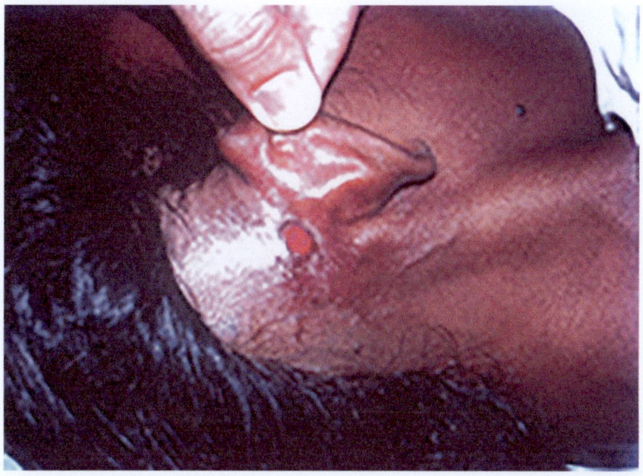

Fig. 33.4 Another patient of a subperiosteal abscess that has ruptured

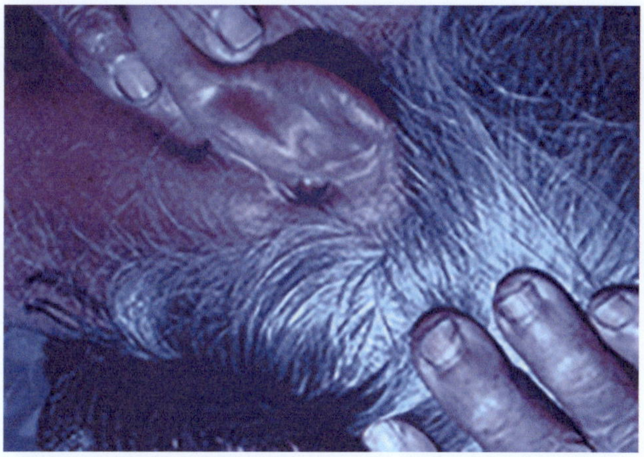

Fig. 33.5 A rare complication of otitis media: a chronic discharging mastoid fistula. This patient was found to have a cholesteatoma

Bezold's Abscess (Fig. 33.6)

Bezold's abscess typically presents deep to sternocleidomastoid muscle, and it reaches there when the pus breaks through the tip of the mastoid process and into the Digastric groove. Bezold's abscess presents with a fluctuant neck mass and otitis media. If left untreated, it can prove fatal as it can involve carotid sheath and the vessels and nerves in it, parapharyngeal space, and mediastinum.

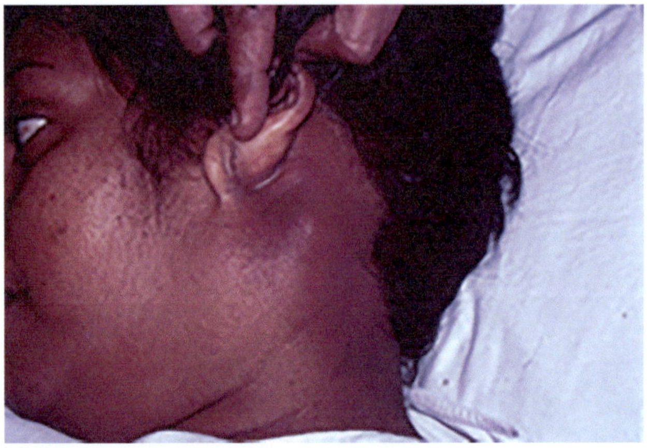

Fig. 33.6 Bezolds abscess in a patient suffering from acute otitis media

Luc's Abscess

Luc's abscess is a collection of purulent secretions under the temporalis muscle. This occurs when the infection tracks along the external auditory canal. Infection can spread to the infratemporal fossa via pneumatized zygomatic arch. The patient will present with induration and tenderness over the temporalis muscle and projection of the upper half of the pinna away from the skull.

High-resolution temporal bone CT scans will demonstrate soft tissue in the middle ear and mastoid cavity, erosion of its cortical bone, and subperiosteal collection of pus.

The treatment modality of choice is surgical drainage with a cortical mastoidectomy along with high dose of appropriate antibiotics. If the patient has acute otitis media, a myringotomy will also need to be performed. Should the patient have a cholesteatoma then a radical, canal wall down mastoidectomy will need to be performed. High-dose antibiotics will also need to be simultaneously administered.

Comment

Though complications of otitis media have declined significantly, they have not disappeared completely. This can be attributed to a variety of reasons such as poor patient compliance with mediation, limited access to health care, patients who are not vaccinated adequately, and lack of recognition of symptoms.

The bacteriology of such infections has not changed. Radiological imaging has played a major role in identifying these conditions and outlining extent of disease. Ideally, the treatment of otitis media involves a multidisciplinary approach, prevent its sequelae, and most definitely avoid complications. This is needed to successfully eliminate disease and its consequences.

References

1. Kangsanarak J, Navacharoen N, Fooanant S, Ruckphaopunt K. Intracranial complications of suppurative otitis media: 13 years' experience. Am J Otol. 1995;16:104–9.
2. Goldstein NA, Casselbrant ML, Bluestone CD, Kurs-Lasky M. Intratemporal complications of acute otitis media in infants and children. Otolaryngol Head Neck Surg. 1998;119:444–54.
3. Nissen AJ, Bui H. Complications of chronic otitis media. Ear Nose Throat J. 1996;75:284–92.
4. Cassano P, Ciprandi G, Passali D. Acute mastoiditis in children. Acta Biomed. 2020;91(1-S):54–9.
5. Wetmore RF. Complications of otitis media. Pediatr Ann. 2000;29:637–46.
6. Pollock RA, Brown LA, Graham MD, House WF, editors. Facial paralysis in otitis media. Disorders of the facial nerve. New York: Raven Press; 1982. p. 221–4.
7. Joseph EM, Sperling NM. Facial nerve paralysis in acute otitis media: cause and management revisited. Otolaryngol Head Neck Surg. 1998;118:694–6.
8. Torok N. Tympanogenic labyrinthitis. Otolaryngol Clin North Am. 1972;5:45–57.
9. Shambaugh GE. Diplacusis: a localizing symptom of disease of the organ of Corti. Arch Otol. 1940;31:160–84.
10. Sheehy JL, Brackmann DE. Cholesteatoma surgery. Management of the labyrinthine fistula—a report of 97 cases. Laryngoscope. 1979;89:78–87.
11. Mandolis S. Complications associated with labyrinthine fistula in surgery for chronic otitis media. Otolaryngol Head Neck Surg. 2000;123:733–7.
12. Vanianinen E. What is the best method of treatment for labyrinthine fistula caused by cholesteatoma? Clin Otolaryngol. 1992;17:258–60.
13. Gacek RR. The surgical management of labyrinthine fistulae in chronic otitis media with cholesteatoma. Ann Otol Rhinol Laryngol. 1974;84(Suppl 10):1–19.
14. Lindsay JR. Suppuration in the petrous pyramid. Ann Otol Rhinol Laryngol. 1938;47:3.
15. Rainer A. Development and construction of pyramidal cells. Arch Ohren Nasen Kehlkupfh. 1938;145:3.
16. Spiegel JH, Lustig LR, Lee KC, et al. Contemporary presentation and management of a spectrum of mastoid abscesses. Laryngoscope. 1998;108:822–8.

34 Intracranial Complications of Otitis Media

Diane Biju, Aishan Patil, Shaila Sidam, Aditi Govil, Kanchan Gupta, Vishal Tyagi, Rosemarie de Souza, and Chris de Souza

Introduction

Complications of suppurative otitis media occur when the natural defense barriers of the middle ear cleft are overcome. Complications should be distinguished from sequelae of otitis media, which occurs as a direct result of the disease process. Sequelae do not present as an acute medical or surgical emergency. Sequelae are limited to the mucoperiosteum lining of the middle ear. An example of a sequelae is tympanosclerosis. Complications occur when the disease process extends beyond the mucoperiosteum of the middle ear. An example is meningitis, sinus thrombosis, etc. These need to be death with swiftly, effectively, and appropriately.

D. Biju
Holy Spirit Hospital, Mumbai, India

A. Patil
Vascular Surgery, Borders General Hospital, Melrose, Scotland, UK

S. Sidam
All India Institute of Medical Sciences, Bhopal, Madhya Pradesh, India

A. Govil
Lilavati Hospital and Research Centre, Mumbai, India

BJ Medical College, Ahmedabad, India

K. Gupta
Lilavati Hospital and Research Centre, Mumbai, India

V. Tyagi
Holy Family Hospital, Holy Spirit Hospital, Mumbai, India

Dept of ENT, VN Desai Hospital, Mumbai, India

R. de Souza
Internal Medicine, BYL Nair Hospital and TNM College, Mumbai, India

C. de Souza (✉)
Faculty SUNY, Brooklyn, NY, USA

LSUHSC, Shreveport, LA, USA

Lilavati Hospital, Holy Family Hospital, Holy Spirit Hospital, Mumbai, India

The incidence of complications of otitis media has declined dramatically with the introduction of antibiotics. There is a clear divide between the era prior to the administration of antibiotics and that after it. The era after it is now known as the era of antibiotics [1–7]. The availability and administration of antibiotics have been responsible for the sharp decline in complications of otitis media. Prior to the antibiotic era, intracranial complications (ICs) occurred in 2.3–4% of cases. With the advent of antibiotics, improved understanding of diseases, advances in radiological imaging, improvements in the standard of living, and improved hygiene, the incidence of complications of otitis media has been greatly reduced to 0.15–0.04%. Mortality decreased from 25% to 8%. These are significant reductions.

From 1928 to 1910 [8–14], 3 years preceding introduction of antibiotics approximately 1 in every 40 days in a General Hospital was spent in treating an intracranial complication of otitis media. Meningitis was found to be the most common health disease followed by sinus thrombosis and brain abscess. Following the introduction of antibiotics, the incidence of complications has declined significantly [15, 16].

Mortality following lateral sinus thrombophlebitis has virtually disappeared, as has the incidence of brain abscess. The factor responsible for this decrease has been attributed to the introduction of antibiotics [17–21]. Purulent meningitis remains the most frequent intracranial complication of otitis media. Though the incidence has substantially reduced, it has not disappeared. In the past, cases of purulent meningitis had 100% mortality. In present times, if this condition is diagnosed early and treated appropriately, the recovery is nearly complete [22–29].

Inappropriate use of antibiotics result in alterations of symptoms and signs leading to patients to present differently as compared to the pre-antibiotic era. Host resistance, early identification of the symptoms, and signs lead to a quick diagnosis, followed by prompt therapy. This can prevent morbidity and mortality. Cardinal symptoms that indicate the

M. V. Goycoolea et al. (eds.), *Textbook of Otitis Media*, https://doi.org/10.1007/978-3-031-40949-3_34

possibility of impending intracranial complications [30–33] are the following:

1. Unrelenting pain. This indicates the possibility of pus under pressure in middle ear cleft leading to likely intracranial complications.
2. Headaches, drowsiness, and visual field defect points toward the diagnosis of brain abscess.
3. Unresolving, persistent, high-grade fever is indicative of the possibility of meningitis or sinus thrombophlebitis being present.

Factors That Influence the Development of Complications [34–38]

The spread of infection from middle ear to adjacent spaces is influenced by a number of factors. These are as follows:

1. The status of the hosts' immunity.
2. Virulence of the infecting organism/organisms.
3. Sensitivity to antibiotics (the adequacy of antibiotic therapy).
4. Integrity of anatomic barriers and the drainage of pneumatic spaces.

The organisms involved in intracranial complications have not changed significantly. *Streptococcus pneumoniae* haemophilus influenzae and moraxella catarrhalis cause most of the acute infections. However, the emergence of antibiotic resistance has changed the way patients now present with complications of otitis media.

Organisms involved in chronic infections are different from those involved in acute infection. Bacteria like pseudomonas aeruginosa are much more commonly isolated in chronic infections.

In immunocompromised persons, microbial infections are more likely to be atypical pathogens.

Anatomical bony barriers such a cellular septae and mucosal folds help retard and delay the spread of middle ear infections into the intracranial cavity. Intracranial extension of acute otitis media (AOM) is seen to occur more frequently when the temporal bone is poorly pneumatized. These anatomical barriers may be eroded by antecedent infections, granulation tissue, and cholesteatoma, thus allowing contamination to spread into the cranial cavity from the middle ear cleft. Trauma to the temporal bone which results in fractures can lead to the creation of passages that allow infection to bypass these natural defenses. Obstruction in drainage in middle ear cleft leads to accumulation of infected secretions which under pressure leads to erosion of natural anatomic barriers, thus opening the way for complications to occur.

Pathway of Spread of Infections in the Middle Ear Cleft [39–46]

Infections can likely spread beyond the middle ear cleft if the infection is uncontrolled or poorly controlled.

Infections can enter the intracranial cavity through one of three mechanisms listed below.

Bone Erosion

Bone erosion is the most frequent cause of spread in cases of otitis media (either acute or chronic OM) in well-pneumatized bones.

In AOM, bone erosion of the cellular septae within the mastoid bone results in coalescent mastoiditis. This causes a buildup of pus which under pressure leads to erosion and thinning of the mastoid bone which then results in either extracranial or intracranial spread of infection. In chronic cases, it is usually caused by cholesteatoma and less commonly caused by chronic osteomyelitis.

Granulations are formed on the bone and function as the last line of defense.

A dehiscent bone barrier and a layer of granulations over neighboring structure are always observed during surgeries for complications of otitis media.

Treatment of such complications implies surgical removal of suppurative, bone eroding focus. Which if not done completely may lead to recurrent or possibly more complications.

Preformed Pathways [47–52]

Direct extension by preformed pathways is seen in acute exacerbations of COM (chronic otitis media) or acute otitis media (AOM).

These pathways are normal anatomic openings in bony walls, such as the oval or round window, internal auditory canal, cochlear aqueduct, or endolymphatic duct and sac. Congenital dehiscence such as a patent suture or a dehiscent floor of the hypotympanum over the jugular bulb can also act as a conduit that serves to spread infections.

A preformed pathway can be created by a fracture, or an inadvertent defect created by previous surgery. A labyrinthine fistula can also serve as a pathway for infection.

The possibility of a preformed pathway should be considered when there is a history of a skull fracture, repeated attack of meningitis, previous surgery on the temporal bone, or previous healed otitis media.

Treatment of complications involves

(a) Treatment of the complication, i.e., treatment of the brain abscess, thrombophlebitis, etc. Intracranial complications involve prioritization of which problem needs to be addressed first.
(b) Surgical closure and sealing of the preformed pathway and.
(c) Surgical drainage of the pus and removal of disease in the temporal bone.

 The complications listed below can either occur singly or can occur simultaneously. The common source from all they occur is located in the ear. Thus, if a patient presents with meningitis and a brain abscess, the physician is obliged to examine the ear carefully to determine if the source is located in the ear. It should be further cautioned that if a patient presents with acute otitis media and meningitis the physician needs to identify the source from where the ear infection was initiated. This could have been from what was thought to be a simple upper respiratory tract infection. Thus the entire ears, nose, and throat along with the other body systems will need to be evaluated equally and carefully.
(d) Aggressive and appropriate antibiotic therapy cannot be overemphasized. Surgical eradication of disease alone will not control the infection that has resulted in the complication.
(e) A multidisciplinary approach. Different specialities need to be involved in order to bring about a successful resolution.

Thrombophlebitis

Infections travel from the lining mucosa of the middle ear and mastoid through intact bone by means of thrombophlebitis. Thrombophlebitis occurs in small venules and then advances to involve larger ones. Brain abscesses have been found to be the consequence of retrograde thrombophlebitis.

A rich network of veins within the temporal bone are in direct communication with extracranial and intracranial veins and cranial diploic veins which can further the spread of the infection. Extracranial and intracranial venous systems are linked via mastoid emissary veins which enter the sigmoid sinus which in turn drain into the superior and inferior petrosal sinuses. This interconnection of dural venous sinuses can lead to sigmoid sinus thrombophlebitis which in turn could result in thrombophlebitis of other venous sinuses.

Complications resulting from acute infections usually start within a week of the infection being initiated. On occasion, it can sometimes occur within a day or two of the infection being contracted. In the presence of thrombophlebitis, surgical findings reveal that the bone of the middle ear cleft is intact. The common complication of coalescent mastoiditis is found to be absent. Thrombophlebitis in addition to causing cerebellar abscesses can also cause meningitis.

Cardinal Symptoms of Impending/Ongoing Intracranial Complications

Complications usually occur within the temporal bone first before shifting outward to cause intracranial complications.

The cardinal symptoms of imminent intracranial complications are as follows:

1. **Persistence of otorrhea**: the pus is foul smelling and thicker and on occasion is blood-stained. Decrease in discharge points toward obstruction in drainage and likely subsequent onset of intracranial complications.
2. **Pain**: patient usually complains of deep boring pain, may be generalized which is usually "the worst headache" they had in their life.
3. **Fever**: High-grade fever that never returns to base line is typical of an intracranial complication.
4. **Altered sensorium, toxemia, photophobia, and irritability**.
5. **Neck stiffness** and generalized malaise are signs indicative of infections advancing toward the cerebrospinal fluid (CSF) space.

The goals of the surgery in the presence of complications of otitis media are as follows:

Correct prioritization of treatment. Commonly both areas, the brain and the ear, will need to be treated simultaneously.

1. The total eradication of disease and the prevention of recurrence of ear disease.
2. Establishment of adequate drainage and ventilation in the temporal bone.
3. Swift, prompt, and adequate treatment of the intracranial complication.

Antibiotics must always accompany surgical intervention as well, for surgery alone will be insufficient in bringing about a cure.

A complete cortical mastoidectomy for the purpose of comprehensive eradication of the disease and the evacuation of pus is carried out. The disease removed is sent for histopathological evaluation, and the pus retrieved is sent for microbiological evaluation.

In AOM, usually high dose of appropriate antibiotics and a cortical mastoidectomy accompanied by myringotomy with ventilation tube insertion tube insertion is sufficient to provide adequate drainage and ventilation.

In chronic disease with cholesteatoma, canal wall down mastoidectomy with a wide meatoplasty is recommended.

Wide meatoplasty provides adequate drainage and allows subsequent examination and cleansing of the mastoid cavity.

Meningitis

Generalized meningitis involves infection and inflammation of the pia arachnoid and the CSF of the subarachnoid space which is continuous for the entire cerebrospinal axis.

In the pre-antibiotic era, meningitis was the most common intracranial complications of otitis media. Recovery from meningitis has improved significantly. Meningitis occurs more commonly in the presence of AOM than COM.

Bacteriology

H. influenzae and *S. pneumoniae* are most commonly identified microorganisms isolated in instances of meningitis caused by otological infections. Streptococcus pneumoniae infections of the meninges are often associated with acute otitis media. Anaerobic organisms are seen in cases of intraventricular rupture of a brain abscess. In cases secondary to otogenic infections, less than 1% of cases demonstrate evidence of polymicrobial infections.

Pathophysiology

Meningitis occurs when infections spread from the ear to the CSF via retrograde thrombophlebitis, bone erosion, and preformed pathways. Infections can also reach the CSF via the labyrinth through the round and oval windows. Infections can also travel through perineural spaces to the internal auditory canal and less frequently via the endolymphatic ducts. Trauma to the ear with resultant fractures, accidental dural tears following otologic ear surgery with resulting CSF leaks can also result in meningitis.

Clinical Presentation

Otogenic causes of meningitis should always be ruled out in all cases of meningitis. Meningitis can occur with or without otorrhoea.

In cases of AOM, the presentation is far swifter. The earliest symptoms are headache, fever, vomiting, photophobia, irritability, and restlessness. Infants may have seizures. As the infection progresses, the headaches increase in intensity, and vomiting becomes more pronounced. Neck stiffness is present and is the signature sign of meningitis.

Brudzinski's sign is the inability to flex the leg without moving the opposite leg (or flexion of the neck resulting in flexion of the hip and knee) and is a sign of meningitis. Kernig's sign, an inability to extend the leg when lying supine with the thigh flexed toward the abdomen, is a specific sign for meningitis.

Management

High-resolution CT scanning is the imaging modality of choice. Bony details are best visualized with CT scanning. High-resolution CT scans of the temporal bone help rule out the presence of congenital car malformations while demonstrating the entire anatomy of the temporal bone.

Magnetic resonance imaging (MRI) (Fig. 34.1) gives better resolution of the brain substance and shows inflammatory changes in the brain and meninges and middle ear fluid. MRI of the brain and surrounding structures and CT scanning of the temporal bone complement each other and are very valuable when assessing a patient who has meningitis.

Lumbar puncture is imperative to identify the causative organism and the source of infection. Cloudy CSF, elevated white blood cell count, low glucose, and high protein point toward meningitis.

Fundoscopic of the examination of the eye has been found to show indistinct disk margins and choking of vessels in meningitis.

Gram-staining of the fluid, confirmation by culture, and sensitivity testing help in the selection of a suitable appropriate antimicrobial drug. A swab should be taken from the ear as well.

Treatment

Antimicrobial drugs are at the core of treatment of meningitis. Meningitis resulting from acute otitis media is usually directed at *H. influenzae* type B with second- or third-generation cephalosporins which cross the blood–brain barrier.

Bactericidal drugs should be preferred over bacteriostatic drugs.

Large amounts of fragments of the inflammatory processes are released that have severe neurologic and auditory sequelae because of rapid bacteriolysis. Glucocorticoids like dexamethasone if given concurrently or before antibiotics have shown to decrease the sequelae of this catastrophic event.

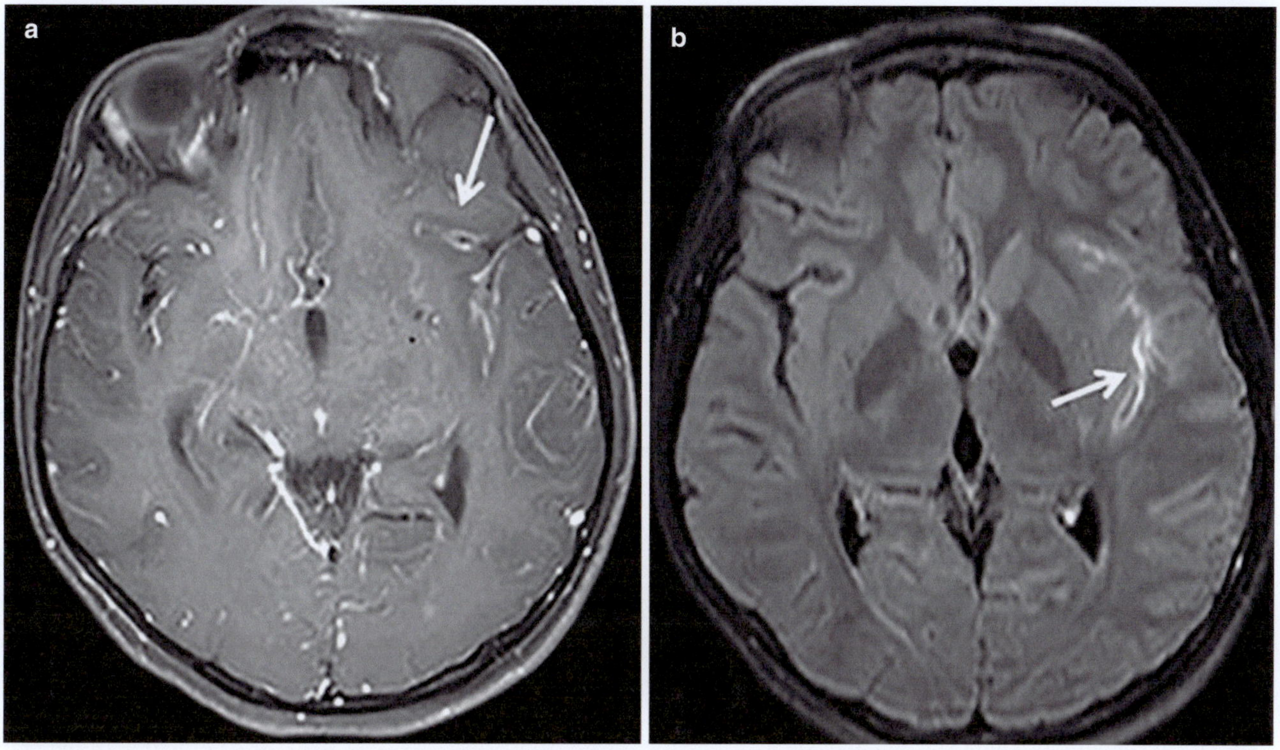

Fig. 34.1 MRI scan of a patient suffering from meningitis as a complication of otits media. (**a**) Axial postcontrast T1 and (**b**) postcontrast FLAIR shows leptomeningeal enhancement in left sylvian fissure (arrow)

These measures have been found to be useful only for meningitis caused by acute otitis media and only if there are no other intracranial complications presents.

Role of Surgery

For the patient of acute otitis media with an intact tympanic membrane who presents with no clinical or radiological evidence of mastoiditis, myringotomy with evacuation of the fluid from the middle ear is sufficient enough treatment for otogenic meningitis.

In situations where mastoiditis is clinically and radiologically evident, cortical mastoidectomy with middle ear exploration needs to be performed. Should the patient present with a history of trauma involving the head and temporal bone accompanied by rapid onset of meningitis, the surgeon should look for a likely fracture in the temporal bone. Once that site has been correctly identified, that communication which was responsible for the causation of meningitis must be repaired to prevent recurrence of meningitis. Radiological evidence in the form of CT scans of the temporal bones will help in accurately demonstrating the site of the fracture. This area should be repaired, and the passage should be sealed off.

Should a cholesteatoma be present then radical mastoidectomy with wide meatoplasty is the surgical modality of choice.

Brain Abscess

A brain abscess is a focal suppurative process within the brain parenchyma and is surrounded by a region of encephalitis.

Brain abscesses secondary to otitis media are seen mostly in children and in the fourth decade [53–60]. The male-to-female ratio has been approximately 3 to 1.

Most of the brain abscesses are associated with infections resulting from cholesteatomas.

Otogenic brain abscesses are more likely to be located in the cerebrum (predominantly in the temporal lobe) than in the cerebellum. But the majority of cerebellar abscesses are associated with middle ear infections, which are more likely to be fatal.

The most important factor in the treatment of brain abscesses depends on swift control of the infection.

Factors implicated in the causes of brain abscesses

1. The immune status of the patient influences the microbiology of brain abscess. Multiple organisms have been reported in brain abscesses. Gram-positive organisms like *Streptococcus* and *staphylococcus* and gram-negative like *Escherichia coli* and *Proteus Miabilis*, *Klebsiella*, and *Pseudomonas* species are typically isolated from brain abscesses. *H. influenzae* is rarely found in otogenic brain abscesses.

2. Brain abscesses are likely to occur when the following conditions are present.
   (a) Contiguous spread of disease to surrounding structures.
   (b) Hematogenous spread from a distant focus like chronic pyogenic lung disease.
   (c) Trauma to the head or cranial/surgery on the ear.

Venous thrombophlebitis rather than direct extension of disease from the ear to the brain is the common cause of otogenic brain abscesses.

Surgical causes, i.e., mastoidectomy when an open mastoid cavity has been created but residual disease persists, can lead to brain abscess.

Pathophysiology

1. Osteitis or granulation tissue causes retrograde thrombophlebitis of dural venous sinuses that terminate in the white matter of the brain, causing encephalitis.
2. This progresses to necrosis and liquefaction of brain tissue (focal suppuration) with surrounding edema.
3. After approximately 2 weeks, an abscess capsule surrounded by granulation tissue forms. It has been observed that encapsulation is more well defined on the cortical side as compared with the ventricular side. This perhaps explains the propensity of abscesses to rupture medially into the ventricular system rather than into the subarachnoid space.

Clinical Presentation

Symptoms usually present for approximately 2 weeks before the brain abscess is fully formed. Brain abscess formation is indicated by the presence of (a) headache, (b) high-grade fever, and (c) focal neurologic deficits. Signs of meningitis are also usually present.

The patient is appears very "toxic" and drowsy and often complains of deep bony pain in the ear. Foul smelling, creamy otorrhea indicates a fulminant, destructive process. Location of the abscess can be predicted by the focal deficits, cerebellar abscesses present with dizziness, ataxia, nystagmus, and vomiting. Seizures are seen in temporal lobe lesions. Papilledema is a late sign seen in stage 3 of abscess formation.

Imaging

In computed tomographic scanning, brain abscess appears a hypodense area surrounded by an area of edema "ring sign." Serial scans can help in assessing the response of the treatment.

MRI (Figs. 34.2, 34.3, and 34.4) is more useful in checking the brain parenchyma and detecting the progress of abscess though it does not help in assessing the temporal bone for which a separate CT scan of the temporal bones may be needed.

Sequalae of Otogenic Brain Abscess

The brain abscess could rupture into the ventricle resulting in death. Brain abscesses can also cause herniation of the brain resulting in death. Brain asceses also can result in seizures, permanent neurologic deficits, and vegetative state.

Management

Management consists of antibiotic therapy and surgical management of the source of infection.

High-dose antimicrobial medication has to be started immediately. The decision to eradicate the infective focus from the ear will need to be performed at the earliest. Some prefer to operate at the earliest citing that once the focus of infection is eradicated, the infection in the brain will respond quickly to the antibiotics administered.

Neurosurgical intervention is required if the abscess is 2.5 cm or bigger.

The decision to excise or drain a brain abscess is controversial as improved radiological imaging and more effective antibiotics have radically improved the outcomes of such complications.

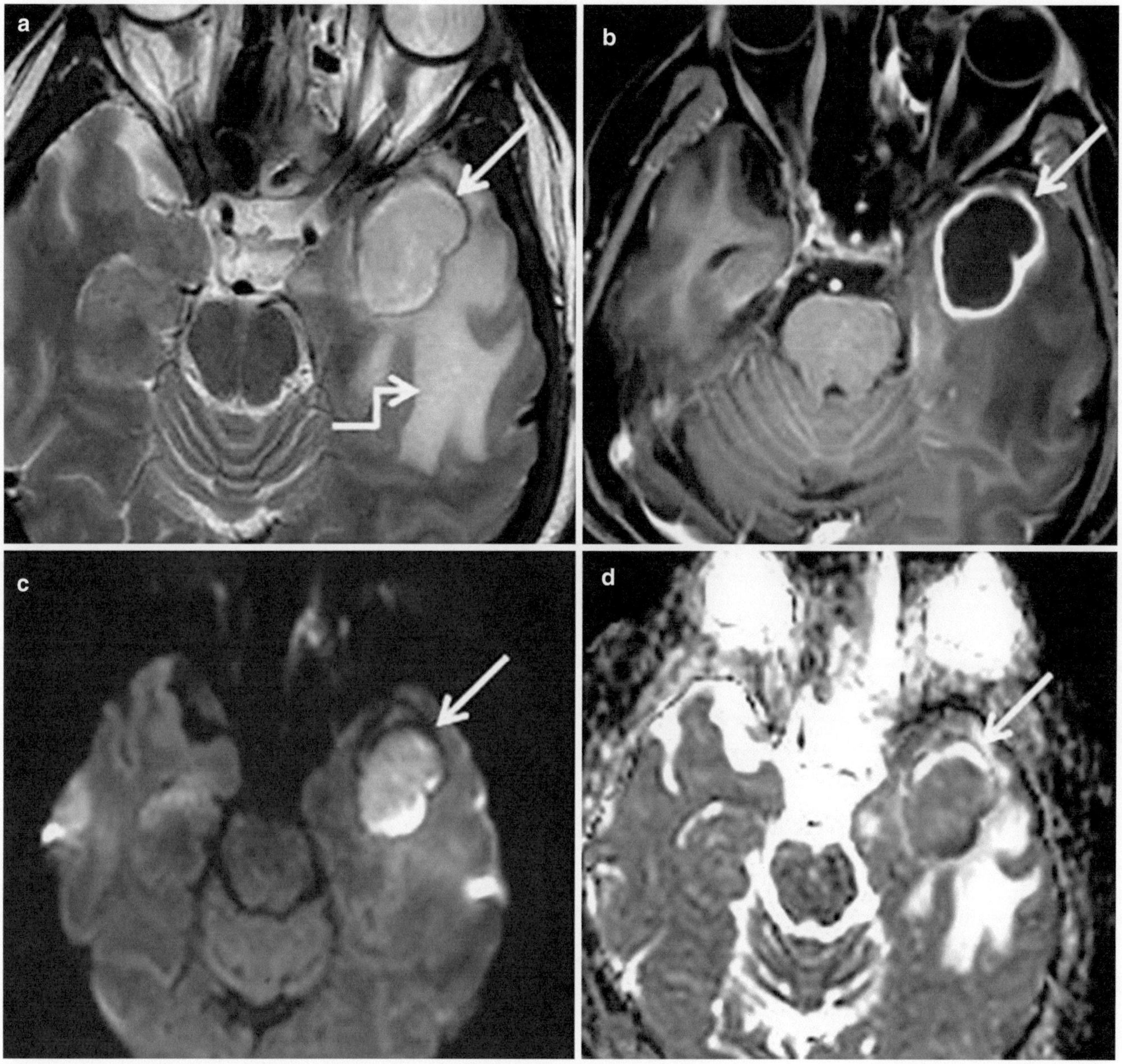

Fig. 34.2 (**a**) Axial T2-weighted image shows well-defined hyperintense lesion (arrow) with hypointense wall and perilesional edema (stepped arrow) in left temporal lobe, (**b**) axial T1W postcontrast image shows rim enhancement (arrow), (**c**) restriction on diffusion-weighted image (arrow), and (**d**) signal drop on ADC (arrow)

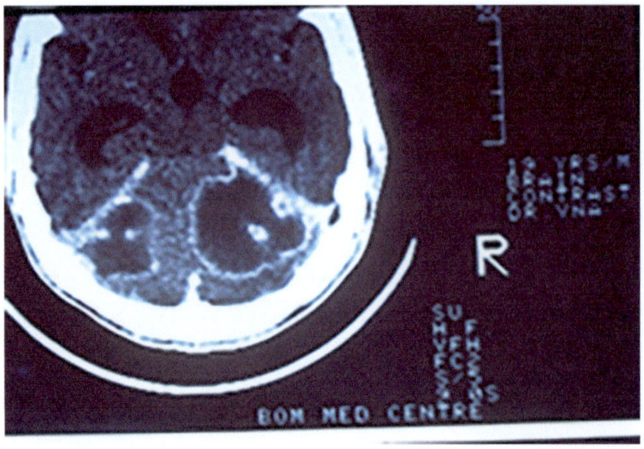

Fig. 34.3 Bilateral brain abscess of otogenic origin

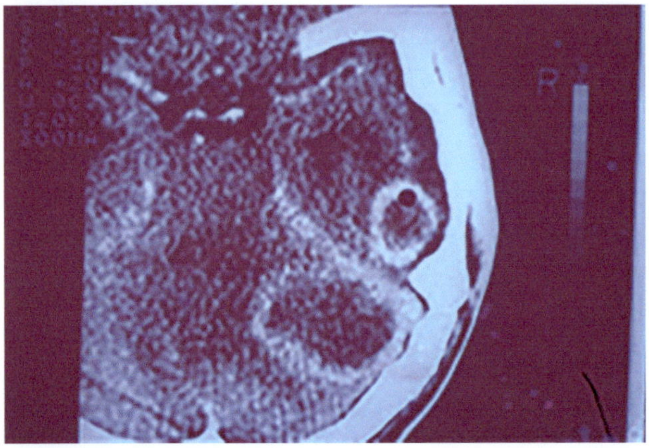

Fig. 34.4 Brain abscess of otogenic origin involving the temporal lobe and the cerebellum

Otogenic Suppurative Thrombophlebitis

The dural venous sinuses are blood vessels located between the endosteal and meningeal layers of dura mater that covers the brain. These venous sinuses receive blood from the cerebral veins and cerebrospinal fluid (CSF) from the subarachnoid space via arachnoid granulations. They drain into the internal jugular vein.

Suppurative thrombophlebitis of the sigmoid sinus is associated with both with acute and chronic otitis media [61–69].

Pathophysiology

Thrombosis occurs after the infection has spread to the intima of the vein. This results in edema resulting in sluggish blood flow in the lumen of the sinus resulting in a thrombus. This infected thrombus increases in size occluding the lumen of the vein. This can embolize downstream causing seeding of infection which can then result in generalized septicaemia and other problems like stroke.

Suppurative thrombus can propagate intracranially or into the jugular vein and onto the right atrium of the heart. Intracranial extension results in brain abscess and thrombophlebitis of other vessels in the cranial cavity. Intracardiac spread results in widespread spreading of infection and fulminant septicemia [70–73].

Bacteriology

Cultures have revealed the presence of polymicrobial infections. The B-hemolytic streptococcus, *Bacteroides* and *Streptococcus* species as well as gram-negative rods are seen. *Pseudomonas* and *Proteus* species have also been isolated.

Clinical Presentation

The patient will be seriously ill and restless and will complain of otalgia. Otalgia is described as a deep, boring pain, which usually heralds a worsening neurologic status. Otorrhea is foul smelling and usually blood-stained.

High-grade fever is a "picket fence" appearance or may be high grade without returning to baseline. Neck stiffness and papilledema are present. If beta-hemolytic streptococci are responsible for the infection, the patient may present with steadily worsening anemia, manifesting in pallor. Proptosis, ptosis, chemosis, and ophthalmoplegia are signs of the thrombus spreading to the cavernous sinus. Griesinger's sign is usually present. Greisinger's sign consists of tenderness, and edema over the mastoid is pathognomonic for suppurative thrombophlebitis of the sigmoid sinus and its cause is thrombosis of the mastoid emissary veins. Extension of the thrombus into the internal jugular vein causes it to become hard, cord-like, and very tender to palpation and results in a stiff neck. The cervical lymph nodes along the internal jugular vein are enlarged and tender. Otitic hydrocephalus is seen in involvement of the torcular and sagittal sinuses.

Imaging

MRI (Figs. 34.5, 34.6, 34.7, and 34.8) is the imaging tool of choice. MRI scans demonstrate venous sinus obstruction, and reversal of blood flow is seen. On gadolinium-enhanced MRI, the delta sign is observed. The thrombus is seen as a soft tissue signal with a bright appearance of the dural walls. It can help in differentiating an early and a late thrombus. The early thrombus is rich in deoxyhemoglobin; hence on the T1 weighted image, it has intermediate density and a low

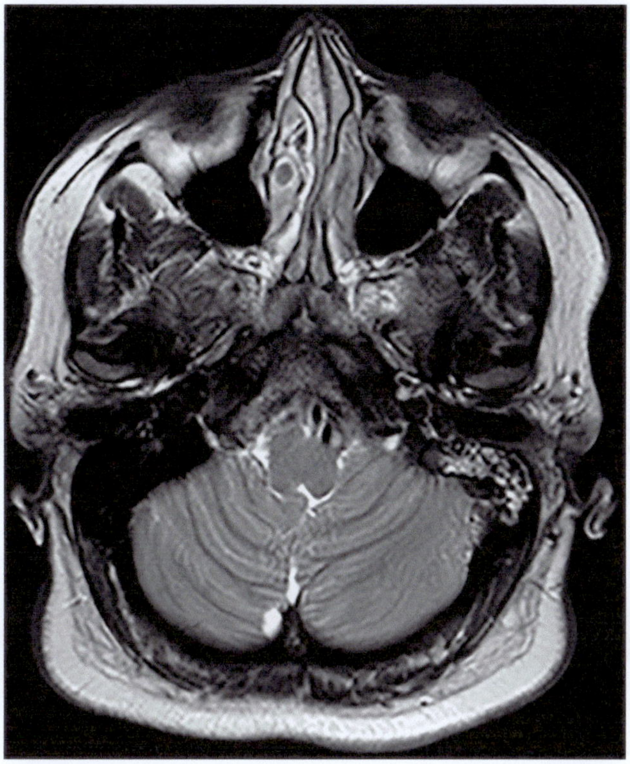

Fig. 34.5 MRI scan showing mastoiditis

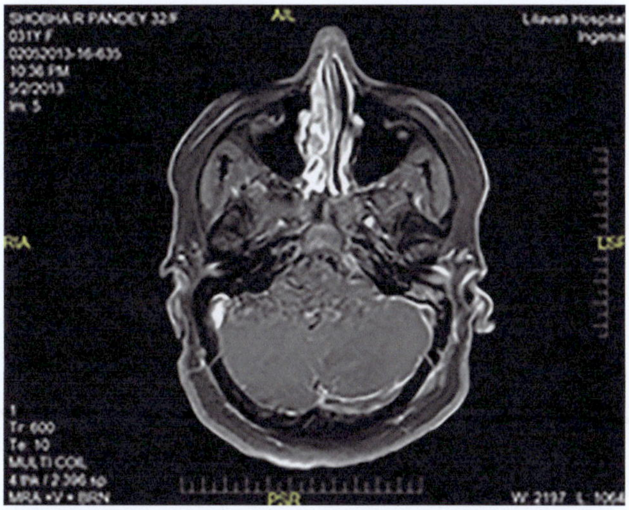

Fig. 34.6 MRI scan showing thrombus on the left side in the transverse sinus

intensity on the T2 image. In a mature thrombus, the clot appears hyperintense on both T1 and T2 images because of the formation of methemoglobin.

CT scans shows the "delta sign" clot surrounded by a high-intensity rim of contrast-enhanced dura.

Cerebral angiography is not indicated as it has a potential to dislodge the thrombus.

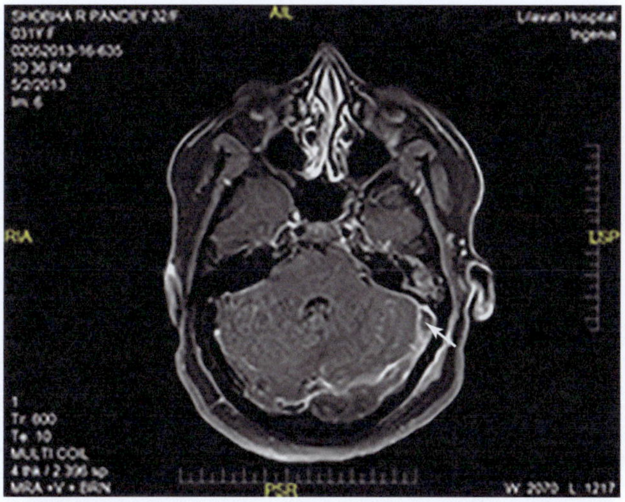

Fig. 34.7 MRI scan demonstrating sigmoid thrombophlebitis with typical "delta" sign

- **Queckenstedt's (or the Tobey–Ayer)** test is used to detect lateral venous sinus thrombosis: a spinal needle is placed in subarachnoid space and attached to a manometer, and the resting CSF pressure is measured. Pressure is applied to the IJV with fingers sequentially and then both at once. The test is considered positive if pressure fails to rise after compression of internal jugular vein (IJV) on the side of the diseased ear and fails to fall when the vein is released with a prompt contralateral response.

A false positive is seen mostly on the left side in cases where one sigmoid sinusis smaller than the other.

False-negative test is observed in cases in which there are well-developed collaterals around the sigmoid sinus through the mastoid emissary vein and the petrosal sinus.

Contraindications to lumbar puncture are high intracranial pressures are also contraindications for the performance of Queckenstedt's test.

With the advent of greatly improved radiological imaging techniques, Queckensted's test is now infrequently performed.

Blood cultures provide important information for the management of the sigmoid sinus thrombophlebitis. The microorganisms can be correctly identified, and the appropriate treatment can be initiated to deal with the infection.

Treatment

Prior to the antibiotic era, surgery on the ear was the focal point of treatment. A mastoidectomy with unroofing of the sigmoid sinus was carried out, and the perisinus abscess, if present, was drained. If the sinus demonstrated a thrombus, it would be removed. Scanty bleeding around the venous

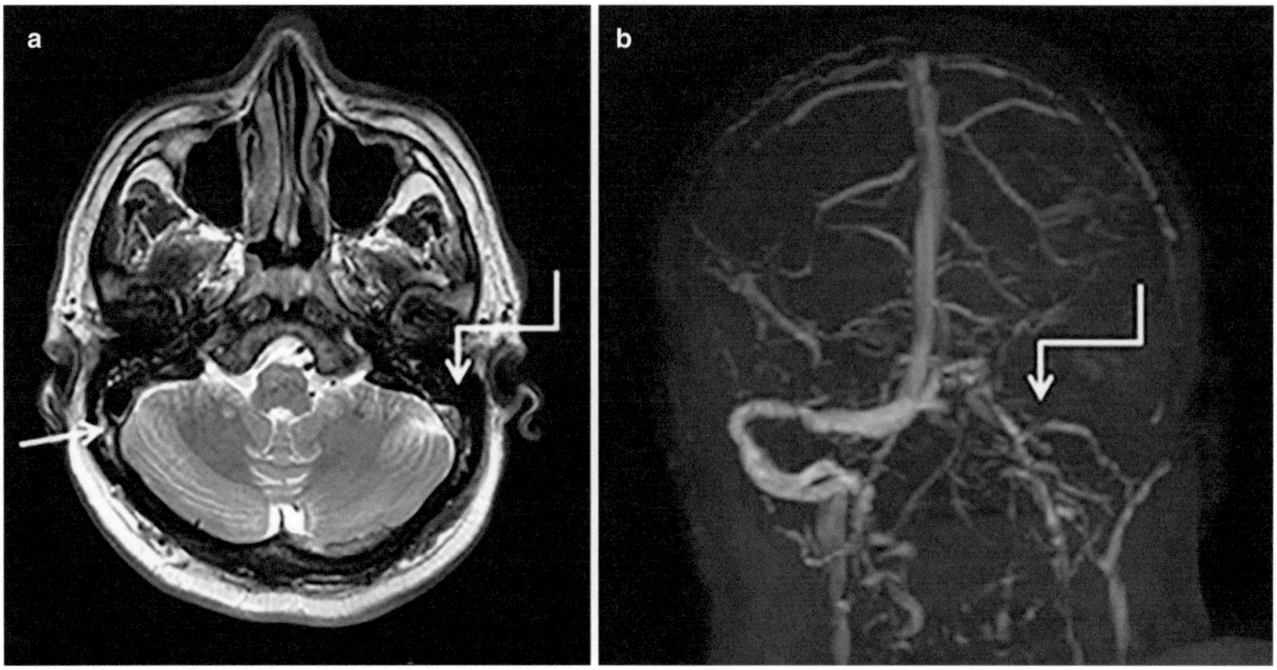

Fig. 34.8 (**a**) Axial T2W image shows the absence of flow void in left transverse sinus (stepped arrow) as compared to normal flow void on right side (arrow); (**b**) TOF venogram shows no flow-related enhancement in left transverse and sigmoid sinuses (stepped arrow)

sinus indicated the presence of an intraluminal clot. In such situations, the sinus should be opened very carefully to avoid inadvertent tearing of the medial dural wall. A tear in the medial dural wall would result in a CSF leak. The entire thrombus should be removed. In advanced thrombus formation, some authors state that the Internal Jugular Vein should be ligated to prevent passage of the thrombus into the heart.

In recent times, such extensive disease is rarely seen. High doses of appropriate antibiotics combined with complete evacuation of the disease from the middle ear and the mastoid is carried out. This should be adequate to halt the progress of disease and prevent worsening of the patient's condition. Drainage of the perisinus abscess and removal of the thrombus are included in the mastoidectomy procedure. Ligation of the internal jugular vein is rarely performed. It is carried out only in situations where the disease is advancing toward the heart in spite of the adequate and appropriate treatment. Anticoagulants are no longer recommended as they lead to increased chances of venous infarction.

Otitic Hydrocephalus

Otitic hydrocephalus or benign raised intracranial tension was first described by Quincke in 1897. It is a syndrome associated with otitis media characterized by intracranial pressure with normal CSF findings. It recovers spontaneously and is frequently associated with sigmoid sinus thrombophlebitis.

Pathophysiology

The precise mechanism underlying the development of otitic hydrocephalus is not known [74–77].

1. Sahs and Joynt [78] postulated that the hydrocephalus is secondary to brain edema as brain biopsies revealed interstitial edema.
2. Weed and Flexner [79] postulated disruption in venous circulation as a cause, since changes in CSF pressure are directly related to intracranial venous pressure.

Clinical Presentation

Patient presents with headache, drowsiness, vomiting, blurring of vision, and diplopia. Acute or chronic otitis media is usually present at the onset of otitic hydrocephalus.

Ophthalmic evaluation reveals the presence of papilledema and sixth cranial nerve palsy. If left untreated, optic atrophy can eventually occur.

Elevated CSF pressures with normal CSF biochemistry are the classic findings of otitic hydrocephalus.

Management

Ear pathology is eradicated, and the increased CSF pressure is assessed and addressed so that the hydrocephalus is reduced.

Drainage of cerebrospinal fluid with shunts have been recommended. Optic sheath decompression can be considered to prevent optic atrophy [80–83]. Medical therapy consists of corticosteroids, mannitol, diuretics, and acetazolamide which are also administered simultaneously.

Subdural Empyema

Collection of pus in the space between the dura mater and the arachnoid membrane is termed subdural empyema [81, 82].

Pathophysiology

The subdural spaces are anatomically confined spaces and can quickly develop into fatal mass lesion. It is a potential space than an actual one. It is divided into compartments by foramen magnum, tentorium cerebelli, base of the brain, and the falx cerebri.

Clinical Presentation

Sudden-onset severe headache is typical of subdural empyema. It is accompanied by fever and vomiting.

The rapid deterioration of the patient's conditions points to the presence of a subdural empyema.

Magnetic resonance imaging is the imaging modality of choice.

It can easily differentiate between epidural and subdural infection.

Multiple, discrete, and loculated subdural collections are seen. Magnetic resonance imaging is advantageous because of the absence of bone artifact, heightened contrast between bone, CSF, and brain parenchyma, as well as because of its multiplanar imaging capability.

Magnetic resonance imaging also allows differentiation of sterile, bloody, and infected collections.

Treatment

Immediate drainage of the abscess with complete removal of the focus of infection within the ear along with simultaneous administration of high-dose intravenous antimicrobial medication forms the core treatment modality.

Lumbar puncture is contraindicated as it may trigger herniation of the cerebellar tonsils.

Epidural (Extradural) Abscess

The epidural (extradural) space is the potential space between the dura mater and the bone of the intracranial cavity. Granulation tissue is seen in direct continuity with the suppurative process. Large accumulations of pus are rare. An epidural abscess usually precedes other intracranial complications, especially sinus thrombophlebitis and brain abscess. Sinus thrombophlebitis is the most complication coexisting with an epidural abscess.

Pathogenesis

Bone reabsorption in coalescent mastoiditis leads to bone giving way, especially in areas of sigmoid sinus, resulting in a pocket of granulation tissue or pus which infects the sigmoid sinus. It is mostly associated with chronic suppurative otitis media without cholesteatoma.

Chronic suppurative otitis media without cholesteatoma is usually associated with granulation tissue that invades the perisinus air cells.

Asymptomatic (silent) extradural granulation tissue if left untreated has the potential to progress into far more serious complications.

MRI is the best radiological imaging modality of choice for the diagnosis of epidural abscesses. Frequently, these epidural abscesses are found as incidental findings during surgery as they are rarely symptomatic unless very large.

Management

The presence of granulation tissue penetrating the bone along the sigmoid sinus indicates the presence of an epidural abscess. The surrounding bone should be opened, and the granulations should be removed and the abscess should be drained. Care should be taken that dura is not punctured as it can lead to CSF leak which can have catastrophic consequences.

How Common Are Intracranial Complications in Recent Times?

Complications have most certainly declined when looking at medical literature in recent times. However, reports advise against complacency. A report by Bales et al. [83] report complications occurring in developed nations where there is access to healthcare. Even in the antibiotic era, intracranial complications of otitis media still occur in developing nations. The reasons cited [84] for these problems are as follows:

1. Many patients do not seek medical care and delay treatment.

2. Poor access to healthcare.
3. Poor compliance with treatment. Patients either take inadequate treatment or stop treatment without the consultation of a medical person.
4. Healthcare centers are often so rudimentary that modern radiological imaging modalities are not available. This in turn impacts diagnosis and eradication of disease. This in turn impairs the detection of complications should they be within the temporal bone or on within the intracranial cavity.
5. Unlike developed nations where healthcare is covered by insurance, developing nations quite often do not have facilities available that are covered by healthcare insurance.
6. A large amount of the population has not received the pneumococcal vaccine. The protection offered by this vaccine is against the pneumococcal serotypes and Hemophilus serotypes. Both these bacteria are frequently implicated in complications caused by otitis media.

In today's times, are complications associated more frequently with acute otitis media or chronic otitis media? Recent literature [85, 86] indicates that chronic otitis media associated with cholesteatoma is the source. Literature cites the indolent manner in which chronic otitis media presents is the reason why patients often defer seeking treatment. This results in a complication which often takes a long time to diagnose causing a delay in treatment [87].

What are the frequently encountered complications in the antibiotic era in developed nations? The literature [88] cites meningitis as the commonest followed by brain abscess. These are the common intracranial complications. Temporal bone complications are subperiosteal abscess. Both intracranial complications and temporal bone complications are frequently associated with cholesteatoma. Though cholesteatoma is associated with a high incidence of complications, acute otitis media [89] when not diagnosed and treated in a timely and appropriate manner can result in an intracranial complications even in a developed nation.

One report [90] puts it very succinctly by stating the following,

(a) Complications of otitis media are still present even in the antibiotic era and in the age of awareness and information.
(b) Male children and adults are frequently affected. Chronic otitis media is responsible for most of the complications, approximately 80% of all intracranial complications.
(c) Acute otitis media causes complications below the age of 15 years. Indolent pediatric chronic otitis media when not correctly diagnosed results in complications.
(d) The most frequently encountered complications were in the order of frequency brain abscess with meningitis (78%), lateral sigmoid sinus thrombosis (13%), empyema (8%), and otitic hydrocephalus 1%.
(e) The organisms detected in these complications are *Proteus mirabilis*, *Pseudomonas aeruginosa*, *Staphylococcus aureus*, *Streptococcus pneumoniae*, and *Streptococcus pyogenes*. These organisms are commonly cited in nearly all literature as being responsible for infections associated with otitis media.

References

1. Cawthorne T. The surgery of the temporal bone. Laryngol Otol. 1953;67:377.
2. Beck J. In: Denker A, Kahler O, editors. Handbuch der Hals-Nassen-Ohr-enheilkunde. Berlin: Springer; 1927.
3. Morand SF. Opuscules de chirurgie. Paris; 1768.
4. Lebert. Ueber Entzundung der Hirn-Sinus. Virchows Arch. 1856;9:381.
5. MacEwen W. Pyogenic infective diseases of the brain and spinal cord. Glasgow: Maclehose; 1893.
6. Korner O. Die Otitischen Erkrankungen des Hirns, der Himhaute und der Blutleiter. Wiesbaden; 1908.
7. Eagleton WP. Brain abscess: its surgical pathology and operative technic. New York: Macmillan; 1922.
8. Shambaugh GE Jr. The surgical treatment of meningitis of otitic and nasal origin. JAMA. 1937;108:696.
9. Lebert. Ueber Gehirnabscesse. Virchows Arch. 1856;10:78.
10. Zaufal E. Operation der Sinusthrombose und Versuche mit Cocain am Gehororgane. Prag Med Wochenschr. 1884;9:474.
11. Lane WA. Middle ear suppurations and their complications. BMJ. 1889;1:998.
12. Ballance CA. Pyemic thrombosis of the lateral sinus. Lancet. 1890;1:1057.
13. Jansen A. Referat die Operations methoden bei den verschiedenen otitischen Gehirnkomplikationen. Verhandl Deutsch Otol Gesellsch. 1895;4:96.
14. Gradenigo G. Sulla leptomeningite circoscritta e sulla paralisi dell'adducente di origine otitica. Gior Accad Med Torino. 1904;10:59.
15. Kopetsky SJ, Almour R. Suppuration of the petrous pyramid. Ann Otol Rhinol Laryngol. 1931;39:996.
16. Eagleton WP. Unlocking the petrous pyramid for localized bulbar meningitis secondary to suppuration of the petrous apex. Arch Otol. 1931;13:386.
17. Courville CB. Intracranial complications of otitis media and mastoiditis in the antibiotic era. Laryngoscope. 1955;63:31.
18. Rosenwasser H, Adelman N. Otitic complications. Arch Otol. 1957;65:225.
19. Lund WS. A review of 50 cases of intracranial complications from otogenic infection between 1961 and 1977. Clin Otolaryngol. 1978;3:495–501.
20. Bluestone CD, Stephenson JS, Martin LM. Ten-year review of otitis media pathogens. Pediatr Infect Dis J. 1992;11(Suppl 8):S7–11.
21. Feinmesser R, Wiesel YM, Argaman M, Gay I. Otitis externa bacteriological survey. ORL J Otorhinolaryngol Relat Spec. 1982;44:121–5.
22. Neely G. Complications of suppurative otitis media, parts 1 and 2. Washington, DC: American Academy of Otolaryngology Head and Neck Surgery; 1978.
23. Schuknecht HF, Reisser C. The morphologic basis for perilymphatic gushers and oozers. Adv Otorhinolaryngol. 1988;39:1–12.

24. Jackler RK, Hwang PH. Enlargement of the cochlear aqueduct fact or fiction? Otolaryngol Head Neck Surg. 1993;109:14–25.
25. Glasscock ME 3rd. The stapes gusher. Arch Otolaryngol. 1973;98:82–91.
26. Hughes GB, Sismanis A, House JW. Is there consensus in perilymph fistula management? Otolaryngol Head Neck Surg. 1990;102:111–7.
27. Glasscock ME 3rd, McKennan KX, Levine SC. Persistent traumatic perilymph fistulas. Laryngoscope. 1987;97(7 Pt 1):860–4.
28. House H. Acute otitis media. A comparative study of the results obtained before and after the introduction of the sulfonamide compounds. Arch Otolaryngol Head Neck Surg. 1946;43:371–5.
29. McLay K. Otogenic meningitis. J Laryngol Otol. 1954;68:140–6.
30. Gower D, McGuirt WF. Intracranial complications of acute and chronic infectious ear disease: a problem still with us. Laryngoscope. 1983;93:1028–33.
31. Habib RG, Girgis NI, Abu el Ella AH, et al. The treatment and outcome of intracranial infections of otogenic origin. J Trop Med Hyg. 1988;91:83–6.
32. Samuel J, Fernandes CM, Steinberg JL. Intracranial otogenic complications: a persisting problem. Laryngoscope. 1986;96:272–8.
33. Roos K, Scheld WM. Acute bacterial meningitis in children and adults. In: Scheld W, editor. Infections of the central nervous system. New York: Raven Press; 1991. p. 335–409.
34. Scheld W. Bacterial meningitis and brain abscess. In: Isselbacher K, et al., editors. Harrison's principles of internal medicine. 13th ed. New York: McGraw-Hill; 1994. p. 2296–309.
35. Nager GT. Mastoid and paranasal sinus infections and their relation to the central nervous system. Clin Neurosurg. 1966;14:288–313.
36. Kaplan R. Neurological complications of infections of the head and neck. Otolaryngol Clin N Am. 1976;9:729–49.
37. Proctor CA. Intracranial complications of otitic origin. Laryngoscope. 1966;76:288–308.
38. Cawthorne T. Otogenic meningitis. J Laryngol Otol. 1939;54:444–70.
39. Neely G. Intratemporal and intracranial complications of otitis media. In: Bailey B, editor. Otolaryngology-head and neck surgery. Philadelphia: Lippincott; 1993.
40. Jacobs R. A prospective randomised comparison of cefotaxime vs ampicillin and chloramphenicol for bacterial meningitis in children. J Pediatr. 1985;107:129–35.
41. Quagliarello V, Scheld W. Bacterial meningitis: pathogenesis. Pathophysiology and progress. N Engl J Med. 1992;327:80–72.
42. Weiner GM, Williams B. Prevention of intracranial problems in ear and sinus surgery: a possible role for cefotaxime. J Laryngol Otol. 1993;107:1005–7.
43. Lebell M. Dexamethasone therapy for bacterial meningitis: results of 2 double blind placebo controlled trials. N Engl J Med. 1988;319:964–6.
44. Odio CM. The beneficial effects of early dexamethasone administration in infants and children with bacterial meningitis. N Engl J Med. 1991;324:1525–31.
45. de Souza CE, Goycoolea M. Complications of otitis media in children. In: de Souza CE, Stankiewicz J, Pellitteri PK, editors. Pediatric otorhinolaryngology head and neck surgery. San Diego, London: Singular. 1999; p. 115–35.
46. Yen P, Chan S, Huang T. Brain abscess with special reference to otolaryngologic sources of infection. Otolaryngol Head Neck Surg. 1995;113:5–22.
47. Meyers E, Ballantine H. The management of otogenic brain abscess. Laryngoscope. 1965;75:273–88.
48. Sennaroglu L, Sozeri B. Otogenic brain abscess: review of 41 cases. Otolaryngol Head Neck Surg. 2000;123:751–5.
49. Stuart E, O'Brien F, McNally W. Some observations on brain abscesses. Arch Otolaryngol Head Neck Surg. 1955;104:542–3.
50. Murthy PS, Sukumar R, Hazarika P, et al. Otogenic brain abscess in childhood. Int J Pediatr Otorhinolaryngol. 1991;22(1):9–17.
51. Kornblut AD. Cerebral abscess—a recurrent otologic problem. Laryngoscope. 1972;82:1541–56.
52. Quijano M, Schuknecht HF, Otte J. Temporal bone pathology associated with intracranial abscess. ORL J Otorhinolaryngol Relat Spec. 1988;50:2–31.
53. Ingham H, Selkon J, Roxy C. Bacteriological study of brain abscesses: chemotherapeutic roles of metronidazole. BMJ. 1977;2:991–3.
54. Brook I. Bacteriology of intracranial abscesses in children. J Neurosurg. 1981;54:484–8.
55. Nissen A. Intracranial complications of otogenic disease. Am J Otol. 1980;2:164–7.
56. Keet PC. Cranial intradural abscess management of 641 patients during the 35 years from 1952 to 1986. Br J Neurosurg. 1990;4:273–8.
57. Maniglia AJ, VanBuren JM, Bruce WB, et al. Intracranial abscesses secondary to ear and paranasal sinuses infections. Otolaryngol Head Neck Surg. 1980;88:670–80.
58. Ward PH, Setliff RC, Long W. Otogenic brain abscess. Trans Am Acad Ophthalmol Otolaryngol. 1969;73:107–14.
59. Buchheit WA, Ronis ML, Liebman E. Brain abscesses complicating head and neck infections. Trans Am Acad Ophthalmol Otolaryngol. 1970;74:548–54.
60. Nalbone VP, Kuruvilla A, Gacek RR. Otogenic brain abscess: the Syracuse experience. Ear Nose Throat J. 1992;71:238–42.
61. Maniglia A, Goodwin J, Arnold J, Ganz E. Secondary to nasal, sinus and orbital infections in adults and children. Arch Otolaryngol Head Neck Surg. 1989;115:1424–9.
62. Williams MR. Open evacuation of pus: a satisfying surgical approach to the problem of brain abscess? J Neurol Neurosurg Psychiatry. 1983;45:697–700.
63. LeBeau J, King S. Surgical treatment of brain abscess and subdural empyema. J Neurosurg. 1973;38:198–203.
64. Brand B, Caparosa RJ, Lubic LG. Otorhinological brain abscess therapy-past and present. Laryngoscope. 1984;94:483–7.
65. Teichgraeber J, Perlee H, Turner J. Lateral sinus thrombosis: a modern perspective. Laryngoscope. 1982;92:744–51.
66. Seid A, Sellars S. The management of otogenic lateral sinus disease at the Groote Schuur Hospital. Laryngoscope. 1973;83:397–403.
67. Wolfowitz BL. Otogenic intracranial complications. Arch Otolaryngol. 1972;96:220–2.
68. Buonanno F, Moody D, Ball M, Laster D. Computed cranial tomographic findings in cerebral sinovenous occlusion. J Comput Assist Tomogr. 1978;2:281–90.
69. Harris T, Smith R, Koch K. Gadolinium DTPA enhanced MR imaging of septic dural thrombosis. J Comput Assist Tomogr. 1989;13:682–4.
70. Doyle WJ, Webster DB. Neonatal conductive hearing loss does not compromise brainstem auditory function and structure in rhesus monkeys. Hear Res. 1991;54:145–51.
71. Fritsch M, Miyamoto R, Wood T. Sigmoid sinus thrombosis diagnosis by contrasted MRI scanning. Otolaryngol Head Neck Surg. 1990;103:451–6.
72. Davison SP, Facer GW, McGough PF, et al. Use of magnetic resonance imaging and magnetic resonance angiography in diagnosis of sigmoid sinus thrombosis. Ear Nose Throat J. 1997;76:436–41.
73. Rizer FM, Amiri CA, Schroeder WW, Brackmann DE. Lateral sinus thrombosis: diagnosis and treatment a case report. J Otolaryngol. 1987;16:77–9.
74. Symonds C. Otitic hydrocephalus. Brain. 1931;54:55–71.
75. Symonds C. Hydrocephalic and focal cerebral symptoms in relation to thrombophlebitis of the dural sinuses and cerebral veins. Brain. 1937;60:531–50.
76. Foley J. Benign forms of intracranial hypertension toxic and "otitic" hydrocephalus. Brain. 1955;78:1–41.

77. Calabresse V, Selhorst J, Harbison J. Cerebrospinal fluid infusion test in pseudotumor cerebri. Ann Neurol. 1978;4:173.
78. Sahs A, Joynt R. Brain swelling of unknown cause. Neurology. 1956;6:791–802.
79. Weed L, Flexner L. The relations of the inracranial pressure. Am J Phys. 1933;105:266–72.
80. O'Connor A, Moffat D. Otogenic hypertension. J Laryngol Otol. 1978;92:767–75.
81. Horton J. Decompression of the optic nerve sheath for vision threatening papilledema caused by dural sinus occlusion. Neurosurgery. 1992;31:203–12.
82. Weingarten K. Subdural and epidural empyema. MR imaging. Am J Radiol. 1989;152:615–21.
83. Baum PA, Dillon WP. Utility of magnetic resonance imaging in the detection of subdural empyema. Ann Otol Rhinol Laryngol. 1992;101:876.
84. Bales CB, Sobol S, Wetmore R, Elden LM. Lateral sinus thrombosis as a complication of otitis media: 10-year experience at the Children's Hospital of Philadelphia. Pediatrics. 2009;123:709. https://doi.org/10.1542/peds.2008-0280.
85. Gendeh HS, Abdullah AB, Goh BS, Hashim ND. Intracranial complications of chronic otitis media: why does it still occur? Ear Nose Throat J. 2019;98(7):416–9.
86. Kirti YK, Yashveer JK. Dilemmas in current management of complicated chronic otitis media. Indian J Otolaryngol Head Neck Surg. 2018;71:1929. https://doi.org/10.1007/s12070-018-1333-4.
87. Govea Camacho LH, Perez Ramirez R, Cornejo Suarez A, et al. Diagnosis and treatment of the complications of otitis media in adults. Case series and literature review. Cirugia y Cirujanos. 2016;84(5):398–404.
88. Abhilash S, Viswanatha B. Lateral sinus thrombosis with pneumocephalus. A rare complication. J Otolaryngol ENT Res. 2019;11(3):166–9.
89. Osama U, Cureoglu S, Hosoglu S. The complications of otitis media; report of 93 cases. J Laryngol Otol. 2000;114:97–100.
90. Krishnan M, Walijee H, Jesurasa A, De S, Sinha A, Sharma R, Donne A. Clinical outcomes of intracranial complications secondary to acute mastoiditis. The Alder Hay experience. Int J Pediatr Otorhinolaryngol. 2020;128(2020):109675.

Basic Imaging and Normal Temporal Bone Sections

35

Marcos V. Goycoolea, Catalina Gutiérrez, and Francisco Chiang

Introduction

For years I dreamed of writing a chapter with horizontal sections, histological sections stained with hematoxylin-eosin, and axial computerized tomographic sections of temporal bones, all at the same levels simultaneously. I felt that this would allow the readers to: (1) acquire a three-dimensional view of the temporal bone, (2) develop an anatomic understanding of the areas involved with disease, and (3) interpret the imagenological studies based on anatomical concepts. With this purpose I contacted Otolaryngologist Catalina Gutiérrez who combines anatomical concepts with computer abilities and our Neuroradiologist Francisco Chiang who performs and interprets our temporal bone studies in our Otolaryngology Department. We tried to keep the sections at the same levels, it worked out well, my dream came true, and we can share it with you.

The chapter describes 18 horizontal sections from superior to inferior. Sections start at the level of the epitympanum (area in which the middle ear cavity extends superiorly above the tympanic membrane) ending at the hypotympanum. The sections are presented without detailed descriptions; however, the structures are clearly labeled.

The anatomical and histological sections are my own and were acquired during my many years at the Department of Otolaryngology at the University of Minnesota directed by Michael M. Paparella. I trained and later worked with Michael Paparella, an inspiration for all of us members of the Department. In fact, all the co-editors of this book have been part of Michael's team.

M. V. Goycoolea (✉)
Department of Otolaryngology, Clínica Universidad de Los Andes, Santiago, Chile

C. Gutiérrez
Hospital Sótero del Río, Santiago, Chile

F. Chiang
Department of Radiology, Clínica Universidad de Los Andes, Santiago, Chile

M. V. Goycoolea et al. (eds.), *Textbook of Otitis Media*, https://doi.org/10.1007/978-3-031-40949-3_35

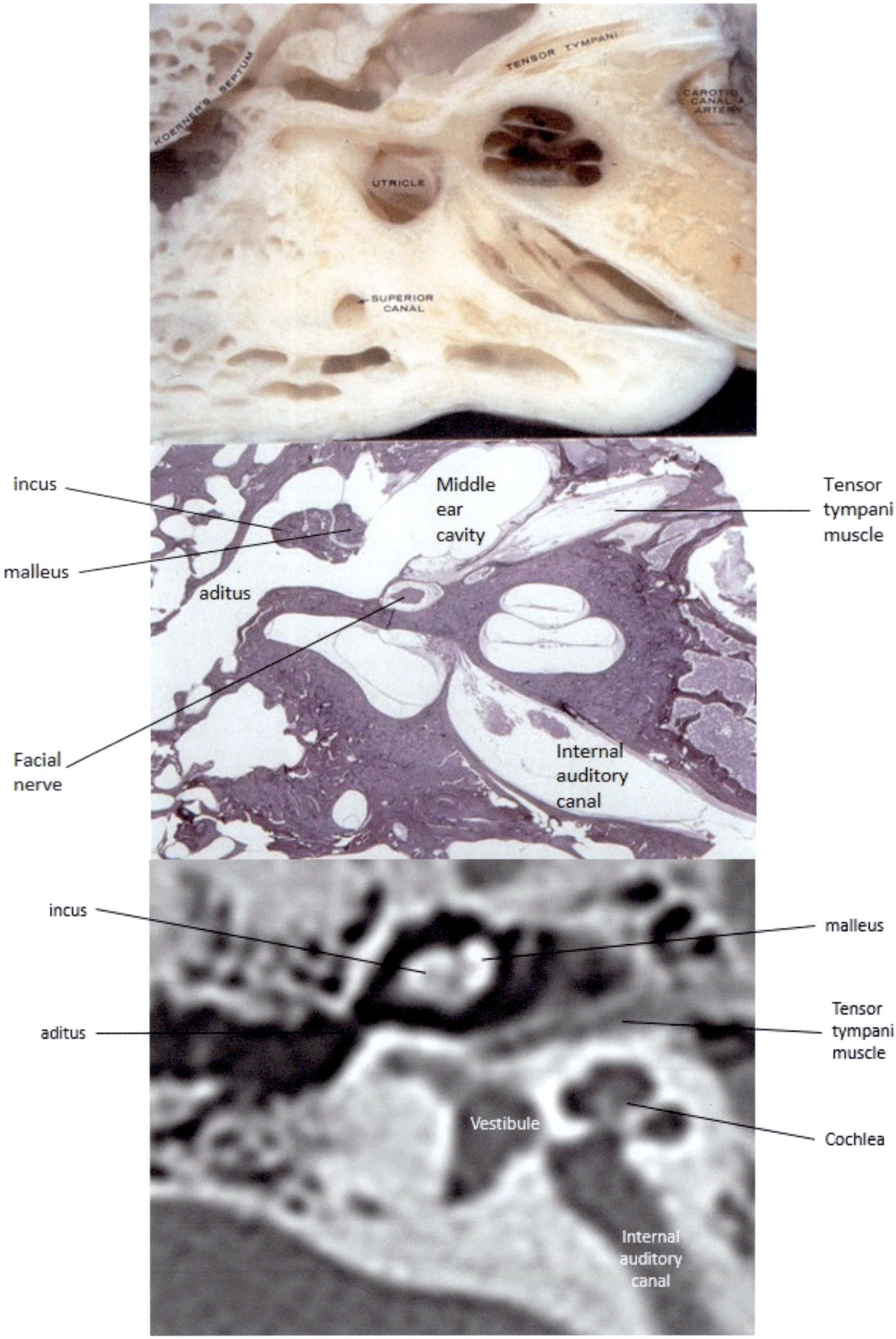
KOERNER'S SEPTUM
TENSOR TYMPANI
UTRICLE
SUPERIOR CANAL
incus
malleus
Middle ear cavity
Tensor tympani muscle
aditus
Facial nerve
Internal auditory canal
incus
malleus
aditus
Tensor tympani muscle
Vestibule
Cochlea
Internal auditory canal

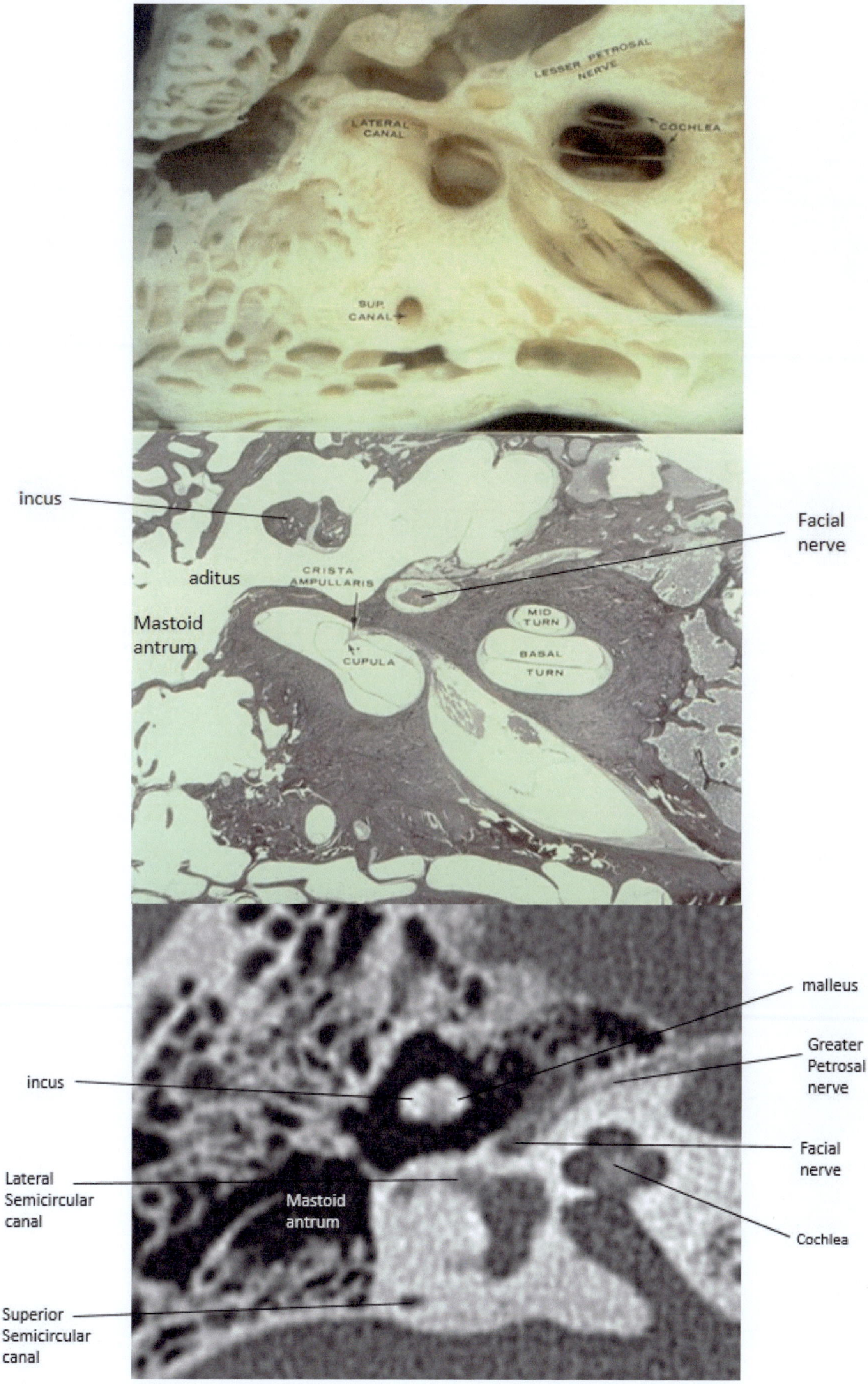
LESSER PETROSAL NERVE
LATERAL CANAL
COCHLEA
SUP. CANAL
incus
aditus
Mastoid antrum
CRISTA AMPULLARIS
CUPULA
Facial nerve
MID TURN
BASAL TURN
malleus
Greater Petrosal nerve
incus
Facial nerve
Lateral Semicircular canal
Mastoid antrum
Cochlea
Superior Semicircular canal

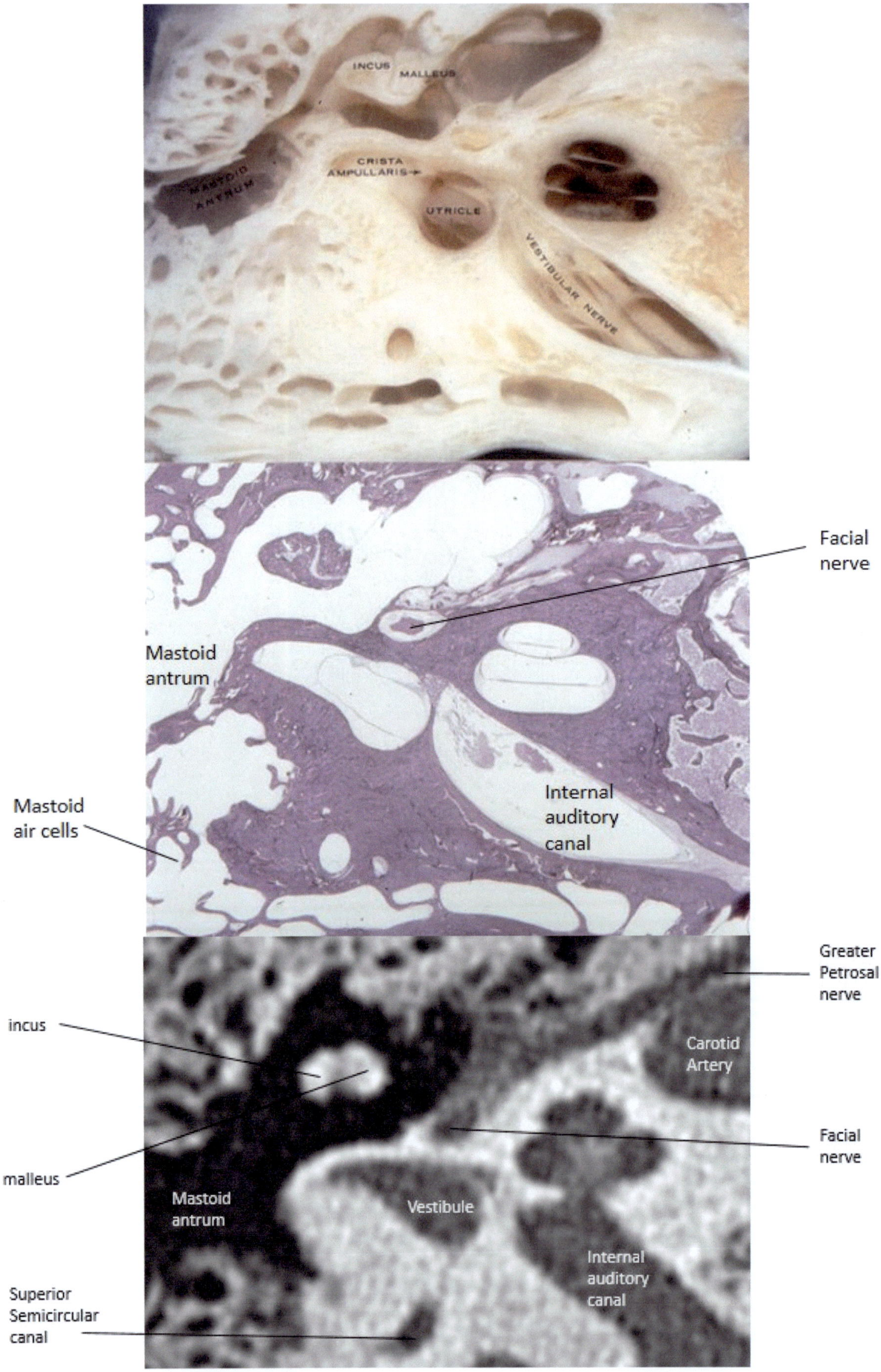
INCUS
MALLEUS
CRISTA AMPULLARIS
MASTOID ANTRUM
UTRICLE
VESTIBULAR NERVE
Facial nerve
Mastoid antrum
Mastoid air cells
Internal auditory canal
Greater Petrosal nerve
incus
Carotid Artery
Facial nerve
malleus
Mastoid antrum
Vestibule
Internal auditory canal
Superior Semicircular canal

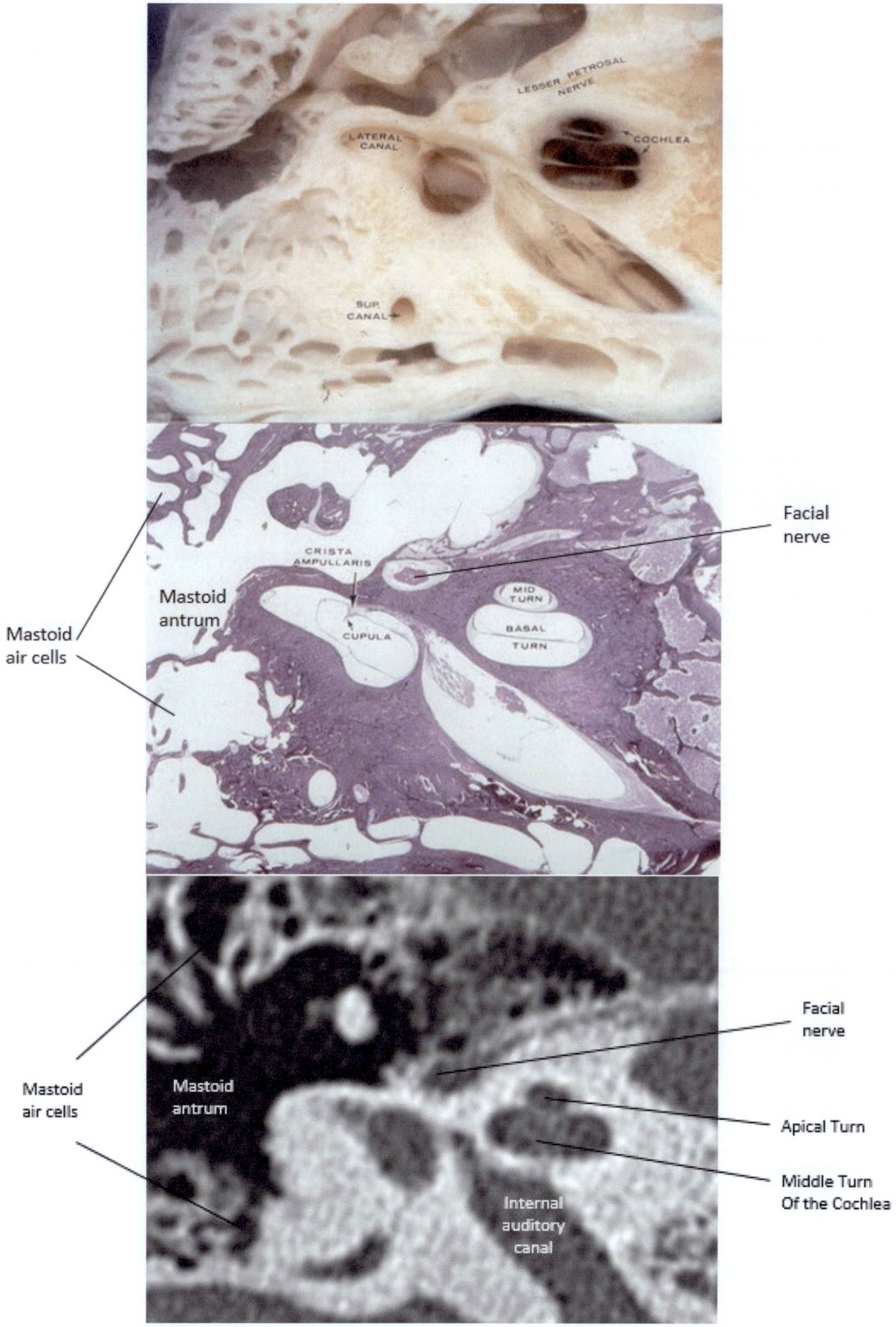
LESSER PETROSAL NERVE
LATERAL CANAL
COCHLEA
SUP. CANAL
Facial nerve
CRISTA AMPULLARIS
Mastoid antrum
MID TURN
Mastoid air cells
CUPULA
BASAL TURN
Facial nerve
Mastoid air cells
Mastoid antrum
Apical Turn
Middle Turn Of the Cochlea
Internal auditory canal

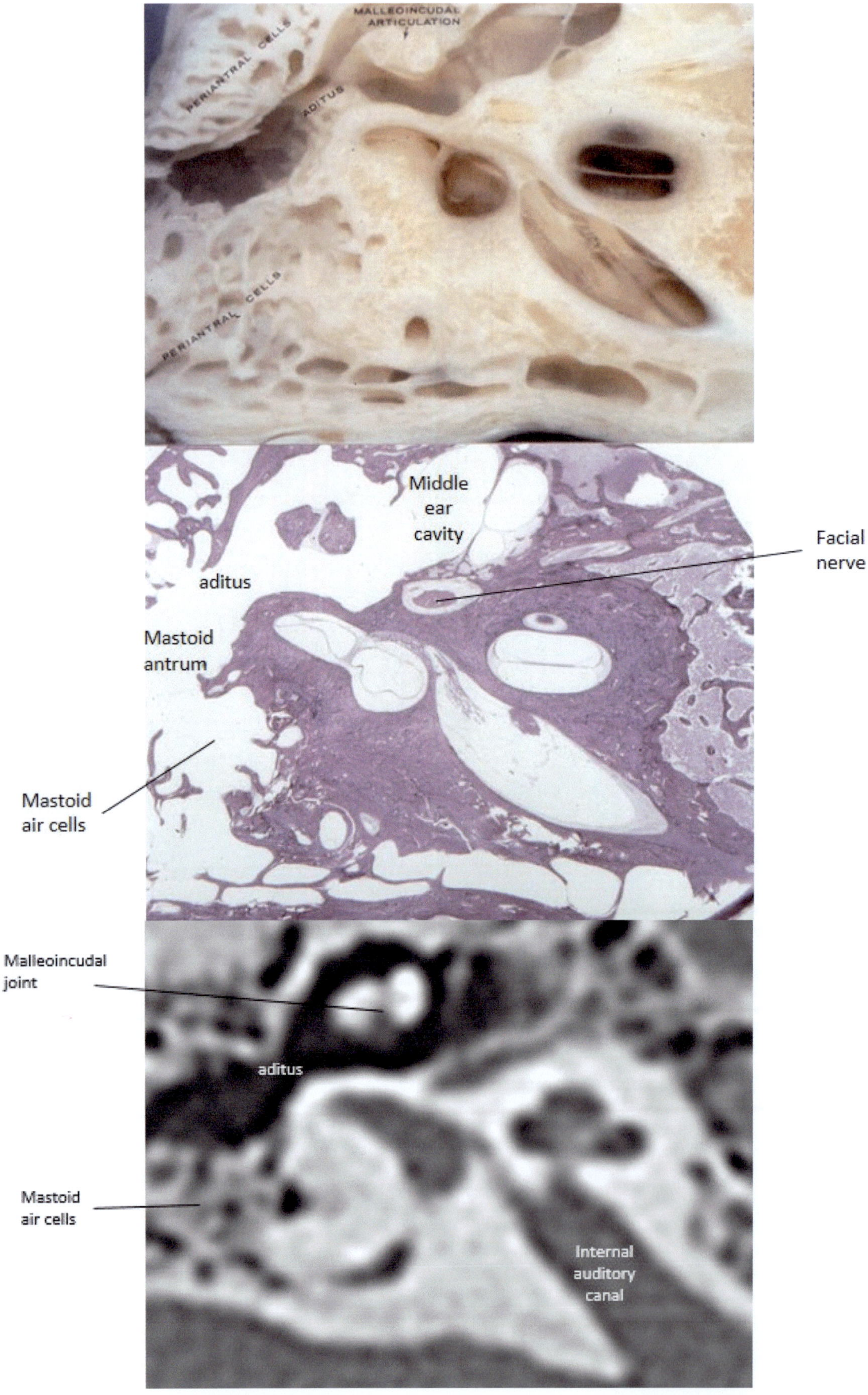
MALLEOINCUDAL ARTICULATION
PERIANTRAL CELLS
ADITUS
PERIANTRAL CELLS
Middle ear cavity
Facial nerve
aditus
Mastoid antrum
Mastoid air cells
Malleoincudal joint
aditus
Mastoid air cells
Internal auditory canal

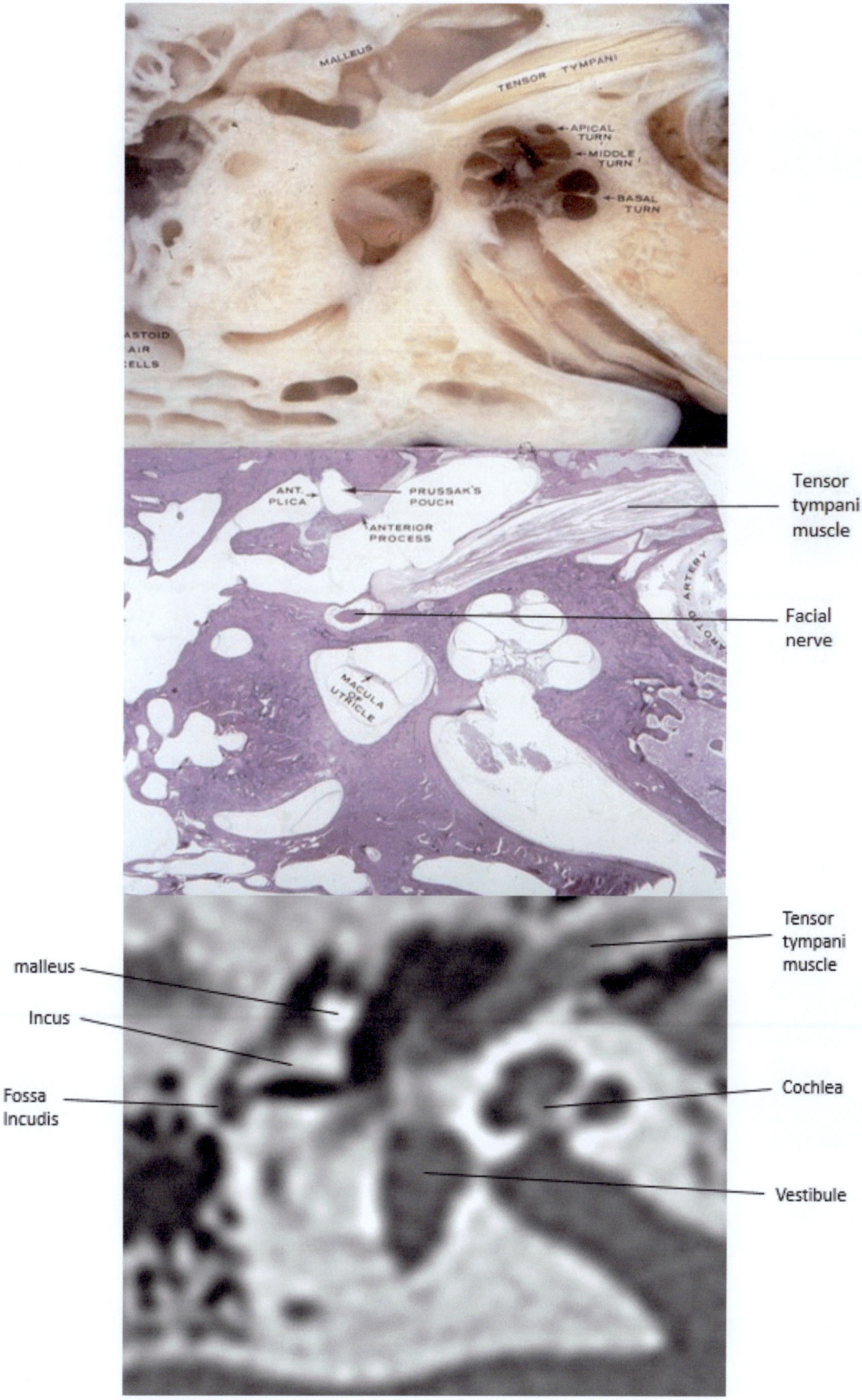
MALLEUS
TENSOR TYMPANI
APICAL TURN
MIDDLE TURN
BASAL TURN
ANT. PLICA
PRUSSAK'S POUCH
ANTERIOR PROCESS
MACULA OF UTRICLE
ARTERY
Tensor tympani muscle
Facial nerve
malleus
Incus
Fossa Incudis
Tensor tympani muscle
Cochlea
Vestibule

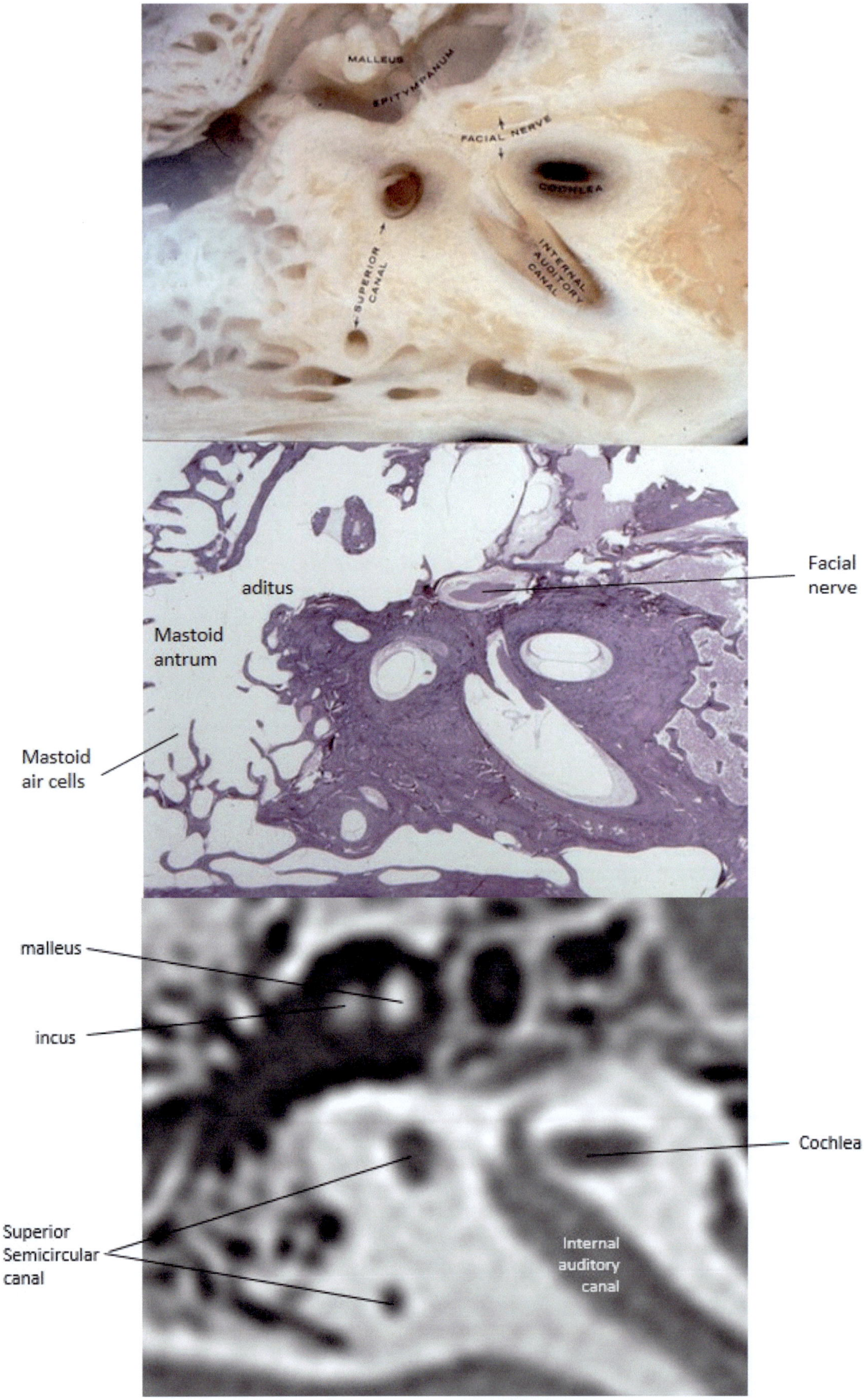
MALLEUS
EPITYMPANUM
FACIAL NERVE
COCHLEA
INTERNAL AUDITORY CANAL
SUPERIOR CANAL
aditus
Facial nerve
Mastoid antrum
Mastoid air cells
malleus
incus
Cochlea
Superior Semicircular canal
Internal auditory canal

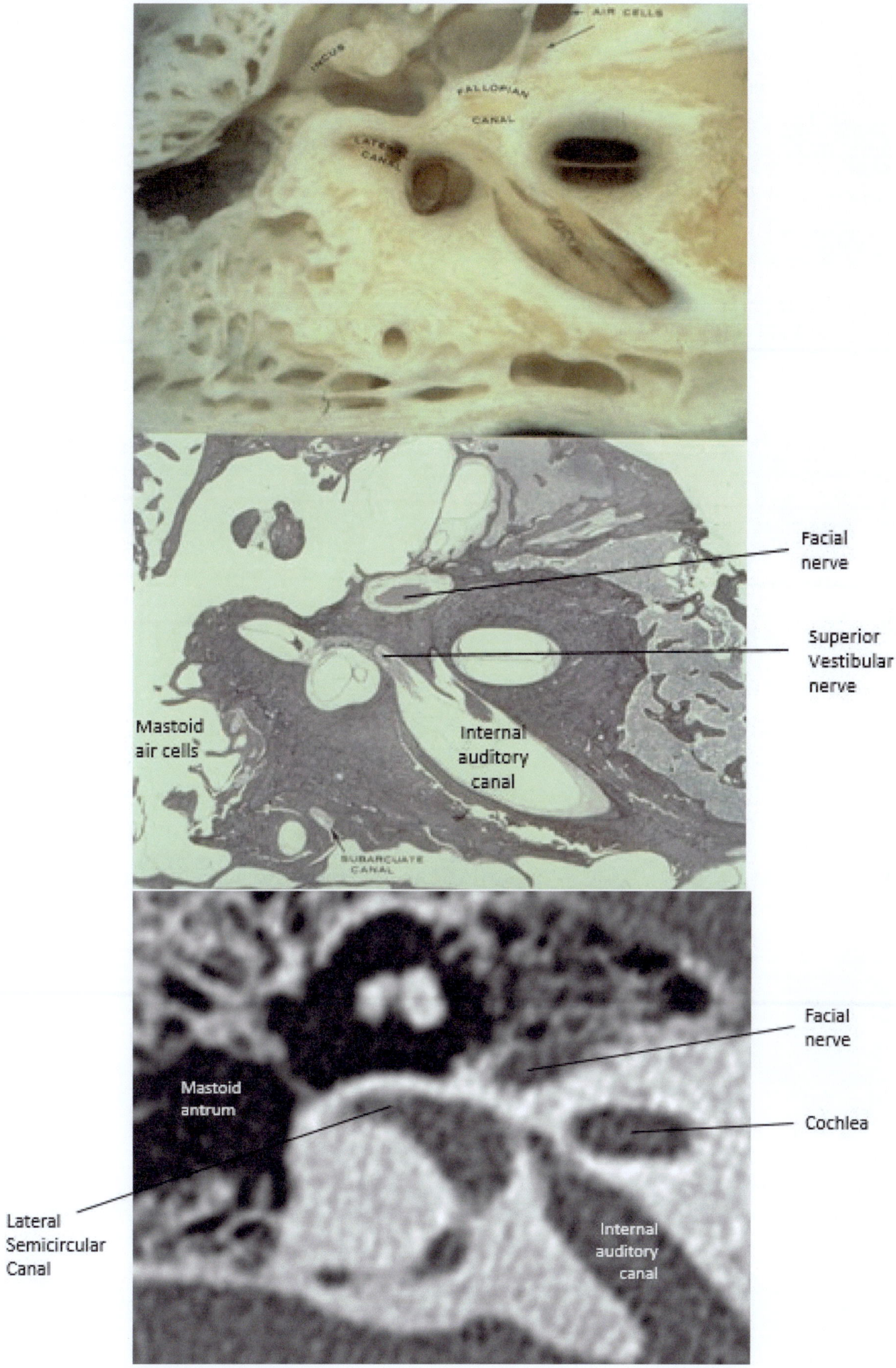
AIR CELLS
INCUS
FALLOPIAN CANAL
Facial nerve
Superior Vestibular nerve
Mastoid air cells
Internal auditory canal
SUBARCUATE CANAL
Facial nerve
Mastoid antrum
Cochlea
Lateral Semicircular Canal
Internal auditory canal

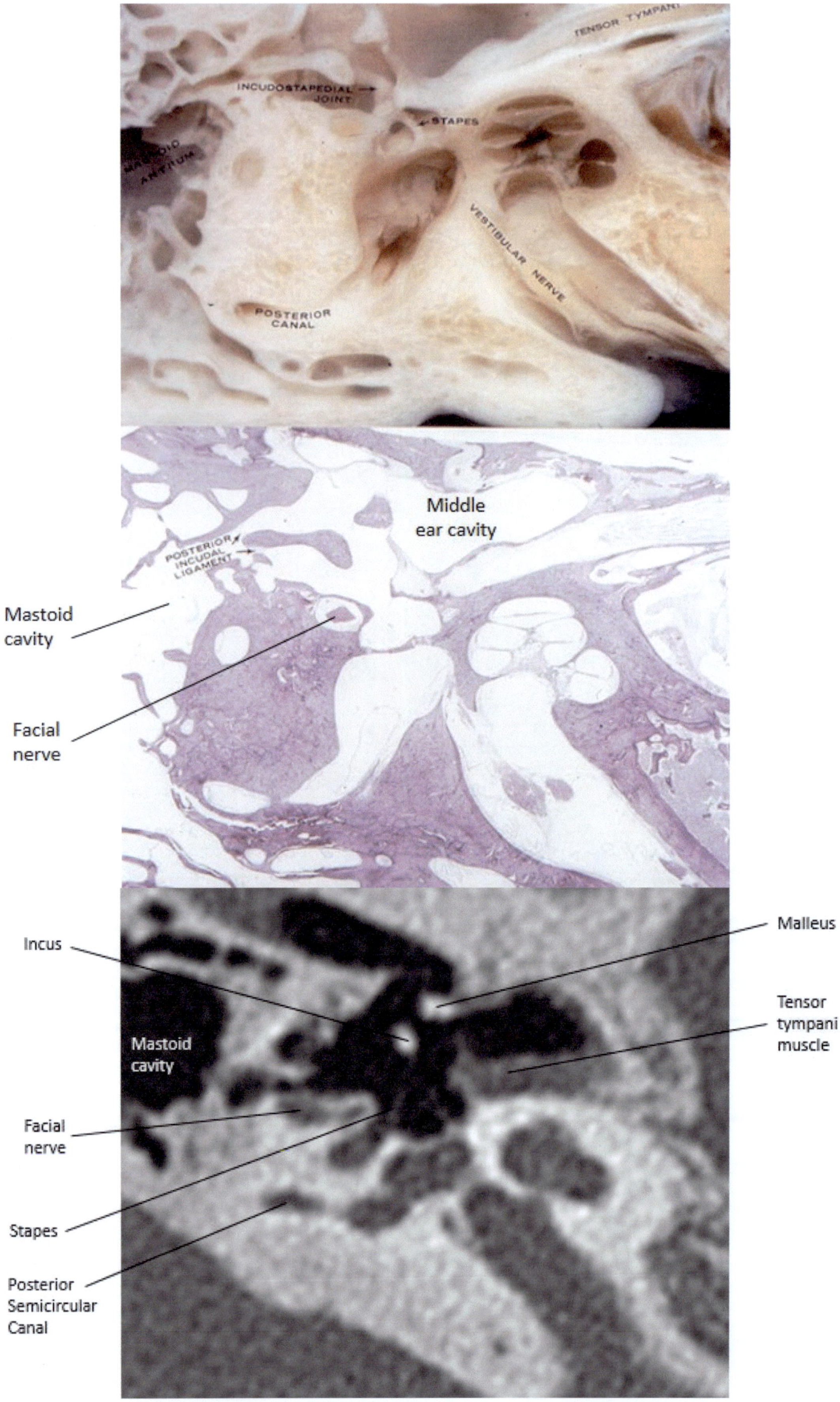
TENSOR TYMPANI
INCUDOSTAPEDIAL JOINT
STAPES
MASTOID ANTRUM
VESTIBULAR NERVE
POSTERIOR CANAL
Middle ear cavity
POSTERIOR INCUDAL LIGAMENT
Mastoid cavity
Facial nerve
Incus
Malleus
Tensor tympani muscle
Mastoid cavity
Facial nerve
Stapes
Posterior Semicircular Canal

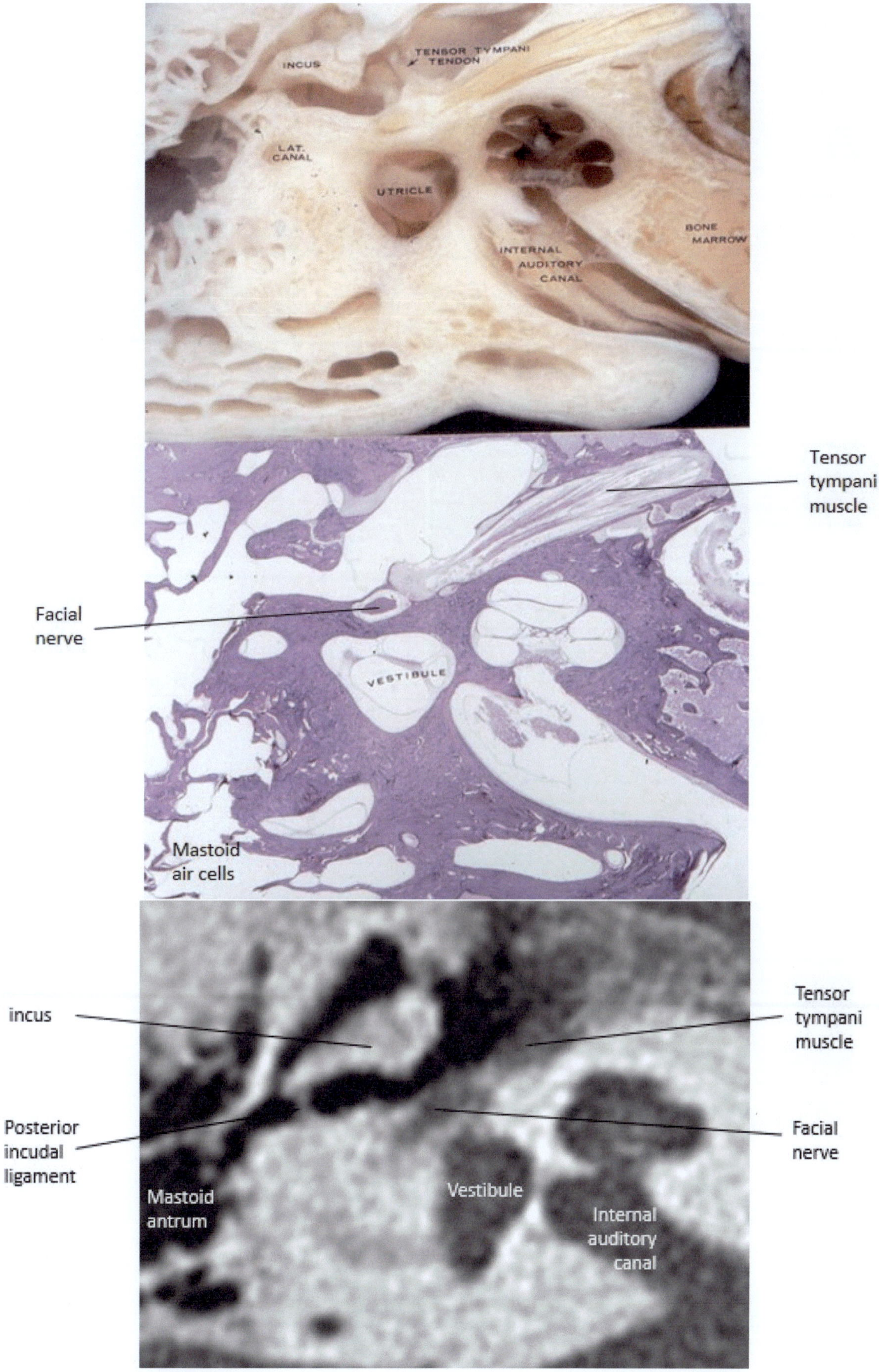
INCUS
TENSOR TYMPANI TENDON
LAT. CANAL
UTRICLE
INTERNAL AUDITORY CANAL
BONE MARROW
Tensor tympani muscle
Facial nerve
VESTIBULE
Mastoid air cells
incus
Tensor tympani muscle
Posterior incudal ligament
Facial nerve
Mastoid antrum
Vestibule
Internal auditory canal

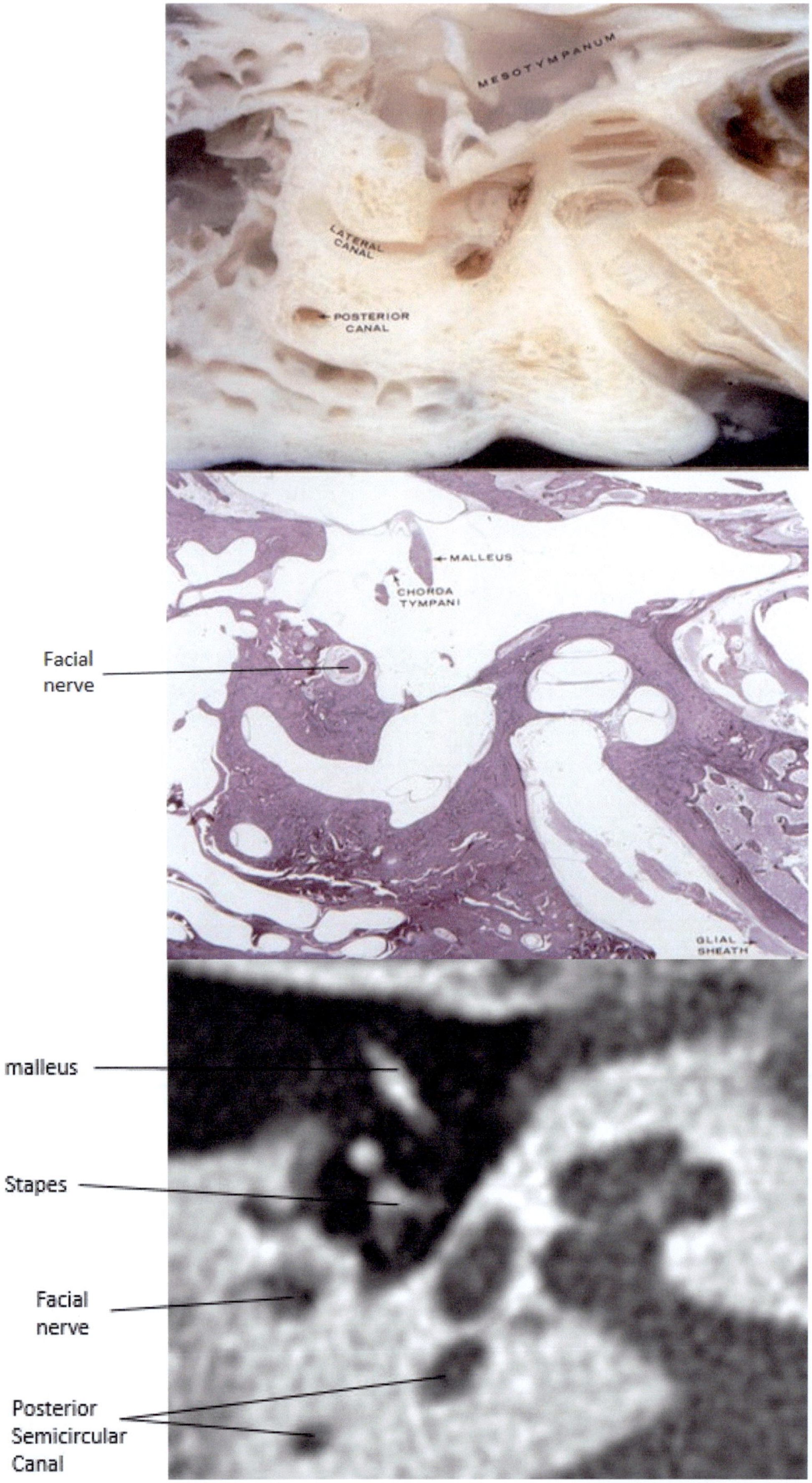
MESOTYMPANUM
LATERAL CANAL
POSTERIOR CANAL
MALLEUS
CHORDA TYMPANI
Facial nerve
GLIAL SHEATH
malleus
Stapes
Facial nerve
Posterior Semicircular Canal

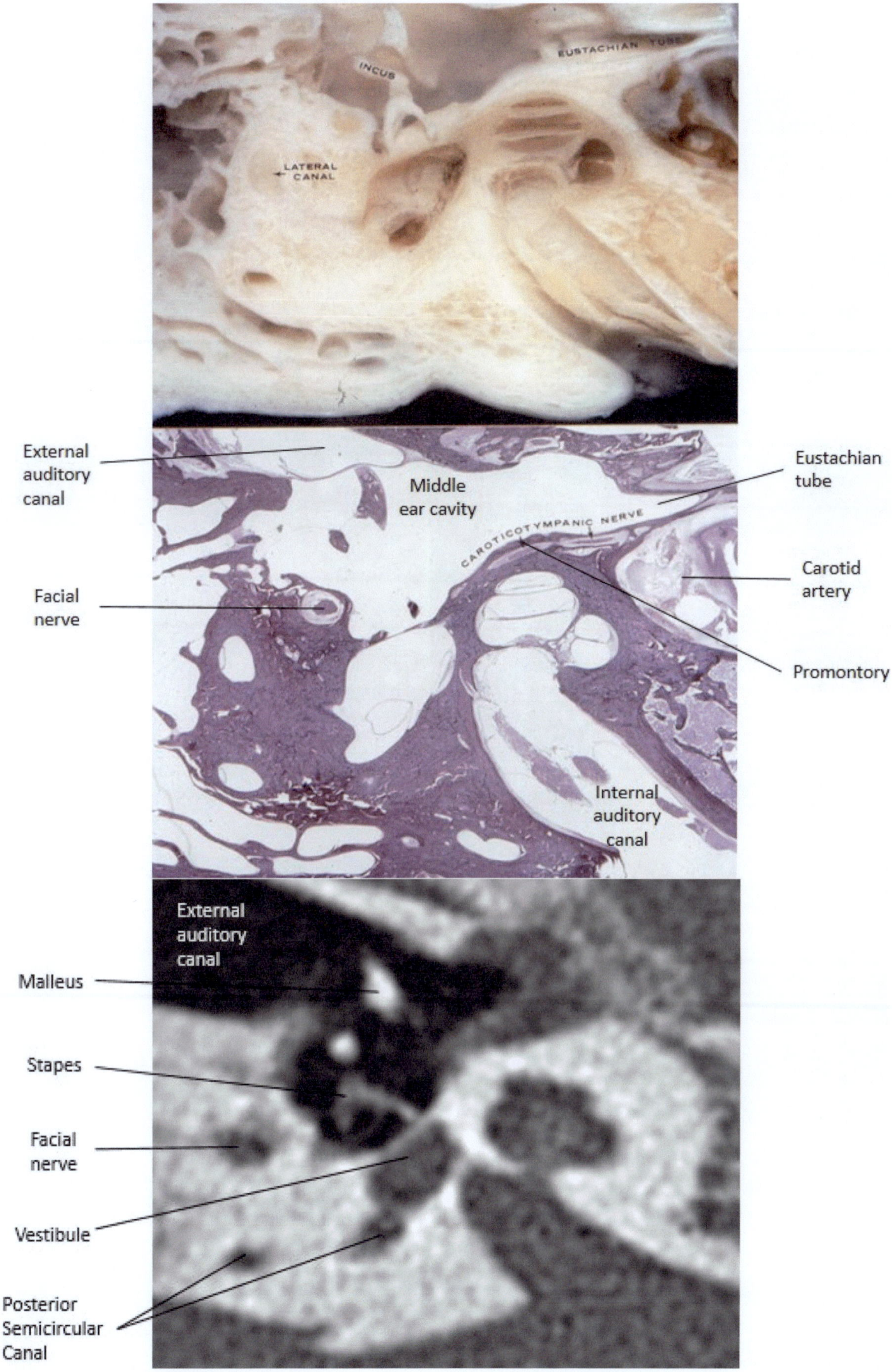
EUSTACHIAN TUBE
INCUS
LATERAL CANAL
External auditory canal
Middle ear cavity
Eustachian tube
CAROTICOTYMPANIC NERVE
Carotid artery
Facial nerve
Promontory
Internal auditory canal
External auditory canal
Malleus
Stapes
Facial nerve
Vestibule
Posterior Semicircular Canal

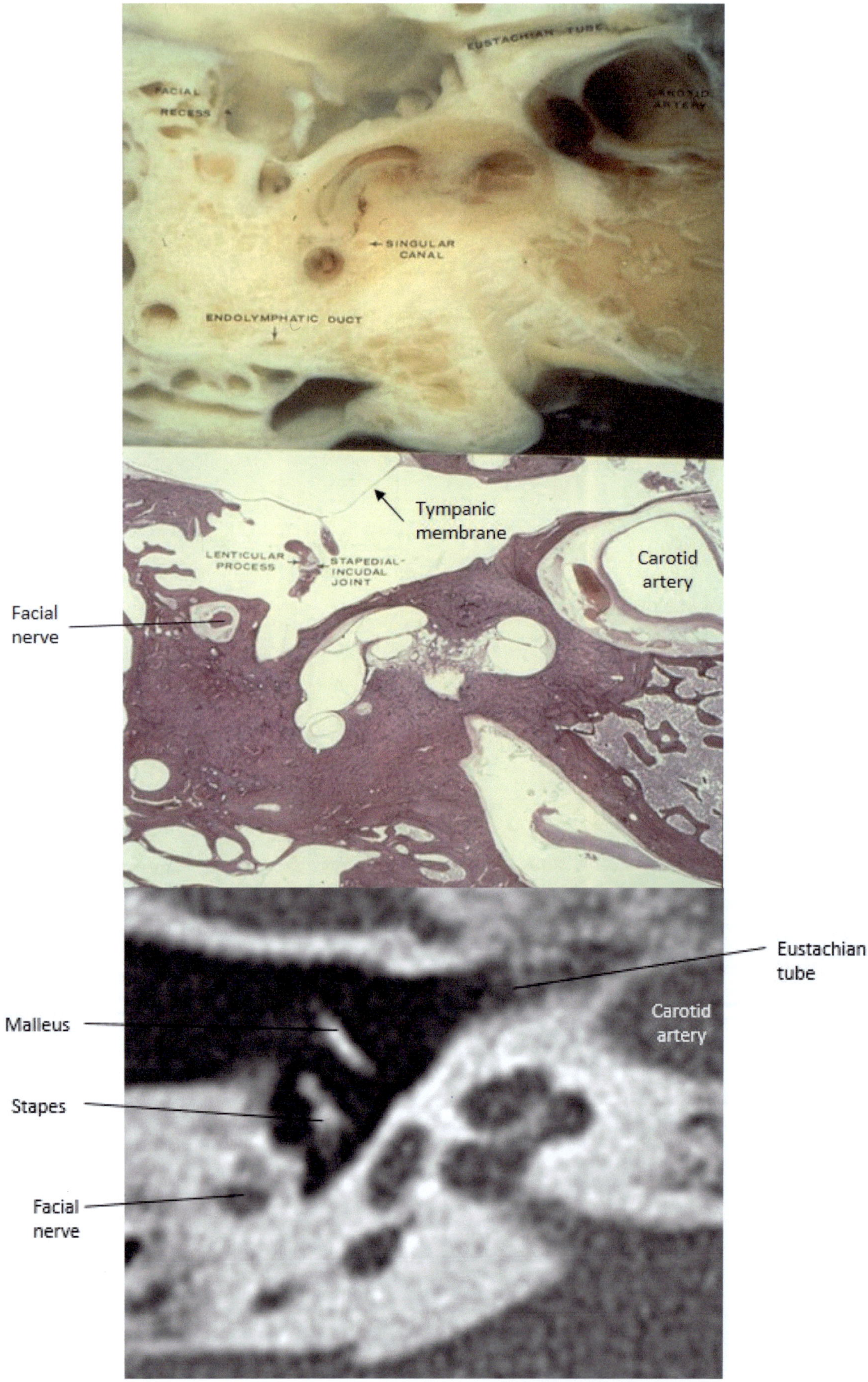
EUSTACHIAN TUBE
FACIAL RECESS
CAROTID ARTERY
SINGULAR CANAL
ENDOLYMPHATIC DUCT
Tympanic membrane
LENTICULAR PROCESS
STAPEDIAL-INCUDAL JOINT
Carotid artery
Facial nerve
Eustachian tube
Carotid artery
Malleus
Stapes
Facial nerve

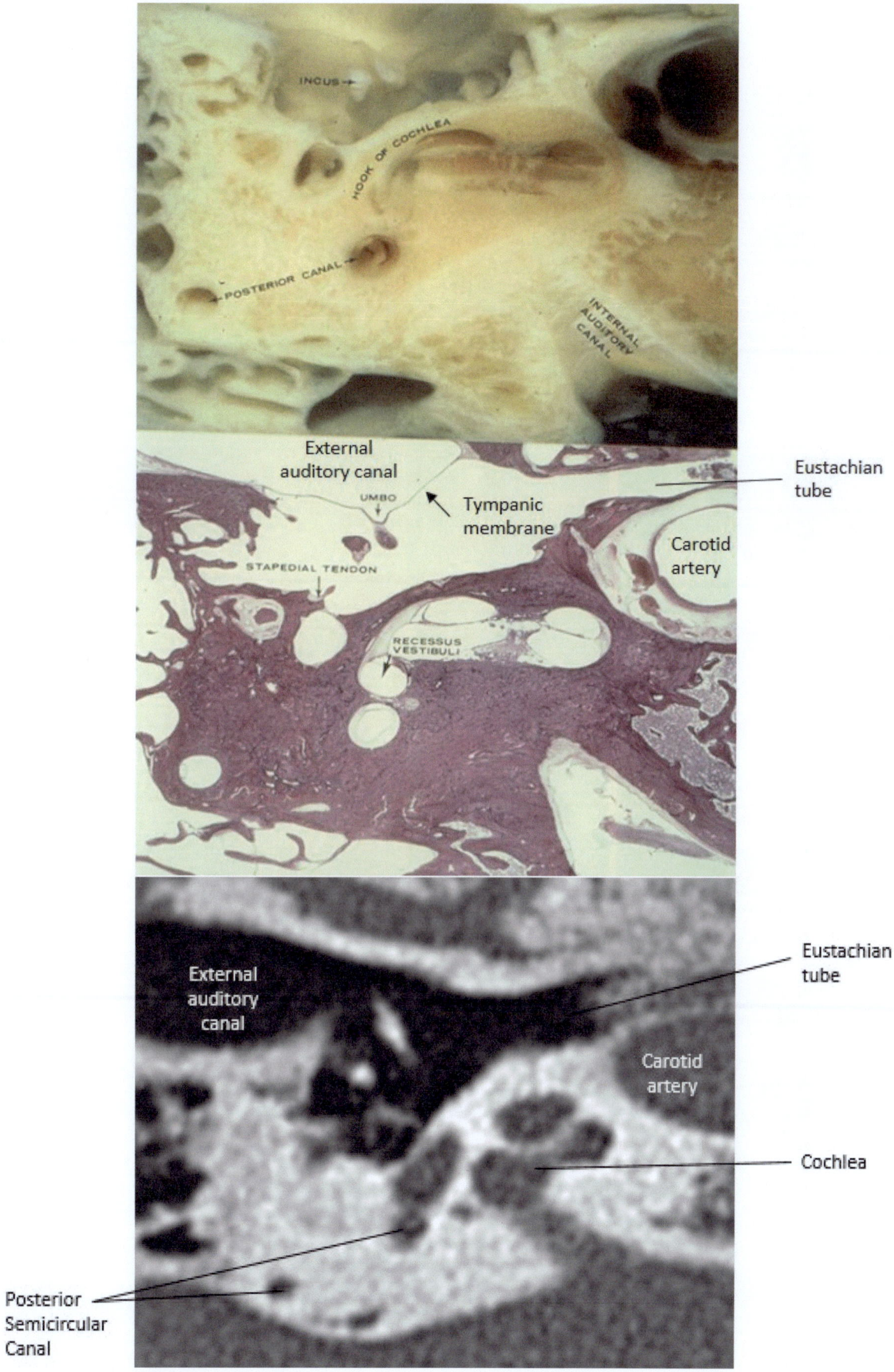
INCUS
HOOK OF COCHLEA
POSTERIOR CANAL
INTERNAL AUDITORY CANAL
External auditory canal
UMBO
Tympanic membrane
Eustachian tube
Carotid artery
STAPEDIAL TENDON
RECESSUS VESTIBULI
Eustachian tube
External auditory canal
Carotid artery
Cochlea
Posterior Semicircular Canal

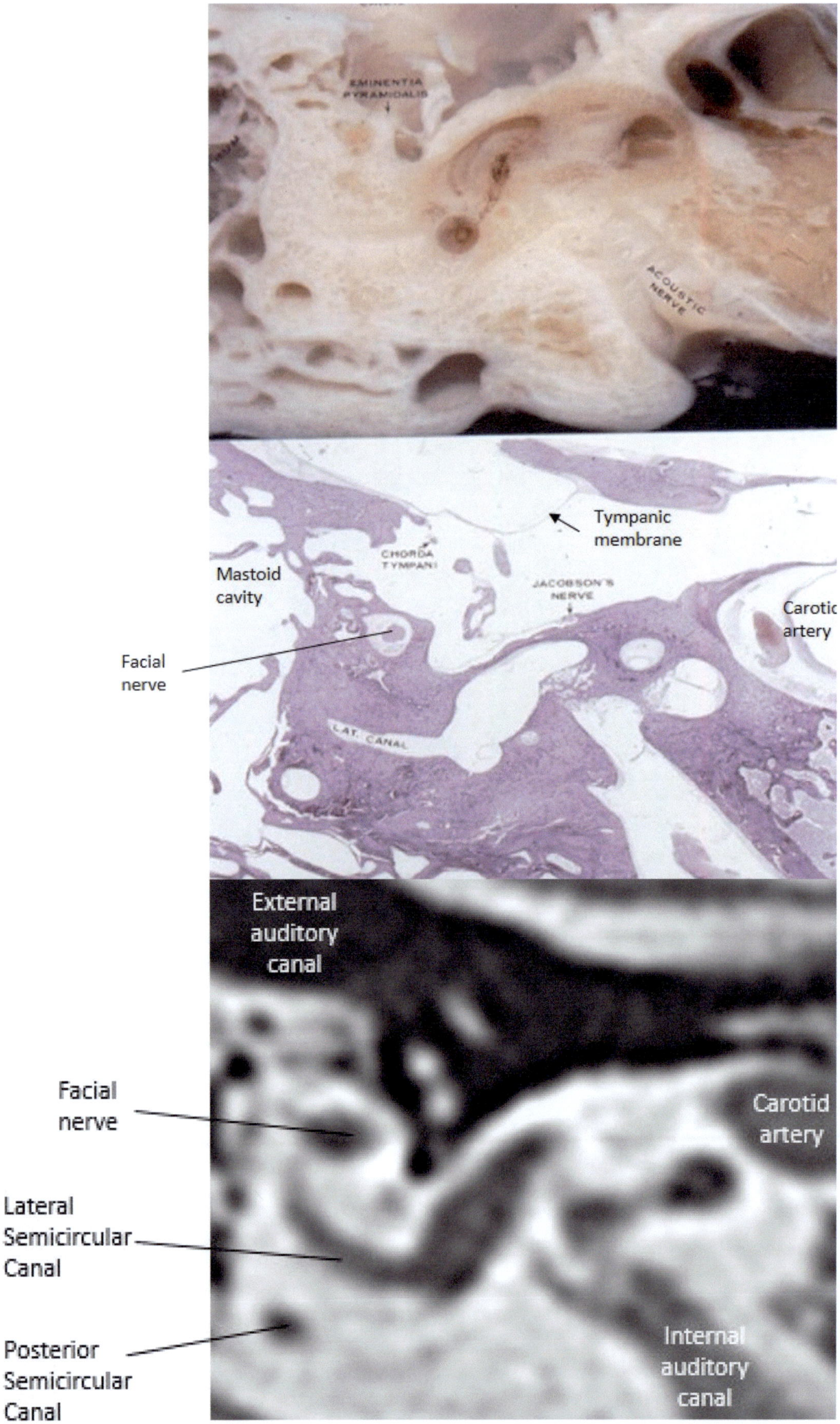
EMINENTIA PYRAMIDALIS
ACOUSTIC NERVE
Tympanic membrane
CHORDA TYMPANI
Mastoid cavity
JACOBSON'S NERVE
Carotic artery
Facial nerve
LAT. CANAL
External auditory canal
Facial nerve
Carotid artery
Lateral Semicircular Canal
Posterior Semicircular Canal
Internal auditory canal

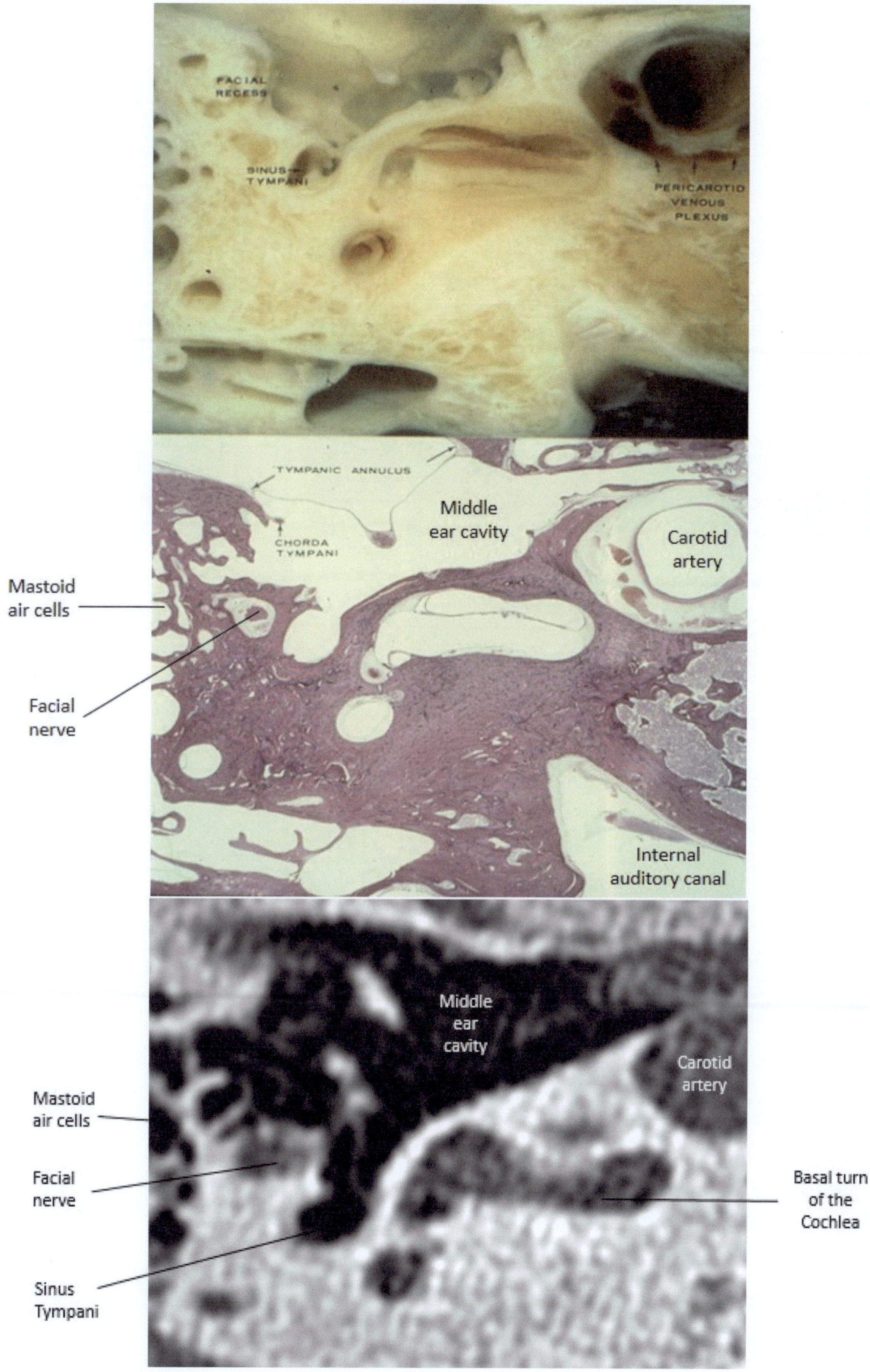
FACIAL RECESS
SINUS TYMPANI
PERICAROTID VENOUS PLEXUS
TYMPANIC ANNULUS
CHORDA TYMPANI
Middle ear cavity
Carotid artery
Mastoid air cells
Facial nerve
Internal auditory canal
Middle ear cavity
Carotid artery
Mastoid air cells
Facial nerve
Sinus Tympani
Basal turn of the Cochlea

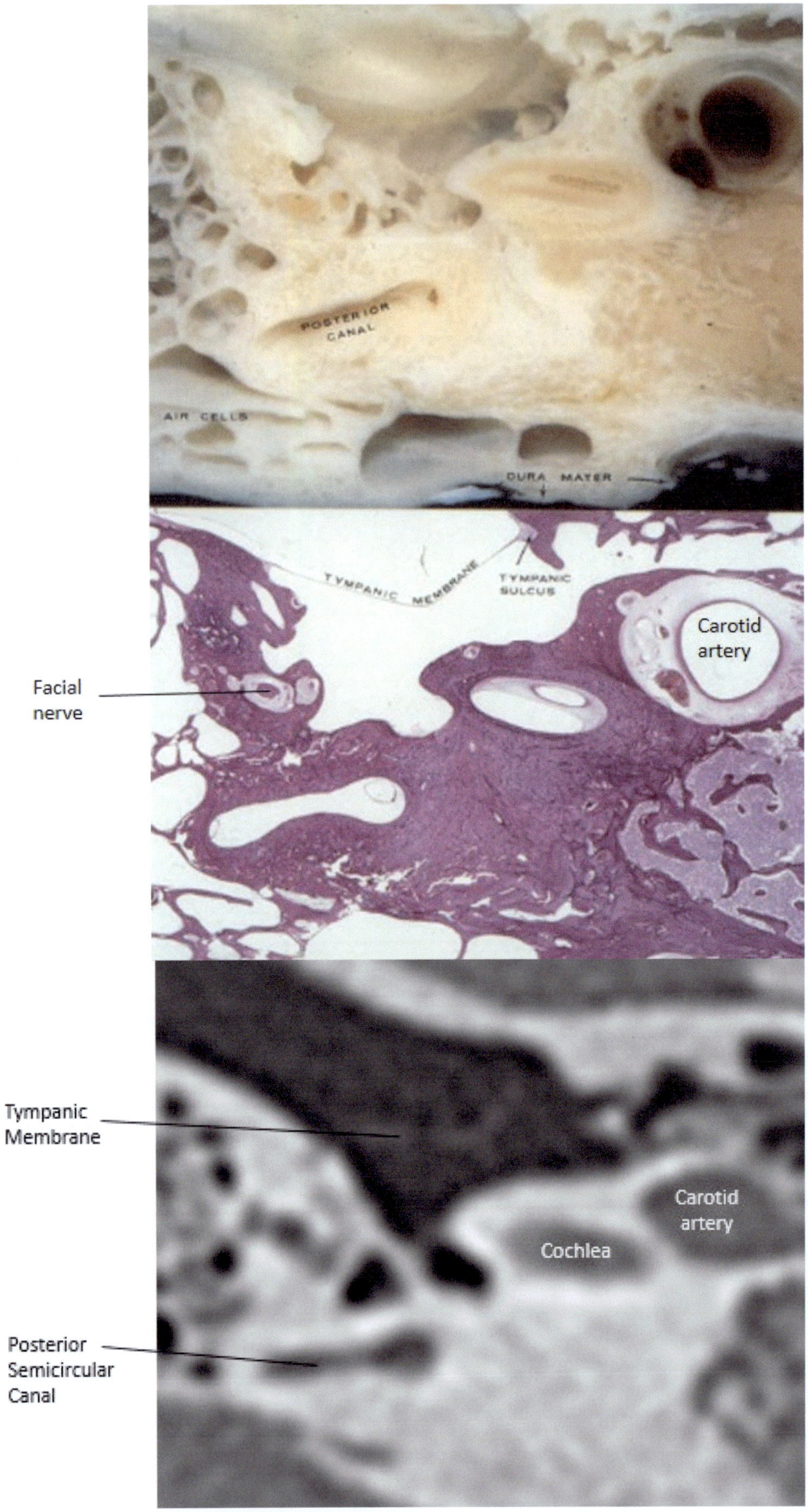
POSTERIOR
CANAL
AIR CELLS
DURA MATER
TYMPANIC MEMBRANE
TYMPANIC
SULCUS
Carotid
artery
Facial
nerve
Tympanic
Membrane
Cochlea
Carotid
artery
Posterior
Semicircular
Canal

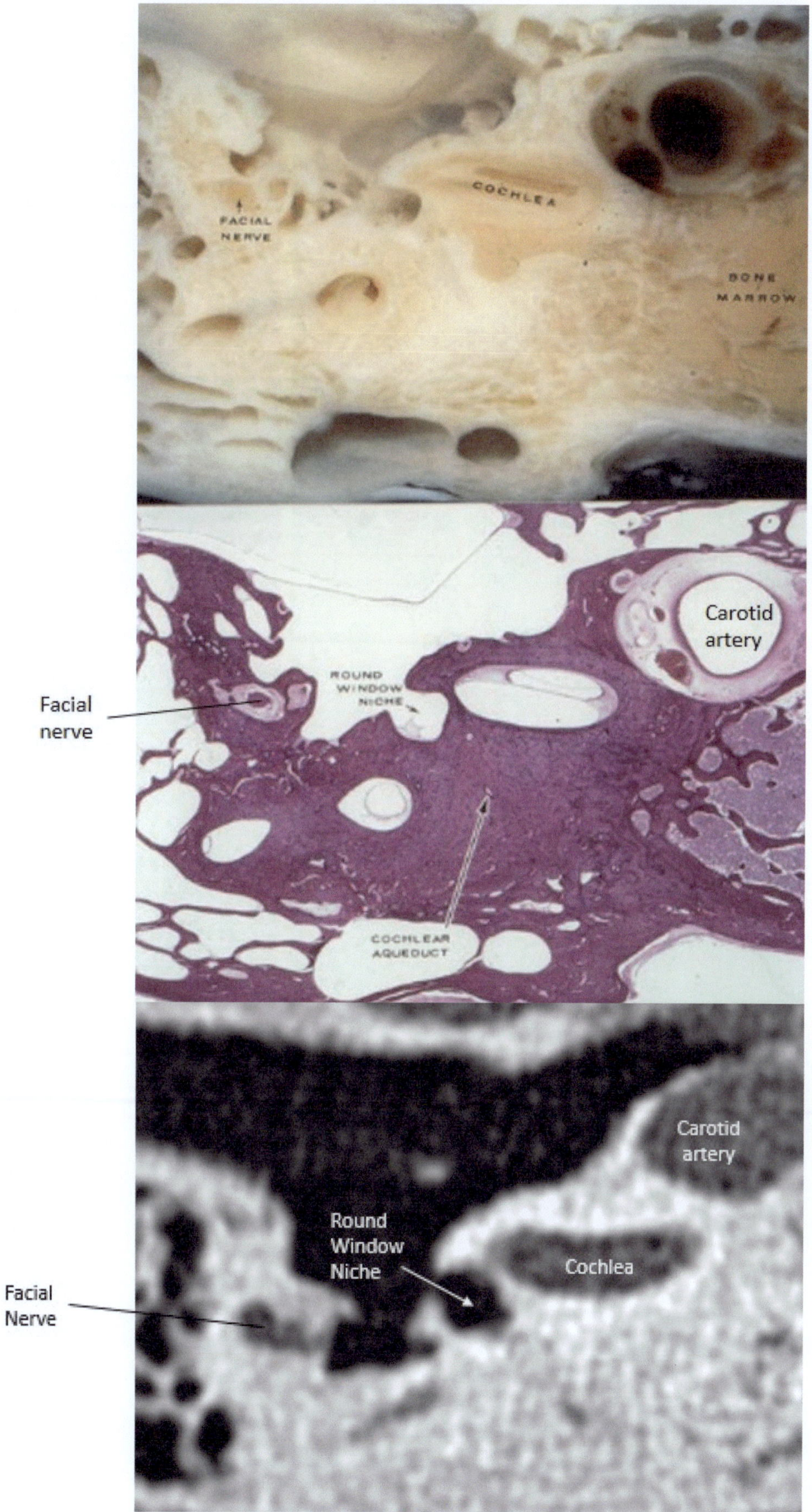
COCHLEA
FACIAL NERVE
BONE MARROW
Carotid artery
ROUND WINDOW NICHE
Facial nerve
COCHLEAR AQUEDUCT
Carotid artery
Round Window Niche
Cochlea
Facial Nerve

Evaluation and Auditory Rehabilitation in Chronic Otitis Media (COM)

36

Byanka Cagnacci Buzo, S. Catherine Catenacci, and G. Raquel Levy

Chronic Otitis Media and its Effects on Hearing

Hearing loss is a major global public health problem, occurring in both developed and developing countries, with more than 466 million people affected worldwide [1]. The causes of hearing loss are varied, but one of the most common is chronic ear infection, especially chronic otitis media (COM). It is estimated that about 164 million cases of hearing impairment may be due to COM. Global incidence rates are estimated at 5% for COM, of which 23% are children [2].

COM is a chronic inflammation of the middle ear with discharge that drains into the ear canal through a perforation in the tympanic membrane and often develops during early childhood. As an after effect, the chronic perforations and scarring of the tympanic membrane provoke hearing deterioration. In addition, the chronic state of inflammation and discharge in the middle ear can lead to erosion of the middle ear bones, worsening hearing loss. Because hearing loss is often established in early childhood, it leads to difficulties in language and speech development, together with associated cognitive development. This again can result in impaired social and emotional abilities, lower educational achievements, and restricted employment opportunities [3]. Because of its long duration and greater severity compared to other types of otitis media, and because most children need louder auditory stimuli than adults to function optimally, it is likely that COM in children hinders cognitive and language development.

During the inflammatory process, COM frequently generates a conductive type of hearing loss. Moreover, the inflammatory process of the middle ear can be detrimental to the inner ear, as shown in histological and animal studies. During the inflammatory process, toxins can cause damage to the round window membrane. This triggers the diffusion of toxins into the inner ear and fluid leakage from the inner ear, resulting in loss of cochlear function, leading to permanent loss as will be discussed below [4].

Assessment of Hearing

The measurement of hearing is exemplified on a graphic called an audiogram, in which the frequencies studied are located on the horizontal axis and the intensity in decibels HTL (hearing threshold level) on the vertical axis. The audiologist enters the symbols corresponding to the threshold hearing of the patient in response of the sound stimuli that are given through earphones (air conduction) or through the bone vibrator (through the bone). The following audiogram shows an audiological examination, in which its air and bone thresholds are within normal limits (Fig. 36.1).

Hearing loss that is reflected in the audiogram in cases of chronic otitis is generally classified as conductive hearing loss, since it is the conductive or transmission system (external auditory canal, eardrum, and intratympanic bones) that is affected. In some cases, there can also be a mixed hearing loss, when, in addition to the eardrum-ossicular system, there is also damage to the inner ear.

In cases of COM with conductive hearing loss, the audiogram shows an altered air conduction, i.e., outside the normal range while the bone conduction is within normal limits. It is important to say that conductive hearing loss is charac-

B. C. Buzo (✉)
Santa Casa de Sao Paulo School of Medical Science Hearing and Speech Science Program, São Paulo, Brazil

Department of Research, Cochlear LATAM, Panamá City, Panamá
e-mail: bcagnacci@cochlear.com

S. Catherine Catenacci · G. Raquel Levy
Department of Otolaryngology, Clinica Universidad de Los Andes, Santiago, Chile
e-mail: ccatenacci@clinicauandes.cl; rlevy@clinicauandes.cl

M. V. Goycoolea et al. (eds.), *Textbook of Otitis Media*, https://doi.org/10.1007/978-3-031-40949-3_36

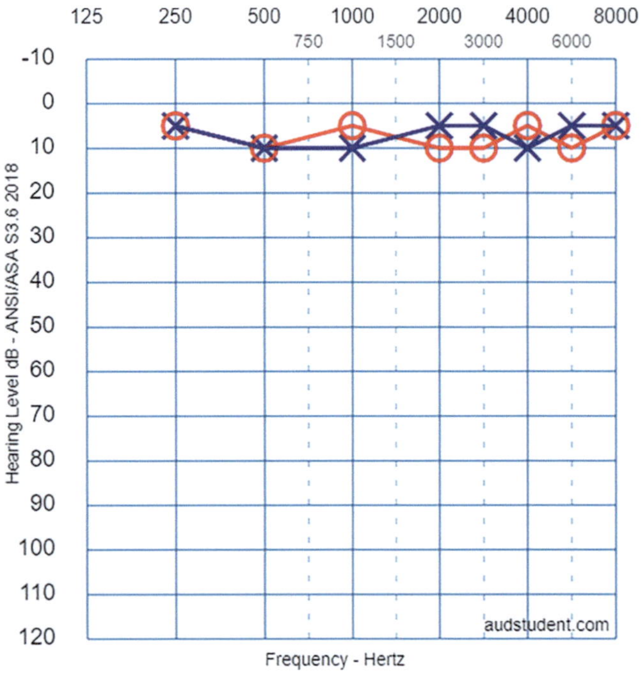

Fig. 36.1 Audiogram and symbols. Audiogram displaying the hearing threshold levels within the normal ranges in accordance with WHO [1]

terized by a difference between air and bone thresholds called air-bone GAP (Fig. 36.2).

Hearing loss is classified by different grades. This classification is given by the average of the air conduction thresholds of 500, 1000, 2000, and 4000 Hz, which we call PTA4 (pure tone average – 4). Thus, conductive hearing loss can be mild (PTA4 = 20 < 35 dB HL), moderate (PTA4 = 35 < 50 dB), until reaching its highest stage, which is moderately severe (PTA4 = 50 < 65 dB HL).

If recurrent infections continue, damage occurs at the inner ear level. In these cases, the bone conduction deterioration begins to increase. Therefore, for air thresholds over 65 dB HL, hearing loss should already be expected to be of the mixed type, which is plotted in the audiograms below (Fig. 36.3).

When we talk about chronic otitis, we refer to a repetitive process over time, a hearing loss that is installed and will probably increase if its cause is not stopped. As previously mentioned, this presents a very complicated scenario for children in the language development stage, if they have long-standing hearing loss. It is urgent to rehabilitate these patients' hearing.

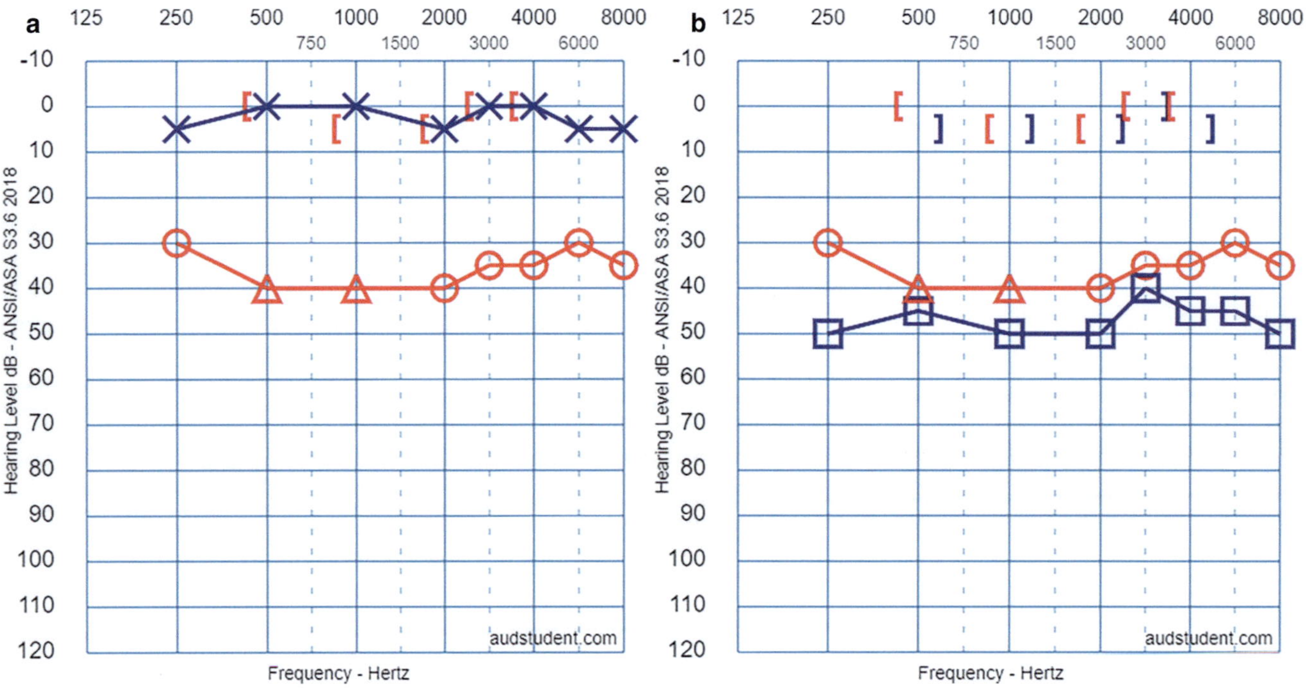

Fig. 36.2 (**a**) Conductive Hearing loss right ear. (**b**) Bilateral conductive hearing loss

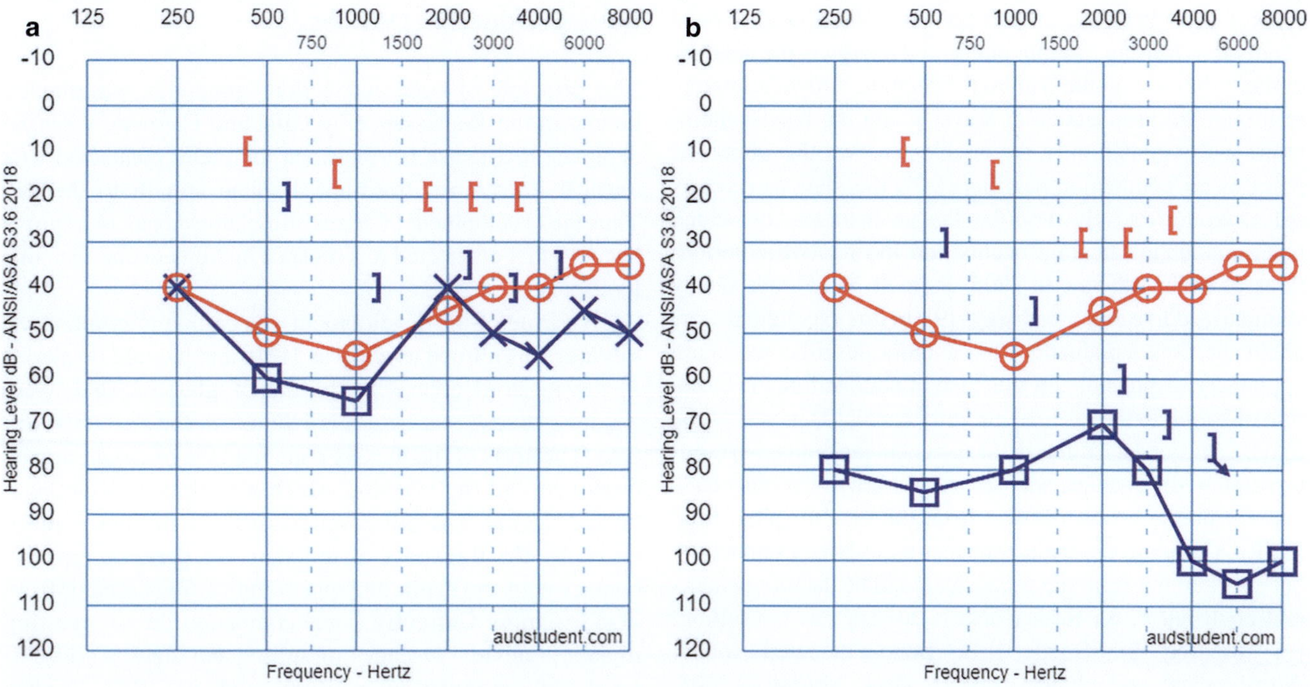

Fig. 36.3 (**a**) Mixed hearing loss left ear, conductive hearing loss right ear. (**b**) Bilateral mixed hearing loss: severe in left ear and moderate in right ear

Thinking About Hearing Rehabilitation

The most logical reasoning for cases of conductive or mixed hearing loss would be the adaptation of a conventional hearing aid. However, we must start with a practical question: What effect can a conventional hearing aid produce in COM cases? Let us remember that the hearing aid has a dome or earmold that is placed in the external auditory canal of the ear that seals it partially or even totally, to transmit the sound toward the middle ear.

Auditory rehabilitation of patients with conductive or mixed hearing loss due to chronic otitis media (COM) can be challenging due to surgical sequelae with anatomical abnormalities and/or susceptibility to infections [5]. In daily clinical practice, patients often find that fluid is leaking to their external auditory canals when attempting to fit a standard hearing aid [6].

Consequently, people with chronic ear infections may have difficulty using traditional hearing aids if they experience fluid drainage from the middle ear into the ear canal. In these cases, this dome or earmold, which is located in the external auditory canal, can become damp with middle ear drainage, creating a humid space that facilitates the proliferation of germs and can lead to external and/or media otitis, compromising the user's hearing performance.

For that reason, it would be necessary to adapt sound conduction devices that do not use the most conventional means for hearing, which is the air conduction. The option would be to use bone conduction. Rehabilitation using bone conduction implants (BCI) has several advantages, as it does not interfere with the local physiology and does not increase the risk of infection. Additionally, it is particularly effective in bypassing dysfunctional middle ear structures and transmitting sound directly to the inner ear. A bone conduction hearing device does not block the ear canal and does not require devices in the external auditory canal, making COM patients highly qualified for the use of this technology.

The ability of the cranial bone to conduct sound has been exploited for a long time, and such sound transmission technology is now quite widespread as we shall see below [7].

Sound Transmission by Bone Conduction

We know that sound is not transmitted in a vacuum; it requires a medium to propagate. This propagation involves a transport of energy, in the form of mechanical waves that spread through matter, in this case, bone.

These vibrations travel in the same direction in which sound propagates. It is a longitudinal wave, which is transmitted in a straight line from the point of origin, and we know that the speed of transmission of it is faster in solid bodies than in less dense bodies.

Multiple physiological mechanisms contribute to bone conduction hearing. Simply put, sound energy is the conduction of vibrations in the skull to the cochlea, which ultimately results in the propagation of waves along the basilar membrane and stimulation of the cochlear nerve: the same end point as air conduction hearing[8]. To this day, research is still ongoing to fully describe the mechanisms by which bone conduction hearing occurs and the relative contributions of each pathway. In 2005, Stenfelt and Goode nicely summarized five major pathways [9]. In this excellent review about the bone conduction, the authors describe five main appliances responsible for this type of conduction: (1) radiation of sound to the external auditory canal, (2) inertia of the middle ear bones, (3) inertia of the cochlear fluids, (4) compression of the cochlear walls (compression of the inner ear), and (5) pressure transmission from the cerebrospinal fluid (CSF). These are the main contributors to bone conduction, but cochlear fluids inertia is considered to be the most important contributor; for further details, we suggest consulting: [9] (Stenfelt S., Goode R.L. Bone-conducted sound: Physiological and clinical aspects. Otol. Neurotol. 2005; 26:1245–1261).

Hence, in the words of Professor Stefan Stenfelt, "direct stimulation of the cochlea by bone-conducted sound is achieved through inertia of the cochlear fluids and compression and expansion of the cochlear space. The first refers to the set of windows (oval window and round window) mainly, and the second, to the movement of the bone surrounding the cochlea that compresses and expands the cochlear space in phase with the bone movement wave" [10].

Under these physical concepts of sound transmission, it is clear that acoustic cochlea stimulation can be achieved by bypassing the outer and middle ear. From this arises the technology of bone conduction devices (BCDs). These devices take advantage of the above mechanisms by converting sound energy into skull vibrations. Since the initial work of Tjellström et al. [11], numerous commercial devices have been introduced, including surgically implanted devices and devices simply superimposed on the skull bone. These devices are intended to assist with auditory rehabilitation for patients with conductive or mixed hearing loss who cannot use conventional air conduction hearing aids or even for patients with single-sided deafness. The ability to use conventional transcranial devices is highly limited by recurrent infections such as chronic otitis externa, previous surgical intervention and altered physiology, microtia or anotia, canal atresia or stenosis, or other anatomical limitations. In the unilaterally deaf population, bone conduction devices direct transcranial signals to the contralateral normal hearing cochlea.

Bone Conduction Devices

This principle of bone conduction stimulation was already known in the Renaissance by Girolamo Cardano, when he demonstrated that a rod between the teeth, connected to a musical instrument, transmitted sound stimuli to the ear. Thus the development of dental stimulators began to improve hearing, first connected to a musical instrument and then to a loudspeaker.

By virtue of the development of a carbon microphone, a vibrator was refined as early as 1950, and it could be placed in the mastoid area with the aid of glasses. They were "audio-glasses" that held this vibrator in the retroauricular area. The arms of the glasses contained the microphone, the amplifier, and the vibrator, which are applied to the bone behind the ear. The effectiveness of these devices is influenced by the thickness of the skin, the pressure exerted, contact with the skull, and any complications arising from skin irritation. Currently, some companies are re-investing in such a device. Decades of subsequent studies corroborated this stimulation pathway and in 1977, Anders Tjellstrom implanted the first bone vibrator onto mastoid [12].

Thus, a bone conduction device is an alternative to a conventional hearing aid for those with outer or middle ear problems. The device transmits sound by bone vibration directly to the cochlea, bypassing the outer and middle ear. This means it is useful for conductive and mixed hearing loss, which the cochlea still works to send sounds to the brain with the aim of achieving aural rehabilitation for patients.

Nowadays, we have several types of bone conduction devices, which allow us to choose the most appropriate fit for each patient, adapting each to their hearing characteristics and needs. They are divided by their amplification characteristics (passive or active), sound transmission (percutaneous or transcutaneous), and technology (electromagnetic and piezoelectric). Moreover, they could be implantable or non-implantable, and osseointegrated or anchored. In the following section, each of them will be presented.

Types of Bone Conduction Devices

Bone conduction devices transform acoustic sound waves into mechanical vibrations, which are conducted to the inner ear through direct contact with the skull. As already mentioned, the contact with the skull can be classified into two main groups: percutaneous devices and transcutaneous devices (Fig. 36.4).

The major difference between the two types is that in percutaneous devices an abutment is surgically positioned on

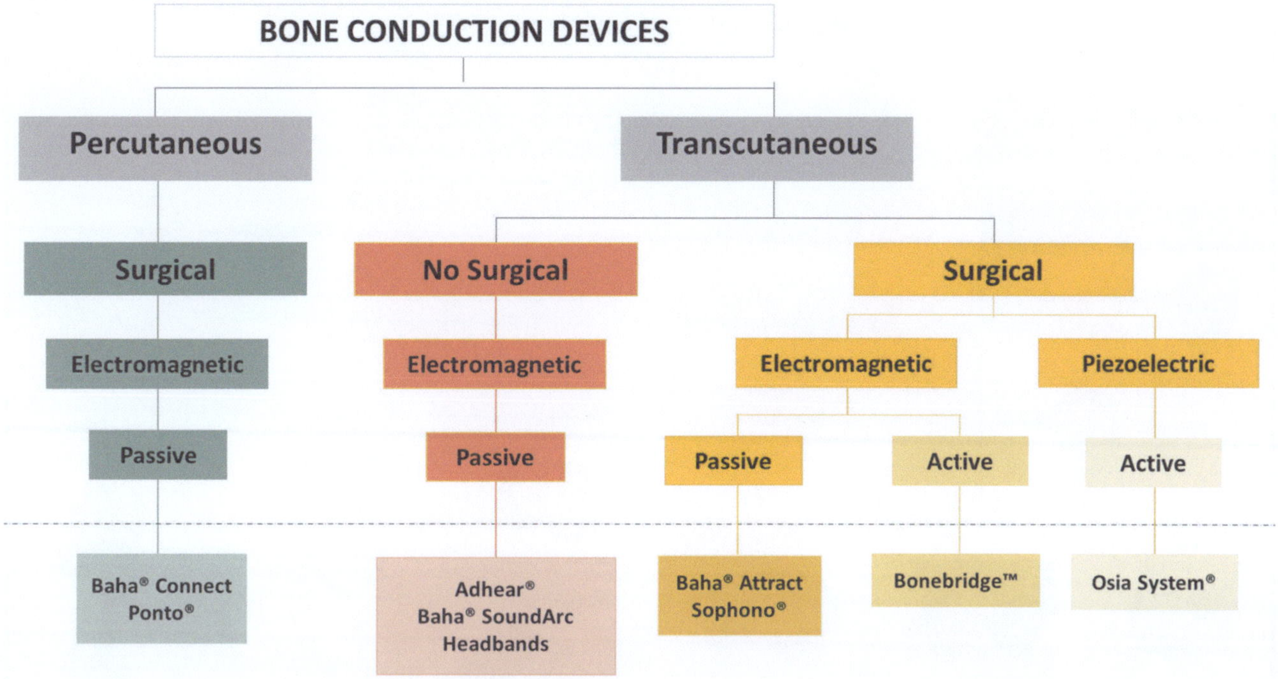

Fig. 36.4 Diagram showing present modalities of bone conduction devices

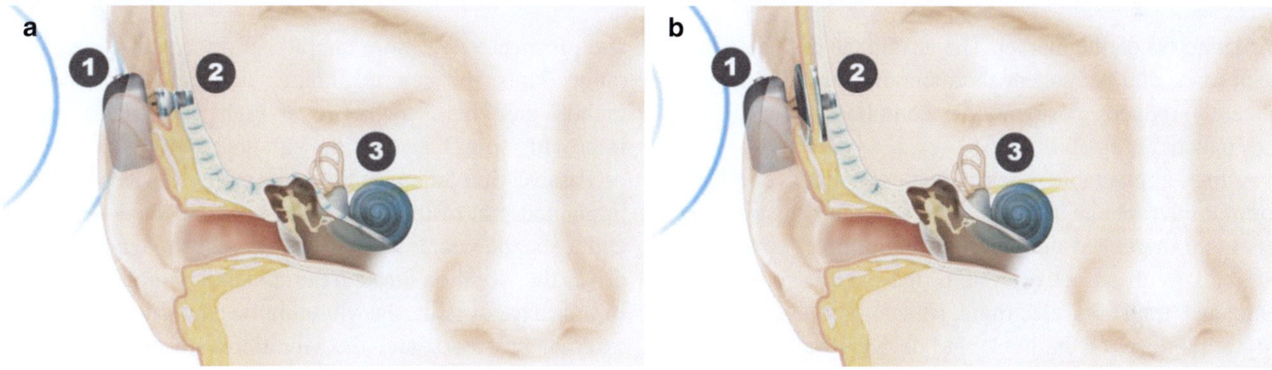

Fig. 36.5 (**a**) Percutaneous device. (**b**) Transcutanous device. (*1*) The sound processors captures sounds in the air. (*2*) The sound processor turns the sound into vibrations and sends them through the abutment (**a**) or magnetic (**b**) connection to the implant. (*3*) The implant transmits the vibrations through the bone directly to your inner ear. *Source: images courtesy of Cochlear®*

the skin connecting the processor to the internal implant, while in transcutaneous devices two magnets will make the connection between the processor and the internal implant (Fig. 36.5).

Percutaneous: Percutaneous implants have a skin-penetrating abutment that transmits sound vibrations very efficiently because it does not suffer from attenuation of the skin and soft tissues of the skull. While the vibration is transmitted more successfully by the skin-penetrating abutment, such a coupling system potentially leads to infections and chronic at the abutment site. Technological improvements tend to reduce infection resistance and skin tolerance [13]. However, its acceptance by some patients remains being psychologically difficult [14].

All percutaneous devices are considered passive, as all vibrations transmitted to the skull are generated by the external processors and from there, transmitted via the abutment to the bone implant within the skull bone. Some of commercial brands are Baha®Connect (Cochlear BAS, Sweden) and Ponto (Oticon Medical AB) (Fig. 36.6).

Transcutaneous: The skin limitations observed with percutaneous devices have led manufacturers to seek a solution for direct energy transmission to the bone with the skin closed. As a result, in 2012, a transcutaneous active implant

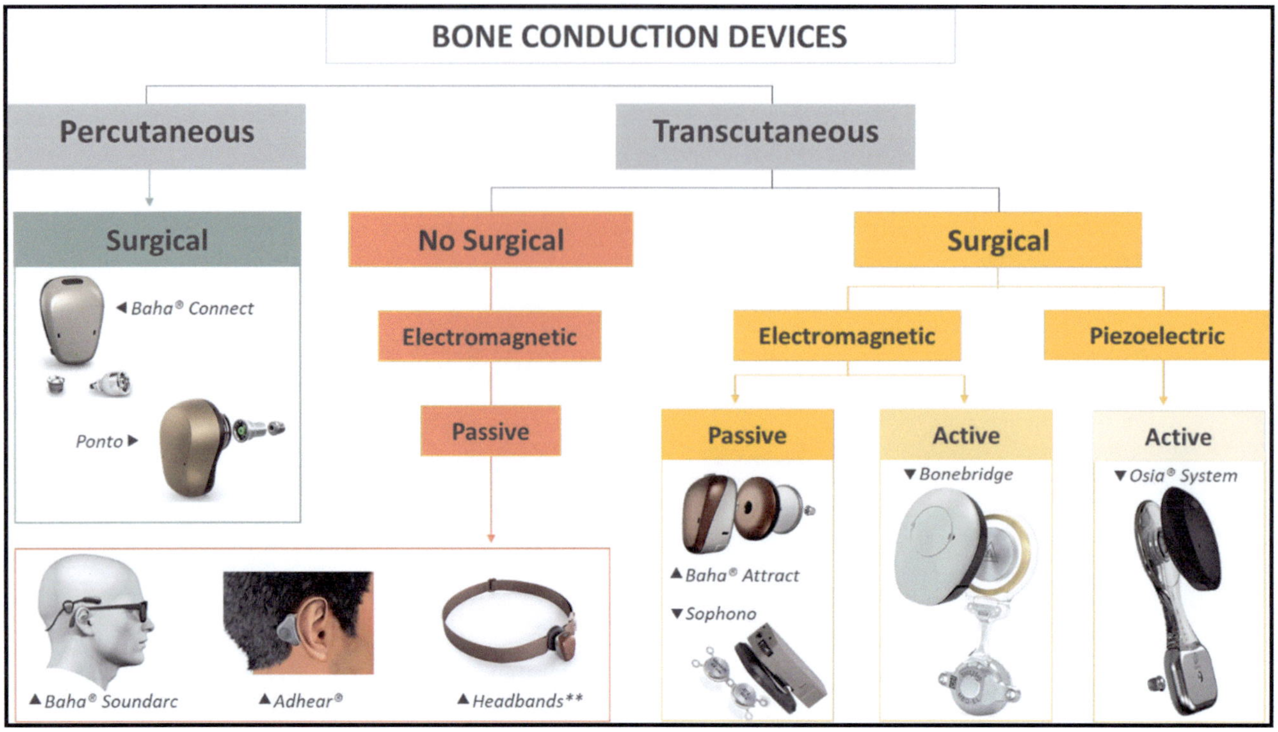

Fig. 36.6 Devices commercial names. ** Headbands are commercially available as *Baha® Start(Cochlear BAS), Alpha 2 sound processor on a headband Sophono® (Medtronic), Ponto Softband (Oticon Medical AB)*

was launched on the market. The advantage of this device is the absence of a permanent abutment in the head, which significantly reduces postoperative complications and facilitates patient acceptability [15].

Active implantable transcutaneous devices contain an external microphone and processor that send electronic signals to an implanted vibrating device in direct contact with the skull. With an active system, the external processor is static and transmits electronic signals. Vibration happens only at the level of the implanted device. Available devices are *Bonebridge (MED-EL)* and *Osia® System (Cochlear BAS)* (Fig. 36.6). Although both are active, the amplification mechanisms are different.

Bonebridge (MED-EL) has a floating mass electromagnetic transducer attached by cortical screws to the cranial bone that transmits vibrations to the bone without soft tissue attenuation. The external processor is fixed to the subcutaneous coil by a magnet that transmits information and energy to the implant. The bone conduction floating mass transducer under closed skin minimizes skin complications and provides direct connection to the bone with greater efficiency compared to external vibrators through closed skin. The great difference between *Osia® System (Cochlear BAS)*and *Bonebridge(MED-EL)*is the *Osia®* has an amplification generated by a piezoelectric system, which is far superior, mainly because of its low impedance at high frequencies and, respectively, more amplification on that frequency range. Thus, the new technology is capable of generating greater gain never achieved at high frequencies, mainly improving speech distinction with noise [16].

Passive implantable transcutaneous devices have an implanted part of the device directly connected to the skull and a separate external part held in place magnetically that drives the vibration through the skin to the implanted device. In a passive system, the vibration occurs at the level of the external processor and the vibrations are transmitted in a transcutaneous manner to the implanted device. Available commercial options are *Baha® Attract (Cochlear BAS)* and *Sophono® (Medtronic)* (Fig. 36.6).

Still, transcutaneous passive devices could be divided in implanted and non-implantable devices: The first generations of bone conduction systems were the passive and non-implantable transcutaneous devices. An external vibrator is held with a headband on the skin behind the ear. In fact, the skin and soft tissues attenuate sound mainly at high frequencies, and this attenuation varies according to the frequency and can attenuate from 8 to 20 dB [17].

The headbands (Fig. 36.6) allow to test the devices, or to use them prior to surgery. This is how pediatric population, while waiting to meet the presurgical anatomical requirements, stimulates their hearing early. It is very important that the child perceives the benefit of these devices and develops an attachment to them. They are commercially available as *Baha® Start(Cochlear BAS), Alpha 2 sound processor on a headbandSophono® (Medtronic),* and *Ponto Softband (Oticon Medical AB).*

For those who need a different nonsurgical option of headbands, *Baha®SoundArc* (Cochlear BAS) (Fig. 36.6) could be an excellent option. It allows high-quality demonstrations, evaluations, and trials with the Baha processors. The *Baha®SoundArc (Cochlear BAS)* was designed to sit above the ears and be worn behind the head, with the Baha sound processor attached to a connector disk just behind the ear.

Finally, instead of headbands it still is available an adhesive nonsurgical solution composed of two parts: the thin adhesive adapter and the audio processor. The adhesive adapter is glued behind the ear in the area where there is no hair. Its commercial name is *Adhear® (MED-EL)* (Fig. 36.6).

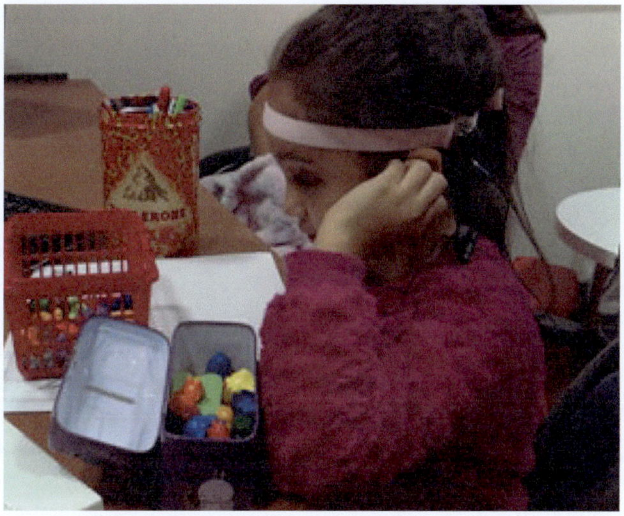

Fig. 36.7 Bone conduction audiometry (in situ)

Evaluation of Bone Conduction Device Candidates

When choosing a bone conduction device, many factors must be considered. Each patient has unique needs that are related to their degree and type of hearing impairment, anatomy, vocational or educational needs, and personal preferences. Finding this information in a consolidated location can be a challenge for patients and providers.

In the evaluation of candidates, several aspects of the audiological and medical indications are analyzed as well as integral aspects to the patient such as age, living environment, lifestyle and work environment, expectations regarding the results, motivation, family support, their education, and the possibility of follow-ups. Candidates for a bone conduction device directly attend the audiology department after being referred by the otolaryngologist. An interview with the audiologist is scheduled so that they can get to know the device and clarify their doubts. The patient wants to see the device, its size, its texture, color options, among others, to imagine their personal appearance while wearing it. Thus, the esthetic factor is very important.

Once these aspects are examined, a test of the bone conduction device is performed, instance in which the patient can test how the bone conduction amplification would work.

Through the programming software, a sound processor anchored to a headband is calibrated and placed around the patient's head, positioning the processor in the mastoid region. This device is calibrated mainly on the basis of previous audiometry and in situ tests (bone conduction audiometry) allowed by the calibration software (Fig. 36.7).

Once the processor is calibrated, the patient is able to feel and experience hearing again through the bone conduction device, although we know that once the patient is operated, the benefit will be greater after.

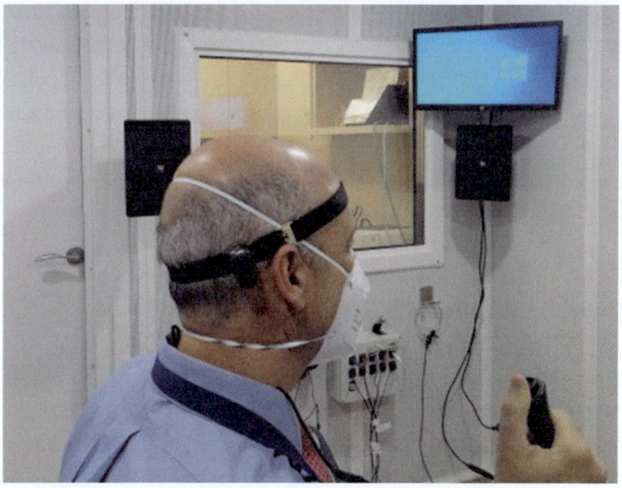

Fig. 36.8 Free-field audiometry to measure functional gain of the speech processor

Candidates for a bone conduction device directly attend the audiology department after being referred by the otolaryngologist. An interview with the audiologist is scheduled so that they can learn about the device and clarify their doubts. The patient wants to see the device, its size, its texture, its color options, among others, to imagine their personal appearance while wearing it, and the esthetic factor is very important.

The final performance of the device is studied in a silent camera with free-field audiometry (Fig. 36.8).

At this time, surgical procedures related to bone conduction implants are minimally invasive with increasingly simplified surgical techniques and a postsurgical period very well tolerated by the patient that allows them to resume his usual activities promptly.

The minimum age for implantation varies according to the device chosen and the ones authorized by the regulatory authority that governs the country. For instance, the minimum age for implanting an active conduction device such as *Osia® System (Cochlear BAS)* according to the FDA in the United States is 12 years and for European countries governed by the EC is 5 years.

Usually, the surgeon requests an ear scanner to verify that the bone thickness of the calotte allows the anchorage of the implant. For example, in the case of the implants which require osseointegration of a titanium implant of 3 or 4 mm, it will require a bone thickness the measures above mentioned. In addition to the ear scanner, routine presurgical examinations will be requested following health condition of each patient.

The initial fitting procedure for the sound processor should be scheduled approximately four weeks after the operation, for example, in *Osia® System or Baha® Attract Systems(Cochlear BAS)*. In the event that the tissue is still too swollen, consider a later fitting. Fitting should be checked in regular intervals as per clinic protocol.

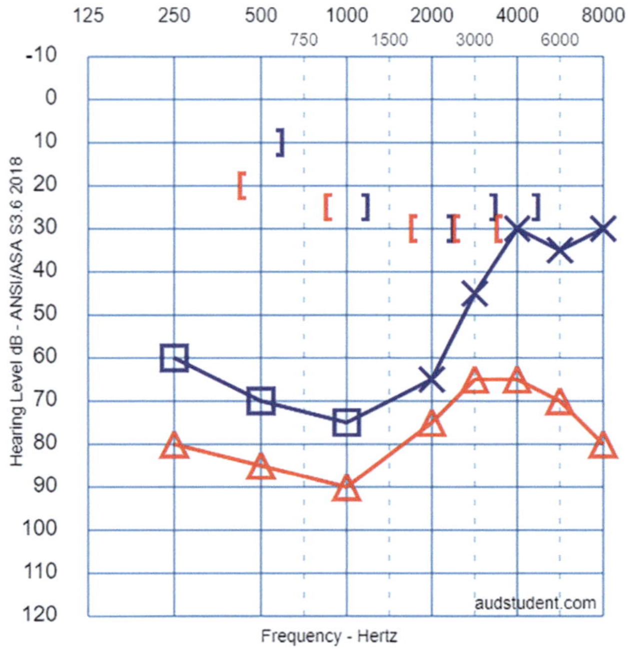

Fig. 36.9 Audiogram shows bilateral mixed hearing loss

Clinical Cases

Case 1: Bone Conduction Device—Passive, Transcutaneous, and Piezoelectric

A 56-year-old woman, with a history of bilateral chronic otitis media since childhood, has undergone several tympanoplasties in both ears. As of now, the right ear has an opaque and scarred eardrum, but it is closed and does not ooze, and she consistently wears a hearing aid in that ear. In the left ear, the eardrum is perforated.

The patient is an active woman who works daily and requires better hearing.

The audiometry shows a mixed hearing loss in both ears (Fig. 36.9), with significant air–osseous gap in the low frequencies and good discrimination of disyllabic words (left ear: 96% at 95 dB and right ear: 88% at 100 dB).

A softband with sound processor test was performed in the left ear, considering direct bone conduction and piezoelectric technology as the best option for the perforated eardrum conditionin this ear.

The patient reported immediate improvement during device testing and underwent left ear surgery on 2018 with a passive, transcutaneous, and piezoelectric bone conduction implant.

Today, in 2022, the patient is still a consistent user of a hearing aid in her right ear and she made an upgrade for the sound processor in her left ear.

The latter processor features innovative speech sound processing and optimal noise handling, which greatly facilitates speech distinction in different sound environments.

Case 2: Bone Conduction Device—Passive, Transcutaneous, and Piezoelectric

This case is that of a 30-year old woman, architect, and very active at work, who consulted an ENT doctor in October 2021. The audiological examination shows mixed hearing loss with an average pure tone of 90 dBs HL in the right ear by air conduction and neurosensorial hearing loss in the left ear (Fig. 36.10).

Physical examination showed microtia of the right ear with stenosis of the external auditory canal. Radiological examinations, on the other hand, showed malformation of the middle ear ossicles.

She reported having undergone cosmetic ear surgery a few years earlier.

We proceeded to test a headband with a sound processor on the patient so that she could feel the performance of the external device, and she reacted positively to the test, stating that no conventional hearing aid previously tested had achieved such audiological performance.

She underwent surgery on her right ear with a *passive, transcutaneous, and piezoelectric bone conduction implant* on December 21, 2021.

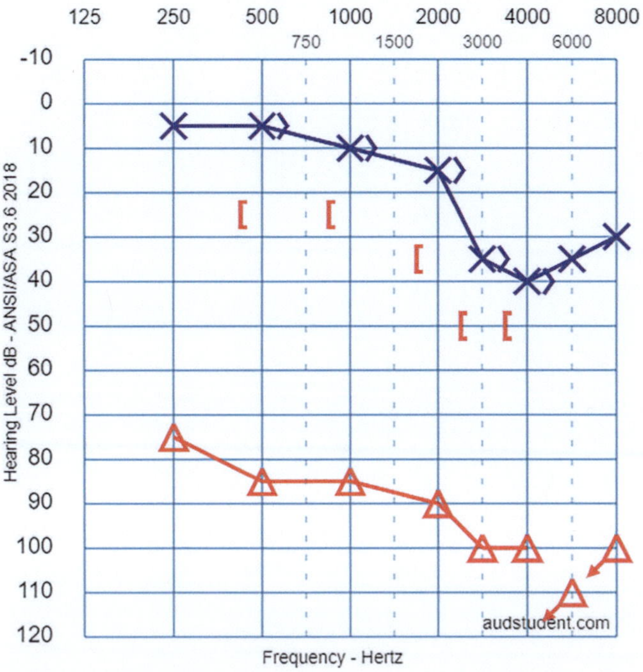

Fig. 36.10 Audiogram, October 2021

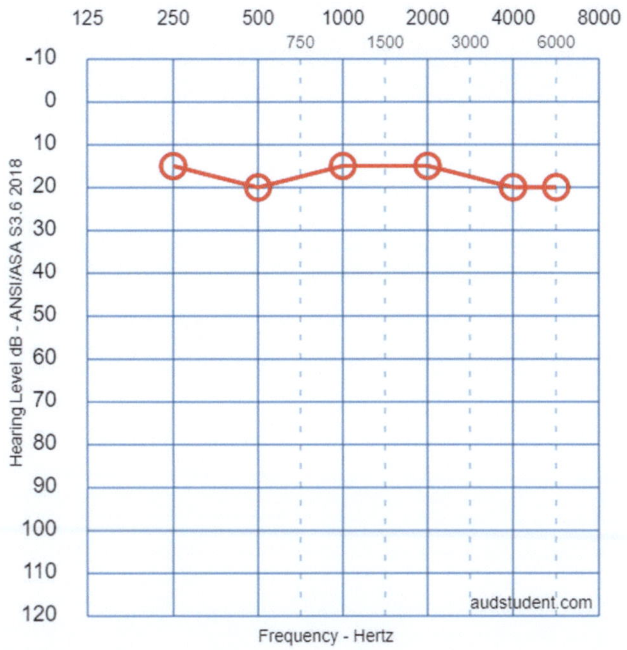

Fig. 36.11 Free-field audiometry with *a bone conduction device*

She is an excellent user of the bone conduction device who has never presented a problem with the adhesion of the magnet and her skin, and her performance in a free-field audiometry is shown in Fig. 36.11 that shows a great improvement at low and high frequencies.

References

1. WHO Deafness and Hearing Loss. https://www.who.int/en/news-room/fact-sheets/detail/deafness-and-hearing-loss. Accessed November 6, 2020.
2. Monasta L, Ronfani L, Marchetti F, et al. Burden of disease caused by otitis media: systematic review and global estimates. PLoS One. 2012;7:e36226. https://doi.org/10.1371/journal.pone.0036226.
3. Kral A, O'Donoghue GM. Profound deafness in childhood. N Engl J Med. 2010;363(15):1438–50. https://doi.org/10.1056/nejmra0911225.
4. Dobrianskyj FM, Rocha DGÍ, Tamaoki Y, et al. Correlation between sensorineural hearing loss and chronic otorrhea. Ear Nose Throat J. 2019;98:482–5. https://doi.org/10.1177/0145561319840573.
5. Håkansson B, Tjellström A, Rosenhall U, Carlsson P. The bone-anchored hearing aid. Principal design and a psychoacoustical evaluation. Acta Otolaryngol. 1985;100(3–4):229–39.
6. Gluth MB, Friedman AB, Atcherson SR, Dornhoffer JL. Hearing aid tolerance after revision and obliteration of canal wall down mastoidectomy cavities. Otol Neurotol. 2013;34:711–4. https://doi.org/10.1097/MAO.0b013e31828daeca.
7. McLarnon CM, Davison T, Johnson IJ. Bone-anchored hearing aid: comparison of benefit by patient subgroups. Laryngoscope. 2004;114(5):942–4.
8. Stenfelt S. Acoustic and physiologic aspects of bone conduction hearing. Adv Otorhinolaryngol. 2011;71:10–21.
9. Stenfelt S, Goode RL. Bone-conducted sound: physiological and clinical aspects. OtolNeurotol. 2005;26:1245–61. https://doi.org/10.1097/01.mao.0000187236.10842.d5.
10. Stenfelt S. Cochlear boundary motion during bone conduction stimulation: implications for inertial and compressional excitation of the cochlea. In: AIP conference proceedings (vol. 1703, no. 1). AIP Publishing; 2015.
11. Tjellström A, Lindström J, Hallén O, Albrektsson T, Brånemark PI. Osseointegrated titanium implants in the temporal bone. A clinical study on bone-anchored hearing aids. Am J Otol. 1981;2:304–10.
12. Mudry A, Tjellström A. Historical background of bone conduction hearing devices and bone conduction hearing aids. In: Implantable bone conduction hearing aids, vol. 71. Karger Publishers; 2011. p. 1–9. https://doi.org/10.1159/000323569.
13. D'Eredità R, Caroncini M, Saetti R. The new Baha implant: a prospective osseointegration study. Otolaryngol Head Neck Surg. 2012;146(6):979–83.
14. Zawawi F, Kabbach G, Lallemand M, Daniel SJ. Bone-anchored hearing aid: why do some patients refuse it? Int J PediatrOtorhinolaryngol. 2014;78(2):232–4.
15. Riss D, Arnoldner C, Baumgartner WD, Blineder M, Flak S, Bachner A, et al. Indication criteria and outcomes with the Bonebridge transcutaneous bone-conduction implant. Laryngoscope. 2014;124(12):2802–6.
16. Goycoolea M, Ribalta G, Tocornal F, Levy R, Alarcón P, Bryman M, Cagnacci B, Catenacci C, Oyanguren V, Vilches I, Briones V, García R. Clinical performance of the Osia™ system, a new active osseointegrated implant system. Results from a prospective clinical investigation. Acta Otolaryngol. 2020;140(3):212–9.
17. Verstraeten N, Zarowski AJ, Somers T, Riff D, Offeciers EF. Comparison of the audiologic results obtained with the bone-anchored hearing aid attached to the headband, the testband, and to the "snap" abutment. Otol Neurotol. 2009;30(1):70–5.

37 Pathogenesis of Chronic Otitis Media and the Continuum: The Basics, Further and Beyond

Sady Selaimen da Costa and Michael M. Paparella

Otitis Media: The Basics

Otitis media (OM) is defined as an inflammatory process (associated or not to infection), in the middle ear cleft (MEC) [1–3]. It might affect the ME as a whole (generalized) or focally. It is one of the most prevalent infectious diseases being associated with an immense social impact worldwide [4]. The morbidity (and even mortality) of this condition still poses a formidable challenge to otolaryngologists, pediatricians, and generalists.

Due to its immense social impact, otitis media has been exhaustively studied, but even so, a consensus on its complete understanding is far from being achieved. Pending questions remain regarding the epidemiology, pathogenesis, and treatment of this condition. Even the classification and definition of otitis media among its different subgroups is very controversial. It is clear the struggle of the authors to agree upon a definitive classification which would only be unquestionable if it could accommodate all features of a given subgroup. As an example, the so-called acute otitis media (AOM), as a rule, would be always associated with a suppurative, purulent, or mucopurulent component. However, in special situations—such as large variations in atmospheric pressure—a typical serous collection can suddenly develop filling completely the middle ear. In the same way, a wide perforation of the *pars tensa* of the tympanic membrane (TM) can arise as a sudden complication in the course of some infectious disease (measles as an example) or as a consequence of a temporal bone trauma [5].

Years ago, an International Study Group was organized to discuss topics related to otitis media. According to the conclusions of this committee, the following classification was proposed [6].

Suppurative Otitis Media
- Acute (AOM)
- Chronic otitis media without cholesteatoma (NCCOM)
- Chronic otitis media with cholesteatoma (CCOM)

Nonsuppurative Otitis Media
- Serous (SOM)
- Secretory (MOM)

The same committee defined chronic otitis media as an inflammatory condition always associated with a perforation of the tympanic membrane (TM) and otorrhea. This definition is quite traditional and has been echoed in many publications around the world [5–10].

Chronologically, acute otitis media is defined as a short duration inflammatory process with a gap between its beginning and resolution no longer than three weeks. This gap is extended to three months when subacute otitis media is considered and the term chronic is reserved only for those cases when, even after three months, the resolution does not ensue.

We will adopt this classification (although we recognize that it is incomplete and subject to well-founded criticism) as a starting point for future discussions. The authors themselves identify its obvious limitations, remembering that this is just another "working" classification widely publicized and, therefore, simple and accessible. It fulfills purely didactic objectives as we seek new operational hypotheses in relation to the pathogenesis of OM. In this sense, several works have demonstrated that the mechanisms involved in the

S. S. da Costa (✉)
Department of Otolaryngology, Head and Neck Surgery, School of Medicine-Universidade Federal do Rio Grande do Sul, Porto Alegre, Brazil

International Hearing Foundation, Minneapolis, MN, USA

American Academy of Otolaryngology and Head & Neck Surgery, Alexandria, VA, USA

Department of Otolaryngology, University of Minnesota, Otopathology Laboratory, Minneapolis, MN, USA

M. M. Paparella
American Academy of Otolaryngology and Head & Neck Surgery, Alexandria, VA, USA

Department of Otolaryngology, University of Minnesota, Otopathology Laboratory, Minneapolis, MN, USA

M. V. Goycoolea et al. (eds.), *Textbook of Otitis Media*, https://doi.org/10.1007/978-3-031-40949-3_37

installation and perpetuation of the ME inflammatory processes are much more complex [2, 11–13].

Despite all its limitations, we will employ this working classification to build up a prototype model of pathogenesis. In this process, we will try to frame all the subgroups (AOM, SOM, MOM, NCOM, and CCOM) in a logical march from normality to chronicity. The problem is that this model, despite being attractive and easy to understand, collapses when confronted with a series of key questions that are extremely relevant and still not completely clarified. To exemplify, in the next paragraphs, we will review, point by point, the traditional concepts just exposed and their pathogenic basis, later opposing them to a second hypothesis born from the work developed by the group from Minneapolis: the so-called *continuum theory* [13].

Acute Otitis Media and Otits Media with Effusion

Acute otitis media (AOM) is a sudden, suppurative infectious process marked by the presence of infected middle ear fluid and inflammation of the mucosa lining the middle ear cleft (MEC). Mechanisms involved in its development include tubal dysfunction (secondary to physiological immaturity, obstruction, or edema resulting from upper airway infections and/or allergy) and aspiration of infected secretions from the rhino pharynx [1, 2].

Eustachian tube (ET) dysfunction, when prolonged, can cause negative pressure in the MEC with the consequent transudation of liquid from the intravascular compartment to the interstitial compartment and from there to the lumen of the MEC. This establishes the so-called serous otitis media or otitis media with effusion (OME) which may be defined as the presence of middle ear fluid without signs of acute infection.

Chronic Otitis Media with and Without Cholesteatoma

The trademark® of chronic otitis media has always been the presence of a tympanic perforation (which until then, who knows how it was produced!) [5, 7–10]. In NCCOM, this perforation can be subclassified as central or marginal. What differentiates the first from the second is the persistence (central) or not (marginal) of an eardrum remnant around the 360° of the perforation. This fibrous ring would theoretically prevent skin from the external auditory canal to migrate through the perforation gaining access to the middle ear. On the other hand, in marginal perforations (where there is a partial or complete absence of this fibrous margin), the perforation itself can work as a gateway to the middle ear (Fig. 37.1).

When not encountering any resistance, the keratinized stratified squamous epithelium from the EAC, fulfilling its renewal cycle, can penetrate the MEC. There, it develops a typical cycle to this type of epithelium when in an ectopic location: it encysts and begins to produce keratin. In other words, it gives rise to the so-called secondary cholesteatoma, secondary to a NCCOM with a marginal perforation. Important to stress that aural cholesteatoma is defined as the presence of exfoliated keratin in any pneumatized area of the temporal bone (Fig. 37.2).

The next question is as obvious as it is pertinent. If there is a secondary cholesteatoma, is there a primary cholesteatoma and, if so, how does it develop? The answer to this question is yes, but its development does not require the presence of a TM perforation since they arise from progressive TM retractions. In this regard, the region of the pars flaccida of the TM, of dimer composition, would be the most prone to suffer a progressive retraction. The evolution of this retraction follows through the stages of simple retraction (the bottom diameter is smaller than the external opening), TM

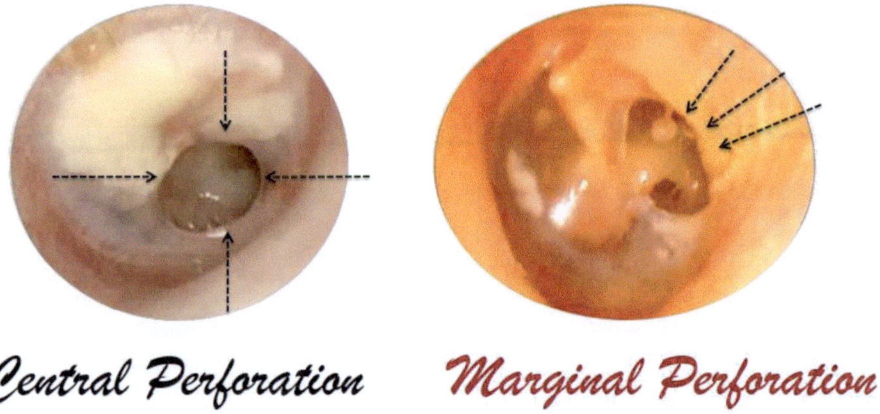

Fig. 37.1 Central X marginal perforations

retraction pocket (the bottom diameter is greater than the external opening making it prone to losing its self-cleaning properties), and cholesteatoma (when accumulation of keratin finally ensues) (Fig. 37.3). The primary cholesteatoma has two main gateways: the TM pars flaccida (attic cholesteatoma) and the TM posterior–superior quadrant (tensa cholesteatoma). Both may extend to other areas of the temporal bone following preexistent pathways created by the unique embryological development of the ME.

Potential Pitfalls of the So-Called Working Classification

All those who are dedicated to the study and care of patients with otitis media will agree that this model, despite being attractive and easy to understand, collapses when confronted with a series of key questions that are extremely relevant and still not completely clarified. In other words, with a few exceptions, we present a classification composed of well-defined (pseudo) subgroups but dissociated from each other and with many "missing links" along the way. For example:

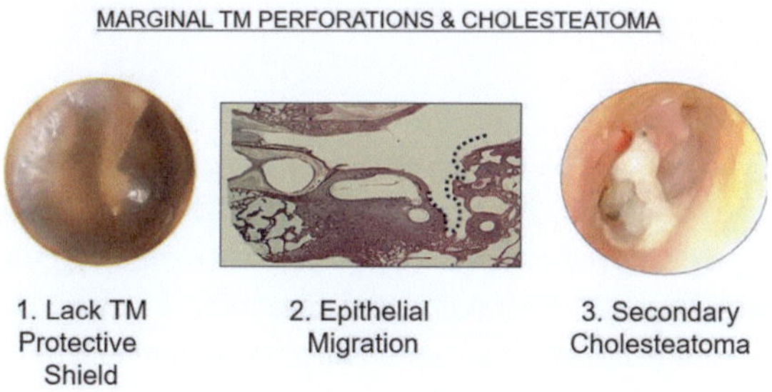

Fig. 37.2 Cholesteatoma following a marginal perforation

- What is the difference between serous and secretory (mucoid) otitis—which, incidentally, are definitions inappropriately used as synonyms or both under the umbrella name of otitis media with effusion?
- What is the connection between the eminently physical process of transudation and the complex inflammation/infection typical of suppurative and secretory (mucoid) otitis media?
- What is the origin of the wide tympanic perforations characteristic of COM (traditionally referred to as a consequence of an acute necrotizing otitis media (a very unusual condition) or induced by a temporal bone trauma that did not spontaneously heal?
- What is the reason for the frequent association between fluid and gross pathological changes within the ME?
- Why are we increasingly exploring ME filled with granulation tissue, cholesterol granuloma, and/or ossicular destruction whose tympanic membranes are intact and with an appearance close to normal?
- Why do studies demonstrate similar histopathological profiles between temporal bones with chronic otitis media and intact and perforated eardrums?
- What is the relationship between compartmentalized hypo-aeration of ME and associated pathological findings?
- Where did the concept of silent chronic otitis media come from?
- In short, there is a number of waiting to be answered questions waiting to be addressed and answered in order to bring a better and more realistic understanding in the pathogenesis of otitis media.

This is particularly true when human and animal temporal bones with OM are studied through the powerful lenses of

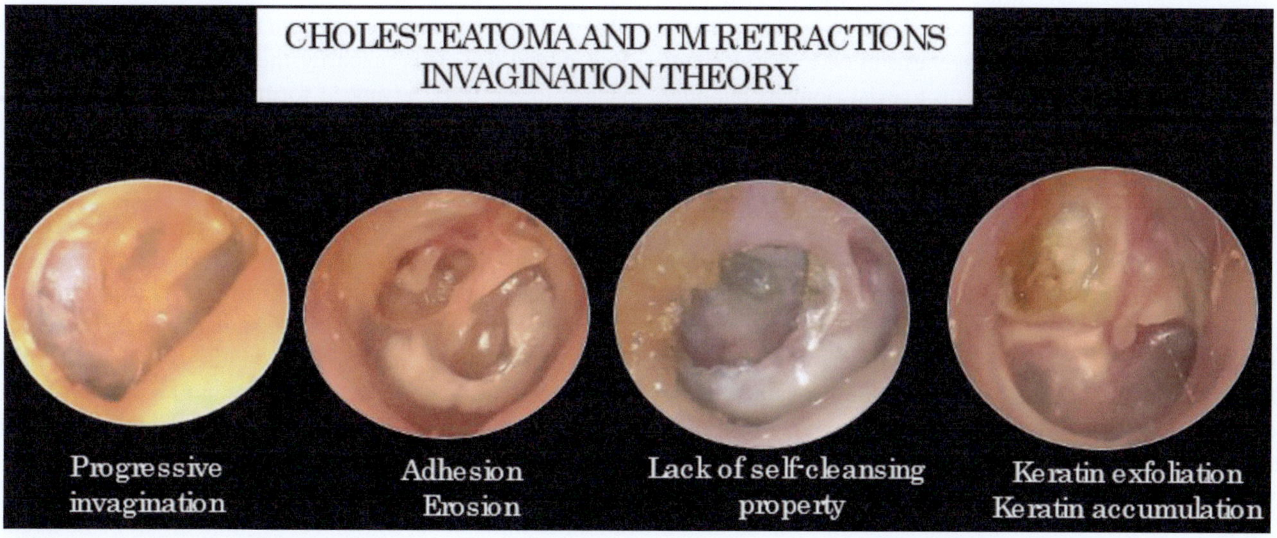

Fig. 37.3 Cholesteatoma following progressive tympanic membrane retractions

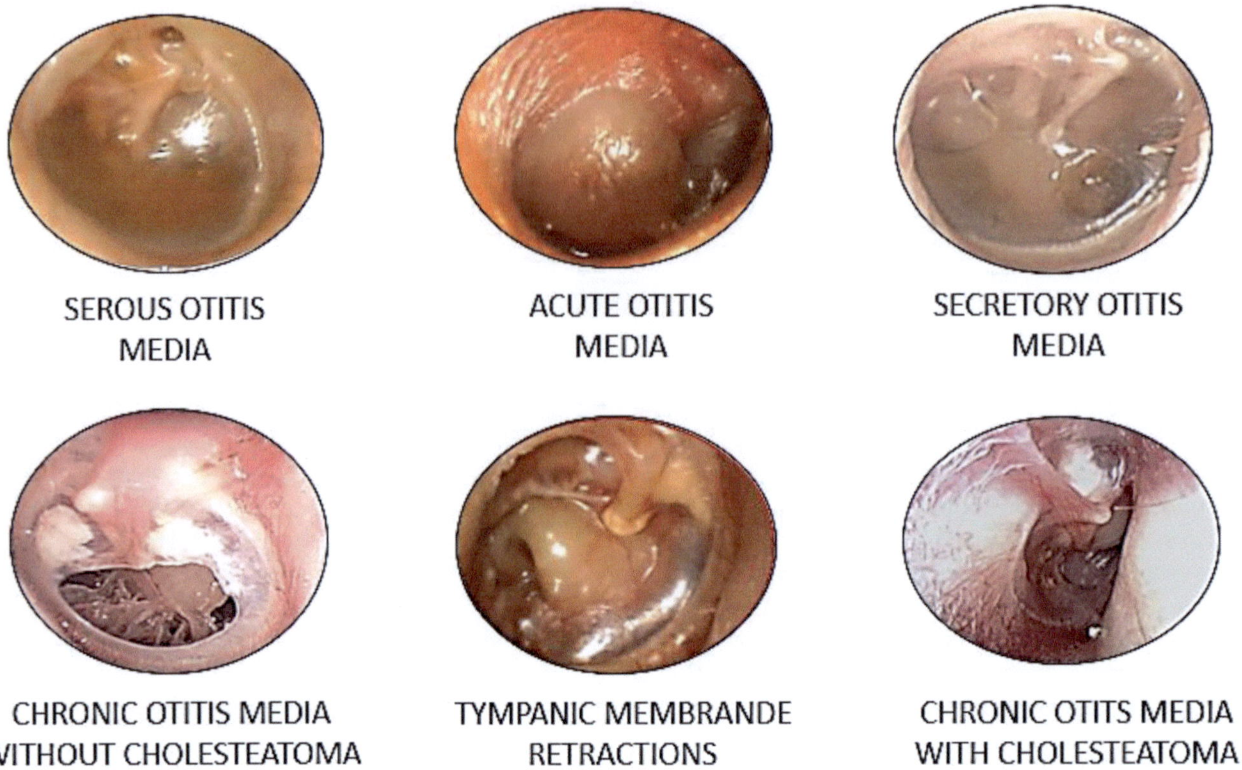

Fig. 37.4 Otitis media continuum

last-generation microscopes by the most talented otopathologists. These studies have shown that the histopathologic boundaries between one form and another are tenuous if not intersected suggesting that we are not dealing with specific and isolated diseases but with one single condition which may evolve through progressive stages. This progression may not be linear, being influenced by cofactors generally linked to the aggressor, the subject, and facilitating or moderating circumstances. Aware of this possibility, in 1970 Paparella and colleagues suggested the hypothesis of the continuum to explain the pathogenesis of OM. According to these authors, the condition seems to exist along a continued series of events in which, after a "triggering off" insult, with early forms progressing to more chronic stages of the disease (serous or purulent OM to seromucoid, mucoid, and, eventually, chronic) (Fig. 37.4).

They also suggested that structural changes in the epithelial and subepithelial spaces of the ME would be responsible for this dynamic behavior. In their first animal model, they obstructed the ET of monkeys to develop experimental OM. After this pioneering experiment, the hypothesis of the "continuum," or that all subgroups of OM (serous, purulent, mucoid, and chronic) represent different phases of the same evolving process, has been tested and confirmed by many elegant and well-designed studies. Independently of the animal model used, they have shown that the histopathologic and biochemical profiles of these subgroups are progressive and, at one time or another, overlapped. To exemplify, in the next paragraphs, we will review, point by point, the traditional concepts just presented, and their pathogenic rationale developed by the group from Minneapolis: the so-called *continuum theory*.

Otitis Media and the Continuum Further

We will dedicate the next paragraphs to detailing how we understand the paths taken by the disease from its earliest stages to the most advanced forms. It is very important to point out that the natural history of this journey can be aborted midway by native defense barriers or by timely and efficient medical intervention.

An initial trigger, in the reversible phase of this whole process, would be functional or mechanical tubal dysfunction (persistent or temporary). Since the ET was unable to balance atmospheric and intratympanic pressures (even with the aid of voluntary maneuvers), middle ear aeration would depend exclusively on the establishment of a pressure gradient between the nasopharyngeal and tympanic extremities of the ET. This gradient would have to be big enough to displace air toward the middle ear. Physiologically, it would be obtained through the constant absorption of gas in the middle ear, which from a closed but ventilated system would be transformed, due to tubal obstruction, into a closed and non-ventilated system. In fact, this pressure regulation mechanism seems to be very common in children [6]. Persistent tubal obstruction would trigger a negative intratympanic pressure cycle that, at first, would try to be compensated by the medial displacement of the tympanic membrane and the consequent decrease in middle ear volume (Fig. 37.5).

Thus, with the contraction of the continent (middle ear space), the intratympanic pressure could be slightly modified up to certain limits. Physiologically, this limit depends on the total volume of the middle ear cleft and the speed with which the tubal obstruction is established. At this moment, the process would reach a critical limit from which a series of events could endanger the anatomical and physiological integrity of the ear:

A. An air bolus would penetrate from the nasopharynx (NF) toward the middle ear potentially carrying on contaminated secretions from the nasopharynx (NF) rich in microorganisms. Once installed in the middle ear, these microorganisms would find a favorable environment for multiplication with the consequent development of acute otitis media (AOM). This same process can be repeated several times as long as the initial triggering factor is not corrected: acute recurrent otitis media with a normal middle ear between attacks (Fig. 37.6).

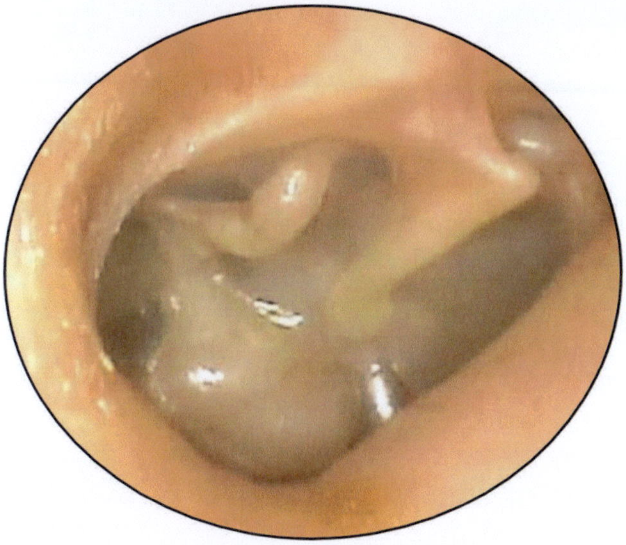

Fig. 37.5 Tympanic membrane retraction due to negative pressure in the middle ear

B. If negative pressure is sustained, the subepithelial space would react in a more or less uniform fashion, with vasodilation of small vessels by vascular engorgement caused by the vacuum increasing its thickness. Consequently, there would be an increase in intravascular hydrostatic pressure and passive plasma outflow from the vessels to the subepithelial space and from there to the lumen of the ME configuring the so-called otitis media with effusion (serous) (Fig. 37.7).

   Since, even in this phase, there is the possibility of the eustachian tube opening, the aspiration of NF secretions could, from time to time, exacerbate this condition—recurrent episodes of AOM with serous otitis media in between (Fig. 37.8).

C. The persistence of fluid in the middle ear associated with subepithelial changes and prolonged hypoxia would expose and damage the middle ear mucosa which in turn would react like any chronically attacked epithelium, that is, going through a process of metaplasia. The epithelium that is normally cuboidal or squamous would change into a secretory epithelium: pseudo-stratified columnar rich in goblet cells and submucosal glands. The mucus actively secreted by these glands would eventually fill the middle ear replacing the serous plasmatic fluid: secretory otitis media, mucoid, or glue ear (Figs. 37.9 and 37.10).

   As we have pointed out, from this stage onward the ME undergoes through a series of biological changes, that is, the epithelium provoked by environmental aggressions engages in an active process of metaplasia. The serous fluid characteristic of SOM (transudate with a low

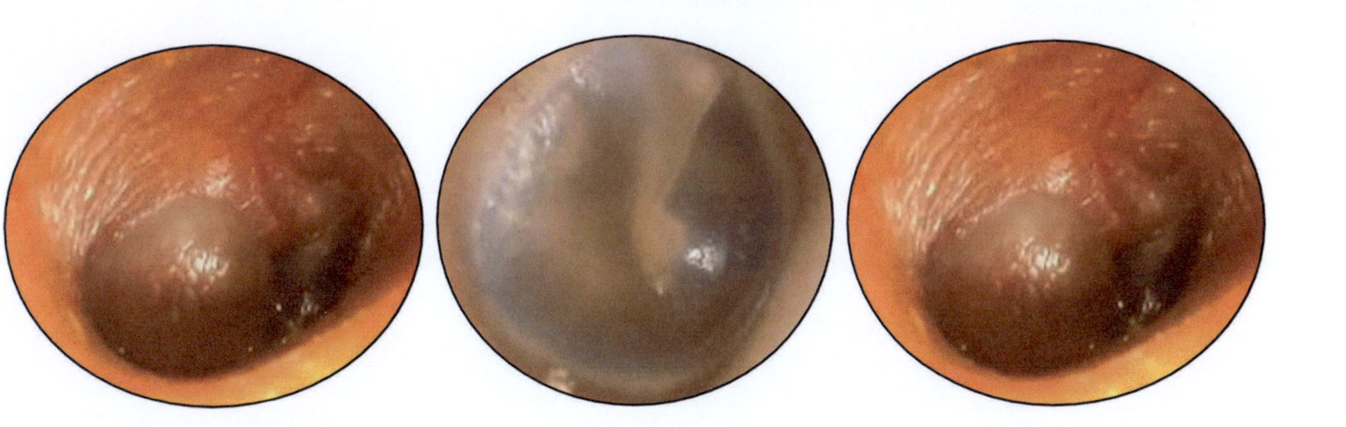

Fig. 37.6 Acute otitis media and normal middle ear in-between

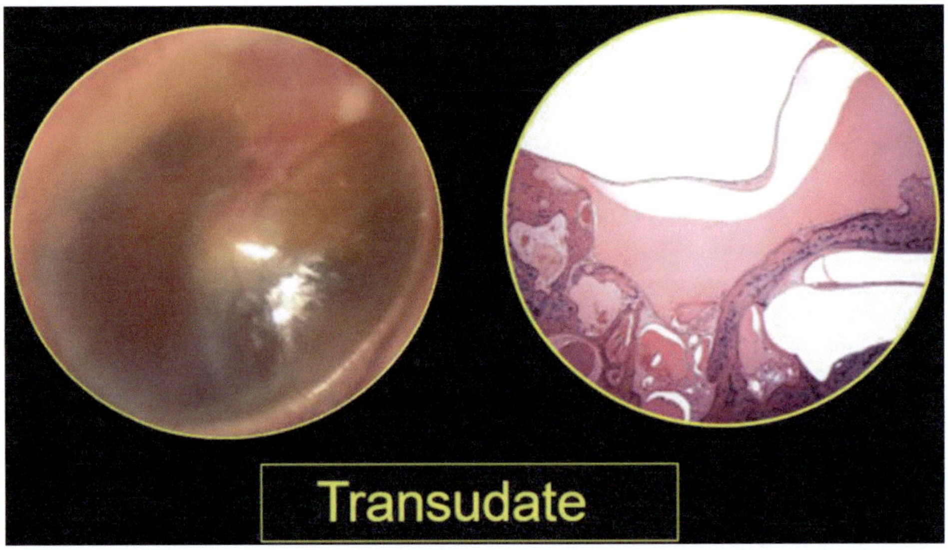

Fig. 37.7 Serous fluid (transudate) filling the middle ear space

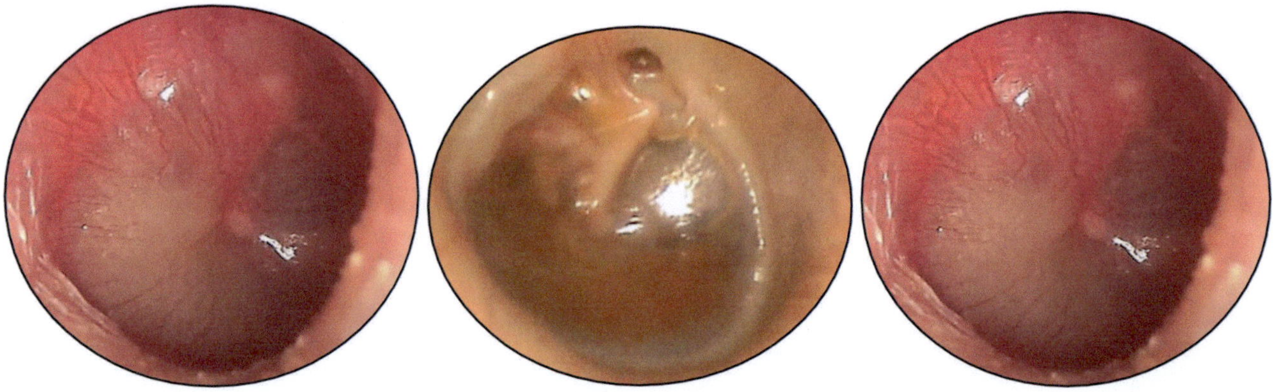

Fig. 37.8 Acute recurrent otitis media with middle ear fluid in-between bouts

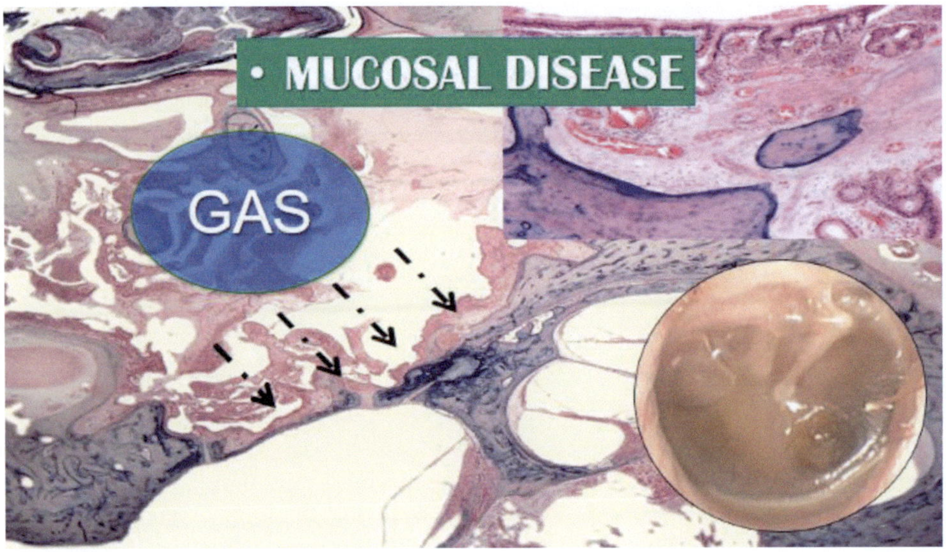

Fig. 37.9 Middle ear undergoing epithelial metaplasia and filled with mucoid fluid. Secretory otitis media.

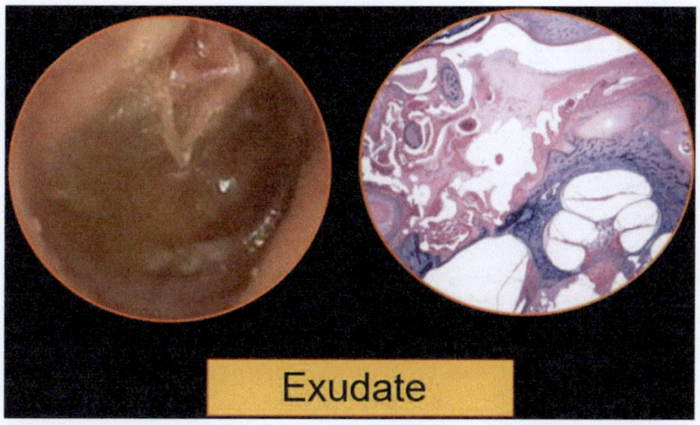

Fig. 37.10 Tympanic membrane retraction, with changes in color typical of secretory otitis media and a temporal bone section with the same findings

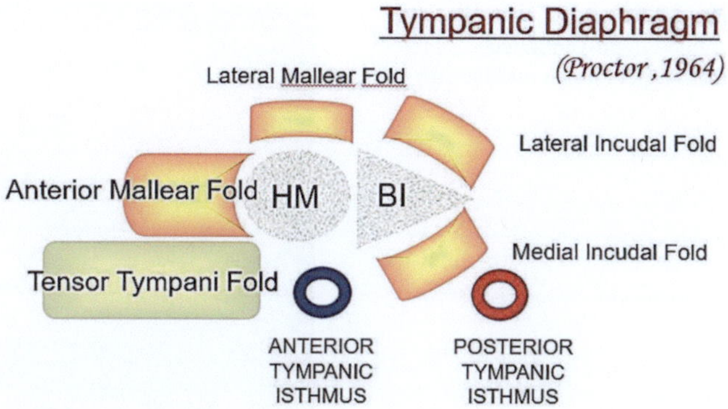

Fig. 37.11 Proctor´s tympanic diaphragm, its components, and main routes of aeration

protein concentration) would be progressively replaced by a mucoid, thick secretion with high levels of proteins (exudate), the transition between one phase and the next is clinically difficult to determine.

Appropriate clinical therapy at any of these stages could permanently reverse them as long as the triggering factors are properly identified and treated (medical treatments or surgery like ventilation tubes insertion). Spontaneous resolution could also occur at this stage.

D. It is possible that in some situations where there is an apparent complete resolution of the process, the inflammation always associated with it can inflict changes in the delicate structures of the ME/mastoid complex (thickening of mucosal folds, ligaments, and tendons) creating closed compartments or true "hypo-ventilated islands" even after the ET function was reestablished.

In fact, Proctor [14] demonstrated that, although the middle ear is ventilated by the ET, the air passages within the ME are narrow. A series of mucosal folds, part of the ossicles and suspensory ligaments, known as the tympanic diaphragm (TD), practically separate the mesotympanum from the epitympanum and mastoid.

The components of this diaphragm are the head of the malleus, the body of the incus, the lateral and medial incudal folds, the anterior and lateral malleolar folds, and the tensor tympani fold (Fig. 37.11).

Only two narrow passages, the anterior and posterior tympanic isthmus, perforate the diaphragm. The anterior isthmus is larger and more consistent, lying medially to the body of the incus, passing between the stapes and the tensor tympani tendon. When a medial incudal fold is present, a small posterior isthmus appears between this fold and the posterior tympanic wall. When this fold does not exist, the tympanic isthmus is a single passage. In less than 10% of cases, the tensor tympani fold may fail to develop, creating an additional passageway between the mesotympanum and the anterior attic. The epitympanum communicates with the mastoid antrum through a small triangular area known as the "aditus ad antrum" [14].

The clinical importance of the TD is that its patency is essential for ventilation of the epitympanum and whole mastoid via aditus ad antrum [14].

The simple edema and thickening of the mucous folds that constantly follow long-term or recurrent SOM, MOM, or even AOM may block these tiny openings sealing the passages of air to the epitympanum and the mastoid with the consequent development of a new cycle of localized negative pressure (Fig. 37.12).

In such circumstances, the negative pressure can reach extreme levels compromising the mucosa and especially the fine endothelial structure of its rich capillary network with consequent micro-bleedings randomly scattered in the ME. As red blood cells break down, cholesterol in the hemoglobin is released and the immune system reacts to the cholesterol as a foreign body, producing an inflammatory response and the consequent formation of cholesterol granulomas (Figs. 37.13 and 37.14).

Another common response of the subepithelial space is the development of granulation tissue (GT) following a process of increasingly thickness due to inflammatory infiltrates, vascular neoformations, and influx of fibroblasts. The formation of GT in the middle ear space begins with a break in the basement membrane of surface epithelial cells. Inflammatory cells in the underlying lamina propria traverse through the broken basement membrane and enter the Iumen of the middle ear space. This rupture may be caused by bacterial toxins, inflammatory mediators produced by ruptured lysozymes, and the accumulation of subepithelial fluid and vacuoles, all of which exert pressure on the surface epithelium [15].

The second step in the formation of GT occurs when a small piece of the lamina propria extrudes through the

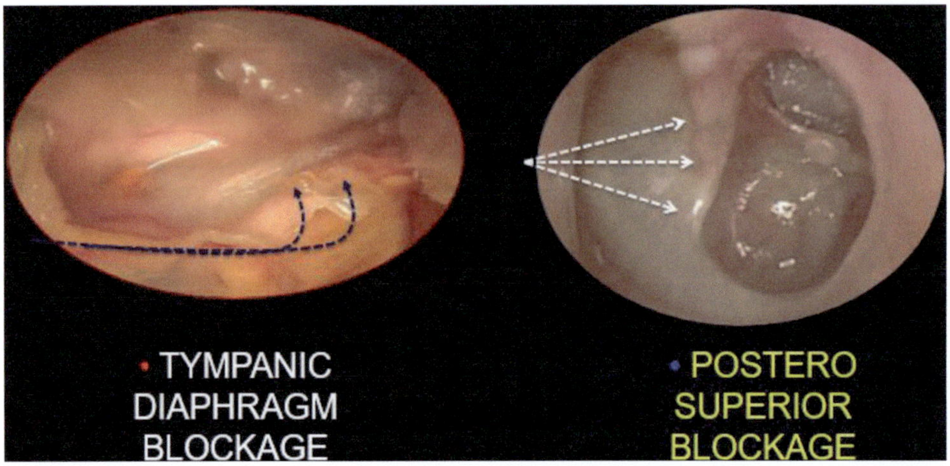

Fig. 37.12 Pathologically created hypo-ventilated micro-spots in the middle ear

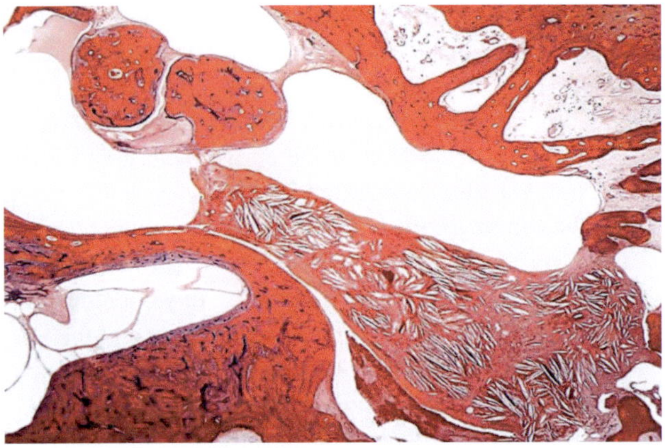

Fig. 37.13 Hematoxylin-eosin-stained histopathology demonstrating numerous cholesterol crystal clefts, surrounding multinucleate giant cells, epithelioid histiocytes, and foamy macrophages, all of which are consistent with a cholesterol granuloma

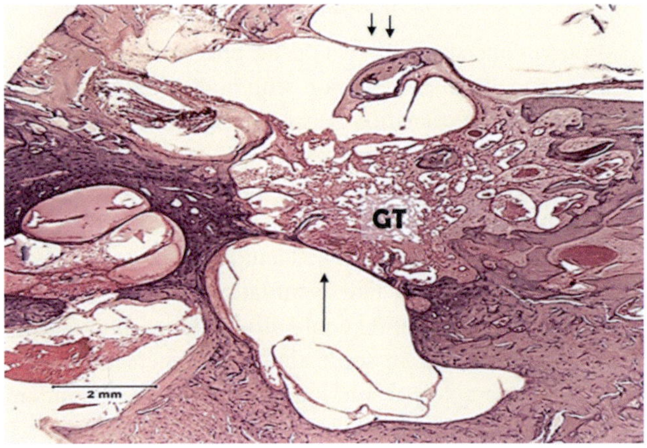

Fig. 37.15 Human temporal bone section showing an intact TM (double arrows); the footplate (single arrow); and a mass of granulation tissues filling the oval window niche and the posterior recesses (GT)

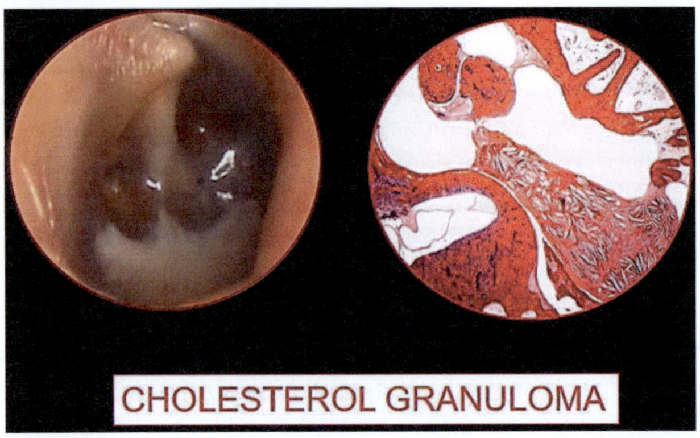

Fig. 37.14 Paparella´s "idiopathic hemotympanum". Patient with a history of long-lasting otitis media with effusion followed by cholesterol granuloma. The TM has a characteristic brownish color and always with some degree of retraction

ruptured area of the epithelial cell surface. If the growth of granulation tissue is vigorous and aggressive, polyps can form (Figs. 37.15 and 37.16). Both cholesterol granulomas and granulation tissue hold the strong potential to

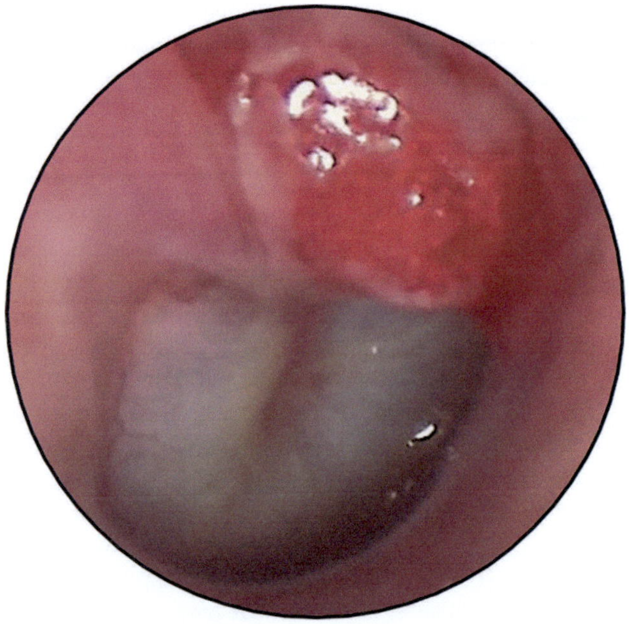

Fig. 37.16 Right ear showing a polyp in a position corresponding to the pars flaccida extending to the external auditory canal.

cause bone and ossicular absorption, especially when stimulated by inflammation, local pressure, and specific cytokeratins.

E. Cholesterol granuloma, granulation tissue, and ossicular erosion are among the most prevalent irreversibly inflammatory pathologic tissue encountered in the ME. The presence of any of these findings (in isolation or any combination) focally or diffusely filling the middle ear cleft in the presence of an intact tympanic membrane configures a condition defined by as "silent chronic otitis media" (SCOM). In these conditions, the intact TM may display a spectrum of changes from grossly abnormal aspect (retracted; atrophic of thickened) to, curiously a near-normal appearance! So, the definition of chronic silent otitis media is the presence of intractable inflammatory-related disease focally or generalized in the ME/mastoid complex associated with a non-perforated TM. This innovative concept confronted the classic definitions of chronic otitis media that required the presence of tympanic perforation (Fig. 37.17). It is important to highlight that the presence of the intact eardrum does not exclude, in most cases, the detection of otitis media, particularly mainly if the diagnosis is supported by a careful history and a good clinical examination. For this reason, and to avoid the overuse of the term, SCOM has been divided in two variants: undetected and undetectable. This distinction is very important, because if the undetected SCOM may be due to a negligent investigation, the undetectable SCOM is a clinical challenge to the physician, who must be aware of the fact that a near-normal TM does not preclude the presence of active and focal pathology in one or more of the ME multiple compartments.

Regarding granulation tissue, it is well known its high prevalence and generalized distribution throughout the entire middle ear/mastoid complex. Only a handful of publications, however, mention the problem of some patients who present with profuse and unremitting purulent otorrhea due to a large masses of granulation tissue. Costa and Cruz [12] observed that the presence of small masses of focal GT strategically distributed in the MEC, especially in the region of the round and oval window niches could be potentially responsible for audio-vestibular symptoms presented by some patients.

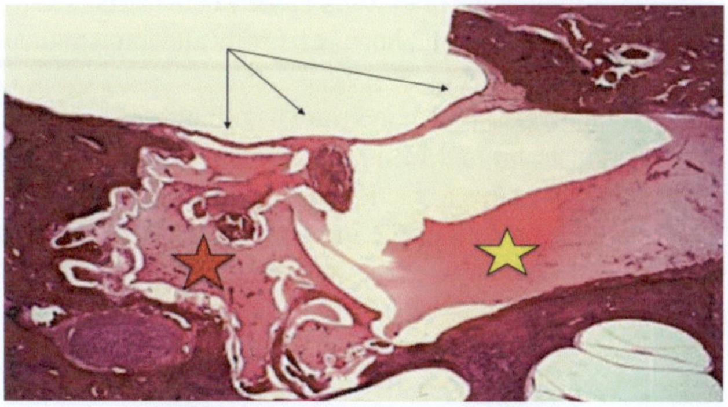

Fig. 37.17 Section of a human temporal bone at mesotympanum level showing the presence fluid filling the anterior mesotympanum (yellow star) concomitant with granulation tissue in the posterior recesses (red star). Notice the presence of an intact TM (black arrows)

In conclusion, GT can cause a series of signals and symptoms like otorrhea, osteitis, ossicular necrosis, conductive and/or sensorineural hearing loss, and other symptoms related to the posterior labyrinth. Granulation tissue may also affect the homeostasis of the ME through at least two mechanisms: (1) its own inflammatory profile and (2) the possibility of blocking transitional areas of the MEC (protympanum, isthmus and aditus), interrupting the natural airflow inside the ME compartments, compromising the ventilation and generating a vicious cycle of additional pathological changes. Next to the presence of effusion in ME, GT is the most prevalent finding in SCOM. Expanding potential clinical Implications of SCOM, there are two important concepts to discuss: (1) hearing loss and bone pathology in COM; (2) interaction between middle and inner ear.

The hearing loss associated with otitis media may appear early or late during the process, varying considerably regarding the type and degree. As for the type, the hearing loss may be conductive, sensorineural, or mixed. As for the degree, depending on how aggressive and the extension of the pathological process, they can vary from mild, moderate losses (usually associated with the conductive type) even severe degrees with severe and profound losses (sensorineural).

As mentioned before, the mechanisms involved in sensorineural hearing losses have been explained based on the biological behavior of the round window, mainly, and the oval one during the inflammatory processes of the MEC. This way, they could behave as true entrance doors for toxins coming from the middle ear to arrive in the inner ear configuring a legitimism interaction between these two compartments. Several studies demonstrate an association of the chronic otitis media to cochlear damage again pointing to the round window as the structure responsible for the transmission of the pathological process to the labyrinth.

Costa et al carried out a study including 150 patients with unilateral chronic otitis media and normal otoscopy and normal hearing in the contralateral ear (CLE). The main outcome measure was bone conduction threshold averages calculated for frequencies of 500, 1000, 2000, 3000, and 4000 Hz, with comparison between the normal ear and the ear with chronic otitis media. Thresholds were examined separately for each frequency. The bone conduction threshold averages for the normal side were lower than those for the ear with chronic otitis media. The threshold shift was statistically significant for each frequency ($P < 0.0001$, Student's t test) clearly showing that chronic otitis media may be associated with a decrease in cochlear function.

On the other hand, it is well established that the conductive losses regarding COM includes a series of changes in the tympanossicular system. Concerning the tympanic membrane, the loss of substance (perforations), the atrophy (and the consequent retraction), and the increase of its rigidity (because of tympanosclerosis plaque) are some of the biggest causes of hearing loss. The ossicles, however, may be affected by ossicular erosion (with the interruption of the chain as a consequence) and ossicular fixation due to tympanosclerosis, osteoneogenesis, and/or fibrosis.

Finally, the mass effects within the MEC by effusion, cholesterol granuloma, cholesteatomas, and granulation tissue can also compromise the vibratory ability of the tympanossicular system. Furthermore, all these changes may be found isolated or in several combinations in the middle ear. For instance, gross erosions of the long process of the incus, as usual, follow the atrophy and retraction of the posterosuperior quadrant of the TM. Nowadays, we believe the ossicular defects are a consequence of active processes of bone reabsorption and not of ossicular necrosis. This theory presupposes the presence and the participation of live cells in the mechanisms of demineralization, erosion, and destruction of the bone. A simply necrotizing bone can remain in situ for several years without suffering reabsorption process.

All those dedicated to middle ear surgery agree that during the step of the exploratory tympanotomy, a series of different pathological findings frequently are revealed cohabiting the ME regardless of the TM status (retracted or perforated). We will return to this relevant topic and expand its clinical and surgical implications later in this chapter.

F. The sum of all these components (effusion, hypoxia, negative pressure, and mucosal metaplasia) completely modifies the environment of the middle ear and its relationships with neighboring structures, and the TM (being the most fragile wall of the ME) is the first to be damaged. Consequently, the pars tensa may undergo sectorial or diffuse atrophy (Fig. 37.18).

Functionally, these patchy atrophic areas could not be clinically relevant; however, if the intratympanic process aggravates or even in the event of a traumatic injury, the atrophic and fragile regions then created could easily rupture creating TM perforations of considerably larger dimensions and more difficult to heal than those seen in previously healthy ears.

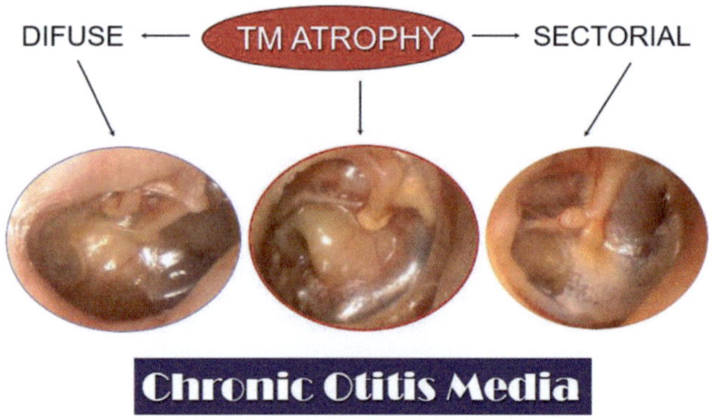

Fig. 37.18 TM displaying different stages of atrophy and sectorial or diffuse retractions

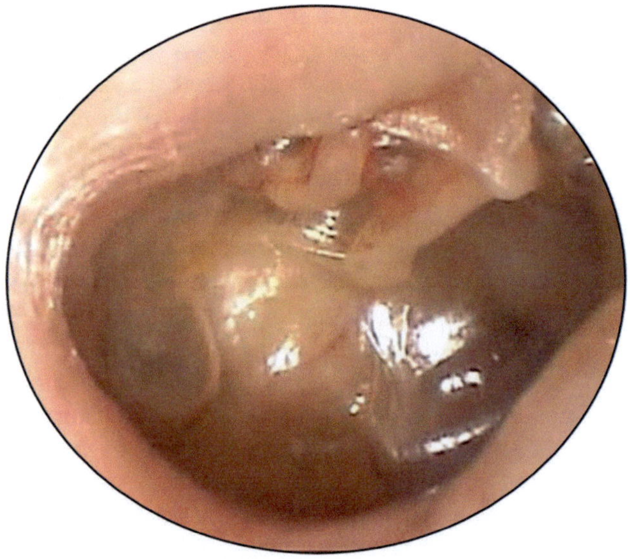

Fig. 37.19 Tympanic membrane atelectasis. The TM can be detached from the promontory after efficient Toynbee or Valsalva maneuver.

Diffuse atrophy could also lead to total TM retraction, with the membrane practically carpeting the structures of the middle ear without, however, firmly attaching to them (TM atelectasis) (Fig. 37.19).

Another possible condition would arise when the retraction is limited to the posterosuperior region. The progression of this retraction may be followed by erosion of the long process of the incus and fixation of this TM segment to the head of the stapes, regardless of the formation of cholesteatomas (myringostapediopexy). Curiously, most patients with natural myringostapediopexy have clinically irrelevant conductive hearing loss as it may work as a type III tympanoplasty (Fig. 37.20).

G. Yet another situation may follow with retraction of large portions of the pars tensa attaching the ossicles and ME mucosa. In such conditions, the possibility of destabilization of ME homeostasis may cause capillary pressure ischemia, necrosis, and progressive atrophy of the TM eventually leading to a loss of its integrity. The large perforations thus generated, as a rule, show clear signs that they were preceded by TM retractions (Fig. 37.21).

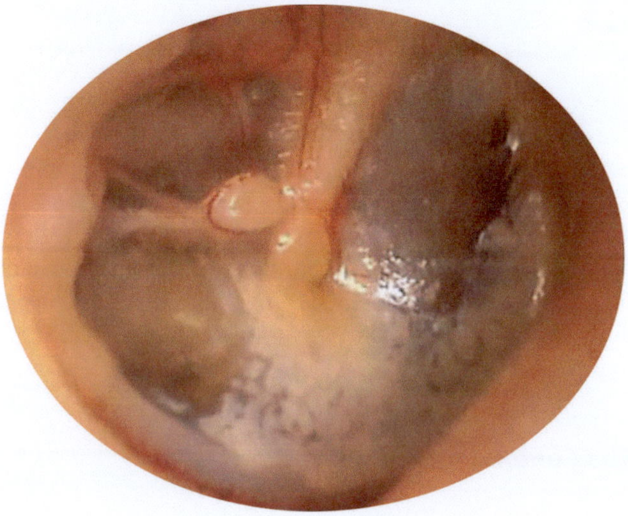

Fig. 37.20 Myringostapediopexy (notice the retraction of the postero-superior portion of the TM with erosion of the long process of incus and attachment of the TM to the head of the stapes.

In any of these situations, the resulting perforation could be central or marginal. In the case of a marginal perforation, there is a chance of the skin from the external auditory canal (EAM) to migrate across it gaining access to the ME and generating a secondary cholesteatoma (Fig. 37.2).

Regarding the flaccid pars, it is well known that its composition renders it prone to retraction which may evolve along stages: simple retraction, retraction pocket, and primary cholesteatoma (Fig. 37.22).

As pointed out before, the same process may develop in posterior–superior quadrant of the TM where the retractions are aggravated by overlapped bouts of infection with consequent irritation and hyperplasia of cells in the basal layer generating streams of squamous cells toward the middle ear.

This sequence of events may not necessarily follow a unidirectional pathway. In fact, it can be modified by several factors extrinsic and intrinsic to the ear, with a deceleration of the inflammatory reaction and formation of tympanosclerosis and bone new bone (Fig. 37.23).

Two last issues that still remain to be addressed are the non-healed traumatic tympanic perforations and those perforations related to acute necrotizing otitis

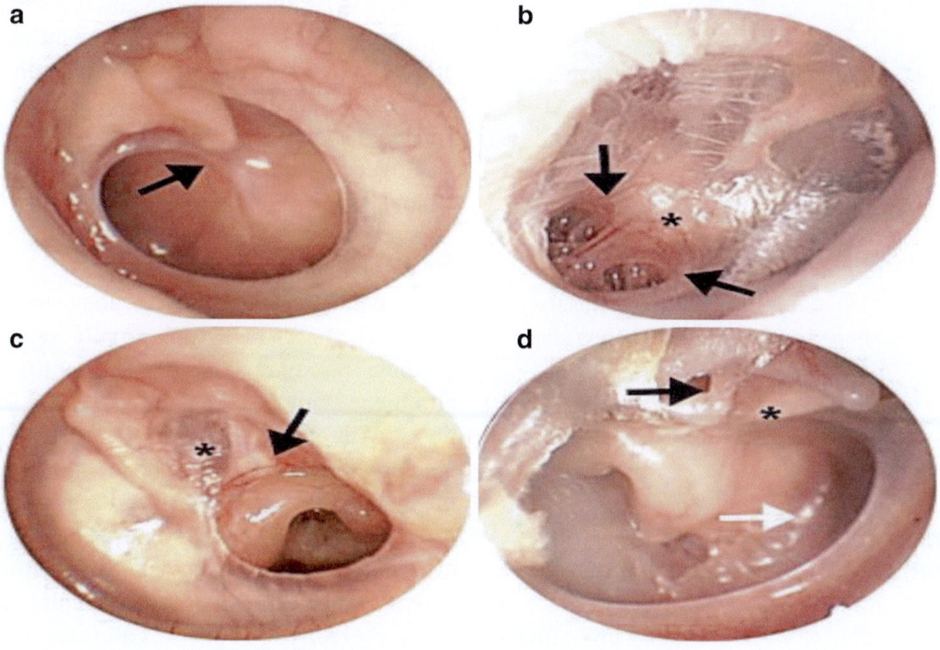

Fig. 37.21 Signs of retraction associated with tympanic perforation. (**a**) Medialization of the malleus handle, including touch in the promontory (black arrow). (**b**) Tympanic remnants lying over the promontory, black arrows are indicating the TM transition from the usual position until the promontory. (**c**) Erosion of the ossicular chain and tympanic remnants over it, with the black arrow pointing to the stapes without the incus (and tympanostapedopexy), showing an area of the eardrum medialized concerning its usual position until it touches the ossicular chain. (**d**) Otoscopy in which the tympanic retraction and perforation are almost indistinguishable: white arrow showing medialization of TM up to the promontory, black arrow pointing MT over the ossicular chain and significant thinning of the incus long process, over the medialized malleus.

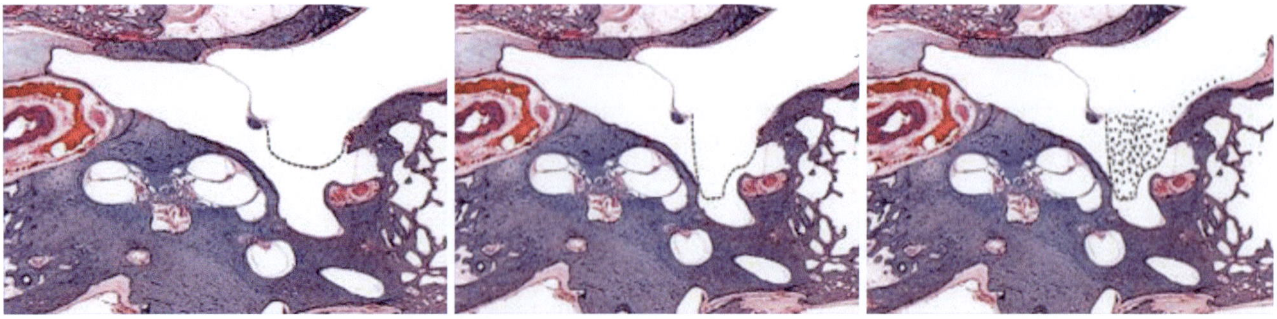

Fig. 37.22 Evolution from simple retraction to retraction pocket and cholesteatoma

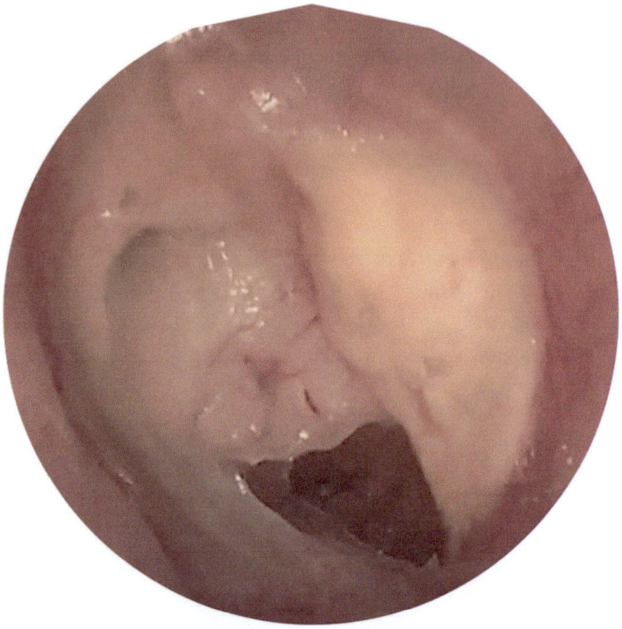

Fig. 37.23 Dry TM perforation with diffuse plaques of tympanosclerosis

media. In these rare situations, TM perforation is usually central and kidney-shaped and associated by few changes in the ME.

Otitis Media: Further

The *Continuum:* An Operational Model for the Pathogenesis of Chronic Otitis Media

As we have discussed above, when we try to mix clinical, pathological, and temporal aspects to obtain a rational classification of otitis media, we do not come up with crystal clear and definitive concepts. On the contrary, interconceptual superpositions are frequent feeding more discussion and controversy.

This difficulty is not limited as an academic issue, but it is also intrinsic to our daily work with deep implications on the clinical set. It is quite common in some patients, even after a complete workup we cannot come to the conclusion of which form of otitis media we are dealing with. This difficulty is due to the constant dynamic behavior verified in this pathological process.

The *Continuum*: Animal Studies

As we mentioned before, the first experiment involving the idea of the *continuum* was carried out by Paparella in 1970 employing the monkey as animal model. Later in 1977, the group by the University of Minnesota presented to the American Otological Society in Boston, the results of longitudinal and parallel animal and human studies that supported this theory. These studies focused on the chemical and pathologic evaluation of three essential components of otitis media: (1) ME effusion; (2) ME epithelium; and (3) ME subepithelial space.

Goycoolea et al. [16] and Junh et al. reported further animal studies demonstrating the *continuum* of events from serous or purulent effusion to mucoid effusion and, finally, becoming chronic or deaccelerating and turning into sequelae. Furthermore, they indicated that acute inflammatory changes are usually seen in patients with purulent otitis media and serous otitis media, whereas chronic inflammatory changes are more severe in temporal bones with mucoid and chronic otitis media. Finally, these studies showed overlaps in histopathologic findings among the various types of otitis media that suggested a steady progression from the acute purulent stages to mucoid and eventually chronic otitis media. Chemical and cellular activity in the effusion, the epithelium, and the middle ear subepithelial space underlies all forms of otitis media, and the extent of involvement in each of these compartments dictated the form of otitis media present in the middle ear cleft.

Recently, Bauer et al. [17] evaluated otoendoscopies of Mongolian gerbils after cauterization of the eustachian tube and found a steady increase in the sequence: effusion, retraction, and cholesteatoma in relation to controls.

The *Continuum*: Human Histopathology Studies

The 1990 human histopathology study was conducted by Yoon et al. [3] revealing that epithelial and subepithelial layers of the mucoperiosteum of the middle ear are actively involved in all stages of otitis media. A very important observation drawn from these and other classic histopathological studies is that that they define chronic otitis media regardless of its association with drumhead perforations, otorrhea, or even prolonged temporal evolutions. More simply, chronic otitis media is defined as a condition associated with, focal or generalized, irreversible tissue pathology within the middle ear cleft.

In his textbook, Schucknecht [18]meticulously describes the profile of chronic otitis media breaking it into two stages: active (increased vascularization of the mucosa and submucosa, acute inflammatory infiltrate, ulcerations of the mucosa, and granulation tissue) and scarred (fibrosis and neo-bone formation). Though all these authors agree that the drumhead perforation (and the otorrhea—its most common clinical manifestation) are included in this group of irreversible pathological findings they are not "*sine qua non*" findings for the definition of this condition.

We agree that those episodes of COM associated with drumhead perforations and otorrhea express themselves more dramatically, but many well-designed histopathological studies, retrospectives in human temporal bones (HTBs), and prospective in animals have demonstrated inflammatory irreversible tissue pathology in the middle ear cleft independently of rigid temporal parameters and, much more importantly, regardless of the presence of a tympanic membrane perforation [2, 11, 12, 19, 20].

With these concepts in mind, we conducted a study in the temporal bone lab of the University of Minnesota with 144 HTB with indisputable inflammatory irreversible tissue pathology (granulation tissue, ossicular changes, cholesteatoma, cholesterol granuloma, tympanosclerosis, and tympanic membrane perforation).

The middle ear cleft was topographically divided into ten different sites, so we mapped it completely in terms of kind and location of pathology. Temporal bones were further divided into two groups: those with intact tympanic membranes (group I) and those with perforated tympanic membranes (group II). Both groups had their findings statistically compared through the chi-square test.

Granulation tissue (97.9% of the temporal bones), ossicular changes (91.6%), tympanosclerosis (24.3%), tympanic membrane perforation (19.4%), cholesterol granuloma (13.8%), and cholesteatoma (10.4%) were the findings most frequently encountered within the HTB.

Surprisingly, the comparative analysis of temporal bones with and without tympanic membrane perforation indicated that both groups were similar. When one considers granulation tissue, ossicular changes and cholesterol granuloma were found in both groups with a difference in frequency not statistically significant. Cholesteatoma and tympanosclerosis were identified more frequently in the temporal bones with tympanic membrane perforations (group II) [2]. The conclusion of our study clearly shows that chronic middle ear inflammation may be underestimated using conventional definitions of COM.

In short, chronic otitis media has been defined under clinical and pathological criteria. Both definitions share some common aspects, but they differ deeply regarding the presence of the TM perforation. We believe that our responsibility is to shift the clinical criteria (very restrictive in our opinion) to the more encompassing and broader field of the pathological definition. Perhaps, aware of this possibility, we will investigate, understand, and work more properly some ear symptoms that appear, at the first sight, obscure, and unexplainable. In our opinion, to neglect these concepts is a big medical mistake. It could be interpreted as we were much more concerned about either plugging or poking holes upon the tympanic membrane than actually disclosing and treating middle and inner ear pathology.

The *Continuum*: Human Clinical Studies

In the above paragraphs, we reviewed a series of studies where the *Continuum* has been consistently replicated in animal models. Strong evidences also pointing to the same direction came from elegant researches employing HTB with otitis media. For obvious reasons, the process cannot be studied longitudinally in the clinical set, since it would be ethically unacceptable to only contemplate the classic evolution of the disease from early stages of serous and mucoid effusion to the development of irreversible inflammatory pathology.

Still the ear surgeon can witness many irrefutable evidences of this march of events whenever performing middle ear and mastoid surgery for COM. It is not rare to find during middle ear exploration a myriad of different pathologies dwelling the same ear: cholesteatoma in the attic and antrum; cholesterol granuloma in the tip of the mastoid and the oval and round window niches; granulation tissue over the posterosuperior quadrant and promontory; thick mucoid fluid in the protympanum and tympanic orifice of the eustachian tube and tympanosclerosis patches all over the TM not rarely involving and fixating the ossicular chain and the cochleariform process (Fig. 37.24).

These findings not only have confirmed that the otitis media inflammation/infection complex is very dynamic but also led to the development of new surgical techniques, especially designed to treat this ongoing process. The prototype

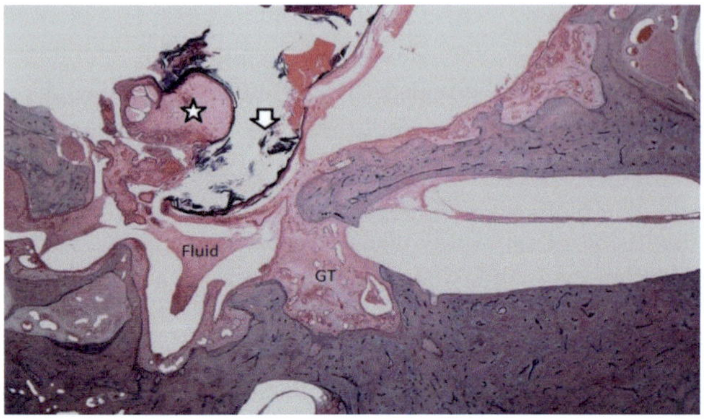

Fig. 37.24 Multiple pathological findings in the middle ear cleft: fluid; granulation tissue (GT) in the round window niche; polyp (star); cholesteatoma (arrow)

of these techniques is the flexible tympanomastoidectomy approach which was described in detail by Costa et al [19]. The so-called *flexible approach* consists in is a stepwise technique designed to methodically and systematically explore all the contents of the middle ear cleft and in the process to disclose, confirm, and treat the disease encountered. We strongly believe that this flexible approach can be best defined as a true pathology-guided, pathogenesis-oriented surgery for the middle ear.

Besides the unequivocal findings during chronic ear surgery, we have pursued other practical alternatives to study the *continuum* in a human model.

For such we decided to transversally investigate the middle ear status of a series of patients with cleft palate [21]. The rationale behind the study was the well-known fact that these patients have a chronic eustachian tube (ET) dysfunction which is not completely corrected by palate reconstruction. As a consequence, the occurrence of middle ear disease among patients with cleft lip and palate or cleft palate only is extremely high [22, 23]. In this population, almost as a rule, there is an anomalous insertion of the elevator and tensor *veli palatine* muscles into the posterior margins of the hard palate. Besides, there is also muscle hypoplasia, which may cause ET dysfunction [24, 25]. As pointed out before, ET tube malfunction, when persistent, may cause a negative pressure in the tympanic cavity, with the resulting transudation of fluid from the intravascular to the interstitial space, and from there to the lumen of the middle ear [26]. This is one of the initial landmarks of the pathogenesis of otitis media [27]. From this point, the subepithelium (and later the epithelium) reacts to the adverse situation, and there is the setup of histological alterations that may become irreversible inside the middle ear, and that will define the next pathologic process [3, 27].

The goal of our study was to describe the pattern of middle ear alterations in 180 patients with cleft of lip and palate or isolated cleft palate followed at a university hospital in the South of Brazil with no previous otologic interventions.

Effusions in the middle ear were present bilaterally in 65 patients (37.6%) and unilaterally in 15. Cholesteatoma (CCOM) was seen in 11 patients (6.4%) and in two patients it was bilateral. Chronic otitis media without cholesteatoma (NCCOM) was observed in nine patients (two of them bilaterally).

When considering the type of abnormality, patients were divided into three main groups taking into account the main finding: effusion, moderate/severe retractions, and chronic otitis media, with or without cholesteatoma. Sixty-seven patients (38.2%) presented middle ear effusions as the main finding, 24 patients (13.3%) presented with moderate to severe retraction as the main finding, and 18 (10%) presented with chronic otitis media, with or without cholesteatoma.

There was a statistically significant association between age and the occurrence of cholesteatoma. The higher the age, the higher the prevalence of the disease (chi-square linear trend, $P = 0.008$). The distribution of NCCOM among different age ranges has also shown a linear association. The higher the age, the higher the prevalence of this condition ($P = 0.003$). Increasing age has also correlated with the presence of retraction pockets on the tympanic membrane ($P < 0.0001$).

The presence of middle ear effusions exhibited a linear association with age. Older patients tended to a lower prevalence of effusions ($P < 0.0001$). Figure 37.25 shows the linear trends in the distribution of the pathologies found: effusions, moderate/severe retractions, CCOM, and NCCOM.

In conclusion, the middle ear findings of a group of patients with theoretically known ET dysfunction supported the concept of the *continuum*: across younger age ranges, there is the predominance of middle ear effusions, whereas in the older patients the prevalence of retractions and chronic otitis media are predominant. Underlined the obvious limitations of our study, we firmly believe that the progression of the severity of the ME findings in the cleft palate population through the years is in close analogy with the findings derived from many well-designed longitudinal animal studies.

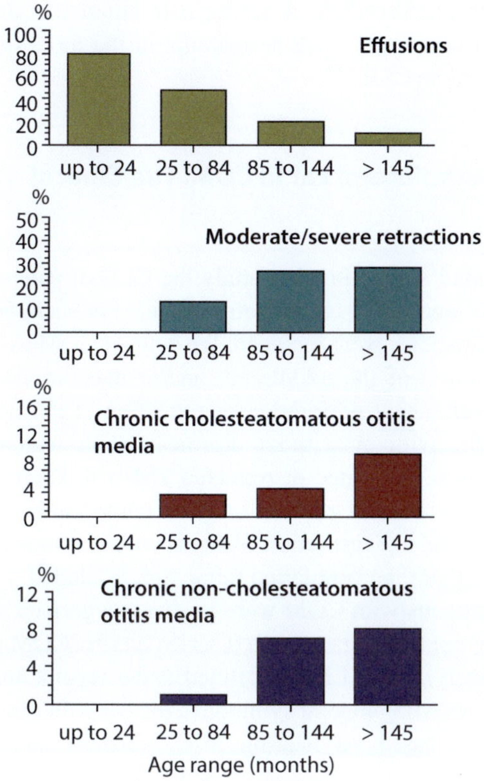

Fig. 37.25 Linear correlation between age range and otologic findings

Otitis Media: Beyond

The Contralateral Ear in Chronic Otitis Media

It is curious to notice that even after such massive evidences, the *Continuum* theory is not so much explored by those who dedicate their best efforts to study COM pathogenesis and natural history. Perhaps one of the reasons for such a paradox is due to the extreme concern of the clinicians in unveiling the secrets of two groups of conditions: otitis media with effusion (OME) and cholesteatomas. These studies have effectively shed light on a number of questions related to the etiopathogenesis, diagnosis, and treatment of these conditions. Notwithstanding, few studies try to establish the right connections existing between these two extremes that, when separately analyzed, seem to follow parallel natural histories. A tacit example of this disconnection is the joint document published by the American Academies of Otolaryngology, Pediatrics and Family Practice in May [28].

These guidelines were published for the sole purpose of informing clinicians of evidence-based methods to identify, monitor, and manage OME in children aged 2 months through 12 years. For such, The American Academy of Pediatrics, American Academy of Family Physicians, and American Academy of Otolaryngology-Head and Neck Surgery selected a subcommittee composed of experts in the fields of primary care, otolaryngology, infectious diseases, epidemiology, hearing, speech and language, and advanced-practice nursing to review the OME guideline.

According to the panel recommendations, "*conditions of the tympanic membrane that generally mandate inserting a tympanostomy tube are posterosuperior retraction pockets, ossicular erosion, adhesive atelectasis, and retraction pockets that accumulate keratin debris. Ongoing surveillance is mandatory, because the incidence of structural damage.*"

It should be noticed that all the above-mentioned conditions are already under the scope of COM (with an honorable mention to "*retraction pockets that accumulate keratin debris*" which literally represents Schuknecht's [18]definition of aural cholesteatoma). The insertion of a ventilation tube at this moment it is not only late but also not anymore indicated, since it will never abort neither abbreviate the natural history of the disease.

In accordance with the *Continuum* theory, OME is the initial step of the process that, when unresolved, may progress to chronic transformation. Although only a percentage of the ears with OME will evolve to COM, our attached question is: once bilateral effusion are reported to be high [29], shouldn't the presence of bilateral COM be also very prevalent?

Therefore, we postulate that the presence of COM in one ear carries a higher risk of coexisting contralateral abnormalities. Based on such reasoning and the limited data available in the literature [30, 31], we have decided to report the characteristics of the contralateral ear (CLE) in COM. To emphasize our concepts and trying to build up overlapped evidences, we carried out three different studies focusing: (1) the cellular level—histology (histopathology of 170 human temporal bones with COM); (2) the anatomy—clinical picture (ME findings of 500 patients with COM and CT scan findings in 75 patients); and (3) the physiology—function (the quantification of the air–bone gap in the CLE of 463 patients with COM).

The Contralateral Ear in COM: The Histopathology

The first study was designed to determine the prevalence of CLE changes in HTB from patients with COM [32]. Secondary objectives included verifying whether the presence of cholesteatoma in the more damaged ear was related to a greater prevalence of CLE changes, and whether there was an association between the findings in the more damaged ear and in the CLE.

We studied 85 pairs of HTB under light microscopy describing all otitis media-related findings (as pointed out before, COM was defined by the presence of irreversible inflammatory alterations in the MEC). The CLE was defined as the normal or the least affected ear.

Our results showed that cholesteatoma was the main pathology in 22.4% of the more damaged ears. The overall prevalence of CLE with alterations was incredibly high (91.8%). We next stratified the CLE changes as slight or significant (with effusion being the mildest form, followed by moderate and severe retractions and TM perforations, the presence of granulation tissue, and cholesteatoma) and still 77.6% were considered to be significant. The chief findings were tissue granulation (81%), effusion (58%), and tympanic membrane retractions (35%) (Fig. 37.26).

Of the 19 donors who had cholesteatoma in the more damaged ear, 7 (36.84%) also exhibited this pathology in the CLE. Granulation tissue was diffuse in 39 (45.9%) samples and focal in 30 (35.3%). Tympanic membrane retractions in the CLE were more prevalent in the pars tensa (43.33%), with nine (30%) ears presenting retraction in the pars flaccida and in both regions for eight (26.67%) cases. Twelve (70.59%) of the retractions in the pars flaccida were moderate to severe, as were 11 (52.39%) of the retractions in the pars tensa.

Of the tympanic membrane perforations observed in the CLE, two (66.67%) were central. All were located in the posterior quadrants of the pars tensa. Of the eight HTB donors presenting perforation in the more damaged ear, two also showed this change in the CLE, showing a bilateral prevalence of 25% (Fig. 37.27).

There was a direct and moderately strong correlation between the extent of granulation tissue in the more damaged ear and the CLE. A strong correlation was observed between the extent of cholesteatoma in the more damaged ear and in the CLE.

The Contralateral Ear in COM: The Clinical Study

Our second study aimed to study the CLE of patients with clinical diagnosis of chronic otitis media. For such, 500 consecutive patients were included. We defined COM as chronic inflammation of the middle ear and/or mastoid associated with a permanent perforation or retraction of the tympanic membrane with or without otorrhea. Cholesteatoma was defined as a perforated or retracted TM with keratin retention, with or without granulation and recurrent inflammation. There was no age restriction. Patients with previous otologic surgery other than ventilation tubes were excluded.

All patients with COM were further categorized as associated or not to cholesteatoma (CCOM and NCCOM groups, respectively). The CLE was defined as the asymptomatic ear or, in cases with bilateral symptoms, the ear with clearly less symptoms based on hearing loss, otorrhea, and overall discomfort.

Otoendoscopy of CLE was reviewed, and the ears were classified as normal or abnormal. All ears were classified by their dominant pathologic findings if more than one finding was present; and these were defined as effusion, retraction, perforation, cholesteatoma, or presence of otitis-derived sequelae (tympanosclerosis). The TM retraction was classified according to a modified Sadé and Berco classification

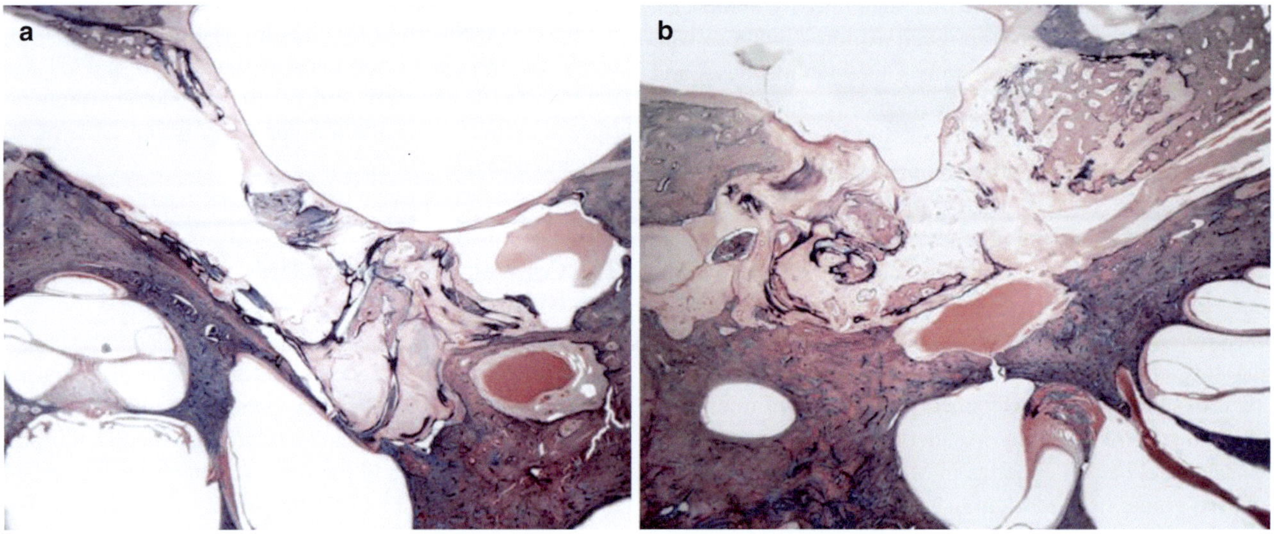

Fig. 37.26 (**a**) Histological section of the right ear with TM retraction, bone erosion, and granulation tissue and tympanosclerosis in the middle ear cleft. (**b**) The contralateral temporal bone with exactly the same profile (hematoxylin-eosin; magnification, X10)

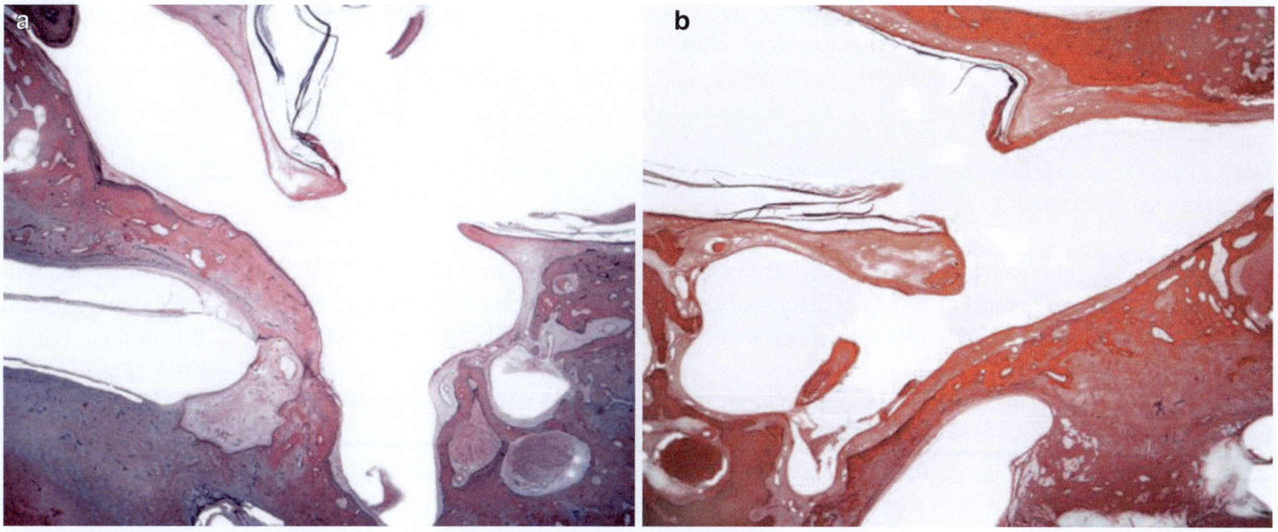

Fig. 37.27 (**a**) Histological section of the most affected ear. There is granulation tissue filling the round window niche and central TM perforation. (**b**) Histological section of the contralateral ear. Central TM perforation (diagonal arrow) and thickening of the middle ear mucosa (vertical arrow) (hematoxylin-eosin; magnification, X10).

Table 37.1 Data about the CLE of each patient were recorded in the specific protocols

Location	Degree	Definition
Pars tensa	Mild (PT1)	Extended to the external third of the middle ear
	Moderate (PT2)	Extended into the middle third of the middle ear
	Severe (PT3)	Extended into the inner third of the middle ear or abutted the promontory and/or the medial wall
Pars flaccida	Mild (PF1)	Minimal medial displacement of the tympanic membrane
	Moderate (PF2)	Medial dislocation of the tympanic membrane with adherence to the malleus
	Severe (PF3)	Medial displacement with adherence and bony erosion
Mixed	Mild/moderate (M1)	Description above
	Moderate/severe (M2)	Description above

Modified from Sadé (1979)

(2006) as from the pars tensa or pars flaccida. The retractions were then further graded as mild, moderate, or severe, according to the criteria shown in Table 37.1.

Overall, only 24.8% of the patients presented with a completely normal CLE. In the 75.2% with abnormalities, the most frequent findings were TM retraction (38.2%), TM perforations (26.2%), cholesteatoma (5.2%), tympanosclerosis (3.6%), and effusion in the middle ear (2.0%). A total of 302 patients (60.4%) presented with NCCOM in the most affected ear, and of this group, 30.1% presented with a normal CLE. In the 69.9% with abnormalities, the most frequent

Table 37.2 Description of the abnormalities found for NCCOM and CCOM separated and together

Videotoscopy	WITH	NCCOM	CCOM
Normal	157	119	38
Mild retraction	112	78	34
Moderate retraction	78	41	37
Severe retraction	32	10	22
Perforation	102	82	20
Cholesteatoma	19	0	19
Total	500	330	170

alterations were TM perforations (30.8%), TM retraction (30.1%), tympanosclerosis (6.0%), and effusion (3.0%). Among patients with CCOM, 16.7% presented with a normal CLE. The most frequent abnormalities in this group were TM retraction (50.1%), TM perforation (19.3%), cholesteatoma (13.3%), and effusion in the middle ear (0.6%). Table 37.2 describes the abnormalities found for NCCOM and CCOM separately and together.

Although all listed abnormalities were undisputable, some of them were mild and possibly not as clinically relevant. Therefore, an effort was made to focus on the more marked levels of disease. For this analysis, we excluded those CLEs with solely the presence of mild retractions, serous effusion, and otitis-derived sequelae (tympanosclerosis); and we still found a total of 55.8% of CLEs with abnormalities; 43.0% in the NCCOM group and 68.6% of CLE in the CCOM group (Table 37.3). The difference between the two groups was statistically significant ($P < 0.0001$).

When we looked only for the presence of retractions on the CLE, we found in the NCCOM group mild retractions in 17.9% of the CLE, moderate retractions in 8.6%, and severe

Table 37.3 Description of the major findings in the CLE (horizontal axis) of patients with COM (NCCOM and CCOM, vertical axis) after excluding normal, mild TM retractions, tympanosclerosis, and effusion in the CLE

Videotoscopy	Moderate retraction	Severe retraction	Perforation	Cholesteatoma	Total
Perforation	26 (20.0%)	11 (8.5%)	93 (71.5%)	0 (0.0%)	130 (100%)
Cholesteatoma	23 (16.9%)	49 (36.0%)	38 (27.9%)	26 (19.2%)	136 (100%)
Total	49 (18.4%)	60 (22.2%)	131 (49.7%)	26 (9.7%)	266 (100%)

Fisher's exact test; $P < 0.0001$

retractions in 3.6%. Interestingly, in the CCOM group, those with cholesteatoma in the most affected ear displayed severe retractions in 24.7% of the CLE, mild retractions in 14.1%, and moderate retractions in 11.2%.

Our results support the conclusion that patients with chronic otitis media in one ear have a high chance of presenting some degree of pathology in the contralateral side. We believe that our findings suggest that chronic otitis media should ideally be approached not as a static pathological incident affecting one ear but rather as an ongoing process which may affect both ears.

The Contralateral Ear in COM: The Functional Study

Our first two studies were able to clearly demonstrate that there is a high prevalence of bilateral COM or, at least, a considerable slice of the population with COM in the main ear that also exhibits gross abnormalities in the CLE. Whether these pathological findings actually may affect the physiology of the tympanossicular system was the predominant question of our third study.

It is well known that COM (even at early stages) may compromise the effectiveness of the vibratory pattern of the TM and/or ossicular chain. As a consequence, a variable degree of conductive hearing loss is almost omnipresent in these patients. The pathogenesis of the hearing loss is related to a combination of many factors which include partial or total loss of vibratory surface of the TM, ossicular chain erosion or fixation.

In order to bring our primary hypothesis to the functional level, we carried out a prospective cross-sectional study of 463 patients with COM to analyze the hearing status of the CLE focusing on the presence of an air–bone gap as an indicator of tympanossicular damage.

We employed the same definitions of COM and the same parameters to determine the main and the CLE as in the clinical study discussed in the sections above. The patients were divided into four categories according to the clinical diagnosis in the main ear: NCCOM ($n = 324$); *pars flaccida* CCOM ($n = 60$); *pars tensa* CCOM ($n = 72$); open CCOM ($n = 7$).

All patients were submitted to PTA, determining air conduction thresholds (AC) at 250, 500, 1000, 2000, 3000, 4000, 6000, and 8000 Hz; bone conduction thresholds (BC); and air–bone gaps (ABG) at 500, 1000, 2000, 3000, and 4000 Hz frequencies. The ABG was calculated using the difference between AC and BC thresholds. For BC thresholds, a bone conduction transmitter placed on the mastoid bone was used. Even for AC and BC, Narrow Band masking noise was applied when needed. In young children, which could arise problems to measure reliable thresholds, playful conditioning (play-conditioned audiometry with supra-aural earphone) was performed. When necessary, the PTA could be concluded after two sessions in order to confirm its results.

The mean ABG variable represented the arithmetic mean of the gaps at the same frequencies. Taking into consideration the magnitude of the mean ABG, it was created three new subcategories: ABG (0–14 dBHL); ABG (15–29 dBHL); and ABG (≥30 dBHL). The mean ABG was further subdivided according to the tested frequencies: low frequencies (500 and 1000 Hz), and high (2000, 3000, and 4000 Hz).

We have compared with the Kruskal–Wallis test the mean ABG and the mean ABG for low and high frequencies in the CLE among the four groups and no differences were found ($P = 0.567$).

In the other hand when we analyzed all CLE for the occurrence of ABG of any magnitude, we found that they were present in almost 30% of the ears (135 CLE or 29.10% with ABG greater than 14 dBHL). There were no statistically significant differences ($P = 0.940$) when we compared through the chi-square test the prevalence of the ABG among the four studied groups (30.3% NCCOM; 22.4% pars flacida cholesteatomas; 29.4% pars tensa cholesteatomas; 34.4% open cholesteatomas)

The conclusions of the functional study are closely related to the histological and clinical ones, i.e., at least one-third of the CLE of patients with COM have a major interference in the tympanossicular system possibly related to inflammatory conditions.

The Contralateral Ear in COM: The Radiologic Study

Previous studies indicate a bilateral tendency of chronic otitis media, and they clearly showed that the contralateral ear can provide the potential pathogenesis in the most affected ear.

The CT scan is an excellent test to evaluate the structures of the temporal bone and the changes resulting from otitis media. In the fourth study of our group, Silva et al (2013) evaluated Temporal Bone Computed Tomography of 75 patients with chronic otitis media. All the exams were requested as part of our preoperative workup, and the main ear in this study was the one booked for surgery. Only the most severe cases of COM are referred for CT examination. Among these are patients with persistent granulation tissue refractory to office treatment, conductive hearing loss above 30 dB or associated with sensorineural hearing loss, suspected complications, and presence of cholesteatomas. Thus, the study population was a convenience sample of patients with COM, five years old or more. A neuroradiologist blinded to clinical information and diagnosis evaluated CT scans. Images were evaluated based on a 38-question protocol focusing on the structures considered to be the most important in the radiological analysis of the temporal bone. Only indisputable findings secondary to COM in the CLE were accounted for: middle ear opacification, epitympanum opacification, gross erosion of the lateral wall of the attic, and mastoid sclerosis or opacification (Figs. 37.28 and 37.29). The results also showed a high prevalence of abnormalities in the CLE (54.7%).

Within the tympanic cavity, the prevalence of some degree of inflammation was 28%, 20%, 18%, and 25% in the mesotympanum, hypotympanum, protympanum, and epitympanum, respectively. Posterior recesses were filled by soft tissue density material in 24% of facial recesses and sinus tympani. Similar findings were observed in the mastoid: 65.3% well-pneumatized mastoids; 6.7% diploic, and 28% sclerotic. Out of these, 6.7% were patients with signs of some form of complication, such as cortical erosion of the

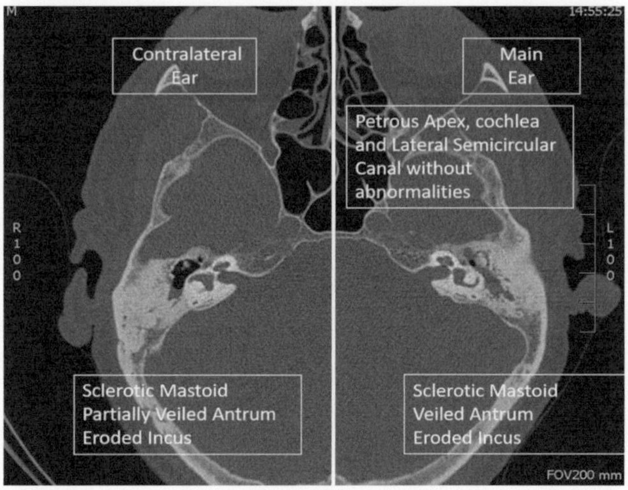

Fig. 37.28 CT scan—axial incidence—radiological findings in the main and contralateral ear in a patient with COM

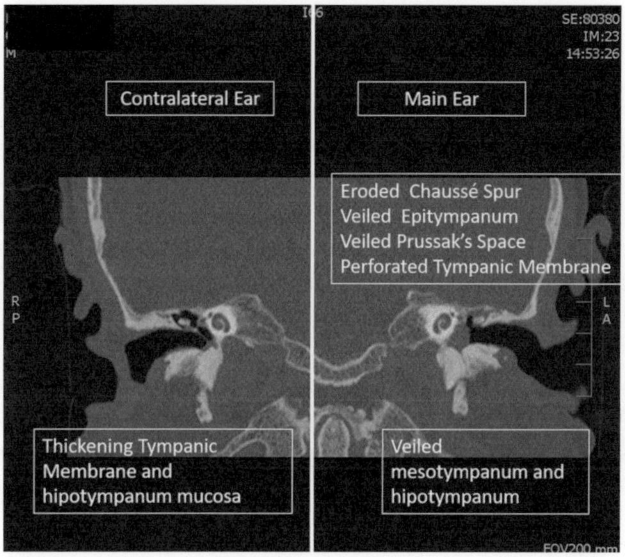

Fig. 37.29 CT scan—coronal incidence—radiological findings in the main and contralateral ear in a patient with COM

mastoid, tegmen erosion, or fistula of the lateral semicircular canal.

Once again, the high prevalence of radiographic findings in the contralateral ears of patients with COM point to the same direction than the clinical, histopathological, and functional studies or the tendency of the disease to affect both ears.

The Contralateral Ear in COM: Tympanic Membrane Perforations Study

TM perforations are the trademark of NCCOM. Their size and location are of paramount importance when surgery is planned and are also key determinants for graft-taking rates. Despite the plethora of new technologies available, the dimensions and location of tympanic membrane (TM) perforations and tympanosclerosis plaques have been subjectively estimated in terms of how they affected the geometry of the four quadrants, since there is a lack of a specific tools that could provide such information.

A careful evaluation of the different aspects of the middle ear environment, especially the integrity of its lateral wall (the TM) and the limitations inherent to the unaided human visual judgment of measurement-related aspects, has pointed to the need of developing an alternative method to more precisely quantify these findings.

This led to the creation of the Cyclops Auris Project, which aimed at the development of quantitative computational methods to assess the spatial relationships between affected tympanic areas and surrounding tissue through the analysis of stored digital video-otoendoscopy.

The Cyclops Auris system was developed specifically as a standalone software tool to be used in the clinical routine for the quantitative analysis of the extension of TM pathologies, implementing a set of mathematical and image processing methods customized for this specific purpose. The software wizard provides a user-friendly and semi-automated solution, where the medical end user has only to intervene where medical judgment is required, such as in the fine-tuning of the determination of the boundaries of the anatomical structures, being all mechanical error-prone tasks performed automatically by the software. The Cyclops Auris also allows the quadrant-wise measurement of the perforated relative area, which was shown to have clinical implications. Finally, Cyclops Auris' features that allow the direct feeding of a database with the measurement results or the export of data in statistical programs friendly formats allow the easy performing of retrospective and prospective studies. A complete description of this tool is beyond the scope of this chapter, but its methodology involves five steps and is summarized in Fig. 37.30.

After validated (2009), the Cyclops Auris was tested on our examination collection encompassing 950 patients with chronic otitis media, without any previous clinical or surgical treatment for whom examinations were acquired bilaterally, totaling 19,000 video-otoscopic recordings. Seven hundred patients were classified as presenting NCCOM, and 166 (16.57%) of them were selected for having bilateral dry TM perforations as the sole alteration. The size and location of these perforations were calculated with the help of the software.

When the Spearman coefficient was applied on the sizes of the major perforation, called principal ear (PE) and the minor perforation, called contralateral ear (CE) of the 166 patients presenting a bilateral pathology, there was found a strong correlation (rS = 0 .79; $P < 0.0001$). When the perforation position of both ears of these patients were compared with the Wilcoxon test ($P < 0.0001$), there was also found a high concordance ($P < 0.0001$).

In a group of patients, the similarity of the size and location of the perforations were so impressive that they could be considered almost as mirror images (Figs. 37.31 and 37.32).

The conclusions of this study again showed that the prevalence of NCCOM is high. Furthermore, in those cases where bilateral perforations were documented, their size and quadrant distribution were strongly correlated. In short, the findings of all the studies briefly presented above point to the

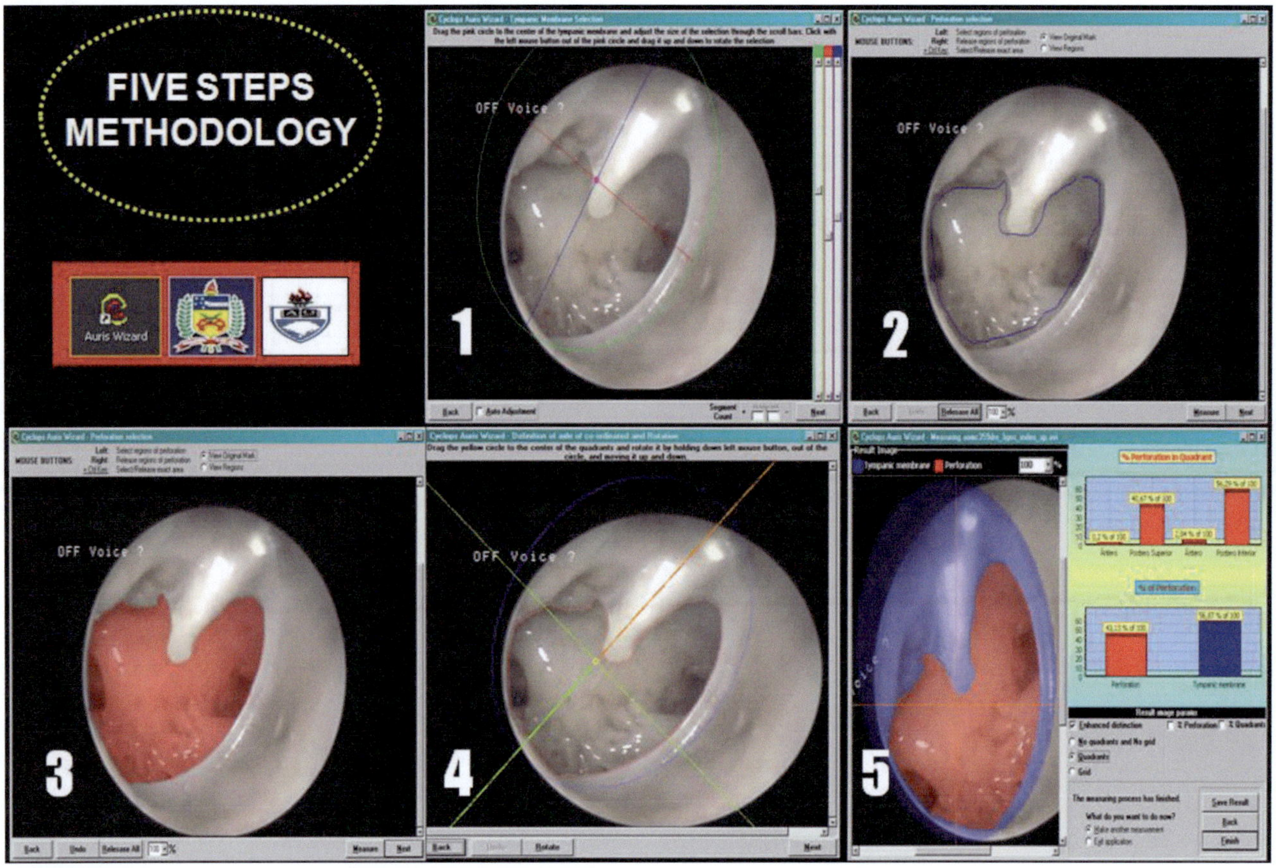

Fig. 37.30 Cyclops Auris: five-step methodology. 1: Opening the file and describing the boundaries of the TM. 2: Selecting the perforation area. 3: Fine-tuning the perforation area. 4: Adjusting the quadrants. 5: Making the measurements

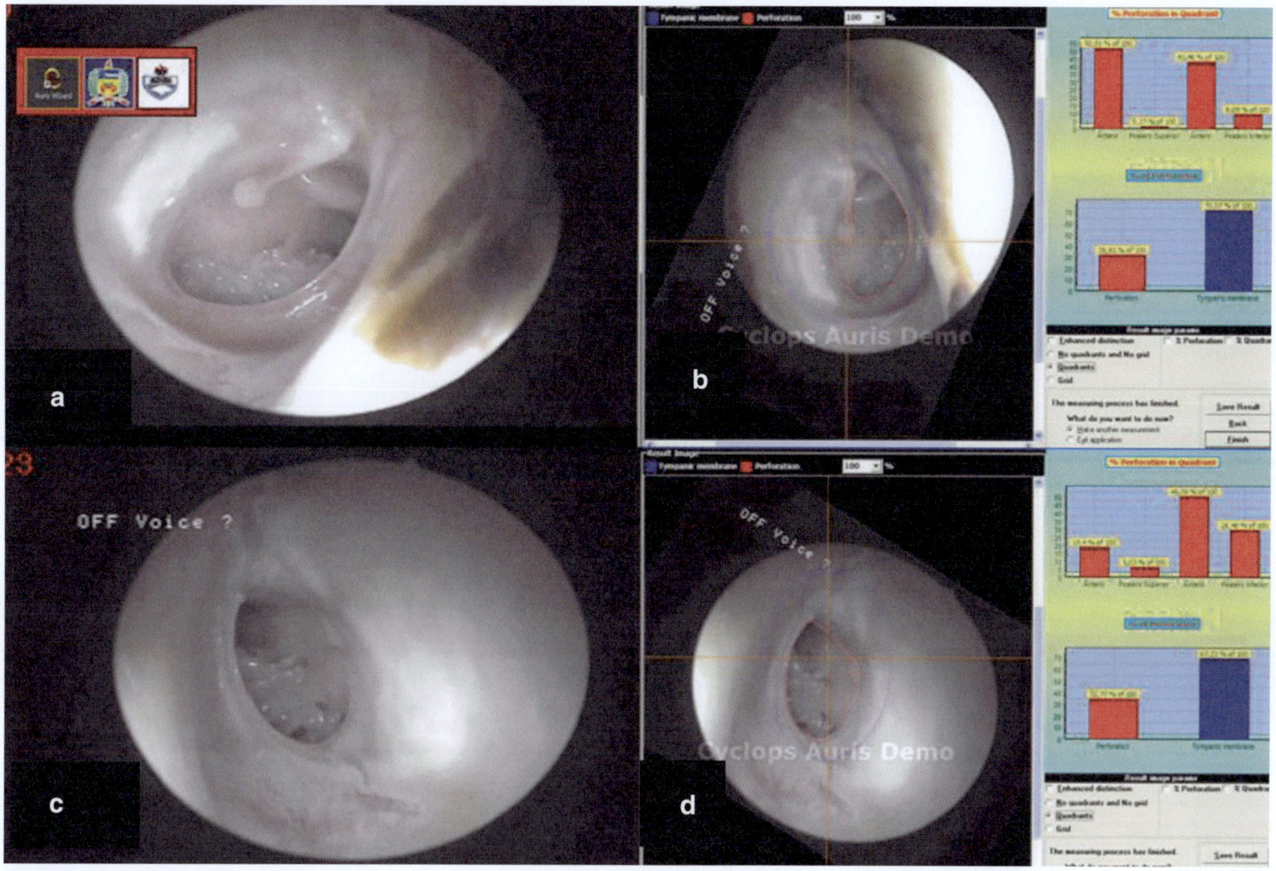

Fig. 37.31 Video-otoscopy and analysis of bilateral perforations. It is easy to notice the resemblance, both in image and the measured parameters. (**a**) Video-otoscopy right ear. (**b**) Measures in the right ear. (**c**) Video-otoscopy left ear. (**d**) Measures in the left ear

same direction overlapping evidences that the bilateral chronic otitis media is much more than a coincidence.

The Contralateral Ear in COM: Discussion and Practical Implications

A close analysis of the history of the procedures designed to treat COM and its complications clearly show that otological surgery gradually evolved during this last century with at least three different phases: preservation of life (the 1853 simple mastoidectomy by Schwartz); anatomical conservation (the 1910 Bondy operation), and hearing improvement (the 1955 tympanoplasty by Wullstein and Zollner). Interestingly, these three phases bring us to current concepts which can be perfectly summarized under the contemporary objectives of chronic ear surgery: elimination of infection, preservation of the normal anatomical contours of the ear and, whenever possible, restoration of hearing function.

In fact, the last objective of COM surgery was set more than 50 years ago! During the same period, there were major advances in the understanding of a variety of ear pathologies. These advances were spread over a variety of fields: from microbiology to the ultra-structure; from physiology to molecular biology; and from the pathogenesis to technological breakthroughs. Essentially, the degree of scientific development from 1955 to 2010 highly exceeds the verified between 1853 (when the simple mastoidecotomy was completely described) and 1955 (when the last objective—hearing restoration—was first proposed).

After all these years, the body of knowledge that has emerged coped with the accumulated experience mandates an important question: Is it possible to come up with a fourth objective in COM surgery? Our answer to that question is YES, IT IS: to interfere and abort the natural history of the disease. The basic precondition for doing so is the correct understanding of the pathogenesis of the condition. In other words, to identify which direction the process will take from the precipitating etiology to the establishment of irreversible tissue pathology or an outburst of a dangerous complication.

The body of studies defines a roughly standard natural history allowing us to forecast and possibly anticipate unfavorable end points, since COM follows what we call a "predictable script." Some interventions along the process are traditional and include:

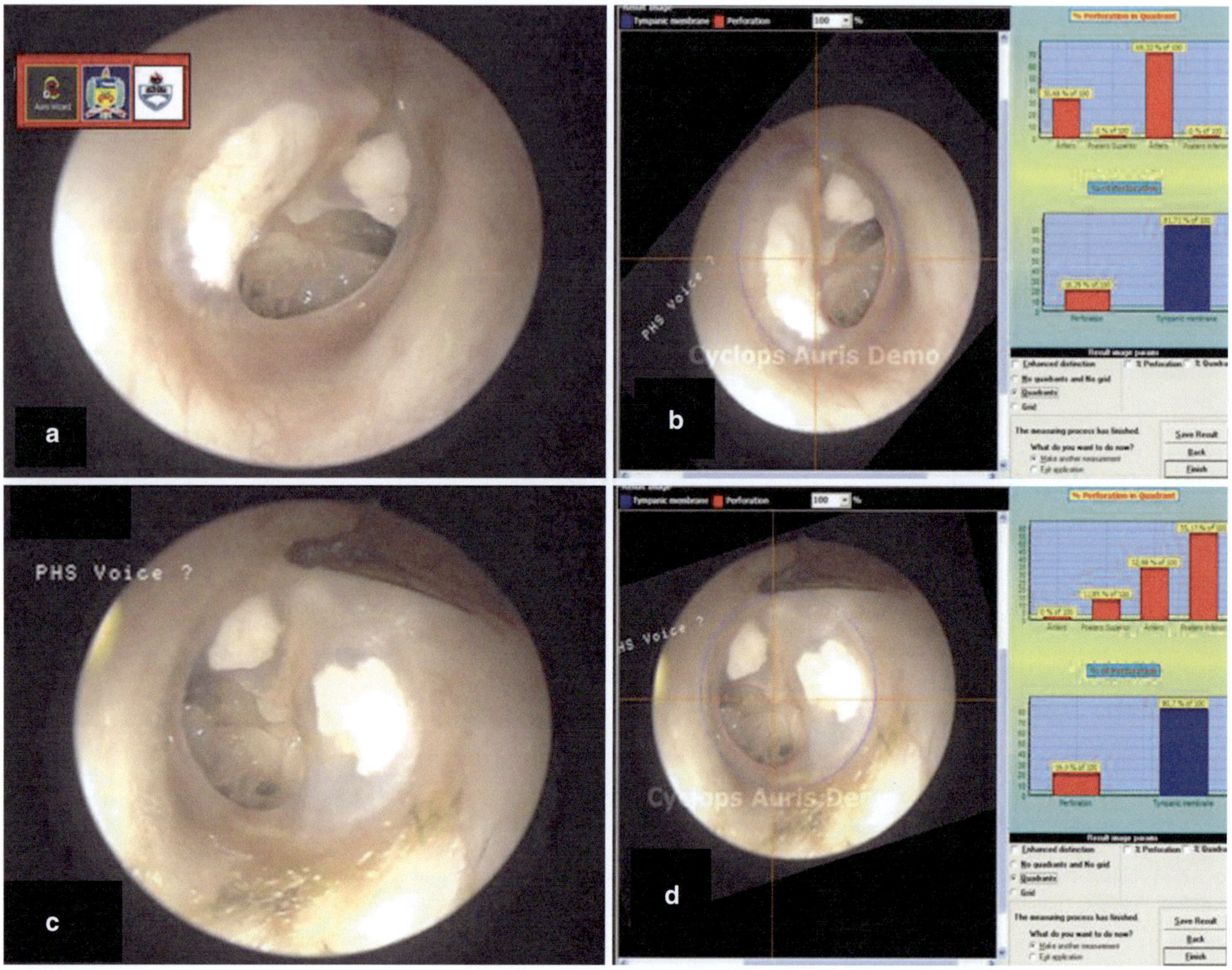

Fig. 37.32 Video-otoscopy and analysis of bilateral perforations. (**a**) Video-otoscopy right ear. (**b**) Measures in the right ear. (**c**) Video-otoscopy left ear. (**d**) Measures in the left ear

1. Identifying and controlling risk factors
2. Clinical treatment during early phases
3. Close and careful follow-up
4. Management of diseases in the neighborhood

With this concept in mind, we advance the discussion to a new level by considering a more vigorous and active intervention in the oligosymptomatic early steps of the disease.

The main dilemma is to appropriately decide between a passive or contemplative attitude or to undertake an early intervention to thwart progressive disease, despite the fact that an intervention is not devoid of intrinsic morbidity! Should one wait for a dry symptomless retraction pocket to become a draining cholesteatoma which then needs major surgery? Or, would a less invasive approach to an earlier stage have been better? Of course, the answers would be simple if we could ensure that this transition would be inevitable! Choosing the best option between these two extremes and targeting the correct timing of intervention implies a very challenging decision, since there is a lack of evidence-based information to support choosing one or other approach. When the clinician is confronted to this borderline situation what should be his next step? Holding back and waiting for an evidence-based solution or venturing into a yet to be proven new alternative technique?

When we take into consideration a patient that comes to our attention hoping to be cured, waiting for the evidences may become too late or no more appropriate. In the other hand, choosing a new technique in the hope of aborting the process may be ineffective and aggressive. The main difficulty when getting to this crossroad is the natural history of the disease itself since it moves freely between different stages, going through phases that are not necessarily unidirectional. Thus, as the active disease relapses for long periods, the silent sequel may emerge in acute outbursts, at times, very close to complications.

In real-life practice, it is frequently impossible to determine the boundaries between subtypes of otitis media since the limits are thin if not overlapped.

We believe the importance of considering the CLE in conjunction with the most affected side in COM cannot be overemphasized. Regardless of the presence of cholesteatoma, the astute analysis of both ears may shed some light into three key aspects of the disease process: where did it come from? (etiology) what is the current condition (established pathology) and, more importantly, how fast and in which direction the disease is marching toward (natural history). The answer to these questions will illuminate and improve the true understanding of the pathogenesis of COM by helping the treatment and the counseling of patients and relatives.

When we take into account the CLE, we can understand the dynamic pathologic process right before our eyes. There are many patients displaying similarity on both sides, at times one step ahead or behind the other.

For example, it is not rare to find a patient with a posterosuperior cholesteatoma in one ear and a severe retraction of the pars tensa in the other, or with a classical pars flacida cholesteatoma in one ear and a deep attic retraction pocket, but still cholesteatoma free in the other (Fig. 37.33a, b).

Precise and critical analysis of both ears plays a key role in the prognostic assessment of each case, since the ear established with COM may predict the likely evolution of the CLE. An aggressive cholesteatoma on one side with massive bony destruction and unfavorable evolution should lead us to more vigilant follow-up care of the CLE.

Another clinical condition in which the analysis of the CLE can be extremely helpful is the one experienced by many patients submitted to tympanotomy with bilateral ventilation tubes. On many occasions, one of the tubes is extruded early and the other remains in situ for prolonged periods of time. Although it is not our routine to remove ventilation tubes, sometimes we consider removal as a response to the patient's anxiety to sum up a routine lifestyle. Analysis of the CLE is critical in determining whether the remaining ventilation tube should be removed. If we find the "extruded" ear with a satisfactory appearance, we may assume that normal physiology has been restored, encouraging removal of the remaining tube, since the CLE suggests no trend toward progression of the disease.

The same holds true for a TM perforation: it is not rare having patients referred to us for tympanoplasty with small- to medium-sized perforations in one ear and TM retractions or effusion in the other. The most relevant problem in this kind of situation is the retraction! The perforation, probably represents what Ingesltedt once called "a God sent ventilation tube" and should preserved as such! (Fig. 37.34a, b).

This situation represents what Costa et al have called the "crystal ball effect" [31]. In other words, the ears should be analyzed as an intrinsically related pair and not as an isolated unit. Frequently, the most affected ear can predict the future status of the contralateral side. The march toward chronicity can then be aborted with the most appropriate treatment.

Finally, an interesting observation regarding TM perforations was noted in our clinical study. It was common to find ears with wide central or marginal perforations associated with badly retracted CLE. Often, there were other clinical findings such as erosion of the long process of the incus, the superstructure of the stapes, and horizontal displacement of the malleus handle. Moreover, some of these cases unveiled remains of squamous epithelium and keratin lying over the promontory and/or ossicular chain (Fig. 37.35a, b).

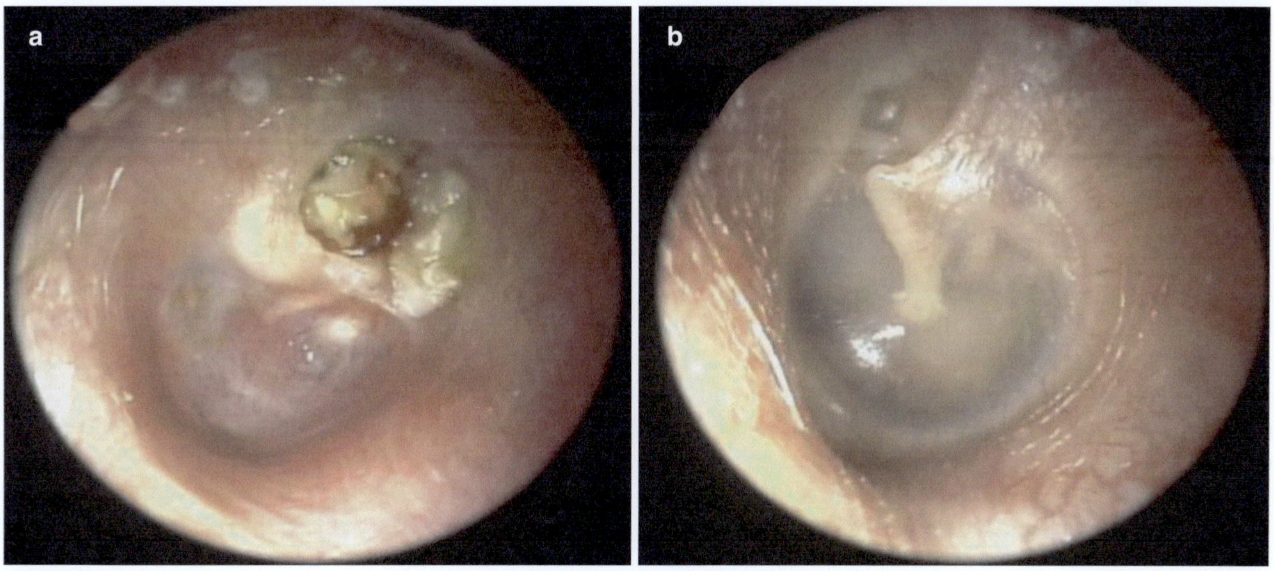

Fig. 37.33 (**a**) Case 559 (right ear): Pars flacida cholesteatoma. (**b**) Case 559 (left ear): CLE with a pars flacida moderate retraction

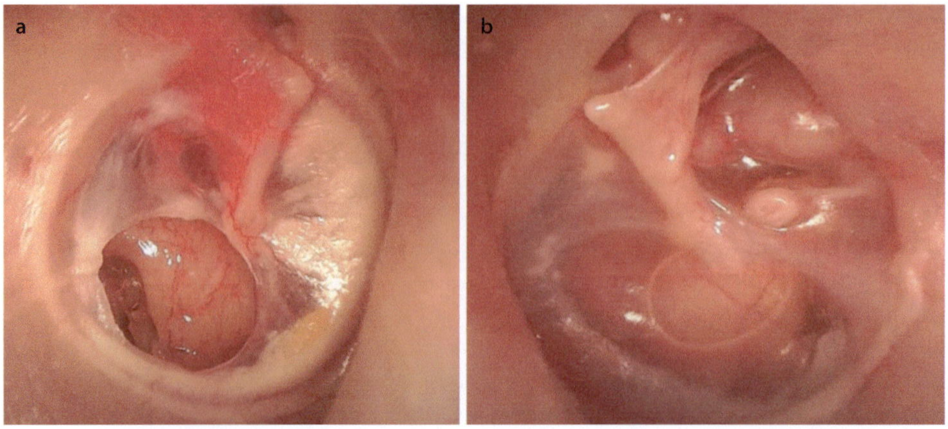

Fig. 37.34 (**a**) Case 401: right ear with a central dry TM perforation. (**b**) Case 401: left ear of the same patient with a TM retraction grade 3–4

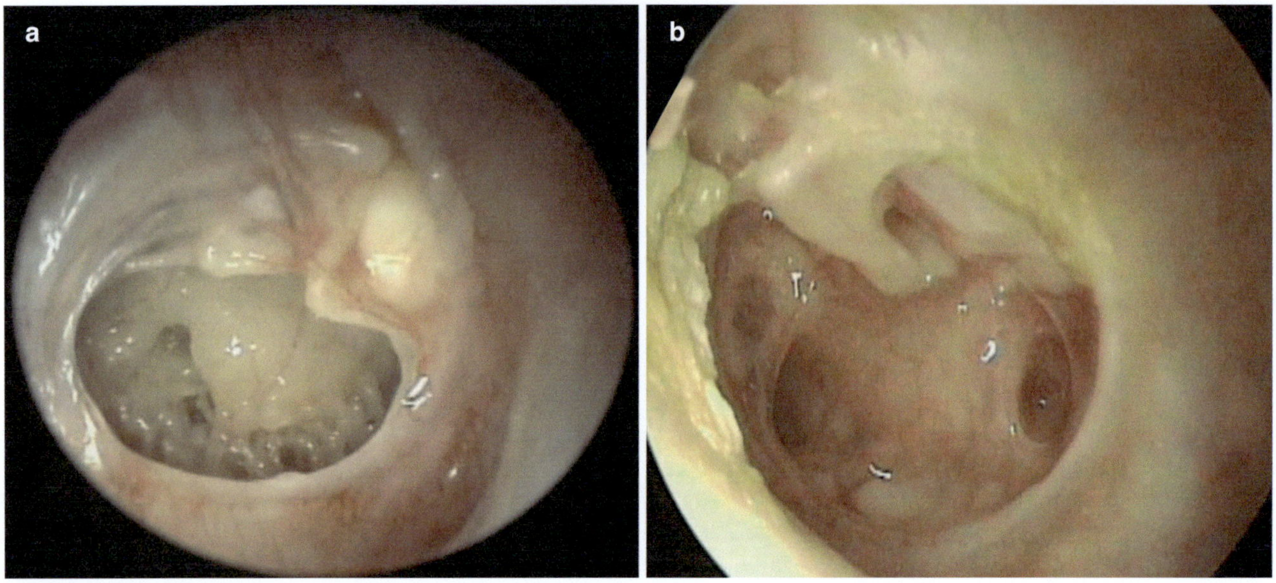

Fig. 37.35 (**a**) Case 563 (right ear): TM perforation. (**b**) Case 563 (left ear): CLE with TM perforation, medial displacement of the malleus and adhesions of the remaining TM to the medial wall of the cleft

This observation gives us some extra insights regarding the origin of the TM perforations. It has long been postulated that TM perforations are a consequence of a series of triggering situations including recurrent acute otitis media, acute necrotizing otitis media, and trauma to the temporal bone, which in our opinion are rare events (as causes of large definitive TM perforations). Nevertheless, we keep seeing patients with the condition on a daily basis. In other words, it seems that the mechanisms traditionally related to the origin of those perforations (i.e., causes) are identified in a much smaller proportion on a daily basis than the number of tympanic perforations that is presented to us (i.e., the consequences). Given this paradox, it is possible to conclude that there must be other mechanisms, which are responsible for the generation of these alterations, or we are faced with a bizarre "missing link" as far as chronic otitis media pathogenesis is concerned.

Our studies supply sufficient information in order to reject missing links, considering additional explanations in the pathogeneses of tympanic perforations. This way, the transition between acute and chronic cases has been explained predominantly through "explosive" mechanisms, that is, any sudden inflammatory or traumatic events that befall a primarily rigid structure. The rupture of the intratympanic homeostasis will induce a series of histological transformations in the mucosa layer of the middle ear, which will modify proportionally according to future aggressions. The adoption of this acute-chronic express or "direct" model of pathogenesis leaves out a series of situations commonly experienced by the otolaryngologist. Historically, some of these events (tympanic retractions, atelectasis, and adhesive otitis media) have been inexplicably set aside this discussion.

The chronic silent otitis media, however, (along with its long list of clinical and pathological explanations) have been neglected due to lack of both information and technological resources for its correct identification and analysis. New studies focused on the specific characteristics of these conditions may provide the necessary information for the elaboration of more realistic and operational concepts of the NCCOM. It is our firm opinion that such findings (when associated with a badly retract CLE) unequivocally point to a mechanism of TM perforation that we term outside-in. In other words, the TM perforation was not created as a sudden and permanent complication of an acute explosive middle ear event (like the so-called necrotizing otitis media or temporal bone traumas) but rather as a final result of an insidious and slowly progressive process of retraction, atrophy, infection, and perforation. According to Sade, pathodynamically these perforations represent the fifth stage of atelectasis and can be revealed only if atelectatic ears are followed systematically for some time. They appear insidiously without an acute otitis media presenting itself and sometimes in the midst of a previous tuft of granulation tissue. Erosion of the ossicles and medialization of the malleus also suggest that a force was exerted over the tympano-ossicular system. The axis of this force was from lateral to medial and obviously a retracted TM preceded the perforation.

Since 1987, we have spent a great deal of our time on researching the pathological profile and the pathogenesis of the NCCOM. The results of our studies, allied to practice, point to NCCOM as a reference in the chapter of inflammatory processes in the middle ear, acting perhaps, as a "link" between the most incipient and advanced forms of otitis media. Summing up, excluding in one extreme AOM and OME and in the other the cholesteatomas, we conceptually refer to the all the inflammatory pathology in-between, as NCCOM. The incidence of tympanic perforation in that context is merely one more detail in the realm of the irreversible tissue alterations that comprise this prevailing disease. We point out that, if the presence of a simple tympanic continuity solution (always) represented a serious medical problem we, "diligent" doctors, would certainly prevent our patients from being inserted, all over the world, millions of ventilation tubes every year.

Again, an apparent paradox takes us to one more question: what is the true morbidity of the tympanic perforations, since a great deal of them is caused by ourselves? The answer to this question involves a series of considerations about the dimension and the location of the perforation, the degree of the associated hearing loss and the intra-tympanic instability directly related to it, and obviously to its impact on the patient's quality.

Analyzing this subject more technically, Costa [2], while studying HTB with COM, noted that the pathological findings within the middle ear cleft were independent of the TM status and some HTB with perforated TM presented less salient inflammatory profiles and with well-established sequelae (tympanosclerosis and bone neoformation). In the light of these findings, the authors concluded that, in these occasions, the tympanic perforation might have worked as a natural ventilation tube, allowing the aeration of the middle ear, thus helping to the inflammatory process to slow down and stabilize.

A broad view of this scenario (at one extreme the ventilation tubes and small perforations and in the other draining ears and highways to epithelial migration), we conclude the existence of two types of perforation: the solution-perforation and the problem-perforation. The former, apparently, soothes, decelerates, or solves the intra-tympanic inflammatory events, while the latter clearly emphasizes them.

In short, retractions of the TM play an essential role either in the development of cholesteatomas and/or some of the TM perforations seen in the daily practice. The natural history of TM retractions may follow one of four destinies: (1) resolve, (2) erode bone and stabilize, (3) perforate, and (4) accumulate keratin and become a cholesteatoma.

As pointed out before, retractions pockets are clearly an element of otitis media and likely represent an early stage of the process of cholesteatoma formation. They may present in a rather innocuous fashion, being asymptomatic, with normal or near-normal hearing and a percentage are thought to evolve to cholesteatoma. The key question here is to single out which of them will cross the thin line between a dry retraction and an active cholesteatoma and so benefit from an early intervention! It is our opinion that definitive surgical indications include conductive hearing loss, accumulation of debris, and keratin or uncontrolled retraction pockets.

References

1. Juhn SK, Paparella MM, Kim LS, Goycoolea MV, Giebink S. Pathogenesis of otitis media. Ann Othol Rhinol Laryngol. 1977;86(4):481–93.
2. Costa SS. Contribution to the study of chronic otitis media. Dissertation (master's degree)—Faculty of Medicine of Ribeirão Preto, USP, 1991.
3. Yoon TH, Schachern PA, Paparella MM, et al. Pathology and pathogeny of tympanic membrane retraction. Am J Otolaryngol. 1990;11:10–7.
4. Bluestone CD. Epidemiology and Pathogenesis of chronic otitis suppurative otitis media: implications for prevention and treatment. Int J Pediatr Otorhinolaryngol. 1998;42(3):207–23.
5. Lopes Filho O. Otites averages chronicles. In: Lopes Filho O, editor. Topics in otorhinolaryngology, vol. 2. São Paulo: Manole; 1978. p. 65–86.
6. Bluestone CD, Kenna MA. Workshop on chronic suppurative otitis media. Ann Othol Rhinol Laryngol. 1988;97:131.
7. DeWeese DD, Saunders WH. Diseases of the middle ear and wastoid. In: DeWeese DD, Saunders DD, editors. Textbook otolaryngology. St. Louis: CV Mosby Co; 1964. p. 378–96.

8. Goin DW. Chronic inflammatory diseases of the middle ear and mastoid. In: English DE, editor. Otolaryngology. A textbook. Hageratown: Harper & Row; 1976. p. 167–75.
9. Hungria H. Otitesmédiascrônicassupurativas. Timpanoplastias. In: Hungria H, editor. Otorrinolariongologia. 5th ed. Rio de Janeiro: Guanabara Koogan; 1988. p. 307–25.
10. Kenna MA. Microbiology of chronic suppurative otitis media in children. Ann Otol Rhinol Laryngol. 1988;97(131):9–13.
11. Costa SS, et al. Temporal bones in chronically infected ears with intact and perforated tympanic membranes. Laryngoscope. 1992;102(11):1229–36.
12. Cruz OLM, Costa SS. Simple chronic otitis media. In: Costa SS, Cruz OLM, Oliveira JAA, editors. Otorhinolaryngology. Principles and practice. Porto Alegre: Medical Arts Publisher; 1994.
13. Paparella MM, Hiraide F, Juhn SK, Kaneco J. Celular events involved in middle ear fluid production. Ann Rhinol Otol Laryngol. 1970;79(4):766–79.
14. Proctor B. The development of the middle ear spaces and their surgical significance. Laryngol Otol. 1964;78(7):631–45.
15. Fishman AJ, Marrinan MS, Roland JT. Repair of the total tympanic membrane perforation: alloderm vs temporalis fascia. Otolaryngol–Head Neck Surg. 2004;131(2):P50.
16. Goyccolea MV, Paparella MM, Carpenter AM. Oval and round window changes in otitis media: an experimental study in the cat. Surg Forum. 1978;29:598–80.
17. Bauer JA, Huve FDC, Oliveira FH, Silva MNLD, Sperling N, Costa SSD. Mongolian Gerbils as a model for the study of cholesteatoma: otoendoscopic as a diagnostic tool. Int Arch Otorhinolaryngol. 2023;26:643–8.
18. Schuknecht HF. The pathology of the ear. Cambridge: Harvard University; 1974.
19. Costa SS et al. Histopathology of chronic otitis media with perforated and non-perforadedtympanic membrane. In: Presented at the Midwinter Meeting of the Association for Research inOtolaryngology. Clearwater, 1989.
20. Meterhoff WL, Kim CG, Paparella MM. Pathology of chronic otitis media. Ann Otol Rhinol Laryngol. 1978;87(6):749–61.
21. CarvalhalLHSK. Otologic findings in patients with cleft lip and palate or isolated clef palate. Dissertation (master's degree) – Faculty of Medicine UFRGS, 2003.
22. Paradise JL, Bluestone CD, Felder H. The universality of otitis media in 50 infants with cleft palate. Pediatrics. 1969;44:35–42.
23. Tasaka Y, Kawano M, Honjo I. Eustachian tube function in OME patients with cleft palate. Acta Otolaryngol (Stockh). 1990;471:5–8.
24. Caldarelli DD. Incidence and type of othopathology associated with congenital palatopharyngeal incompetence. Laryngoscope. 1978;88:1970–84.
25. Fara M, Dvorak J. Abnormal anatomy of the muscles of the palato-pharyngeal closure in cleft palates. Plast Reconst Surg. 1970;46:488–96.
26. Doyle WJ. Functional Eustachian tube obstruction and otitis media in a primate model. Acta Otolaryngol (Stockoh) Suppl. 1984;414:52–7.
27. Sadé J, Air A. Middle ear and auditory tube: middle ear clearance, gas exchange and pressure regulation. Otolaryngol Head and Neck Surg. 1997;116:499–524.
28. American Academies of Otolaryngology, Pediatrics and Family Practice. Clinical practice guidelines: otitis media with effusion. Otolaryngol Head Neck Surg. 2004;130:S95–S118.
29. Casebrant M, Brostoff LM, et al. Otitis media with effusion in preschool children. Laryngoscope. 1985;95:428–36.
30. Chalton R, Stearns M. The incidence of bilateral chronic otitis media. J Laryngol Otol. 1984;98:337–9.
31. Vartiainen E, Kansanen M, Vartiainen J. The contralateral ear in patients with chronic otitis media. Am J Otol. 1996;17:190–2.
32. Rosito LPS, Costa SS, Scharchen PA, et al. Contralateral ear inchronic otitis media: a histologic study. Laryngoscope. 2007;117:1810–4.

Chronic Otitis Media Without Cholesteatoma

38

Fábio André Selaimen, Mauricio Noschang Lopes da Silva, and Sady Selaimen da Costa

Introduction

Otitis media is defined as an inflammatory process, infectious or not, focal or generalized, located in the middle ear cleft [1]. Because of its high prevalence and multiple clinical presentations, otitis media generates high social costs and gets directly or indirectly expensive. In the same way, the family suffering caused by the otitis media is absolutely immeasurable—the pain, the discomfort, the hearing loss, the moral damage of an ear with chronic fluids and foul smell, the psychological trauma of a child who is unable to enjoy the fun of a single dive (or at least a single bath unsupervised), the complications, and unfortunately, the death, are still problems faced by otorhinolaryngologists in their daily office routine. Thus, even with extreme scientific advances, otitis media contradicts all expectations and is, still in the third millennium, a global health public problem far away from being equated [2].

Definitions

Chronic otitis media (COM) can be defined under different aspects: the clinical, the temporal, and the histopathological [3].

From the eminent *clinical* point of view, it is characterized as an inflammatory condition associated with wide and persisting perforation of the tympanic membrane (TM) and otorrhea.

Chronologically, it refers to an inflammatory process of the middle ear, which does not last less than 3 months.

F. A. Selaimen (✉) · M. N. L. da Silva
Hospital de Clínicas de Porto Alegre, Porto Alegre, Brazil

Instituto Gaúcho de Otorrinolaringologia, Porto Alegre, Brazil

S. S. da Costa
Hospital de Clínicas de Porto Alegre, Porto Alegre, Brazil

Instituto Gaúcho de Otorrinolaringologia, Porto Alegre, Brazil

Universidade Federal do Rio Grande do Sul, Porto Alegre, Brazil

Histopathologically, it has been defined as an inflammatory process of the middle ear associated with irreversible tissue changes. Still, from the histopathological aspects, this inflammatory process may even dispense from tympanic perforation and chronic otorrhea for its characterization. However, it will always be associated with irreversible clinical tissue damage.

While acute otitis media (AOM) presents an inflammatory process that develops abruptly, and the resolution comes quickly and thoroughly, COM is usually associated with insidious, persistent, and, mainly, destructive inflammatory situations. It is subclassified into two major groups: non-choleseatomatous chronic otitis media (NCCOM) and cholesteatomatous chronic otitis media (CCOM) [4, 5]. As their names reveal, the fundamental difference between these two groups is the presence of the cholesteatoma, which on its own would place a degree of increased aggressiveness to this condition. The present chapter describes and discusses only the NCCOM and its variations.

Etiology

Some of the main situations that trigger the installation of a chronic inflammatory process in the middle ear are recurrent otitis media, acute necrotizing otitis media (ANOM), and trauma. In addition, social-economical and geographical factors also influence the incidence of the disease.

Repeated Otitis Media

The NCCOM may originate from a repeated outbreak of acute otitis media (AOM) [6–9], either because of inappropriate treatment or conditions that ease the re-infection. Risk factors for repetitive AOM are selective immune deficiency, allergy, and eustachian tube dysfunction, among others. Understanding these factors and the correct treatment is vital to prevent the process from becoming chronic. In case the outbreak happens many times, the possibility of weakening

M. V. Goycoolea et al. (eds.), *Textbook of Otitis Media*, https://doi.org/10.1007/978-3-031-40949-3_38

of the TM increases, with the consequent manifestation of degenerative mucous changes, such as epithelial dysplasia and interstitial fibrosis. This cycle will make it easy to establish the chronicity of the infection or the functional and morphological consequences [10–12].

Acute Necrotizing Otitis Media (ANOM)

The NCCOM may also develop after an outbreak of necrotizing AOM [13]. Most of the time, the ANOM affects children and young people with a systemic acute or toxic disease like scarlatina, pneumonia, measles, or any other acute and feverish disease. The otologic infection often goes unnoticed until we have otorrhea, which is usually profuse and requires regular microscopic aspiration. If this is not done, the diagnosis will be postponed until the next appointment with the physician. A typical characteristic of this entity is the erosion of the TM in the early stages of the disease, happening at the same time the patient begins to complain about pain and the beginning of the otorrhea. The otoscopy will reveal, very soon, a perforation of great dimensions different from that seen in common suppurated AOM with small and little granulation tissue around.

Trauma

Another possible etiology for a tympanic perforation, and thus the characterization of an NCCOM, is the trauma over the TM. The most common traumas are barotrauma (atmosphere pressure variation), explosion, and foreign bodies (cotton swabs, keys, and pens). Most often, the damaged TM heals spontaneously, mainly in children. However, in substantial losses, the healing may not happen and result in a perforation. Thus, an open door for contamination will be formed, from the external auditory canal into the middle ear.

Upper Airway Infections

Repeated upper airway infections, associated or not to allergic conditions, are a possible risk factor for COM [14]. Chronic tonsillitis can collaborate with impaired middle ear homeostasis, usually associated with eustachian tube dysfunction. Adenoid hypertrophy can promote obstruction of the ostium of the eustachian tube and can be associated with contamination of the region, mainly in children [15, 16]. Allergic and infectious rhinitis and sinusitis have also been associated with generating favorable conditions for middle ear contamination through mechanisms similar to those in tonsillitis.

Fungal Otitis Externa

Especially in countries with a tropical climate and also considering a predilection for certain seasons of the year, external fungal otitis can be quite frequent. In some cases, they can lead to partial necrosis of the TM and generate a tympanic perforation, often permanent. Prompt recognition of this condition and, consequently, appropriate treatment may reduce the risk of irreversible damage to the TM.

Social-Economical and Geographical Factors

Malnutrition, inadequate hygiene, low quality of living, and high population density are factors that, from the epidemiological point of view, are associated with a higher incidence of middle ear infection. The incidence of COM is higher in countries with a low development level.

Clinical Forms

While CCOM is unequivocally characterized due to the presence of squamous epithelium in the middle ear (or other pneumatized areas of the temporal bone), NCCOM presents a greater variety of clinical presentations [4].

Although it is impossible to subdivide with absolute precision the clinical phases of a disease as complex as COM, it is necessary to establish some parameters for didactic and research purposes to organize the study. Thus, the clinical entities described below as separate diseases may often present points of intersection between them or simply coexist in the same ear. For example, a retraction may course with effusion, or a tympanic perforation may result from a retraction.

Retractions

It is proposed that TM retractions result from the middle ear and mastoid deventilation. Starting in a dysfunctional eustachian tube, the sustained negative pressure in the middle ear ends up collapsing the most fragile wall of the system, that is, the TM [11, 16–18]. Retractions are classified according to their location and degree.

The study of retractions should also consider the presence of effusion, involvement of the ossicular chain, or other bone erosions (posterosuperior wall, lateral wall of the attic). In the clinical evaluation, in addition to the otoscopic findings at the first consultation (degree and location), it is essential to analyze the hearing status and to follow evolution over time. The instability of the retraction, with recurrent granulation or otorrhea, is also crucial in deciding on the (surgical) management of the retraction.

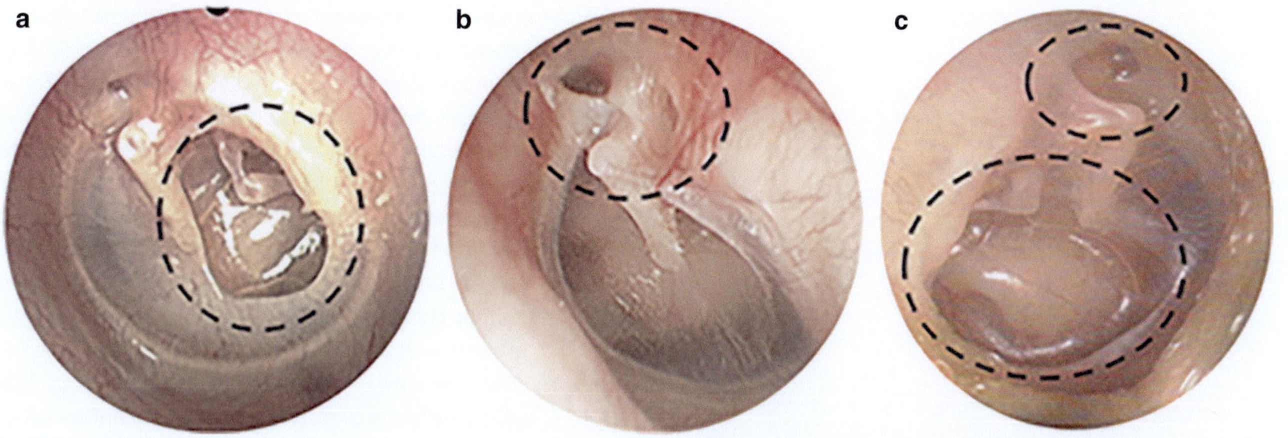

Fig. 38.1 Retractions according to localization. (**a**) *Pars tensa* retraction. (**b**) *Pars flaccida* retraction. (**c**) Two-route retraction

We suggest the reader refer to the specific chapters about TM retractions available in this book. In Fig.38.1, we illustrate the three types of retractions according to localization: *pars tensa*, *pars flaccida*, and two-route retractions.

Perforations

Tympanic membrane perforations are defined as a lack of integrity of the tympanic membrane (TM), which can result from different etiologies and require different treatments. They are part of a spectrum of diseases known as chronic otitis media (COM). Historically, tympanic perforations are divided into *central*, that is, if there are TM borders in all 360° of the perforation, and *marginal*, if there is a lack of any of the perforation edges [4, 5].

In our group, after many years of studies and publications on this subject, we currently prefer to classify perforations as ***outside-in*** (or retraction-perforation) or ***inside-out*** (without associated retraction or explosive), as we will see below. We strongly recommend that the reader to refer to chapter **Tympanic Membrane Perforations and Tympanoplasty: New Profiles, New Strategies**.

In short, the ***inside-out*** are the ones not associated with retraction, that is, an "explosive" perforation. This group of perforations, whose proposed etiology is related to acute events (acute suppurative otitis media, traumatic perforations, and external otitis with partial necrosis of the tympanic membrane), is understood as an "accident." They are previously healthy middle ears, which possibly have suffered aggression at a specific moment, be it traumatic, inflammatory, or infectious, generating tympanic perforation as a permanent sequel. Disruption of intratympanic homeostasis, caused by an acute mechanism, will modulate a series of histological transformations in the mucous lining of the middle ear, which would change permanently, characterizing COM. Figure 38.2 illustrates an *inside-out* perforation.

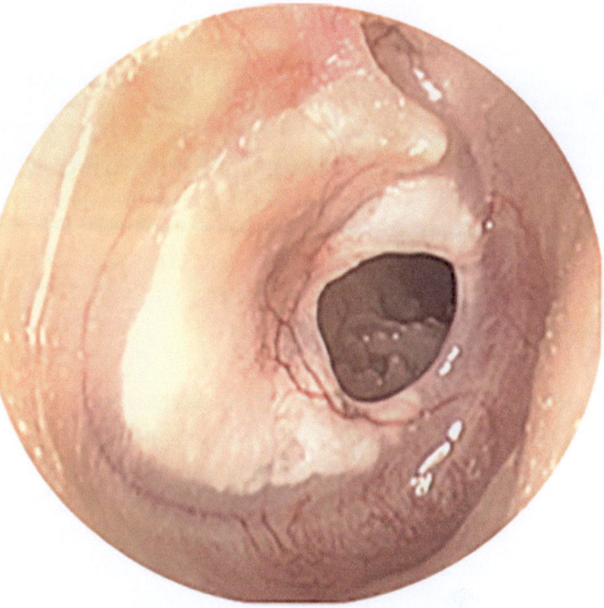

Fig. 38.2 Inside-out perforation, without signs of TM retraction

On the other hand, the ***outside-in*** perforations (Fig.38.3) refer to the ones associated with retraction signs. Those signs are (a) medialization of the malleus handle, (b) tympanic remnants over the promontory, (c) tympanic remnants over the ossicular chain, and (d) erosion of the ossicular chain. It represents an alternative pathogenesis model in which a progressive retraction would lead to perforation. The pressure self-generated by the retracted TM against the structures of the middle ear (ossicles, promontory) induces ischemia of the capillaries of the membrane and, consequently, the necrosis of a part of it. It is reaching the apex of this process that the retraction will turn into a perforation.

Thus, the pathogenesis proposed for this group of perforations is very similar to that of tympanic retractions, involving a negative pressure mechanism (probably from auditory

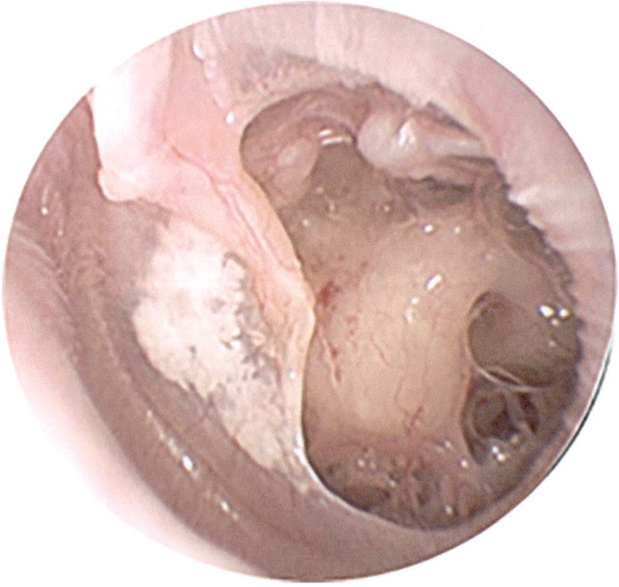

Fig. 38.3 Outside-in perforation, with signs of TM retraction

tube dysfunction) and an entire altered middle ear homeostasis, which would be responsible for the progressive retraction until perforation.

Chronic Silent Otitis Media

Although NCCOM is traditionally associated with tympanic perforations and otorrhea, histopathological studies in animals and human beings are unanimous in demonstrating pathological tissue with irreversible inflammatory changes in the middle ear despite the presence of perforations in the tympanic membrane. Based on evidence like this, Paparella et al. [19] created the term *chronic silent otitis media,* referring to the inflammatory pathologies in the middle ear with veiled and disguised progression. Thus, it is important to highlight that the presence of a normal TM does not exclude, in many cases, the detection of otitis media.

This way, aiming to avoid the inappropriate use of the term chronic silent otitis media (CSOM), it was divided into two variants: *undetected* and *undetectable*. This distinction is crucial since the *undetected* CSOM may be due to a primary failure during the otolaryngologic investigation; on the other hand, the *undetectable* CSOM is a challenging diagnosis to the physician, who must be aware of the fact that an asymptomatic ear, apparently normal, may shelter an active and focal pathological process.

In 1991, Costa studied 144 human temporal bones with irreversible inflammatory changes (granulation tissue, ossicular changes, cholesteatomas, cholesterol granuloma, tympanosclerosis, and tympanic membrane perforations) [2]. The temporal bones were divided into two groups: those with intact tympanic membrane (group I) and those with tympanic membrane perforations (group II). The more frequent findings in these temporal bones were granulation tissue (in 97.9%), ossicular changes (in 91.6%), tympanosclerosis (in 24.3%), tympanic membrane perforations (in 19.4%), cholesterol granuloma (in 13.8%), and cholesteatomas (in 10.4%). There were tympanic membrane perforations in 28 temporal bones (19.4%), while 116 bones presented intact membranes. Surprisingly, the comparative analysis of the temporal bones with or without tympanic membrane perforations indicated that the groups were similar: granulation tissue, ossicular changes, and cholesterol granuloma were found in both groups, and the differences in frequencies were not meaningful. However, cholesteatomas and tympanosclerosis were identified more frequently in temporal bones with tympanic membrane perforations (group II).

Clinical Implications and Physiopathogenesis Evolved from the Concept of the Chronic Silent Otitis Media

Frequencies and Distribution of the Granulation Tissue

The high frequencies and generalized distribution of the granulation tissue throughout the entire middle ear cleft in temporal human bones with or without tympanic perforations seem to be very important [3, 15, 20–22]. A lot has been written about the CCOM. However, a few publications mention the problem of some patients who, although do not present cholesteatomas, complain of profuse and continuous purulent otorrhea. The origin of this otorrhea is the granulation tissue that practically fills up the middle ear and, not rarely, extends to the mastoid. This type of otitis cannot be considered a synonym of the *simple* chronic otitis media (a term widely used in medicine to name an otitis media case that is not associated with cholesteatomas), since it carries a morbidity similar to the one in the cholesteatomas itself. In a panel about mastoidectomies, Paparella, Caparosa, and Glasscock were unanimous in pointing to the granulation tissue as the primary pathologic condition that most frequently conducted this procedure.

Lau and Tos [23] named this condition granulomatous NCCOM, recommending, in these situations, the tympanomastoidectomy whenever an aggressive conservative therapy (with frequent cleaning, local and systemic antibiotic therapy) does not succeed in controlling the inflammatory process after three months. Proctor [24] recommended tympanomastoidectomy in patients with chronic otorrhea, who are resistant to the clinical treatment, despite the presence of cholesteatoma in the middle ear. Paparella et al. [25] and Costa and Cruz [26] claim that the presence of small masses of focal granulation tissue strategically distributed in the middle ear cleft (mainly in the region of the round window niche) is responsible for hearing loss.

In conclusion, the granulation tissue is an almost unique characteristic of the histopathological profile of chronic otitis media. Its clinical importance originated from the possibility of generating, even in isolation, a series of signals and symptoms like otorrhea, osteitis, ossicular necrosis, conductive and sensorineural hearing loss, and disturbs related to the posterior labyrinth. Besides that, its pathogenicity does not end itself since the presence of granulation in transitional areas of the middle ear cleft (protympanum, isthmus and *aditus ad antrum*) interrupts the airflow. Thus, a vicious cycle of additional pathological changes is established.

Interaction Between Middle and Inner Ear

Various studies show the connection between chronic otitis media and cochlear damage. Paparella et al. [27], English et al. [28], Dumich and Harner [29], Walby et al. [30], and Paparella [1, 31] all of them indicated the relationship between chronic otitis media and sensorineural hearing loss. Paparella et al. [27] investigated the pathology of sensorineural hearing loss caused by otitis media. Also, Goycoolea et al. [32] and Walby et al. [30] published this subject. Their work points to the round window membrane as responsible for transmitting the pathological process to the labyrinth. The anatomy and localization of the round window niche predispose to the accumulation of pathology in the presence of otitis media.

Dysventilation of the Middle Ear Cleft and the Development of Otitis Media

Several studies point out that dysventilation is the most important factor in the pathogenesis of otitis media. Therefore, the regions deprived of O_2 tend to suffer pathological alterations more frequently. To corroborate this hypothesis, studies with patients and with temporal bone dissections have also led us to believe that sites of ventilation obstruction (in certain sections or compartments of the middle ear) may influence chronic otitis media pathogenesis [16, 33–35]. Those obstructions might be due to anatomic, physiologic, or even pathologic variations that result in compartmental pathologic processes [16].

With this information, we can more appropriately investigate, understand, and work with some otological symptoms that seem, at first sight, obscure, and inexplicable. Neglecting those concepts would be a tremendous medical mistake, which suggests that we are more interested in provoking or sealing perforations in the tympanic membrane rather than diagnosing and treating pathologic conditions of the middle or inner ear.

Ossicular Pathology of the Chronic Otitis Media

The hearing loss associated with otitis media may appear early or late during the process, varying considerably regarding the type and degree. As for the type, the hearing loss may be conductive, sensorineural, or mixed [36]. As for the degree, depending on how aggressive and the extension of the pathological process, they can vary from mild or moderate losses (usually associated with the conductive type) in the majority of cases. However, some cases may course with severe and profound losses (sensorineural).

As mentioned before, the mechanisms involved in sensorineural hearing losses have been explained based on the biological behavior of the round window, mainly, and the oval one during the inflammatory processes of the middle ear [37, 38]. This way, they can be understood as gateways for toxins from the middle ear toward the inner ear, characterizing the interaction between these two compartments. Furthermore, several studies demonstrate an association of the chronic otitis media to cochlear damage, again pointing to the round window as the structure responsible for the transmission of the pathological process to the labyrinth.

On the other hand, the conductive losses regarding COM include a series of changes in the tympano-ossicular system. Concerning the tympanic membrane, the loss of substance (perforations), the atrophy (and the consequent retraction), and the increase of its rigidity (because of tympanosclerosis plaque) are some of the most often causes of hearing loss. The ossicular system, however, can also be compromised by ossicular erosion (with the interruption of the sound transmission as a consequence), as ossicular fixation, due to tympanosclerosis or fibrosis.

Finally, the effects of mass in the middle ear cleft (caused by liquid, cholesterol granuloma, cholesteatomas, or granulation tissue) may damage the ossicles and compromise the vibratory capacity of the tympano-ossicular system. Thus, conductive hearing loss is generated or majored.

Considering the dynamic nature of COM, all those changes may present themselves isolated or in combinations at the middle ear. For instance, as usual, gross erosions of the long incus process follow the atrophy and retraction processes of the posterosuperior quadrant of the tympanic membrane. Likewise, the oversized perforations, the cholesteatomas, and the granulation tissue may cause ossicular destructions and, consequently, significant hearing damage [39–41]. The long-term active inflammatory processes [42] of the middle ear may course with tympanosclerosis with fibrosis of the ossicular chain.

Costa et al. [43] studied specifically the ossicular pathology of 132 temporal human bones with COM and pathologies in 91, 6% of the subjects. These changes varied from simply the erosion of the ossicular cortical to complete destruction. According to the authors, the ossicular damage caused by the pathological process was incus (91%), followed by the stapes (69, 4%) and the malleus (54, 2%).

Surprisingly, the comparative analysis of the temporal bones with and without perforations of the tympanic membrane indicated that the groups were similar concerning the ossicular pathology (prevalence, localization, and mainly damaged ossicles). These findings again call our attention to the large number of COM cases that might be underdiagnosed. In this context, the correct diagnosis can only be confirmed through an exploratory tympanostomy. This procedure is an irreplaceable tool for these patients once all irreversible changes in the middle ear are not evident.

Thus, the exploratory tympanostomy is added to the propaedeutic and therapeutical resources of the otologist as a minor surgical procedure [44]. It is safe and extremely useful because it allows the direct visualization of the middle ear, revealing, confirming, and frequently treating pathological conditions. The accurate knowledge of the nature and extension of the lesions will then determine the following surgical steps.

The numbers are still similar when we compare these findings with clinical studies concerning the ossicular changes. Austin [45] noticed the interruption of the ossicular chain in 50% of his patients that were submitted to tympanoplasty because of COM. Tos [46] found interruption in the ossicular chain in 50% of the ears that underwent surgery dry and in 80% of the surgery patients with otorrhea. Sadéand Halevy [37], when revising their cases of tympanoplasties and tympanomastoidectomies, observed lesions in the ossicular chain in 84% of the ears with CCOM and 83% of the ears with NCCOM. We must emphasize that these studies, as eminently clinical, functionally classified the ossicular pathologies. Small erosions in the ossicular surfaces were probably not considered. Thus, only ossicular in discontinuity, destroyed, or amputated were considered pathological.

We believe the ossicular defects result from active processes of bone reabsorption and not ossicular necrosis. This theory presupposes the presence and participation of immune cells in the mechanisms of demineralization, erosion, and destruction of the bone. An ossicle without blood supply can remain in situ for several years without suffering the reabsorption process, as we can testify in the ossicular reconstruction techniques. The mechanism through which bone reabsorption occurs in the chronic otitis media is not entirely understood [47].

Ruedi [12] and Tumarkin [48] suggested that bone reabsorption would happen because of the pressure done by the cholesteatomas over the ossicular surface. Sadé and Berco [38] and Thomsen [49] noticed that the eroded ossiculars were invariably surrounded by an inflammatory reaction and suggested that the inflammation was the cause of the ossicular reabsorption. It has demonstrated that the tissue of the granulation adjacent to the ossicles is capable of producing a variety of enzymes and mediators that accelerate the ossicular reabsorption. These include lysosomal enzymes that accelerate ossicular reabsorption. However, the dominant cell in the process of bone reabsorption is still controversial. While some studies reveal the presence of osteoclasts in bone destruction, others point to the mononuclear cells as the responsible ones for the situations. There is evidence that mastocytes function in the mechanisms of bone reabsorption because these cells increase in several pathologies like, for example, osteoporosis and chronic periodontal destructive disease.

Pathogenesis of Non-Cholesteatomatous Chronic Otitis Media

Considering such a complex disease, with so many faces and a high level of complexity, searching for the only trigger of this series of events, its pathological results, and multiple clinical consequences seems an unachievable task. In other words, our opinion is that searching for a unique explanation for a disease with so many facets and nuances could be seen as exaggerated optimism or scientific naiveness [5].

On the other hand, a brief (but careful) review of the medical literature shows that this theme has been approached two ways equally unsatisfying: the unsuitable simplification (which ignores controversial evidences and elects the acute necrotizing otitis media as the starting point of all of those processes) and the inconsistent generalization (which hides a number of frailties and many hypotheses incompletely tested under the broad name “multifactorial”).

Perhaps, many restrictions to the discussion about the pathogenesis of this disease are imposed by vices originated by either, and in this case, objective but distorted definitions or excluding didactic classifications (also known as “working” classifications). An additional complicating factor in this sense is the difficulty of selecting specific clinical and pathological characteristics in this complex realm that allow the development of representative subgroups of the active disease, sequels, and complications. Besides that, the natural history of the disease conspires against our intention to dispose of it in those subgroups and transits freely among those stages, going through courses that are not necessarily unidirectional. Thus, as the active disease relapses for long periods, the silent sequel may emerge in outbreaks that get more and more acute and, at times, very close to complications.

Some proposed triggers for developing the chronic inflammatory process in the middle ear are the suppurative acute otitis media (repetitive or inappropriately treated), the necrotizing ones, the temporal traumas, and the insidious infections of the upper airways. It is widely spread that these situations can be molded negatively by various unfavorable social, geographical, and economic co-factors.

Whatever origin they might have, the pathology of the TM acts as open doors to middle ear cleft contamination. These ways of contamination include fundamentally one intrinsic route (nasopharynx—Eustachian tube—middle ear) and another extrinsic (external ear, middle ear cleft—middle ear). In the first model, leaking and loss of middle ear pneumatic space (usually guaranteed by the integrity of the tympanic membrane) facilitate the aspiration of contaminated secretions of the nasopharynx (through the eustachian tube) to the middle ear. In the second one, the direct infection of the middle ear through externally contaminated fluids is a joint event and obviously facilitated by small and medium perforations.

Contrariwise to what has been exposed in earlier paragraphs, daily practice shows us that these triggering situations (acute otitis media, recurrent acute otitis media, and trauma) are infrequent events. Nevertheless, otorhinolaryngological clinics care daily for many patients with tympanic perforations. In other words, it seems that the mechanisms traditionally related to the origin of those perforations (that is, causes) are identified in a much smaller proportion daily than the number of tympanic perforations presented to us (that is, the consequences). Given this paradox, it is possible to conclude that there must be other mechanisms responsible for the generation of these alterations, or we are faced with a bizarre "missing link" in otitis media pathogenesis.

Our studies supply sufficient information to reject missing links, considering additional explanations in the pathogenesis of NCCOM. This way, the transition between acute and chronic cases has been explained through predominantly "explosive" mechanisms, that is, any sudden inflammatory or traumatic events that befall a primarily rigid structure. The rupture of the intratympanic homeostasis will mold a series of histological transformations in the mucosa layer of the middle ear, which will modify proportionally according to future aggressions.

Adopting this acute-chronic express or "direct" model of pathogenesis leaves out a series of situations commonly witnessed by the otorhinolaryngologist. Historically, some of these events (tympanic retractions, atelectasis, and adhesive otitis media) have been inexplicably set aside in this discussion. Still, the chronic silent otitis media (along with its long list of clinical and pathological explanations) have been disregarded, not due to negligence, but due to a lack of information and technological resources for correct identification and analysis. New studies focused on the specific characteristics of these conditions may provide the necessary information for elaborating more realistic and operational concepts of NCCOM. For many years, we have seen two entities being studied as if they were different conditions: otitis with effusion (serous, secretory, and acute) and cholesteatoma. Studies have brought light to several questions related to etiopathogenesis, diagnosis, and treatment of those conditions. Notwithstanding, it is necessary to establish the right connections between these two extremes.

Since 1987, we have spent much of our time researching the pathological profile and the pathogenesis of NCCOM. The results of our studies, allied to practice, point to NCCOM as a reference in the chapter related to inflammatory processes in the middle ear. Perhaps, it acts as a "link" between the most incipient and advanced forms of otitis media. In short, at one extremity (the beginning), there are acute, serous, and secretory otitis media cases. On another end, there are cholesteatomas. Finally, we can understand all the pathology described in this chapter, conceptually as NCCOM, being the link between both.

The tympanic perforation in that context is merely one detail more in the realm of the irreversible tissue alterations that comprehend this prevailing disease. We point out that if a simple tympanic continuity solution (always) represented a severe medical problem, we, "diligent" and zealous doctors, would undoubtedly prevent our patients from being introduced, all over the world, millions of ventilation tubes every year. So, one more time, an apparent paradox takes us to one more question: what is the actual morbidity of the tympanic perforations, since a great deal of them is caused by us? The answer to this question involves a series of considerations about the dimension and the localization of the perforation, the degree of the hearing loss, and the intratympanic instability directly related to it, and obviously to its impact on the quality of life of the patient in question.

Analyzing this subject more technically, Costa et al. [2], while studying temporal bones of humans who had chronic otitis media, noted that besides the activity and aggressivity of the pathological findings revealed in the interior of the middle ear cleft, regardless of the tympanic integrity, some of the temporal bones with perforated tympanic membrane presented inflammatory profiles less salient and with well-established sequels (tympanosclerosis and bone neoformation). In light of these findings, the authors stated that, in these cases, the tympanic perforation might have worked as a natural ventilation tube, allowing the aeration of the middle ear and, thus, collaborating with the deceleration and stabilization of the inflammatory process.

A broad view of this scenario (on one extremity, the ventilation tubes and the small perforation in the injured ear, and on the other, the secretory ears and fast lanes to migration of epithelial tissue to the middle ear), we conclude the existence of two types of perforation: the solution perforation and the problem perforation. The former soothes, decelerates, or solves the intratympanic inflammatory events, while the latter clearly emphasizes them.

References

1. Paparella MM. Current concepts in otitis media. Henry Ford Hosp Med J. 1983;31(1):30–6.
2. Costa SS. Contribuiçãoaoestudo da otitemédiacrônica. Dissertação de mestrado. Faculdade de Medicina de Ribeirão Preto, USP; 1991.
3. Juhn SK, Paparella MM, Kim LS. COL.: Pathogenesis of otitis media. Ann Otol Rhinol Laryngol. 1977;86:481–93.
4. Dornelles C, Costa SS, Laux M, Weber R. Estudocomparativo da dissolução de trêsdiferentesmarcas de colágenoutilizadas-emtécnicascirúrgicasotológicas. Rev Bras de Otorrinolaringol. 2003;69(6):744–51.
5. Dornelles C, Hemb L, Schweiger C, Matter R, Smith M, Schimdt L, Costa SS. Epidemiologia dos pacientespediátricos do ambulatório de otitemédiacrônica no Hospital de Clínicas de Porto Alegre (AOMC-HCPA). Rev Bras de Otorringol. 2004;71(4):536–46. no prelo
6. Linden A, Roithman R. Ossicular chain reconstruction: a combined prosthesis with organic and synthetic material. Laryngoscope. 1991;101:436–7.
7. Matter R, Schweiger C, Hemb L, Smith M, Schmidt L, Dornelles C, Costa SS. Estudo da orelha contralateral na otitemédiacrônica, empacientespediátricos. Revista do HCPA. 2003; www.hcpa.ufrgs.br
8. Meyerhoff WL, Giebink GS, Shea DA. Silent otitis media: an animal study. Ann Otol Rhinol Laryngol. 1984;93:136–9.
9. Palva T, Northrop C, Ramsay H. Effect of amniotic fluid cellular content on attic aeration pathways. Histologic observations on infants aged 2–4 months. Am J Otol. 2000;21(1):62–70.
10. Schmidt V, Dornelles C, Weber R, Schimdt L, Dall'Igna D, Carvalhal L, Kruse L, Costa SS. Perdaauditivacondutiva na otitemédiacrônica com perfuração central ou marginal. Pesquisa: Logos e Praxis. Unidade de Pesquisa do Instituto de Cardiologia; 2002. p. 220.
11. Sheehy JL, Linthicum FH Jr, Greenfield EC. Chronic serous mastoiditis, idiopathic hemotympanum and cholesterol granuloma of the mastoid. Laryngoscope. 1969;79(7):1189–217.
12. Ruedi L. Cholesteatosis of attic. Laryngol Otol. 1958;73:593–609.
13. Paparella MM, Hiraide F, Juhn SK. COL.: Cellular events involved in middle ear fluid production. Ann Otol Rhinol Laryngol. 1970a;79:766–79.
14. Eggston A, Wolff D. Histopathology of the ear, nose and throat. Baltimore: Williams e Wilkins; 1947.
15. Paparella MM, Meyerholff WL. Clinical significance of granulation tissue in chronic otitis media. In: Sadé J, editor. Cholesteatoma and mastoid surgery. Proceedings of the second international conference. Amsterdam: Kluger; 1982. p. 387–95.
16. Proctor B. The development of the middle ear spaces and their surgical significance. J Laryngol Otol. 1964;78:631–47.
17. Proctor B. Attic-Aditus block and the tympanic diaphragm. Ann Otol Rhinol Laryngol. 1971;80:271–5.
18. Tos M. Upon the relationship between secretory otitis in childhood and its sequellae in adults. J Laryngol Otol. 1981;98:1011–22.
19. Paparella MM, Shea D, Meyerhoff WL, Goycoolea MV. Silent otitis media. Laryngoscope. 1980;90(7):1089–98.
20. Giebink GG, Ripley ML, Shea DA, Wright PF, Paparella MM. Clinical histopatological correlations in experimmental otitis media: implications for silent otitis media in humans. Pediatr Res. 1985;19(4):389–97.
21. Jaisinghani VJ, Paparella MM, Schachern PA. Silent intratympanic membrane cholesteatoma. Laringoscope. 1998;108:1185–9.
22. Paparella MM, Koutroupas S. Exploratory timpanotomy revisited. Laryngoscope. 1982;92:531–4.
23. Lau T, Tos M. Long-Term results of surgery for chronic granulating otitis. Am J Otolaryngol. 1986;7:341–5.
24. Proctor B. Chronic otitis media and mastoiditis. In: Paparella MM, Shumrick DA, Gluckman JL, Meyerhoff WL, editors. Otolaryngology. 3rd ed. Philadelphia: WB Saunders Co.; 1991. p. 1349–78.
25. Paparella MM, Goycoolea MV, Bassiouni M, Koutroupas S. Silent otitis media. Clinical applications. Laryngoscope. 1986;96(9):978–85.
26. Costa SS, Cruz OLM. Exploratory tympanotomy. OperTechn in Otolaryngol Head and Neck Surg. 1996;7:20–5.
27. Paparella MM, Oda M, Hiraide F, Brady D. Pathology of sensorio neural hearing loss in otitis media. Ann Otol Rhinol Laryngol. 1972;81:632–47.
28. English GM, Northern JL, Fria TJ. Chronic otitis media as a cause of sensorineural hearing loss. Arch Otolaryngol. 1973;98:18–22.
29. Dumich PS, Harner SG. Cochlear function in chronic otitis media. Laryngoscope. 1983;93(5):583–6. https://doi.org/10.1002/lary.1983.93.5.583.
30. Walby AP, Barrera A, Schucknecht HF. Cochlear pathology in chronic suppurative otitis media. Ann J Otol Rhinol Laryngol. 1983;92(25):3–19.
31. Paparella MM. Quiet labyrinthine complications from otitis media. J LaryngolOtol. 1983;8:53–8.
32. Goycoolea MV, Paparella MM, Carpenter AM. Oval and round window changes in otitis media. Potential pathways between middle and inner ear. Laryngoscope. 1980;90:1387–91.
33. Sadé, J. (ed.) Secretory otitis media and its sequellae;1979.
34. Sadé J, Fuchs C, Luntz M. Shrapnell membrane and mastoid pneumatization. Arch Otolaryngol Head Neck Surg. 1997;123(6):584–8.
35. Scheibe AB, Smith MM, Schmidt LP, Schmidt VB, Dornelles C, Carvalhal LHSK, Kruse L, Costa SS. Estudo da orelha contralateral na otitemédiacrônica: "Efeito Orloff". Rev Bras Otorrinolaringol. 2002;68(2):245–9.
36. Sudhoff H, Liebehenz Y, Aschenbrenner J, Euteneurer S, Ebmeyer J, Bernal-Sprekelsen M, Stark T, Dazert S. Expression of osteoclast stimulating and differentiating factors in a murine model of localized inflammatory bone resorption. Laryngorhinootologie. 2004;83(1):14–9.
37. Sadé J, Halevy A. The aetiology of bone destructioninchronic otitis media. J LaryngolOtol. 1974;88(2):139–43.
38. Sadé J, Berco E. Bone destruction in chronic otitis media: a histopathological study. J LaryngolOtol. 1974;88:413–22.
39. Tos M. Manual of middle ear surgery. Stuttgart, NY: Thieme; 1993.
40. Tos M. Pathology of the ossicular chain in various chronic middle ear diseases. J Laryngol Otol. 1979;93:769–80.
41. Yoon TH, Paparella MM, Schachern PA, Lindgren BR. Morphometric studies of the continuum of otitis media. Ann Otol Laryngol. 1990;99:23–7.
42. Costa RAC.Citocinas, Sinalização e MorteCelular. Site RNA Society, 2002.
43. da Costa SS. Otites médias - aspectos gerais. In: Cruz OLM, da Costa SS, editors. Otologia Clínica e Cirúrgica. 1st ed. Rio de Janeiro: Revinter; 1999. p. 137–61.
44. Chole RA, Frush DP. Quantitative aspects of Eustachian tube epithelium during vitamin A deprivation and reversal. In: Sadé, editor.

Proceedings of the 2nd International conference cholesteatoma and mastoid surgery. Amsterdam: Kluger; 1982.
45. Austin DF. Ossicular reconstruction archives of otolaryngology. Arch Otolaryngol. 1971;94(6):525–35.
46. Tos M, Falbe Hansen J Jr. Tympanoplasty on only hearing ears. J Laryngol Otol. 1975;89(10):1057–64. https://doi.org/10.1017/s0022215100081366. PMID: 1202116
47. Friedmann I. Comparative pathology of otitis media: experimental and human. II. The histopathology of experimental otitis with particular references to experimental cholesteatoma. J Laryngol Otol. 1955;69:588–601.
48. Tumarkin A. Attic cholesteatoma. J Laryngol Otol. 1958;72:610–9.
49. Thompsen J. Bone resorption in chronic otitis media. In: McCabe BF, Sade J, Abramson M, editors. Cholesteatoma: first international conference. Birmingham Ala: Aescupulus Publishing Co.; 1977. p. 136.

39 Tympanic Membrane Perforations and Tympanoplasty: New Profiles, New Strategies

Fábio André Selaimen, Mauricio Noschang Lopes da Silva, Tiago Isamu Saiguchi Murakami, and Sady Selaimen da Costa

Introduction

Tympanic membrane perforations are defined as a lack of integrity of the tympanic membrane (TM), which can result from different etiologies and require different treatments. They are part of a spectrum of diseases known as chronic otitis media (COM) [1, 2].

The COM, in turn, can be defined in several ways. From a clinical point of view, it is typically characterized as an inflammatory condition usually associated with otorrhea. Chronologically, it refers to an inflammatory process in the auditory cleft, which lasts no less than three months. Finally, histologically, perhaps the most comprehensive definition describes it as an inflammatory process of the middle ear associated with irreversible tissue alterations [2, 3].

For many decades, didactically, tympanic perforations have been classified as *central* or *marginal*. The *central* ones are those with tympanic membrane borders around 360° of the perforation, while *marginal* ones lack tympanic borders in any region around the perforation [4–6]. Such classification gained relevance in the literature due to the possibility of the formation of secondary cholesteatoma, which comes from the epithelial migration of the external acoustic meatus (EAC). The absence of protection from the tympanic annulus would be the determining factor in this case because, when present, it would act as an anatomical barrier to the migration of EAC epithelium toward the middle ear [3, 4].

It is imperative to remember that the currently most used COM classifications emerged between the 1950s and 1970s. Back then, the instruments available for evaluation were flagrantly less developed and accurate. Otomicroscopy, endoscopy (straight or angled), computed tomography (CT), and nuclear magnetic resonance have revolutionized the evaluation of COM. As a result, the comprehension of the disease and its etiopathogenesis are being reformed, while the classifications for didactic and research purposes have not yet completed their renewal cycle.

Today, we can have a broader and deeper view of the disease. For instance, our group has been engaged, over the past 20 years, in the studies of COM. The accumulated knowledge and the instruments that arose over those years are the main factors contributing to this deeper view. Namely, the tools are:

- The high-resolution otoendoscopy.
- The capture devices that allow the recording and exhaustive reanalysis of each otoscopy.
- The computerized methods for measuring and locating perforations.

Among all the aspects that a disease as complex and still little understood as COM presents, we consider etiopathogenesis to be the most relevant. Looking at the present, that is, the established pathology, we seek to understand the past (etiology) and try to modify the future (prognosis).

We believe that the current classification of tympanic perforations does not allow for such a broad approach to the disease. In other words, the current categorization system only considers the established pathology at the time of its assessment. At the same time, an evolutionary view could be more productive in terms of allowing the understanding of the disease globally.

In this chapter, we will approach not only the traditional aspects of tympanic perforations, such as the anatomy and biology of the tympanic membrane, but also new concepts arising from studies by our group and recently published. Further in this chapter, we will address clinical treatment and general concepts related to the surgical treatment applied to pathogenesis. We remember that surgical techniques can be found in specific chapters in this book.

F. A. Selaimen (✉) · M. N. L. da Silva
Hospital de Clínicas de Porto Alegre, Porto Alegre, Brazil

Instituto Gaúcho de Otorrinolaringologia, Porto Alegre, Brazil

T. I. S. Murakami
Pontifícia Universidade Católica do Rio Grande do Sul, Porto Alegre, Brazil

S. S. da Costa
Hospital de Clínicas de Porto Alegre, Porto Alegre, Brazil

Universidade Federal do Rio Grande do Sul, Porto Alegre, Brazil

M. V. Goycoolea et al. (eds.), *Textbook of Otitis Media*, https://doi.org/10.1007/978-3-031-40949-3_39

Brief Anatomical and Physiological Summary Applied to Pathogenesis

Anatomy and Biology of the Tympanic Membrane

The middle ear is a three-dimensional, small, and complex compartment whose primary function is transmitting sound from the air environment to the liquid environment of the inner ear. It begins with the capture of air acoustic waves, followed by the vibratory stimulus of the tympanic-ossicular system. Finally, it is completed by transmitting the waves to the vestibular scale of the cochlea via the oval window. The TM defines the lateral limit of the tympanic cavity, having the capture and the beginning of the sound transmission process as the primary function. The mechanism is primarily based on the difference in area between the TM and the stapes footplate. The ossicular chain conducts the sound pressure captured in the tympanic membrane to the footplate of the stapes, which has a considerably smaller area, thus concentrating the energy [7].

The approximate dimensions of the TM are 8 mm wide, 9–10 mm high, and 0.1 mm thick. Shrapnell [8], considering structural properties and mobility, divided the TM into two portions: one named *pars flaccida* (PF), superior, and the other as *pars tensa* (PT), inferior. The anatomical landmarks that divide PF and PT are the anterior and posterior malleolar ligaments, which are the extension of the tympanic ring. The ring, at the level of the tympanic spines, extends toward the lateral process of the malleus. The PT, in turn, was subdivided into four quadrants: the anterosuperior (AS), the anteroinferior (AI), the posterosuperior (PS), and the posteroinferior (PI), which are illustrated in a normal TM in Fig. 39.1.

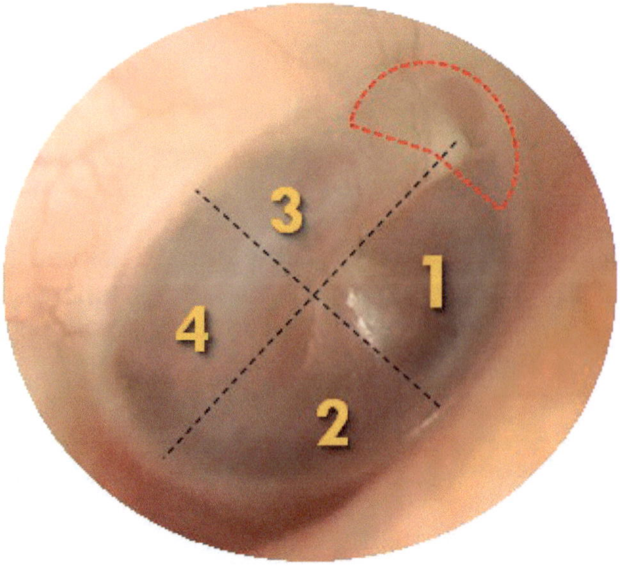

Fig. 39.1 TM considered normal—right ear. In red, the *pars flaccida* is delimitated. The black dotted lines show the separation of the *pars tensa* into quadrants: (1) anterosuperior; (2) anteroinferior; (3) posterosuperior; (4) posteroinferior. Image from own collection

The TM consists of three layers: an outer layer of keratinized squamous epithelium, a fibrous middle layer of mesodermal origin, and an inner endodermal mucosal layer. The membrane is approximately 130 μm thick, with the squamous layer measuring about 30 μm, the lamina propria about 100 μm, and the mucous layer 1 μm or less [7, 8].

The **outer epidermal layer** of TM is formed by a stratum corneum, a granular layer, a spinous layer, and a basal layer. Basal cells undergo cell division and migrate upward to replace dead and desquamated horny cells. The exact control mechanism that regulates this growth needs to be clearly understood. Studies have shown the presence of epidermal growth factors and fibroblast growth factors that are believed to promote the healing of tympanic membrane perforations. The epidermal layer also has migratory properties responsible for the ear's self-cleaning ability [7].

The human TM epidermis migrates centrifugally to the periphery, preferably in a posterosuperior direction, at a rate of about 131 μm/day, with a higher migratory speed in the umbo region. There is also a centripetal movement of the epithelium, which is speculated to be important in the healing process. Studies using cultures of fetal tympanic membranes have confirmed this unique feature. However, the exact cellular mechanism responsible for this migratory function is not clearly understood.

The epidermal layer also contains Langerhans cells, which are involved in the immune response as antigen-presenting cells, T lymphocytes, and mast cells. Thus, the tympanic membrane may present an immune response and, therefore, be part of the defense mechanism of the ear.

The **middle layer**, also called the lamina propria, has different composition depending on its location on the tympanic membrane. The lamina propria in Shrapnell's membrane, or *pars flaccida*, consists of a network of loose connective tissue, disorganized collagen and elastic fibers, and a network of blood vessels and nerves, internally and externally. The presence of elastic fibers explains the flaccidity of Shrapnell's membrane. There are also abundant histamine-filled mast cells in the *pars flaccida*. This finding, again, may be associated with primary or secondary hypersensitivity reactions with direct repercussions on the pathogenesis of otitis media.

In the *pars tensa*, the lamina propria consists of a subepidermal layer of loose connective tissue containing an internal network of blood vessels and nerve fibers. This layer, however, is composed of well-organized fibers, with radial fibers being the outermost and circular fibers being the innermost. This unique arrangement of fibers seems essential in the vibratory capacity of the tympanic membrane. It has critical reflections in understanding tympanic retractions and perforations, since the PS quadrant has particularities that differentiate it from the rest of PT and PF.

Specific Characteristics of the Posterosuperior Quadrant

This division mentioned before classically establishes the PF as the most sensitive area to retractions and, consequently, to the formation of primary cholesteatoma. However, recent studies indicate a very similar frequency in the formation of PF and PT cholesteatoma. With this information, and based on anatomical findings described below, we could begin to understand the PS quadrant as a transition between PT and PF since it has characteristics that sometimes resemble one region, sometimes the other.

The tympanic annulus consists of a thickening of the TM periphery, and it is inserted in the tympanic sulcus. In the PT, this combination between annulus and sulcus confers firmness and consistency to the region. However, as the tympanic annulus detaches from the sulcus, it goes toward the lateral process of the malleus, forming the anterior and posterior malleolar ligaments. Consequently, in the PF, there is no tympanic annulus. Thus, the TM is more malleable, filling the Rivinus notch and being attached directly to the scutum [9].

The tympanic sulcus, in its posterior region, is divided into two portions, separated, in most cases, by the emergence of the chorda tympani nerve. Inferior to the nerve, the sulcus maintains its characteristics identical to the inferior and anterior quadrants. It is well defined, with a depth between 0.5 and 0.9 mm, evident borders, and a stable surface. Above the nerve, the tympanic ring is no longer located within the sulcus but passes along the medial face of the posterior bone wall in 93% of the temporal bones studied by Paço et al. [9]. From that point on (the emergence of the chorda tympani nerve), the tympanic ring progressively becomes detached from the sulcus, which, in turn, progressively becomes shallower until it disappears. Topographically, the emergence of the chorda tympani nerve marks the limit of the posterosuperior quadrant. These characteristics confer less tension on the TM in the PS quadrant compared to the AS, AI, and PI quadrants. Figure 39.2 schematically shows such characteristics:

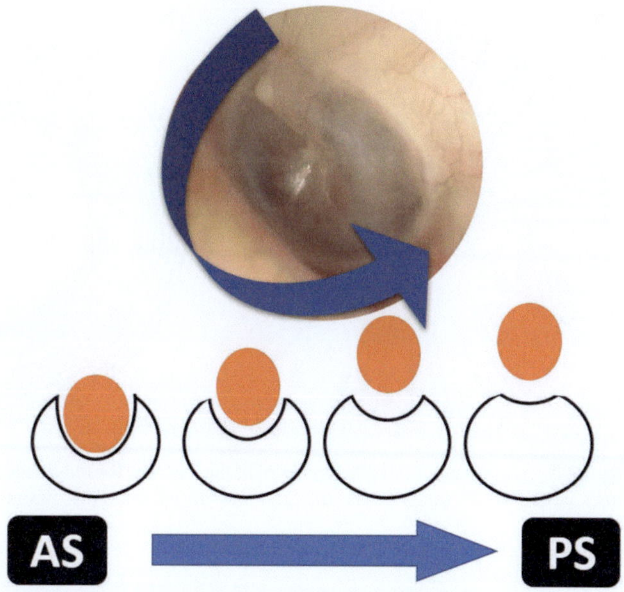

Fig. 39.2 Insertion of the ring (fibrous) in the tympanic sulcus (bone). In orange, the tympanic ring is represented. In black, the bone sulcus (groove). Progressively, when moving away from the anterior quadrants and reaching the PS, the sulcus will become shallower, and the annulus, in turn, more superficial and less adhered to the bone

Another point we deem essential to highlight about the PS quadrant concerns the histology of the TM in this region about its middle layer (lamina propria). In PT, the lamina propria consists of collagen types II and IV and is connected to the malleus handle and the tympanic bone. It consists of two layers, one radially oriented and the other circular in shape. The radial fibers (stratum radiatum) are attached to the manubrium of the malleus and run radially to the annulus. Meanwhile, the circular fibers (stratum circulare) are arranged concentrically with insertion into the manubrium. The latter are located medially in relation to the former.

In turn, the PS quadrant presents some peculiarities compared to the other portions of the PT, which would give it a greater chance of atrophy and consequent retraction in this region in case of negative pressure in the middle ear. First, the region does not have a developed circular fibrous layer, as mentioned in the previous paragraph (Fig. 39.3). In addition, its vascularization is more abundant, allowing greater penetration of collagenase-producing inflammatory cells, which have a more significant potential for destroying collagen fibers, which are already less dense by nature.

Furthermore, we must remember the anatomy of the PS quadrant, also characterized by peculiarities that increase susceptibility to the formation of retraction pockets in the region. Initially, a combination of the malleus handle, the subiculum of the promontory, and the tympanic annulus give the region anatomical accidents that culminate in reducing the distances and spaces for aeration in the region. The presence of the ossicular chain in this quadrant is yet another factor that differentiates it from the others because while the rest of the middle ear is filled only with air, the PS quadrant is full of structures competing for space. An occasional negative pressure in the middle ear could make the malleus medialize to the point of approaching, even more, the promontory, carrying the TM with it and, consequently, touching the subiculum of the promontory and the ossicular chain. Together with the greater flaccidity of the TM and the tym-

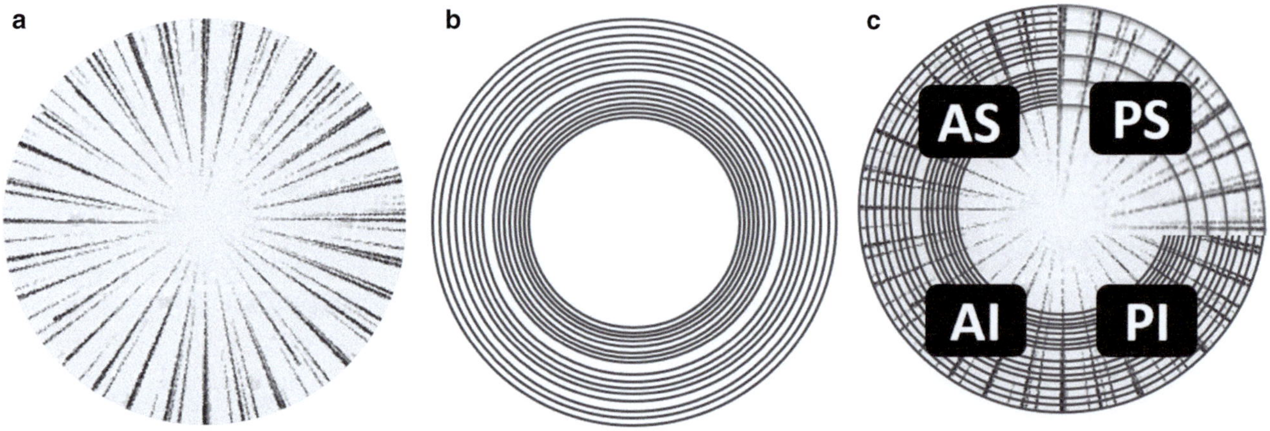

Fig. 39.3 Arrangement of collagen fibers in the TM. (**a**) Radial fibers, (**b**) concentric fibers, and (**c**) arrangement in the four quadrants of the *pars tensa*, where the PS quadrant has the least amount of concentric fibers

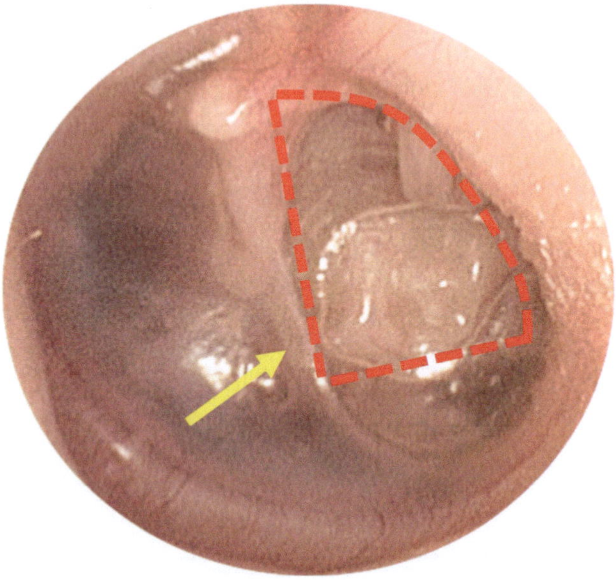

Fig. 39.4 Compartmentalization of the PS quadrant. The yellow arrow shows the point of major proximity between the TM (malleus umbo) and the promontory (subiculum). Negative pressure can make the malleus medialize, and, therefore, the TM will collapse over the promontory, isolating the PS quadrant from the ventilation routes

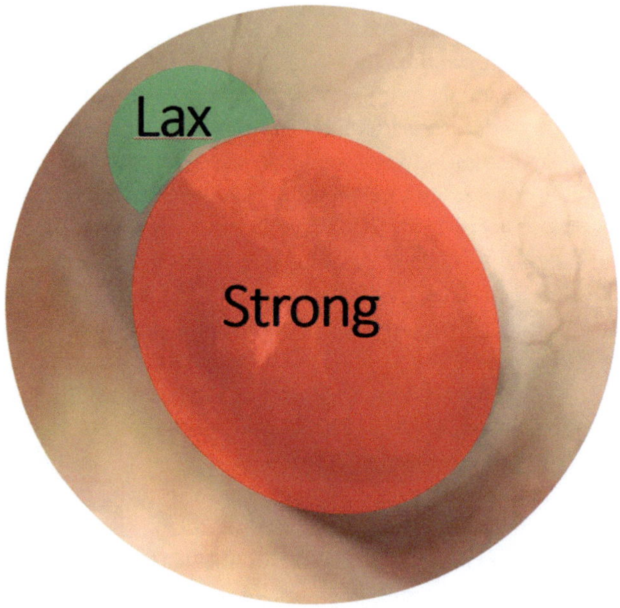

Fig. 39.5 Classic description of PT as robust and PF as weak (susceptible to retractions). We consider this division insufficient given the current knowledge of the anatomy and biology of TM

panic ring less inserted in the sulcus, there would be a compartmentalization of the region (Fig. 39.4), isolating it from the aeration routes originating from the mastoid via the aditus ad antrum, and the auditory tube, via the protympanum and mesotympanum.

Given all those peculiarities of the PS quadrant, we understand it as a transition between the *pars tensa* and the *pars flaccida*, as illustrated in Figs. 39.5 and 39.6.

Healing of the Tympanic Membrane

For a perfect understanding of tympanic membrane regeneration processes, we also need to review some concepts about epithelial migration. Two types of epithelial migration are known. One is centrifugal movement from the umbo, which occurs at a rate of approximately 0.07 mm per day. In addition, studies have shown several areas of mitotic activity dispersed in the eardrum, which suggests the existence of

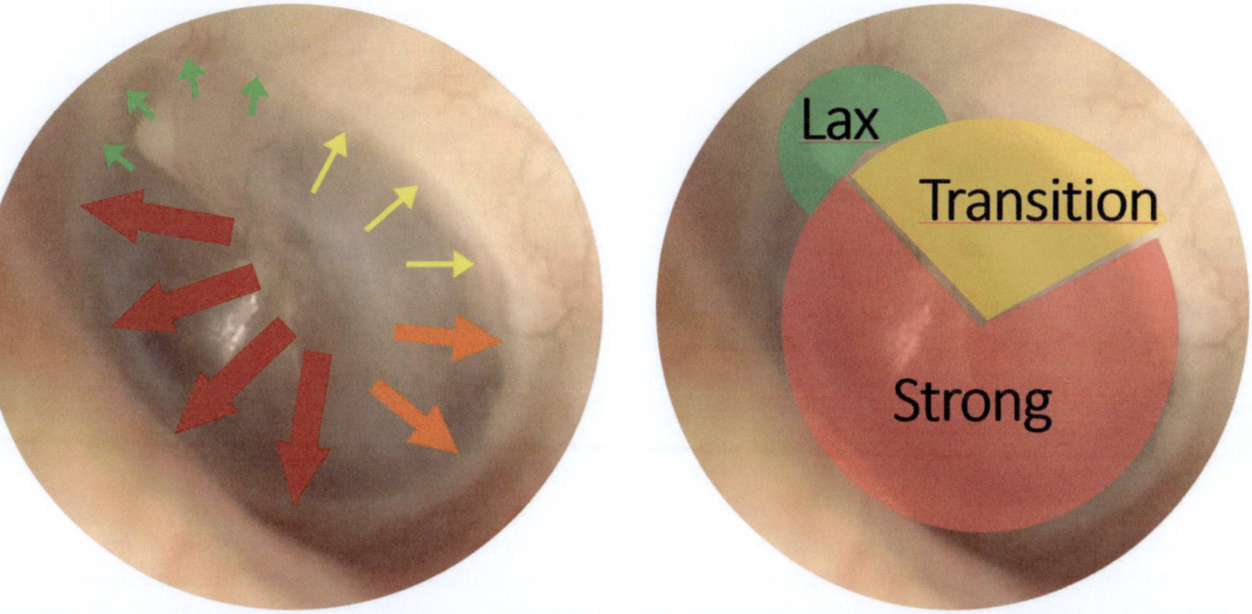

Fig. 39.6 TM firmness and tension in each quadrant, from the knowledge described in this section. Red arrows mark extreme tension, with a transition to green ones with less tension

multiple centers that generate this movement. This cell migration, called "keratin dispersion," aims to remove keratin, cerumen, and foreign bodies in the external ear.

A second migratory pattern is a centripetal movement which, in turn, seems essential for tympanic perforations' healing. Unlikely the wound healing in other tissues, mitotic activity is not confined to the wound edge only but rather the entire pars tensa of the tympanic membrane, with more significant activity around the tympanic ring and 2 mm from the edge of the lesion and, to a lesser extent, around the manubrium of the malleus. This distant migratory process is also suggested by the lack of proliferation of basal cells at the edge of the lesion, contrary to any other tissue where this cellular activity is intense.

Several studies have demonstrated the importance of F-actin microfilaments, a cytoskeletal contractile protein, in the migration of the squamous epithelium. Furthermore, this protein is abundant in the basal epithelial layer, suggesting that this layer plays an essential role in epithelial migration and consequent sealing of tympanic perforations.

The healing process traditionally involves the stages of hemostasis, inflammation, proliferation, remodeling, and contraction. First, platelets adhere and aggregate to injured cells in the wound, leading to vasoconstriction and thrombus formation. This event is followed by the formation of an inflammatory exudate composed of neutrophils, macrophages, and cytokines, with subsequent conversion of the fibrin matrices of the lesion into glycosaminoglycans and proteoglycans. At this point, when we talk about the healing of other tissues, fibroblasts proliferate, and collagen is deposited in the wound, with the consequent formation of granulation tissue matrices, which allows the spread of epithelialization.

In the tympanic membrane, however, studies have shown that epithelial regeneration precedes fibrous proliferation. Immediately after perforation, there is retraction of the edges of the pars tensa, followed by hemostatic and inflammatory changes. Epithelial hypertrophy and advancement of the edges of the lesion are early events and can be seen only 48 hours after the insult. Layers of squamous epithelium migrate in an attempt to cover the perforation in the first place. Only at a second moment does the proliferation of the fibrous component of the lamina propria begin. The hypertrophy of the wound edges reduces the dimensions of the tympanic continuity solution, which is quickly followed by the proliferation of other layers of the epithelium. These events are analogous to grafts' "bridge" function in chronic otitis media surgery. In these situations, the graft acts as a substitute for the stratum corneum, over which currents of epithelialization slide in order to repair the perforation.

The lateral (epithelial) and medial (mucosal) tympanic layers regenerate during this process. On the contrary, the structure of the lamina propria remains fragile, consisting only of a few disorganized fibers and a few fibroblasts. Thus, in some situations, the process can lead to forming a practically dimeric tympanic membrane (lateral and medial layers only).

Efforts are being made to unravel the biomolecular secrets of tympanic membrane healing. Animal studies have demonstrated the presence of epidermal growth factor (EGF) and primary growth factors—basic fibroblast growth factor (bFGF) in the tympanic membrane as early as three days after perforation. Growth factors are cytokines that regulate cell proliferation and differentiation. Receptors corresponding to these factors are also being discovered in animal models, suggesting that both may play relevant roles in TM perforation repair processes.

Symptoms

The cardinal symptoms of tympanic perforation are otorrhea and hearing loss. Other less frequent symptoms are otalgia, dizziness or vertigo, and, very rarely, facial paralysis. Right now, it is essential to point out that every patient with tympanic perforation will present two situations that may alternate with a relatively high frequency: infected and noninfected perforation. Such distinction is of fundamental importance to be recognized by the otorhinolaryngologist, since it may require clinical treatment and change planning, counseling, and surgical prognosis. Figure 39.7 illustrates the situation described above.

Hearing Loss: The patient with noninfected perforation will mainly report hearing loss symptoms. The main component is conductive due to the lack of area in the TM to capture the sound wave for consequent concentration in the footplate of the stapes and sound amplification. However, in some cases, the sensorineural component may also be present, configuring mixed hearing loss. One hypothesis for the existence of the sensorineural component would be cell death due to the migration of toxins to the inner ear, via the round window membrane, during infectious episodes. The intensity of the conductive loss is closely related to the degree of middle ear injury, and a conductive loss no higher than 20 dB typically indicates the integrity of the ossicular chain. On the other hand, erosion of the ossicles, particularly of the long process of the incus, or its fixation, usually produces hearing losses of 30 dB or more.

Otorrhea: It is the most common manifestation of chronic otitis media, occurring primarily during perforation infection periods. Short-term, intermittent mucoid drainage usually denotes a simple perforation without major pathological findings. Once the clinical treatment is carried out, the infection will resolve, and, consequently, the otorrhea will stop. On the other hand, chronic, constant, purulent, bloody, and bad-smelling otorrhea, which continues despite treatment and clinical management, is usually associated with significant middle ear and mastoid pathologies.

Otalgia: Pain is not frequently associated with tympanic perforations but may be present in cases of infectious exacerbation. Still, when present, it requires a careful approach. Concomitant external otitis should be ruled out, sometimes due to self-sensitization of the EAC skin or suppurative complications such as abscesses, although rare when the cholesteatoma is absent.

Vertigo: Reports of vertigo episodes associated with middle ear pathology, with or without cholesteatoma, represent chemical irritation (serous labyrinthitis) or pyogenic invasion (purulent labyrinthitis) of the labyrinth. Concerning TM perforations, it can be present when there is very exuberant inflammation of the middle ear, with granulation tissue and pus generating an extension of the inflammatory process into the inner ear. In any of these circumstances, assessment must be carried out promptly and treatment instituted as soon as possible.

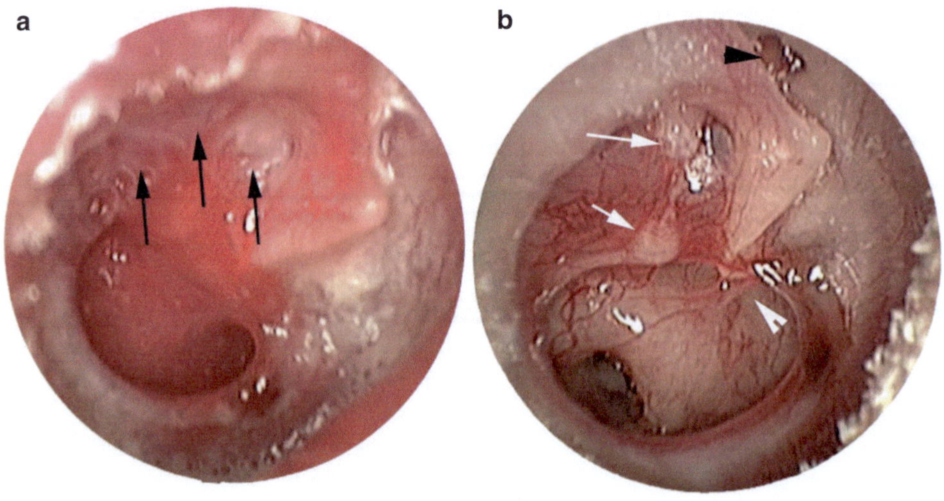

Fig. 39.7 Tympanic perforation in two different moments. (**a**) When infected, with an appearance that may suggest a cholesteatoma. Note the hyperplastic mucosa and the accumulation of epithelium in the posterosuperior quadrant (black arrows). (**b**) After clinical treatment and without infection. The absence of mucosal hyperplasia makes it possible to visualize the ossicular chair, with an erosion of the long crus of the incus (long white arrow) and myringostapediopexy (short white arrow). It also allows for identifying signs of retraction, such as medialization of the malleus handle (white arrowhead) and attic retraction (black arrowhead)

Facial Nerve Paralysis or Paresis: The finding of progressive or complete peripheral facial paralysis associated with COM indicates the involvement of the nerve in its tympanic-mastoid segment until proven otherwise. It is infrequent to occur in perforations and other clinical forms without cholesteatoma. In these rare situations, surgery must be performed immediately. Thus, the pathological process can be completely evacuated, and the path of the seventh cranial nerve can be thoroughly explored from the geniculate ganglion to the stylomastoid foramen.

Clinical Assessment

Otoscopy

Otoscopy is the major step in evaluating tympanic perforations, and the otorhinolaryngologist must obtain as much information as possible during the TM inspection. Therefore, it is essential to use technologies such as otomicroscopy, otoendoscopy, and, of course, to adequately prepare the patient for the examination and subsequent recording.

If present, otorrhea must be entirely aspirated, and epithelial debris and desquamation of the external acoustic meatus must be completely removed. If present in TM or EAC, granulation tissue may require focal cauterizations, followed by antibiotics and topical corticosteroids. Granulation can sometimes hide underlying pathologies, especially cholesteatoma associated with perforation. Figure 39.8 shows a tympanic perforation in one ear with granulation in a risk area, as it could hide a possible posterior epitympanic cholesteatoma. In this case, the otorrhea could be perpetuated both by the granulation continuously secreting or by the possible cholesteatoma hidden by it. It undoubtedly needs to be treated to obtain the proper diagnosis.

Fungal co-infection (Fig. 39.9) should be treated whenever identified, especially before surgical procedures, as closing the EAC at the end of surgery and during the postoperative period could boost the proliferation of the fungus. Sometimes, the identification is quite obvious, with the presence of hyphae in the EAC before the aspiration (Fig. 39.9a) or also adhered to the TM and inside the middle ear through the perforation (Fig. 39.9b). At other times, the signs may be more subtle, such as lumpy otorrhea or refractory to antibacterial treatment.

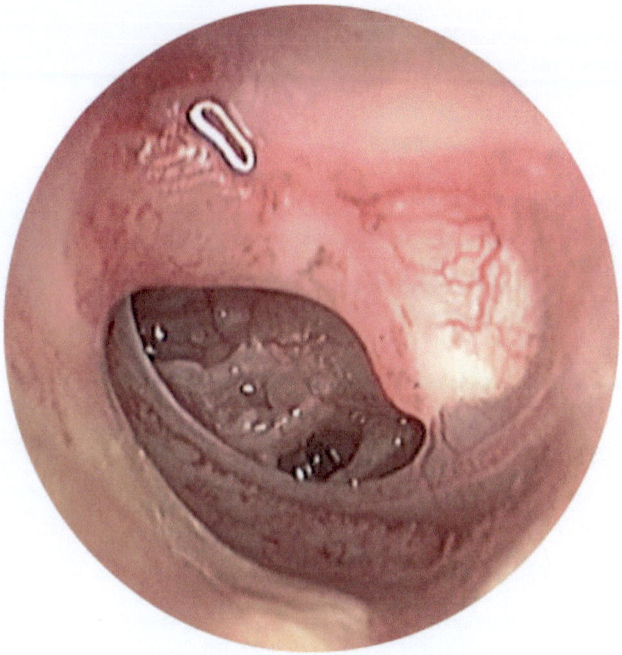

Fig. 39.8 Granulation tissue on the edges of the tympanic perforation extends to the AS quadrant and the attic region. Therefore, the treatment of granulation is fundamental, not only as part of the clinical improvement but also for adequate preoperative evaluation

Fig. 39.9 Fungal infection in COM. (**a**) Hyphae filling the EAC before aspiration. (**b**) Hyphae adhered to the TM and infested the middle ear through the perforation

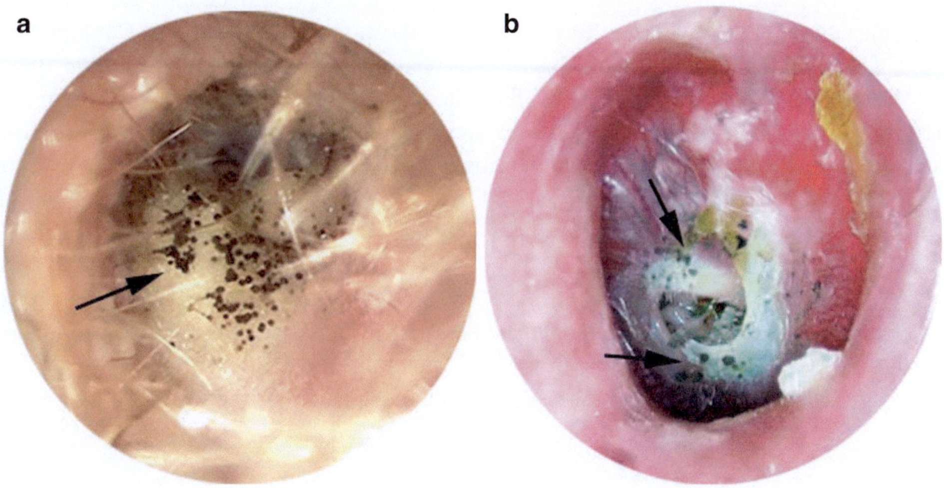

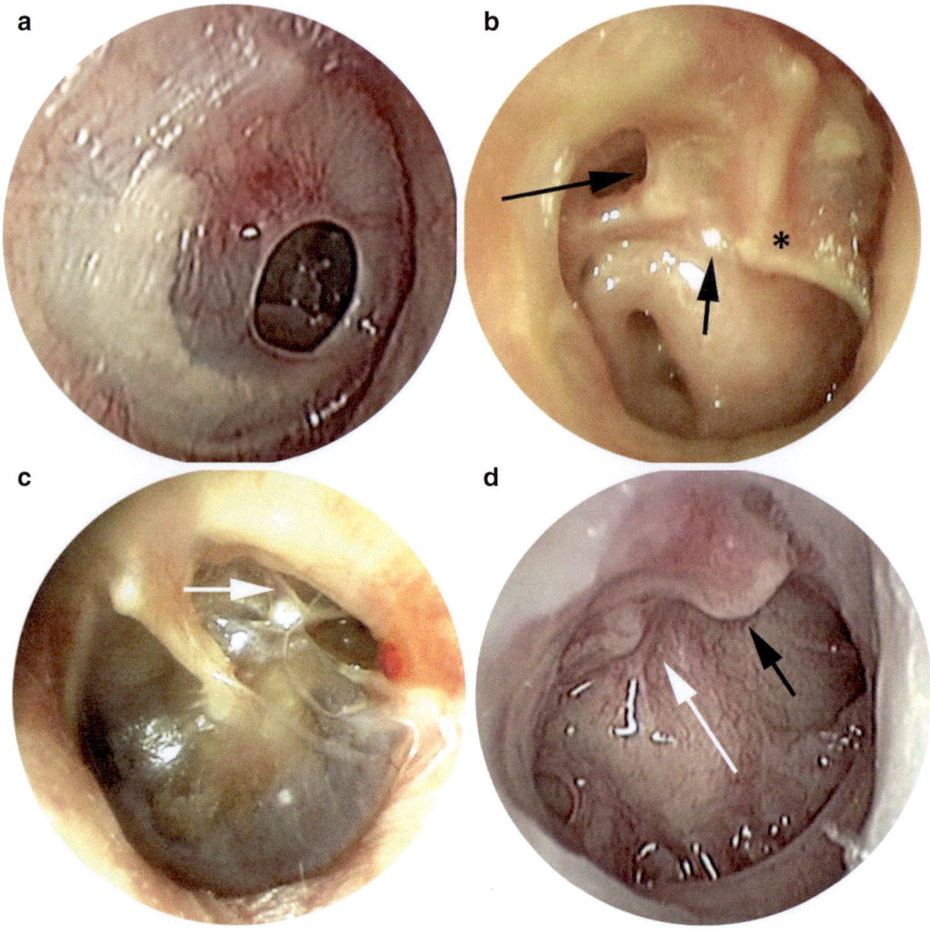

Fig. 39.10 Signs of retraction before perforation. (**a**) No signs of retraction. (**b**) Medialization of the malleus handle, including touching the promontory (asterisk); tympanic membrane touching the promontory (short black arrow), and tympanic membrane adhering to the ossicular chain (long black arrow). (**c**) Erosion of the long crus of the incus and tympanic membrane touching the ossicular chain, including myringostapediopexy (white arrow). (**d**) Medialization and amputation of the malleus handle (black arrow); tympanic membrane adhered to the promontory (white arrow) and ossicular chain

The presence of signs of retraction that occurred prior to tympanic perforation must also be evaluated. In this task, otoendoscopy is indispensable, with the objective of image magnification, better lighting, and consequent detailing of the characteristics pursued. The following signs are considered suggestive of the previous retraction: (1) medialization of the malleus handle; (2) tympanic remnants over the headland; (3) tympanic remnants over the ossicular chain, and (4) ossicular chain erosion. Figure 39.10 illustrates those signals, which will be better discussed later in this chapter.

We suggest the reader refer to the chapter Office Examination in Chronic Otitis Media to complement the steps of evaluation and registration of otoscopy.

Size and Location

The analysis of the total affected area (TM perforation size) and the location according to the TM quadrants is also a relevant factor in the assessment. The posterior quadrants of the TM are more subject to retractions and, consequently, to retractions-perforations. This fact is due to a set of anatomical and physiological factors of the PS quadrant, which have already been described and make the proper location of the disease in TM important, including for surgical planning.

Developed in partnership with the Federal University of Rio Grande do Sul and the Federal University of Santa Catarina, the Cyclops Auris Wizard software is used in our group to determine the size of tympanic perforation, as well as the location in each quadrant. The program is easy to use and intuitive, allowing its use by medical students until experienced otologists after brief training. Measurements are in relative size, initially taking into account the percentage of perforated area in a reason to the total area of the TM. Subsequently, each quadrant's relative percentages of perforation are provided in relation to the total perforated area. Figure 39.11 shows the result of a measurement.

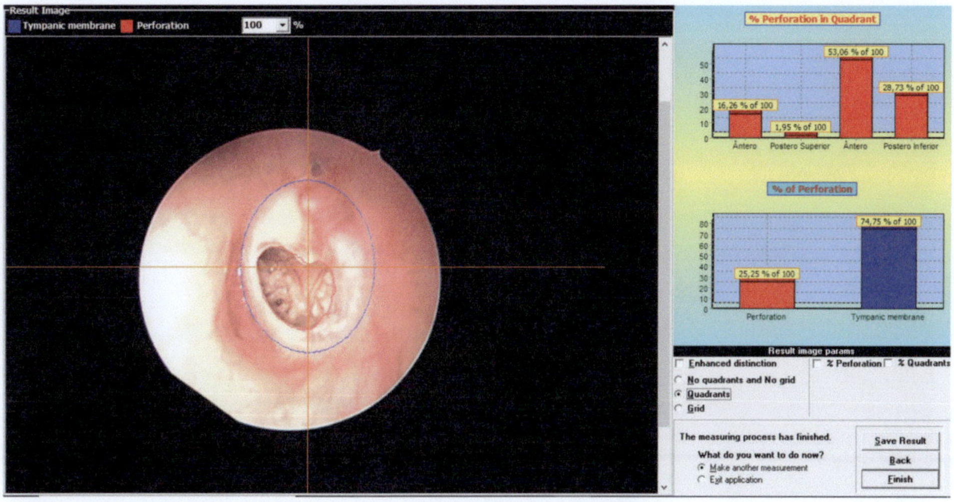

Fig. 39.11 Result of a TM perforation measurement with the Cyclops Auris Wizard

Audiological Evaluation

Acumetry should be routinely performed with a tuning fork at 512 Hz. The otologist can never do without acumetry, especially during preoperative evaluations. A conductive loss pattern is expected, and sometimes mixed loss can be identified. If the otologist suspects deep sensorineural loss, it is essential to share this information with the audiologist.

Tonal and vocal audiometry is indicated in all patients with tympanic perforation. Similar to otoscopy, proper ear preparation is necessary before audiometry. The presence of accumulated debris or otorrhea in the EAC and granulations in the middle ear or mucosal hyperplasia may overestimate the conductive component of the patient in question.

Hearing loss will be characteristically conductive in patients with tympanic perforation. The degree of loss will be influenced by factors such as perforation size, perforation location, presence of tympanosclerosis, and ossicular chain involvement, whether due to mucosal adherence or ossicular erosion.

We can come across a mixed hearing loss with relative frequency, with the sensorineural component also in a variable degree. The etiology of sensorineural loss seems to be related to chronic inflammation, leading inflammatory mediators to the inner ear (via round window), and consequent cochlear cell destruction. It is an essential factor in patient counseling, as the conductive component can often be improved with surgery, whereas the sensorineural component cannot. Very pronounced bone pathway asymmetries should be investigated for possible retrocochlear etiologies.

Radiological Evaluation

We do not indicate ear computed tomography (CT) as a routine in evaluating patients with tympanic perforation. Central, dry perforations, without signs of associated retraction or other signs described below, may dispense with radiological evaluation. However, several situations may require CT imaging in COM without cholesteatoma.

It is essential to emphasize the gain in quality that CT has gained in recent years; as the resolution has increased considerably, the radiation used in the exam has also decreased. Today, an image of poor quality, with low resolution and coarse cuts, is unacceptable. In addition, the availability of coronal, axial, and sagittal oblique sequences is essential. Thus, the microscopic structures of the middle ear and mastoid are detailed. We also recommend reading the specific chapter.

Despite adequate clinical management and expected care by the patient, a perforation that keeps discharging requires tomographic evaluation to evaluate the mastoid cells. The filled mastoid cells can indicate the presence of accumulated secretion, granulation tissue, or cholesterol granuloma, which can act as a permanent source of bacteria and biofilms, perpetuating the mesotympanum's inflammation. Often, mastoidectomy associated with tympanoplasty will be indicated in these cases.

Conductive hearing losses greater than expected for the patient's otoscopy also require investigation through imaging examination. In a simplified way, an air–bone gap (ABG) above 25 dB will require investigation by high-resolution tomography. Not only can we find ossicular chain erosions

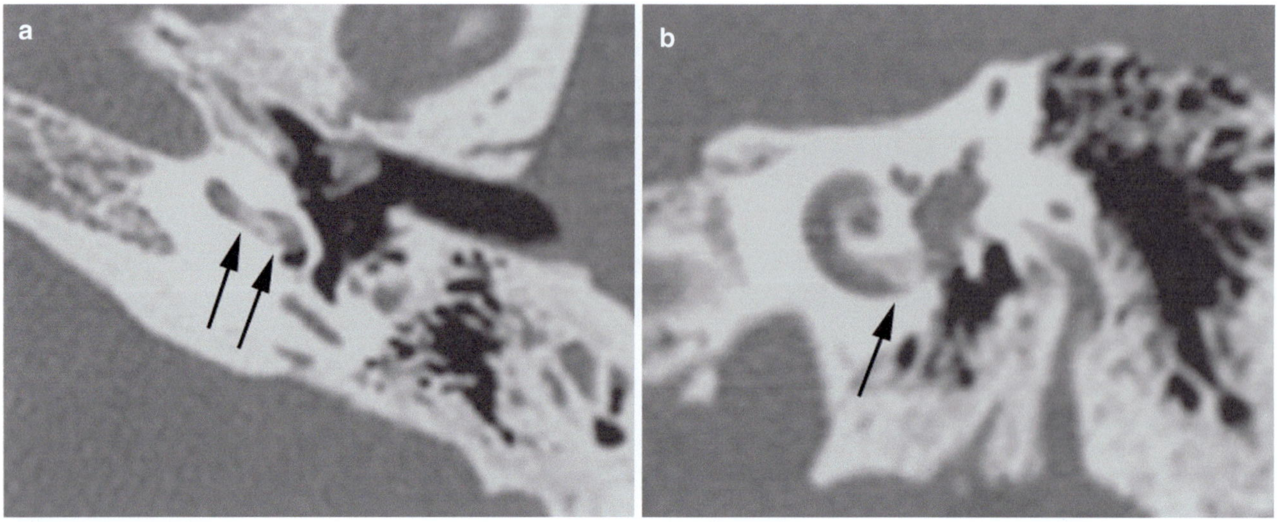

Fig. 39.12 Labyrinthitis ossificans. (**a**) Axial section shows calcification of the basal turn of the cochlea in a patient with COM without cholesteatoma (black arrows). (**b**) Oblique sagittal view from the same patient, showing better detail of the calcification (black arrow)

(sometimes not visualized in otoscopy), but also ossicular chain fixations and tympanosclerosis can be seen.

A sensorineural component is also a warning sign for investigation through imaging. In rare cases, chronic otitis media, even if not cholesteatomatous, can affect the inner ear, with intracochlear calcification and cell injury. This situation, known as labyrinthitis ossificans, can be seen in Fig. 39.12. In addition, asymmetric sensorineural hearing loss may require further investigation with nuclear magnetic resonance.

- Quick Tips: When to perform image in TM perforation?
  - A TM perforation that never gets dry
  - Conductive hearing loss greater than 25 dB
  - Sensorineural hearing loss
  - Asymmetric sensorineural hearing loss

Classification

Central *Versus* Marginal: The Traditional Classification

Historically, tympanic perforations are divided into **central**, that is, if there are TM borders in all 360° of the perforation, and **marginal**, if there is a lack of any of the perforation edges (Fig. 39.13). This classification gained relevance in the literature due to the potential effect of secondary cholesteatoma formation from a marginal perforation. According to this theory, there would be migration of epithelium from the EAC toward the interior of the middle ear, allowed by the absence of anatomical protection provided by the tympanic annulus. However, such a theory is not consensual, being challenged daily in the daily practice of otologists and already criticized in the literature.

Still, the classification according to the borders of the perforation can be contested in other respects. Indeed, the most relevant would be the need for more practical applicability of the classification in therapeutic procedures. Even after decades of using the current division, we have still not been able to identify any indication for clinical or surgical treatment, which is modified if perforation is central or marginal.

Studies on the subject, primarily focused on surgical results, have not demonstrated relevant differences between a central and a marginal perforation. In addition to very heterogeneous and discordant results, no publication has yet been able to indicate a change in conduct according to the type of perforation. We can find publications comparing techniques and associating success rates to patient age, tympanoplasty graft material, graft position, use of preoperative medications, endoscopic or microscopic approach, as well as smoking, otorrhea, state of the mucosa, ossicular chain, and contralateral ear (CLE), among others. Studies looking for differences in the perforation closure rate according to the current classification—central or marginal—did not find significant differences.

Added to this is the fact that the current classification does not have any prognostic value, especially in the medium and long term, and, inevitably, we conclude that the classification used so far is quite deficient. At this point, it is worth remembering that the classification was developed many decades ago, even before the popularization of microscopes and, more recently, endoscopes in clinical practice.

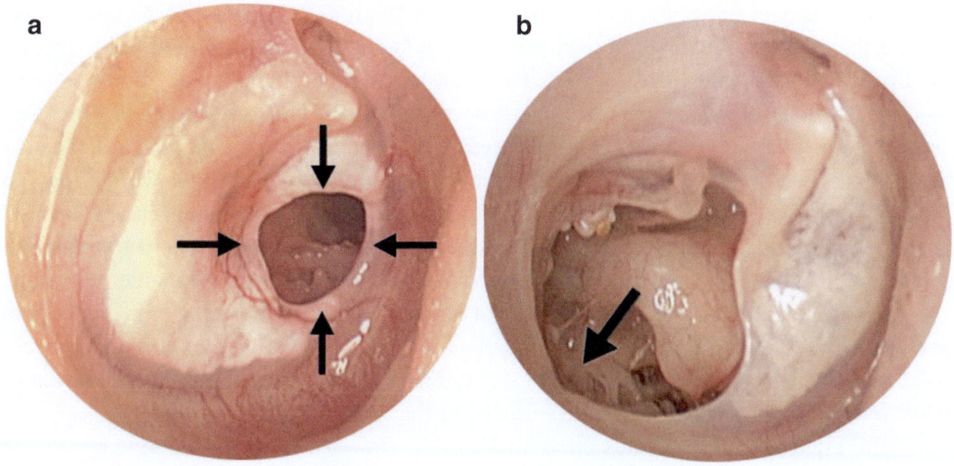

Fig. 39.13 Traditional classification of tympanic perforations. (**a**) Central perforation, with 360° borders (black arrows). (**b**) Marginal perforation, with the absence of tympanic edges in part of the perforation (black arrow)

The view provided by the otoscope, without angulation, and with limited amplification, often blocks the view of essential points of the middle ear anatomy. The most evident and consensually perceived factor is difficulty visualizing the anterior tympanic borders in patients whose external acoustic meatus is tortuous. With the routine use of otoendoscopy, the perforation previously considered marginal can often be reclassified as central, since the borders, hidden by the tortuosity of the EAC, can now be visualized.

This technological evolution allowed many improvements while performing an otoscopy: angled vision, full HD amplification of the image, the possibility of proximity from the structures (often almost in direct contact with the tympanic membrane), and, finally, the recording of the otoscopy. This way, allowing the successive and exhaustive reanalysis of the otoscopies, new perspectives have emerged for assessing COM.

Today, we evaluate parameters that we consider undoubtedly more relevant than the mere presence, or absence, of tympanic borders around the perforation. The anatomy of the EAC, the size and location of the TM perforation, the presence of tympanosclerosis, and the presence or absence of signs of tympanic retraction before perforation are the main parameters that we must consider in the evaluation of the disease.

Therefore, we currently prefer to classify perforations as **outside-in** (or retraction-perforation) or **inside-out** (without associated retraction or explosive), as we will see below.

Inside-Out *Versus* Outside-In: A Look Over the Pathogenesis

The proposed pathogenesis for tympanic perforations, classically, involves a series of trigger situations in which an acute event would lead to a chronic condition (perforation). Acute suppurative otitis media, traumatic perforations, and external otitis (with partial necrosis of the tympanic membrane), among others, are the etiologies usually described for the genesis of chronic otitis.

For this reason, the transition between acute and chronic conditions is explained by predominantly "explosive" mechanisms, that is, some sudden inflammatory or traumatic event affecting a previously healthy structure. Disruption of intratympanic homeostasis, caused by an acute mechanism, will modulate a series of histological transformations in the mucous lining of the middle ear, which would change permanently, characterizing COM. We can call this model the "direct line" between the acute (trigger situations) and the chronic (tympanic perforation).

However, clinical practice shows us that we receive many more patients with tympanic perforations than we can explain through this model. In other words, it seems that the mechanisms traditionally related to the origin of these perforations (the causes) are identified in everyday life in a much smaller proportion than the number of perforated TM that reach us (the consequences). It is evident in clinical practice that the otologist observes several patients with tympanic perforations. However, we rarely witness an acute event (recurrent acute otitis media, external otitis, and trauma) that could justify the chronic condition. Faced with this paradox, one can conclude that other mechanisms must be responsible for generating an expressive number of perforations.

Furthermore, the adoption of this "express" or "direct line" acute–chronic pathogenesis model disregards a daily situation witnessed by otorhinolaryngologists. Historically, events such as tympanic retractions, atelectasis, and adhesive otitis media, among others, have been inexplicably placed on the sidelines of this discussion. It is as if, in theory, tympanic membrane retractions were a chapter of chronic otitis media, while perforations would be in another (entirely separate) chapter.

From what has been exposed in this chapter so far, considering the technological evolution, the accumulated knowledge acquired over the years, and the successive reflections around the paradoxes exposed above, we pursue other ways of classifying tympanic perforations. Thus, based on the detailed analysis of otoscopy, we began to value findings suggestive of tympanic retractions **associated** with perforations. Thus, we sought to understand a second model of pathogenesis for tympanic perforations, which associates and shows a critical intersection between the knowledge referring to retractions and the tympanic perforations.

The observed retraction characteristics associated with perforation are (a) medialization of the malleus handle, (b) tympanic remnants over the promontory, (c) tympanic remnants over the ossicular chain, and (d) erosion of the ossicular chain. Figure 39.14 illustrates these findings.

When we find zero or one of the characteristics mentioned above, we consider the perforation not associated with retraction, that is, an "explosive" perforation. This group of perforations, whose proposed etiology is the express model (acute leading directly to chronic), we convention to call "inside-out," that is, from the middle ear to out, in an imagined explosive process. Of course, the nomenclature is intended to translate a process (acute condition leading to chronic) and not a specific etiology. Etiologies may be not only acute otitis media or recurrent acute otitis media but also external ear processes such as fungal or bacterial infections that lead to necrosis of part of the TM.

In other words, they are previously healthy middle ears, which possibly have suffered aggression at a specific moment, be it traumatic, inflammatory, or infectious, generating tympanic perforation as a permanent sequel. The absence of signs of the previous retraction would be the mark of an "explosive" process or, in other words, punctual in time, characterizing the opposite of the subsequently mentioned group.

In the second group, there are the perforations with two or more retraction characteristics associated with the perforation. It represents an alternative pathogenesis model in which a progressive retraction would lead to perforation. The pressure self-generated by the retracted TM against the structures of the middle ear (ossicles and promontory) induces ischemia of the capillaries of the membrane and, consequently, the necrosis of a part of it. It is reaching the apex of this

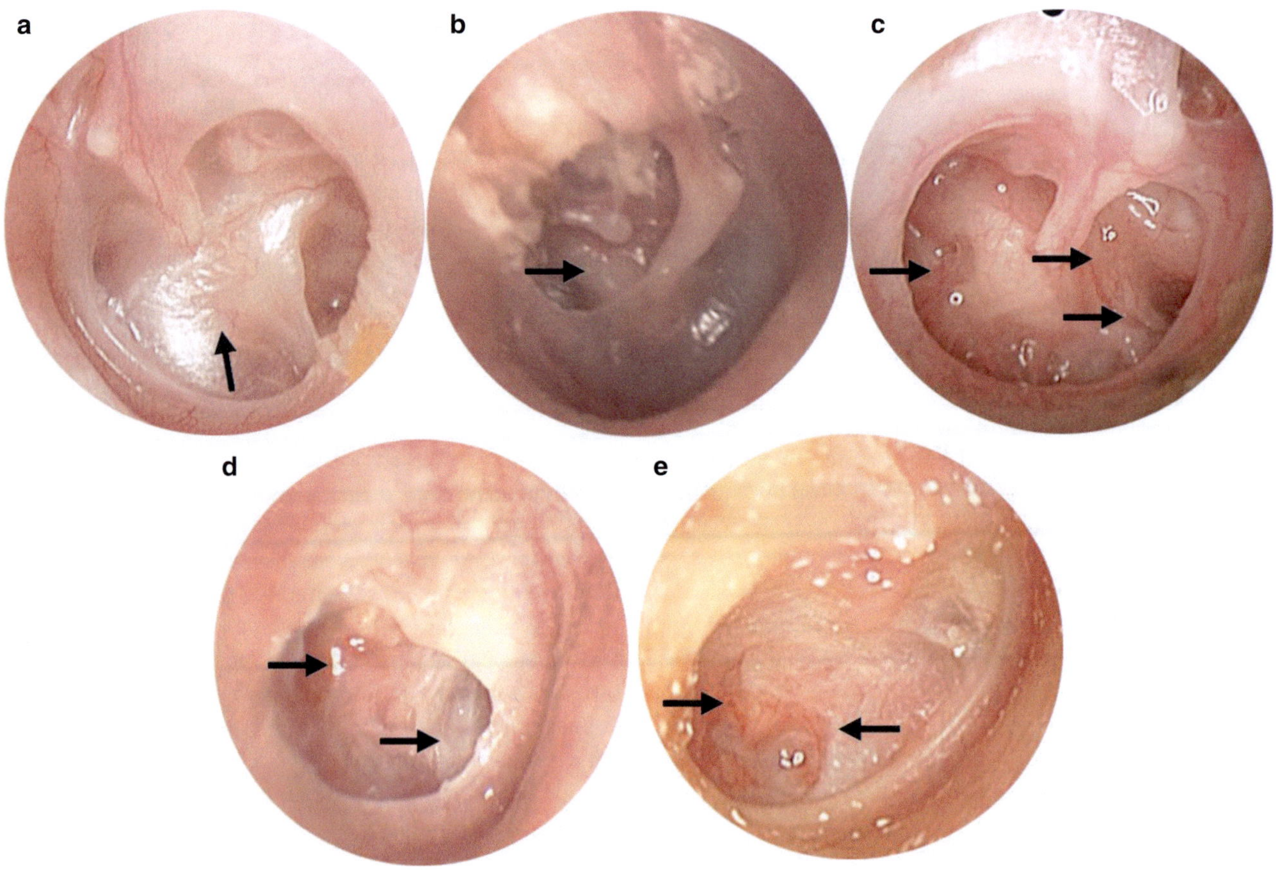

Fig. 39.14 Signs of retraction. (**a**) Bridge between the healthy TM and the one attached to the promontory. (**b**) More accentuated brightness over the promontory because the TM has adhered to it in the PS quadrant. (**c**) Brighter and smoother middle ear mucosa, suggesting atelectasis with subsequent loss of the lateral epithelial layer of the TM. (**d**) Epithelium in the proliferation phase on the promontory. (**e**) Transition between MT adhered to the promontory with its epithelialized lateral layer and, more posteriorly, with a mucosal appearance

process that the retraction will turn into a perforation. Of course, a different type of perforation than mentioned in the previous paragraph. The illustrated signs (of the previous retraction) would be the marks left by this long process of progressive retraction, which we conventionally call outside-in. Thus, the pathogenesis proposed for this group of perforations is very similar to that of tympanic retractions, involving a negative pressure mechanism (probably from auditory tube dysfunction) and an entire altered middle ear homeostasis, which would be responsible for the progressive retraction until perforation.

In a study by Selaimen and collaborators (2020), the analysis of 1003 ears divided according to the above criteria into inside-out and outside-in showed very different parameters for each group. We will now present the main results, through which we will be able to understand the reasons that lead us to consider the proposed classification more representative of the pathogenesis.

Initially, observing the functional criterion, not only the tritonal mean thresholds on airway conduction (AC), but also the bone conduction (BC), and air–bone gap (ABG) were all higher in the outside-in group, with statistical significance, demonstrating that functionally they are the most affected ears. Also, the duration of symptoms was longer in the outside-in group, which included patients with a higher mean age.

When analyzing the contralateral ear (CLE), the inside-out group showed a significant majority of normal CLE. On the other hand, the outside-in group had a much higher rate of altered CLE. This difference occurred especially at this group's expense of more retractions and cholesteatomas. CLE has been studied for decades, with ample evidence that it is an excellent predictor of main ear behavior. Thus, understanding COM as a bilateral disease, such findings corroborate the theory that, while the inside-out group represents the previously healthy ears, the outside-in represents chronically dysfunctional ones.

Finally, analyzing the differences between the groups in size and location of the perforation, the inside-out group had smaller and more anterior perforations. In comparison, the outside-in group included larger and more posterior perforations. Still, marginal perforations are found almost exclusively in the outside-in group, in agreement with a study by Rosito et al., which indicated that these perforations almost always result from the previous retraction.

In summary, based on these otoscopic signs of the previous retraction in tympanic perforation—or their absence—we believe we can differentiate a previously healthy ear from a chronically dysfunctional one. Furthermore, this classification of tympanic perforations seems to make more sense since it brings inferences about the etiopathogenesis of the disease. Table 39.1 summarizes the main differences between the types of perforations. Figure 39.15 illustrates three inside-out perforations, while Fig. 39.16 exemplifies three outside-in perforations.

Obviously, this distinction will lead to changes in treatment proposals, especially in surgical aspects. On the one

Table 39.1 Summary of characteristics according to the new classification of tympanic perforations

	Inside-out	Outside-in
Size	Smaller	Bigger
Location	More likely anterior quadrants	More likely posterior quadrants
Hearing (AC and BC)	Higher thresholds	Lower thresholds
Hearing (ABG)	Smaller gap	Bigger gap
Tympanic borders	Central (almost always)	About half marginal
Contralateral ear (CLE)	More normal ears	More abnormal ears

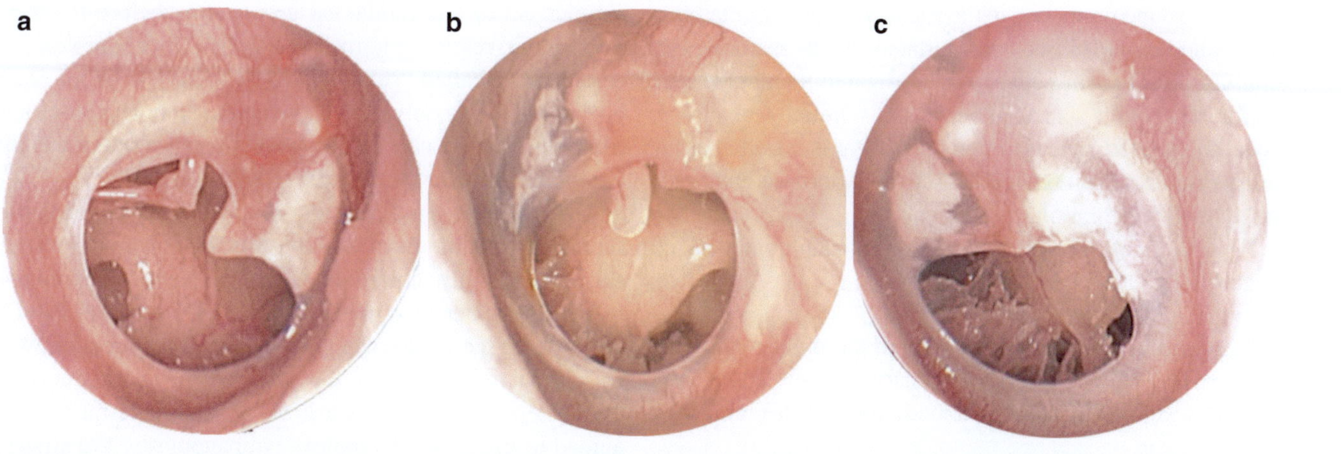

Fig. 39.15 Three examples of **inside-out,** or explosive, perforations (with no associated retraction). We did not see any of the described signs of retraction. (**a**) Perforation in quadrants AI, PI, and PS, with intact ossicular chain and without medialization of the malleus or tympanic membrane over the ossicular chain or promontory. (**b**) Perforation in all quadrants, sparing part of the AS, also with no signs of retraction. (**c**) Perforation in the AI and PI quadrants, without malleus medialization or other signs of the previous retraction

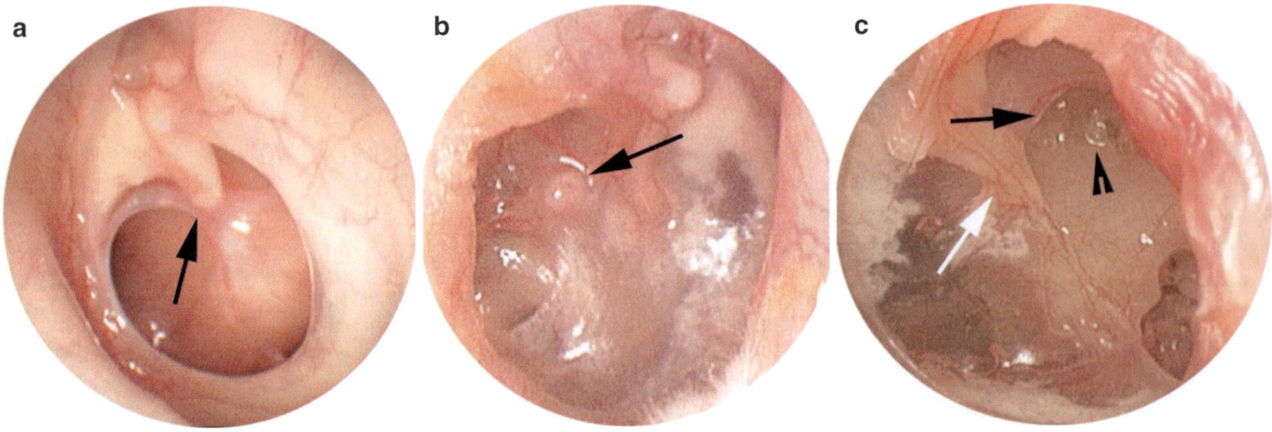

Fig. 39.16 Three examples of outside-in perforation, or perforation-retractions. (**a**) Medialization of the malleus manubrium, including touching the promontory with a TM bridge to the promontory (black arrow). (**b**) Erosion of the long incus crus with tympanostapedopexy (black arrow) and clear medialization of the TM in the posterior quadrants. (**c**) Medialization of the malleus manubrium (white arrow), tympanic membrane bridge between the malleus and the facial nerve (black arrow), and ossicular chain erosion—only the stapes footplate is present, without superstructure (black arrowhead)

hand, the inside-out perforations represent normal middle ears in terms of aeration and physiology, but which suffered an "accident on the way," resulting in a tympanic perforation. On the other hand, outside-in perforations translate the end of a chronic process into a middle ear with altered physiology; they represent a chronic otitis media in its essence. Indeed, the processes to restore normality will need to be much more detailed in the second group of tympanic perforations.

Surgical Treatment

Principles of Treatment Applied to the Pathogenesis

The aim and physiological principle of tympanoplasties are to restore sound protection to the round window by obtaining an air-filled cavity, closed but ventilated, and by restoring the amplifier mechanism between the tympanic membrane and the footplate of the stapes. In other words, initially, obtaining a healthy, aerated, mucosa-lined middle ear is essential as an indispensable condition for subsequently proceeding with the ossicular restoration.

Regardless of the technique used, the main objectives of surgery for COM are as follows:

1. Removal of all diseased tissue from the middle ear, with complete elimination of inflammatory and infectious processes and the consequent obtaining of a dry and safe middle ear.
2. Preservation or reconstruction of the middle/outer ear complex.
3. Restoration of the mechanisms that conduct sound.

These objectives can be achieved in a single step or staged over two procedures. In the latter situation, the first surgery is performed to control the infection and recover tympanic integrity. The so-called "second stage" aims to reestablish the connection between the tympanic membrane and the endocochlear fluids, that is, the reconstruction of the ossicular chain.

The effort to differentiate the etiopathogenesis of each type of perforation has as its main objective the individualization of the treatment applied to each case. If the previous classification fails to present any practical applicability in the treatments, be it central or marginal perforation, the new parameters aim to improve the planning and execution of the treatment. The look at the past (etiology) helps us to understand the present (type of tympanic perforation) in order, fundamentally, to be able to plan the future (treatment and prognosis).

The handling of inside-out perforation seems to be much simpler. Since the middle ear was healthy before tympanic perforation, restoring normality can be a less complex process. The so-called "simple" tympanoplasty, with the interposition of fascia only, may be sufficient in most perforations from this group. **Later in this book, there's a specific chapter for the surgical technique step-by-step**.

On the other hand, outside-in perforation, which represents the physiology of a previously dysfunctional middle ear, will certainly require more surgical steps to restore normality. If the negative pressure in the middle ear persists, it may lead to the recurrence of neotympanum retraction, with or without recidivism of the perforation. Therefore, additional steps may be necessary, which is the reason why we agreed to call this a "complex" tympanoplasty. **We suggest reading the specific chapter later in this book**, but in summary, outside-in perforations may require the following associated procedures:

- The use of more resistant grafts, such as cartilage associated with the temporal fascia (double graft), thus preventing future retraction.
- The insertion of a concomitant ventilation tube, thus ensuring adequate ventilation in the immediate and midterm postoperative periods.
- Lateralization of the malleus (most likely including sectioning the tendon of the tensor tympani), thus allowing air circulation from the eustachian tube throughout the entire middle ear.
- Cleaning of epithelium adhered to the promontory (and often occupying posterior recesses), thus preventing the formation of a cholesteatoma in the future.
- The use of angled optics to inspect posterior recesses, hypotympanum, and supratubal recess.
- Ossicular chain reconstruction since ossicular erosion is more frequent in this group of perforations.
- Procedures aimed at improving eustachian tube function.

Preoperative Preparation

Almost all patients with tympanic perforation will, at some point, have an active infection with purulent discharge from the ear. As we mentioned earlier in the evaluation, the infection must also be controlled in the preoperative preparation to maximize the chances of success with graft vitality.

Counseling

We doctors are sometimes taken by an unjustified arrogance, and we judge the destiny of our patients without, many times, offering them a more comprehensive explanation of what we intend to accomplish. This conduct, which would be deplorable itself, constitutes an additional risk for the doctor, who faces a growing wave of medico-legal problems.

As soon as we indicate the surgery, it is our routine to meet with the patient and his family in a frank conversation and accessible language to make them aware of the characteristics of the disease, its natural history, and possible consequences. We take advantage of this moment to present our surgical vision plan, its possible complications, and a preview of the postoperative evolution and care. After explaining to the patient, we digitally sent the preoperative and postoperative instructions (including the care that will be taken in the 30 days after the surgery), as well as the informed consent form.

Thus, wholly informed about the nature of his problem, the patient can weigh the pros and cons of the proposed therapy and maturely decide on his own destiny. Also, after this consultation in which the procedure was indicated, a preoperative consultation will be carried out, in which the patient and their family members will be able to bring new questions from the initial conversation and the reading of the terms sent to them.

Hospital Admission

The patient is admitted to the hospital on the day of the procedure. Routinely, we keep the patient hospitalized for one day after the procedure, especially those who come from other cities or states.

Surgical Center

In addition to the technical aspects (not discussed in this section), a series of small details must be observed in the operating room, and we will explain them below.

Patient: The patient must be positioned with the head at the foot of the table and tied firmly to it, as the surgeon may often request lateral decubitus for better visualization of structures in each surgical procedure. The patient's head should be brought as close as possible to the surgeon, taking care not to project the shoulder superiorly in such a way as to impede its movements. The head must be positioned in extension, resting on a roller that keeps it stable.

The operating table should be positioned with the patient's head slightly above the plane of the feet (anti-Trendelenburg position), as this measure may help to reduce bleeding in the operative field. The surgeon's chair should go under the surgical table, at the height of the patient's head, taking care that the base of the table does not impede the approximation of the chair and, consequently, cause discomfort to the surgeon (and a big backache!).

The surgeon must feel comfortable and at ease in the operating room. Therefore, the surgeon must maintain an upright posture throughout the surgery, sitting on an adjustable stool with support in the lumbar region and bringing the operating microscope closely.

Surgical instruments: The surgeon must be familiar with the instruments that will be used. The material used in otologic surgery is extremely delicate, especially compared to other surgical instruments. Thus, in the vast majority of surgical centers in general hospitals, breaking delicate materials (hooks, Rosens, needles) is, unfortunately, a routine.

Our group agreed to standardize instrument boxes for all otological surgeries. Thus, we could separate the cruder materials (Weitlaner, scalpel) from the delicate material (Rosens, needles, hooks), the latter being placed in custom-made boxes. Such boxes allow the material to be safely sterilized and not break during transportation and the sterilization process itself.

Often, for reasons beyond our control, we are forced to perform delicate surgeries outside our "natural habitat" and with a paramedical team that is also unknown to us. In these situations, arriving at the operating room well in advance is prudent, thus enabling a review of the instruments available and a complete check of the microscope, motors, pens, and drills.

Preparing the Surgical Field

It will be discussed in the surgical technique chapter, step-by-step.

Traditional Techniques and Access Approaches

Currently employed tympanoplasty techniques involve repairing the tympanic membrane defect by placing a graft over or under the edges of the perforation. The graft acts as a bridge, allowing regeneration of the squamous epithelium of the external ear, on its lateral side, and of the middle ear mucosa, on its medial side.

The two surgical techniques traditionally used are the underlay, which positions the graft below the tympanic remnant (medial technique, by Austin), and the overlay, which positions the graft above the remnant (lateral technique, by Sheehy). Furthermore, there is the possibility of performing the surgery with the inlay graft, that is, at the same level as the tympanic membrane. Trained otologists get nearly identical results. In our group, we have preferably used the Austin technique, reserving Sheehy's for exceptional situations.

Regarding the approaches, we can describe four techniques:

- Transcanal: surgeon works in the microscope with visualization through the ear specula, which can be fixed to the table with the holder, or by the surgeon's nondominant hand.
- Endaural: through the incisions of Lempert I, II, and III and positioning of the self-static retractors.
- Retroauricular: incision in the retroauricular sulcus and anterior bending of the pinna.
- Endoscopic: more modernly, through the use of endoscopes, transcanal tympanoplasty expanded its possibilities of use with this tool.

In our group, we prefer the retroauricular approach, as it provides wider exposure and, therefore, the greater possibility of handling possible trans-operative unforeseen findings. Below, we list the necessary criteria for the use of the transcanal approach:

- First surgery
- Favorable EAC
- COM without cholesteatoma
- Tympanic perforation in the posterior quadrants
- Air–bone gap less than 25 dB
- All perforation borders are visible preoperatively without the use of the endoscope.

When the patient does not meet all these criteria, which happens in most patients who come to our offices, the retroauricular access route will be preferred.

Postoperative Care

At the end of the skin suture, we insert gauze in the EAC and place a compressive dressing to avoid excessive edema in the external acoustic meatus and the retroauricular surgical wound.

Finally, the procedure must be described still in the operating room before the patient leaves. Then, the prescription and dressings must be performed by the surgeon, who must accompany the patient to the recovery room and remain there until making sure that the patient recovers well from the anesthesia and the functions of the seventh cranial nerve are maintained.

The surgeon's responsibility is to personally assess the patient and prescribe his medication at the bedside the morning after the procedure. At this moment, there is the opportunity to explain the surgical procedure details to the patient, who is already awake. The compressive dressing can be removed the day after surgery, and the patient is usually discharged. Instructing the patient to avoid wetting the operated ear until the healing process is complete is essential. He is also instructed that when he sneezes or coughs, he should do so with his mouth open and avoid any effort that increases pressure in the ear (Valsalva type). A common reaction after ear surgeries is the perception of clicking and the discreet drainage of a clear secretion. It must be informed to the patient as typical from the postoperative. In one week, the patient should be reevaluated. Subsequently, visits will be scheduled according to the postoperative evolution.

References

1. Bezold F. Cholesteatom, Perforation der Membranaflaccida und Tubenverschluß. Z Hals NasenOhrenheilk. 1890;20:5–29.
2. Bluestone CD, Kenna MA. Introduction: definitions and goals of the workshop. Ann Otol Rhinol Laryngol. 1988;97(Suppl. 2):7.
3. Bluestone CD. Epidemiology and pathogenesis of chronic suppurative otitis media: implications for prevention and treatment 1. Int J Pediatr Otorhinolaryngol. 1998;42:207–23.
4. da Costa SS, de Dornelles CC, Netto LFS, Braga MEL. Aspectosgerais das otitesmédias. In: da Costa SS, Cruz OLM, de Oliveira JAA, editors. Otorrinolaringologia: Princípios e Prática. 2nd ed. Artmed; 2006.
5. da Costa SS, de Dornelles CC. OtiteMédiaCrônicanão-colesteatomatosa. In: da Costa SS, Cruz OLM, de Oliveira JAA, editors. Otorrinolaringologia: Princípios e Prática. 2nd ed. Porto Alegre: Artmed; 2006. p. 289–308.
6. da Costa SS, Rosito LPS, de Dornelles CC, da Costa LM. Otite MédiaCrônicaNãoColesteatomatosa. In: Neto SC, de Junior JFM, Martins RHG, da Costa SS, editors. Tratado de Otorrinolaringologia e Cirurgia Cervicofacial. 2nd ed. São Paulo: Editora Roca; 2011. p. 99–121.
7. Zorzetto NL. Anatomia da orelha. In: da Costa SS, Cruz OLM, de Oliveira JAA, editors. Otorrinolaringologia: Princípios e Prática. 2nd ed. Porto Alegre: Artmed; 2006. p. 23–60.
8. Shrapnell HJ. On the form and structure of the membrane timpani. London Med Gazette. 1832;10:120–4.
9. Paço J, Branco C, Estibeiro H. The posterosuperior quadrant of the tympanic. Otolaryngol: Head Neck Surg. 2009;140(6):884–8.

Ossicular Pathology in Chronic Otitis Media

40

Cemil Kayaalp, Henrique Furlan Pauna, Rafael C. Monsanto, Hamed Sajjadi, Michael M. Paparella, and Sebahattin Cureoglu

Embryology

The middle ear ossicles derive from the first and second branchial arches: the Meckel's cartilage (first arch) forms the malleus and incus, and the Reichert's cartilage (second arch) forms the apophysis of the malleus and the incus [1–3].

Anatomy

The middle ear sound conducting apparatus is composed by the tympanic membrane and the ossicular chain. The tympanic membrane is a thin, multilayered tissue, supported by the bony tympanic ring, which separates the external ear from the middle ear. The middle ear cavity is encapsulated in the auditory bulla and may be categorized into three compartments: (a) the attic, which contains the head of the malleus, incudo-malleolar joint, and the short process of the incus; (b) the mesotympanum, which is the space located medially to the tympanic membrane; and (c) hypotympanum, located inferiorly to the inferior limit of the tympanic annulus. The chain is comprised by three ossicles (malleus, incus, and stapes) that are connected by synovial joints (malleo-incudal and incudo-stapedial). The ossicular chain conducts the mechanical sound wave from the tympanic membrane to the cochlea, being also responsible for amplifying the sound intensity to provide adequate stimulation of the cochlear hair cells [4, 5].

The malleus is divided into head (caput mallei), neck (collum mallei), short process (procesus brevis), and handle (manubrium mallei). The anatomic portions of the incus are body (corpus incudis), short process (crus breve), and long process (crus longum), which is capped with the lenticular apophysis. The stapes is divided into head (caput stapedis), anterior and posterior crus, and footplate (basis stapedis). The air pressure changes caused by the sound wave are detected by the malleus, which is loosely connected to the tympanic membrane along the manubrium and more tightly at the umbus (Fig. 40.1). Two middle ear muscles are attached to the ossicular chain: the *tensor tympani*, which is located in a bone canal adjacent to the bony eustachian tube, and the stapedial muscle, located at the pyramidal eminence. The *tensor tympani* muscle tendon emerges into the middle ear at the cochleariform process and attaches to the lateral portion of the handle of the malleus. Although the exact role of the *tensor tympani* muscle in the hearing physiology is still under debate, it provides stability to the ossicular chain, being responsible for maintaining the conical shape of the tympanic membrane by pulling the malleus medially. The tendon of the stapedial muscle, which is the smallest muscle of the human body, emerges into the middle ear through the pyramidal eminence, attaching to the neck of the stapes. The stapedial muscle has a major role in the hearing, acting as the effector component of the acoustic middle ear reflex [4, 5].

The main arteries supplying the middle ear are the carotico-tympanic branches (from the vertical portion of the internal carotid artery), the inferior tympanic artery (ITA) (branch of the ascending pharyngeal artery), the stylomastoid artery (SMA) (posterior auricular artery branch), the superficial petrosal artery (SPA), and superior tympanic artery (STA) (branches of the middle meningeal artery), subarcuate artery, a branch of the meatal segment of anterior inferior cerebellar artery (AICA), anterior tympanic artery (ATA) and deep auricular artery (from the internal maxillary artery), and the eustachian tube artery [6].

Two main branches from the anterior tympanic artery supply the malleus. However, the handle of the malleus is less well supplied, and it seems that the mucosal capillary network might be of high importance for its vascular supply.

C. Kayaalp · R. C. Monsanto · M. M. Paparella · S. Cureoglu (✉)
Otopathology Laboratory, Department of Otolaryngology, University of Minnesota, Minneapolis, MN, USA
e-mail: cureo003@umn.edu

H. F. Pauna
Hospital Universitário Cajuru, Curitiba, PR, Brazil

H. Sajjadi
Stanford University, School of Medicine, San Jose Ear & Sinus Medical Center, Los Gatos, CA, USA

M. V. Goycoolea et al. (eds.), *Textbook of Otitis Media*, https://doi.org/10.1007/978-3-031-40949-3_40

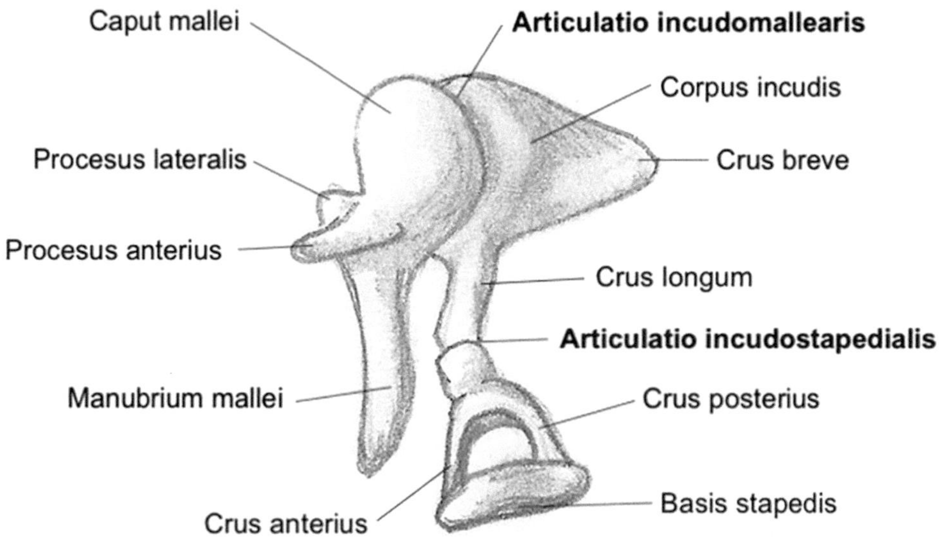

Fig. 40.1 Anatomical representation of the ossicular chain, medial view

Three small arteries are related with the bloody supply of incus. One comes from the superior branch of the anterior tympanic artery and goes into the body of the incus close to its articulation with the malleus. The second branch, which supplies the body and the long process of the incus, is a long, tortuous vessel that passes through a mucosal fold from the anterior tympanic artery to the lateral side of the incus. A third, smaller branch, comes via a mucosal fold from the posterior branch of the anterior tympanic artery. Intraosseous vessels might be extremely thin at the long process of the incus. Infectious or inflammatory conditions may obliterate (partially or totally) these vascular channels, leading to an important decrease in the mucosal blood supply to the ossicular chain.

The main blood vessel supplying the stapes comes from the stylomastoid artery. The arterial supply of the footplate comes from inferior tympanic arteries, but also from the stylomastoid artery. The blood supply to the head of the stapes arises from intraosseous vessels. The crura and the footplate, however, might be completely devoid of intraosseous blood vessels, and the blood supply may depend entirely on the mucosal arterioli and capillaries. Thus, as compared to the other two ossicles, the stapes seems to be more prone to ischemia [7].

When the tympanic membrane and ossicles receive the sound wave, the mechanical energy is transmitted to the fluid-filled inner ear through the oval window. The differences in the acoustic impedance between air in the middle ear and the liquid-filled inner ear, that could compromise the propagation of the sound wave, are bypassed by several adaptative mechanisms. The difference in the area between the tympanic membrane and the footplate, in addition to the difference in the length of the malleus and the long process of the incus, provides amplification of the signal intensity [5]. Additionally, the curvature of the TM is also responsible for a minor pressure gain [8, 9]. The mechanical energy transmitted to the inner ear is then finally transformed in an electrical impulse through a synergic action from the outer and inner hair cells at the Organ of Corti and later transmitted to the central nervous system [5].

Diagnosis

Stapedial reflex: Any obstruction in the transmission of the sound to the inner ear may end up in reduced or absent acoustic reflex.

The introduction of *high-resolution computed tomography (HRCT)* has been a turning point in the evaluation of temporal bone abnormalities. It has high sensitivity and specificity in diagnosing abnormalities affecting the ossicular chain [10]. Although 3-D reconstruction of HRCT scans have been proposed as a potential tool in evaluating potential ossicular chain abnormalities, they do not provide a precise estimate of erosion of the middle ear structure. With a HRCT scan, it is possible to detect erosion of the malleus and the incus in most cases, allowing an adequate preoperative surgical planning (Fig. 40.4). Erosion of the stapes and the malleus handle, however, may not adequately seen in most of these scans, as erosion of these structures are not detected in one-third of the cases [11].

Spiral computed tomography imaging is an important diagnostic method for bone erosion and can provide essential information for surgery. It seems superior to conventional computed tomography in the preoperative assessment of the presence of ossicular chain abnormalities in patients with COM [12].

Cone beam computed tomography (CBCT) is another imaging test that can be used in the assessment of ossicular chain abnormalities. Studies demonstrated that the CBCT has a higher accuracy as compared with the other CT modalities due to the primary voxel size. Nonetheless, there seems to be a limitation in the evaluation of smaller structures, such as the head or the crura of the stapes [13].

Optical coherence tomography (OCT) creates coherent infrared light waveforms. It is a noninvasive, noncontact imaging modality. It is like an optical US based on light rather than sound or radiofrequency with no radiation. The use of long wavelength light allows it to penetrate the scattering medium. OCT may aid in the diagnosis and management of otitis media, especially when interpreted alongside physical exam and otoscopy findings.

Optical Coherence Tomography-Doppler Vibrometer (OCT-DV) is a new and novel technique and not restricted to measurements on the surface of the tympanic membrane and is able to measure the vibration of any optically reflecting structure in the middle ear. OCT-DV measurements are spatially resolved, and complex cases of conductive hearing loss that involve fixations or discontinuities at multiple locations may be better characterized by considering motion at different points in the ossicular chain [14, 15]. Umbo velocity measurements are a more direct measure of the dynamic state of the middle ear ossicles and are less influenced by the compliance of the tympanic membrane [16, 17].

Pathology of the Ossicles

The middle ear space should be well aerated to enable ossicular function. Especially, pneumatization of the round window membrane is a prerequisite for ossicular reconstruction in order to reestablish hearing back. The ossicular chain transmits the sound into the inner ear. Under normal conditions, sound is transmitted to the oval window membrane at an earlier phase than to the round window membrane.

The discontinuity of the sound due to ossicular pathologies such as fixation, dislocation, or resorption will lead to a conductive hearing loss. To restore sound transmission, ossiculoplasty may be required following the eradication of middle ear cleft pathologies. Such pathologies can be cholesteatoma (Fig. 40.2), granulation tissues (Fig. 40.3), cholesterol granuloma, atelectasis (Fig. 40.4), or tympanosclerosis (Fig. 40.5). If an ossicular erosion is suspected in a case with chronic otitis media, each ossicle should be evaluated independently during surgery (Fig. 40.6). In addition, tensor tympani and stapedial muscles should be assessed to rule out any calcification.

Throughout the course of chronic otitis media, osseous changes including osteitis, necrosis, reabsorption, and osteoneogenesis can occur in the middle ear cleft [18] (Fig.40.7). The bony involvement parallels the severity of the pathologic inflammatory process in the middle ear. In the generalized form of the chronic active otitis media, although all three ossicles can show chronic changes, the lenticular process of incus, which is the most involved, being followed in frequency by the stapes suprastructure, body of incus, and then the malleus (Fig. 40.8) [18].

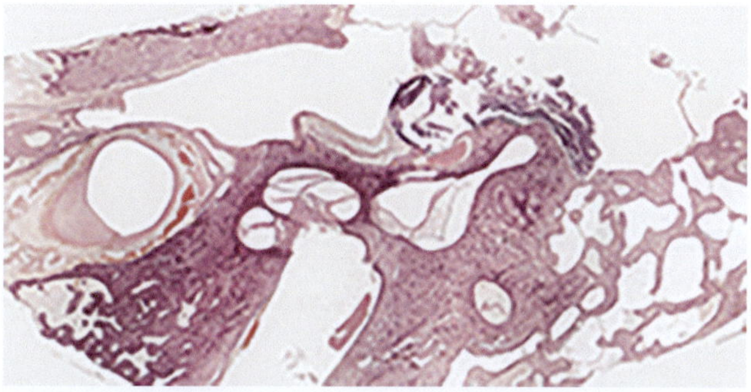

Fig. 40.2 A 59-year-old male with diffuse encephalopathy had a history of mixed-type hearing loss. Histopathologic analysis showed chronic otitis media with attico-antral cholesteatoma. Note the erosion of Fallopian canal

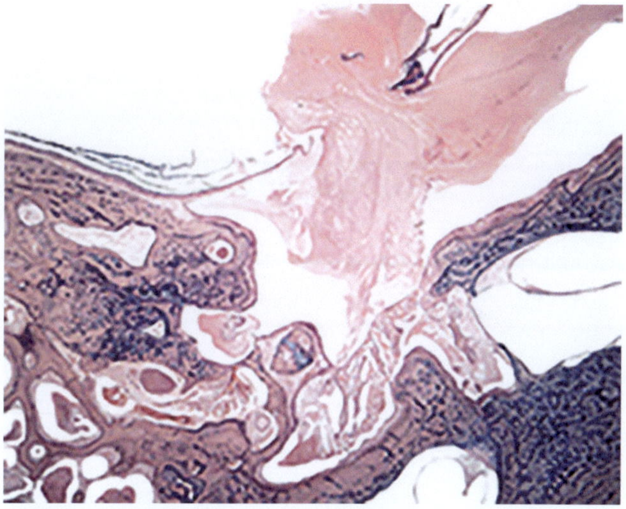

Fig. 40.3 Histopathologic section showed chronic otitis media with granulation tissue, which was located at the round window niche, and actively draining from the perforated tympanic membrane

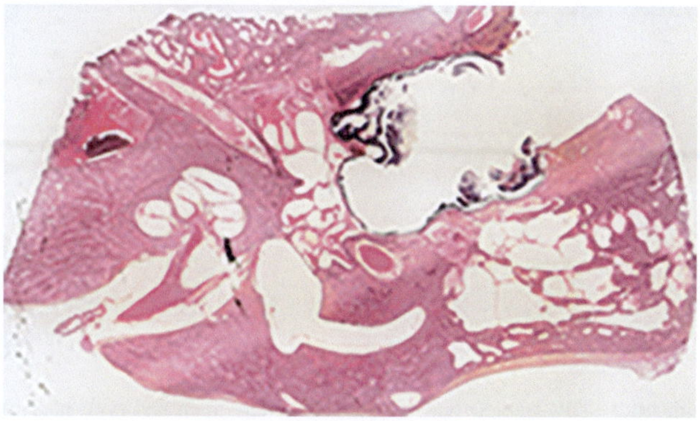

Fig. 40.4 A 83-year-old patient with carcinoma of bladder showed retraction pocket and cholesteatoma with erosion of the ossicular chain in the middle ear

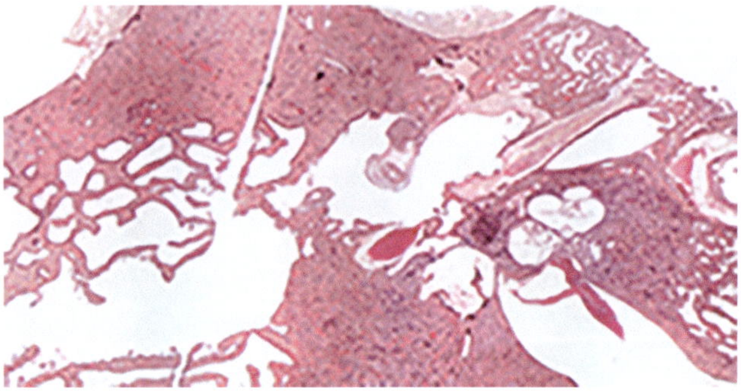

Fig. 40.5 A 73-year-old female had a history of bilateral chronic otitis media. Histopathologic analysis showed tympanosclerosis, especially around the incus

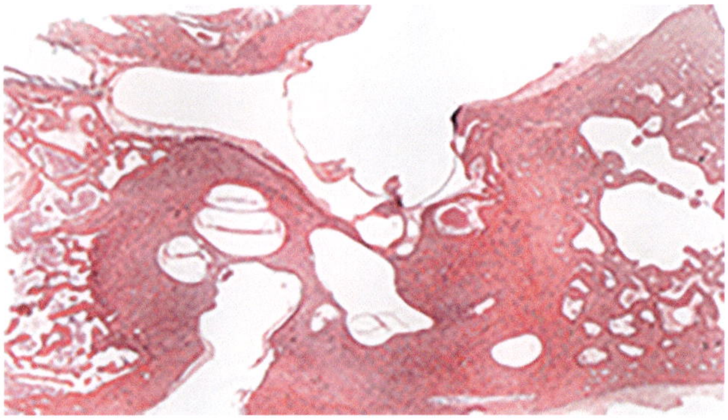

Fig. 40.6 This was a 50-year-old patient with metastatic breast carcinoma. Histopathologic evaluation showed retraction pocket with the erosion of incus and carcinoma involvement of the petrous apex

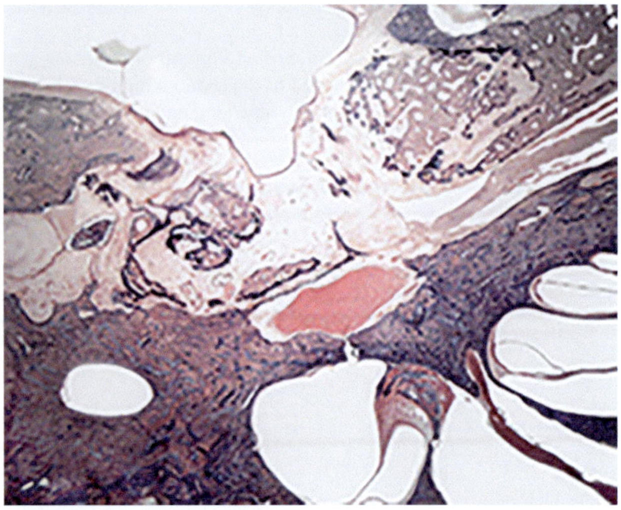

Fig. 40.7 This patient had a history of bilateral mixed-type hearing loss due to chronic otitis media with new bone formation, ossicular erosion, fibrocystic changes, and tympanic membrane retraction

Granulation tissue is the most common pathology encountered in chronic ears. It consists of vascularized connective tissue with a component of acute inflammatory exudation.

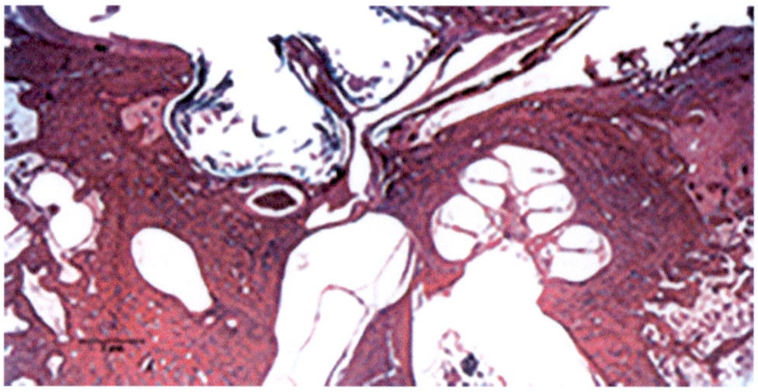

Fig. 40.8 Chronic otitis media with cholesteatoma caused erosion of incus and stapes ending up with conductive hearing loss

The most common sites for granulation tissue are the epitympanum, mesotympanum, round window niche, and mastoid antrum [18, 19]. During the formation of granulation tissue, the mucous membrane is thickened by edema, submucosal fibrosis, and infiltration with chronic inflammatory cells. Later, mucosal edema may progress to the formation of polyps [20]. With maturation, granulation tissue becomes more fibrous and less cellular with increased collagen and reticular formation [18]. This pathologic growth may lead to adhesion, fixation, and/or resorption of the ossicles in the middle ear [20]. Furthermore, this activity, if unchecked, may lead to serious complications, such as inflammation of the inner ear [21].

Cholesteatoma (Fig. 40.9a, b) may cause erosion of the ossicular chain by several mechanisms including the pressure exerted by the cholesteatoma mass, osteoclastic activities, or enzymatic activities. Even after a radical cleaning of cholesteatoma during surgery, residual cholesteatoma can occur in 7–50% of cases [22, 23]. Residual cholesteatoma can be found in inaccessible areas such as around the arch of the stapes, the sinus tympani, oval window area, retrolabyrinthine, and the perifacial regions [24]. Therefore, the removal of all accessible mastoid air cells and the pathologic tissue hidden in the inaccessible areas are necessary for reliable eradication of cholesteatoma. It has also noted that many innocent-looking mucosal changes at a considerable distance from cholesteatoma can contain squamous epithelium [25].

Tympanosclerosis is observed as a submucosal whitish onion-like lamellar deposit in the middle ear. It usually is a consequence of chronic otitis media and starts with collagen deposition or fibrosis in the subepithelial extracellular matrix of the middle ear or tympanic membrane. Then, it is followed by fusion of collagen fibers into a homogenous mass and later the deposition of extracellular calcium and phosphate crystals appear [26]. Usually, no suppuration is seen with tympanosclerosis. Because tympanosclerosis will diminish the perfusion of the mucosa and ossicles, it will eventually cause devitalized bone. This might be the under-

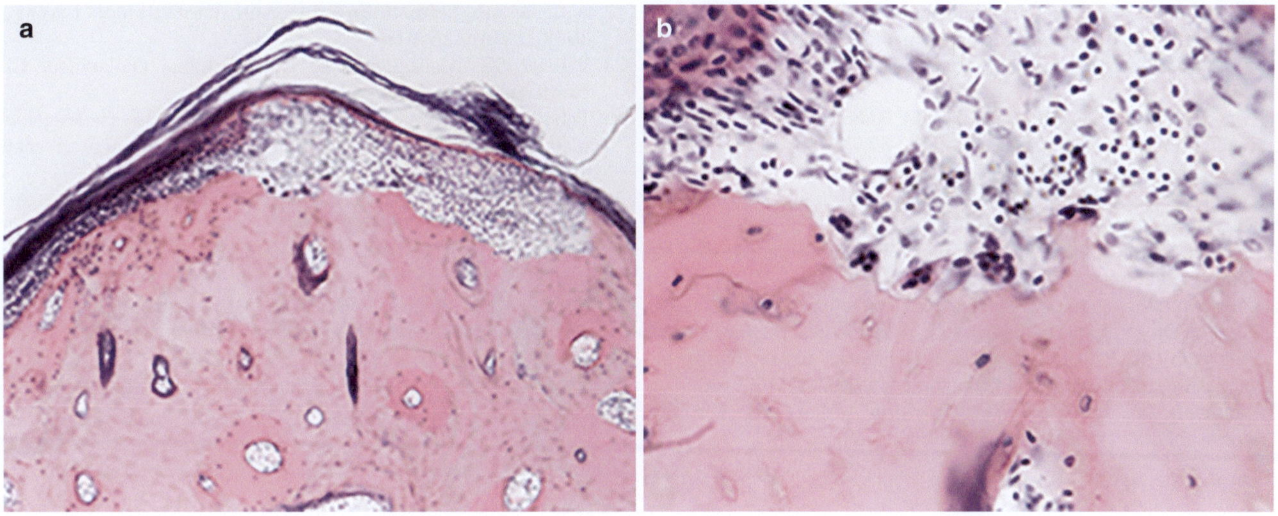

Fig. 40.9 (**a**) This was a 94-year-old male patient with a hx of total deafness at the age of 12 years. A cholesteatoma was found in the middle ear eroding the ossicles. (**b**) High magnification showed macrophages

lying pathogenesis of failure of revision surgeries in cases with residual hearing loss due to tympanosclerosis. Otoscopic examination shows white plaques in the tympanic membrane and nodular appearance within submucosa of the middle ear.

If tympanosclerosis is localized in the tympanic membrane, it may not affect the hearing. If the ossicular chain is involved, it will cause air–bone gap and may require ossicular reconstruction [27]. If the stapes is involved, a staged surgery including first myringoplasty and reconstruction of malleo-incudal fixation before releasing the fixation of stapes will be performed. If the fixation is observed at the stapedial muscle level, stapes movement may be provided by just cutting the stapedial tendon. Rarely, the head of the malleus may be fixed in the attic due to tympanosclerosis or calcification process (Fig. 40.5).

If the ossicles are intact but the tympanic membrane is perforated, the intensity of hearing loss will be linearly proportional to the size of perforation [28]. If the ossicular disruption is combined with a perforated tympanic membrane, the hearing loss may be around 35–40 dB. However, the ossicular disruption under an intact tympanic membrane will reflect the sound back to the external ear canal with ending up a maximal conductive hearing loss of 55–60 dB. If ossicular resorption is associated with a retracted tympanic membrane that attaches to the stapedial supra-structure, relatively a better hearing is observed due to the uninterrupted conductivity of the sound to the inner ear [29].

References

1. Anthwal N, Thompson H. The development of the mammalian outer and middle ear. J Anat. 2016;228:217–32.
2. Chapman SC. Can you hear me now? Understanding vertebrate middle ear. Front Biosci. 2011;16:1675–92.
3. O'Gorman S. Second branchial arch lineages of the middle ear of wild-type and Hoxa2 mutant mice. Dev Dyn. 2005;234:124–31.
4. Fuchs JC, Tucker AS. Development and Integration of the ear. Curr Top Dev Biol. 2015;115:213–32.
5. Luers JC, Huttenbrink KB. Surgical anatomy and pathology of the middle ear. J Anat. 2016;228:338–53.
6. Nager GT, Nager M. LXXXIII the arteries of the human middle ear, with particular regard to the blood supply of the auditory ossicles. Ann Otol Rhinol Laryngol. 1953;62:923–49.
7. Hamberger C-A, Wersall J. Vascular supplyof the tympanic membrane and the ossicular chain. Acta Oto-laryngol. 1964;57:308–18.
8. Killion MC, Dallos P. Impedance matching by the, combined effects of the outer and middle ear. J Acoust Soc Am. 1979;66:599–602.
9. Tonndorf J, Khanna SM. The role of tympanic membrane in middle ear transmission. Ann Otol Rhinol Laryngol. 1970;79:743–53.
10. Singh R, Rai R, Singh P, Sethi S, Ahluwalia APS, Choudhary G. High-resolution computed tomography (HRCT) in pediatric and adult patients with unsafe chronic suppurative otitis media (CSOM) and its surgical correlation. J Family Med Prim Care. 2020;9:4067–73.
11. Fuse T, Aoyagi M, Koike Y, Sugai Y. Diagnosis of the ossicular chain in the middle ear by high-resolution CT. ORL J Otorhinolaryngol Relat Spec. 1992;54:251–4.
12. Naghibi S, Seifirad S, Adami Dehkordi M, Einolghozati S, Ghaffarian Eidgahi Moghadam N, Akhavan Rezayat A, Seifirad S. Comparison of conventional versus spiral computed tomography with three dimensional reconstruction in chronic otitis media with ossicular chain destruction. Iran J Radiol. 2016;13:e9018.
13. Guldner C, Diogo I, Bernd E, Drager S, Mandapathil M, Teymoortash A, Negm H, Wilhelm T. Visualization of anatomy in normal and pathologic middle ears by cone beam CT. Eur Arch Otorhinolaryngol. 2017;274:737–42.
14. Matthews TJ, Adamson R. Optical coherence tomography: current and future clinical applications in otology. Curr Opin Otolaryngol Head Neck Surg. 2020;28(5):296–301.
15. Rosowski JJ, Nakajima HH, Merchant SN. Clinical utility of laser-Doppler vibrometer measurements in live normal and pathologic human ears. Ear Hear. 2008;29:3–19.
16. Nakajima HH, Ravicz ME, Merchant SN, Peake WT, Rosowski JJ. Experimental ossicular fixations and the middle ear's response to sound: evidence for a flexible ossicular chain. Hear Res. 2005;204:60–77.

17. Rosowski JJ, Nakajima HH, Hamade MA, Mahfoud L, Merchant GR, Halpin CF, Merchant SN. Ear-canal reflectance, umbo velocity, and tympanometry in normal-hearing adults. Ear Hearing. 2012;33:19–34.
18. Meyerhoff WL, Kim CS, Paparella MM. Pathology of chronic otitis media. Ann Otol Rhinol Laryngol. 1978;87:749–60.
19. Jaisinghani VJ, Paparella MM, Schachern PA, Le CT. Tympanic membrane/middle ear pathologic correlates in chronic Otitis media. Laryngoscope. 1999;109:712–6.
20. Paparella MM, Sipila P, Juhn SK, Jung TTK. Subepithelial space in Otitis media. Laryngoscope. 1985;95:414–20.
21. Paparella MM, Sugiura S. The pathology of suppurative labyrinthitis. Ann Otol Rhinol Laryngol. 1967;76(3):554–86.
22. Edelstein DR, Parisier SC. Surgical techniques and recidivism in cholesteatoma. Otolaryngol Clin North Am. 1989;22:1029–40.
23. Veldman JE, Braunius WW. Revision surgery for chronic otitis media: A learning experience: report on 389 cases with a long-term follow-up. Ann Otol Rhinol Laryngol. 1998;107(6):486–91.
24. Parisier SC. Management of cholesteatoma. Otolaryngol Clin North Am. 1989;22:927–40.
25. Palva T, Makinen J. Why does middle ear cholesteatoma recur?Histopathologic observations. Arch Otolaryngol (Stockh). 1987;104:487–94.
26. Sorensen H, True O. Histology of tympanosclerosis. Acta Otolaryngol. 1972;73(1):18–26.
27. Javia LR, Ruckenstein MJ. Ossiculoplasty. Otolaryngol Clin North Am. 2006;39(6):1177 89.
28. Mehta RP, Rosowski JJ, Voss SE, O'Neil E, Merchant SN. Determinants of hearing loss in perforations of the tympanic membrane. Otol Neurotol. 2006;27(2):136–43.
29. Paparella MM, Jung TK. Experience with tympanoplasty for atelectatic ears. Laryngoscope. 1981;91:1472–7.

41 Tympanic Membrane Retractions: Pathophysiology, Classification, and Management

Inesangela Canali, Letícia Petersen Schmidt Rosito, and Caroline Catherine Lacerda Elias

Tympanic membrane (TM) retractions are defined as a medialization of its position toward the promontory. Anatomically, they can be pars flaccida (PF) or pars tensa (PT) of TM and may be sectoral or diffuse. By definition, retractions that have a diameter of the outer opening smaller than that of the inner part are known as retraction pockets, having less self-cleaning capacity. Atelectasis refers to a diffuse medialization of the TM, while adhesive otitis media occurs when the TM is adhered to the promontory [1].

Histologically, TM is formed by an outer layer of keratinized squamous epithelial tissue, an inner layer of cuboidal mucosal epithelium, and a middle layer (lamina propria) formed by fibrous connective tissue. The posterosuperior portion of the PT has a thinner lamina propria and also an increase in vascular supply, which makes it more susceptible to rupture of its collagen fibers during inflammatory processes, thus making it more likely to retract. The same occurs in FP, for having a thinner lamina propria and lack of the fibrocartilaginous ring in the Rivinus notch [2].

I. Canali (✉)
Department of Otolaryngology, Pontifical Catholic University, Porto Alegre, Rio Grande do Sul, Brazil

Federal University of Rio Grande do Sul, Porto Alegre, Rio Grande do Sul, Brazil

L. P. S. Rosito
Federal University of Rio Grande do Sul, Porto Alegre, Rio Grande do Sul, Brazil

Department of Otolaryngology—Head and Neck Surgery, Porto Alegre Clinica's Hospital, Porto Alegre, Rio Grande do Sul, Brazil

C. C. L. Elias
Federal University of Rio Grande do Sul, Porto Alegre, Rio Grande do Sul, Brazil

Department of Otolaryngology, Hospital Nossa Senhora da Conceição, de Porto Alegre (GHC), Porto Alegre, Rio Grande do Sul, Brazil

Pathogenesis of Tympanic Membrane Retractions

The TM has a natural elasticity that allows its shape and position to vary according to the pressure variations of the middle ear (OM) with the environment. A healthy TM is capable of equalizing certain pressure variations, however, when the pressure gradient exceeds the capacity of this equalization, a positive or negative pressure is installed. In normal situations, this pressure variation is corrected by active or passive opening of the eustachian tube. Sustained negative pressures make the TM elastic fibers lose elasticity and thickness and retract more easily [1].

Classically, there are three described mechanisms that regulate OM pressure: (a) equalization of OM and environmental pressures through the eustachian tube; (b) gas exchange through the mucosa of the OM; and (c) pressure control mechanism of the ventilated spaces of the mastoid.

Auditory Tube

When pathological conditions are installed, determining permanent occlusion of the auditory tube (AT), the negative pressure, in a vicious cycle, will tend to progressively increase, causing TM retraction [3]. In addition, there may be cavity transudation of intravascular fluid to the interstitial space and from there to the lumen of OM [4]. Sustaining this negative pressure can also lead to histopathological changes in the epithelium and subepithelium of the auditory cleft, leading to the occurrence of TM retractions and atelectasis which, in the absence of restraining factors, could evolve and culminate in the formation of cholesteatomas. This sequence of events is known as the continuum theory, proposed by Paparella and collaborators to explain the pathogenesis of chronic otitis media [5].

Although the term tube dysfunction is usually used in cases of AT obstruction, it also encompasses situations in which it is pathologically open (patent tube) [3]. Studies have

M. V. Goycoolea et al. (eds.), *Textbook of Otitis Media*, https://doi.org/10.1007/978-3-031-40949-3_41

shown that patent AT can also result in changes in OM. Some patients who present this alteration develop the habit of sniffing constantly and repeatedly (sniffers) to alleviate the uncomfortable symptoms presented [6]. This maneuver, despite providing temporary comfort from symptoms, as it tends to close the tube, can lead the patient to overcorrect, creating conditions similar to the functional obstruction of AT. Thus, this habit results in a high negative pressure in the OM, which can lead to the occurrence of TM retraction and its possible subsequent pathological evolution [7].

Gas exchange Through the Middle ear Mucosa

The gas exchange that takes place between the tympanic cavity and the mastoid with the mucosal microcirculation is another important factor in the regulation of pressure in OM. The direction of gaseous diffusion is implicated in differences in the partial pressure of gaseous components in the auditory cleft. Inflammatory processes that influence mucosal thickness and blood flow in the tympanic cavity have a direct effect on the rate of diffusion. In general, when the mucosa is healthy, there is an equal gas exchange rate so that oxygen and nitrogen are absorbed in the same way that carbon dioxide is expelled. However, the thicker and more vascularized the mucosa, the greater the rate of gas diffusion [4].

It is believed that when the AT remains occluded, a negative pressure would set in, with a predominance of carbon dioxide over oxygen and causing thickening of the OM mucosa, vasodilation with serous transudation, and mucosal metaplasia in the tympanic cavity, with an increase in the number of glandular structures, ultimately resulting in an accumulation of fluid in the ME in an attempt to equalize the pressure difference. Thus, the accumulation of fluid in the tympanic cavity would be the last way to regulate the pressure [8]. According to Bunne et al. [9], this hypothesis has been questioned for several reasons. Among them is the fact that it is based on the assumption that gas is continuously absorbed by the mucosa of the OM, but studies have shown that transmucosal gas transport is bidirectional, and that the pressure in the tympanic cavity can be maintained equal to that of the environment, or even be positive, without tubal opening in healthy ears. Thus, these findings support the hypothesis that gas exchange is an important mechanism for pressure regulation in OM, while AT serves as an escape valve for excessively positive pressures and also to equalize excessively negative pressures [8, 9].

Middle Ear Complex: Mastoid and Middle Ear Ventilation Pathways

The pneumatization of the mastoid, which starts in the thirty-third week of gestation and continues until 8–9 years of age, could also influence pressure maintenance in OM. This pressure depends not only on a functioning AT but also on the gas exchange existing in the auditory cleft mucosa, which, in turn, is related to the degree of pneumatization of the mastoid. A well-pneumatized mastoid would have greater capacity to compensate for pressure changes than an eburnean mastoid [10].

In addition to AT, other anatomical factors would play an important role in the ventilation of middle ear (ME) spaces and in the pathogenesis of retractions, especially those located in the epitympanum.

The anatomy of the OM and the mastoid and their airways have been described since the end of the 19th century. Proctor in 1964 and after Palva and Johnson were the first to describe the airways of the tympanic cavity and their implications for OM diseases [11–13]. In recent decades, the use of endoscopes in ear surgeries has made it easier for surgeons to explore anatomical spaces that were not so well visualized with the use of a microscope alone.

A series of mucous folds, ligaments, and part of the ossicles make up the so-called tympanic diaphragm, practically separating the mesotympanum from the epitympanum and the mastoid. Two narrow passages cross this diaphragm: the anterior and the posterior tympanic isthmus. The anterior isthmus is more consistent, lying medially to the body of the incus, passing between the stapes and the tendon of the tensor tympani muscle. When the medial incudal fold is present, a small posterior isthmus appears between this fold and the posterior tympanic wall [12, 14, 15]. Figure 41.1 shows the two main ventilation pathways to the epitympanum, as mentioned above.

Right ear: A, posterior view; B, anterior view. A schematic drawing representing the two independent aeration routes of the epitympanum. The major aeration route (red arrow) passing through the isthmus for the large upper unit (epitympanic compartments, antrum, and mastoid cells); the second independent aeration route (yellow arrow) for the smaller lower unit (Prussak's space) passing through the posterior pouch between the tympanum and the posterior malleolar ligamental fold. PES, posterior epitympanic space; AES, anterior epitympanic space; in, incus; Hma, malleus head; imlf, incudomalleolar lateral fold; mlf, malleolar lateral fold; is, tympanic isthmus; st, stapes; cp, cochleariform process; et, eustachian tube; pml, posterior malleolar ligament; aml, anterior malleolar ligament; tf, tensor fold; PS, protympanic space; tt, tensor tympani; Prs, Prussak space; hm, malleus handle; ps, posterior spine.

Eustachian tube is the direct ventilation route to the mesotympanum and hypotympanum, while the epitympanic region receives ventilation from the tube through the tympanic isthmus which, in normal ears, are physiologically open [16, 17].

The obstruction of the tympanic isthmus, however, is observed in several OM pathologies such as TM retractions

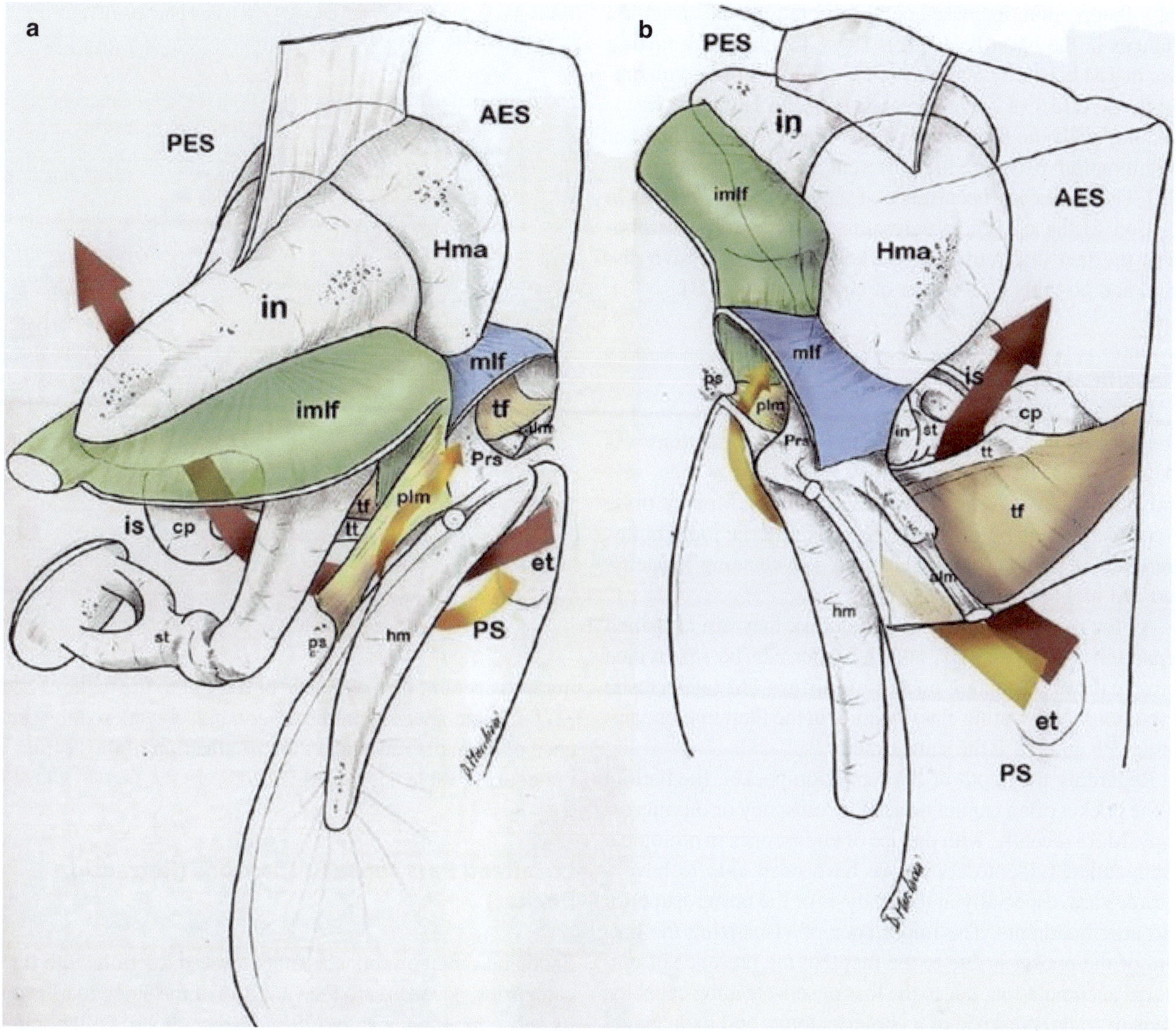

Fig. 41.1 Anatomy of middle ear folds and the two main ventilation routes [19]. Right ear: (**a**) posterior view; (**b**) anterior view

and cholesteatomas. Marchioni et al. described in their endoscopic studies the presence of anatomical blocks in the ventilation pathways. These blocks could cause poor sectorial (epitympanic) ventilation of the OM, which they called the "selective epitympanic dysventilation syndrome"[18]. This syndrome is characterized by the presence of normal eustachian tube function, complete epitympanic diaphragm, and total isthmus block [19]. Thus, these individuals have normal aeration of the mesotympanum and hypotympanum, while the attic and mastoid have poor ventilation and, consequently, a negative pressure is installed and perpetuated, which can trigger the evolution to a retraction bag or attic cholesteatoma. They also observed that, even in the absence of isthmus blocks, if the Prussak space does not have enough airways for the adjacent spaces and the OM mucosa presents an inflammatory process, negative pressures can also set in [20]. It is believed that once these hypoventilation microfoci are created, adhesions between the inner layer of the TM and the mucoperiosteum of the ossicles and OM are formed, being the precursors of the perimatrix of a future cholesteatoma, regardless of the reestablishment of OM ventilation [21].

Inflammationand Formation of Retractions—Histopathology

Inflammatory processes, such as acute otitis media or the presence of persistent effusion in OM, through inflammatory mediators and cytokines, can structurally affect the mucosal histology of OM and TM [1]. The main histological features observed in the more advanced stages of retraction pockets are usually: loss of the collagen fibrous double layer in the lamina propria, increased keratinization, chronic subepithelial inflammation, increased cell proliferation, and structural changes in the basal layer [22]. These findings may favor a loss in TM elasticity and plasticity, making it more vulnerable to the effect of negative pressures [23]. However, histopathologically, no differences were observed in the degree of inflammation between the different degrees of retraction [22]. The increasing occurrence of these histological signs in relation to the clinical progression of retractions corroborates the fact that retraction pockets are a progressive disease, and possibly a precursor of cholesteatoma [23].

Classification

The first and best known classification of TM retractions was proposed by Sadé and Berco, in 1976 [24]. Since then, several authors have described its variations [25]. Most of these classifications encompass the following criteria: topography, presence of ossicular chain erosion, self-cleaning property, and TM mobility.

As for the location of the retractions, they are classified separately by PF and PT, and the latter can be subdivided into localized (retraction pocket) or diffuse TM (atelectasis) retractions. No existing classification in the literature encompasses PF and PT at the same time.

Regarding the depth of the retraction pocket, the bottom of the pocket often cannot be seen by otoscopy or otomicroscopy. More recently, with the use of endoscopes in otological examination (videotoscopy), we have been able to have a clearer view, especially in the analysis of the posterosuperior and attic quadrants. The importance of visualizing the bottom of the pocket is due to the fact that the presence of epithelial accumulation, due to the loss of self-cleaning capacity, leads us to the presence of a cholesteatoma, and its management is distinct from retraction [1].

Another criterion to be analyzed is the presence of bone erosion, which may be from the long branch of the incus and stapes suprastructure, when there is involvement of the posterosuperior quadrant and the scutum (attic lateral wall) and/or the malleus head and incus body, when there is attical involvement. These erosions commonly cause a conductive hearing loss, even if clinically insignificant, as demonstrated in previous studies by our research group [26].

Pars Flaccida Retractions

The three most used classification systems for PF are described in Table 41.1:

Initially, Sadé et al. proposed three stages for the retractions, in which the graduation increases, being able to be dry or humid and with the bone limits of the attic intact or not [24]. Later, Tos et al. published a new classification also taking into account the adherence of the TM to the malleus head [27]. Characon et al., on the other hand, considered the presence of TM adherence and the visualization of the bottom of the pocket (Table 41.1) [28].

Table 41.1 Staging of pars flaccida retraction pockets [25]

Stage	Sadé	Tos	Charachon
1	Micro-metula: retraction is very small and noticed only if looked for	Pars flaccida is dimpled and is more retracted than normal	Mobile retraction pocket
II	Metula: an obvious, easily observed RP, resting on the malleus neck. Often, some of the scutum around it is missing	The retraction pocket is adherent to the malleus head	Fixed, fundus is visible regardless of the atticotomy size
III	Macro-metula: large RP with erosion of the scutum and visible head of malleus	The retraction pocket may be hidden. There may also be associated erosion of the outer attic wall (scutum)	Fixed, fundus is not visible, regardless of the atticotomy size
IV	NA	There is a definite erosion of the outer attic wall. The fundus cannot he clearly seen	NA

NA, not applicable; *RP* retraction pocket

Localized Pars Tensa Retractions (Retraction Pocket)

Sadé and collaborators classified these retractions into three categories, according to the visibility of the stock market and its self-cleaning capacity [29]. Charachon and collaborators proposed the classification for PT applying the same mobility criteria of MT that were applied to PF [28]. In 1998, Gersdorff et al. proposed a classification similar to that of Charachon, but with modifications granted by the use of the endoscope, the last two stages culminating in the presence of cholesteatoma [30]. These classifications are described in Table 41.2.

Generalized Pars Tensa Retractions (Atelectasis)

Sadé and Berco proposed stages for grading atelectasis, according to the medial extent of PT retraction (Fig. 41.2) [24]. This classification served as a model for future classifications and modifications by several authors (Table 41.3).

In 2000, Dornhoffer et al. proposed a modification in the Sadé classification, with the last stage being attributed to the failure to visualize the entire extension of the TM by otomi-

Table 41.2 Staging of retraction pockets located in the pars tensa [25]

Stage	Sadé	Charachon	Gersdorff
1	Fundus can be easily seen, self-cleaning	Mobile, can be aspirated by Valsalva or politzer even if adheres to incus	Mobile can be aspirated by valsalva or politzer even if adheres to incus
II	Fundus can be easily seen, not self-cleaning, but its debris can be easily aspirated in totality	Fixed, visible fundus with erosion of incus	IIa: Fixed, fundus is visible by microscope IIb: Fixed, fundus is visible by otoendocope
III	Large RP tilled with infected keratin debris	Fixed, fundus not visible but still self-cleansing	Fixed, fundus not visible by otocndoscope
IV	NA	NA	Stage III + accumulation keratin debris
V	NA	NA	Cholesteatoma with purulent otorrhea

NA not applicable; *RP* retraction pocket

Table 41.3 Staging of generalized pars tensa retractions[25]

Stage	Sadé	Domhoffer	Erasmus
I	TM slightly retracted	Mild retraction of the tympanic membrane	TM atrophic but not adherent
II	TM retracted and touching the incus or stapes	Retraction to the incus or stapes, the so-called myringo-incudo-stapedopexy	TM adherent to the promontory
III	TM touching the promontory	Involvement down to the promontory	TM adherent to the incus or stapes
IV	TM adherent to the promontory	The full extent or depth of the retraction cannot be adequately visualized by micro-otoscopy	Adherent to ossicles with RP but without cholesteatoma
V	Perforated TM	NA	RP with cholesteatoma or breakthrough

AM not applicable, *TM* tympanic membrane

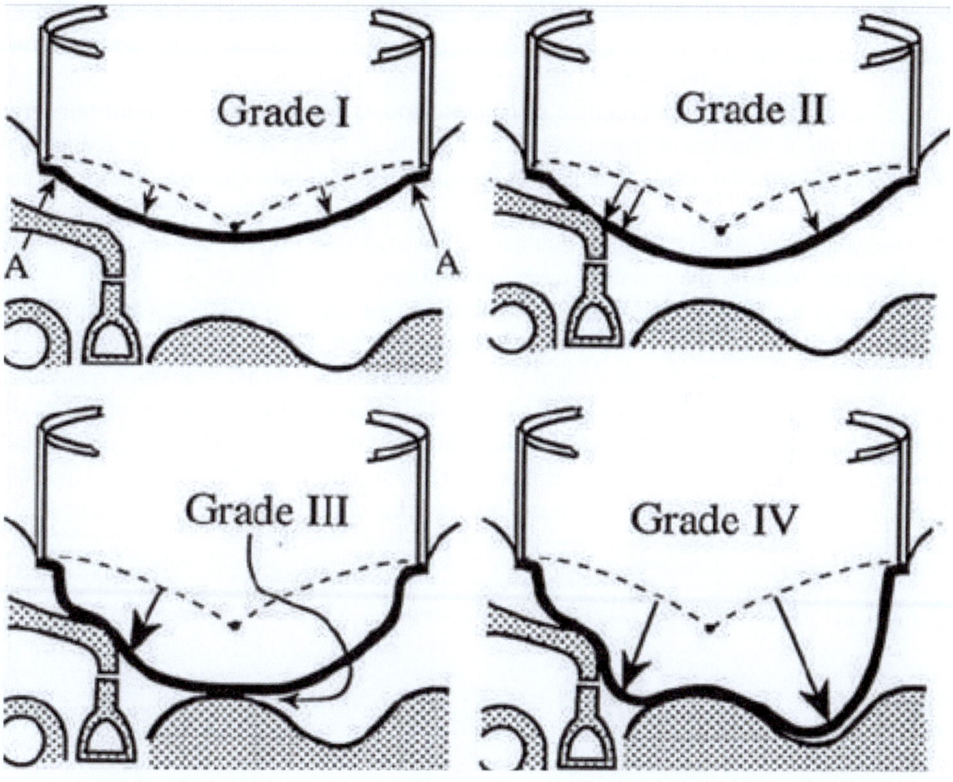

Fig. 41.2 Grades of tympanic membrane retractions [24]

croscopy, as they consider that this is the most effective way to assess the existence of epithelial accumulation in retraction. They also evaluated the mobility of TM at each stage of their graduation [31].

Borgstein et al. (2007), proposed a new classification, which they called "The Erasmus Atelectasis Classification" due to the need for a more current systematization that takes into account the assessment of children [32]. While in the Sadé classification, the retraction of the TM along the headland is a more severe degree than the retraction along the ossicular chain, in the Erasmus classification, the opposite occurs.

However, little is discussed about the applicability and reproducibility of the classifications. In 2012, James et al.

published endoscopically evaluating existing staging systems (Tos for PF and Sadé and Erasmus for PT) [33]. They also compared the latter two with an analysis they proposed evaluating multiple variables involved in PT retractions: (0) normal; (1a) retraction without touching the ME structures; (1b) touch the headland; (2a) touch the anvil; (2b) retraction enveloping anvil; (3a) partial erosion of the anvil; (3b) complete erosion of the anvil; (4) bottom of the bag not visualized; (5) accumulation of keratin medial to the anulus (potentially removable); (6) presence of granulation tissue in the retraction; and (7) cholesteatoma. They observed that the interobserver and intraobserver agreements were very weak, especially for PF and for the Erasmus classification of PT. The Sadé classification, on the other hand, showed a moderate inter- and intra-observer correlation and the characterization with the proposed variables showed a more robust correlation [33].

Each rank, as seen above, prioritizes certain aspects for its ranks. We observed that in addition to them not being in agreement with each other, and they tend to systematically divide the retractions according to the regions of the TM affected, in PF and PT, and not analyze the TM globally, none of them takes into account the degree of hearing loss for their graduations. In addition, the last stages of some classifications represent the presence of cholesteatoma. We know that the distinction of a severe retraction, starting the formation of epithelial debris with a cholesteatoma, is often a challenge.

The concept of staging assumes that each stage is different from the other by the variables described and that each graduation is a prognostic indicator and must have different management. However, unlike established staging systems already established in medicine, such as the TNM classification for malignant tumors, the existing retraction classifications in the literature are not clear indicators of prognosis, much less of management, mainly because there is no unified staging system. In this way, currently the existing classifications serve much more like an instant demonstration of the retractions at a given moment than as a prognosis or as definitions of conduct.

In our studies regarding TM retractions, they have been classified according to the Sadé and Berco classification, modified by our group. Mild retractions were considered when there was a medialization of the TM onto the promontory without contact in this, or in the ossicular chain; moderate retractions were considered when there was a contact of the TM on the ossicular chain or in the promontory or in the scutum, and severe retractions when there was erosion of the ossicular chain or bone limits. We believe that the mild retractions behave like normal ears and so we consider for study and classification only ears with moderate and severe retractions.

TM was divided into PF (atticus) and PT (posterior and anterior quadrant). Each region was analyzed, and the following degrees of severity were noted:

PF: (1) normal or mild retraction, without contact onto the scutum; (2) contact with the scutum (retraction in the attical lateral wall without contact with the malleus neck and/or ossicle heads or erosion); (3) erosion of the scutum (attical lateral wall); and (4) erosion of the malleus head or incus body (Fig. 41.3)

PT—posterior quadrant (PQ): (1) normal or slight medialization of the TM without contact in the promontory or in the ossicular chain; (2) contact with the long process of the incus or with the promontory; (3) erosion of the long process of the incus; and (4) erosion of the stapes superstructure (Fig. 41.4)

Grade 2 was considered moderate retraction, while Grade 3 and 4 severe for both PF and PT (PQ).

PT—anterior quadrant (AQ): 1, normal; 2, contact with the promontory (Fig. 41.5)

Grade 2 was considered moderate retraction.

The presence or not of adhesions of TM to the ossicular chain or promontory, analyzed in many classifications, how-

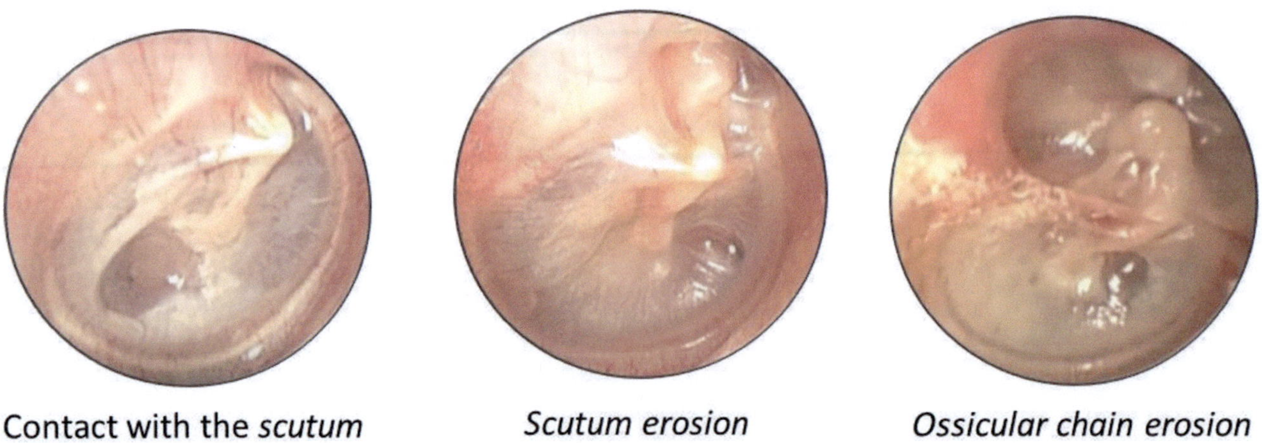

Fig. 41.3 Classification of moderate and severe pars flacida retractions

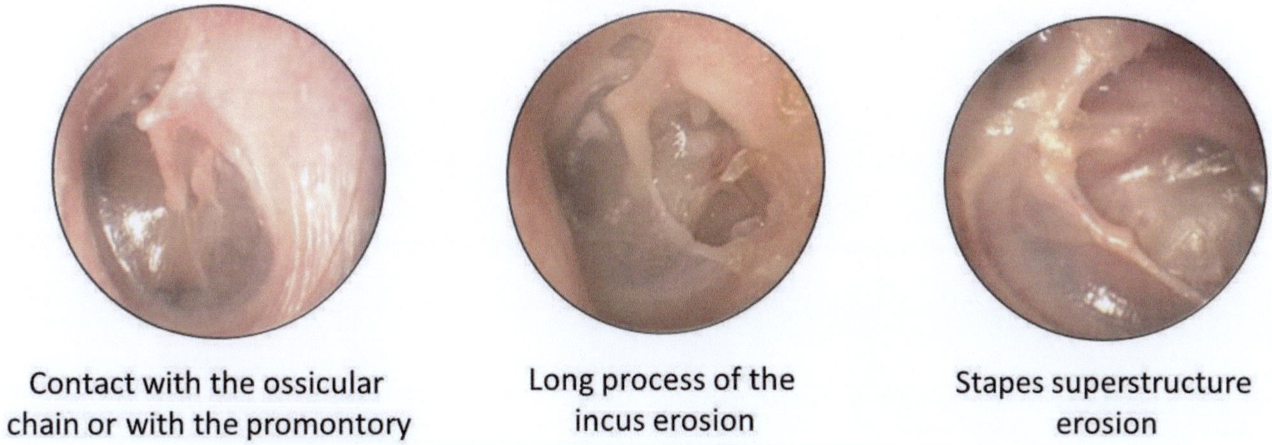

Fig. 41.4 Classification of moderate and severe pars tensa retractions (posterior quadrant)

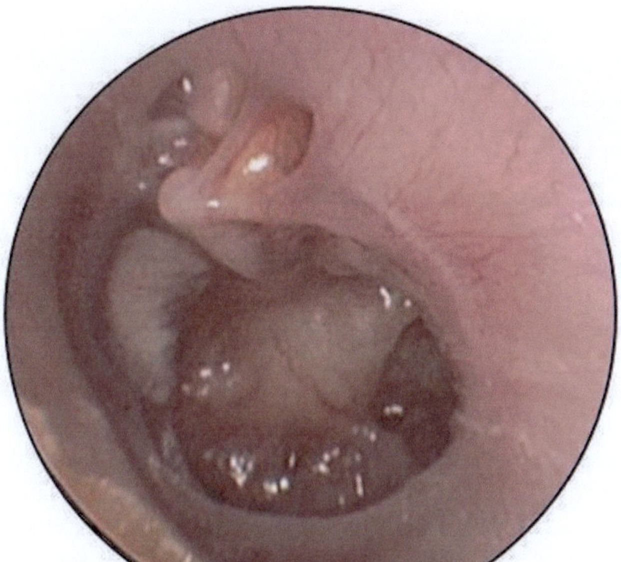

Fig. 41.5 Classification of moderate and severe pars tensa retractions (anterior quadrant)

ever, remains a challenge. The lack of standardization in the technique used for its evaluation, the intra- and inter-individual differences in the performance of the Valsalva maneuver, the difficulty of the pediatric population, and the lack of correlation between the data observed clinically and those found during surgery after the use of protoxide make its evaluation extremely difficult and of little use [34]. It appears that the presence of erosions of the ossicular chain and the accumulation of epithelial debris in the retraction (cholesteatoma) are the main indicators of severity (Fig. 41.6).

In a retrospective cohort, 661 ears with moderate and severe TM retractions were analyzed, corresponding to 24.5% of 2200 patients with COM. When analyzing the exclusive alterations of each area, it was observed that 64% of the ears presented retraction in more than one area (PF and PT) at the same time, while 24.9% presented isolated PF retraction, 10.6% presented isolated posterior quadrant (PT) retraction, and only 0.3% presented isolated anterior quadrant retraction. These findings suggest that, although didactic, the current classifications do not describe the retractions globally and, therefore, are not able to present us with an accurate clinical diagnosis.

The prevalence of PF isolated retractions observed in our study can be explained by the pathophysiology of middle ear ventilation pathways. The blocking of the tympanic diaphragm, due to the retraction itself or due to an inflammatory process, with thickening of the mucosa, can cause poor ventilation in the middle ear, creating the selective epitympanic dysventilation syndrome, or even global, as the negative pressure is present and other areas of TM are affected [16, 18]. The PF retraction would therefore be a consequence of the blockage of the epitympanic diaphragm by a preexisting retraction in the PQ. As the ventilation of the mesotympanum would be more easily restored, either by resolving the inflammatory processes of the middle ear or restoring the functioning of the auditory tube, the blockages of the anterior and posterior isthmus, which compartmentalize the epitympanic space, could be more difficult to resolve naturally. It was observed in the transoperatory that such isthmus is routinely obliterated in the attic cholesteatomas, either by fibrosis or by granulation tissue. Thus, retractions would occur concurrently in both regions most of the time and because ventilation in the middle ear has a greater tendency to spontaneously reestablish, changes in PQ would resolve more easily, explaining the higher prevalence of retractions in the PF when seen isolated. The most frequently observed

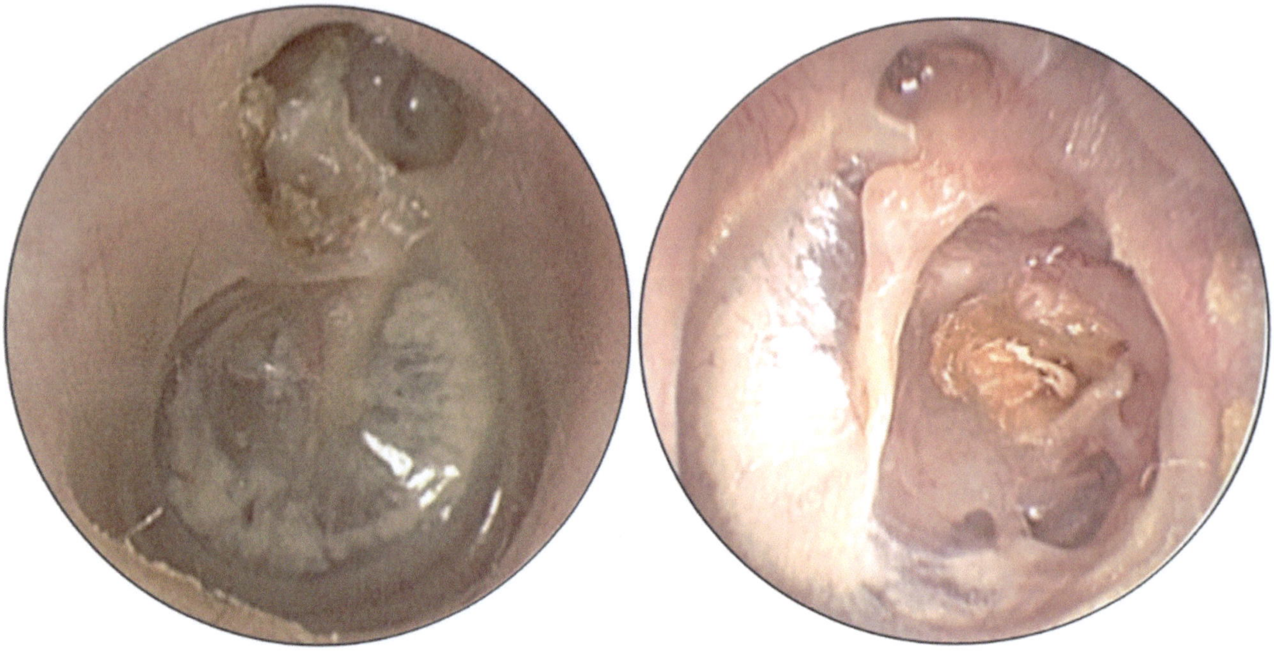

Fig. 41.6 This figure shows, respectively, a right ear with an atical retraction and a left ear with atical and posterior retraction with ossicular erosion, both with the accumulation of epithelial debris in the retraction (cholesteatoma).

alteration in the PF was the erosion of the scutum, whereas, in PQ, it was the erosion of the incus, suggesting that PQ retractions would be more frequently associated with conductive hearing loss. Another study by our group has shown that incus erosion is the alteration associated with larger air-bone gaps (ABGs) in posterior mesotympanic cholesteatomas when compared with posterior epitympanic [35].

Regarding the audiometric pattern of these ears, few studies correlated the degree of retraction and the severity of hearing loss. Cassano and Cassano evaluated 45 ears of children with varying degrees of TM retraction severity, based on the Sadé's classification. They observed that in grades I and II, the average hearing threshold was less than 10 dB HL in 68.7% of ears and greater than 20 dB HL in 18.7%. In grade III, the average hearing threshold was less than 10 dB HL in 29.1% and greater than 20 dB HL in 25%. In those with grade IV, no one had an average threshold of less than 10 dB, and the threshold was greater than 20 dB HL in 80% [36].

In our study, we also demonstrated that 72% of the ears had an ABG lower than 20 dB HL, and only 5% had an ABG greater than 40 dB HL. These findings meet those in the literature [36, 37].

We found that the pure tone average (PTA) ABG median was greater when the posterior quadrants were involved, exclusively or not. This can be explained by the ossicular chain involvement in this region. It is well known that chronic otitis media can compromise the TM's effectiveness and/or the ossicular chain's vibratory pattern. Therefore, a variable degree of conductive hearing loss is almost omnipresent in these patients. The pathogenesis of hearing loss is related to several factors, including partial or total vibratory TM surface loss, and ossicular chain erosion or fixation.

We observed a significant correlation between the severity of retraction and the worsening of AC and ABG threshold, only for PT. These findings indicate that ABG measure is not influenced by even more severe PF involvement. However, the severity of ossicular erosion in the posterior quadrants was predictive of an increase in the ABG and worsening of an AC.

The retractions were systematically classified in the literature, according to the region of TM affected by PF and PT. In our study, we analyzed the behavior of retractions in all areas of TM, and we observed that the majority of retractions had an association with affected regions. Jesic et al. showed that the combination of PF and PT retractions in the same ear was a predictor of a long incus process and stapes superstructure erosion [38]. However, the ABG's PTA was not a predictor of ossicular chain erosion. This corroborates with the existing data, which shows no correlation between hearing thresholds and the stages of retraction [36–38].

Only a few studies have investigated the magnitude of hearing loss in specific cases of myringostapediopexy (retraction limited to the posterosuperior region, in which erosion of the long process of the incus and fixation of the

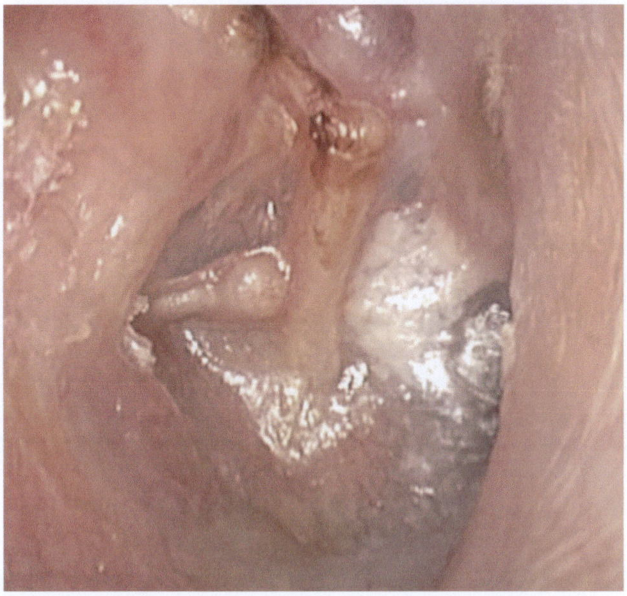

Fig. 41.7 A right ear with myringostapediopexy

affected tympanic segment to the stapes head occurs, regardless of cholesteatoma formation—Fig. 41.7) [39]. A study by our research group evaluated conductive hearing loss in this condition [26]. The tritonal average of the ABG was 18.46 dB HL. Fifty-three percent of the patients had an ABG equal to or lower than 25 dB HL at all frequencies. The analysis of tritonal PTA revealed that 85% of all ears with natural myringostapediopexy had conductive hearing loss equal to or lower than 25 dB HL. In the study done by Mills, 31 ears presented the PTA of the ABG were less than 20 dB HL in 77% of the ears, and only 3.2% had an ABG greater than 40 dB HL [40]. These findings suggest that these cases are similar to a type III tympanoplasty in relation to hearing loss.

The significant repercussions of the degree of hearing loss in these cases, especially of the ABG, depend on the decision whether the patient will benefit from early intervention or not.

Few studies in the literature have compared the degree of severity of retractions in children and adults. TM retraction may be associated with a conductive hearing loss, especially when the posterosuperior quadrant is compromised [1, 41]. The difference in prevalence of cholesteatoma in children and adults has already been demonstrated in previous studies, with the posterior mesotympanic cholesteatomas being more prevalent in the first group [42, 43]. The severity of hearing loss is comparable in these two age groups as demonstrated in studies on cholesteatomas [42, 43]. However, there are no studies that compare the severity of hearing loss in children and adults in the former stages of cholesteatomas such as in tympanic retractions.

In a study of our group, 47% of the samples were children, and we evaluated the differences between children and adults based on the location of the retractions, their severity, and the degree of the associated air–bone gap (ABG). We found a higher prevalence of retractions involving the PT in children, isolated or not, and of isolated PF retractions in adults. These findings are consistent with the literature, wherein most retractions located in the PT in pediatric patients, which is also the most frequent site of acquired cholesteatomas in the current population. PF retractions, on the other hand, seem to be more prevalent in adults [33, 37]. In a previous study by our group, we also found that acquired cholesteatoma exhibited the same pattern with respect to their location; posterior mesotympanics were more prevalent in children, and posterior epitympanic (attical) in adults [42, 43]. Likewise, we had already observed in another previous study, involving patients with ME cholesteatoma, that when present, both moderate and severe TM retraction and cholesteatoma in the contralateral ear tend to follow the same pathway of cholesteatoma formation in the main ear. These findings reaffirm the important role played by TM retractions in the pathogenesis of cholesteatoma [21].

We also observed that, as the age of the patients increases, the prevalence of attical (PF) retractions also increases progressively, and the opposite occurs for the prevalence of retractions located in the PQs (PT), irrespective of their association with attical impairment, whose frequency decreases as the age increases. The explanation for such findings would be that, in childhood, for reasons mainly related to the dysfunction of the auditory tube and the occurrence of gas exchange through the hyperplastic mucosa of the ME, the maintenance of the negative pressure sustained in the auditory cleft would be the main cause of TM retraction and its preferred location in PT. However, as the retraction of the PT persists, the medialization of the manubrium of the malleus, hyperplasia of the mucosa of the ME, and the presence of the secretion plugs could determine the obliteration of the tympanic isthmus, contributing to the epitympanic dysventilation syndrome and, thus, resulting in the concomitant occurrence of attical retraction. The changes that lead to PT retraction would be easier to resolve over time. The functioning of the auditory tube can improve as the child grows. Likewise, recurrent otitis media and upper airway infections are also becoming less frequent, consequently reducing the inflammatory processes in the ME mucosa. However, the compartmentalization of the epitympanum, with persistence of the isthmus blockage and appearance of fibrosis, is not a process that would resolve so easily on its own, thereby persisting over the years. This could explain the higher prevalence of isolated PF retractions and, consequently, posterior epitympanic cholesteatomas, in adults [1, 44].

We also observed that there was no difference between children and adults regarding the severity of isolated retractions of both PT and PF, demonstrating that the severity of the retraction can already be established at earlier ages. In our study, there was no difference in the ABG size between children and adults, regardless of the area of TM involvement. The management of the moderate and severe tympanic membrane retractions will be discussed in a separated chapter.

Management of Retractions

Managing TM retractions is one of the most exciting topics for otologists. Many controversies associated with this condition are based on the difficulty in understanding the pathophysiological characteristics, which make some TM retractions remains stable in the long term and others easily destabilize, possibly evolving with epithelial flow.

The difficulty is based on the fact that most patients are asymptomatic and hearing loss is, in most cases, small, even in cases where there is ossicular chain erosion [31]. The great dilemma is usually: should the surgical intervention be early, being prophylactic, or should the intervention be postponed until the development of cholesteatoma or hearing loss? The answers to this question are divergent.

Behavior of Retractions

The natural history of TM retractions is that they can follow one of four destinations: (1) resolution, (2) stabilization, (3) perforation, and (4) keratin accumulation with cholesteatoma formation.

Mechanisms responsible for the progression of retractions continue to be debated. Tubal dysfunction, impairing middle ear ventilation, remains an important factor in the evolution to cholesteatoma. Primary acquired cholesteatoma tend to be the most frequent and originate, in most cases, as a result of the progression of a pars flaccida (PF) retraction pocket medially and depth toward the epitympanum, or of a retraction pocket of the posterosuperior quadrant toward the mesotympanum [11, 20, 42, 43, 45].

Experiments in guinea pigs, conducted by Chole et al., demonstrate the development of cholesteatoma from TM retractions. In their studies, they observed that the ET cauterization in gerbils resulted in cholesteatoma in 40–75% of the ears after 16 weeks of obstruction [46]. They also demonstrated that infection by Pseudomonas Aeruginosa made cholesteatoma present a more aggressive behavior, with faster growth, when compared to noninfected ones. The sustained inflammatory process of the middle ear (ME) mucosa leads to a change in gas transmission blocking the auditory cleft, adding to the processes mentioned above [47].

We believe, therefore, that the inflammatory factors that break the stability of the retractions are essential for this evolution.

There is a dearth of literature on the natural history of retractions and their evolution. This can be attributed to the fact that monitoring these ears is time-intensive, and there is a consequent loss of patients to follow-up. Although there are many studies on retractions, they are not subject to comparisons, since the inclusion criteria are not the same and the classifications are different, and, therefore, are not in agreement with one other.

Management

The progression to cholesteatoma and hearing loss are two main concerns regarding retraction pockets and should and must be taken into account when defining their management [41, 44]. Also we have to take in account the presence of recurrent infections, the state of the contralateral ear, and the ET function.

Different managements have been proposed in the treatments of retractions, including: observational treatment, insertion of ventilation tubes, excision of the retraction pocket associated with tympanoplasty with fascia and/or cartilage graft, and tympanomastoidectomy. Ossiculoplasty may be necessary, depending on the status of the ossicular chain and hearing loss. When observational treatment is indicated, careful surveillance must be performed, with serial clinical and audiometric evaluations every six months [25].

In a meta-analysis, conducted by Nankivell and Pothier, on the treatment of retraction pockets, 71 patients were included [48]. No statistically significant benefit was obtained from cartilage tympanoplasty, on observational conduct, in relation to disease progression and hearing loss. They also observed that there was no benefit from the insertion of ventilation tube associated with cartilage graft, when analyzing the hearing improvement [48].

Despite all the controversies regarding the management of retractions, there are two situations in which surgical intervention is somehow indicated, without question: when there is keratin in the retraction pocket (cholesteatoma) and when there is significant hearing loss [14, 33].

It is needed to correlate the severity of otoscopic findings with the degree of conductive hearing loss in order to define the need for an early surgical intervention for each case. Whether the surgical intervention must be early, prophylactic, or should be postponed until the development of epithelial accumulation (cholesteatoma) or significant hearing loss is debatable. Perhaps this question is even more pertinent in the pediatric population, since children tend to have a higher prevalence of recurrent infections and, probably, longer periods of instability and otorrhea. In addition, identifying the location of the retraction (preferably involving the posterior quadrant) precisely on the ossicular chain would help determine the degree of risk of hearing loss, based on our previous study, or development of later mesotympanic cholesteatomas, which are generally associated with greater hearing impairment and more frequent recurrences [42, 43]. On the other hand, mild tympanic retraction can be solved without surgery; especially in the case of children, in whom it evolves to resolution in 35% of affected ears [36, 49].

The significant repercussions of the degree of hearing loss in these cases, especially of the air–bone gap (ABG), depend on the decision whether the patient will benefit from early intervention or not. As described in the literature, we know that stapes superstructure erosion is one of the main predictors of poor surgical results; therefore, the probability of a favorable postsurgical outcome is uncertain in patients with small ABG.

A review of studies on surgical indication and hearing results of ossiculoplasty revealed that the minimum preoperative ABG required ranges from 24 to 27 dB HL. The American Academy of Otolaryngology Committee on Hearing defines treatment success as conductive hearing loss equal to or lower than 20 dB HL [50]. The rates of treatment success ranged from 47% to 86.9% with total ossicular reconstruction prosthesis (TORP) and from 50% to 84.6% with partial ossicular reconstruction prosthesis (PORP) [51–53].

The literature often shows better audiometric results with PORP than with TORP. However, a meta-analysis comparing the two groups showed better outcomes with TORP [31]. All studies agree that the presence of stapes determines a better prognosis in the results of ossiculoplasty [53]. Although the stapes superstructure does not provide additional audiometric gain, it promotes better stabilization and fixation of the prosthesis [54]. Thus, reconstruction of the ossicular chain, and tympanoplasty, would not be justified in retraction cases with an ABG lower than 25 dB HL, especially in patients with stapes erosion. However, factors such as the presence or progression to cholesteatoma and the frequency of ear infections must be considered when monitoring therapies.

It is important to emphasize that, in the management, especially of the attic retractions, the reestablishment of the ventilation pathways to the epitympanum is important in order to promote direct ventilation to the attic region and prevent the recurrence of the retraction pocket and formation of cholesteatoma [11, 20].

Finally, we believe that management should be individualized for each patient, considering not only the topographical and momentary description of the severity of the retraction but also evaluating the hearing in each case, as well as the degree of stability of these ears, and the state of the contralateral ear.

References

1. Alper C, Olszewska E. Assessment and management of retraction pockets. Otolaryngologia Polska. 2017;71(1):1–21.
2. Seibert JW, Danner CJ. Eustachian tube function and the middle ear. Otolaryngol Clin N Am. 2006;39(6):1221–35.
3. Bluestone CD. Eustachian tube function: physiology, pathophysiology, and role of allergy in pathogenesis of otitis media. J Allergy Clin Immunol. 1983;72(3):242–51.
4. Doyle WJ, Seroky JT, Alper CM. Gas exchange across the middle ear mucosa in monkeys. Estimation of exchange rate. Arch Otolaryngol Head Neck Surg. 1995;121(8):887–92.
5. Paparella MM, et al. Cellular events involved in middle ear fluid production. Ann OtolRhinolLaryngol. 1970;79(4):766–79.
6. Magnuson B, Falk B. Diagnosis and management of eustachian tube malfunction. Otolaryngol Clin N Am. 1984;17(4):659–71.
7. Asawapittayanont P, et al. Tubal function tests with optional myringotomy detect Eustachian tube closing failure in acquired pars flaccida retraction cholesteatoma. Auris Nasus Larynx. 2017;44(1):65–9.
8. Levy D, et al. Direct demonstration of gas diffusion into the middle ear. Acta Oto-Laryngol. 1995;115(2):276–8.
9. Bunne M, et al. Variability of Eustachian tube function: comparison of ears with retraction disease and normal middle ears. Laryngoscope. 2000;110(8):1389–95.
10. Licameli GR. The eustachian tube. Update on anatomy, development, and function. Otolaryngol Clin N Am. 2002;35(4):803–9.
11. Marchioni D, et al. Prevalence of ventilation blockages in patients affected by attic pathology: a case-control study. Laryngoscope. 2013b;123(11):2845–53.
12. Palva T, Northrop C, Ramsay H. Aeration and drainage pathways of Prussak's space. Int J PediatrOtorhinolaryngol. 2001;57(1):55–65.
13. Palva T, Ramsay H. Incudal folds and epitympanic aeration. Am J Otolaryngol. 1996;17(5):700–8.
14. Costa S, et al. Otitesmédias: aspectosgerais. In: Cruz O, Costa S. (org.). Otologiaclínica e cirúrgica. Rio de Janeiro: Revinter, 2000. pp. 137–161.
15. Maniu A, et al. Anatomical variants of tympanic compartments and their aeration pathways involved in the pathogenesis of middle ear inflammatory disease. Clujul Med. 2013;86(4):352–6.
16. Marchioni D, et al. The contribution of selective dysventilation to attical middle ear pathology. Med Hypotheses. 2011;77(1):116–20.
17. Palva T, Ramsay H. Epitympanic diaphragm in the new-born. Int J PediatrOtorhinolaryngol. 1998;43(3):261–9.
18. Marchioni D, et al. Selective epitympanic dysventilation syndrome. Laryngoscope. 2010b;120(5):1028–33.
19. Marchioni D, et al. Endoscopic evaluation of middle ear ventilation route blockage. Am J Otolaryngol. 2010a;31(6):453–66.
20. Marchioni D, et al. Endoscopic anatomy and ventilation of the epitympanum. Otolaryngol Clin N Am. 2013a;46(2):165–78.
21. Rosito LPS, et al. The role of tympanic membrane retractions in cholesteatoma pathogenesis. BioMed Res Int. 2018;2018. (online edition)
22. Shunyu NB, et al. Histological and immunohistochemical study of pars tensa retraction pocket. Otolaryngol Head Neck Surg. 2011;145(4):628–34.
23. Urík M, et al. Histological analysis of retraction pocket pars tensa of tympanic membrane in children. Int J PediatrOtorhinolaryngol. 2016;86:213–7.
24. Sade J, Berco E. Atelectasis and secretory otitis media. Ann OtolRrhinolLaryngol. 1976;85(2 Suppl 25 Pt 2):66–72.

25. Alzahrani M, Saliba I. Tympanic membrane retraction pocket staging: is it worthwhile? Eur Arch Oto-Rhino-Laryngol. 2014;271(6):1361–8.
26. Schmidt B, et al. Myringostapediopexy: is it a natural type III tympanoplasty? OtolNeurotol. 2013;34(1):79–82.
27. Tos M, Stangerup SE, Larsen P. Dynamics of eardrum changes following secretory otitis. A prospective study. Arch Otolaryngol Head Neck Surg. 1987;113(4):380–5.
28. Charachon R. Classification of retraction pockets. Rev LaryngolOtolRhinol. 1988;109:205–7.
29. Sade J, Avraham S, Brown M. Atelectasis, retraction pockets and cholesteatoma. Acta Oto-Laryngol. 1981;92(5–6):501–12.
30. Bours AF, Decat M, Gersdorff M. Our classification of tympanic retraction pockets. Acta Oto-Rhino-LaryngolBelg. 1998;52(1):25–8.
31. Dornhoffer JL. Surgical management of the atelectatic ear. Am J Otol. 2000;21(3):315–21.
32. Borgstein J, et al. The Erasmus atelectasis classification: proposal of a new classification for atelectasis of the middle ear in children. Laryngoscope. 2007;117(7):1255–9.
33. James AL, et al. Tympanic membrane retraction: an endoscopic evaluation of staging systems. Laryngoscope. 2012;122(5):1115–20.
34. Canali I, et al. Assessment of Eustachian tube function in patients with tympanic membrane retraction and in normal subjects. Braz J Otorhinolaryngol. 2017;83(1):50–8.
35. Rosito LPS, et al. Hearing impairment in children and adults with acquired middle ear cholesteatoma: audiometric comparison of 385 ears. OtolNeurotol. 2015;36(8):1297–300.
36. Cassano M, Cassano P. Retraction pockets of pars tensa in pediatric patients: clinical evolution and treatment. Int J PediatrOtorhinolaryngol. 2010;74(2):178–82.
37. Borgstein J, Gerritsma TV, Bruce IA. Erosion of the incus in pediatric posterior tympanic membrane retraction pockets without cholesteatoma. Int J PediatrOtorhinolaryngol. 2008;72(9):1419–23.
38. Jesic SD, et al. Pars tensa retractions without cholesteatoma in children: predictors for ossicular chain destruction, air conduction thresholds, and postoperative retractions. OtolNeurotol. 2014;35(6):997–1002.
39. Monsell EM. New and revised reporting guidelines from the Committee on Hearing and Equilibrium. American Academy of Otolaryngology-Head and Neck Surgery Foundation, Inc. Otolaryngol Head Neck Surg. 1995;113(3):176–8.
40. Mills RP. Management of retraction pockets of the pars tensa. J LaryngolOtol. 1991;105(7):525–8.
41. Canali I, et al. Audiometric pattern in moderate and severe tympanic membrane retraction. OtolNeurotol. 2021a;42(6):e716–23.
42. Rosito LPS, et al. Cholesteatoma growth patterns: are there audiometric differences between posterior epitympanic and posterior mesotympanic cholesteatoma? Eur Arch Oto-Rhino-Laryngol. 2016a;273(10):3093–9.
43. Rosito LS, et al. Classification of cholesteatoma according to growth patterns. JAMA Otolaryngol Head Neck Surg. 2016b;142(2):168–72.
44. Canali I, et al. Critical analysis of moderate and severe retractions in the pars tensa and pars flaccida of the tympanic membrane. Braz J Otorhinolaryngol. 2023;89:114–21.
45. Jackler RK, Santa Maria PL, Varsak YK, Nguyen A, Blevins NH. A new theory on the pathogenesis of acquired cholesteatoma: Mucosal traction. Laryngoscope. 2015;125:S1–S14.
46. Wolfman DE, Chloe RA. Experimental retraction pocket cholesteatoma. Annals of Otology, Rhinology Laryngology. 1986;95:639–44.
47. Kania R, Portier F, Lecain E, Marcusohn Y, Ar A, Herman P, Huy PTB. Experimental model for investigating trans mucosal gas exchanges in the middle ear of the rat. Acta Oto Laryngologica. 2004;124:408–10.
48. Nankivell PC, Pothier DD. Surgery for tympanic membrane retraction pockets. Cochrane Database of Systematic Reviews. 2010;7:CD007943.
49. Cutajar J, Nowghani M, Tulsidas Mahtani B, Hamilton J. The Natural History of Asymptomatic Deep Pars Tensa Retraction. The journal of internacional advanced otology. 2018;14:10–4.
50. Iñiguez-Cuadra R, et al. Type III tympanoplasty with titanium total ossicular replacement prosthesis: anatomic and functional results. OtolNeurotol. 2010;31(3):409–14.
51. Fong JCW, et al. Titanium versus autograft ossiculoplasty. Acta Otolaryngol. 2010;130(5):554–8.
52. Vincent R, et al. Ossiculoplasty in intact stapes and malleus patients: a comparison of PORPs versus TORPs with malleus relocation and silastic banding techniques. OtolNeurotol. 2011;32(4):616–25.
53. Yu H, et al. PORP vs. TORP: a meta-analysis. Eur Arch Otorhinolaryngol. 2013;270(12):3005–17.
54. Alaani A, Raut VV. Kurz titanium prosthesis ossiculoplasty-follow-up-statistical analysis of factors affecting one ear hearing results. Auris Nasus Larynx. 2010;37(2):150–4.

Temporal Bone Cholesteatoma: The Full Picture

42

Sady Selaimen da Costa, Leticia Petersen Schimdt Rosito, Mauricio Noschang Lopes da Silva, and Fábio André Selaimen

Introduction

Middle ear cholesteatomas are one of the most intriguing otologic diseases, and their treatment demands a meticulous and complete analysis of many different facets. As a rule, the main discussion always narrows down (mistakenly) to the surgical technique. Over the years, countless congresses, symposiums, and meetings have been organized on five continents with the aim of discussing advances in the understanding of this disease. As we mentioned earlier, the focus of these debates emphasizes the following hierarchy:

1. **THE SURGICAL TECHNIQUE or how do we do it?**
2. **THE SURGICAL TIMING or when to do it?**
3. **THE SURGICAL REATIONALE or why do we do it?**
4. **WHAT DOES ORIENT OUR DECISIONS or the theoretical basis!**

We believe that the best and most complete way to approach this condition is to reverse this order. Thus, in our opinion, the priority should be rearranged as follows:

1. **WHAT DOES ORIENT OUR DECISIONS or the theoretical basis!**
2. **THE SURGICAL REATIONALE or why do we do it?**
3. **THE SURGICAL TIMING or when to do it?**
4. **THE SURGICAL TECHNIQUE or how do we do it?**

Thus, as at the base of a pyramid, the broad theoretical base will support our therapeutic decisions, defining more securely why, when, and how to treat. Not infrequently and in very special situations, surgery may not be the best option at a given time. Likewise, it is necessary to better and more thoroughly understand the natural history of the disease and its pathogenesis (masterfully defined by MM Paparella as the "journey between the etiology and the established pathology"). This is the best way to propose a set of rational strategic actions throughout the process that may abort its evolution and the potential risks of complications. We always like to paraphrase the famous British neurosurgeon Henry Marsh:

> *It is often said it takes three months to learn how to do an operation, three years to learn when to do it, and 30 years to learn when not to do it.*

The Expression

The German anatomist Johannes Mueller used the word "cholesteatoma" for the first time, in 1838 [1]. The root of this word means *chole* (from cholesterol); *steato from fatty tissue), and oma (ending meaning tumor in biology)*, that is, a tumor in which fatty tissue and cholesterol crystals are present. Etymologically, this term is completely incorrect since cholesteatomas originates from the keratinized stratified squamous epithelium of the tympanic membrane (TM) and/or external auditory canal (EAC) and does not have cholesterol crystals or fat in its composition and, in addition to its tumor nature being largely debatable.

S. S. da Costa (✉)
School of Medicine - Federal University of Rio Grande do Sul, Porto Alegre, Brazil

Hospital de Clínicas de Porto Alegre, Porto Alegre, Brazil

International Hearing Foundation, Minneapolis, MN, USA

American Academy of Otolaryngology—Head and Neck Surgery, Alexandria, VA, USA

L. P. S. Rosito
School of Medicine - Federal University of Rio Grande do Sul, Porto Alegre, Brazil

Hospital de Clínicas de Porto Alegre, Porto Alegre, Brazil

M. N. L. da Silva · F. A. Selaimen
Hospital de Clínicas de Porto Alegre, Porto Alegre, Brazil

M. V. Goycoolea et al. (eds.), *Textbook of Otitis Media*, https://doi.org/10.1007/978-3-031-40949-3_42

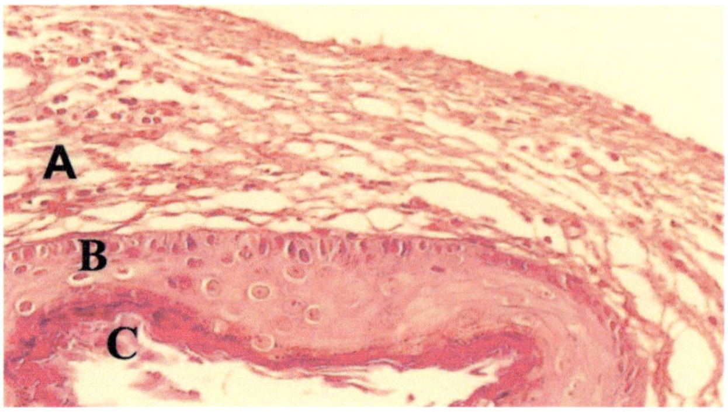

Fig. 42.2 Digitized image of slide, with cross section of the cholesteatoma, stained with hematoxylin-eosin. We can see its three constituent parts: (**a**)—perimatrix, (**b**)—matrix, and (**c**)—cystic content

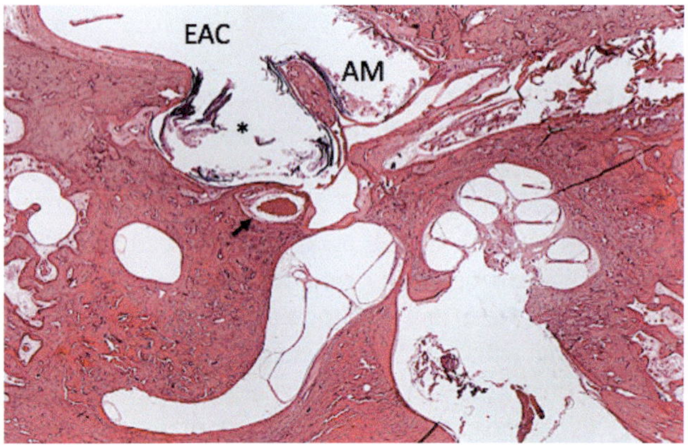

Fig. 42.1 Human temporal section (left ear) showing a middle ear cholesteatoma filling the posterior mesotympanum. (* cholesteatoma; black arrow: facial nerve; *EAC* external auditory canal, *AM* anterior mesotympanum)

Other names have been suggested through the years such as *pearly tumor*, by Cruveilhier (1829), margaritoma (Craigie 1891), *epidermal cholesteatoma* (Cushing 1922), *epidermoid* by Critchley and Ferguson (1928), and keratoma by *Shuknecht*, in 1974 (apud [1]). All these terms, although more adequate and descriptive, have not become popular in the medical literature and the word cholesteatoma definitely has been enshrined among otologists.

The Definition

Friedmann defined cholesteatomas in 1959 [2], as cystic structures covered by stratified squamous epithelium, resting on a fibrous stroma of variable thickness, which may contain some elements of the original mucous lining.

More simply, Schuknecht, in 1974 [3], defines them as accumulation of exfoliated keratin inside the middle ear or any pneumatized area of the temporal bone, arising from a keratinized stratified squamous epithelium.

Ferlito et al. [4] describes the cholesteatoma as an epidermoid cyst, of independent and progressive growth, with destruction of the adjacent tissues, especially the bone tissue, with a tendency to recur (Fig. 42.1).

Informally, we tend to simplify by referring to cholesteatomas as "skin in the wrong place!" Macroscopically, it is a round or oval cystic lesion with variable shape and size; histologically, it may be broken into three main components: (1) the matrix—keratinized stratified squamous epithelium; (2) the perimatrix—a rich network of connective tissue, collagen fibers, and inflammatory cells; and (3) the cystic content—keratin and epithelial rests (Fig. 42.2).

Epidemiology and Risk Factors

It is estimated that over 20 million people worldwide are afflicted with chronic otitis media (COM). Of these, one-fourth (about five million) have a cholesteatoma [5], although the overall number of cases of acquired cholesteatoma seems to be in decline [6, 7]. The annual incidence of cholesteatoma is reported as 3 per 100,000 in children and 9.2 per 100,000 adults. Males slightly outnumber females in a ratio of 1.4:1, and cholesteatomas that present in the middle ear are more frequently found in persons younger than 50 years of age [8, 9]. Caucasian persons show the highest prevalence, but cholesteatoma is infrequently found in Inuit, Native American, and Asian populations [10]. Several reports reviewed by Jennings et al. evaluated familial clustering and inheritability of cholesteatoma and found that incomplete penetrance exists and may depend on a combination of environmental and genetic factors for the formation of an acquired cholesteatoma. Jennings also states that evidence from syndromic cases suggests genes controlling ear morphology may be risk factors for congenital or acquired cholesteatoma formation [11]. Syndromes where a diagnosis of cholesteatoma has been reported finding include Turner syndrome [12–14], Treacher Collins syndrome[15], Down syndrome [16–19], and focal dermal hypoplasia [20]. Numerous reports of patients presenting with cleft palate and cholesteatoma [21–27] have been presented with the rate of incidence approaching 6% in that population [26]. When compared to children who did not develop a cleft palate, those with a cleft palate face a 100–200 times greater likelihood of developing a cholesteatoma [22, 26]. Additionally, a link between allergic rhinitis and the development of cholesteatoma was recently discovered in that patients with allergic rhinitis presented with a significantly lower 10-year cholesteatoma disease-free rate [28].

At the Chronic Otitis Media Outpatient Clinic at Hospital de Clínicas de Porto Alegre (AOMC-HCPA), 2603 patients were diagnosed with COM in follow-up. Of those, 638 (24.51%) presented cholesteatoma, which was bilateral in 17.1%. The mean age was 34, 49 years, and 53.5% were female. Also, most patients were 18 years or older (63.8%). Concerning the cholesteatoma growth patterns, the anterior epitympanic was 1.9%, the posterior epitympanic (PEC) was 32.9%, the posterior mesotympanic (PMC) corresponded to 33.7%, two-route cholesteatoma was 14.8%, and open cholesteatoma (or indeterminate) was 16.7%.

Classification

Cholesteatomas are classified as congenital or acquired. The former can be found in five temporal bone regions; in turn, the acquired can be subdivided into primary or secondary (Table 42.1).

Congenital cholesteatomas (CCs) were defined by Derlacki and Clemis [29] as a conglomerate of epithelial remnants found in ears with intact tympanic membranes and usually without a previous history of infections. According to Valvassori [30], they can be found in four regions of the temporal bone: tympanic-mastoid, petrous apex, cerebello-pontine angle, and jugular foramen. There is still a fifth location, described by Sobol [31], who reported the existence of small epithelial pearls between the layers of the tympanic membrane.

If the congenital nature of some cholesteatoma is quite clear, there is much debate about the origin of acquired cholesteatomas. Conceptually, they have been dichotomized into two groups: primary and secondary. The former would result from progressive tympanic retraction, which, at some point, loses its self-cleaning properties and starts to accumulate desquamated epithelium and keratin. On other hand, secondary cholesteatomas would arise from the migration (invasion) of the external auditory canal epithelium into the middle ear through a marginal perforation of the tympanic membrane. Once inside the middle ear, a standard biological behavior would follow: it would encyst and start producing keratin [32]. Today, our understanding that the division of cholesteatomas into these two models, although being quite didactic and easy to understand, is vastly operationally incomplete. We will expand on this discussion in specific sections of this chapter.

Table 42.1 Classification of temporal bone cholesteatomas

Congenital	Acquired	From the external auditory canal
Eardrum-mastoid	Primary	
Petrous pyramid	Secondary	
Cerebellar point angle		
Jugular foramen		
Intratympanic		

Meyerhoff and Truelson [33] tried to classify cholesteatomas according to their pathophysiology, location, ossicular defects, and presence of complications, also dividing them into congenital and acquired, the latter being primary, secondary, or tertiary.

Tos [34] proposed an otoscopic classification, dividing cholesteatomas into:

1—Attic.
2—Pars Tensa I (marginal disease).
3—Pars Tensa II (central disease).

In 1993, the same author proposed another classification, based on the site of origin of the cholesteatoma, which he considers an important factor for the surgical procedure and for the prognosis. This taxonomy presents three categories:

1—Attic cholesteatoma—a retraction of the pars flaccida or Shrapnell's membrane, extending from the attic, passing through the aditus, and eventually reaching the antrum, mastoid, or tympanic cavity.
2—Cholesteatoma of the sinus tympani—posterosuperior retraction or perforation of the pars tensa, extending to the tympanic sinus and posterior recesses.
3—Cholesteatoma of the pars tensa—retraction and total adhesion of the pars tensa of the tympanic membrane (TM) involving the tympanic orifice of the eustachian tube (ET).

Saleh and Mills [35] proposed another classification, according to the sites affected by cholesteatoma, characterized as follows:

S1—If the cholesteatoma is restricted to the place where it started.
S2—when the disease extends to another location.
S3—if it affects three locations.
S4—if installed in four locations.
S5—for cases in which the first affected site and, in addition to this, four or more are involved.

These same authors distinguish seven locations used for this classification: attic and antrum, middle ear, mastoid, ET, labyrinth, and middle fossa.

Saleh and Mills [35] also present a classification of the condition of the ossicular chain, based on the descriptions of Wullstein [36] and [37], through the following score:

0—intact ossicular chain.
1—Incus is eroded and with discontinuity of the ossicular chain.
2—Incus and stapes superstructure are eroded.
3—Malleus head and incus are absent, and the stapes superstructure is eroded.

As for preoperative complications, Saleh and Mills [35] classified cholesteatoma as:

C0—when there are no complications.
C1—for the occurrence of one complication.
C2—for the existence of two or more.

As complications, the authors consider lateral semicircular canal (LSC) fistula, facial paralysis, total sensorineural hearing loss (SHL), sinus thrombosis, and intracranial invasion.

Finally, in 2017, a task force of international researchers was assembled with the aim of standardizing these classifications and proposing pathogenesis models. The conclusions were published in the Journal of International Advances in Otolaryngology—EAONO/JOS Joint Consensus Statements on the Definitions, Classification and Staging of Middle Ear Cholesteatoma [38]. The clinical classification suggested in the final consensus of this group contemplates the division of congenital and acquired cholesteatomas and ratifies pathogenesis models (Fig. 42.3).

Among the conclusions of this consensus and in order to simplify the extent of cholesteatoma, they propose the so-called STAM system dividing the middle ear and mastoid space into four sites: difficult access sites (S), tympanic cavity (T), attic (A), and mastoid (M). The difficult access sites (S) include S1, the supratubal recess (also called the anterior epitympanum or protympanum), and S2, the sinus tympani. The posterior border of the attic is the posterior end of the incus short process or the fossa incudis. The mastoid includes the antrum and mastoid cells (Fig. 42.4).

The EAONO/JOS also proposed a very encompassing staging system that applies to four types of middle ear cholesteatoma (pars flaccida cholesteatoma, pars tensa choles-

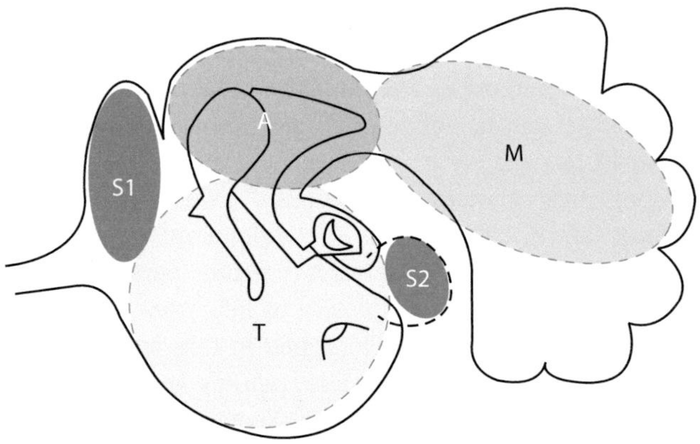

Fig. 42.4 Divisions of the middle ear space using the STAM system

Fig. 42.3 Schematic drawing of the clinical classification of middle ear cholesteatoma

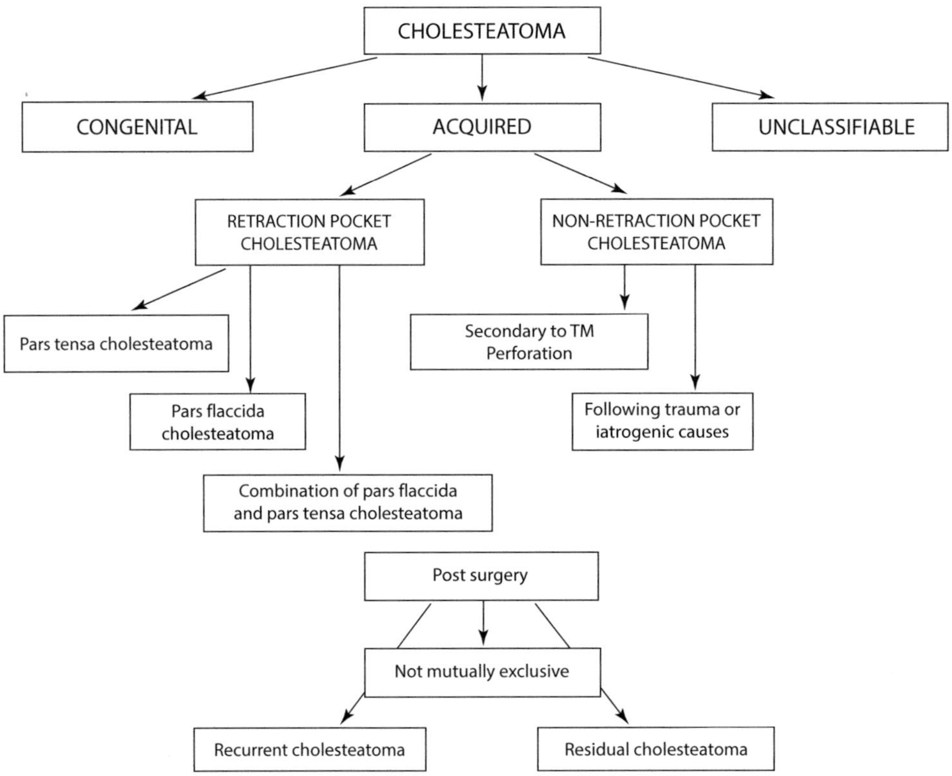

Table 42.2 The EAONO/JOS staging system applies to four types of middle ear cholesteatoma

Stage I: Cholesteatoma located in the primary site*
*The site of cholesteatoma origin, i.e., the attic (A) for pars flaccida
Cholesteatoma; the tympanic cavity (T) for pars tensa cholesteatoma, congenital cholesteatoma, and cholesteatoma secondary to a tena perforation
Stage II: Cholesteatoma involving two or more sites
Stage III: Cholesteatoma with extracranial complications or pathologic conditions including
Facial palsy,
Labyrinthine fistula: with conditions at risk of membranous labyrinth,
Labyrinthitis,
Postauricular abscess or fistula,
zygomatic abscess,
Neck abscess,
Canal wall destruction: more than half the length of the bony ear canal,
Destruction of the tegmen: with a defect that requires surgical repair, and
Adhesive otitis: total adhesion of the pars tensa.
Stage IV: Cholesteatoma with intracranial complications including
Purulent meningitis,
Epidural abscess,
Subdural abscess,
Brain abscess,
Sinus thrombosis, and
Brain herniation into the mastoid cavity
The staging system does not apply to petrous bone cholesteatoma

teatoma, congenital cholesteatoma, and cholesteatoma secondary to a tensa perforation). This system is summarized in Table 42.2 [38].

Histopathology

Cholesteatoma, macroscopically, is a round or oval cystic lesion with variable configuration and size. Ferlito et al. [4] characterized cholesteatoma as an epidermoid cyst, with independent and progressive growth, with destruction of the adjacent tissues, especially bone, with a tendency to recur.

The advent of transmission electron microscopy made possible many advances in the knowledge of cellular structure. Using this instrument, in 1972, Lim and Saunders [39] presented a detailed histological description of cholesteatomas. They described that cholesteatoma has a keratinized stratified squamous epithelium, with four layers identical to those of normal epidermis (basal, spinous, granulosa, and cornea), Langerhans cells (in greater numbers than in normal epidermis), and keratohyaline granules. They called this epithelium the matrix of the cholesteatoma. They also observed the presence of a connective tissue, containing collagen fibers, fibrocytes, and inflammatory cells, which was called perimatrix, which was in contact, in most cases, with a layer of scaly or cylindrical ciliated cells, remnants of the original mucosa of the middle ear. In some cases, although the perimatrix was absent at optical microscopy, it was present when studied with the transmission electronic microscope, showing itself to be extremely thin, with practically absent collagen fibers and containing crystals of calcium carbonate. The cystic content was formed by accumulated keratin, epithelial debris, and inflammatory compounds.

This tripartite structure, matrix, perimatrix, and cystic content, is well illustrated in Fig. 42.5 and will be detailed below:

Perimatrix

Paludetti et al. [40] described the perimatrix as a mass of granulation tissue or inflamed subepithelial connective tissue. According to Milewski et al. [41], the growth of a cholesteatoma would require angiogenesis in the connective tissue of the perimatrix, and that cells and substances of the healing cascade could have an important role in the development and growth of cholesteatomas. These processes would involve the fibroblastic growth factor b (b-FGF), which, according to these authors, could stimulate the production of collagenase. They also suggested that the persistence of inflammation would cause a permanent healing process in the perimatrix, the proliferation of fibroblasts (granulation tissue), and epithelium (matrix).

Ferlito et al. [4] describe the perimatrix as the most peripheral portion of the cholesteatoma, consisting of granulation tissue or inflammatory subepithelial connective tissue, with lymphocytes, histiocytes, and neutrophils. Sprekelsen et al. [42] state that the matrix and perimatrix, in normal or pathological tissues, are formed by type IV collagen, tenascin, fibronectin, b-FGF, and metalloproteinases (MMP). According to Jacob et al. [43], the increase in the proliferation of the cholesteatoma matrix would be the result of the inflammation process, suggesting that the perimatrix would be the main factor in the development of cholesteatomas.

Hamzei et al. [44] analyzed 21 cholesteatomas, through polymerase chain reaction (PCR), immunohistochemistry, and histology, with the aim of investigating the factors of stimulation and differentiation of osteoclasts present in cholesteatomas, using the skin of the external acoustic meatus as a control. Immunohistochemical analysis demonstrated an increase in osteoclast precursor cells and macrophages in cholesteatomas. The perimatrix analysis demonstrated that, in this region of the cholesteatoma, there are all the necessary factors for osteoclastogenesis and for the stimulation of bone reabsorption.

Briefly, we like to define the perimatrix as a rich inflammatory network that surrounds the cholesteatoma. It represents an authentic "battlefield" which may play interesting

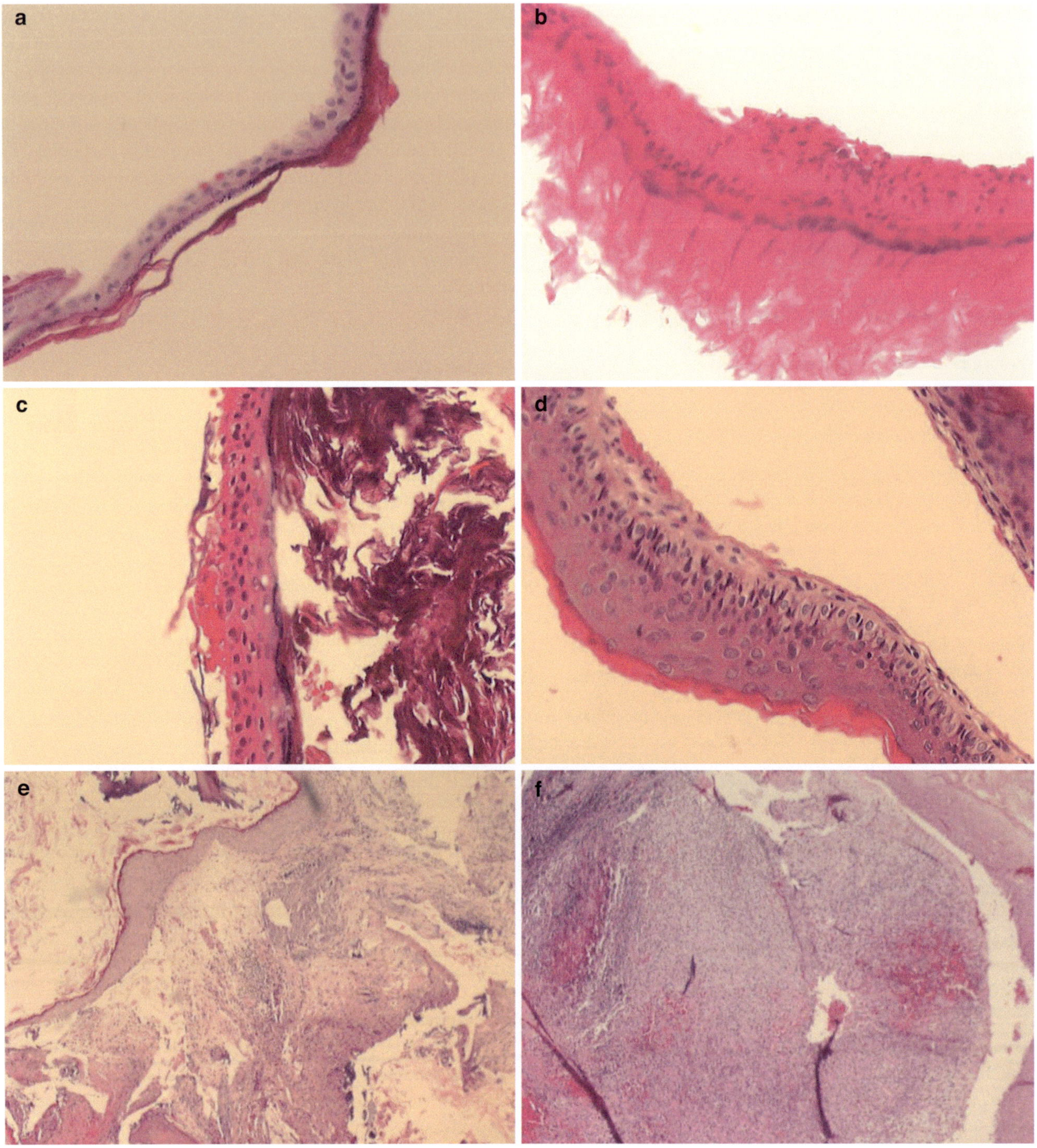

Fig. 42.5 (**a**) Stratified squamous epithelium, keratinized, with an average of three layers of cells. Missing perimatrix. (**b**) Stratified squamous epithelium, keratinized, with an average of six layers of cells. Narrow, fibrotic perimatrix, with rare lymphocytes. Absence of granulomas. (**c**) Stratified squamous epithelium, keratinized, with an average of four layers of cells. Very narrow perimatrix, without fibrosis and without inflammatory infiltrate. (**d**) Stratified squamous epithelium, keratinized, with an average of six layers of cells. Narrow and delicate perimatrix, without fibrosis and with a very discreet inflammatory infiltrate. (**e**) Stratified squamous epithelium, keratinized, with an average of 12 layers of epithelial cells. The perimatrix exhibits dense fibrosis, accentuated chronic inflammatory infiltrate, and is delimited in its deep plane by simple cuboidal epithelium. (**f**) Stratified squamous epithelium, keratinized, with an average of 13 layers of epithelial cells showing epithelial hyperplasia. Perimatrix shows discreet fibrosis with accentuated inflammatory infiltrate and neutrocytic exudation, being delimited in its deep plane by simple cuboidal epithelium. Absence of granulomas

and antagonistic roles in this dynamic process: at times smoothing the paths for the aggression of the highly proliferative epithelium and sometimes helping the native mucosa to wedge the invasion.

Matrix

The cholesteatoma matrix consists of keratinized stratified squamous epithelium characterized by the presence of intercellular bridges and by a regular arrangement of the various cell layers. It is made up of five components:

Basal layer or stratum germinative—composed of columnar epithelium, formed of cubic cells, which exhibit an enlarged nucleus with a hyperchromatic and basophilic appearance.

Stratum spinosum or malpighian layer—composed of larger cells, still relatively cylindrical in shape, which become polyhedral in the more superficial layers.

Stratum granulosum or granular layer—cells become progressively flattened, containing keratohyaline and hyperchromatic granules in the cytoplasm.

Stratum lucidon—often goes undetected.

Stratum corneum—with a hyperkeratotic and scaly appearance, in which the keratin lamellae form the cystic content.

Acquired cholesteatomas are sometimes accompanied by glandular metaplasia. If the cholesteatoma sac ruptures, keratin is released in the subepithelial layer, resulting in a foreign body-type reaction. Osteoclasts are frequently observed at the interface of the cholesteatoma matrix and the subjacent bone tissue [4].

Cystic Content

The cystic contentis composed of well-differentiated anucleate keratinocytes and laminar keratin masses [45, 46].

All cholesteatomas, whether acquired or congenital, present practically the same morphological characteristics. However, due to their different formation mechanism, some of them may present particularities. According to Ferlito et al. [4], the matrix would be thicker in the acquired form than in the congenital form, and this would generally be composed of 15 cell layers, while the congenital form would only present five cell layers. However, Dornelles et al. [45], studying acquired cholesteatomas, found an average number of eight cell layers in the matrix. Another histopathological variation observed by Ferlito et al. [4] was that in congenital cholesteatoma, contrary to the acquired one, normally it presents few inflammatory signs, being generally absent the glandular structures of the perimatrix. Another difference would be the dendritic cells, identified in greater numbers in the squamous epithelium of congenital cholesteatomas. The method used to identify dendritic cells was immunohistochemistry, using the S-100 protein as a specific marker. This marker can be useful in the histopathological diagnosis of cholesteatoma [47].

In short, the histological diagnosis of cholesteatoma is performed through the identification of its components: perimatrix, matrix, and cystic component. The ultrastructural characteristics of cholesteatomas are similar to those of normal epidermis. In particular, Langerhans cells were found in the spinosum layer, between the keratinocytes, and Merkel cells in the germinal layer. Scanning electron microscopy showed the presence of corneocytes in the form of hexagonal disks, organized in regular columns, with each column surrounded by six others [4].

In Fig. 42.5, some cross-sectional images of acquired cholesteatomas can be seen, showing the great variability in the thickness of the perimatrix, as well as its histological components.

Biology of Cholesteatoma

The study of cells, in optical and electron microscopy, can give the misleading impression that these are static structures. However, on the contrary, many processes and movements are constantly happening in the cellular intimacy, occurring more quickly in some tissues, slower in others. It is easy to understand that, as cells differentiate, they simultaneously acquire certain structural and physiological characteristics.

Epithelia are tissues with limited life, with constant renewal, due to continuous mitotic activity. The speed of this cell replacement is variable, ranging from two to 50 days, depending on the tissue considered [48].

The connective tissue, which constitutes the cholesteatoma perimatrix, presents a more complex growth process, since it is formed by several types of cells— fibroblasts, macrophages, mast cells, plasmocytes, and leukocytes—separated by abundant intercellular material. The richness of this material is one of its most important characteristics. It consists of two parts: one with a defined microscopic structure—connective fibers—and the other unstructured— fundamental amorphous substance [48]. For all this complexity, it is to be expected that the process of renewing this tissue is quite elaborated.

There are hypotheses that chronic otitis media with cholesteatoma (CCOM) could be the result of uncontrolled cell proliferation [4] comprising a series of complex and dynamic events involving cellular and extracellular components with alterations in their biological behavior, such as dysregulation of keratinocytes [49], which show hyperproliferative growth and alterations in cell differentiation. However, it is not known for sure whether this lack of control is caused by defects in genes that control proliferation, by cytokines released from inflammatory cells, or by other yet unknown mechanisms [1]. Therefore, determining the existence of defects in its biology, biochemistry, and genetics is critical to understanding its pathogenesis.

As previously described, the capacity for invasion, migration, change in differentiation, proliferation, and recurrence of cholesteatomas is very similar to neoplasms; however, there is reluctance among researchers to accept the inclusion of cholesteatomas in this category [50, 51]. For cholesteatomas to be considered a neoplastic lesion, evidence of genetic instability is required; this can be manifested through changes in the DNA or specific chromosomal abnormalities. In 1995, Shinoda and Huang [52] detected the p53 protein in cholesteatomas, suggesting that these could be tumors. However, Desloge et al. [51] demonstrated that there were no alterations in the DNA, thus discarding this hypothesis.

As the cited researches do not indicate any genetic instability of these lesions, we must investigate another possible reason for the development of the cholesteatoma, being necessary to ask about the origin of its characteristic keratinized squamous epithelium. To study this issue, many investigations using immunohistochemical analysis have been carried out to compare the location of differentiating markers in cholesteatomas and in the skin of the external auditory canal. Due to the properties presented by cytokeratins, they have been considered by many investigators as one of the best instruments for this purpose [49, 53, 54].

Cytokeratins are proteins that constitute one of the two categories of intermediate filaments, located in the cytoplasm of epithelial cells; they have 20 subclasses, and their expression depends on the type of epithelium and its stage of differentiation [55]. Pereira [56], Albino et al. [50], and Kim and Chung [57] reported that the matrix of cholesteatomas expresses cytokeratin 16 (CK16) in the suprabasal layers, and the expression of this protein filament is characteristic of hyperproliferative epithelia. Leperque et al. [58] describe that CK16 does not appear in the normal epithelium, except in areas under pressure and friction, or in the epithelium lining the hair follicles. According to Broekaert et al. [59], CK16 is expressed in specific regions, such as the tympanic annulus and the medial and inferior regions of the external acoustic meatus. Pereira et al. [60] state that the cholesteatoma has a cytokeratin pattern similar to that of the external acoustic meatus and the epithelial layer of the tympanic membrane. The presence of CK16 in the cholesteatoma matrix could indicate its hyperproliferative behavior, similar to that of hyperproliferative epidermal diseases, even if the histological aspect of the cholesteatoma is the same as that of the normal epidermis. According to Albino et al. [50], the cholesteatoma is formed as a result of the attempt to repair an injury, which could explain the presence of CK16, characterizing this epithelium as immature with a predominance of cell proliferation. Kujipers et al. [54] analyzed the pattern of cytokeratins and suggested that the cholesteatoma matrix is not the result of a metaplastic change. In their study, they found an epithelium similar to that of the tympanic membrane and the skin of the external auditory canal, but in different stages of proliferation, depending on the degree of inflammation present.

A characteristic sign of cholesteatomas is infiltration of the perimatrix by cells of the immune system. Piltcher [61], in his thesis on cytokines in chronic otitis media with effusion, states that, in addition to the already known risk factors, such as tubal dysfunction and infections, much research on otitis media has been directed to the study of the different components of the inflammatory response. The key issue is whether inflammation should be considered only as a defense process or whether it plays a role in the perpetuation of CCOM. Milewski [62]suggested that inflammatory cytokines, fibroblasts, and macrophages would be responsible for the origin, growth, and bone destruction of cholesteatomas. Several cytokines and growth factors could be involved in the mechanism of proliferation and development of the cholesteatoma epithelium [63, 64]. Tomita [65] states that there are several hypotheses that growth factors and cytokines, present in cholesteatomas, induce the activation of genes, such as *c-myc,* causing the deregulation of cell proliferation. Sudhoff et al. [66] investigated the distribution and expression of tumor growth factor (TGF-alpha), epithelial growth factor (EGF-R), and *c-myc oncogene*in normal middle ear epithelial cells and in cholesteatomas. These factors were found in the matrix of cholesteatomas, but not in normal cells. In addition to the autocrine regulation of the epithelium, through the production of epithelial growth factor (EGF), cholesteatoma hyperproliferation could depend on the interaction of the subepithelial tissue and the inflammatory changes that occur in this pathology. Sudhoff et al. [67] investigated the expression and location of growth factors in angiogenesis in 22 cholesteatomas, in comparison with the normal epidermis of the external auditory canal and the normal middle ear mucosa to identify some growth factors involved in the pathogenesis. of cholesteatomas. These researchers found, in normal skin and mucosa, 5.3 ± 1.2 vessels/mm^2, while in the cholesteatoma group there were 21.1 ± 11.7 vessels/mm^2, and this average varied according to the degree of inflammation in the perimatrix: 9.0 ± 3.5 vessels/mm^2 in grade I, 19.2 ± 3.6 vessels/mm^2 in grade II and 31.7 ± 9.4 vessels/mm^2 in grade III. They also reported a decrease in type IV collagen and laminin in the basement membrane in cholesteatoma compared to controls.

A common feature in the pathogenesis of various types of cholesteatomas is the presence of bacteria which could promote a critical bond between the cholesteatoma and the host, preventing the newly formed epithelium from completing its differentiation process, which would leave it in a quiescent state, minimally proliferative, without being migratory or invasive at this stage [68]. Interactions between inflammatory cells and the cholesteatoma epithelium could be responsible for inducing the aberrant biological characteristics of this pathology.

Chole and Faddis [68] studied, by transmission electronic microscopy, 24 human cholesteatomas and 22 Mongolian squirel (gerbil). Of the samples from humans, 16 showed histological findings consistent with biofilm bacteria, while in the gerbil material, 21 showed evidence of this bacteria. This finding could be related to the activity of cholesteatomas, mainly with persistent or recurrent infections and their resistance to topical and systemic antimicrobials. The authors suggested that the cholesteatoma matrix is an ideal medium for the development of a mixed microbiological biofilm. These authors also state that bacteria with biofilm are resistant to antibiotics by mechanisms different from those used by planktonic bacteria; however, the exact mechanism of resistance of bacterial colonies in biofilm is unknown.

The studies published so far present many data regarding the biology of cholesteatomas, but many doubts persist. As previously mentioned, cholesteatomas present neoplastic characteristics (invasion, migration, and change in differentiation), but, so far, no indication of genetic instabilities in their structure has been found, a fact that rules out the possibility of classifying them as neoplasms. Another property that seems constant in cholesteatomas is their hyperproliferative activity, perhaps residing here as a possible answer to their characteristics of aggressiveness and uncontrolled growth. In addition to this fact, the stimuli of the immune response, represented by cytokines related to the inflammatory cells of the perimatrix, represent a strong candidate for the role of main actor in this intricate network of mechanisms. All these hypotheses lead us to consider the complexity involved in the biology of cholesteatomas and, consequently, the tangle of events related to their pathogenesis.

Animal Models

Several animal models have already been used for the experimental study of acquired cholesteatoma, among which we can mention rabbits, chinchillas, guinea pigs, rats, and Mongolian gerbils [69]. However, the gerbil seems to be the currently preferred animal model since it spontaneously develops aural cholesteatomas [70]. Also, those cholesteatomas are similar to the humans, concerning the epithelial and subepithelial linings of the middle ear and the destructive characteristics of the gerbilline cholesteatoma [71].

In addition to the spontaneous cholesteatomas, numerous methods were tried to develop the disease in animal models. Numerous substances, such as talcum powder and fibrina, dimethyl-benzanthrancene (a chemical carcinogen widely used for experimental purposes), propylene glycol, have been used [69]. Schmidt and Hellstrom [72, 73] performed a perforation in the posterosuperior quadrant of the tympanic membrane of rats and weekly introduced dimethylbenzanthracene for four consecutive weeks. After survival from 1 to 8 weeks, the authors observed the invagination of highly desquamative stratified squamous epithelium through the perforation in 89.5% of the animals, and in 47% of these there was complete epithelization of the middle ear. The authors observed the permanence of the inflammatory process and the presence of purulent secretion throughout the experiment.

In other animal models, where cholesteatomas were also induced, different methods were employed ranging from the inoculation of bacteria and upper respiratory infections [74, 75], obstruction of the eustachian tube (ET) [76, 77], skin grafts placed in the middle ear [78], and external auditory canal (EAC) ligation [79, 80].

The rate which experimentally induced cholesteatomas was high, varying from 39% [81] to 100% [82], with a wide range of results between them, depending on the animals and the protocol used. Bauer et al. [83] introduced the use of otoendoscopy to the gerbilline model, through which the authors evaluated the development and the characteristics of pars flaccida retraction pocket and cholesteatoma in Mongolian gerbils after the obliteration of the eustachian tube, compared to a control group. At the end of the 16-week follow-up, cholesteatoma was present in 34.2% of the ears in the intervention and in 20.6% in the control group ($p = 0.197$).

The lowest positivity rates, regardless of protocol, were generally obtained in cases where the survival period was short (e.g., 2 weeks, 0 positivity; [81]) or the irritant agent concentration was low (e.g., propylene—10% glycol, 12.5% positivity; [84]). In cases where the survival period was longer (e.g., 5 months), the positivity obtained reached 87.5% [81]; in parallel, in cases where the concentration of the stimulating agent was high (e.g., 90% propylene glycol), the positivity obtained reached 100% [85].

Furthermore, in animal models where the eustachian tube was obstructed, the tendency toward greater positivity in relation to the presence of cholesteatomas, with greater survival, was clearly observed [76, 77]. Wolfman and Chole [76, 77] obtained the formation of cholesteatomas with an increasing percentage with a greater survival, in up to 75% of the animals, in a model in the Mongolian gerbil with obstruction of the eustachian tube and consequent retraction of the tympanic membrane. Huve et al. [82] compared the incidence and the histopathological aspects of spontaneous and the two most used induced Mongolian gerbils' models of cholesteatoma (EAC obliteration and the ET cauterization). It was observed that the incidence of cholesteatoma in Mongolian gerbils after EAC obliteration was significantly higher than that observed after ET cauterization, which in turn was significantly higher than the spontaneous occurrence of the disease in the control group (100%, 52.9% and 16.7%, respectively, $p < 0.0001$).

Despite this apparent relationship between the development of cholesteatomas and middle ear ventilation deficiency, Meyerhoff et al. [86], in an animal model in chinchillas, using 60% propylene glycol and placing a ventilation tube (VT) in the bulla, demonstrated that, despite ventilation of the middle ear, cholesteatomas developed in 66.6% of the animals. They concluded that negative pressure is not necessarily a primordial factor for the development of cholesteatomas, following this protocol.

Some animal models were presented, where an attempt was made to inhibit the formation of cholesteatomas induced by the use of propylene glycol. This attempt was unsucccesful when cyclophosphamide [87], isotretinoin [88], and hyaluronic acid [89] were used. Wright et al. [90] used 60% propylene glycol in the bula of chinchillas that had ventilation tubes, and the application was repeated two more times. In these animals, after the third application of propylene glycol, 5% 5-fluorouracil was placed on the lateral surface of the tympanic membrane, and this application was repeated twice more. After 4 weeks of survival, it was observed that the use of 5-fluorouracil prevented the formation of cholesteatomatous cysts in all 16 temporal bones studied. However, microscopic invasions of epithelium on the medial surface of the tympanic membrane were observed in four studied ears, and three of them had tympanic membrane perforation.

The same methodology employed in the study resulted in intense hyperplasia of the epithelial and connective layers of the tympanic membrane and cholesteatomas in 60–70% of the animals, when 5-fluorouracil was not used [86, 91]. The antimetabolic action of 5-fluorouracil apparently has an effect on reducing epidermal proliferation, and retinoic acid also seems to have an effect on epidermal keratinization and on glandular secretory activity. Metaplasia and keratinization of the middle ear epithelium were observed by Chole and Frush [92], in rats fed with a diet low in vitamin A, and its supplementation led to a normalization of these epithelial alterations. Furthermore, a study carried out in cell culture of specimens of human cholesteatomas, obtained in surgeries, demonstrated the inhibitory effect of retinoic acid on their proliferation [93], different from the experimental results obtained by Jove et al. [88] with isotretinoin, which is a synthetic analog of retinol (vitamin A). White et al. [89] used hyaluronic acid with the aim of reducing connective tissue hyperproliferation, which, together with the inflammatory process, is believed to be one of the main factors involved in the pathogenesis of acquired cholesteatomas. Sixty propylene glycol was placed in the chinchillas' bula and, after the third injection, a viscous solution of 1.5% hyaluronic acid was placed laterally to the tympanic membrane, and the application was repeated six more times. After a four-week survival, the presence of cholesteatomas was observed in approximately 70% of the animals that received propylene glycol, regardless of the use of hyaluronic acid or not. Pownell et al. [87] used cyclophosphamide systemically in chinchillas for 14 days, and on days 5, 8, and 11 the animals received bilateral applications of propylene glycol. After a four-week survival, the presence of cholesteatomas was observed in 50% of the animals. In this animal model, cyclophosphamide, which has an anti- inflammatory and immunosuppressive action, did not seem to inhibit the formation of cholesteatomas.

Studies related to epithelial migration in the pathogenesis of acquired cholesteatomas were mostly related to the invagination of the squamous epithelium, through discontinuities of the basement membrane in the pars flaccida of the TM or to the migration of squamous cells from the external auditory canal and/or tympanic membrane, through perforations secondary to chemical necrosis.

Hueb [94] performed an experimental study on epithelial migration patterns and acquired cholesteatomas in chinchillas. The objective was to establish a new animal model, based on the pathogenesis of epithelial migration by intentional tympanic perforation, in the presence of a tissue irritant, with evaluation of the presence and remission of the effects of the inflammatory process. Through mechanical perforation of the tympanic membrane, a modified collagen membrane was introduced into the left middle ear, without occluding the eustachian tube or introducing infectious agents (15 animals and 3 subgroups). This membrane consisted of type B bovine collagen, succinyl chloride, and butyl isocyanate. After sacrifice (8, 10, and 12 weeks of life) and proper preparation and staining of the sections with hematoxylin and eosin, migration of squamous cells through the perforation and formation of cholesteatoma was observed in 53.5% of the animals. Migration occurred through tympanic perforation, collagen membrane, organized effusion, and granulation tissue, all functioning as a "facilitating bridges." In some animals, there was closure of the tympanic perforation through the migration of squamous epithelium cells over the organized effusion. Cholesteatomas formed most frequently in the region of the anterior tympanic bulla, occasionally in the epitympanic region. The mean thickness of the squamous epithelium and keratin layer in the cholesteatoma region was greater than that observed for the anterior and posterior regions of the external auditory canal and tympanic membrane.

The demonstration of these data suggested that, in the region of cholesteatomas, the squamous epithelium proliferated and produced keratin more intensely than in its regions of origin, certainly stimulated by the irritating factor of the membrane components, in addition to not being subject to structural limitations and functional aspects of the regions of origin. Epithelial migration, occurring in areas of granulation tissue and/or inflammatory process, suggested a direct relationship between cause/stimulus and cholesteatoma. In addition to the importance of the inflammatory process in stimulating and "bridging" the migration of the epithelium, it was observed that the granulation tissue is responsible for bone erosion in otitis. It was also observed that the formation of granulation tissue occurred due to an intense cellular infiltration of the inflammatory fluid in the middle ear (immature granulation tissue) with secondary epithelialization of the mucosa in these areas (mature granulation tissue). These findings corroborate epithelial migration as being involved in the genesis of acquired cholesteatomas and also demonstrate the fundamental participation of the inflammatory fluid in the origin of the granulation tissue and its importance in the association between the inflammatory process/granulation tissue/cholesteatomas.

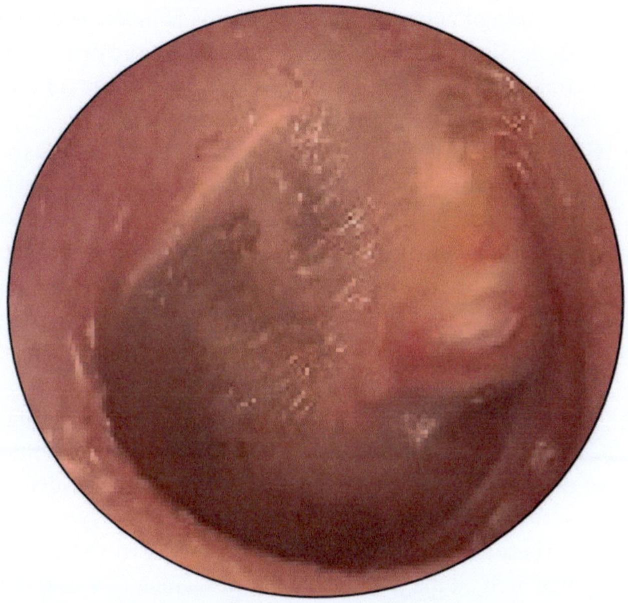

Fig. 42.6 Digital otoscopy of congenital cholesteatoma as a whitish mass in the anterior aspect of the tympanic membrane

Etiopathogenesis

Ferlito [4] describes that three predisposing conditions would be necessary for the development of a cholesteatoma: (a) the meeting of two different epithelia in the middle ear cleft; (b) chronic destruction of the submucosal layer of the middle ear by infectious and inflammatory processes; and (c) the healing process or proliferation phase.

The mechanisms underlying the etiopathogenesis of acquired cholesteatoma remain a subject of competing hypotheses with, basically, six main theories (Table 42.3), which have generated controversy for over 100 years.

Congenital

The theory of congenital cholesteatomas (Fig. 42.6), according to which they would arise from nests of epithelial cells, which over the years would multiply until the formation of an epithelial tumor, was proposed by Korner and Virchow (apud Eggston 1959), in the nineteenth century, and supported by Cushing and McKenzie, as reported in Jackler [95], during the first half of the twentieth century.

Table 42.3 Main hypotheses for the etiopathogenesis of cholesteatomas

Hypothesis	Author	Year
Congenital cholesteatomas	Korner and Virchow	1863
Metaplasia	Wendt	1873
Migration	Habermann	1889
	Bezold	1889
Invagination	Bezold	1908
Hyperplasia	Manasse	1917
Implantation	Schoer	1958

Cawthorne [96] reported a series of nine temporal bone cholesteatomas associated with facial paralysis. In 1963, the same author reported a case of a young man affected by a cholesteatoma in the middle ear, behind an intact tympanic membrane, suggesting that it would be a form of cholesteatoma originating from embryonic remains. Delarcki and Clemis [29] presented 10 cases of patients with this type of cholesteatoma. The diagnostic criteria postulated by these authors were:

- presence of intact tympanic membrane,
- the absence of a history of otitis media, otorrhea, or otologic procedure.

Levenson [97] altered the definition by Clemis and Derlacki by admitting the congenital origin in some selected cases with a positive history for the presence of otitis. In fact, the relationship between congenital cholesteatoma and otitis media is controversial. Some hypotheses were formulated:

- Congenital cholesteatoma develops regardless of whether there is otitis media or not. The finding by Derlacki and Clemis of the relationship between congenital cholesteatoma and the absence of a history of otitis media could be due to chance due to the small number of patients included in the study. There is no concrete evidence that previously reported cases of congenital cholesteatomas did not have a past history of otitis media in childhood.

- The origin of congenital cholesteatoma is independent of otitis media, but when cholesteatomas are large or occupy a strategical location blocking the aeration of the middle ear or mastoid, they can cause otitis media.
- Congenital cholesteatoma would be the result of a perforation of the tympanic membrane or otitis media. All patients with congenital cholesteatoma would have to present a previous history of otitis media or tympanic membrane perforation. If this hypothesis were true, the so-called congenital cholesteatoma would not be congenital but acquired. This hypothesis is the least likely.

Levenson et al. [97], studying 37 children with congenital cholesteatomas of the middle ear, suggested that they could have originated from an epithelioid formation (EF), identified in the latero-supero-anterior portion of the tympanic cavity. These embryonic structures are derived from the first branchial arch, at the junction of the eustachian tube and the middle ear. According to this theory, the epithelioid formation, which is always present during embryonic development, should regress from the 33rd week of gestation. The persistence of EF would shelter the niche that formed the congenital cholesteatoma. Karmody [98] performed a systematic analysis on children's temporal bones in order to histologically document the origin of congenital cholesteatomas (CCs). Characteristic histological findings of this form of cholesteatoma were found in two patients. In both cases, the masses were asymptomatic, located in the anterosuperior quadrant of the tympanic cavity. Current studies relate the persistence of epidermoid formation with the development of congenital cholesteatomas [99–101].

Regarding other locations in the temporal bone, Gacek [102] proposed that cholesteatomas of the petrosal apex would be born from the foramen lacerum, which would be a favorable area for the persistence of epithelial remains, which would later trigger the formation of epidermoid cysts. Reeves [103] indicated previous trauma as a possible seeding element of ectopic epithelium in these situations. Souza and Costa [104], reviewing 30 cases of epidermoid lesions of the cerebellopontine angle, found no history of significant trauma in any of them.

Implantation

The introduction of stratified squamous epithelium in the middle ear can give rise to the so-called post-traumatic cholesteatoma. The triggering event of this condition can be classified as traumatic or iatrogenic. Indeed, Sheehy [33] reports the formation of small pearls of cholesteatomas on the tympanic membrane as one of the frequent complications of tympanoplasties that use the placement of the graft above the perforation (overlay). Regarding myringotomy with placement of a ventilation tube (VT), the cholesteatoma originating from this procedure is a relatively rare complication (Fig. 42.7). One of the hypotheses refers to the development of a cholesteatoma due to the implantation of epithelial cells in the middle ear, resulting from cell migration through the myringotomy, or from the displacement of a small TM flap to the middle ear during the procedure. Another hypothesis refers to the induction of cholesteatoma after VT removal, with a retracted tympanic membrane, due to the persistence of negative pressure in the middle ear.

McKennan and Chole [105] point out some singularities of post-traumatic cholesteatomas:

1. Late onset—patients usually develop cholesteatomas years after the original trauma.
2. Atypical development.
3. Large proportions—as these patients usually have a negative history of otitis media, the mastoids are well pneumatized, which apparently would allow extensive growth of the cholesteatoma, before it manifests itself clinically.
4. Open surgical techniques must be used in the treatment of these pathologies due to their size.
5. There is an increased risk of CSF leaks.

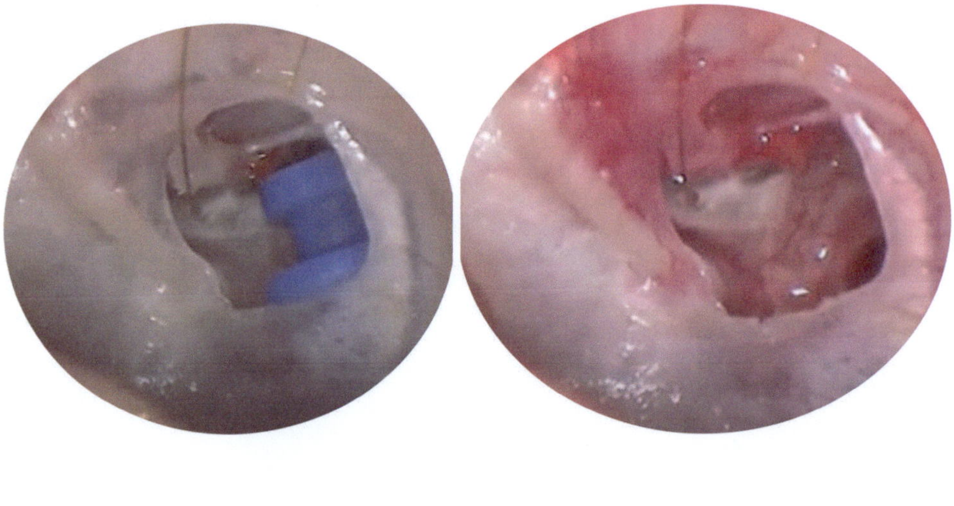

Fig. 42.7 Digital otoscopy of cholesteatoma due to implantation caused by placement of a ventilation tube. Clear presence of implanted epithelium islands in the promontory mucosa

Metaplasia

Wendt, in 1873 [106], was the first proponent of the theory related to epithelial metaplasia as a possible causative agent of cholesteatomas. His theory was based on the observation that the epithelium of the respiratory tree can undergo squamous metaplasia when exposed to chronic infection and trauma. This hypothesis received new impetus after some works carried out years later by Birrel [107] and Sadé [108] which pointed in this direction. Sadé [109] performed biopsies of the middle ear mucosa of children with otitis, finding islands of keratinized squamous epithelium. Chole and Frush [92] observed that vitamin A deprivation in rats led to keratinization of the tympanic mucosa.

Still, although Friedmann [2], Birrel (1958), Schechter [110], and others agree that the middle ear epithelium can undergo metaplastic transformation to stratified squamous epithelium, there is little evidence that it will become keratinized [111].

Van Blitterswijk [112] suggested the metaplastic origin of cholesteatomas from observations on the pattern of keratinocyte differentiation and expression of cytokeratins. However, Broekaert [113] and Vennix [49] related this differentiation and expression of "ectopic" cytokeratins to the hyperproliferative characteristic associated with the modulator effect of the middle ear mesenchyme, and not to a metaplastic process.

Migration

Epithelial migration, whether originating from the external auditory canal or the tympanic membrane, is considered by numerous investigators as the most common cause involved in the pathogenesis of acquired middle ear cholesteatomas [94]. This theory was initially postulated by Habermann [114] and Bezold [115] simultaneously, being based on a well-known pathological phenomenon, namely the epithelization suffered by sinuses and fistulous tracts. Thus, the cholesteatoma would be produced by the migration of squamous epithelium originating from the EAC into the middle ear cleft, which would arrive there through a breach in the TM (Figs. 42.8 and 42.9). These considerations are based on clinical observations of cholesteatomas in the presence of tympanic membrane retractions and/or perforations and on studies on the greater similarity between the patterns of cytokeratin found in cholesteatomas with those found in the external auditory canal and tympanic membrane [78, 112, [116, 117].

This would occur despite the migratory direction of the EAC epithelium in humans in the opposite direction to the middle ear, that is, from the malleus umbo to the external acoustic meatus. The factors responsible for the inversion of

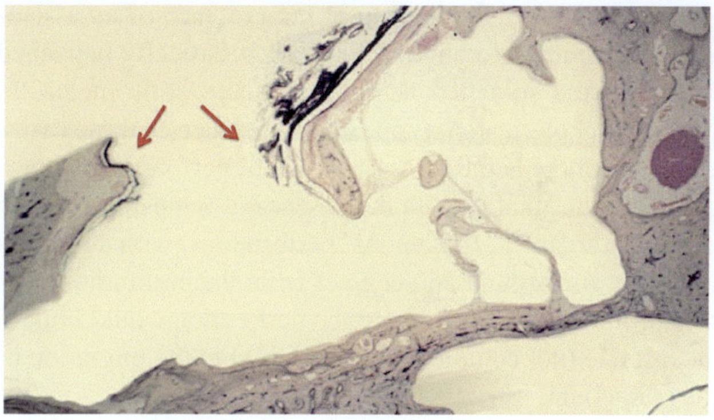

Fig. 42.9 Photomicrograph of a human temporal bone showing a perforation of the anterior aspect of the tympanic membrane and a migratory flow of epitelium and keratine toward the middle ear (arrows)

Fig. 42.8 Otoendoscopy with a central and a marginal tympanic perforation. In the last, note the epithelium of the external auditory canal (EAC) migrating through the tympanic perforation

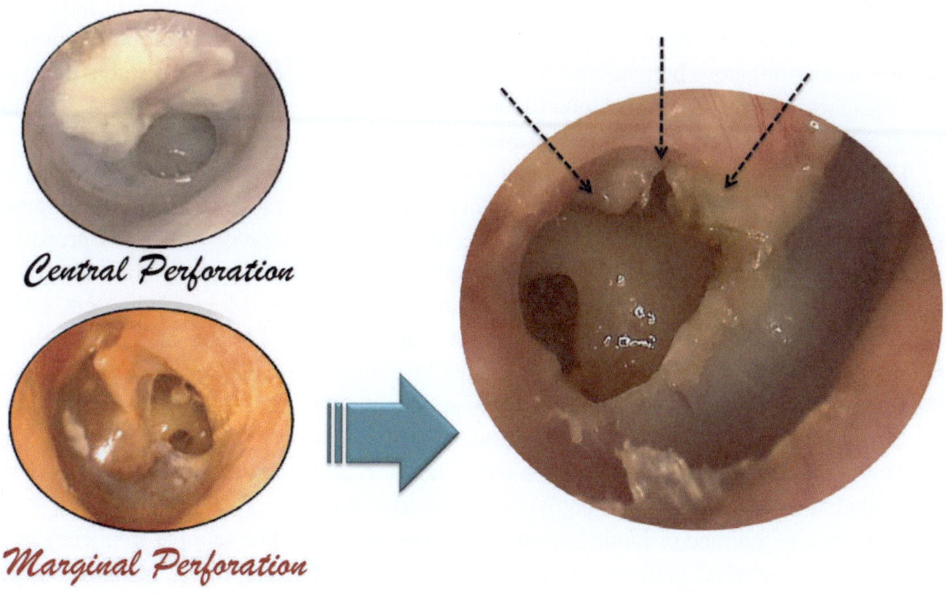

this migratory flow, as well as those that would lead to the appearance of a cholesteatoma and not just the pure and simple epithelialization of the middle ear, have not yet been well determined.

Data obtained from studies in humans are not suggestive of hyperproliferation of the normal epidermis in patients with cholesteatoma [118] or even of changes in the pattern of epithelial migration in patients with unilateral cholesteatoma (Mori arty et al., 1991). Following this line of reasoning, it is assumed that, for cells to migrate from the external auditory canal and/or tympanic membrane and epithelialize the middle ear, a stimulus and a bridge are needed. Additionally, for the development of cholesteatoma, changes in the tympanic membrane (perforation or retraction) would be prerequisites.

Hyperplasia

Initially, it was believed that migration of the epithelium to the middle ear would develop in the presence of an associated tympanic perforation. This is what basically happened following the so-called necrotizing acute otitis media, in which the cholesteatoma appeared years later. In these cases, the gates for epithelial invasion would be perforations known as "marginal," that is, with the absence of tympanic remnant in a given segment. In "central" perforations (with a residual tympanic rim around 360 degrees from the perforation), the ring of fibrosis created around the perforation would impose an obstacle (not completely insuperable) to the migration of the epithelium.

Despite being ingenious, this theory is not able to justify the presence of cholesteatomas in other situations. The incidence of necrotizing otitis seen in daily practice does not equal the number of new cases of detected cholesteatomas. Furthermore, as Tos [119] argued well, very rarely necrotizing otitis is observed causing tympanic perforations in the region of Schrapnell's membrane. The need for tympanic rupture as an obligatory prerequisite for the development of cholesteatomas began to be questioned and theories trying to prove the exact opposite began to be formulated.

The EAC skin close to the tympanic membrane is extremely active. Acanthosis and hyperkeratosis are particularly prevalent in the vicinity of the attic, with cellular activity occurring primarily in the basal cell layer, being intensified by middle ear infections [110]. Ruedi [120] demonstrated this fact by experimentally irritating the middle ear mucosa and stimulating basal cell hyperreactivity. As a result, he obtained the formation of streams of squamous cells toward the middle ear from the EAC and, subsequently, cholesteatoma.

Although the evidence for basal cell proliferation and subepithelial tissue invasion is unequivocal, it would require the basement membrane or lamina to either invaginate with the invading epithelial cells or undergo microruptures to allow the epithelial cells to proliferate into adjacent tissues and subsequently reconstruct itself. For Chole and Tingling [121], this last hypothesis would be the most likely. According to these authors, the basement membrane is made up of glycoproteins and collagen. To provoke its rupture, specific collagenases would be necessary. Apparently, not only inflammatory processes but also the epithelial cells themselves can secrete these enzymes. Loss of the basal lamina leads to the emergence of the contact guidance phenomenon, originally described by Giacometti [122] and demonstrated in the ear by Lim et al. [39]. Due to this phenomenon, the loss of the basement membrane would stimulate the basal cells to form pseudopodia toward the subepithelial tissue, which in turn would originate epithelial cones and finally cholesteatomas. However, there are studies that do not confirm the relationship between cholesteatoma expansion and distortions in the basal lamina [49]. The hyperproliferative phenotype is not homogeneous across all cholesteatomas. An increased expression of non-epidermal cytokeratins was observed in the peripheral portions of the cholesteatoma, in the region where there is direct contact with the inflammatory process of the middle ear mesenchyme. Lim [123] reported the presence of inflammatory cells in the mucous–cutaneous junction of the cholesteatoma, relating the invasive phenotype of the cholesteatoma to the inflammatory stroma, and not to characteristics inherent to the squamous epithelium. On the other hand, in the more central regions of the cholesteatoma matrix, the hyperproliferative condition is less marked. This indicates that, after the matrix develops, there is a tendency for the return of the original, non-hyperplastic phenotype.

Perforations in the tympanic membrane in dry, uninfected ears can remain for years without any sign of epidermal growth in the middle ear. Vennix [49] evaluated, through histological sections, the transition between the epidermis and the epithelium of the middle ear. In this study, smooth transitions were found between the two epithelia, suggesting the existence of stable mucosal–cutaneous junctions. The disorganization of these junctions, concomitant with hyperproliferation of keratinocytes and formation of inflammatory tissue, would be related to the pathogenesis of cholesteatomas. Thus, the development of an underlying inflammatory and/or infectious process would be necessary for the tympanic perforation to evolve into a middle ear cholesteatoma.

More studies are still needed in order to satisfactorily evaluate, at the molecular level, the middle ear cholesteatoma–mesenchyme interface.

Invagination

The relative frequency of cholesteatomas located in the attic and aditus ad antrum associated with defects in Shrapnel's membrane stimulated interest in the emergence of a theory for its pathogenesis that could justify the preference of this pathology to occupy such regions.

Bezold [124] described a theory relating ET dysfunction to cholesteatoma formation, called the invagination theory. Malfunction of the tube function would generate a negative pressure inside the middle ear, effusion, and retraction of the TM, mainly in the pars flacida, which would result, after an infectious and inflammatory stimulus, in the development of cholesteatoma. Wolfman and Chole [76, 77] obtained experimental evidence of cholesteatomas secondary to tympanic retractions. When using guinea pigs whose auditory tubes had been blocked with electrocautery, they found cholesteatomas in 75% of the animals sacrificed 16 weeks after the initial insult. Cassano et al. [125] 52, in a study that included 40 ears of children with tympanic retractions not submitted to any treatment, observed, after 2 years of follow-up, the progression of severe retractions to cholesteatoma in 20% of the cases.

Sadé et al. [126], in a cohort involving 215 ears with tympanic membrane retractions, observed the incidence of cholesteatoma in only one ear with pars tensa retraction pocket (2%) and in only two ears with moderate and severe retraction in the pars flaccida (2%). This study, however, analyzed retractions of different degrees of severity and with very variable follow-up times. Some clinical studies, however, have failed to demonstrate this evolution accurately. This is probably due to the low incidence of this pathology and the difficulty in guaranteeing the follow-up of these patients for long periods. Thus, other alternatives designed to test this appealing hypothesis are needed.

The invagination theory can be conceptually summarized in the following steps (Figs. 42.10 and 42.11):

- Middle ear negative pressure.
- Retraction and invagination of the pars flaccida or segments of the pars tensa.
- Stage of simple retractions (the diameter of its external opening remains larger than its bottom).
- Stage of "bottle-shaped" retraction pockets (the diameter of the bottom of the pocket is wider than its opening).
- Loss of the self-cleaning properties of the pocket.
- Keratin accumulation, infection, and expansion.

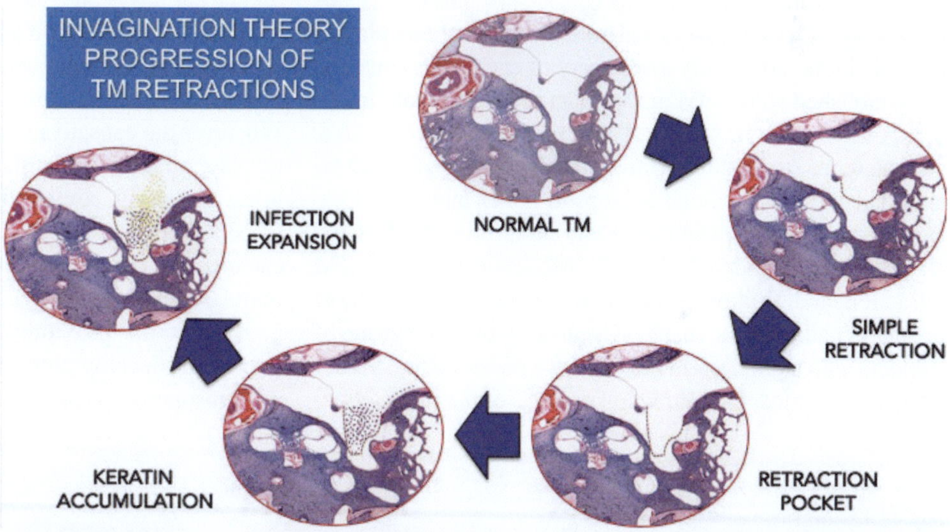

Fig. 42.10 Steps in the invagination theory—histopathology

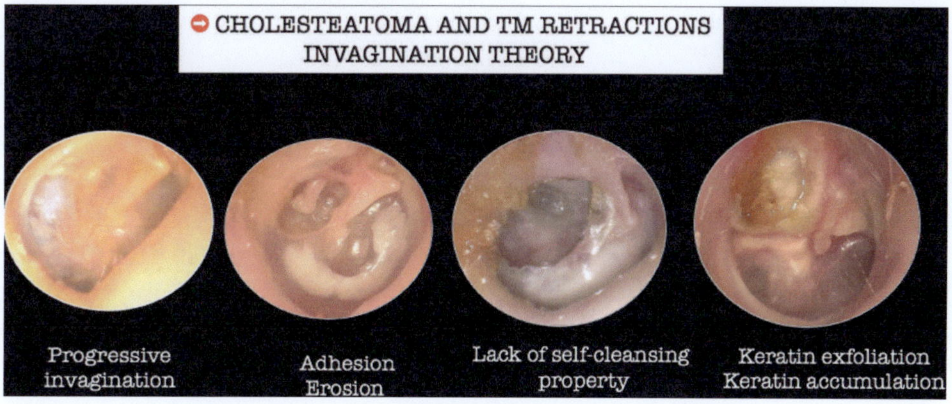

Fig. 42.11 Steps on the invagination theory—otoendoscopy

Pathophysiology

Since 2008, we have been indirectly studying the pathogenesis of chronic otitis media by examining the contralateral ear (CLE). Our observations have systematically showed a high prevalence of alterations in the CLE in clinical (Costa et al.), histopathological (Rosito et al.), functional (Silveira Netto et al.), and radiological (Noschang et al.) studies. Moreover, our results demonstrate that the frequency of alterations in the CLE was even higher in patients with COM with cholesteatoma. All our findings point to the same direction or the disease's tendency to affect both ears. Costa et al. stressed the importance of studying the diseased ears in pairs to understand the dynamic pathological process at presentation. Therefore, the maxim "you will be in my shoes tomorrow" was used by those authors to emphasize that the ears should be analyzed as an intrinsically related pair and not as an isolated unit. In doing so, frequently the first affected ear might predict the future status of the CLE. Regardless of the presence of cholesteatoma, the astute analysis of both ears may shed light into three key aspects of the disease process: where did it come from? (etiology), what is the current condition? (established pathology), and, more importantly, how fast and in which direction is the disease progressing? (natural history). Precise and critical analysis of both ears plays a key role in the prognostic assessment of each case, since the ear established with COM may predict the likely evolution of the CLE. One of our studies [127] changed our perspective, and the focus was redirected from the main ear (with cholesteatoma) to the CLE in an attempt to better understand the earlier steps of the condition. Only about one-third of the CLEs were considered normal. Moderate-to-severe TM retraction and cholesteatoma were undoubtedly the most prevalent pathological changes. Analyzing only the group of subjects with alterations in the CLE, we observed that 95.8% of them presented with retraction or signs of previous retraction (outside-in perforations), or progression of these retractions (cholesteatoma) in the CLE (Fig. 42.12).

Interestingly, our results showed that there was a strong association between growth patterns of cholesteatomas in the main ear and the location of TM retractions in the CLE (Fig. 42.12). Therefore, it seems plausible to infer that these retractions retrospectively represent the initial phases of cholesteatoma formation in the main ear.

The mechanisms responsible for progressive TM retraction leading to cholesteatoma formation are still debated. ET dysfunction resulting in impaired middle ear ventilation has been indicated as an important factor. Cauterization of the ET in gerbils resulted in retraction of the PF and cholesteatoma in 75% of the animals [76, 77]. Paradoxically, studies have shown that a patent ET can also result in middle ear alterations. This finding can be easily picked up during the clinical exam under magnification and the use of dynamic otoscopy (Toynbee and Valsalva maneuvers, swallowing and sniffing). In our experience, patulous ET as a main cause of middle ear cholesteatomais much more common than one could expect, but, still, receives very little attention from the literature. One interesting feature of this type of cholesteatoma is the association with well-developed mastoids suggesting that the middle ear has been aerated during childhood [128].

Middle ear inflammation, leading to changes in the mucosa and subepithelial space, also may explain the increased gas loss rate—Ars et al. [129]—(Fig. 42.13). Whatever the causative mechanism, negative pressure seems to play, at least, an initial role in TM retractions since it brings in closer contact the TM and middle ear structures (especially those projecting more laterally into the middle ear: neck of the malleus; long process of the incus and the dome of the promontory).

Besides the proximity to these structures, why do the retractions develop preferentially in the pars flaccida and the posterosuperior aspect of the pars tensa? As its name sug-

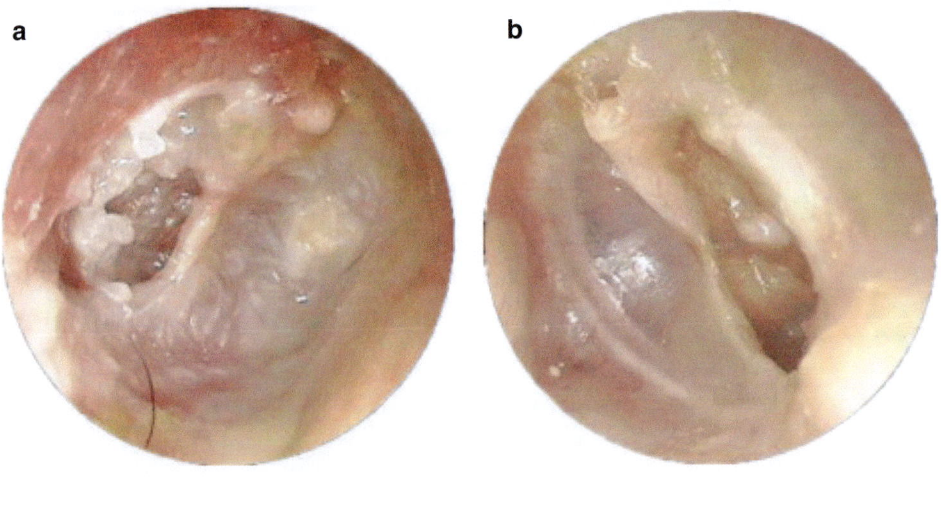

Fig. 42.12 (**a**) Right ear showing a pars tensa cholesteatoma in the posterosuperior sector of the tympanic membrane. (**b**) Left ear of the same patient with a severe retraction at the same location

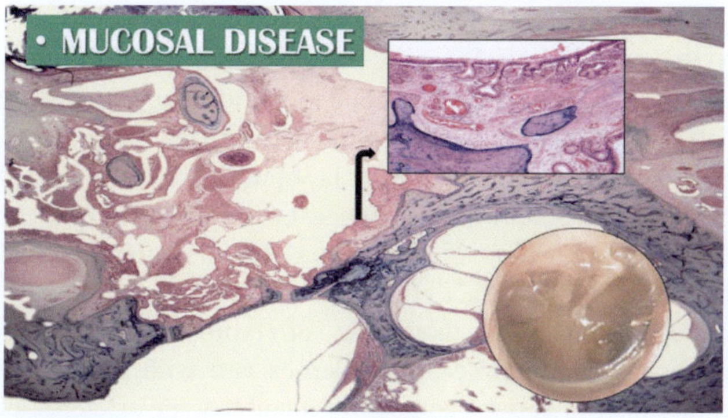

Fig. 42.13 Histologic view in a middle ear with thickened mucosa, associated with middle ear inflammation and effusion

gests, the pars flaccida possess higher elastic properties, allowing it to be drawn in more easily. It is composed of three layers, with epithelial layers similar to the pars tensa but a thicker and less organized connective tissue layer in-between. Furthermore, the pars flaccida is the only part of the TM that has been shown to contain mast cells. Mast cells are known to secrete a number of pro-inflammatory cytokines and proteinases. Mast cell migration into epithelium is seen in cholesteatoma but has not been observed in normal skin from any other anatomic site [95]. Additionally, the lateral aspect of the Prussak space is represented by the Shrapnel membrane (PF), and its medial and inferior aspects are formed respectively by the neck and the short process of the malleus. The superior limit is the fold of the lateral malleolar ligament, which also represents the floor of the lateral malleolar space; this ligament inserts laterally on the medial wall of the scutum. The anterior aspect of the Prussak space is bounded by a thin, membranous fold among the tympanic membrane and the anterior malleolar ligament fold, which inserts laterally on the tympanic membrane and medially on the neck and long process of the malleus. The posterior wall is represented by a large posterior pocket (the posterior pocket of von Tröltsch), which is the main route of ventilation. This posterior pocket is bounded laterally by the pars tensa and pars flaccida of the TM and medially by the posterior malleolar ligament fold. This posterior pocket develops in a posterior–inferior direction and opens at the most cranial portion of mesotympanum, so, in most people, ventilation of the Prussak space occurs through the communication with the mesotympanum (the only ventilation route that is separated from the epitympanic upper unit). This ventilation route is narrow, especially compared with the ventilation routes through tympanic isthmus, which aerates the upper epitympanic compartment and is wider. For these reasons, the possibility of anatomic reduction of the passage until the closing of the posterior pocket is plausible, especially the presence of thick and viscous secretions within the Prussak space that could cause a chronic sectorial dysventilation associated with a retraction of the Sharpnell membrane and its adhesion with the malleus neck [130].

Regarding the posterosuperior quadrant retraction of the TM, some extra considerations are needed. The tympanic annulus (that is absent in the pars flaccida) consists of a thickening of the TM periphery, and it is firmly inserted in the tympanic sulcus. In the PT, this combination between annulus and sulcus confers firmness and consistency to the region. However, as the tympanic annulus detaches superiorly from the sulcus, it goes toward the lateral process of the malleus, forming the anterior and posterior malleolar ligaments. Consequently, in the PF, there is no tympanic annulus. Thus, the TM is more malleable, filling the notch of Rivinus and being attached directly to the scutum. The tympanic sulcus, in its posterior region, is divided into two portions, separated, in most cases, by the emergence of the chorda tympani nerve. Inferior to the nerve, the sulcus maintains its characteristics identical to the inferior and anterior quadrants. It is well defined, with a depth between 0.5 and 0.9 mm, evident borders, and a stable surface. Above the nerve, the tympanic ring is no longer located within the sulcus but passes along the medial face of the posterior bone wall in 93% of the temporal bones studied by Paço et al. [131]. From that point on (the emergence of the chorda tympani nerve), the tympanic ring progressively becomes detached from the sulcus, which, in turn, progressively becomes shallower until it disappears.

Topographically, the emergence of the chorda tympani nerve marks the boundaries ofthe posterosuperior quadrant. These characteristics bring less tension on the TM in the PSquadrant compared to the other quadrants.

Another issue that we deem essential to highlight about the PS quadrant concerns the histology of the TM in this region. The middle layer of the PT (the lamina propria) consists of collagen types II and IV and is connected to the malleus handle and the tympanic bone. It consists of two layers, one radially oriented and the other circular in shape. The radial fibers (stratum radiatum) are attached to the manubrium of the malleus and run radially to the annulus. Meanwhile, the circular fibers (stratum circulare) are arranged concentrically with insertion into the manubrium. The latter are located medially in relation to the former [132, 133].

In turn, the PS quadrant presents some peculiarities compared to the other portions of the PT, which would give it a greater chance of atrophy and consequent retraction in this region in case of negative pressure in the middle ear. First, the region does not have a developed circular fibrous layer. In addition, its vascularization is more abundant, allowing greater penetration of collagenase-producing inflammatory cells, which have a more significant potential for destroying collagen fibers, which are already less dense by nature.

Besides the composition of the TM in these two segments, we postulate that the site of the obstruction is related to the creation of hypo-ventilated micro-spots within the middle ear cleft.

As we have mentioned before, regarding the posterosuperior quadrant of the PT a decreased middle ear pressure leads to a medial displacement of the TM and the handle of the malleus toward the dome of the promontory [134]. The medialization of the malleus handle, the prominence of the dome and subiculum of the promontory, and a less than firm attachment to the tympanic annulus reduce the distances and spaces in the PS quadrant creating a theoretically hypo-ventilated micro-spot isolated from the aeration routes. Furthermore, the presence of the ossicular chain (with attached tendons and mucosal folds) completes a scenario of multiples structures competing for space [82].

In relation to PF retraction, the tympanic isthmus seems to have a crucial role. We believe that, once created, these micro-spots may become stable through tight fibrous adhesions between the inner mucosal layer of the TM and the mucoperiosteum of the ossicles and middle ear (which may become the precursor of the future cholesteatoma perimatrix), regardless of the reestablishment of ME ventilation.

As pointed out by Jackler [95], although a middle ear vacuum could initiate TM retraction, it cannot credibly be the sustaining force for progressive growth of the cholesteatoma pouch. The epitympanum, aditus, and antrum become blocked early in the course of the disease and subsequently fill with mucous and/or inflammatory tissues; creation of a vacuum due to gas reabsorption is impossible under these circumstances. We still argue whether the TM retraction per se is enough to cause cholesteatoma formation. We believe that other factors that can disrupt the stability of the retraction are essential. Sudhoff and Tos [135], after observing the retraction of both the PT and the PF in some children, proposed a four-step concept for the pathogenesis of cholesteatoma that combines the retraction and proliferation theories: (i) the retraction pocket stage; (ii) proliferation of the retraction pocket, subdivided into cone formation and cone fusion; (iii) expansion of cholesteatoma; and (iv) bone resorption. On the other hand, Jackler et al. [136] proposed the theory of mucosal traction, which is based on the premise that the squamous pouch is drawn inward by the interaction of opposing motile surfaces of middle ear mucosa.

After observing thousands of tympanic retractions through powerful microscope lenses and with the use of endoscopes at various angles, we found that the existence of typical retraction pockets (the base larger than the external opening) in addition of being rare, were found almost exclusively in the region of the PF. Even so, through the serial follow-up of several patients, we were able to clearly observe the transition of many retractions (without the bottleneck appearance) into cholesteatomas (Fig. 42.14). Without exception, in all these cases the accumulation of epithelial debris and keratin was always associated with an inflammatory (infectious) process in frank activity. We conclude that TM retractions can become unstable through two mechanisms: either by spontaneous and natural accumulation of epithelium (true retraction pocket and natural accumulation), or, more commonly, by epithelial hyperproliferation triggered by an acute inflammatory process (hyperactive retraction and inflammation-hyperplasia) (Figs. 42.14 and 42.15).

We have followed patients with gross tympanic retractions who, after spending several years practically asymptomatic, suddenly present a drastic destabilization in their clinical picture with the appearance of drainage typical of cholesteatoma. It is clear under these circumstances that the catalyst for this change was an acute inflammatory trigger (Fig. 42.16).

Finally, through serial observations over time, we began also started to notice the presence in the external auditory canal of currents of epithelial desquamation that systematically march toward areas of previous TM retraction or perfo-

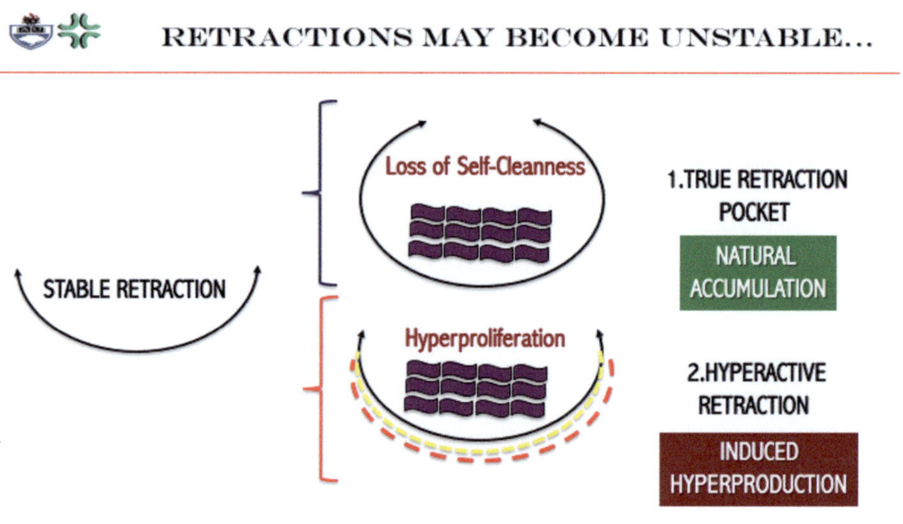

Fig. 42.14 Possible mechanisms causing instability in a retracted TM: (1) spontaneous and natural accumulation of epithelium (true retraction pocket and natural accumulation), and (2) epithelial hyperproliferation triggered by an acute inflammatory process (hyperactive retraction and inflammation-hyperplasia)

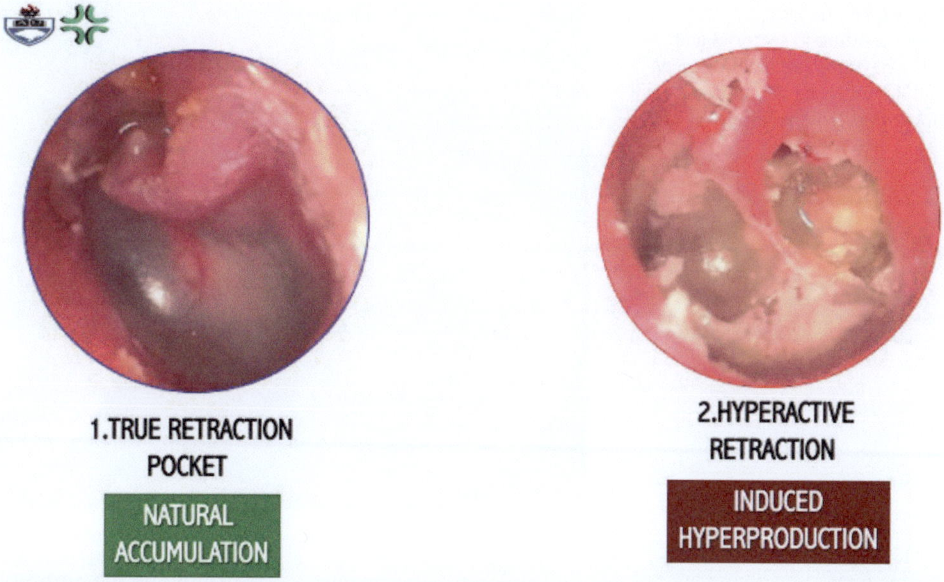

Fig. 42.15 Clinical example of possible mechanisms causing instability in a retracted TM: (1) spontaneous and natural accumulation of epithelium (true retraction pocket and natural accumulation), and (2) epithelial hyperproliferation triggered by an acute inflammatory process (hyperactive retraction and inflammation-hyperplasia)

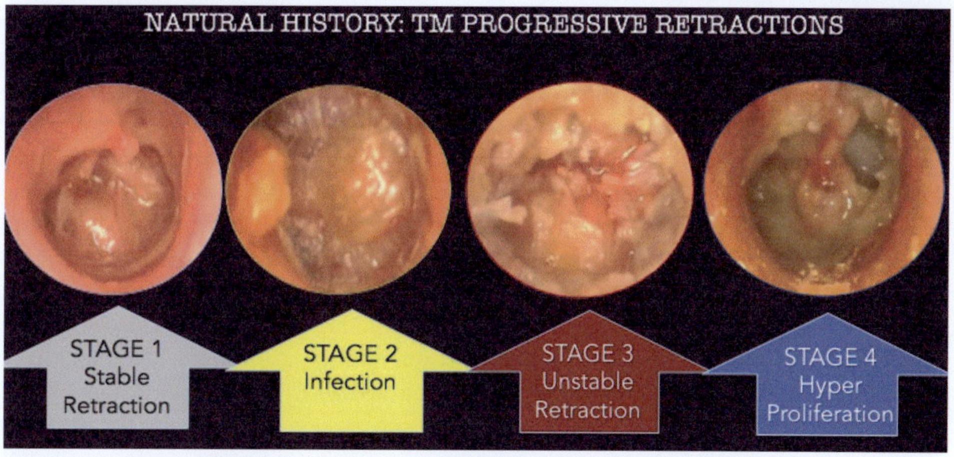

Fig. 42.16 Serial images of the right ear of a patient followed for many years. Notice the transition from a stable dry retraction, to acute otitis media, instability, and finally hyperproliferation

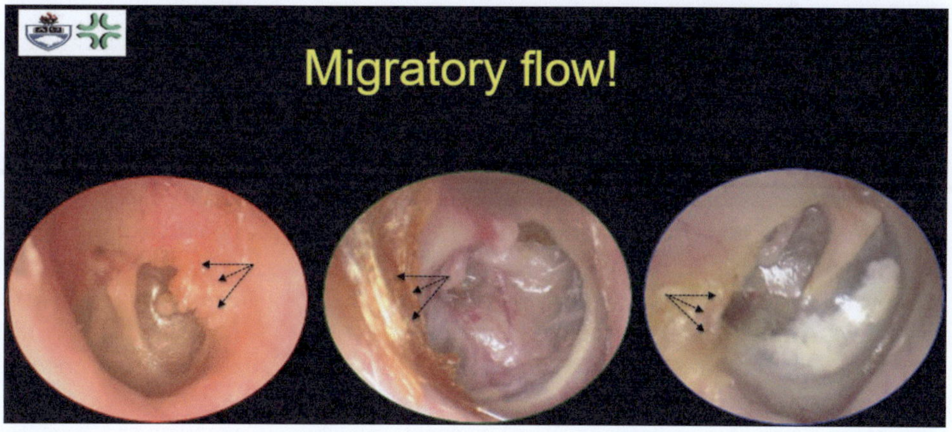

Fig. 42.17 Images corresponding to sectorial and diffuse tympanic retraction and the presence of a uniform flow of peeled epithelium

ration (Figs. 42.17 and 42.18). During the careful removal and under microscopy of these sheets of epithelial rests, we can notice that they systematically extend around the tympanic annulus and invade the middle ear and its posterior recesses. It is difficult to know if this epithelial migratory flow is made in one direction or the other (EAC-middle ear or middle ear-EAC), but it seems very plausible to us that it is toward the middle ear in a potential attempt to repair a damage inflicted on the tympanic membrane (perforation or retraction).

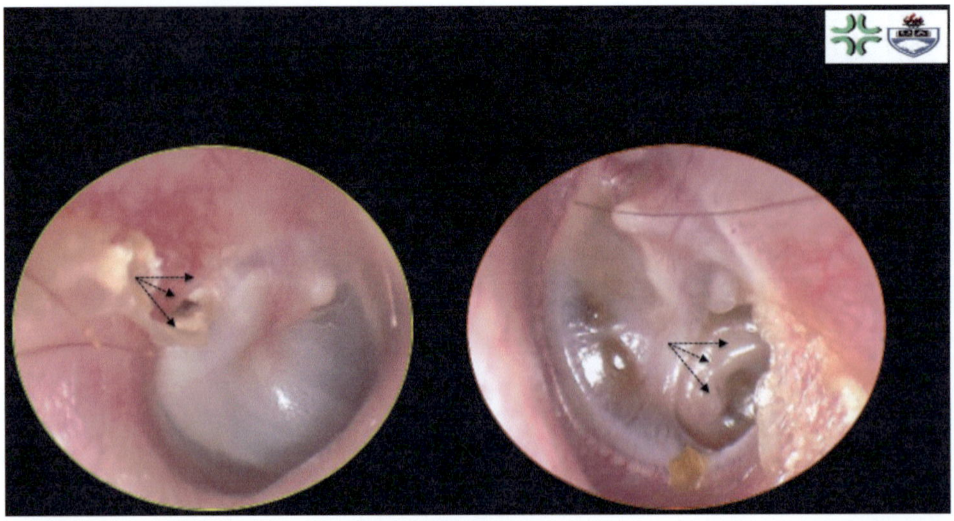

Fig. 42.18 Images corresponding to sectorial and diffuse tympanic retraction and the presence of a uniform flow of peeled epithelium

In short, the existence of congenital and implantation cholesteatomas is indisputable. Regarding the mechanism of pathogenesis of other acquired cholesteatomas, the only point of convergence in all theories is that TM retractions were almost universally implied in the first stages of its development. We do not exclude the role of cellular hyperplasia or even epithelial migration in the process, but our thousands of observations and experiments endorse the essential role of TM retraction at least in the earlier phases of cholesteatoma pathogenesis. In the intimacy of this tiny nutshell space, a whole universe of biological events is set into motion frequently, driving the retraction to a self-determining outcome. It also seems clear that the transition from a previously stable retraction to an active cholesteatoma always requires the presence of an acute inflammatory trigger.

Cholesteatoma Growth Pathways

Most cholesteatomas assume typical growth patterns, according to their site of origin and related anatomical structures and, when in expansion, they follow sinuous paths, between mucous folds, ligaments, and ossicles. Migration routes of cholesteatomas tend to follow vestigial planes created in embryogenesis. It is not uncommon for multiple cholesteatoma sacs to occur in the same ear, involving two, even three growth routes simultaneously. While the vast majority of cholesteatomas follow one or more routes, others assume a different growth pattern. This probably occurs due to anatomical variations of the mucous folds and ligaments, which tend to channel and guide the growth of cholesteatomas.

Jackler [95] proposed a widely accepted classification with three main routes followed by the disease:

(a) Posterior epitympanic (PEC): this is the most common route. It starts from an invagination of Shrapnell's membrane penetrating posteriorly through Prussak's space, following the embryological path of the saccule medius. This route passes through the superior incundal space, lateral to the body of the incus, crossing the aditus ad antrum, and entering the mastoid. These cholesteatomas can reach the mesotympanum by dipping through the floor of Prussak's space into the posterior space of Von Trölscht (Fig. 42.19).
(b) Posterior mesotympanic (PMC): the posterosuperior portion of the pars tensa retracts toward the mesotympanum, forming a sac extending to the antrum via the posterior tympanic isthmus and inferior incundal space. The surgical inaccessibility of the posterior tympanic recess makes it difficult to completely remove cholesteatomas located in this area. Unlike the posterior epitympanic pathway, the extension of these cholesteatomas to the mastoid passes medial to the malleus and incus, following the embryological course of the posterior and superior pouchs (Fig. 42.20).
(c) Anterior epitympanic pathway (AEC): the anterior epitympanic pathway arises from a retraction of the tympanic membrane anterior to the malleus head, following the path of the saccule anticus. Cholesteatomas in this area may go unnoticed during surgical exploration if the region anterior to the malleus head is not adequately explored. Since the lower limit of the epitympanum is related to the horizontal portion of the facial nerve (FN) and the geniculate ganglion, facial nerve dysfunction may occur in these lesions. Anteroinferior extension into the supratubal recess is common and the mesotympanum is reached via the anterior space of Von Tröltsch (Fig. 42.21).

Depending on the route followed by the cholesteatoma, the associated hearing loss will be early or late. The most commonly encountered growth patterns are summarized in Table 42.4.

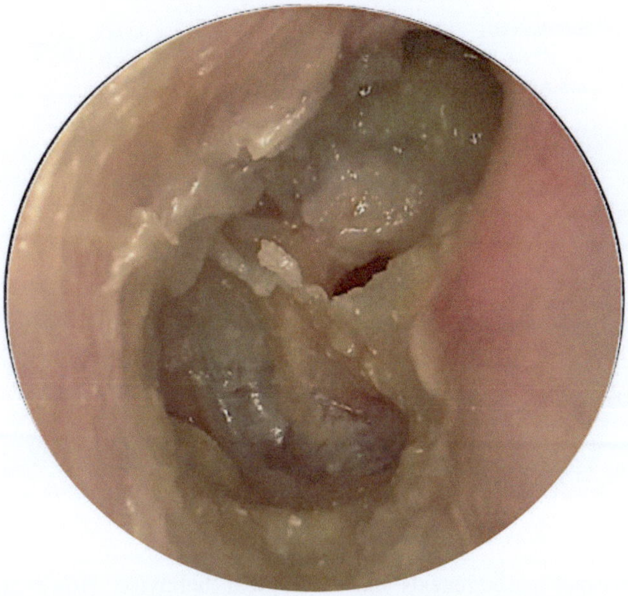

Fig. 42.19 Posterior epitympanic cholesteatoma in the left ear

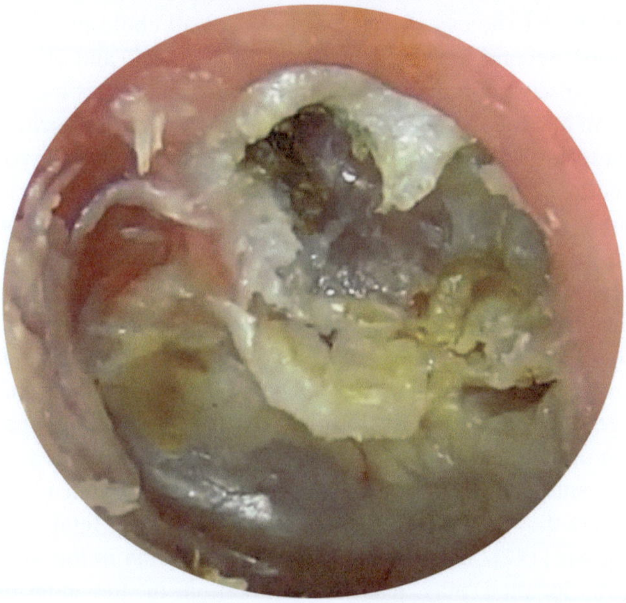

Fig. 42.20 Posterior mesotympanic cholesteatoma in the left ear

A few years ago, with the aim of making an inventory of our cases we carried out a cross-sectional comparative study of 638 ears with middle ear cholesteatoma and no history of ear surgery treated at our institution searching for the prevalence of each traditional growth patterns (flaccida or PEC; tensa or PMC; anterior epitympanic). In our study, we observed a similar prevalence of 34.3% for PEC and 33.8% for PMC. These findings were in agreement with those of a previous report that found a prevalence of 45% for pars tensa and 41% for attic cholesteatomas [138].

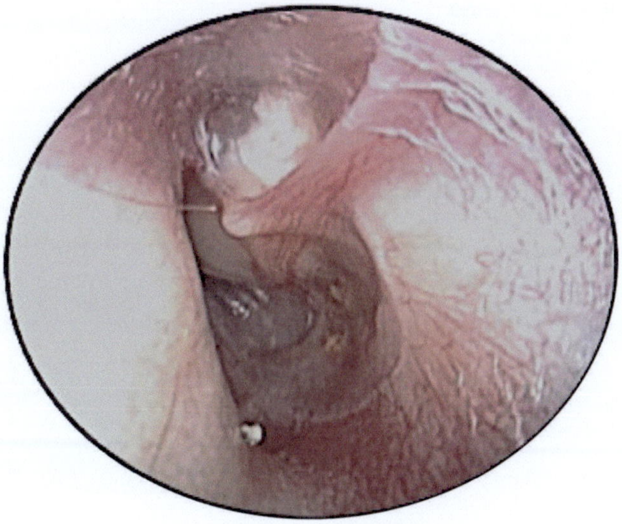

Fig. 42.21 Anterior epitympanic cholesteatoma in the left ear

Table 42.4 Growth patterns of middle ear cholesteatomas

1. Posterior epitympanic
(a) Epitympanum → Prussak space → upper → incudal spaceaditus → antrum → mastoid
(b) Von Troltsch space → middle ear
2. Posterior mesotympanic
(a) Posterosuperior quadrant posterior → tympanic isthmus → inferior → incudal space aditus → mastoid
(b) Posterior–superior quadrant → recess of the facial → tympanic sinus.
3. Anterior epitympanic
Epitympanum → anterior → epitympanum supratubal recess → Von Tröltsch's previous space → middle ear

However, 124 of the cholesteatomas (30.0%) could not be classified as PEC, PMC, or anterior epitympanic. We observed that, in 57 ears (13.8%), both the pars flaccida and the pars tensa were involved, so we termed them 2-route cholesteatomas. Finally, in 67 ears (16.2%), no precise growth pattern could be identified by videotoscopy. We classified these cholesteatomas as undetermined [139]. In view of these findings, we have changed our classification, currently including the three traditional routes described by Jackler [137] incorporating two new elements: (1) two routes; (2) open or undetermined. Figure 42.22 shows our classification and the prevalence of each route in our series.

Regarding age groups, PEC was more prevalent in adults, whereas AEC and PMC were more prevalent in children (in fact, AEC was exclusively found in this age group). The prevalence of two routes and undetermined cholesteatoma was similar between both age groups [139].

When we analyze the cholesteatomas which predominantly involved the pars tensa, the classification among authors is a bit different. While Jackler considered only PMC

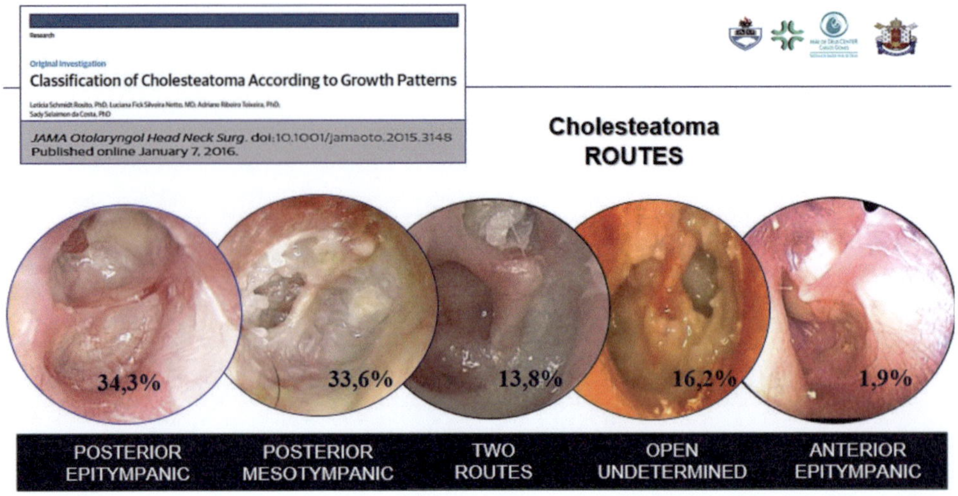

Fig. 42.22 Current classification of cholesteatoma routes and their prevalence

as originated from the posterior sector of the pars tensa, Tos divided the pars tensa cholesteatoma into two variants:

- Sinus (which is the equivalent to PMC);
- Tensa (open according to our classification).

We agree with the posterior mesotympanic concept because it refers to a typical route of extension in which, in contrast to posterior epitympanic, the mastoid progression of cholesteatoma typically passes medial to the malleus and incus, and the sinus tympani and facial recess are generally involved. What is the clinical relevance of this progression? First, it grows over the most delicate part of the ossicular chain (long process of incus and incudostapedial joint) causing early conductive hearing loss. Second, the extension for the posterior recesses makes the complete surgical removal a very laborious and complicated task.

When the entire area of the middle ear is affected by the cholesteatoma, however, it is difficult to determine precisely whether the disease is the result of a complete pars tensa atelectasis or whether it is a posterior mesotympanic or even a posterior epitympanic cholesteatoma that has advanced to other compartments. For such reasons, we preferred to classify unknown cases as undetermined or open.

One may ask: What's the importance of tracking the routes of middle ear cholesteatomas formation? We firmly believe that the correct knowledge of the paths followed by cholesteatomas extremely helpful in the pathophysiological understanding of the disease and also during the preoperative planning and selection of most appropriated surgical approach.

One last issue regarding the classification of cholesteatomas is that their sites of origin and progression routes that remain to be addressed are regarding the AEC. The classification of cholesteatomas into congenital and acquired is useful since it separates two types of cholesteatoma with distinct pathogenesis and biological behavior. However, sometimes it is difficult to clinically determine whether the cholesteatoma is congenital or acquired. First, congenital cholesteatoma is rare, accounting for approximately 4% of childhood cholesteatomas and 2–5% of all cholesteatomas [140]. Second, the classic definition by Derlacki and Clemis [29] of congenital cholesteatomas as a pearly mass medial to an intact tympanic membrane and no history of otorrhea, tympanic membrane perforation, or previous otologic procedures have been questioned mainly because middle ear infection in children is almost universal [97]. In our study, we found a prevalence of 1.9% of AEC and all of them in children. Furthermore, all the contralateral ears were healthy [139]. For these reasons, we hypothesize that the few EAC in our series could be, indeed, not acquired but congenital (even when associated with retraction and drainage). Corroborating this hypothesis, it is well known that the most prevalent location of congenital cholesteatomas is the anterosuperior quadrant of the mesotympanum [141] where they arise from epidermoid residues of the fetal middle ear [142]. The growing of a cholesteatoma in this specific location may lead to obliteration of the anterior segment of the tympanic isthmus (which in healthy ears is an open structure [130]) followed by pars flaccida retraction.

Bone Erosion

As we have pointed out before, ossicular erosion is one of the most frequent consequences of the progression of cholesteatoma, and the pattern and impact of this damage depend on its origin and the pathways in which cholesteatoma develops. Partial or total ossicular erosion is observed in approximately 80% of patients with cholesteatoma [143]. The two main factors probably involved in cholesteatoma-related ossicular erosion are chronic inflammation, which leads to cytokine release and osteoclast activation, and pressure necrosis, caused by the cholesteatoma mass [144].

While the PEC arises in the pars flaccida and progresses laterally to the head of the malleus and body of incus, the PMC grows directly over the fragile long process of the incus, erodes serially the incudostapedial joint, the suprastructure of the stapes reaching the footplate and oval window. These distinctive growth patterns can lead to different levels of hearing impairments, even including inner ear damage and sensorineural loss.

In order to verify whether the hearing impairment caused by PEC differed from that caused by PMC, we conducted a cross-sectional study including 264 ears of patients with cholesteatoma, who had not been subjected to ear surgery [139]. When the air–bone gaps (ABG) were compared, the mesotympanic group had greater thresholds at 500, 2000 Hz, and a greater pure-tone average ($p = 0.003$, $p = 0.03$, and $p = 0.02$, respectively). PMC showed greater air–bone gaps thresholds at the speech frequencies than posterior epitympanic cholesteatoma. Moreover, the two growth patterns were very similar with regard to all other audiometric parameters analyzed in this study [139].

Our results agree with those of several other studies that showed that incus was the most affected ossicle [143–145]. This may be due to the incus mass, its prominent bone marrow, and mainly, due to exposure and fragility of the long process. Martins et al. [146] showed that the erosion of each ossicle contributes to the increase in ABG in a graded and independent manner. The same authors also showed that the status of incus has the most statistically significant association with ABG [146]. Maresh et al. [147] compared primary and secondary acquired cholesteatomas (according to the authors, attic and mesotympanic cholesteatomas, respectively) and found that malleus erosion is more prevalent in the former and stapes erosion in the latter. The prevalence of incus erosion did not differ between the groups. Our results, however, showed a greater prevalence of incus erosion in MPC. This was expected since the PMC cholesteatoma grows just over the incus and its erosion can also explain the greater ABG in this group of patients. We must consider, however, that the ABG differences between PEC and PMC could be underestimated since sometimes the cholesteatoma cyst may itself serves as a bridge to transmit the soundwave from the remnants of the TM to the footplate the so-called columellar effect of the cholesteatoma a phenomenon that could underestimate the potential size of the ABG, especially when the disease is located in the posterior mesotympanum.

Bone absorption is stimulated by a variety of factors, including inflammation, local pressure, specific cytokeratin, and keratin [8, 9]. The enzymatic concept, in which enzymes of epithelial origin are considered responsible for bone destruction, was defined by Abramson [148–150], who demonstrated the presence of collagenases and hydrolases in cholesteatomas, a hypothesis later confirmed by Thompsen [151]. Ken and Gordon (1972), indicated that collagenase may be involved in bone resorption, but not as an isolated factor. Ferlito et al. [4] suggested that the destructive property of cholesteatomas, bone erosion, is caused by collagenase production by components of squamous and fibrous epithelial tissue. It has not yet been well demonstrated whether mineralized bone can be absorbed by collagenase. To the hypothesis of bone resorption by biochemical action, exclusively exercised by collagenolytic enzymes, other agents were later incorporated, such as tumor necrosis factor (TNF), interleukins (IL-1 α), and prostaglandins (PGE_2) [93, 152, 153].

Imai et al.[154] found that a significantly larger number of osteoclasts were observed on the eroded bone adjacent to cholesteatomas than in unaffected areas, and that fibroblasts in the cholesteatoma perimatrix expressed RANKL. Also, the concentrations of interleukin-1β, interleukin-6, tumor necrosis factor α, and prostaglandin E2 were increased in cholesteatomas compared with normal skin. Furthermore, interleukin-1β was expressed in infiltrating inflammatory cells in the cholesteatoma perimatrix [154].

Sangal et al. [155] explored the hypothesis that genetic predisposition for inflammation can influence the development and severity of cholesteatoma. Patients with cholesteatoma exhibited a homozygous CARD8 C10X mutation status 1.95 times higher (29.41% vs. 9.52%) than control population. Although this does not prove that homozygous CARD8 mutation status is causal, it can suggest it as a predisposing factor for cholesteatoma. This result remains an intriguing finding that warrants further investigation. In addition, the potential effect of these mutations on the progression of cholesteatoma (considered by those authors as the severity of bone erosion) was also studied. Mutant CARD8 genotypes exhibited significantly greater levels of bone erosion compared to patients without CARD8 mutations. These results suggest that the host inflammatory state exerts a significant influence on the progression of cholesteatoma bone destruction [155].

Bacteriology

Inherent to the formation and progression of cholesteatoma is the colonization by bacteria within the middle ear and the formation of biofilm that aids in the persistence of inflammation. Numerous pathogens, including Gram-positive, Gram-negative, and various fungal elements, have been identified in the middle ear in association with cholesteatoma tissues. Significant difficulty exists when attempting to treat these elements as delivery of systemic antibiotics is hampered by the lack of blood flow to the lesion and the fact that topical antibiotics may not penetrate as deep as necessary to eradicate pathogens that may be the root cause of the general inflammatory stimulus that leads to the progression of cholesteatomas. Advanced infection can progress to significant complications such as cavernous sinus thrombosis, meningitis, brain abscess, and mastoiditis.

The microbial flora of chronic otitis media is different from that found in acute otitis media. The bacterial agent, which causes the initial process of acute otitis media with perforation of the tympanic membrane and otorrhea, is generally not the same as that isolated in the chronic infection of the middle ear and mastoid that accompanies cholesteatoma. Thus, the recommended antibiotic therapy for acute otitis media may not be effective in cases of chronic suppurative otitis media with cholesteatoma.

The aerobic bacteria most commonly isolated in cases of chronic suppurative otitis media with cholesteatoma are *P. aeruginosa,* S. *aureus, Proteus sp., K. pneumoniae, and E. coli.* Among the anaerobic organisms found are *Bacteroides*, *Peptostreptococcus, Clostridium,* and *Bacteroides sp.* [156]. In many cases, mixed floras are found. Kenna and Bluestone [157] evaluated the bacteriology of CCOM in 36 children. *Pseudomonas aeruginosa was* the most common bacteria, present as the sole pathogen in 31% of cases and in 67% of polymicrobial cultures. Most recently, Fujikawa et al. [158] found a large difference in the colonization of the COM with and without cholesteatoma, also suggesting that *S. aureus* infection is involved in cholesteatoma progression.

Acquired cholesteatoma frequently becomes chronically infected, and the biofilm colonization of the middle ear seems to be responsible for resistance to topical and systemic antimicrobial agents [68]. Increased bacterial retaining and biofilm formation are histologically found in association with massive entrapment of keratin and keratinocyte proliferation resulting in an expanding matrix with osteoclasts recruitment and bone erosion [68]. Galli et al. [159] found a high rate of bacterial biofilm evidence (81.3%) in cholesteatoma, even though the causal relationship remains unclear. The authors hypothesize the keratinized matrix of cholesteatoma and the destruction of the ciliated epithelium of the respiratory tract may represent an ideal substrate for biofilm colonization and survival.

In clinical practice, cultures of middle ear secretions are rarely performed in uncomplicated cases, as the treatment of CCOM is essentially surgical. Identification of the germ is only clinically important in cases with complications, such as abscesses or meningitis. However, antibiotic therapy is useful as an adjuvant treatment, both preoperatively and perioperatively, in order to reduce the risks of postoperative infection.

Clinical Picture and Preoperative Workup

A careful analysis of the symptoms and signs allows physicians to determine the need for surgery, its urgency, and the anticipated results. We always discuss with our fellows, residents, and medical students that the art of taking a good medical history can never be overemphasized. Especially when dealing with a disease that has the possibility to recur as one of its trademarks (like the cholesteatoma). It is mandatory to conduct a careful interview with the patient and/or his family focusing three key periods along the timeline:

1. **Today (the present).**
2. **Yesterday (the past).**
3. **Tomorrow (the future).**

The ideal preoperative workup encompasses the art of history taking, a complete ENT physical examination and important ancillary tests (audiology, imaging, etc.). The workup should guide the physician to three distinct temporal moments equally important (Fig. 42.23):

1. **Today: The diagnosis.**
2. **Yesterday: The etiology.**
3. **Tomorrow: The prognosis.**

This information will permit the clinician to design a rational therapeutic plan which will make possible:

1. **Today: To treat established disease.**
2. **Yesterday: To manage etiologic factors trying to avoid recurrences.**
3. **Tomorrow: To abort the natural history and future complications.**

Signs and Symptons

General Information

In 2016, we carried out a study aimed to determine the prevalence of cholesteatoma in patients with chronic otitis media and describe clinical, audiological, and surgical characteristics. For such, we designed a cross-sectional and prospective cohort analysis including 1710 patients with chronic otitis media, treated between August 2000 and June 2015, without prior surgery. Detailed clinical history, videotoscopy, and audiometry were performed, in addition to review of medical records to search for surgical data. Of the 1710 patients with COM evaluated in the study, cholesteatoma was present in 419 (24.5%). The mean age of patients was 34.49, standard deviation (SD) 19.8, and 53.5% were female. White patients

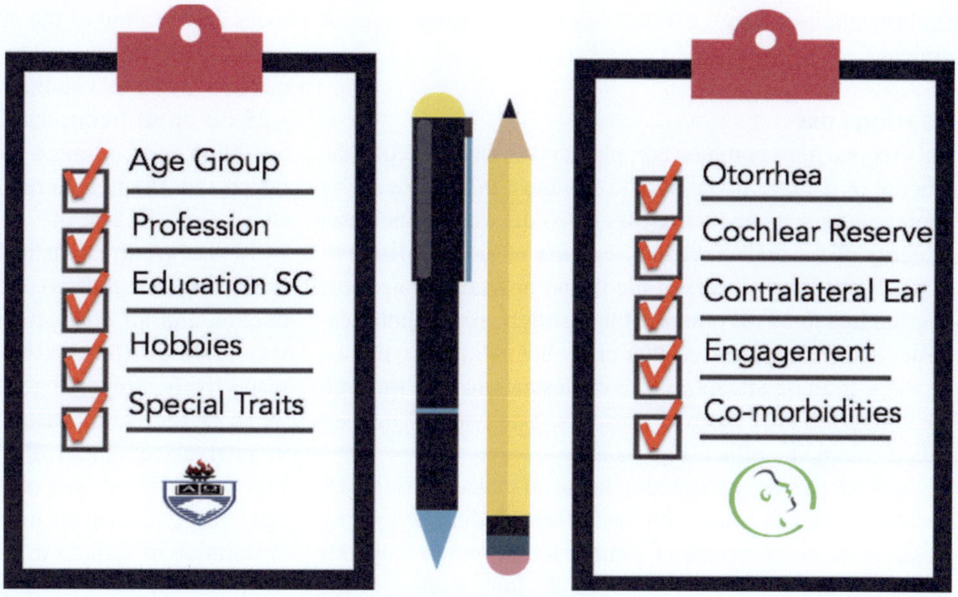
Age Group
Profession
Education SC
Hobbies
Special Traits
Otorrhea
Cochlear Reserve
Contralateral Ear
Engagement
Co-morbidities

Fig. 42.23 Individual characteristics to be researched during the clinical consultation of a patient with chronic otitis media and cholesteatoma

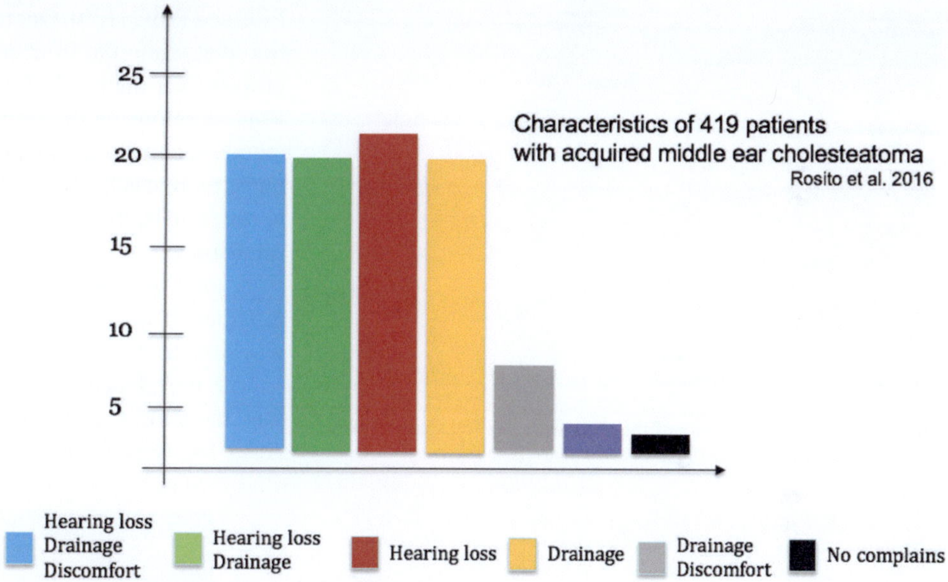

Fig. 42.24 Frequency of the chief complaints of patients with cholesteatoma at the time of first evaluation

accounted for 86.5% of the study population and 5.9% were Black. Adults corresponded to 63.8%. Cholesteatoma was identified in the right ear was in 234 patients (55.8%). The prevalence of cleft palatects in this population was 4.3%.

In the contralateral ear evaluation, only 150 of them (36.1%) were normal and cholesteatoma was identified in 71 (17.1%). The duration of symptoms was longer in patients with changes in the contralateral ear than in those with normal contralateral ear (mean of 14.99 and 11.69, respectively; $p = 0.007$). There was no difference in the prevalence of cholesteatoma in the contralateral ear between children and adults ($p = 0.20$) and between patients with and without palate malformation ($p = 0.19$).

The main complaints of patients at the time of the first evaluation in this service are shown in Fig. 42.24. Hypoacusis, with or without otorrhea, was the main complaint of 84.4% of the study population, and otorrhea was observed in 87%. There were no differences regarding the main complaint when we compared cholesteatomas classified by the route of formation ($p = 0.27$).

Otorrhea

This is the most common manifestation of chronic otitis media, especially cholesteatoma. It is important to ask about its duration, frequency, character, and bad smell. Long-lasting, constant, purulent, or bloody malodorous otorrhea is always associated with significant disease in the middle ear and mastoid. Mucoid discharge of short duration, on-and-off drainage, may denote a simple perforation with no major pathologic findings. It is not infrequent, though, that some cholesteatomas may evolve silently without typical drainage.

Hearing Loss

This second most common complaint is closely related to the amount of damage in the middle ear; thus, in the absence of cholesteatoma, a conductive loss of 20 dB usually indicates integrity of the ossicular chain. Erosion of the ossicles (particularly the long process of the incus) or fixation raises the hearing loss to 30 dB or more. Interestingly, some cholesteatomas can destroy the ossicular chain but still preserve good hearing. In these situations, the cholesteatoma can transmit the sound from the external ear to the oval window in a so-called columellar effect (Fig. 42.25).

Another perplexing situation is the so-called myringostapediopexy (which is a pre-cholesteatoma finding defined by Costa et al. as a retraction limited to the posterosuperior region, in which there is erosion of the long process of the incus and fixation of the affected TM to the head of the stapes). A study conducted by our group found that 53% of the patients with this condition presented with an air–bone gap ≤25 dB at all frequencies. This finding suggests that such condition may mimic a surgical type III tympanoplasty in which the TM is repaired and advanced to the head of the stapes (Fig. 42.26a, b).

In the group of patients included in our cohort study [139], 92.41% underwent audiometry. Regarding bone conduction and air conduction thresholds, the tritonal average was 17.08 dB (SD 16.16 dB) and 46.35 db (SD 22.34 dB), respectively. Regarding gap sizes, the tritonal average is 29.84 db (SD 13.61 dB). The size of the air–bone (grouped in intervals of 20/20 dB) in tritonal average is shown in Fig. 42.27. There was no correlation between gap size and age of the patient at the time of evaluation ($R = 0.03$; $p = 0.55$) or duration of symptoms ($R = 0.08$; $p = 0.13$).

In another study of our group, we aimed to investigate the potential differences in the hearing impairment caused by PEC and PMC [139]. Our rationale was based on the assumption that while the PEC arises in the pars flaccida and progresses over the head of the malleus and body of incus, the PMC develops on the fragile incus long process, erodes the incudostapedialjoint, and may compromise the oval window niche more easily. These distinct growth patterns could lead to different hearing impairments, even including sensorineural damage.

A total of 264 ears were analyzed in this study. Patient distribution according to the cholesteatoma growth pattern was similar: 50.4% had PEC and 49.6% had PMC.

The prevalence of BC PTA thresholds above 25 dB was low and similar between the two groups. According to the AC PTA, only 20% of the ears had normal hearing. The

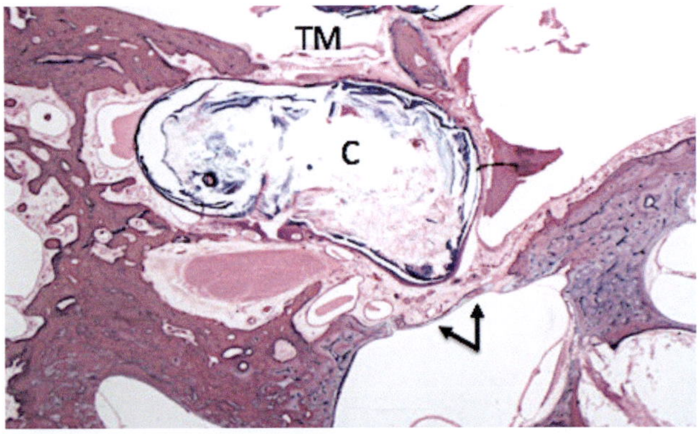

Fig. 42.25 Columellar effect of the cholesteatoma (c), spanning from the tympanic membrane (MT) to the footplate (black arrows)

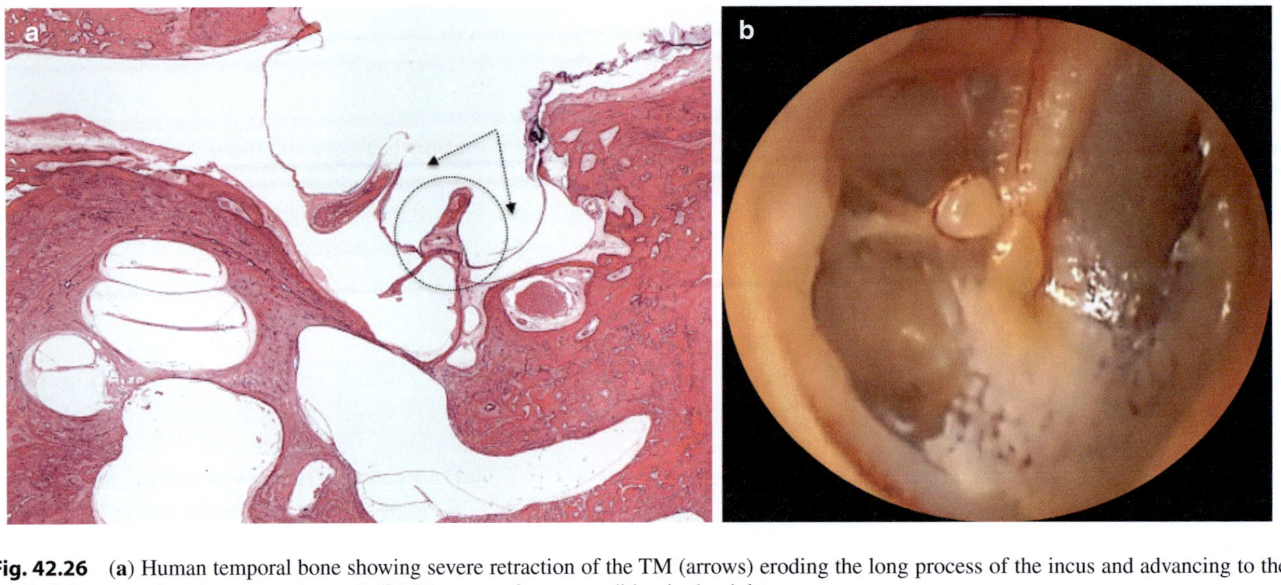

Fig. 42.26 (**a**) Human temporal bone showing severe retraction of the TM (arrows) eroding the long process of the incus and advancing to the head of the stapes (myringoestapedopexy). (**b**) Otoscopy of same condition in the right ear

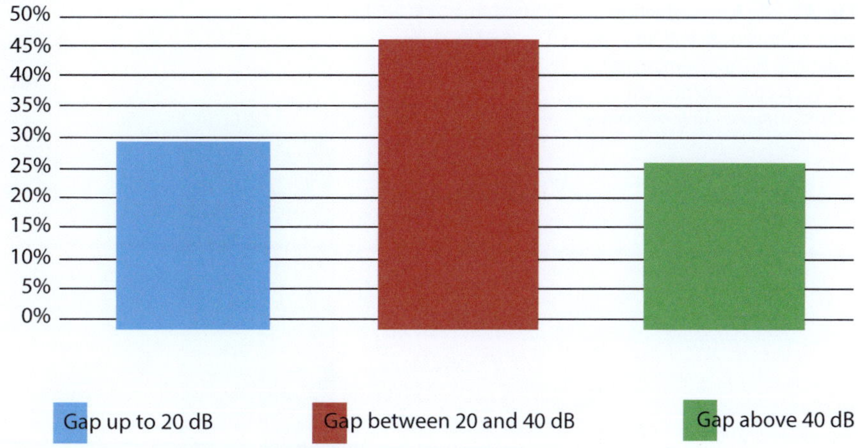

Fig. 42.27 Prevalence of the air–bone difference sizes in tritonal average

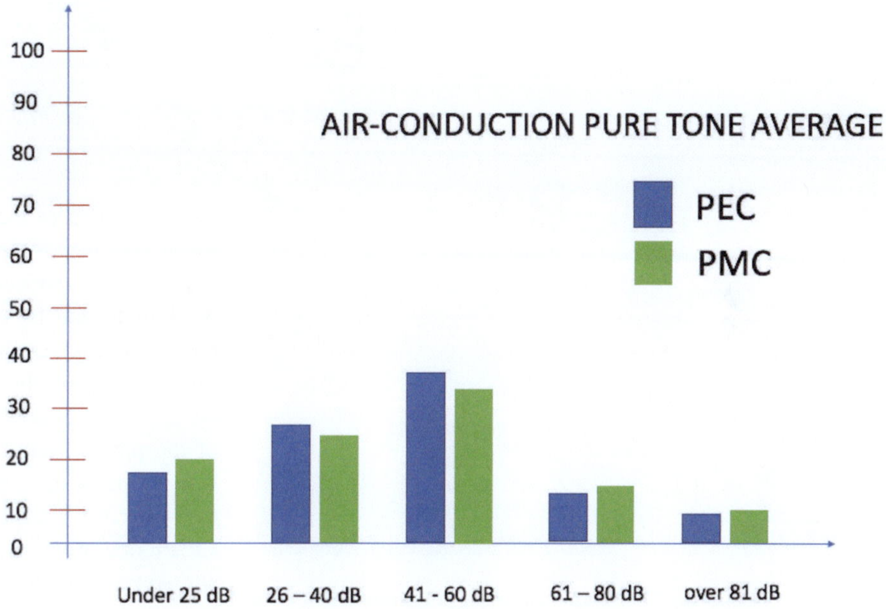

Fig. 42.28 Comparison of hearing loss degree between epitympanic and mesotympanic cholesteatomas

majority of them had at least moderate hearing loss. No difference was found between the PEC and PMC groups for degree of hearing loss, and the means of the AC PTA and the medians of the BC PTA were similar between the PEC and PMC groups. The results of ABG PTA, however, showed that the thresholds were greater in the PMC group (Figs.42.28 and 42.29).

An issue that has recently gained attention is additional sensorineural hearing loss due to chronic otitis media. While the conductive loss can be minimized through surgery, sensorineural hearing loss constitutes a permanent after effect, attenuated only through the use of a hearing aid. However, a few groups have reported a decrease in sensorineural function in these patients as well. Some years ago, we evaluated the occurrence of sensorineural hearing loss in patients with this disease. We reviewed the files of patients with unilateral chronic otitis media. One hundred and fifty patients met the inclusion criteria: normal otoscopy and normal hearing in the contralateral ear. The main outcome measure were bone conduction threshold averages calculated for frequencies of 500, 1000, 2000, 3000, and 4000 Hz, with comparison between the normal ear and the ear with chronic otitis media. Thresholds were examined separately for each frequency. The bone conduction threshold averages for the normal side were lower than those for the ear with chronic otitis media. The threshold shift was statistically significant for each frequency ($p < 0.0001$, Student's t test). There were differences between the groups when analyzed for age (500 and 1000 Hz) or the presence of cholesteatoma (1000 Hz). This study shows that chronic otitis media is associated with a decrease in cochlear function. The association was even greater when cholesteatoma was present. A variety of studies show the connection between COM and cochlear damages. Paparella et al. [160, 161], English et al. [162], Dumich and Harner [163], and Walby et al. [164] have demonstrated an association of the COM with cochlear damage, pointing to the round

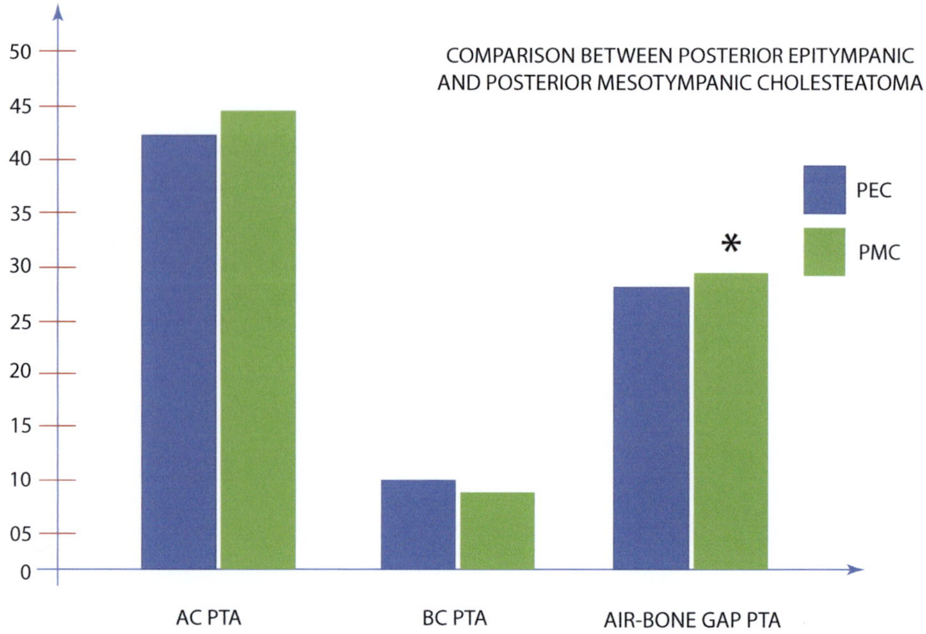

Fig. 42.29 Air conduction, bone conduction, and air–bone gap PTAs comparison between epitympanic and mesotympanic cholesteatomas

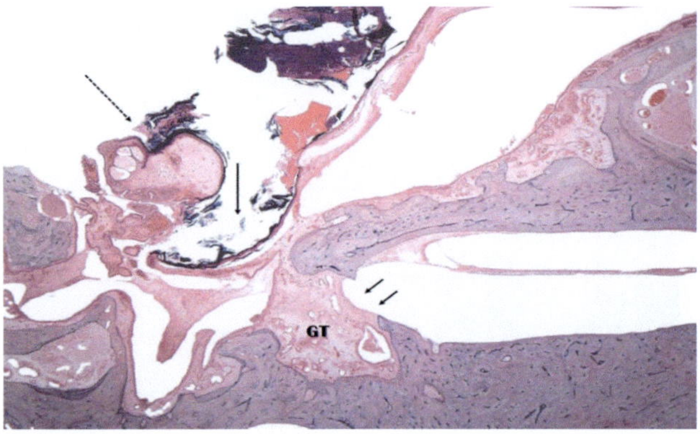

Fig. 42.30 Human temporal section showing a polyp protruding to the EAC (dashed arrow), a cholesteatoma underneath it (solid arrow), and granulation tissue filling the round window niche in close proximity with the round window membrane (small solid arrows) which is slightly ballooned

window as the structure responsible for the transmission of the pathological process to the labyrinth (Fig. 42.30). The anatomy and localization of the round and oval window niches predispose to pathology in the presence of otitis media. This way, they could behave as true entrance doors for toxins coming from the ME to arrive in the inner ear, configuring a legitimism interaction between these two compartments.

Vertigo

Continuous true vertigo in the presence of a cholesteatoma represents a labyrinthine irritation or a fistula in a semicircular canal until proven otherwise.

Labyrinthine fistula (LF) is one of the most common complications associated with cholesteatoma and represents an erosive loss of the endochondral bone overlying the labyrinth. The loss of the overlying protective bone allows pressure or mass-induced motion of the underlying endosteum, perilymph, and by contiguity, the endolymphatic compartment, evoking vestibular and sometimes auditory symptoms. The etiology of cholesteatoma-induced LF in some patients is still poorly understood. Cholesteatoma growth pattern, age of the patient, and time of the disease are possible factors that influence the site of bone erosion and aggressiveness of the disease, which may lead to development of LF. Preoperative detection of LF is of great importance to ear surgeons. LF may not be associated with any specific symptom or sensorineural hearing loss (SHL) before surgery; nevertheless, proper management is essential to prevent poor outcome. [165].

In 2018, our group conducted a study to evaluate patients with cholesteatoma in order to identify possible risk factors or clinical findings associated with labyrinthine fistula [166]. Secondary objectives were to determine the prevalence of labyrinthine fistula in the study cohort to analyze the role of computed tomography and to describe the hearing results after surgery of those patients where a PF was identified. For such, we carried out a retrospective cohort study including patients with an acquired middle ear cholesteatoma in at least one ear with no prior surgery, who underwent audiometry and tomographic examination of the ears or surgery at our institution. As a result, we analyzed a total of 333 patients, of which 9 (2.7%) had labyrinthine fistula in the lateral semicircular canal (LSC) (Fig. 42.31). As in our service, most patients with LF are routinely submitted to open tympanomastoidectomy, so, whenever identified during the surgery, they were classified according to the degree

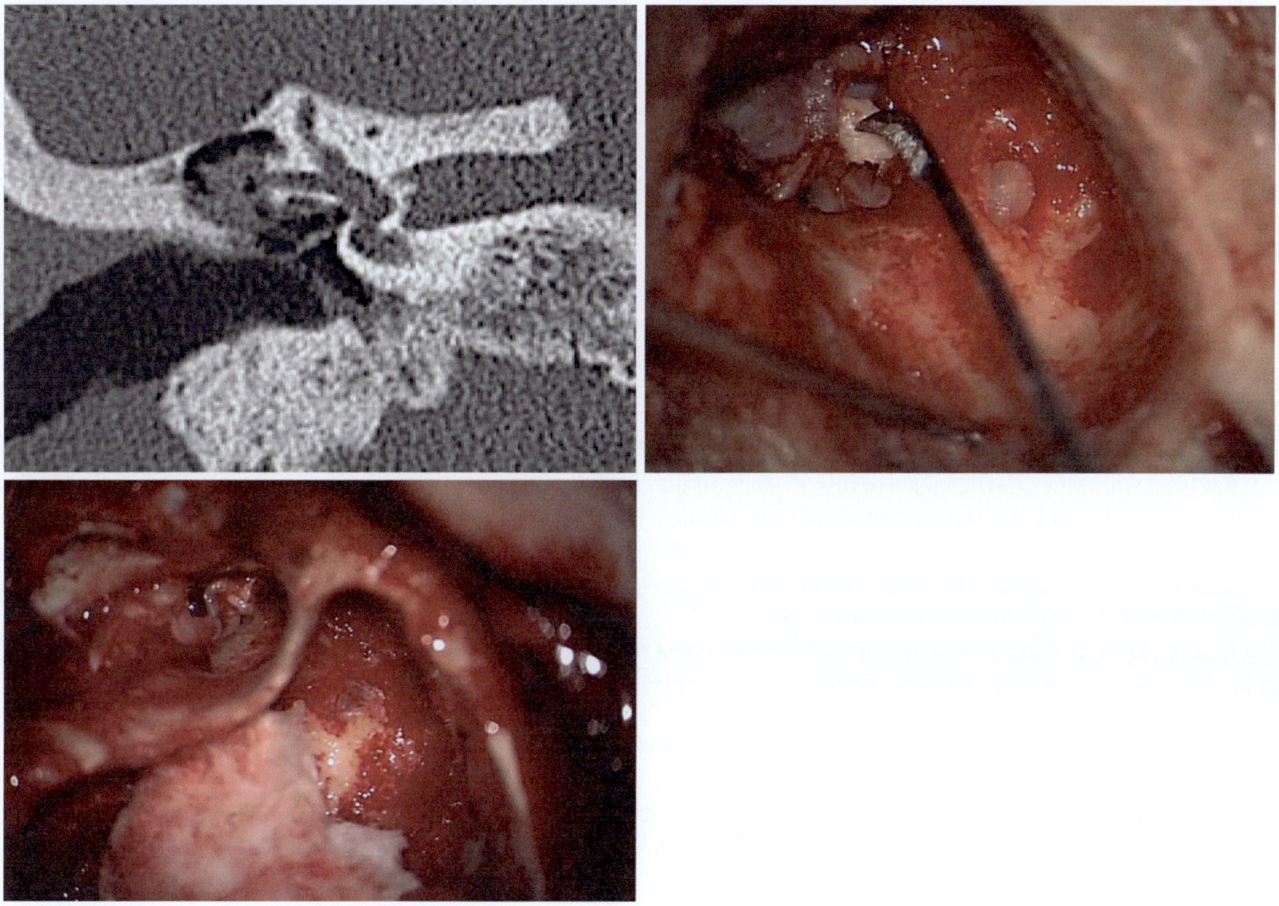

Fig. 42.31 CT scan image showing a cholesteatoma filling the antrum and eroding the lateral semicircular canal. Transoperative image of same finding with the membranous labyrinth ballooning thorugh the bone

Table 42.5 Modified intraoperative classification of Dornhoffer and Milewski

Type	Description
TYPE I	Perilymphatic membrane covered with bone, i.e., blue line only
TYPE II	Perilymphatic membrane exposed
TYPE I	Perilymphatic membrane eroded onto organs or cholesteatoma inside the labyrinth

of labyrinth involvement, as described in Table 42.5 (modified from [167]). We only considered as LF the Stages II or III.

In eight patients, the fistula was first identified on image studies and confirmed at surgery (Fig. 42.31).

Interestingly, in patients with posterior epitympanic and two-route cholesteatomas, the prevalence was 5.0%; and in cases with remaining cholesteatoma growth patterns, the prevalence was 0.6% ($p = 0.16$). We think that this big difference can be explained by the fact that whenever the attic is primarily involved in the growth of a cholesteatoma, its natural expansion is toward the antrum, where it comes in contact with the most projecting limb of the posterior labyrinth or the LSC. The prevalence ratio for labyrinthine fistula between patients who reported vertigo before the surgery was twice as many as those who did not report.

CT is important in the preoperative identification of LF. In previous studies, CT showed 50% sensitivity in the diagnosis of LF. However, more recent studies have reported sensitivity between 85% and 100%, owing to high-resolution CT and thinner cuts (0.5 mm slices) [168–170].

CT is also able to predict the presence of a membranous fistula versus a bone fistula with sensitivity of 66% and specificity of 71% [170].

In our study population [166], high-resolution CT identified LF in all patients, which was confirmed at surgery. The high sensitivity and specificity in our study can be explained by the selection criteria, since we only included patients with LF Type II or Type III with evident bone erosion.

Currently, it has been our policy that a CT scan is mandatory for all patients prior to cholesteatoma surgery for the analyses of anatomic landmarks, disease extension, and mastoid pneumatization, and subsequently, selection of the optimal surgical technique.

Paralysis or Paresis of the Facial Nerve

Currently, paralysis or even paresis of the facial nerve (FN) are uncommon complications of cholesteatoma with an incidence ranging from 1% to 3.4% [171–173] but whenever present (partial or complete) it demands immediate attention and prompt treatment since any delay can lead to irreversible tragic sequelae and, also, other differential diagnosis must also be considered (tumor or an acute aggressive infection).

As pointed out by Psillas and Constantinidis [174], FP to cholesteatoma may have several causes and mechanisms injuring the nerve alone or in association: osteitis, bony erosion, direct pressure, or compression resulting from edema and inflammation of the nerve caused by bacteria or neurotoxic substances, secreted from the cholesteatoma matrix.

It has been shown that the facial nerve fills 35–65% of the fallopian canal (Fig. 42.32); the remaining portion is filled with extra neural blood vessels and connective tissue, without leaving any empty space [175]; thus, edema secondary to infection can easily affect the neural transmission.

It is very plausible that the structure of the fallopian canal could also play an important role in facilitating earlier neural damage. Thus, channels that present marked dehiscence are likely to render the nerve more vulnerable exposing the neural tunnel to toxins and potential compression from its periphery (Fig. 42.33).

Direct pressure on the facial nerve due to cholesteatoma has also been reported; however, FP was expected only after blockage of more than 50% of facial nerve fibers. In slowly evolving facial palsy, the most likely etiology is erosion of the fallopian canal with compression of the facial nerve (Fig. 42.34) (Psillas and Constantinidis) [174].

Pain

Pain is not a common complaint, so, when present, it should be approached carefully. An associated external otitis, an expanding mass of cholesteatoma, or a suppurative complication must be ruled out.

Polyps

The finding of a polyp in the external auditory canal (EAC) is often thought to be a manifestation of inflammatory middle ear disease. Also known as aural polyp (AP), it is usually characterized as a soft to rubbery reddish mass (1) within the external auditory canal, therefore, lateral to the tympanic membrane (Figs. 42.30, 42.35, and 42.36).

The type of chronic otitis media (COM) that first comes to mind for most otologists as the underlying cause for AP is cholesteatoma. Previous studies in the last decades estimated a great variability of cholesteatoma as the final diagnosis for polyps, with prevalence ranging from 25% to 88% [176].

We have carried out a cross-sectional study with patients with unilateral or bilateral aural polyps. A total of 2432 patients were evaluated, and 133 (5.4%) showed a polyp in the external auditory canal. CCOM (58%) and NCCOM (28.3%) were responsible for 86.3% of all polyps evaluated, and the majority of diagnoses were established through surgery (76.5%). Furthermore, we have found that symptoms associated with polyps and their aspect do not reveal the most probable etiologies making imaging exams, biopsy, and surgery necessary steps in aural polyp investigation. Concerning MEC, the frequency of the routes of formation was: 12 PEC, 12 PMC, 7 two-routes (both the pars flaccida

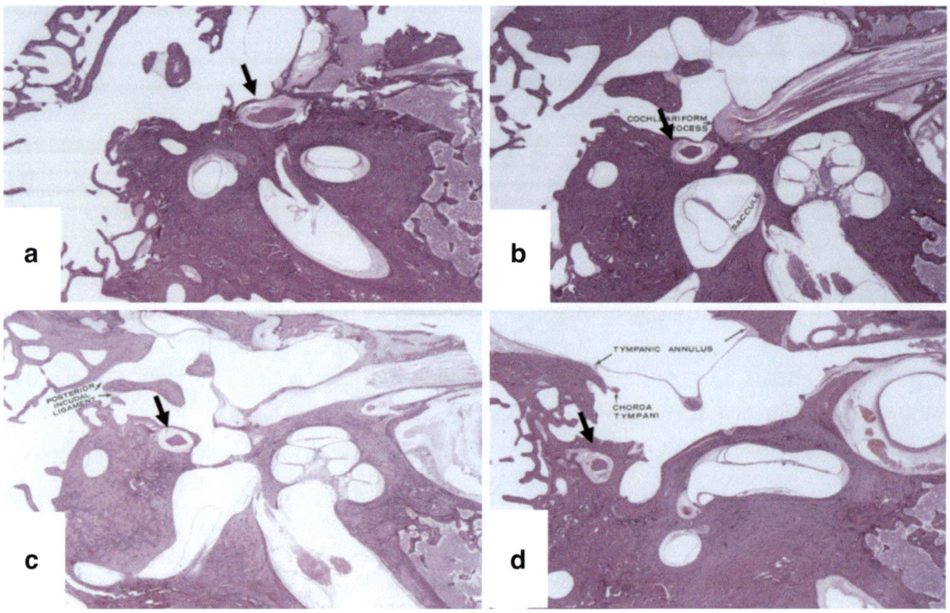

Fig. 42.32 Temporal bone sections with a normal anatomy. The facial nerve is found inside the fallopian canal (arrows) which is completely surrounded by bone. (**a**) Facial nerve inside the fallopian canal (**b**) Facial nerve and its relationship with the cochleariform process (**c**) Facial nerve and its relationship with the incus (**d**) Facial nerve in a view of the mesotympanum

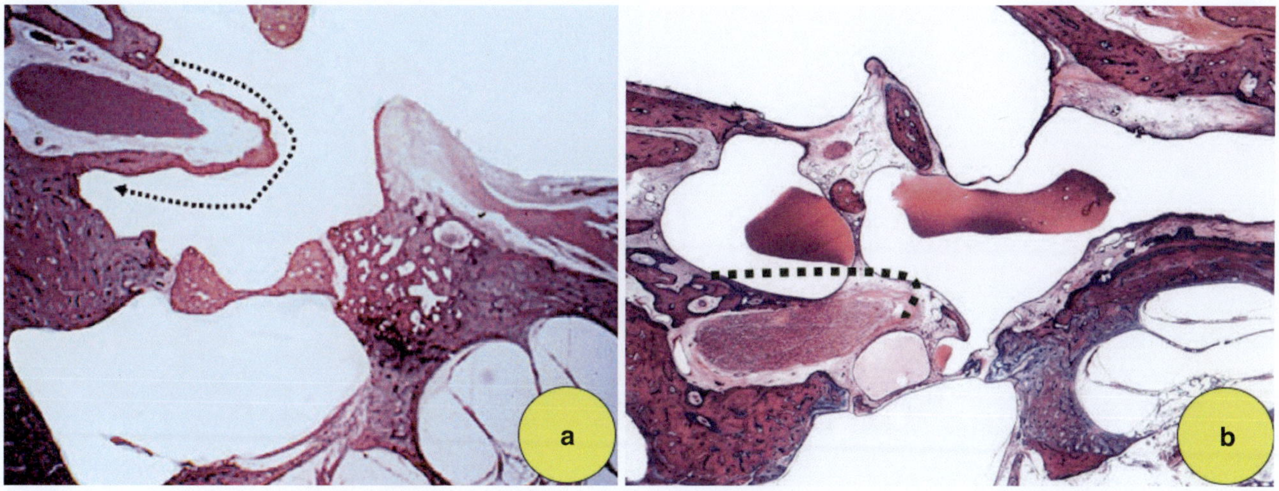

Fig. 42.33 (**a**) Temporal section at the level of the mesotympanum showing a prolapsed but not dehiscent facial nerve (dashed thin black line). (**b**) Temporal bone section showing a dehiscent facial nerve at the same level prolapsing over the oval window niche

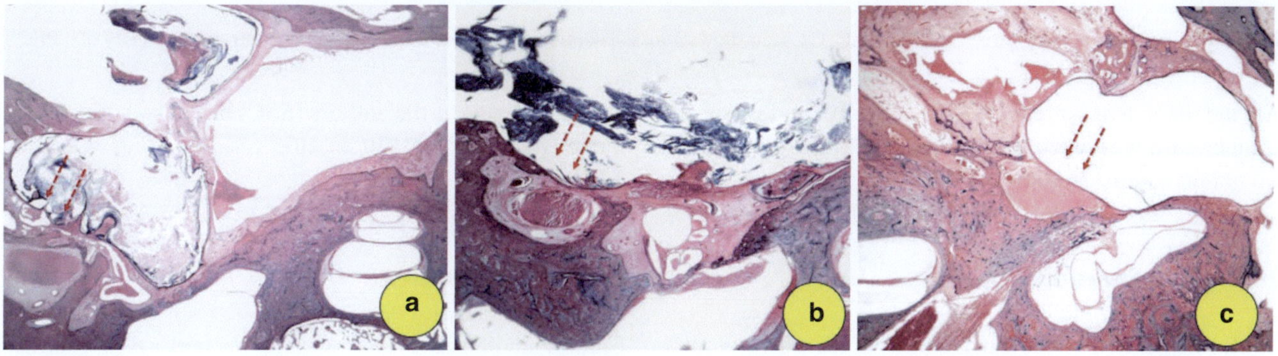

Fig. 42.34 (**a**) A cholesteatoma occupying the posterior recess of the mesotympanum destroying the incus and suprastructure of the stapes but set apart from the facial nerve by a dense layer of bone (red dashed arrows). (**b**) A massive cholesteatoma eroding the facial canal, but the nerve is not yet compressed (red dashed arrows). (**c**) A massive cholesteatoma eroding the facial canal and compressing the facial nerve (red dashed arrows).

Fig. 42.35 Right ear showing the presence of an inflammatory polyp protruding in the EAC pre (**a**) and post (**b**) cauterization with trichloroacetic acid

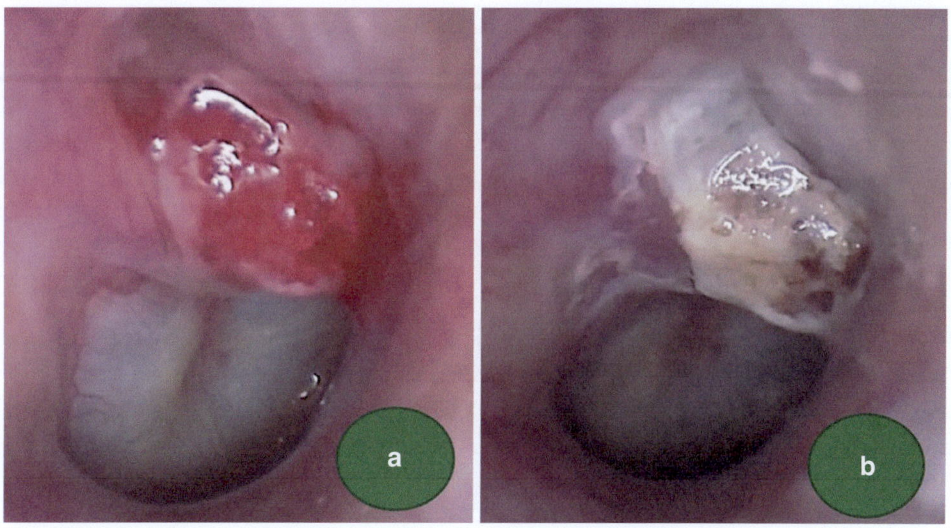

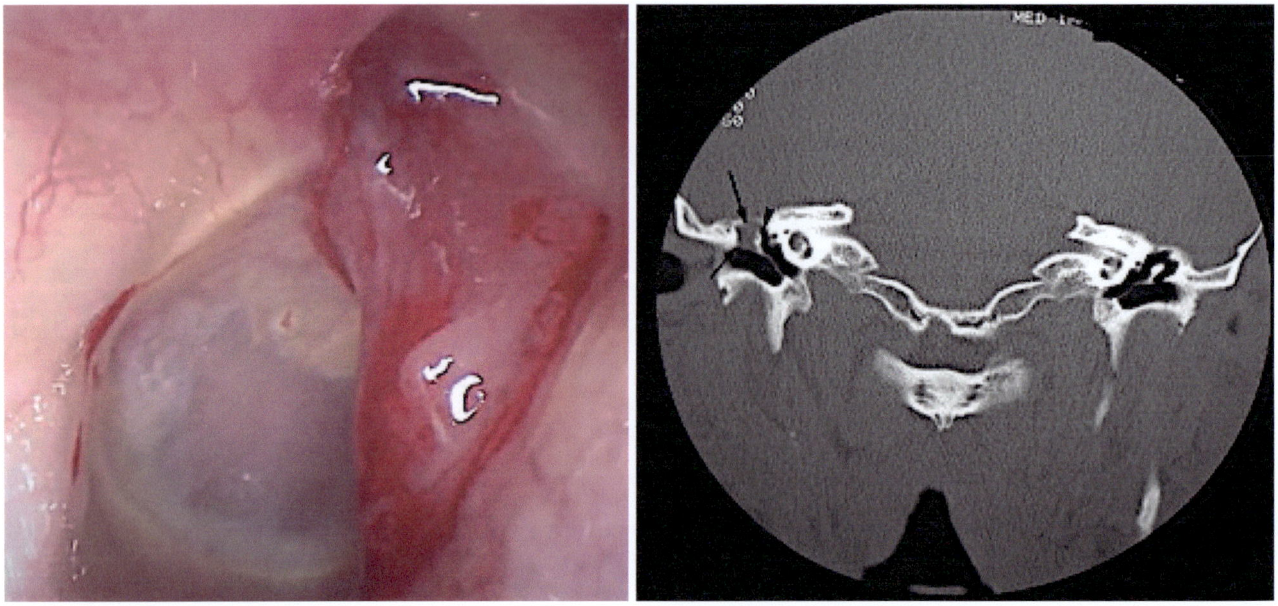

Fig. 42.36 Right ear polyp protruding to the EAC. CT scan shows a mass lateral to the neck and head of malleus (arrows) typically of a PEC

and the pars tensa are involved), and 10 undetermined. Another case was classified as congenital, and five patients had not undergone surgery.

Otologic Evaluation

Careful inspection of the ear includes at least an examination under magnification with the surgical microscope. An otoendoscope can be helpful in reaching hidden recesses of the temporal bone in follow-up of an open cavity. This tool is of particular importance in cases presenting a pars flaccida cholesteatoma. Sometimes, even the otomicroscopy may overlook a silent erosion of the scutum due to the straight field of vision of the microscope. The endoscope penetrating deeper in the ear canal will never miss a finding like this (Fig. 42.37a, b).

The whole 360° of the TM should be inspected, but special care is dedicated to the pars flaccida, the area near the attic, and the posterosuperior quadrant. Besides discharge (discussed earlier), one should note the pattern of perforation and the status of mucosa in the middle ear. A test for fistula should be used when vertigo or dizziness is present. A patch test and a test of the ET, with rare exceptions, are excluded from the authors' workup.

During the otomicroscopy, the canal should be meticulously cleansed all secretions, debris, and cerume. Special attention should be paid to the pars flacida area where not rarely small perforations may be covered by dried crusts. In this regard, one of the authors (SSC) has an aphorism which incites to "never trust in an attic cerume" (Figs. 42.38 and 42.39a, b).

Hearing Evaluation

Careful audiometric tests should be performed routinely. These findings must be compared with those of the basic tests with tuning forks performed by the otologist. The audiometric battery should include pure-tone bone/air conduction thresholds, speech-reception levels, and speech discrimination scores. Results of these more sophisticated tests must always coincide with results of the tuning fork test. Because the authors rarely order a test of ET function in their routine, tympanometry and tests of acoustic reflex are performed only in the presence of an intact TM. Erosion of the ossicles (particularly the long process of the incus) or fixation raises the hearing loss to 30 dB or more. Interestingly, some cholesteatomas can destroy the ossicular chain but still preserve good hearing. In these situations, the cholesteatoma can transmit the sound from the external ear to the oval window in a so-called columellar effect (Fig. 42.25).

Radiologic Evaluation

The imaging evaluation of patients with COM is not always necessary and should be adapted according to clinical find-

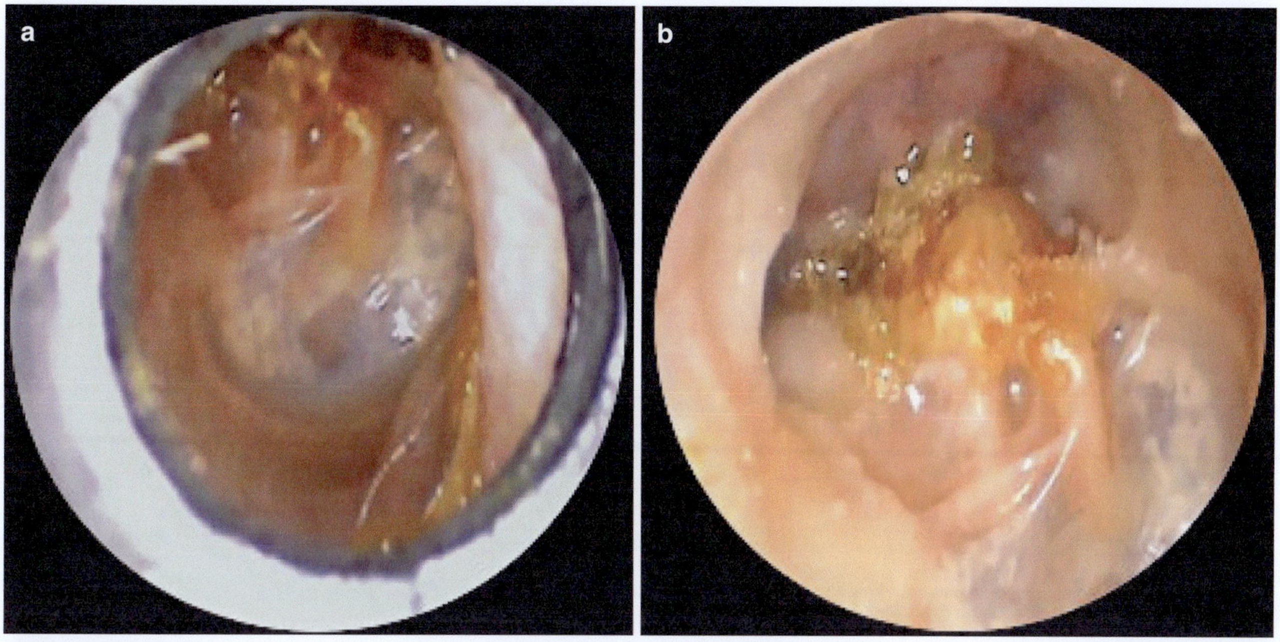

Fig. 42.37 (**a**) Tympanic membrane visualized through the microscope. (**b**) The same ear examined with the aid of a 30° endoscope. The extension of the pars flaccida retraction is fully appreciated

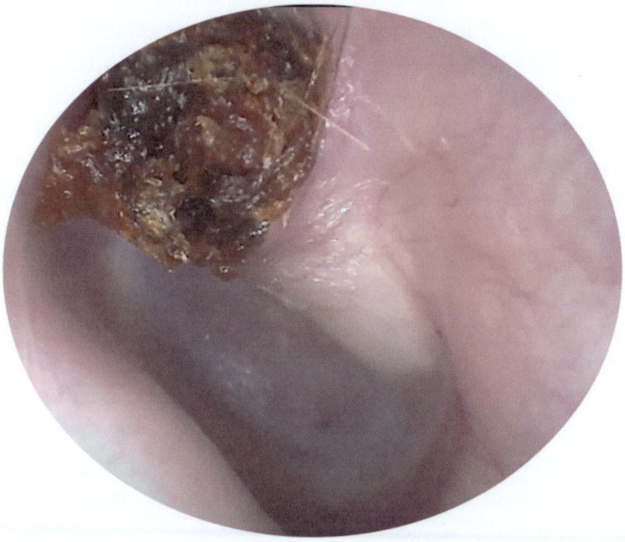

Fig. 42.38 A crust placed superiorly in the fundus of the EAC preventing the inspection of the TM pars flacidda. Notice a whitish mass extending through the posterior pouch of Von Troeltsch to the mesotympanum

ings. In the authors' routine, they dispense with further investigations in patients without cholesteatoma and who present with dry, central perforation and good hearing (small air–bone gap).

A CT scan is mandatory for all with marginal perforations, retraction pockets, an air–bone gap of >25 dB, and all cholesteatomas, regardless its size. Of course, also there's no doubt about ordering CT when we are facing large cholesteatomas, gross bony erosions, exuberant granulation tissue filling the external canal and preventing visualization of structures within the middle ear, chronic silent otitis media, unilateral marked hearing loss, suspicion of malignancy of the temporal bone, or presence of complications.

For cholesteatoma evaluation and planning of the surgery, including the surgical technique, the authors developed a checklist for the CT scan, which will be analyzed both in the axial and coronal plans. Also, the plane of Pöschl (in the same plane as the superior semicircular canal) must be available for the surgeon in the planning. Our checklist is detailed in Table 42.6.

Our group published an interesting case report, which emphasizes the role of the CT in the surgical planning [177]. Figure 42.40 shows a typical posterior mesotympanic cholesteatoma, with an air–bone gap compatible with the disease. The authors firmly believe that, at the present time, there is no reason to perform cholesteatoma surgery without ordering a CT scan. This way the images of the same patient (Fig. 42.41) show an ectopic carotid artery, which leads to an anatomical obstruction of the eustachian tube. We can conclude that there was a clear relationship between the displacement of the carotid artery, the obstruction of the ET, middle ear gas deprivation, and the further retraction of the TM leading to cholesteatoma formation. It appears unequivocal that the sealing of the protympanum by the artery led to TM invagination, keratin accumulation, and infection.

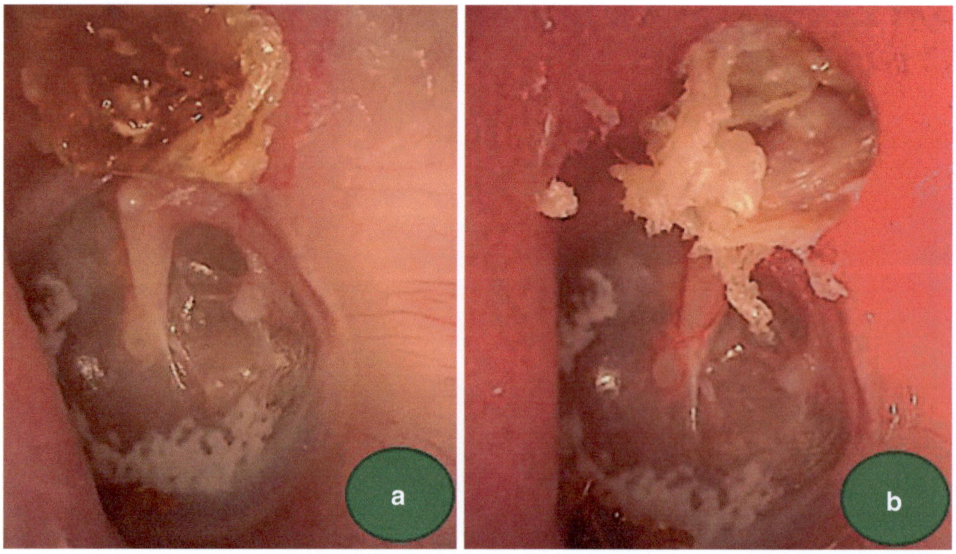

Fig. 42.39 (**a**) A crust placed superiorly in the fundus of the EAC preventing the inspection of the TM pars flacidda. (**b**) After careful removal with the aid of a microscope and adequate instrumentation, the opening of typical pars flaccida cholesteatoma is identified

Table 42.6 Checklist cholesteatoma evaluation on CT

• Degree of mastoid pneumatization
• Erosion of the lateral wall of the attic
• Course of the facial nerve
• Ossicular chain status
• Tegmen timpani and dural dehiscence
• Anatomical variations
• Integrity of bony labyrinth (fistulas)
• Relation to the great vessels (jugular bulb and carotid artery)
• Position of the lateral sinus
• Aeration of the protympanum

In conclusion, through the analysis of one single case, two important concepts emerge:

1. ET dysfunction may play a decisive role in the pathogenesis of COM, at least in the earlier phases of the process;
2. Temporal bone CT scan is affirmed as an extremely important step in surgical planning. It has the ability to show the extent of the disease, to influence the surgical technique employed, and it can help an informed surgeon anticipate intraoperative difficulties.

Magnetic resonance imaging (MRI) has improved cholesteatoma detection rates considerably in the past decade and can be ordered in specific situations. Accurately predicting disease location and extension is essential for staging, planning, and preoperative counseling. Also, considering the second-look for wall-up tympanomastoidectomies, MRI improved sensitivity and specificity and may allow the surgeon to confidently monitor patients, therefore avoiding unnecessary surgery. While the CT is not able to differentiate granulation tissue from cholesteatoma, in the MRI the former enhances intensely with gadolinium on T1-weighted images, while the last does not enhance with gadolinium.

Regardless of the site of origin or etiologic basis, cholesteatomas do not enhance with gadolinium unless infiltrated by granulation tissue. This is a helpful differential diagnostic point that distinguishes these pathologic conditions from other retrotympanic masses, such as paragangliomas or schwannomas.

Cholesterol granuloma on CT scan is nonspecific and similar to that of typical granulation tissue. Magnetic resonance imaging is diagnostic because extracellular methemoglobin within the lesion results in a bright signal in all spin-echo pulse sequence.

There is a specific chapter about the Radiologic Evaluation in COM later in this book, where this issue will be larged explored.

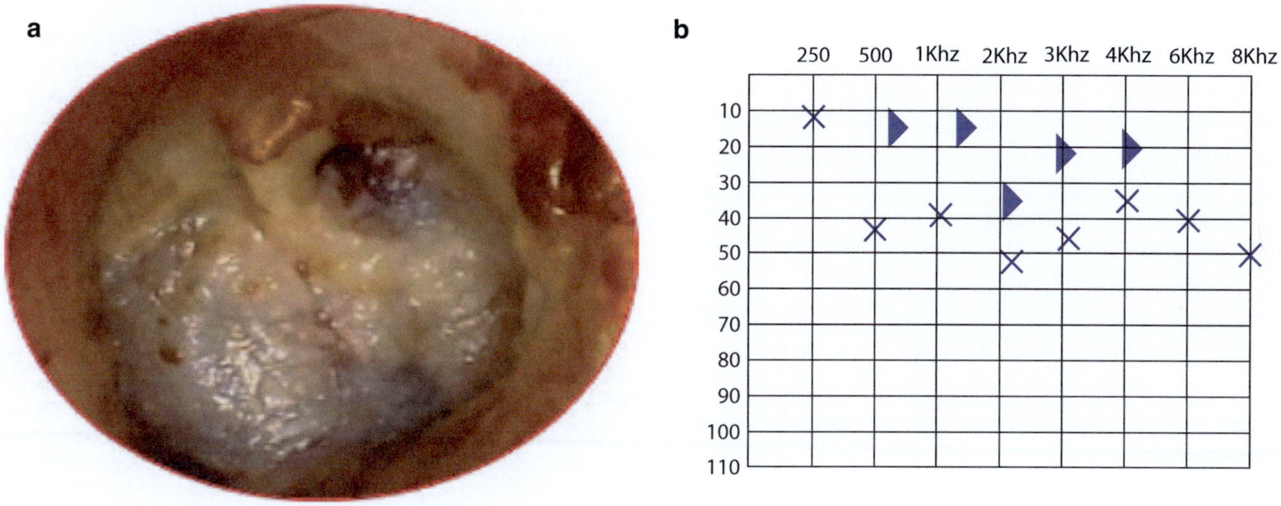

Fig. 42.40 (**a**) Posterior mesotympanic cholesteatoma. (**b**) Audiogram of the same patient, with an air–bone gap compatible with the ossicular chain destruction

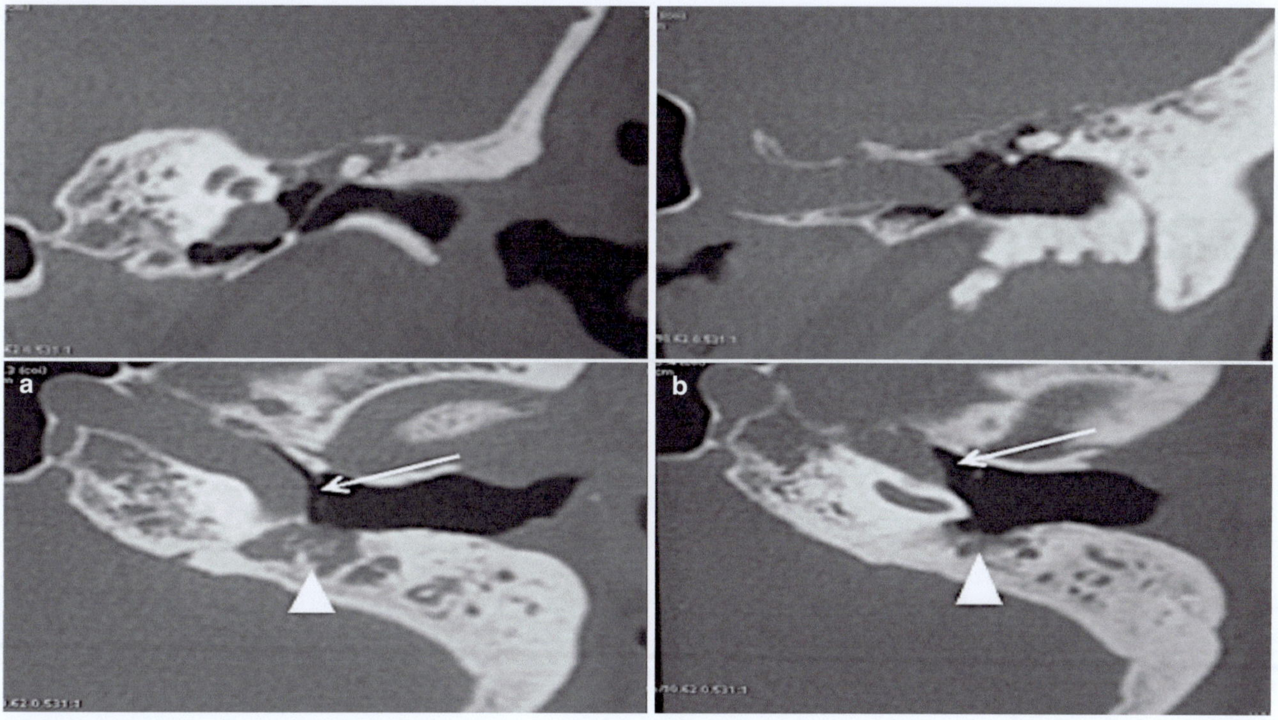

Fig. 42.41 The ectopic carotid artery causing an obstruction of the eustachian tube. (**a**) Ectopic carotid artery (long white arrow) blocking the eustachian tube. Posterior recesses filled with soft tissue density material (white arrow head). (**b**) the same, showing the relationship with the cochlea

Complications

Complications of otitis media can be divided into intratemporal and extratemporal and are processed by three basic mechanisms:

(a) extension by preformed spaces,
(b) bone erosion;
(c) osteothrombophlebitis.

These complications will be studied in a specific chapter.

Treatment

The treatment of chronic cholesteatomatous otitis media is essentially surgical. The primary objective is the complete eradication of the disease, providing the patient with a dry ear and safe from complications. The secondary objective, but no less important, is the preservation or improvement of the function of the tympanossicular system, when this is possible [178, 179].

This subject will be extensively explored in later chapters of this book.

References

1. Cruz OL, Costa SS. Clinical and surgical otology. EdRevinter; 1999.
2. Friedmann I. Epidermoid cholesteatoma and granuloma. Ann OtolRhinolLaryngol. 1959;68:57–9.
3. Schuknecht HF. The pathology of the ear. Cambridge: Harvard University; 1974.
4. Ferlito O, Devaney KO, Rinaldo A, Milroy C, Wenig B, Iurato S, Mccabe BF. Clinicopathological consultation ear cholesteatoma versus cholesterol granuloma. Ann OtholRhinolLaryngol. 1997;106:79–85.
5. Aquino JE, Cruz Filho NA, de Aquino JN. Epidemiology of middle ear and mastoid cholesteatomas: study of 1146 cases. Braz J Otorhinolaryngol. 2011;77:341–7. https://doi.org/10.1590/S1808-86942011000300012.
6. Bennett M, Warren F, Jackson GC. Congenital cholesteatoma: theories, facts and 53 patients. Otolaryngol Clin N Am. 2006;39:1081–94. https://doi.org/10.1016/j.otc.2006.08.001.
7. Shohet JA, De Jong AI. The management of pediatric cholesteatoms. Otolaryngol Clin N Am. 2002;35:841–51. https://doi.org/10.1016/S0030-6665(02)00052-X.
8. Olszewska E, Wagner M, Bernal-Sprekelsen M, et al. Etiopathogenesis of cholesteatoma. Eur Arch Otorhinolaryngol. 2004a;261:6–24. https://doi.org/10.1007/s00405-003-0623-x.
9. Olszewska E, Wagner M, Bernal-Sprekelsen M, Ebmeyer J, Dazert S, Hildmann H, Sudhoff H. Etiopathogenesis of cholesteatoma. Eur Arch Otorhinolaryngol. 2004b;261(1):6–24.
10. Barath K, Huber AM, Stampfil P, et al. Neuroradiology of cholesteatomas. AJNR Am J Neuroradiol. 2011;32:221–9. https://doi.org/10.3174/ajnr.A2052.
11. Jennings BA, Prinsley P, Philpott C, et al. The genetics of cholesteatoma. A systematic review using narrative synthesis. Clin Otolaryngol. 2017;43:55–67. https://doi.org/10.1111/coa.12900.
12. Bois E, Nassar M, Zenaty D, et al. Otologic disorders in Turner syndrome. Eur Ann Otorhinolaryngol Head Neck Dis. 2017;135:21–4. https://doi.org/10.1016/j.anorl.2017.08.006.
13. Hall JE, Richter GT, Choo DI. Surgical management of otologic disease in pediatric patients with Turner syndrome. Int J PediatrOtorhinolaryngol. 2009;73:57–65. https://doi.org/10.1016/j.ijporl.2008.09.022.
14. Lim DBN, Gault EJ, Kubba H, et al. Cholesteatoma has a high prevalence in Turner syndrome, highlighting the need for earlier diagnosis and the potential benefits of otoscopy training for paediatricians. Acta Paediatr. 2014;103:e282–7. https://doi.org/10.1111/apa.12450.
15. Mann W, Al-Nawas B, Wriedt S. Cholesteatoma of the hypotympanum in a patient with Treacher Collins syndrome. Auris Nasus Larynx. 2014;41:101–4. https://doi.org/10.1016/j.anl.2013.05.005.
16. Bacciu A, Pasanisi E, Vincenti V, et al. Surgical treatment of middle ear cholesteatoma in children with Down syndrome. OtolNeurotol. 2005;26:1007–10. https://doi.org/10.1097/01.mao.0000185042.46523.9b.
17. Nash R, Possamai V, Maskell S, et al. Canal wall reconstruction and preservation in the surgical management of cholesteatoma in children with Down's syndrome. Int J PediatrOtorhinolaryngol. 2014;78:1747–51. https://doi.org/10.1016/j.ijporl.2014.07.038.
18. Paulson LM, Weaver TS, Macarthur CJ. Outcomes of tympanostomy tube placement in children with Down syndrome—a retrospective review. Int J PediatrOtorhinolaryngol. 2014;78:223–6. https://doi.org/10.1016/j.ijporl.2013.10.062.
19. Suzuki C, Ohtani I. Bone destruction resulting from rupture of a cholesteatoma sac: temporal bone pathology. OtolNeurotol. 2004;25:674–7. https://doi.org/10.1097/00129492-200409000-00005.
20. Büchner SA, Itin P. Focal dermal hypoplasia syndrome in a male patient. Report of a case and histologic and immunohistochemical studies. Arch Dermatol. 1992;128:1078–82. https://doi.org/10.1001/archderm.1992.01680180072008.
21. Djurhuus BD, Skytthe A, Faber CE, Christensen K. Cholesteatoma risk in 8593 orofacial cleft cases and 6989 siblings: a nationwide study. Laryngoscope. 2015;125:1225–9. https://doi.org/10.1002/lary.25022.
22. Harris L, Cushing SL, Hubbard B, et al. Impact of cleft palate type on the incidence of acquired cholesteatoma. Int J PediatrOtorhinolaryngol. 2013;77:695–8. https://doi.org/10.1016/j.ijporl.2013.01.020.
23. Imbery TE, Sobin LB, Commesso E, et al. Long-term otologic and audiometric outcomes in patients with cleft palate. Otolaryngol Head Neck Surg. 2017;157:676–82. https://doi.org/10.1177/0194599817707514.
24. James AL, Papsin BC. Some considerations in congenital cholesteatoma. CurrOpinOtolaryngol Head Neck Surg. 2013;21:431–9. https://doi.org/10.1097/MOO.0b013e328364b457.
25. Kopcsányi G, Vincze O, Bagdán V, et al. Retrospective analysis of tympanoplasty in children with cleft palate: a 24-year experience. II. Cholesteatomatous cases. Int J PediatrOtorhinolaryngol. 2015;79:698–706. https://doi.org/10.1016/j.ijporl.2015.02.020.
26. Kuo CL, Lien CF, Chu CH, et al. Otitis media with effusion in children with cleft lip and palate: a narrative review. Int J PediatrOtorhinolaryngol. 2013;77:1403–9. https://doi.org/10.1016/j.ijporl.2013.07.015.
27. Lau CC, Loh KK, Kunaratnam N. Middle ear diseases in cleft palate patients in Singapore. Ann Acad Med Singap. 1988;17:372–4.
28. Kuo CL, Shiao AS, Wen HC, et al. Increased risk of cholesteatoma among patients with allergic rhinitis: a nationwide investigation. Laryngoscope. 2017;128:547–53. https://doi.org/10.1002/lary.26220.
29. Derlacki EL, Clemis JD. Congenital cholesteatoma of the middle ear and mastoid. Ann OtholRhinolLaryngol. 1965;74:706–27.

30. Valvassori GE. Benign tumors of the temporal bone. Radiol Clin N Am. 1974;12:533–42.
31. Sobol SM. Intramembranous and mesotympanic cholesteatomas associated with an intact tympanic membrane in children. Ann Othol. 1980;98:312–7.
32. Costa SS, Hueb MM, Ruschel C. Chronic cholesteatomatous otitis media. In: Cruz OL, Costa SS, editors. Clinical and surgical otology. Ed. Revinter; 1999.
33. Meyerhoff WL, Truelson J. Cholesteatoma staging. Laryngoscope. 1986;96:935–9.
34. Tos M. Incidence, etiology and pathogenesis of cholesteatoma in children: a long-term study of results. OtholRhinolLaryngol. 1988;40:110–7.
35. Saleh HA, Mills RP. Classification and staging of cholesteatoma. Clin Otolaryngol. 1999;24:355–9.
36. Wullstein H. Theory and practice of tympanoplasty. Laryngoscope. 1956;66(8):1076–93. https://doi.org/10.1288/00005537-195608000-00008.
37. Austin DF. Types and indications of staging. Arch Otolaryngol. 1969;89(2):235–42. https://doi.org/10.1001/archotol.1969.00770020237005.
38. Yung M, Tono T, Olszewska E, Yamamoto Y, Sudhoff H, Sakagami M, Mulder J, Kojima H, İncesulu A, Trabalzini F, Özgirgin N. EAONO/JOS Joint Consensus Statements on the Definitions, Classification and Staging of Middle Ear Cholesteatoma. J Int Adv Otol. 2017;13(1):1–8. https://doi.org/10.5152/iao.2017.3363.
39. Lim DJ, Saunders WE. A cquired cholesteatoma: light and electron microscopic observations. Ann Otol. 1972;81:2–12.
40. Paludetti G, Alamadori G, Ottaviani F, Rosignoli M, Rossodivita M, D'Alatri L. Ultrastructural aspects of cholesteatoma of the middle ear. Acta Otorhinolaryngol Ital. 1989;9(2):169–80.
41. Milewski C, Fedorowski A, Stan AC, Walter GF. Basic fibroblast growth factor (b-FGF) in the perimatrix of cholesteatoma. HNO. 1998;46(9):804–8.
42. Sprekelsen BM, Ebmeyer J, Anonopoulos A, Sudhoff H. Basement membrane alterations in the middle ear cholesteatoma. Acta OtorEsp. 2001;52:330–5.
43. Jacob R, Welkoborsky HJ, Mann W. Epithelium-stroma interaction in cholesteatoma of the middle ear. Laryngorhinootologie. 2001;80(1):11–7.
44. Hamzei M, Ventriglia G, Hagnia M, Antonopolus A, Bernal-Sprekelson M, Dazert S, Hildmann H, Sudhoff H. Osteoclast stimulating and differentiating factors in human cholesteatoma. Laryngoscope. 2003;113(3):436–42.
45. DornellesC, CostaSS, MeurerL, CoelhoA, Cursino, A. Correlation between clinical inflammation and perimatrix thickness of acquired cholesteatomas. HCPA On-Line Magazine, 2004. www.hcpa.ufrgs.br.
46. Cristina Dornelles, Sady S. da Costa, Luíse Meurer, Cláudia Schweiger. Some considerations about acquired adult and pediatric cholesteatomas. Rev. Bras. Otorrinolaringol. 2005;71(4). https://doi.org/10.1590/S0034-72992005000400023.
47. Frankel S, Berson S, Godwin T, Han JC, Parisier SC. Differences in dendritic cells in congenital and acquired cholesteatomas. Laryngoscope. 1993;103(11 Pt 1):1214–7. doi: https://doi.org/10.1288/00005537-199311000-00002.
48. Junqueira LC, Carneiro J. Basic histology. Rio de Janeiro: Publisher Guanabara; 1985.
49. Vennix PP, Kuijpers W, Peters TA, Tonnaer EL, Ramaekers FC. Keratinocyte differentiation in acquired cholesteatoma and perforated tympanic membranes. Arch Otolaryngol Head Neck Surg. 1996;122:825–32.
50. Albino AP, Reed JA, Bogdany JK, Sassoon J, Desloge RB, Parisier SC. Expression of p53 protein in human middle ear cholesteatomas: pathogenetic implications. Am J Otol. 1998a;19(1):30–6.
51. Desloge RB, Carew JF, Finstad CL, Steiner MG, Sassoon J, Levenson MJ, Staiano-Coico L, Parisier SC, Albino AP. DNA analysis of human cholesteatomas. Am J Otol. 1997;18(2):155–9.
52. Shinoda H, Huang CC. Expressions of c- jun and p53 proteins in human middle ear cholesteatoma: relationship to keratinocyte proliferation, differentiation and programmed cell death. Laryngoscope. 1995;105(11):1232–7.
53. Bujia J, Schiling V, Holly A, Stammberger M, Kastenbauer E. Hyperproliferation-associated keratin expression in human middle ear cholesteatoma. Acta Otolaryngol. 1993;113:364–8.
54. Kuijpers W, Vernnix PP, Peters TA, Ramaekers FC. Squamous metaplasia of the middle ear epithelium. Acta Otolaryngol. 1996;116:293–8.
55. Moll R, Franke VW, Schiller DL. The catalog of human cytokeratins: patterns of expression in normal epithelia, tumors and cultured cells. Cell. 1982;31:11–24.
56. Pereira CSB. Analysis of studies on the expression of cytokeratins in acquired cholesteatoma. Masters dissertation. Faculty of Medical Sciences of Santa Casa de São Paulo; 1997.
57. Kim CS, Chung JW. Morphologic and biologic changes of experimentally induced cholesteatoma in Mongolian gerbils with anticytokeratin and lectin study. Am J Otol. 1999;20(1):13–8.
58. Lepercque S, Broekaert D, Van Cowwenberge P. Cytokeratin expression patterns in the human tympanic membrane and external ear canal. Eur Arch Otorhinolaryngol. 1993;250:78–81.
59. Broekaert D, Coucke P, Lepercque S, Ramaekers F, Van Muijen G, Boedts D, Leigh I, Lane B. Immunohistochemical analysis of the Cytokeratin expression in middle ear cholesteatoma and related epithelial tissues. Ann OtholRhinolLaryngol. 1992;101:931–8.
60. Pereira CSB, Almeida CIR, Viana MR. Immunoexpression of cytokeratin 16 and nuclear antigen Ki-67 in acquired middle ear cholesteatoma. Rev Bras Otorhinolaryngol. 2002;68(4):453–60.
61. Piltcher O. A new experimental model for the investigation of otitis media with effusion and its application in the study of cytokines during the different phases of this disease. Doctoral thesis. Faculty of Medical Sciences of Santa Casa de São Paulo, 2000.
62. Milewski C. Role of perimatrix fibroblast in development of acquired middle ear cholesteatoma. The hypothesis. HNO. 1998;46(5):494–501.
63. Aumente PO, Bujía J, Kim C, Jiménez Giménez J, López VP. Estudiocuantitativo de la presencia de interleucina-1 e interleucina-6 en elcolesteatoma de oído medio [A quantitative study of the presence of interleukin-1 and interleukin-6 in cholesteatoma of the middle ear]. Acta OtorrinolaringolEsp. 1996;47(4):259–62.
64. Bujia J, Kim C, Ostos P, Kastenbauer E, Hultner L. Role of interleukin 6 in epithelial hyper proliferation and bone resorption in middle ear cholesteatomas. Eur Arch Otorhinolaryngol. 1996b;253(3):152–7.
65. Tomita S. Molecular aspects of cholesteatoma—immunoexpression of cell cycle controlled proteins: p53, BAX and BCL-2. SP Doctoral Thesis. School Paulista de Medicina, 2000.
66. Sudhoff H, Borkowski G, Bujia J, Hildmann H. Immunhistochemis tryUntersuchungen von MittelohrschleimhautrestenimCholesteatom. HNO. 1997;45(8):630–5.
67. Sudhoff H, Dazert S, Gonzales AM, Borkowski G, Park SY, Baird A, Hildmann H, Ryan AF. Angiogenesis and angiogenic growth factors in middle ear cholesteatoma. Am J Otol. 2000;21:793–8.
68. Chole RA, Faddis BT. Evidence for microbial biofilms in cholesteatomas. Arch Otolaryngol Head Neck Surg. 2002;128:1129–33.
69. Yamamoto-Fukuda T, Takahashi H, Koji T. Animal models of middle ear cholesteatoma. J Biomed Biotechnol. 2011;2011:394241. https://doi.org/10.1155/2011/394241.
70. Chole RA, Henry KR, McGinn MD. Cholesteatoma: spontaneous occurrence in the Mongolian gerbil Merionesunguiculatis. Am J Otol. 1981;2(3):204–10.

71. Chole RA, Chiu M. Ultrastructure of middle earmucosa in the mongolian gerbil. MerionesunguiculatusActa Oto-Laryngol. 1985;100(3–4):273–88.
72. Schmidt SH, Hellstrom S. Experimental cholesteatoma in the rat. Acta Otolaryngol. 1994a;114(4):430–4.
73. Schmidt SH, Hellstrom S. Experimental cholesteatoma in the rat. Acta Otolaryngol (Stockh). 1994b;114:430–4.
74. Friedmann I. The comparative pathology of otitis media,experimental and human—II. The histopathology of experimental otitis of the guinea-pig with particular reference to experimental cholesteatoma. J LaryngolOtol. 1955a;69(9):588–601.
75. Friedmann I. Comparative pathology of otitis media: experimental and human. II. The histopathology of experimental otitis with particular references to experimental cholesteatoma. J LaryngolOthol. 1955b;69:588–601.
76. Wolfman DE, Chole RA. Experimental retractionpocket cholesteatoma. Ann OtolRhinolLaryngol. 1986a;95(6I):639–44.
77. Wolfman DE, Chole RA. Experimental retraction pocket cholesteatoma. Ann OtholRhinolLaryngol. 1986b;95:639–44.
78. Vennix PPCA, Kuijpers W, Peters TA, Tonnaer ELGM, Ramaekers FCS. Growth and differentiation of meatal skin grafts in the middle ear of the rat. Arch Otolaryngol—Head Neck Surg. 1994;120(10):1102–11.
79. McGinn MD, Chole RA, Henry KR. Cholesteatoma.Experimental Induction in the Mongolian Gerbil, MeirionesUnguiculaus. Acta Otolaryngol (Stockh). 1982a;93:61–7.
80. McGinn MD, Chole RA, Henry KR. Cholesteatona. Experimental induction in the Mongolian gerbil, *Merionesunguiculatus*. Acta Otolaryngol. 1982b;93:61–7.
81. Wright CG, Meyerhoff WL, Burns DK. Middle ear cholesteatoma: an animal model. Am J Otolaryngol. 1985a;6(5):327–41. https://doi.org/10.1016/s0196-0709(85)80010-7.
82. Huve FDC, Bauer JA, Selaimen FA, Silva MNLD, Costa SSD. Experimental cholesteatoma: a comparison between spontaneous and induced models. Braz J Otorhinolaryngol. 2023;89(1):73–8. https://doi.org/10.1016/j.bjorl.2021.09.003.
83. Bauer JA, Huve FDC, Oliveira FH, Silva MNLD, Sperling N, Costa SSD. Mongolian Gerbils as a model for the study of cholesteatoma: otoendoscopic as a diagnostic tool. Int Arch Otorhinolaryngol. 2022;26(4):e643–8. https://doi.org/10.1055/s-0041-1740159.
84. Vassalli L, Harris DM, Gradini R, Applebaum EL. Propylene glycol-induced cholesteatoma in chinchilla middle ears. Am J Otolaryngol. 1988;9(4):180–8. https://doi.org/10.1016/s0196-0709(88)80026-7.
85. Huang CC, Shi GS, Yi ZX. Experimental inductionof middle ear cholesteatoma in rats. Am J Otolaryngol. 1988;9(4):165–72. https://doi.org/10.1016/s0196-0709(88)80024-3.
86. Meyerhoff WL, Wright CG, Gerken GM. Effects of middle ear ventilation on Cholesteatoma development in experimental animals. Acta Otolaryngol (Stockh). 1990;110:1990.
87. Pownell PH, Wright CG, Robinson KS, Meyerhoff WL. The effect of cyclophosphamide on development of experimental cholesteatoma. Arch Otolaryngol Head Neck Surg. 1994;120(10):1114–6.
88. Jove MA, Vassalli L, Raslan W, Applebaum EL. The effect of isotretinoin on propylene glycol-induced cholesteatoma in chinchilla middle ears. Am J Otolaryngol. 1990;11:5–9.
89. White SJ, Wright CG, Robinson KS, Meyerhoff WL. Effect of topical hyaluronic acid on experimental cholesteatoma. Am J Otolaryngol. 1995;16:312–8.
90. Wright CG, Bird LL, Meyerhoff WL. Effect of 5-fluorouracil in cholesteatoma development in an animal model. Am J Otolaryngol. 1991;12:133–8.
91. Masaki M, Wright CG, Lee DH, Meyerhoff WL. Experimental cholesteatoma. Epidermal ingrowth through Tympanic membrane following middle ear application of propylene. Glycol Acta Otolaryngol (Stockh). 1989;108:113–21.
92. Chole RA, Frush DP. Quantitative aspects of Eustachian tube epithelium during vitamin A deprivation and reversal. In: Sadé, editor. Cholesteatoma and mastoid surgery, 1982. Proceedings of the 2nd International Conference. Amsterdam: Kluger; 1982.
93. Minotti AM, Kountakis SE, Leighton WR, Cabral FR. Effects of extracellular calcium on cholesteatoma migration and adhesion in vitro. Otolaryngol Head Neck Surg. 1996;115(5):458–63.
94. Hueb MM. Acquired cholesteatoma: experimental advances in understanding its pathogenesis. Doctoral Thesis, Faculty of Medicine of the University of São Paulo, 1997.
95. Jackler RX. The surgical anatomy of cholesteatoma. Otolaryngol Clin N Am. 1989;22(5):883–96.
96. Cawthorne T, Griffith A. Primary cholesteatomata of the temporal bone Arch Otolaryngol. 1961;73:252–61. https://doi.org/10.1001/archotol.1961.00740020260002. PMID: 13691781.
97. Levenson MJ, Michaels L, Parisier SC. Congenital cholesteatomas in children and embryologic correlations. Laryngoscope. 1988;98:949–55.
98. Karmody CS, Byahatti SV, Blevins N, Valtonen H, Northrop C. The origin of congenital cholesteatoma. Am J Otol. 1998;19(3):292–7.
99. Huang J, Yi Z, Lin G. Altered cytokeratin expression of the epidermoid formation in the tympanic cavity of human fetuses. Chung Hua Erh Pi Yen Hou Ko TsaChih. 1996;31(2):72–4.
100. Jaisinghani VJ, Paparella MM, Schachern PA. Silent intratympanic membrane cholesteatoma. Laryngoscope. 1998;108:1185–9.
101. Kayhan FT, Mutlu C, Schachern PA, Le CT, Paparella MM. Significance of epidermoid formations in the middle ear in fetuses and children. Arch Otolaryngol Head Neck Surg. 1997;123(12):1293–7.
102. Gacek RR. Diagnosis and management of primary tumors of the petrous apex. Ann OtholRhinolLaryngol. 1975;84(Suppl. 18):1–20.
103. Reeves DL. Epidermoid [mixed] tumors of the central nervous system. J Neurosurg. 1976;26:21–4.
104. Souza CE, Souza R, Costa SS, et al. Cerebellopontine angle epidermoid cysts: a report on 30 cases. J Neurol Neurosurg Psychiatry. 1989;52:986–90.
105. MacKennan KX, Chole RA. Post-traumatic cholesteatoma. Laryngoscope. 1989;99:779–82.
106. Wendt H. Desquamative Entzündung des Mittelors Arch Heilk. 1873;14:428.
107. Birrell JF. Cholesteatosis of the attic. J LaryngolOthol. 1958;72:620–5.
108. Sadé J. The metaplastic and congenital origin of cholesteatoma. Acta Otolaryngol. 1983;96:119–29.
109. Sadé J, editor. Secretory otitis media and its sequelae. New York, Edinburgh, London: Churchill Livingstone; 1979.
110. Schechter G. A review of cholesteatoma pathology. Laryngoscopy. 1969;79:1907–20.
111. Ruedi L. Cholesteatosis of the attic. J LaryngolOtol. 1958;72:593.
112. Blitterswijk CA, Grote JJ, Lutgert RW, Hesse Ling SC, Out CJ, Muijen GNP, Fransen JAM. Cytokera tin patterns of tissues related to cholesteatoma pathogenesis. Ann OtholRhinolLaryngol. 1989;98:635–40.
113. Broekaert D, Van Oostveldt P, Coucke P, Reyniers P, Kluyskens P, Gillis E. Differentiation of nuclei during keratinization in middle ear cholesteatoma. DNA cytophotometry completed by computerized image analysis. Acta Otolaryngol. 1988;105(1–2):90–9. https://doi.org/10.3109/00016488809119450.
114. Haberman J. ZurEntstehung des Cholesteatoms des Mittelohrs. Arch Ohrenheilk. 1889;27:42–50.
115. Bezold FC. Perforation of the membrane saggy Shrapnell und Tubernverschluss. Zeitschr für Ohrenheilk. 1980;20:5–28.
116. Chao WY, Huang CC. An immunocytochemical study of cytokeratin expression in human middle ear cholesteatoma. Arch

Otorhinolaryngol. 1989;246(1):37–42. https://doi.org/10.1007/BF00454132.
117. Youngs R, Rowles P. The Spatial Organization of Keratinocytes in acquired middle ear cholesteatoma resembles that of external auditory canal skin and Pars Flacci da. Acta Otolaryngol (Stockh). 1990;1990(110):115–9.
118. Aberg B, Edström S, Johannesson A, Larko O. Evaluation of epidermal hyperproliferation in patients with cholesteatoma. Am J Otol. 1991;12:93–6.
119. Tos M. Upon the relationship between secretory otitis in childhood and its sequelae in adults. J LaryngolOthol. 1981;98:1011–22.
120. Ruedi L. Cholesteatoma formation in the middle in animal experiments. Acta Otolaryngol. 1959;50:233–42.
121. Chole RA, Tingling SP. Basal lamina breaks in the histogenesis of cholesteatoma. Laryngoscope. 1985;95:270–5.
122. Giacometti L. Cells in motion. Primate Netus. 1968;6:3–9.
123. Lim DJ, DeMaria TF. Panel discussion: pathogenesis of otitis media. Bacteriology and immunology Laryngoscope. 1982;92(3): 278–86. https://doi.org/10.1288/00005537-198203000-00011.
124. BezoldF.Textbook of otology; 1908.
125. Cassano M, Cassano P. Retraction pockets of pars tensa in pediatric patients: clinical evolution and treatment. Int J Pediatr Otorhinolaryngol 2010;74(2):178–182. doi: https://doi.org/10.1016/j.ijporl.2009.11.004. Epub 2009 Dec 3. PMID: 19962200.
126. Sadé J, Avraham S, Brown M. Atelectasis, retraction pockets and cholesteatoma. Acta Otolaryngol. 1981;92(5–6):501–12. https://doi.org/10.3109/00016488109133289.
127. Rosito LP, da Silva MN, Selaimen FA, Jung YP, Pauletti MG, Jung LP, Freitas LA, da Costa SS. Characteristics of 419 patients with acquired middle ear cholesteatoma. Braz J Otorhinolaryngol. 2017;83(2):126–31. https://doi.org/10.1016/j.bjorl.2016.02.013.
128. Monsell EM, Harley RE. Eustachian tube dysfunction. Otolaryngol Clin N Am. 1996;29(3):437–44.
129. Ars B, Wuyts F, Van de Heyning P, Miled I, Bogers J, Van Marck E. Histomorphometric study of the normal middle ear mucosa. Preliminary results supporting the gas-exchange function in the postero-superior part of the middle ear cleft. Acta Otolaryngol. 1997;117(5):704–7. https://doi.org/10.3109/00016489709113463.
130. Marchioni D, Piccinini A, Alicandri-Ciufelli M, Presutti L. Endoscopic anatomy and ventilation of the epitympanum. Otolaryngol Clin N Am. 2013;46(2):165–78. https://doi.org/10.1016/j.otc.2012.10.002.
131. Paço J, Branco C, Estibeiro H, Oliveira E, Carmo D. The posterosuperior quadrant of the tympanic membrane. Otolaryngol Head Neck Surg. 2009;140(6):884–8. https://doi.org/10.1016/j.otohns.2009.01.009.
132. Lim DJ. Structure and function of the tympanic membrane: a review. Acta OtorhinolaryngolBelg. 1995;49:101–15.
133. Lim DJ. Tympanic membrane: electron microscopic observations, part II: Pars flaccida. Acta Otolaryngol. 1968;66:515–32.
134. Bhide A. Etiology of the retraction pocket in the posterosuperior quadrant of the eardrum. Arch Otolaryngol. 1977;103(12):707–11. https://doi.org/10.1001/archotol.1977.00780290043004.
135. Sudhoff H, Tos M. Pathogenesis of sinus cholesteatoma. Eur Arch Otorhinolaryngol. 2007;264(10):1137–43. https://doi.org/10.1007/s00405-007-0340-y. Epub 2007 May 30
136. Jackler RK, Santa Maria PL, Varsak YK, Nguyen A, Blevins NH. A new theory on the pathogenesis of acquired cholesteatoma: mucosal traction. Laryngoscope. 2015;125(Suppl 4):S1–S14. https://doi.org/10.1002/lary.25261. Epub 2015 May 25
137. Jackler RK. Experimental evidence against middle ear oxygen absorption. Laryngoscope. 1985;95(10):1281–2. https://doi.org/10.1288/00005537-198510000-00031.
138. Black B, Gutteridge I. Acquired cholesteatoma: classification and outcomes. OtolNeurotol. 2011;32(6):992–5. https://doi.org/10.1097/MAO.0b013e3182255874.
139. Rosito LP, Teixeira AR, Netto LS, Selaimen FA, da Costa SS. Cholesteatoma growth patterns: are there audiometric differences between posterior epitympanic and posterior mesotympanic cholesteatoma? Eur Arch Otorhinolaryngol. 2016;273(10):3093–9. https://doi.org/10.1007/s00405-016-3918-4.
140. Potsic WP, Korman SB, Samadi DS, Wetmore RF. Congenital cholesteatoma: 20 years' experience at the Children's Hospital of Philadelphia. Otolaryngol Head Neck Surg. 2002;126(4): 409–14. https://doi.org/10.1067/mhn.2002.123446. PMID: 11997782
141. Kazahaya K, Potsic WP. Congenital cholesteatoma. Curr Opin Otolaryngol Head Neck Surg. 2004;12(5):398–403. https://doi.org/10.1097/01.moo.0000136875.41630.d6.
142. Nevoux J, Lenoir M, Roger G, Denoyelle F. Ducou Le pointe H, Garabédian EN. Childhood cholesteatoma. Eur Ann Otorhinolaryngol Head Neck Dis. 2010;127(4):143–50. https://doi.org/10.1016/j.anorl.2010.07.001. Epub 2010 Aug 11
143. Chole RA. The molecular biology of bone resorption due to chronic otitis media. Ann N Y Acad Sci. 1997;830:95–109.
144. Dornelles C, Schmidt Rosito LP, Meurer L, da Costa SS, Argenta A, Alves SL. Hystology findings' correlation between the ossicular chain in the transoperative and cholesteatomas. Braz J Otorhinolaryngol. 2007;73(6):738–43. https://doi.org/10.1016/S1808-8694(15)31169-1.
145. Durko M, Kaczmarczyk D. Proliferation activity and apoptosis in granulation tissue and cholesteatomain middle ear reoperations. Folia Morphol (Warsz). 2004;63(1):119–21.
146. Martins O, Victor J, Selesnick S. The relationship between individual ossicular status and conductive hearing loss in cholesteatoma. OtolNeurotol. 2012;33(3):387–92. https://doi.org/10.1097/MAO.0b013e3182487fb0.
147. Maresh A, MartinsOF, Victor JD, Selesnick SH. Using surgical observations of ossicular erosion patterns to characterize cholesteatoma growth. OtolNeurotol. 2011;32(8):1239–42. https://doi.org/10.1097/MAO.0b013e31822e5b5d.
148. Abramson M. Collagenase in the mechanisms of action of cholesteatoma. Ann OtholRhinolLaryngol. 1971;80(3):414.
149. Abramson M. Collagenolytic activity in middle ear cholesteatoma. AnnOtol. 1969;78:112–25.
150. Abramson M, Huang CC. Localization of collagenase in human middle ear cholesteatoma. Laryngoscope. 1976;86:771–91.
151. Thompsen J. Bone resorption in chronic otitis media. In: McCabe BF, Sade J, Abramson M, editors. Cholesteatoma: first international conference. Birmingham, Alabama: Aescupulus Publishing Co; 1977. p. 136.
152. Hansen T, Unger RE, Gaumann A, Hundorf I, Maurer J, Kirkpatrick J, Kriegsmann J. Expression of matrix-degrading cysteine proteinase cathepsin K in cholesteatoma. United States Canadian AcadPathol. 2001;14(12):1226–31.
153. Kurihara A, Toshima M, Yuasa R, Takasaka T. Bone destruction mechanisms in chronic otitis media with cholesteatoma: specific production by cholesteatoma tissue in culture of bone-resorbing activity attributable to interleukin-1 alpha. Ann OtolRhinolLaryngol. 1991;100(12):989–98.
154. Imai R, Sato T, Iwamoto Y, Hanada Y, Terao M, Ohta Y, Osaki Y, Imai T, Morihana T, Okazaki S, Oshima K, Okuzaki D, Katayama I, Inohara H. Osteoclasts modulate bone erosion in cholesteatoma via RANKL signaling. J Assoc Res Otolaryngol. 2019;20(5):449–59. https://doi.org/10.1007/s10162-019-00727-1.
155. Sangal N, Yan J, Pryor J, Elias ML, Joseph B, Ulloa L, Jyung RW. Association of CARD8 activating polymorphism with bone erosion in cholesteatoma patients. Laryngoscope. 2021;131(2):E605–11. https://doi.org/10.1002/lary.28741.
156. Brook I. Aerobic and anaerobic bacteriology of cholesteatoma. Laryngoscope. 1981;91(2):250–3. https://doi.org/10.1288/00005537-198102000-00012.

157. Kenna MA, Bluestone CD, Reilly JS, Lusk RP. Medical management of chronic suppurative otitis media with cholesteatoma in children. Laryngoscope. 1986;96:146–51.
158. Fujikawa T, Tanimoto K, Kawashima Y, Ito T, Honda K, Takeda T, Sonobe A, Aoki N, Bai J, Tsutsumi T. Cholesteatoma has an altered microbiota with a higher abundance of staphylococcus species. Laryngoscope Investig Otolaryngol. 2022;7(6):2011–9. https://doi.org/10.1002/lio2.934. eCollection 2022.
159. Galli J, Calò L, Giuliani M, Sergi B, Lucidi D, Meucci D, Bassotti E, Sanguinetti M, Paludetti G. Biofilm's role in chronic cholesteatomatous otitis media: a pilot study. Otolaryngol Head Neck Surg. 2016;154(5):914–6. https://doi.org/10.1177/0194599816630548.
160. Paparella MM, Oda M, Hiraide F, Brady D. Pathology of sensorineural hearing loss in otitis media. Ann OtolRhinolLaryngol. 1972;81(5):632–47. https://doi.org/10.1177/000348947208100503.
161. Paparella MM, Schachern PA, Choo YB. The round window membrane: otologicalobservations.AnnOtolRhinolLaryngol.1983;92(6 Pt 1):629–34. https://doi.org/10.1177/000348948309200619.
162. English GM, Northern JL, Fria TJ. Chronic otitis media as a cause of sensorineural hearing loss. Arch Otolaryngol. 1973;98(1):18–22. https://doi.org/10.1001/archotol.1973.00780020022006.
163. Dumich PS, Harner SG. Cochlear function in chronic otitis media. Laryngoscope. 1983;93(5):583–6. https://doi.org/10.1002/lary.1983.93.5.583.
164. Walby AP, Barrera A, Schuknecht HF. Cochlear pathology in chronic suppurative otitis media. Ann OtolRhinolLaryngol Suppl. 1983;103(Suppl):1–19.
165. Rosito LPS, Sperling N, Teixeira AR, Selaimen FA, da Costa SS. The role of Tympanic membrane retractions in cholesteatoma pathogenesis. Biomed Res Int. 2018;2018:9817123. https://doi.org/10.1155/2018/9817123.
166. Rosito LPS, Canali I, Teixeira A, Silva MN, Selaimen F, Costa SSD. Cholesteatoma labyrinthine fistula: prevalence and impact. Braz J Otorhinolaryngol. 2019;85(2):222–7. https://doi.org/10.1016/j.bjorl.2018.01.005.
167. Dornhoffer JL, Milewski C. Management of the open labyrinth. Otolaryngol Head Neck Surg. 1995;112(3):410–4. https://doi.org/10.1016/S0194-59989570275-X.
168. Gomaa MA, Abdel Karim AR, Abdel Ghany HS, Elhiny AA, Sadek AA. Evaluation of temporal bone cholesteatoma and the correlation between high resolution computed tomography and surgical finding. Clin Med Insights Ear Nose Throat. 2013;6:21–8. https://doi.org/10.4137/CMENT.S10681.
169. Sethom A, Akkari K, Dridi I, Tmimi S, Mardassi A, Benzarti S, Miled I, Chebbi MK. Apport de la tomodensitométrie dans le bilanpréopératoire de l'otitemoyennechroniquecholestéatomateuse. A propos de 60 cas [Preoperative CT Scan in middle ear cholesteatoma]. Tunis Med. 2011;89(3):248–53.
170. Stephenson MF, Saliba I. Prognostic indicators of hearing after complete resection of cholesteatoma causing a labyrinthine fistula. Eur Arch Otorhinolaryngol. 2011;268(12):1705–11. https://doi.org/10.1007/s00405-011-1545-7.
171. Ikeda M, Nakazato H, Onoda K, Hirai R, Kida A. Facial nerve paralysis caused by middle ear cholesteatoma and effects of surgical intervention. Acta Otolaryngol. 2006;126(1):95–100. https://doi.org/10.1080/00016480500265950.
172. Quaranta N, Cassano M, Quaranta A. Facial paralysis associated with cholesteatoma: a review of 13 cases. OtolNeurotol. 2007;28(3):405–7. https://doi.org/10.1097/01.mao.0000265189.29969.c4.
173. Siddiq MA, Hanu-Cernat LM, Irving RM. Facial palsy secondary to cholesteatoma: analysis of outcome following surgery. J LaryngolOtol. 2007;121(2):114–7. https://doi.org/10.1017/S0022215106003227.
174. Psillas G, Constantinidis J. Facial palsy secondary to Cholesteatoma: a case-series of 14 patients. Audiol Res. 2023;13(1):86–93. https://doi.org/10.3390/audiolres13010008.
175. Ozkul Y, Songu M, Onal K, Imre A, Arslanoglu S, Horoz E, Bayrak F, Pinar E. Effect of surgical intervention on middle-ear cholesteatoma with associated facial paralysis. J LaryngolOtol. 2017;131(2):113–6. https://doi.org/10.1017/S0022215116009804.
176. Alice Lang Silva, Fábio André Selaimen , Isabel Saorin Conte, Marcela Lehmkuhl Damiani, Luciana Lima Martins Costa, Letícia Petersen Schmidt Rosito, Sady Selaimen da Costa. Aural polyps: what's behind them? Scripta Scientifica Medica, 2021;53(2):62–7 Medical University of Varna.
177. Costa SS, Silva MN, Rosito LP, Selaimen FA. Um caso, duas lições: artériacarótida interna aberrantecausandocolesteatomaadquirido [One case, two lessons: an aberrant internal carotid artery causing acquired cholesteatoma]. Braz J Otorhinolaryngol. 2014;80(5):453–4. https://doi.org/10.1016/j.bjorl.2014.05.021.
178. Costa SS, de Souza LCA, Andrade MI. Procedures on the storm—reviewing the nomenclature. Rev Bras Otor. 1991a;57(4):170–9.
179. Costa, SSda, Paparella MM, Shachern P, Yoon TH. Chronic silent otitis media: a clinical-pathological study; a preliminar report. Rev bras otorrinolaringol. 1997: 57(2);81–4, abr.-jun.
180. Aberg B, Edstrom S, Bagger-Sjoback D, Kindblom LG. Morphologic development of experimental cholesteatoma. Arch Otolaryngol Head Neck Surg. 1993;119:272–5.

Progresses in Cholesteatoma Research

43

Immunobiology and Genetics of Middle Ear Cholesteatoma

H. Sudhoff and M. Schürmann

This chapter will elucidate and focusses on the molecular and immunobiology of middle ear cholesteatoma. Even though there are various reasons cholesteatoma progression, e.g., physical cues like pressure changes [1–3] or chemical cues [4], we want highlight the contribution of biological cues. More specifically, we want to concentrate on the role the immunology and genetics that are major contributors during the pathogenesis of cholesteatoma. We will review their impact on its pathogenesis, progression, and recurrence after surgery.

Middle ear cholesteatoma generally reveals a severe tissue damage with frequent bacterial infections and biofilm formation. This is closely linked to the remodeling and restoration of structural and functional integrity of middle ear compartment. This process features analogous patterns to wound healing and is led by inflammatory mediators orchestrating the immune pattern within the middle ear spaces. A major contributor of inflammatory mediators are cells residing in cholesteatoma tissue. Infectious cues initiating the exaggerated inflammation in cholesteatoma tissue play a pivotal role. Specific receptors recognizing these cues are major players to its pathogenesis. Subsequently, pathways and mechanisms lead to the expression targets typical for an inflammatory state. In addition, the role certain immunoregulatory molecules in middle ear cholesteatoma is highlighted. The expression, localization, and role of the corresponding component will be analyzed.

The second part will analyze with the genetics of cholesteatoma. Even though there are a few reports of familial clustering of cholesteatoma suggesting a genetic predisposition, but to date no genetic susceptibility loci have been clearly identified. The possible connection between genetic alterations, e.g., the DNA content, mutations, and epigenetics and cholesteatoma disease will be discussed. Moreover, we will describe the possible role of oncogenes and their regulation by, e.g., miRNAs in cholesteatoma tissue.

It has been proposed that the development of cholesteatoma is due to the altered control of cellular proliferation, which tilts the balance toward the aggressive, invasive growth of squamous epithelium into middle ear. However, whether the cause of this is an altered control of genes that control proliferation, or cytokines released from infiltrating inflammatory cells or another mechanism, is still unknown.

Novel insights into the molecular basis of cholesteatoma will enable improved treatment strategies. Possible molecular-based targets will be presented and discussed.

Inflammation in Middle Ear Cholesteatoma

Immunregulatory Cell Populations in Cholesteatoma Tissue

Due to its highly inflamed subepithelial connective tissue, middle ear cholesteatoma is characterized by a severe infiltration of inflammatory cells. Compared to external auditory canal skin, Hussein et al. found that the majority of immune regulatory cells are upregulated [5].

The major representatives of myeloblast-derived immune cells in cholesteatoma tissue are macrophages [5] that mainly reside in the cholesteatoma perimatrix [6]. Therefore, a known the natural mechanism to induce apoptosis in chronically inflamed tissue macrophages is absent. In accordance, the amount of these cells is four times upregulated [5]. Interestingly RNA-seq comparison of tissue-resident macrophages obtained from middle ear tissue of patients with and without cholesteatoma exhibited characteristics of chronic inflammation and cell survival of macrophages residing in cholesteatoma tissue [7]. Around 20% of the phagocytes in cholesteatoma tissue are CD1+ Langerhans' cells [5]. Likewise, these cells are normally localized in the stratum spinosum and are predominantly localized in the cholesteatoma matrix [8]. In contrary, the amount of Langerhans cells

H. Sudhoff (✉) · M. Schürmann
Department of Otorhinolaryngology, Head and Neck Surgery, Klinikum Bielefeld, Medical Faculty OWL, Bielefeld University, Bielefeld, Germany

M. V. Goycoolea et al. (eds.), *Textbook of Otitis Media*, https://doi.org/10.1007/978-3-031-40949-3_43

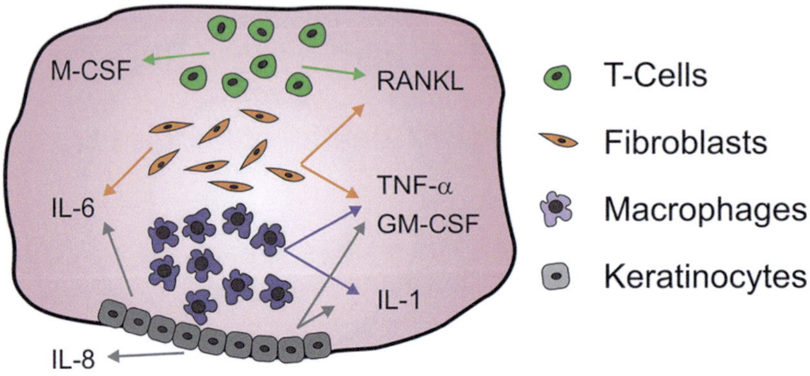

Fig. 43.1 The most important cells in cholesteatoma immunochemistry and their secretion of cytokines upregulated in cholesteatoma tissue. T-cell, macrophages, fibroblasts, and keratinocytes are the most prominent immunomodulatory cells in the cholesteatoma niche. Their upregulated secretion of certain cytokines enables the exaggerated inflammatory level found in cholesteatoma tissue

was not significantly different from regular ear canal skin [9]. Another myeloid cell type, the mast cells, is abundant and threefold to sevenfold increased as compared to regular tissue [10]. These cells are found within the perimatrix usually close to the epithelium [11]. The elevated numbers of mast cells at sites of chronic inflammation have been reported for decades. Their powerful immune regulatory properties are associated with persistent inflammation of the affected sites [12]. The presence of mast cells was shown to correlate to the degree of bone destruction on cholesteatoma patients [13]. Other myeloid cell types, like dendritic cells, were found much less frequent in cholesteatoma tissue compared to macrophages [14]. Similarly, myeloid-derived neutrophils, even though they are the most abundant leucocytes in blood, are rarely observed in cholesteatoma tissue [15].

Among the lymphocytes present in cholesteatoma tissue, CD3+ T lymphocytes are the most abundant variant [5]. Reactivity with anti-CD3 and anti-CD6 antibodies revealed an abundant infiltration of T lymphocytes beneath the squamous epithelium of cholesteatoma [16]. A number of studies have attempted to delineate a Th1/Th2 paradigm of inflammatory events in cholesteatomas and found that according to their expression profile the Th1 cells are dominant [11, 17]. B lymphocytes were only occasionally detected via anti-CD19 and anti-CD22 antibodies [16] or CD20 immunohistochemistry[5] . Fibroblasts, which were traditionally described as a quiescent cell mainly responsible for growth factor secretion and extracellular matrix production. Today, fibroblasts are more and more appreciated as an active player in the tissue-resident immune system [18]. Keratinocytes are the most abundant single cell type in cholesteatoma tissue. In skin keratinocytes establish a physical barrier. Recently, they are viewed as active sentinels shaping, amplifying, and regulating immune via secretion of various cytokines, chemokines, and growth factors [19]. They are also responsible for hyperproliferative inflammatory skin diseases [20]. Even though the immunomodulatory potential of these two cell types is not comparable to that of, e.g., macrophages, their extremely high density in the perimatrix and matrix, respectively, of cholesteatoma tissue needs to be mentioned [21]. Taken together, the four cell types, mast cells, macrophage, T lymphocytes, fibroblasts and keratinocytes, are the most frequently found immune regulatory cells in cholesteatoma tissue (Fig. 43.1).

Cues initiating the Inflammation in Cholesteatoma

PAMP

To understand immunochemistry behind the highly inflamed state of cholesteatoma, we first want to describe the external inputs, which primarily triggers the immune response leading to all the subsequent initiation of antigen-specific adaptive immune response and release of inflammatory cytokines or chemokines. The major triggers of this process, associated with the innate immune system, are the pattern recognition receptors (PRRs). PRRs can be divided into two groups, the pathogen-associated molecular pattern (PAMPs), which are classified as small molecular motifs conserved within a class of microbes and the damage-associated molecular patterns (DAMPs), recognizing components of cells that are released during damage of the cell membrane. It is known cholesteatoma tissue is frequently accompanied by a bacterial infection. This triggering infection seem to be an initiating factor for the development of acquired cholesteatoma [22]. Culture-based bacterial detection methods showed that the two dominant bacterial species are *Pseudomonas aeruginosa* (around 30%) and *Staphylococcus aureus* (around 20%) [23, 24]. Recent sequencing-based studies revealed a higher diversity [25] but again the most abundant species were *Pseudomonas aeruginosa* followed by *Staphylococcus aureus*. The relations between Gram (+) and Gram (−) bacteria are comparable [26]. Systemic antibiotics are ineffective in clearing the bacterial infection of cholesteatoma. Bacteria most often are assembled in the form of biofilms [27, 28]. Interestingly, biofilm presence is positively correlated to cholesteatoma recurrence [29]. Other PAMP providing microbes like fungi are rare [23, 30], and their presence not frequently associated to cholesteatoma manifestation [31]. Viral infections are unlikely to play a role in PAMP generation altering the immune response. Taken together, the bacteria infection with Gram (−) germs like *Pseudomonas aeruginosa*, producing the PAMP lipopolysaccharide (LPS), and Gram (+) bacteria, e.g., *Staphylococcus aureus* generating the PAMPs lipoteichoic acid and peptidoglycan. These three molecules are the main contributors of PAMPs in cholesteatoma tissue. Particularly, LPS might directly promote cholesteatoma progression, since it is present in higher concentration in chronic otitis media with cholesteatoma than those without cholesteatoma [32]. The concentration was 85 ± 6.5 ng/ml in purulent and 0.003 ± 0.5 ng/ml in nonpurulent cholesteatoma tissue [32]. Significantly higher concentrations of LPS were detected in samples from patients with cholesteatoma showing bone resorption compared with cholesteatoma without bone resorption [32]. Studies employing animal models of cholesteatoma have demonstrated that the infection with *Pseudomonas aeruginosa* leads to an acceleration of cholesteatoma growth and bone resorption [33]. Additionally, LPS was demonstrated to stimulate the growth of epidermal cells of cholesteatoma [34]. Therefore, PAMPs can directly be linked to the clinical parameters of cholesteatoma disease (Fig. 43.2).

DAMP

The second class of PRR agonists, DAMPs (damage-associated molecular patterns), comprises molecules released after membrane damage of cell dying cells (necroticpyroptosis, necroptosis) [35]. Cholesteatoma is closely related to an abundant tissue damage. Hence, various DAMPs are upregulated in cholesteatoma tissue. One of these is the head shock proteins (HSPs). HSP60 and HSP70 appeared to be localized in the cytoplasm of keratinocytes in all layers of the epithelium of cholesteatoma [36]. Both HSPs were not labeled in the epidermis of the external ear canal skin or normal facial skin [36]. Ho and colleagues confirmed that the immune reactivity of HSP27 was significantly stronger in cholesteatomas than in postauricular skin and localized to keratinocytes [37]. The authors linked HSP27 to the activation of cell migration, angiogenesis, and proliferation in epithelial cells and hence the growth of cholesteatoma. Another class of DAMPs in cholesteatoma tissue is the S100 proteins. Two independent DNA chip analyses showed that S100A7A, S100A8, S100A9,S100A12, and S100A2 and are upregulated in cholesteatoma compared to auditory canal skin and that the expression of S100A9 and S100A8 was particularly high [38, 39]. As a neural crest-specific protein, the expressions are confined to epithelial cells and macrophages. Interestingly, extracellular S100A8/S100A9 is strongly associated with inflammatory diseases [40]. As related to the middle ear, elevated S100A8 and S100A9 gene expressions were detected in inflamed middle ear epithelium suggesting a role in the pathogenesis of chronic inflammatory state [41]. The high-mobility group protein B1 (HMGB1) is upregulated in cholesteatoma compared to normal auditory skin [42]. It is known, that HMGB1 is overexpressed in chronically inflamed middle ear pathologies [43]. Particularly LPS is able to induce HMGB1 release into the extracellular space [44] and thus play a role in the progression of the inflammation present in the LPS-rich cholesteatoma tissue. An additional DAMP associated with cholesteatoma is prostaglandin (PEG). PEGs are synthesized by cyclooxygenase-2 (COX-2), which increases prostaglandin levels in inflammation. COX-2 mRNA is heavily upregulated in cholesteatoma matrix [45]. Not surprisingly, PGE2 was upregulated in cholesteatoma as compared to adjacent skin or even granulation tissue, which is known to express high levels of PEG2 [46,

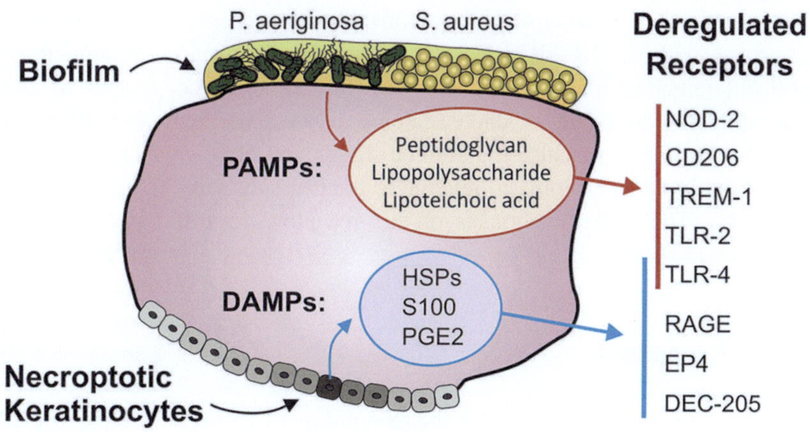

Fig. 43.2 PRR-induced inflammatory reaction in cholesteatoma tissue. Dying keratinocytes and bacterial biofilms generate different DAMP and PAMP, respectively, which act on the cells residing in cholesteatoma tissue. Cholesteatoma cells show deregulation of various PRRs, this amplifies the initiated inflammatory reaction even more

47]. Since the production of PEG by the cyclooxygenase 2 (COX2) is closely linked to the intrinsical level of inflammation of tissue [48]. Interestingly, PEG2 is known to be active in bone resorption [49] and stimulates the proliferation of epidermal cells of cholesteatoma [34]. DAMPs HSP60, HSP70, HSP27, S100A8, S100A9, HMGB1, and particularly PEG2 modulate the innate immune response via PRR and hence play a pivotal role in the establishment of the exaggerated inflammatory pathway contributing to the pathogenesis of cholesteatoma (Fig. 43.2).

Receptors Recognizing the Initial Cues and Initiating the Inflammatory Response

DAMP Receptors

Besides this external stimuli, pathological changes on the cellular level also lead to the high level of inflammation in cholesteatoma tissue. For example, the receptor for advanced glycation end-product (RAGE) is a major receptor for DAMPs [50]. In general, the interaction between RAGE and its ligands leads by intracellular signaling to a translocation of NF-κB and AP-1 and subsequent proinflammatory gene expression. RAGE signaling has been mainly studied as a pathogenetic factor of chronic inflammatory diseases [51]. RAGE is upregulated in cholesteatoma compared to normal auditory skin [42]. We assume that this sensitizes cholesteatoma tissue to the corresponding DAMPs antigens. RAGE ligands S100A12 [52], S100A7 [53], S100A8/A9 [54], and HMGB1 [55] are additionally upregulated in cholesteatoma tissue. Szczepanski et al. could demonstrate that this fatal combination of receptor and agonist correlation leads to signaling of the HMGB1/RAGE pathway, contributing to cholesteatoma pathogenesis [42]. The DAMP PEG2 is recognized by the four prostaglandin receptors EP1-EP4. Comparative investigations between skin and cholesteatoma tissue demonstrated that the proinflammatory receptors EP-1-EP3 are slightly upregulated. Contrarily, the EP4 receptor was significantly downregulated in cholesteatoma tissue on the protein and mRNA level [56]. The EP4 receptor interferes with the NF-kB signaling and acts hereby in an anti-inflammatory manner [57]. This will further reinforce the inflammatory state in cholesteatoma tissue. Another receptor DEC-205 was also found to be significantly higher expressed in cholesteatoma in relation to control skin samples [58]. The exact antagonists of this receptor are still unknown [59].

PAMP Receptors

The most prominent receptors for the recognition of PAMPs are the Toll-like receptors family which comprises 10 different receptors in humans with TLR-1, TLR-2, TLR-4, and TLR-5 recognizing PAMPs derived from bacteria. In chronic inflammation, sustained signaling of TLRs is the characteristic. Any divergence of TLR signaling from the native and healthy state plays an unfavorable role in this pathologic condition [60]. TLR-2 and TLR-4 are expressed in their microenvironment in acquired cholesteatoma [61]. TLRs immunohistochemistry revealed positive reactivity within the matrix as well as the perimatrix cholesteatoma [61]. The expression was increased within the epithelial cells of cholesteatoma matrix [62]. A significant upregulation of TLR-2 and TLR-4 was observed in cholesteatoma as compared with different control samples without any inflammation [63], mucosa from patients with cholesteatoma [64], or external auditory canal skin [62]. The relatively weak expression of these receptors in regular skin may also suggest the important role of these two TLR in the pathogenesis of cholesteatoma. TLR-2 recognizes bacterial PAMPs like peptidoglycan from Gram (−) bacteria and lipoteichoic acid deriving from Gram (+) prokaryotes present in cholesteatoma tissue. In addition various upregulated DAMPs e.g. HMGB1 [65], HSP27 [66], and HSP70 [67] are able to increase the degree of inflammation. The role of the TLR-4 is even more profound and was already widely investigated [68]. In accordance, TLR-4 is significantly upregulated in acquired cholesteatoma tissue [68]. This upregulation of TLR-4 alone is playing a distinct role as drivers of inflammatory environment and cholesteatoma progression [69]. Notably, TLR-4 upregulation is further augmented by recognition of the PAMP LPS derived from Gram (−) bacteria highly present in cholesteatoma [32]. Also Gram (+) bacteria play a role in the immune response [70]. TLR-4 pathway is also activated by nearly all DAMPs upregulated in this inflamed lesion, e.g., HSP27 [66], HSP60 [71], HSP70 [67], HMGB1 [65], and S100A8/S100A9 [72, 73]. The initial triggering [73] of the TLR-4 by PAMPs and DAMPs results in a vicious circle. It is known that HMGB1 enhances the proinflammatory activity of LPS by promoting the phosphorylation of MAPK p38 through RAGE [74]. Likewise, the DAMP HSP70 frequently found in cholesteatoma tissue further aggravates the response of TLR4 to the bacterial LPS [75]. Besides the enhanced inflammatory responses, TLR-4 is most linked to osteoclastogenesis and bone destruction in cholesteatoma tissue [14, 64]. This is further promoted through TREM-2-modulated TLR4 signaling [14] enhanced by Gram (−) bacterial infection [76]. The expression level of TRIM-2 was upregulated in cholesteatoma and positively correlated to the severity of bone destruction [14]. High concentration of LPS,TLR-4, and TREM-2 in cholesteatoma tissue severely stimulates osteoclastogenesis. In vitro experiments demonstrate that the emergence and hyperproliferation of keratinizing epithelium, another clinical feature of cholesteatoma, is directly linked to TLR4 expression in the perimatrix and in the presence of LPS [77].

Apart from the TLR receptors, the NOD-2 receptor recognizes bacterial-derived PAMPs. It is a general sensor for peptidoglycan derived from Gram (+) as well as Gram (−) bacteria [78]. Different studies showed that NOD-2 is expressed in the cholesteatoma on a significantly higher level as compared to skin [79, 80]. Further bioinformatic analysis of the corresponding regulation of genes in the interaction network of the NOD-2 receptor showed that the entire network was upregulated. Therefore, the corresponding innate immune signaling mediation is involved in the pathogenesis of cholesteatoma [80]. NOD-2 is already linked to further chronic inflammatory diseases [81]. PRR CD206 and Mincle are expressed on a higher level in cholesteatoma tissue in comparison to external auditory canal skin [82]. They are capable to sense PAMPs derived from bacteria and induce inflammatory cell signaling. Until now, their role in cholesteatoma development was not further investigated, but their high expression emphasizes the importance of the innate immune response in chronic inflammation common in cholesteatoma development. The triggering receptor is expressed on myeloid cells-1 (TREM-1) [58].TREM-1 is also able to exacerbate the inflammation by positively modulating signaling pathways induced by PRRs, such as TLRs or NOD-2 [83]. Additionally, TREM-1 can directly interact with various DAMP, [84, 85] additionally fueling inflammation.

Pathways of the Initial Immune Response

The mentioned PRR initiate the expression of proinflammatory mediators. For all the PRR, the nuclear translocalization and promotor bind the two transcription factors nuclear factor 'kappa-light-chain-enhancer' of activated B-cells (NF-κB) and Activator protein 1 (AP-1), which are the driving force behind this pattern. Accordingly, the activity of AP-1 was shown to be upregulated compared to skin derived from the ear [86, 87]. Immunohistochemical analysis revealed a predominant localization in the nuclei of the keratinocytes of cholesteatoma matrix [88]. Until now, no further investigations were undertaken to gain a deeper insights into the regulatory mechanisms of the AP-1 network in cholesteatoma tissue. Contrarily, the NF-κB network of cholesteatoma was investigated much deeper. Likewise to Ap-1, different studies verified an upregulation of NF-κB in cholesteatoma tissue compared to normal skin. NF-κB was mainly distributed in the epithelium of the cholesteatoma matrix [89, 90]. In accordance with the abundance of PAMP, DAMP, and PRR, the binding activity of NF-κB to its promotor region was significantly time higher in middle ear cholesteatoma tissue [91]. In vitro experiments demonstrated that cells derived from the cholesteatoma perimatrix showed an enhanced excitability for the pathway involved in NF-κB activation when compared with the same cell type isolated from the dermis of auditory canal skin [69]. Several reasons were described to explain this overexcitability of the NF-κB pathway. There is a strong upregulation of id1 in cholesteatoma matrix [92] and perimatrix [93]. Because id1 potentiates the activation of NF-κB [94]. Another reason might be that the expression of Bcl10, proven to activate the NF-κB pathway [95]. This was significantly higher in cholesteatoma compared to controls [58]. The NF-κB pathway might also be hypersensitive in cholesteatoma because the expression of CYLD, a deubiquitinating enzyme that inhibits activation of the NF-κB, is significantly lower in cholesteatoma tissue [96]. This study also showed that the CYLD expression was negatively correlated to the activity of NF-κB. Notably, the overexcitability of NF-κB in cholesteatoma tissue emphasizes the dominant role of NF-κB pathway in the establishment of its inflammatory microenvironment.

After expression of proinflammatory targets by these transcriptional factors, the translated proteins are further processed by different mechanisms. One of these mechanisms, the inflammasome, seems to play an important role in cholesteatoma disease. The inflammasome is a multiprotein complex that promotes proteolytic cleavage and maturation and secretion of proinflammatory cytokines interleukin 1β (IL-1β) and interleukin 18 (IL-18). Inflammasome activation is initiated by different types of cytosolic PRRs upregulated in cholesteatoma-like NOD-2 [79, 80] as well as AIM2 [97], IFI16 (IFN-inducible protein 16) as well as pyrin. Upon activation, it is assembled to huge complex comprising several hundred of proteins. These proteins are upregulated upon LPS induced middle ear inflammation [98]. Therefore, they are expressed on a higher level in cholesteatoma compared to different control tissues and localized in the matrix keratinocytes and infiltrating macrophages [80, 97, 99]. This complex serves as a scaffold for caspase-1, which is known to be also upregulated in cholesteatoma [97, 99]. Caspase-1 is subsequently cleaved and hence activated to cleave the precursors of IL-1β and IL-18. The inflammasome is able to cleave Gasdermin D, enabling pore formation in the cell membrane and release DAMPs into the extracellular space and further aggravating the inflammatory state.

Inflammatory Mediators Released upon Initial Inflammation

All the signaling mechanisms described above establish a proinflammatory environment characteristic for cholesteatoma. The cells residing in the cholesteatoma niche will start to secrete inflammatory mediators including the prostaglandins, already mentioned above in their role as DAMP, but also cytokines such as chemokines, interleukins, lymphokines, and tumor necrosis factors. Cytokines are produced by a broad range of cells residing in cholesteatoma tissue, e.g., macrophages, T lymphocytes, mast cells, epidermal cells, or fibroblasts. These molecules amplify the inflammatory signal and transmit it back into the extracellular space. These mediators will modulate the inflammatory response, and regulate the maturation, growth, and responsiveness of particular cell populations. Extracellular signaling through cytokines expressed upon the initial immune response are able to induce the secretion of cytokines into the extracellular space and induce further inflammatory signaling in a paracrine or autocrine manner. In the following subchapter, we want to explain the expression and role of different cytokines highly expressed in cholesteatoma tissue.

Probably, the most prominent cytokine the tumor necrosis factor alpha (TNF-α) is known as a potent inducer of inflammation and apoptotic cell death. It is strongly expressed upon activation of the transcription factors NF-κB and AP-1. Hence it is not surprising that TNF-α can be induced in, e.g., monocytes after incubation with cholesteatoma debris containing high levels of LPS [100]. It is not surprising that there is a strong correlation between TNF-α and severity of infection in acquired cholesteatoma [101]. In vivo the expression level of TNF-a was compared to different tissue types and was found to be significantly higher in tissue from cholesteatoma [101–104]. Even the serum level of TNF-α was increased in patients with cholesteatoma than those without inflammatory middle ear diseases [105, 106]. In cholesteatoma, the expression of TNF-α is widely distributed. It was localized in the connective tissue and particularly in macrophages residing in the cholesteatoma perimatrix [104]. Notably, cholesteatoma matrix and perimatrix express high levels of TNF-α [103]. In accordance with these in vitro studies, epidermal cholesteatoma cells produced higher amounts TNF-α than regular keratinozytes [107, 108]. Cholesteatoma keratinocytes expressed higher levels of TNF-α than their healthy auditory canal skin counterparts, which results in a positive feed forward loop further enhancing the already upregulated TNF-α concentration [108]. TNF-α was also found in the tissue adjacent to bone resorption areas in human and experimental middle ear cholesteatomas, where it was localized to mononuclear cells, macrophages, fibroblasts, osteoblasts, and osteoclasts [109]. Interestingly, TNF-α was demonstrated to stimulate osteoclast formation in vivo [110]. In vitro TNF-α stimulated monocytes to form multinucleated cells expressing osteoclast marker and was capable of stimulating macrophages to produce acid phosphatase and collagenase leading to bone resorption [109] (Fig. 43.3). In alignment with this mechanism, several studies found that the TNF-α levels in cholesteatoma patients with bone destruction were higher than in those without bone destruction [101, 105, 111–113]. TNF-α is also able known to promote the proliferation, protein synthesis, and terminal differentiation of basal keratinocytes, resulting in another clinical feature of cholesteatoma disease, the accumulation of keratin debris [104]. Utilizing the supernatant of cholesteatoma cells Kato and co-workers could demonstrate that TNF-α compromised ciliary activity and mucociliary clearance of the Eustachian tube in the guinea pigs [114]. Clinically, this would further aggravate the situation of the middle ear cavity. In contrast to role of TNF-α, the density of the TNF-α receptor could not be correlated with the degree of inflammation or bone destruction present in the acquired middle ear cholesteatoma [115].

Another important group of cytokines is interleukin 1-alpha and interleukin 1-beta (IL-1α and IL-1β). They are both ligands of the two IL-1 receptors (IL-1-R) inducing pro-

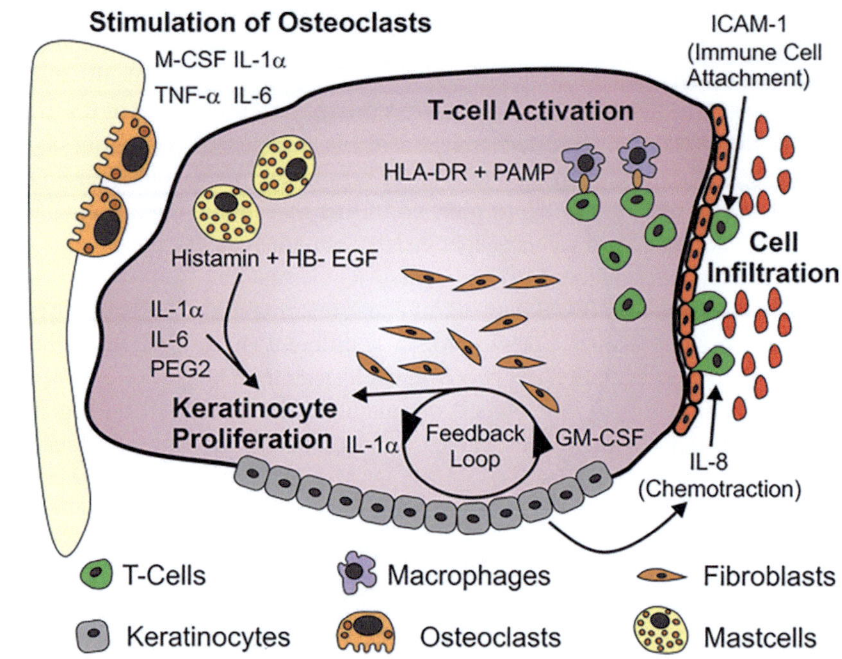

Fig. 43.3 The contribution of different inflammatory modulators to the pathogenesis of cholesteatoma disease. Shown are the pathogenic symptoms characteristic for cholesteatoma disease (bold letters) right next to their modulators upregulated in cholesteatoma tissue

inflammatory immune responses. IL-1 s are produced predominantly by macrophages but also by epithelial cells widely present in cholesteatoma tissue. Their expression is induced by the transcription factor NF-κB induced upon stimulation with, e.g., PAMPs, DAMPs, or TNFs. According to this, it is not surprising that IL-1α as well as IL-1β are upregulated in cholesteatoma compared to healthy middle ear epithelium [116], normal skin [46, 101], auditory canal skin [103, 117] and even tissue from otitis media patients [102]. Corresponding to the common of IL-1 s expression in epithelial cells, immunohistochemistry [116, 118] and in situ hybridization [17] demonstrated that all cellular layers of cholesteatoma epithelium stained strongly and uniformly for Il-1 alpha and IL-1 beta. In the stroma of the cholesteatoma intensely IL-1 s-positive cells belonging to the monocyte macrophage lineage were detected by immunohistochemistry and in situ techniques [46, 118]. In alignment with these observations in vitro experiments demonstrated that keratinocytes but not fibroblasts secreted an enhanced amount of IL-1α as well as IL-1β when compared to the same cell derived from auditory canal skin [119]. Apart from the elevated expression of IL-1 s, the corresponding Interleukin-1 receptor (IL-1R) were 3 times upregulated in cholesteatoma and cholesteatoma keratinocytes compared to the same cell in regular aural skin [120]. Adding to that the upregulation of the IL-1 s the interleukin-1 receptor antagonist (IL-1-RA) showed an elevated concentration in skin samples [117]. Further IL-1α stimulates keratinocytes and macrophages, abundantly present in cholesteatoma tissue, to secret additional IL-1α. All this will positively enhance the already robust pro-inflammatory IL-1 signaling in the already heavily inflamed cholesteatoma tissue. IL-1α stimulates osteoclast formation [110] and is correlated to the expression of MMP-9 in cholesteatoma tissue [121]. IL-1 signaling is suggested to play an aggravating role in cholesteatoma induced bone resorption. Several studies could prove a positive correlation between IL-1α and bone resorption [111, 112, 122]. Even though IL-1α is known to stimulate proliferation in fibroblastic [123] and epidermal cells [124] no correlation between IL-1α and proliferation marker cell nuclear antigen could be detected [121].

Cytokine IL-6 is also increased in cholesteatoma tissue [46, 103] as compared to regular skin [46]. IL-6 was mainly localized in cholesteatoma epithelium as well as subepithelial stroma [103]. Studies comparing cholesteatoma keratinocytes with skin keratinocytes demonstrated, that this elevated expression was preserved even after in vitro cultivation [114, 125].The corresponding IL-6 receptors were mainly found in the epidermis of inflamed cholesteatoma [126]. Downstream of the IL-6 receptors are the activating STAT3 transcriptional factor and the inhibitory SCOS3 proteins. Fanglei et al. found that STAT3 is overexpressed, while SOCS3 is downregulated in cholesteatoma epithelium [127] and that STAT3 and SOCS3 were even negatively correlated in the middle ear cholesteatoma. In accordance, the phosphorylated STAT3, the activated form of the transcriptional factor, was significantly higher in cholesteatoma epithelium than in external auditory canal skin. This is suggesting that abnormal IL-6 signaling in the middle ear cholesteatoma may be involved in hyperproliferation and antiapoptosis of cholesteatoma epidermal cells and hence promotes its formation. Several in vivo studies detected a correlation between IL-6 activity in cholesteatoma and bone erosion [103, 112, 122] . Even correlation between IL-6 serum level and bone erosion was ascertained in cholesteatoma patients [128]. Only a single study was not able to link pSTAT3 to the degree of bone destruction [129]. Notably, IL-6 was also proven to negatively influence the middle ear clearance by inhibiting the ciliary activity in a guinea pig model [114].

The chemokine IL-8 also known as CXCL-8 is also expressed in cholesteatoma tissue and might play a role in cholesteatoma progression. Expression of IL-8 is significantly higher in cholesteatoma tissue [79] or external auditory canal skin or postauricular skin [130]. This is in accordance with the upregulation of id1 in cholesteatoma, which is known to positively regulate IL-8 via different molecular mechanisms [93]. The localization of IL-8 was confined to the basal and suprabasal cell layer of the cholesteatoma matrix [131]. This is resembled in the in vitro situation, where another study compares the expression of cholesteatoma cells to normal skin cells. They described an elevated expression of IL-8 stayed under culture conditions in keratinocytes but absent in fibroblasts [119]. Cholesteatoma keratinocytes reacted to an increase secretion of IL-8 upon stimulation with TNF-α compared to their healthy counterparts [108]. Since TNF-α is highly expressed in cholesteatoma microenvironment, the in vivo situation of high IL-8 expression in keratinocytes might be further increased by TNF-α sensitivity. Since IL-8 is commonly expressed in inflamed cholesteatoma tissue, e.g., via HMGB1/RAGE upregulated in cholesteatoma [42]. As it mainly acts on neutrophils that are infrequent in cholesteatoma tissue, its role in generation of infiltrate and/or pathogenesis is not fully understood.

The cytokine granulocyte-macrophage colony-stimulating factor (GM-CSF) can be initial induced through PRR. It is not surprising that the expression level of GM-CSF of cholesteatoma epithelial tissue is higher in comparison to normal external auditory meatal skin epithelial tissue [132, 133]. Beyond that it is located in the peribasal area, in some suprabasal cells of the epithelium, and in the inflammatory connective tissue, especially in the monocytes and fibroblasts [133]. Particularly its association with fibroblasts might be of importance for cholesteatoma development since its well documented role in proliferation, protein synthesis, and terminal differentiation of keratinocytes [133].

Interestingly, in normal wound healing, the expression of IL-1 s in keratinocytes results in an induction of GM-CSF in dermal fibroblasts which further increases the expression ofIL-1 s in keratinocytes. This positive feedback loop, which results in health restoration of the epithelial barrier during in normal wound healing, might be spin out of control in the case of cholesteatoma tissue. Because the PRR-induced overexpression of IL-1 s in cholesteatoma keratinocytes [119] and GM-CSF in cholesteatoma fibroblasts might tilt the equilibrium in this feedback loop. In accordance to that in vitro studies showed that fibroblasts derived from healthy skin showed a much weaker expression of GM-CSF after stimulation by IL-1α and/or IL-1β compared to cholesteatoma fibroblasts [134]. The less prominent macrophage colony-stimulatingfactorandthemacrophage-colony-stimulating factor were found to be overexpressed in cholesteatoma specimens compared to normal external meatal skin [135]. It was found to be located in the cholesteatoma perimatrix and is released from activated T-cells in response to the inflammatory process [135]. Since M-CSF is essential for osteoclast formation [136], it can be assumed that its role in the pathogenesis is linked to the promotion of osteolytic properties of cholesteatoma.

Besides all these cytokines are released by various cells upon PRR stimulation, mast cells frequently found in cholesteatoma tissue release not only cytokines but also various other inflammatory mediators via degranulation upon stimulation of their PRR. One of these mediators is histamine an organic compound involved and able to increase blood flow and vessel permeability. Another one is Heparin which is of particular interest in cholesteatoma disease, since it enhances the activity of heparin-binding EGF-like growth factor (HB-EGF) . HB-EGF is the predominant growth factor in the epithelialization required for cutaneous wound healing [137]. Compared to normal post auricular skin, HB-EGF is upregulated in cholesteatoma, where it is suspected to play a major role in the excessive growth of epithelium and even bone resorption [138].

The signaling most excessively investigated pathway is the RANK-RANKL-OPG system. Briefly, the RANK-RANKL-OPG system is the major modulator of bone resorption. The receptor activator of nuclear factor κ B (RANK) positively regulates osteoclast differentiation and activation upon binding of its ligand (RANKL), while osteoprotegerin (OPG) on the other side is a decoy receptor for RANKL and hence negatively regulates the osteolysis. RANKL-positive cells and/or the ratio of RANKL/OPG in cholesteatoma were significantly higher than that in external meatal skin [139, 140] postauricular skin [141] normal skin [142], auditory canal skin, and even granulation tissues [139]. The expression of RANKL and RANK was localized mainly in the fibroblasts [46, 140] and CD4-positive activated T-cells [89, 135] in the perimatrix and in the cholesteatoma epithelium [143]. Clinically the increased RANKL expression positively correlated with inflammatory markers [144], cholesteatoma progression [143], and osteolysis [145]. Interestingly, few patients showed an upregulation of OPG-positive cells [140] in their cholesteatoma matrix, which was demonstrated to negatively correlated with the of degree of bone resorption [145]. The expression of OPG in the matrix of cholesteatoma might put resistance against the osteolytic RANKL signaling in some cholesteatoma patients. In vitro data on cholesteatoma epithelia cells suggests that this pathogenic expression of RANKL is induced by stimulation of the TLR4 by LPS [146]. In agreement with this, a TLR4 knockdown in an animal model of acquired cholesteatoma reduced the amount of osteoclast formation [64]. In contrast to this, clinical data showed no correlation between RANKL expression and bacterial infection of the cholesteatoma [147]. It can be assumed that this contradiction is partly caused by the low prevalence of Gram (−) bacteria in this study (only 15%). In most cases, the induction of RANKL expression in cholesteatoma is probably rather linked to the high concentration of DAMP able to stimulate TLR4 signaling anyway. Another way to stimulate the expression of RANKL was detected by another research group. They found that microRNA miRNA-17 was present in the exosomes of cholesteatoma keratinocytes and is able to upregulate the expression of RANKL in fibroblasts and thereby promote osteoclast differentiation. Hence, they concluded that miRNA-17 secreted by keratinocytes in patients with middle ear cholesteatoma can upregulate the expression of RANKL in fibroblasts and induce osteoclast differentiation and bone destruction [148].

Apart from bone destruction, the deposition of extracellular matrix is another pathogenic character of cholesteatoma. The cytokine transforming growth factor beta 1 (TGF-β1) is one of the major inducers of ECM deposition. It was demonstrated that the expression of TGF-β1 in cholesteatoma is upregulated compared to that in normal post aural skin [149]. The expression of TGF-β1 was localized in fibroblastic as well as in lymphoid cell residing in the perimatrix [150]. Additionally, the negative regulator of TGF-β1 signaling Smad7 was significantly reduced, and the positive regulator pSMAD2 was enhanced in cholesteatoma epithelial and stromal cells in relation to the same cell types derived from tissue of the retro auricular skin [151]. This upregulation of TGF-β1 signaling can be linked to the expression of tenascin, fibronectin, and collagen fibrils characteristic for stromal fibrosis [150]. Another interesting study demonstrated that not only fibronectin but also its embryonic form generated by alternative splicing that bears the extra domain A-positive fibronectin (EDA-FN) correlated with the localization of TGF-β1 and another positive regulator of TGF-β1 signaling SMAD3 [152]. Since it is known, that EDA-FN expression is induced via TGF-β1 signaling after wound injury [153], this correlation is not surprising. Unfortunately,

EDA-FN is an endogenous ligand for TLR-4 and will therefore further enhance the TLR-4-driven inflammatory state of cholesteatoma tissue. This will lead to a further recruitment of Th1 cells known for their ability to secrete high amount of EDA-FN upon TGF-β1 stimulation [154]. All this will lead to another positive feedback mechanism perpetuating the devastating exaggerated inflammatory state in cholesteatoma tissue. Apart from this ECM-based pathogenesis, TGF-β1 also induces tissue degeneration. For example, a positive correlation between metalloproteases-1 (MMP-1) and TGF-β1 could be detected in cholesteatoma but not in skin of external auditory meatus [155]. Another major enzyme in cholesteatoma-induced tissue degradation the MMP-9 was induced in external ear canal skin keratinocytes by TGF-β1 derived from cholesteatoma debris and granulation tissue extract [156]. In contrast to that, this correlation between MMP-9 and TGF-β1 expression could not be verified in patient-derived tissue homogenates [157].

Reactive oxygen species (ROS) play a substantial role in the immunochemistry of the cholesteatoma. ROS are known to be related to chronic inflammation and immune response [reviewed in [158]]. Their functions comprise direct antimicrobial activity against bacteria and parasites as well as redox-regulation of immune signaling and induction of inflammasome activation. In chronic inflammation, high doses and/or inadequate removal of ROSs result in oxidative stress, which may damage to biological macromolecules and results in the release of DAMPs, one of the basics roots of cholesteatoma pathogenesis [22]. In addition to this, oxidative stress directly activates NF-κB further aggravating the inflammatory state in cholesteatoma reviewed in [159].

Studies investigating the oxidative status in cholesteatomas demonstrated that a high level of oxidation is present in cholesteatoma. For example the general oxidative stress and antioxidant enzyme imbalance was more severe in cases of chronic otitis media with cholesteatoma compared to the non-cholesteatoma groups [160]. Studies focusing on specific components of the ROS system found, that myeloperoxidase (MPO) was more intense and more often present in cholesteatoma patients compared to chronic otitis medium cases [161]. Usually MPO generates hypochlorite by oxidizing chlorite, which will kill bacteria and other pathogens. However, excessive presents of this hypochlorite may also cause oxidative damage in host tissue further accelerating DAMP induced inflammation. In addition to that the osteolysis might be directly enhanced by oxygen-derived free radicals, which act as intermediaries in the formation and activation of osteoclasts in vivo [162]. Beyond this upregulation of oxidative enzymes, the depletion of enzymatic antioxidants (e.g., superoxide dismutase, catalase, and glutathione peroxidase) was observed in cholesteatoma [163]. However, a relationship between activity of enzymatic antioxidants and the extent of bone erosion was not found.

Indirect Immunoregulatory Molecules

Additional to the described inflammatory regulators, many molecules exist, which are able to indirectly modulate the immunochemistry in the cholesteatoma niche. Since the infiltration with immunoregulatory hematopoietic cell, a major event in the establishment of the inflammatory niche of cholesteatoma disease, the inducer of this process was investigated in deeper detail. In general, the attraction and differentiation of these cells are mediated by the cytokines and chemokines expressed through the mechanisms explained above. The transendothelial migration of the T-cell, abundantly found in cholesteatoma tissue, is mainly induced via the intracellular adhesion molecule- 1 (ICAM-1) expressed on the endothelium of cholesteatoma tissue. An enhanced expression of ICAM-1 was detected in vessels of acquired cholesteatoma compared to normal skin [164], normal external ear canal skin, normal tympanic membrane, normal facial ski, [165], or congenital cholesteatoma [101]. Further studies demonstrated a correlation between the inflammatory states, namely, the expression of TNF-α and the upregulation of ICAM-1 [101]. The molecule lymphocyte function-associated antigen 1 (LFA-1) is known as a ligand of ICAM-1 and plays a key role in the process by which T-cells leave the bloodstream to enter the tissues. Studies found that LFA-1 numerous LFA-1-positive cells could be detected in the stroma of inflamed acquired cholesteatomas [165] and that their number was significantly upregulated compared to uninflamed congenital cholesteatoma [101]. Hence, another vicious cycle of self-enhancing inflammation might be present in cholesteatoma, in which the enhanced recruitment of T-cells into the tissue leads to an increase in inflammation, upregulation of ICAM-1, and resulting in even more T-cell migration into the cholesteatoma stroma.

T-cells play a key role in the progression of inflammation in cholesteatoma disease, the role of Human Leukocyte Antigen – DR isotype (HLA-DR) was also more closely investigated in the context of the cholesteatoma disease. In general, HLA-DR functions as MHC class II cell surface receptor presenting, e.g., bacterial antigens to T-cells. HLA-DR is upregulated in cholesteatoma tissue [11, 166] and abundantly expressed in macrophages present in the perimatrix of cholesteatoma tissue [61]. In case of Langerhans cells residing in the cholesteatoma epithelium, the expression could be detected [166, 167] but was not significantly upregulated [168]. This emphasize once more the inferior role that Langerhans cell play in the immunochemistry of cholesteatoma disease. Anyhow the high expression of HLA-DR on macrophages in combination with the abundancy of, e.g., bacterial antigens results in the activation of the frequently found T-cells and is thought to be the source of the immunologically activated state of the infiltrating cells observed in cholesteatoma tissue [169]. Macrophage and T lymphocytes are the most frequent form all blood cells in cholesteatoma tissue. It can be assumed that the antigen presentation of macrophages to T lymphocytes is the most frequent immune regulatory event in cholesteatoma tissue.

Genetics of Cholesteatoma

There are reports of familial clustering of cholesteatoma suggesting a genetic predisposition [170], but to date no genetic susceptibility loci have been clearly identified [171]. A first systematic review about the genetics of cholesteatoma has found a small body of evidence of a heritable component for its etiology [172].

Investigations regarding the DNA content demonstrated that in only one out of 10 cholesteatoma specimen, an abnormal aneuploid DNA content was found, whereas all six postauricular skin specimens had a normal euploid DNA content [172]. A more recent study comprising a greater cohort detected normal euploid DNA content on all investigated 54 specimens [173]. Two studies, aiming on the evaluating of the copy number alterations of chromosomes 3, 7, 8, and 17, found that different degrees of aneusomy were found for all chromosomes except for chromosome 3. They also were able to associate this copy number alterations with the elevated proliferative rate and the aggressiveness of the lesion [174]. When examined the telomeres of cholesteatoma tissue, their length was shorter in congenital cholesteatoma compared to normal external ear canal skin from the same patient. But for acquired cholesteatoma, their telomere length was almost the same as in the corresponding normal external ear canal skin [175].

On the levels of the genetic code, few linkages between acquired cholesteatoma and genetic alteration were identified (Fig. 43.4). A polymorphisms in TLR2(Arg753Gln) was significantly higher in patients with chronic otitis media and different types of mucosal changes in patients with chronic otitis media were correlated to this polymorphism [176]. Also mutations in the CARD8 gene, which do result in an activation of NF-κB in the context of inflammation, were investigated. It was proven that cholesteatoma patients had a twofold and significantly higher incidence of this CARD8 homozygous TT polymorphism. Unfortunately, cholesteatoma patients with this homozygous polymorphism suffered under a greater bone erosion [177]. Genetic investigations in the context of cytokines in cholesteatoma disease showed that the 86 bp variable number tandem repeat VNTR polymorphism in the IL-1RA gene was altered. The IL-1RA allele frequency distribution was significantly lower in cholesteatoma and led to an increased odds ratio for patients to develop cholesteatoma [178]. In another study, the exome of affected and unaffected individuals in families affected by cholesteatoma was sequenced to identify variants in coding DNA that co-segregate with the phenotype [179]. Two of the variants identified were predicted to have a high functional impact, both are rare, loss-of -function variants. A premature stop codon was identified in EGFL8, and a frameshift mutation was identified in BTNL9. Additional nonsynonymous (amino acid changing) missense mutations have been identified. But so far, this mutation could not functionally linked to inflammation and/or pathogenesis of cholesteatoma.

Another cause of the inflammatory dysregulation present in cholesteatoma tissue might lay in epigenetic alterations. It can be assumed that the tissue memory effect in cholesteatoma cells, in regards to their inflammatory response, reflects an epigenetic adaptation of the cells to the chronic inflammation present in the cholesteatoma niche. It is known that acetylation of histone H3 at the promoters of multiple cytokines and chemokines subsequent to initial inflammation results in the increased recruitment of NF-κB to these regions in a self-enforced positive feedback loop [180]. By

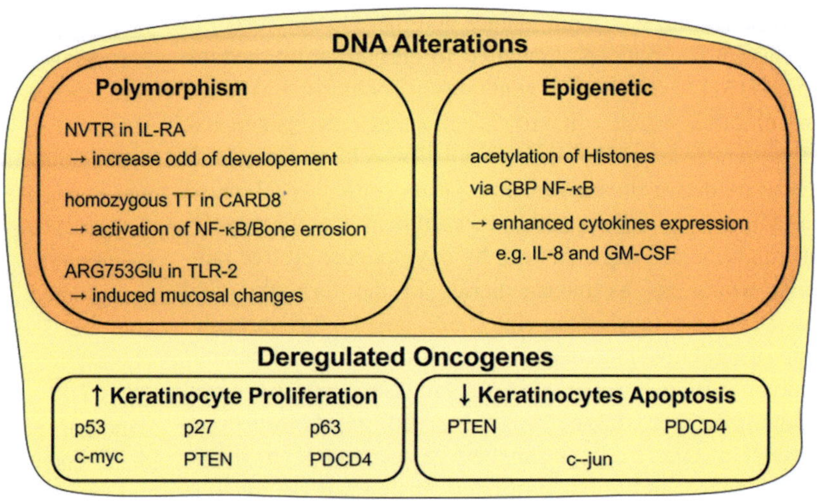

Fig. 43.4 The various aspects of the genetics in a cholesteatoma cell. Inside the schemed nucleus (orange) are the alteration on the DNA level and their relation to cholesteatoma disease. In the cytoplasm (beige) are the deregulated oncogenes and their influence on keratinocyte proliferation and apoptosis depicted

similar means, NF-κB mediates the activation of histone H3 and H4 acetylation reviewed in [181] by DAMPs or PAMPs is able to increase the expression of, e.g., GM-CSF [182] observed in cholesteatoma tissue. Additionally, para- and autocrine mechanisms in cholesteatoma tissue via IL-1β might led to epigenetic changes in cholesteatoma cells as well. This can be caused by the fact IL-1β is able to drive the rapid acetylation of histones via CBP/p300, which is known to acetylate the histones at the promoter of IL-8 [183]. Indeed, the epidermal stem cells present in cholesteatoma tissue represent a good storage medium for epigenetic memories, since they hand their inflammatory memory down to their offspring during the repopulation of the cholesteatoma. Similar mechanisms were already observed for other inflammatory diseases and epidermal stem cells of the skin, respectively [184].

Oncogenes also might play a role in the pathogenesis of cholesteatoma, since they are known to cause survival and proliferation in cells normally designated for apoptosis (Fig. 43.4). The expression of p53, famous for its role in progression through the cell cycle, was found to be 9–20 times higher in cholesteatoma than in normal post auricular skin or tympanic membrane [185]. Further studies showed that the p53 protein was not only overexpressed in cholesteatoma tissue but also localized in the nucleus of keratinocytes in the granular layer of cholesteatoma epithelium, where it further enhances their proliferation [86]. In the same study, a likewise upregulation of c-jun, an oncogenic transcription factor, was proven for cholesteatoma tissue. Similar to p53 the c-jun protein was mainly localized in keratinocytes of the basal and spinous layers of the epithelium. Another oncogene c-myc, known for being linked to the control of growth and differentiation, is upregulated in cholesteatoma compared to atheroma and to normal skin [186]. Hence, it is also subjected to play a role in the pathogenesis of cholesteatoma disease. Investigations utilizing in situ hybridization found that 10 out of 15 cholesteatoma cases showed enhanced frequency of c-myc and likewise to [174] aneuploidy of chromosome 8, the chromosome to which the c-myc gene is localized [187]. They concluded that the deregulating c-myc expression in cholesteatoma might be related to the enhanced c-myc copy number. Another study focused on the localization of c-myc and detected the protein in the nucleus of cholesteatoma epithelium, where it is able to effectively enhance the expression of various genes related to epithelial proliferation. In contrast to that, it was only in an inactive state and localized in the cytoplasmatic region in normal skin [188]. The tumor suppressor p27 was significantly downregulated fivefold in cholesteatoma tissue [189]. Since alterations of p27 levels in keratinocytes can influence their proliferative state, the investigators suggested that the altered p27 levels in cholesteatoma may contribute to the pathology in cholesteatoma. Another study was able to detect an enhance expression of p63, belonging to the p53 gene family, in cholesteatoma tissue [190]. Since p63 is involved in multiple functions during skin growth and development, they concluded that this finding might be linked to the excessive epithelial cell growth characteristic for middle ear cholesteatoma. The tumorsupressor PTEN and PDCD4 were found to be greatly reduced in 3 of 4 cholesteatoma samples. This could be linked to their regulatory miRNA-21, which was upregulated 4.4 fold in cholesteatoma [191]. In accordance with that, another study detected that let-7a downregulates the expression of miRNA-21 and that this mechanism resulted in the suppression of proliferation and induction of apoptosis in keratinocytes derived from cholesteatoma presumably through PTEN and/or PDCD4 [192]. Additional studies could link the expression of PTEN to miRNA-802 [193]. They found a direct link between the enhanced NF-κB signaling, miRNA-802 expression, miR-802 induced repression of PTEN, and the promotion of keratinocyte cell proliferation. They concluded that the NF-κB/miR-802/PTEN signaling pathway plays an important role in the development of cholesteatoma.

Discussion

This chapter of the book illustrates the complex and multilayered immunoregulatory network of cholesteatoma disease. Similar to many chronical inflammations, the chronic form of otitis media is able to severely change the finely tuned immunochemical interplay initially designed to protect our body. We described how long-term exposure of the middle ear to tissue damage (DAMPs) and infections (PAMPs) can overload its innate immune system and cause long time tissue stress, which results in an exaggerated immune reaction in the middle ear.

We described numerous predispositions making the immune system of some chronic otitis media patients go out of course. It might start with an upregulation of some PRRs, which can result in an oversensitive response to the present DAMPs and PAMPs. This results in an increase inflammatory output of the cells present in the middle ear. Subsequently, much too many immune cells, mainly mast cells macrophages and T-cells, are recruited to the side. These cells are potent immune regulators and further raise the level of various immunoregulatory extracellular signals resulting in an additional tightening of the highly inflammatory state of cholesteatoma. This mechanism, which can already be described as vicious circle, can be intensified by cholesteatoma characteristics. On one hand, the acceleration of proliferation and cell death in the matrix generates more and more DAMPs, and on the other hand, the high concentrations of PRRs like RAGE and TLR-4 are able to further enhance the DAMP driven output. Furthermore, positive feedback loops do exist in the middle ear under this condition of heavy chronic inflammation. They are capable to tip the equilibrium of the immunochemistry of cholesteatoma tissue even more out of balance. The most prominent are the self-induced expression of cytokine like TNF-α highly expressed in cholesteatoma tissue, the self-enhancing interplay between IL-1β and GM-CSF in the keratinocytes/fibroblast network, or the NF-κB driven acetylation of histones driving cytokine expression paracrinely enabling further NF-κB activation. In the end of this disturbed tissue homeostasis, an exaggerated expression of paracrine signaling related to the wound healing process is able to further boost the proliferation of epidermal cells, the most prominent symptom of cholesteatoma development and osteoclast maturation and activation and subsequent bone erosion. Hence, this highlights mechanisms, designed to protect the middle ear in the case of the otitis media, are able to turn from a protector into an aggressor during prolonged inflammation and the concomitant tissue stress.

Conclusions and Future Work

The only medical treatment of cholesteatoma is a surgical intervention. It is known that the probability of cholesteatoma recurrence is highly depended on the radicalism of the surgical treatment [194]. Besides this, the recurrence is often correlated to the high level of inflammation [195]. Therefore, a reduction in the inflammatory burden is most favorable for the postsurgical therapy.

As described, one source of this inflammation is PAMPs. Hence, postsurgical application of antibiotics is commonly utilized to reduce the abundancy of PAMPs. Unfortunately, the infection of cholesteatoma tissue is most often present in the form of a biofilm [29, 196, 197]. Hence, the applied antibiotics do not completely eradicate the infection and are only able to reduce the bacterial load for a short time. The release of DAMPs from the inflamed and decomposing tissue always goes along with cholesteatoma disease and thus is hard to prevented. Anyhow, a specific approach might be the selective inhibition of COX-2, which is upregulated in cholesteatoma tissue, by nonsteroidal anti-inflammatory drugs. This will reduce the synthesis of the DAMP PEG and hence reduce the inflammatory state. A more direct approach would be to aim on the main gate to inflammatory signaling inside cholesteatoma tissue, the PRRs. Clinical relevance of RAGE inhibition in inflammatory disease is being demonstrated in emerging clinical trials investigating novel small-molecule RAGE inhibitors [198]. The TLR4, probably the major driver of the exaggerated cholesteatoma inflammation, might be blocked by antagonists, which were clinically investigated already like Eritoran [199] or TAK-242 [200]. We think that the postsurgical topical application of these noncytotoxic substances might significantly decrease cholesteatoma recurrence. Downstream of PRRs lays the multilayered inflammatory landscape. Its high level of inflammation exacerbated itself through numerous positive feedback loops. Because of the diversity of targets found on the level of extracellular signaling, a therapy based on molecular strategies seems unfavorable. Thus, anti-inflammatory drug with broad spectrum was investigated. The popular drug dexamethasone showed good results in in vitro models [146]. In clinical trials, the topical application of dexamethasone postsurgery was also able to perform well and reduced the recurrence rate. Unfortunately, long-term application of these substances is not possible, since it will lead to infections of the middle ear. But topical treatment of the operation side with steroids directly after surgery is common in cholesteatoma surgery to reduce the inflammation at least for a short period of time. At the end of the inflammatory cascade described in this chapter arise the symptoms of cholesteatoma disease, amely, hyperproliferation of epidermal cells and bone resorption. In the past, different approaches were made to induce apoptosis in epidermal cells by heavy cytotoxic drugs usually applied on cancer patients [201, 202]. But the activated oncogenes described above, who drive the proliferation of cholesteatoma epidermal cells, might offer a target for more sophisticated molecular-based treatment strategies, which are applied nowadays in up to date cancer research.

We hope that this chapter will help the readers to gain a better insight into cholesteatoma pathogenesis, the primary root of the progression, and recurrence of cholesteatoma disease. A profound understanding of the links between inflammation, wrongly coined innate immune system, and extracellular signaling is needed. This may lead to novel pharmaceutical strategies enable to interrupt these pathways. Eventually, it would improve cholesteatoma treatment, thus enabling the preservation of middle ear function for many cholesteatoma patients.

References

1. Ohta S, Sakagami M, Suzuki M, Mishiro Y. Eustachian tube function and habitual sniffing in middle ear cholesteatoma. Otol Neurotol. 2009;30:48–53. https://doi.org/10.1097/MAO.0b013e31818de5b3.
2. Magnuson B. Tubal closing failure in retraction type cholesteatoma and adhesive middle ear lesions. Acta Otolaryngol. 1978;86:408–17. https://doi.org/10.3109/00016487809107520.
3. Yamamoto-Fukuda T, Akiyama N, Kojima H. L1CAM-ILK-YAP mechanotransduction drives proliferative activity of epithelial cells in middle ear cholesteatoma. Am J Pathol. 2020;190:1667–79. https://doi.org/10.1016/j.ajpath.2020.04.007.
4. Nguyen KH, et al. Possible participation of acidic pH in bone resorption in middle ear cholesteatoma. Laryngoscope. 2014;124:245–50. https://doi.org/10.1002/lary.23883.

5. Hussein MR, Sayed RH, Abu-Dief EE. Immune cell profile in invasive cholesteatomas: preliminary findings. Exp Mol Pathol. 2010;88:316–23. https://doi.org/10.1016/j.yexmp.2009.12.006.
6. Negri B, Schilling V, Bujia J, Schulz P, Kastenbauer E. Immunotype findings in macrophages in aural cholesteatomas. Eur Arch Otorhinolaryngol. 1992;249:87–90. https://doi.org/10.1007/BF00186453.
7. Fang L, et al. Analysis of inflammatory and homeostatic roles of tissue-resident macrophages in the progression of cholesteatoma by RNA-Seq. Immunol Investig. 2021;50(6):1–13. https://doi.org/10.1080/08820139.2020.1781161.
8. Akdogan V, Yilmaz I, Canpolat T, Ozluoglu LN. Role of Langerhans cells, Ki-67 protein and apoptosis in acquired cholesteatoma: prospective clinical study. J Laryngol Otol. 2013;127:252–9. https://doi.org/10.1017/S0022215112003180.
9. Liu L, Li Z, Hu M. Langerhans cells and human aural cholesteatoma. Zhonghua Er Bi Yan Hou Ke Za Zhi. 1995;30:33–6.
10. Albino AP, Reed JA, Bogdany JK, Sassoon J, Parisier SC. Increased numbers of mast cells in human middle ear cholesteatomas: implications for treatment. Am J Otol. 1998;19:266–72.
11. Ottaviani F, Neglia CB, Berti E. Cytokines and adhesion molecules in middle ear cholesteatoma. A role in epithelial growth? Acta Otolaryngol. 1999;119:462–7. https://doi.org/10.1080/00016489950181008.
12. Metz M, et al. Mast cells in the promotion and limitation of chronic inflammation. Immunol Rev. 2007;217:304–28. https://doi.org/10.1111/j.1600-065X.2007.00520.x.
13. Berger G, Hawke M, Ekem JK. Bone resorption in chronic otitis media. The role of mast cells. Acta Otolaryngol. 1985;100:72–80. https://doi.org/10.3109/00016488509108590.
14. Jiang H, et al. TREM-2 promotes acquired cholesteatoma-induced bone destruction by modulating TLR4 signaling pathway and osteoclasts activation. Sci Rep. 2016;6:38761. https://doi.org/10.1038/srep38761.
15. Banco B, et al. Canine aural cholesteatoma: a histological and immunohistochemical study. Vet J. 2014;200:440–5. https://doi.org/10.1016/j.tvjl.2014.03.018.
16. Schilling V, Bujia J, Negri B, Schulz P, Kastenbauer E. Immunologically activated cells in aural cholesteatoma. Am J Otolaryngol. 1991;12:249–53. https://doi.org/10.1016/0196-0709(91)90001-v.
17. Bujia J, et al. Quantitative analysis of interleukin-1-alpha gene expression in middle ear cholesteatoma. Laryngoscope. 1996;106:217–20. https://doi.org/10.1097/00005537-199602000-00021.
18. Van Linthout S, Miteva K, Tschope C. Crosstalk between fibroblasts and inflammatory cells. Cardiovasc Res. 2014;102:258–69. https://doi.org/10.1093/cvr/cvu062.
19. Jiang Y, et al. Cytokinocytes: the diverse contribution of keratinocytes to immune responses in skin. JCI Insight. 2020;5(20):e142067. https://doi.org/10.1172/jci.insight.142067.
20. Benhadou F, Mintoff D, Del Marmol V. Psoriasis: keratinocytes or immune cells—which is the trigger? Dermatology. 2019;235:91–100. https://doi.org/10.1159/000495291.
21. Kuo CL, et al. Updates and knowledge gaps in cholesteatoma research. Biomed Res Int. 2015;2015:854024. https://doi.org/10.1155/2015/854024.
22. Maniu A, et al. Molecular biology of cholesteatoma. Roman J Morphol Embryol. 2014;55:7–13.
23. Ricciardiello F, Cavaliere M, Mesolella M, Iengo M. Notes on the microbiology of cholesteatoma: clinical findings and treatment. Acta Otorhinolaryngol Ital. 2009;29:197–202.
24. Xu F, Kong W, Peng J, Gu H, Zheng H. Analysis of main pathogenic bacteria and drug sensitivity in patients with chronic suppurative otitis media and middle ear cholesteatoma in China. Biotechnol Lett. 2020;42:1559–66. https://doi.org/10.1007/s10529-020-02880-7.
25. Weiss JP, Antonelli PJ, Dirain CO. Microbiome analysis of cholesteatoma by gene sequencing. Otol Neurotol. 2019;40:1186–93. https://doi.org/10.1097/MAO.0000000000002355.
26. Minami SB, et al. Microbiomes of the normal middle ear and ears with chronic otitis media. Laryngoscope. 2017;127:E371–7. https://doi.org/10.1002/lary.26579.
27. Gu X, Keyoumu Y, Long L, Zhang H. Detection of bacterial biofilms in different types of chronic otitis media. Eur Arch Otorhinolaryngol. 2014;271:2877–83. https://doi.org/10.1007/s00405-013-2766-8.
28. Kaya E, et al. Investigation of the presence of biofilms in chronic suppurative otitis media, nonsuppurative otitis media, and chronic otitis media with cholesteatoma by scanning electron microscopy. Sci World J. 2013;2013:638715.
29. Lampikoski H, Aarnisalo AA, Jero J, Kinnari TJ. Mastoid biofilm in chronic otitis media. Otol Neurotol. 2012;33:785–8. https://doi.org/10.1097/MAO.0b013e318259533f.
30. Attallah MS. Microbiology of chronic suppurative otitis media with cholesteatoma. Saudi Med J. 2000;21:924–7.
31. Singh GB, Solo M, Kaur R, Arora R, Kumar S. Mycology of chronic suppurative otitis media-cholesteatoma disease: an evaluative study. Am J Otolaryngol. 2018;39:157–61. https://doi.org/10.1016/j.amjoto.2017.12.001.
32. Peek FA, et al. Lipopolysaccharide concentration and bone resorption in cholesteatoma. Otol Neurotol. 2003;24:709–13. https://doi.org/10.1097/00129492-200309000-00002.
33. Jung JY, et al. P. aeruginosa infection increases morbidity in experimental cholesteatomas. Laryngoscope. 2011;121:2449–54. https://doi.org/10.1002/lary.22189.
34. Sugita T, Huang CC, Abramson M. The effect of endotoxin and prostaglandin E2 on the proliferation of keratinocytes in vitro. Arch Oto-Rhino-Laryngol. 1986;243:211–4. https://doi.org/10.1007/BF00470624.
35. Lotze MT, et al. The grateful dead: damage-associated molecular pattern molecules and reduction/oxidation regulate immunity. Immunol Rev. 2007;220:60–81. https://doi.org/10.1111/j.1600-065X.2007.00579.x.
36. Shinoda H, Huang C-C. Heat shock proteins in middle ear cholesteatoma. Otolaryngol Head Neck Surg. 1996;114:77–83.
37. Ho KY, et al. Upregulation of phosphorylated HSP27, PRDX2, GRP75, GRP78 and GRP94 in acquired middle ear cholesteatoma growth. Int J Mol Sci. 2013;14:14439–59. https://doi.org/10.3390/ijms140714439.
38. Macias JD, Gerkin RD, Locke D, Macias MP. Differential gene expression in cholesteatoma by DNA chip analysis. Laryngoscope. 2013;123(Suppl. S5):S1–S21. https://doi.org/10.1002/lary.24176.
39. Klenke C, et al. Identification of novel cholesteatoma-related gene expression signatures using full-genome microarrays. PLoS One. 2012;7:e52718. https://doi.org/10.1371/journal.pone.0052718.
40. Austermann J, Spiekermann C, Roth J. S100 proteins in rheumatic diseases. Nat Rev Rheumatol. 2018;14:528–41. https://doi.org/10.1038/s41584-018-0058-9.
41. Hong W, et al. Expression of calcium-binding proteins S100A8, S100A9 and S100A12 in otitis media. Int J Pediatr Otorhinolaryngol. 2017;101:30–6. https://doi.org/10.1016/j.ijporl.2017.07.025.
42. Szczepanski MJ, et al. Molecular signaling of the HMGB1/RAGE axis contributes to cholesteatoma pathogenesis. J Mol Med (Berl). 2015;93:305–14. https://doi.org/10.1007/s00109-014-1217-3.
43. Bellussi LM, et al. High-mobility group box protein 1 expression in inflammatory diseases of the middle ear. Int J Immunopathol Pharmacol. 2017;30:168–73. https://doi.org/10.1177/0394632017698713.
44. Wu CX, Sun H, Liu Q, Guo H, Gong JP. LPS induces HMGB1 relocation and release by activating the NF-kappaB-CBP signal transduction pathway in the murine macrophage-like cell

line RAW264.7. J Surg Res. 2012;175:88–100. https://doi.org/10.1016/j.jss.2011.02.026.
45. Catli T, et al. Quantitative measurement of m-RNA levels to assess expression of cyclooxygenase-II, inducible nitric oxide synthase and 12-lipoxygenase genes in middle ear cholesteatoma. Eur Arch Otorhinolaryngol. 2014;271:1471–5. https://doi.org/10.1007/s00405-013-2614-x.
46. Imai R, et al. Osteoclasts modulate bone erosion in cholesteatoma via RANKL signaling. J Assoc Res Otolaryngol. 2019;20:449–59. https://doi.org/10.1007/s10162-019-00727-1.
47. Jung TT, Juhn SK. Prostaglandins in human cholesteatoma and granulation tissue. Am J Otol. 1988;9:197–200.
48. Dubois RN, et al. Cyclooxygenase in biology and disease. FASEB J. 1998;12:1063–73.
49. Abramson M, Moriyama H, Huang CC. Histology, pathogenesis, and treatment of cholesteatoma. Ann Otol Rhinol Laryngol Suppl. 1984;112:125–8. https://doi.org/10.1177/00034894840930s421.
50. Seong SY, Matzinger P. Hydrophobicity: an ancient damage-associated molecular pattern that initiates innate immune responses. Nat Rev Immunol. 2004;4:469–78. https://doi.org/10.1038/nri1372.
51. Rouhiainen A, Kuja-Panula J, Tumova S, Rauvala H. RAGE-mediated cell signaling. Methods Mol Biol. 2013;963:239–63. https://doi.org/10.1007/978-1-62703-230-8_15.
52. Nakashima A, et al. Effect of circulating soluble receptor for advanced glycation end products (sRAGE) and the proinflammatory RAGE ligand (EN-RAGE, S100A12) on mortality in hemodialysis patients. Clin J Am Soc Nephrol. 2010;5:2213–9. https://doi.org/10.2215/CJN.03360410.
53. Lei H, Li X, Jing B, Xu H, Wu Y. Human S100A7 induces mature Interleukin1alpha expression by RAGE-p38 MAPK-Calpain1 pathway in psoriasis. PLoS One. 2017;12:e0169788. https://doi.org/10.1371/journal.pone.0169788.
54. Hermani A, De Servi B, Medunjanin S, Tessier PA, Mayer D. S100A8 and S100A9 activate MAP kinase and NF-kappaB signaling pathways and trigger translocation of RAGE in human prostate cancer cells. Exp Cell Res. 2006;312:184–97. https://doi.org/10.1016/j.yexcr.2005.10.013.
55. Ibrahim ZA, Armour CL, Phipps S, Sukkar MB. RAGE and TLRs: relatives, friends or neighbours? Mol Immunol. 2013;56:739–44. https://doi.org/10.1016/j.molimm.2013.07.008.
56. Wang S, Xie L, Zhang Y, Xu P, Liu A. Expression of prostaglandin E2 receptors in acquired middle ear cholesteatoma. Clin Exp Otorhinolaryngol. 2018;11:17–22. https://doi.org/10.21053/ceo.2017.00304.
57. Gobec M, Prijatelj M, Delic J, Markovic T, Mlinaric-Rascan I. Chemo-sensitizing effects of EP4 receptor-induced inactivation of nuclear factor-kappaB. Eur J Pharmacol. 2014;742:81–8. https://doi.org/10.1016/j.ejphar.2014.08.039.
58. Kim MG, et al. Increased expression of Dec-205, Bcl-10, Tim-3, and Trem-1 mRNA in chronic otitis media with cholesteatoma. Acta Oto-Laryngol. 2014;134:475–80. https://doi.org/10.3109/00016489.2013.878474.
59. Shrimpton RE, et al. CD205 (DEC-205): a recognition receptor for apoptotic and necrotic self. Mol Immunol. 2009;46:1229–39. https://doi.org/10.1016/j.molimm.2008.11.016.
60. Hamidzadeh K, Christensen SM, Dalby E, Chandrasekaran P, Mosser DM. Macrophages and the recovery from acute and chronic inflammation. Ann Rev Physiol. 79:567–92. https://doi.org/10.1146/annurev-physiol-022516-034348.
61. Szczepanski M, et al. Toll-like receptors 2, 3 and 4 (TLR-2, TLR-3 and TLR-4) are expressed in the microenvironment of human acquired cholesteatoma. Eur Arch Otorhinolaryngol. 2006;263:603–7. https://doi.org/10.1007/s00405-006-0030-1.
62. Byun JY, Cha CI, Yeo SG, Lee SK, Cho JS. Expression of toll-like receptor 2 and toll-like receptor 4 in cholesteatoma. Korean J Otolaryngol Head Neck Surg. 2006;49:482–7.
63. Hirai H, et al. Expression of toll-like receptors in chronic otitis media and cholesteatoma. Intl J Pediatr Otorhinolaryngol. 2013;77:674–6. https://doi.org/10.1016/j.ijporl.2013.01.010.
64. Si Y, et al. TLR4 drives the pathogenesis of acquired cholesteatoma by promoting local inflammation and bone destruction. Sci Rep. 2015;5:16683. https://doi.org/10.1038/srep16683.
65. Yu M, et al. HMGB1 signals through toll-like receptor (TLR) 4 and TLR2. Shock. 2006;26:174–9. https://doi.org/10.1097/01.shk.0000225404.51320.82.
66. Jin C, et al. Human myocardium releases heat shock protein 27 (HSP27) after global ischemia: the proinflammatory effect of extracellular HSP27 through toll-like receptor (TLR)-2 and TLR4. Mol Med. 2014;20:280–9. https://doi.org/10.2119/molmed.2014.00058.
67. Asea A, et al. Novel signal transduction pathway utilized by extracellular HSP70: role of toll-like receptor (TLR) 2 and TLR4. J Biol Chem. 2002;277:15028–34. https://doi.org/10.1074/jbc.M200497200.
68. Nagel J, et al. Stem cells in middle ear cholesteatoma contribute to its pathogenesis. Sci Rep. 2018;8:6204. https://doi.org/10.1038/s41598-018-24616-4.
69. Schurmann M, et al. Stem Cell-Induced Inflammation in Cholesteatoma is Inhibited by the TLR4 Antagonist LPS-RS. Cells. 2020;9 https://doi.org/10.3390/cells9010199.
70. Branger J, et al. Role of Toll-like receptor 4 in gram-positive and gram-negative pneumonia in mice. Infect Immun. 2004;72:788–94. https://doi.org/10.1128/IAI.72.2.788-794.2004.
71. Swaroop S, Sengupta N, Suryawanshi AR, Adlakha YK, Basu A. HSP60 plays a regulatory role in IL-1β-induced microglial inflammation via TLR4-p38 MAPK axis. J Neuroinflammation. 2016;13:1–19.
72. Ehrchen JM, Sunderkotter C, Foell D, Vogl T, Roth J. The endogenous Toll-like receptor 4 agonist S100A8/S100A9 (calprotectin) as innate amplifier of infection, autoimmunity, and cancer. J Leukoc Biol. 2009;86:557–66. https://doi.org/10.1189/jlb.1008647.
73. Vogl T, et al. Mrp8 and Mrp14 are endogenous activators of Toll-like receptor 4, promoting lethal, endotoxin-induced shock. Nat Med. 2007;13:1042–9. https://doi.org/10.1038/nm1638.
74. Qin YH, et al. HMGB1 enhances the proinflammatory activity of lipopolysaccharide by promoting the phosphorylation of MAPK p38 through receptor for advanced glycation end products. J Immunol. 2009;183:6244–50. https://doi.org/10.4049/jimmunol.0900390.
75. Triantafilou M, Triantafilou K. Heat-shock protein 70 and heat-shock protein 90 associate with Toll-like receptor 4 in response to bacterial lipopolysaccharide. Biochem Soc Trans. 2004;32:636–9. https://doi.org/10.1042/BST0320636.
76. Wu M, et al. TREM-1 amplifies corneal inflammation after Pseudomonas aeruginosa infection by modulating Toll-like receptor signaling and Th1/Th2-type immune responses. Infect Immun. 2011;79:2709–16. https://doi.org/10.1128/IAI.00144-11.
77. Schurmann M, et al. Chronic inflammation of middle ear cholesteatoma promotes its recurrence via a paracrine mechanism. Cell Commun Signal. 2021;19:25. https://doi.org/10.1186/s12964-020-00690-y.
78. Girardin SE, et al. Nod2 is a general sensor of peptidoglycan through muramyl dipeptide (MDP) detection. J Biol Chem. 2003;278:8869–72. https://doi.org/10.1074/jbc.C200651200.
79. Lee HY, Park MS, Byun JY, Kim YI, Yeo SG. Expression of pattern recognition receptors in cholesteatoma. Eur Arch Otorhinolaryngol. 2014;271:245–53. https://doi.org/10.1007/s00405-013-2402-7.

80. Leichtle A, et al. NOD-like receptor signaling in cholesteatoma. Biomed Res Int. 2015;2015:408169. https://doi.org/10.1155/2015/408169.
81. Inohara N, et al. Host recognition of bacterial muramyl dipeptide mediated through NOD2. Implications for Crohn's disease. J Biol Chem. 2003;278:5509–12. https://doi.org/10.1074/jbc.C200673200.
82. Kim SH, et al. Expression of C-type lectin receptor mRNA in chronic otitis media with cholesteatoma. Acta Otolaryngol. 2017;137:581–7. https://doi.org/10.1080/00016489.2016.1269196.
83. Arts RJ, Joosten LA, van der Meer JW, Netea MG. TREM-1: intracellular signaling pathways and interaction with pattern recognition receptors. J Leukoc Biol. 2013;93:209–15. https://doi.org/10.1189/jlb.0312145.
84. Denning NL, et al. Extracellular CIRP as an endogenous TREM-1 ligand to fuel inflammation in sepsis. JCI insight. 2020;5 https://doi.org/10.1172/jci.insight.134172.
85. Fu L, et al. Identification of extracellular actin As a ligand for triggering receptor expressed on myeloid cells-1 signaling. Front Immunol. 2017;8:917. https://doi.org/10.3389/fimmu.2017.00917.
86. Shinoda H, Huang CC. Expressions of c-jun and p53 proteins in human middle ear cholesteatoma: relationship to keratinocyte proliferation, differentiation, and programmed cell death. Laryngoscope. 1995;105:1232–7. https://doi.org/10.1288/00005537-199511000-00018.
87. Liang C-F, Zhao K, Fan S-H. Expression of c-fos and c-jun gene proteins in cholesteatoma of middle ear and its significance. Chinese J Clin Oncol Rehab. 2006;13:289.
88. Huang CC, Chen CT, Huang TS, Shinoda H. Mediation of signal transduction in keratinocytes of human middle ear cholesteatoma by ras protein. Eur Arch Otorhinolaryngol. 1996;253:385–9. https://doi.org/10.1007/BF00168488.
89. Xia M, et al. Expression and significance of nuclear factor-kappa B ligand and correlation factor in the tissue of otitis media with cholesteatoma. J Clin Otorhinolaryngol Head Neck Surg. 2007;21:315–7.
90. Hao, Y., Li, K., Wang, J.-T. & Ma, M. Expression of NF-κB and caspase-3 in middle ear cholesteatoma and its clinical significance [J]. J Shanxi Med Univ 2011;4.
91. Xu Y, Tao ZZ, Hua QQ, Wang XX, Xiao BK. Expression and activation of nuclear factor-kappaB in middle ear cholesteatoma. Chinese J Otorhinolaryngol Head Neck Surg. 2006;41:455–9.
92. Zhang QA, Hamajima Y, Zhang Q, Lin J. Identification of Id1 in acquired middle ear cholesteatoma. Arch Otolaryngol Head Neck Surg. 2008;134:306–10. https://doi.org/10.1001/archotol.134.3.306.
93. Fukudome S, et al. Regulation of the angiogenesis of acquired middle ear cholesteatomas by inhibitor of DNA binding transcription factor. JAMA Otolaryngol Head Neck Surg. 2013;139:273–8. https://doi.org/10.1001/jamaoto.2013.1750.
94. Yang Y, Liou HC, Sun XH. Id1 potentiates NF-kappaB activation upon T cell receptor signaling. J Biol Chem. 2006;281:34989–96. https://doi.org/10.1074/jbc.M608078200.
95. Zhou H, et al. Bcl10 activates the NF-kappaB pathway through ubiquitination of NEMO. Nature. 2004;427:167–71. https://doi.org/10.1038/nature02273.
96. Byun JY, Yune TY, Lee JY, Yeo SG, Park MS. Expression of CYLD and NF-kappaB in human cholesteatoma epithelium. Mediat Inflamm. 2010;796315 https://doi.org/10.1155/2010/796315.
97. Zhang C, Chen M, Chi Z. Cytokine secretion and pyroptosis of cholesteatoma keratinocytes mediated by AIM2 inflammasomes in response to cytoplasmic DNA. Mol Med Rep. 2021;23 https://doi.org/10.3892/mmr.2021.11983.
98. Kariya S, et al. NLRP3 inflammasome expression in lipopolysaccharide-induced otitis media. Acta Otolaryngol. 2018;138:1061–5. https://doi.org/10.1080/00016489.2018.1515499.
99. Kariya S, et al. Activation of NLRP3 inflammasome in human middle ear cholesteatoma and chronic otitis media. Acta Otolaryngol. 2016;136:136–40. https://doi.org/10.3109/00016489.2015.1093171.
100. Iino Y, Toriyama M, Ogawa H, Kawakami M. Cholesteatoma debris as an activator of human monocytes. Potentiation of the production of tumor necrosis factor. Acta Otolaryngol. 1990;110:410–5. https://doi.org/10.3109/00016489009107462.
101. Akimoto R, Pawankar R, Yagi T, Baba S. Acquired and congenital cholesteatoma: determination of tumor necrosis factor-alpha, intercellular adhesion molecule-1, interleukin-1-alpha and lymphocyte functional antigen-1 in the inflammatory process. J Oto-rhino-laryngol Rel Spec. 2000;62:257–65. https://doi.org/10.1159/000027756.
102. Yetiser S, Satar B, Aydin N. Expression of epidermal growth factor, tumor necrosis factor-alpha, and interleukin-1alpha in chronic otitis media with or without cholesteatoma. Otol Neurotol. 2002;23:647–52. https://doi.org/10.1097/00129492-200209000-00007.
103. Marenda SA, Aufdemorte TB. Localization of cytokines in cholesteatoma tissue. Otolaryngol Head Neck Surg. 1995;112:359–68.
104. Yan S-D, Huang C-C. Tumor necrosis factor alpha in middle ear cholesteatoma and its effect on keratinocytes in vitro. Ann Otol Rhinol Laryngol. 1991;100:157–61.
105. Sastry KV, Sharma SC, Mann SB, Ganguly NK, Panda NK. Aural cholesteatoma: role of tumor necrosis factor-alpha in bone destruction. Am J Otol. 1999;20:158–61.
106. Chodynicki S, Soroczynska J, [TNF alpha in serum of patients with cholesteatoma]. Polish Otolaryngol. 1994;48:279–81.
107. Zhou X-N, Van De Water TR. The effect of target tissues on survival and differentiation of mammalian statoacoustic ganglion neurons in organ culture. Acta Otolaryngol. 1987;104:90–8.
108. Hilton CW, Ondrey FG, Wuertz BR, Levine SC. Interleukin-8 production in response to tumor necrosis factor-alpha by cholesteatoma keratinocytes in cell culture. Laryngoscope. 2011;121:372–4. https://doi.org/10.1002/lary.21352.
109. Schmid H, Dort J, Fisch U. Long-term results of treatment for children's cholesteatoma. Otol Neurotol. 1991;12:83–7.
110. Sakuma Y, et al. Crucial involvement of the EP4 subtype of prostaglandin E receptor in osteoclast formation by proinflammatory cytokines and lipopolysaccharide. J Bone Miner Res. 2000;15:218–27. https://doi.org/10.1359/jbmr.2000.15.2.218.
111. Artono Surarto B, Purnami N, Hutahaen F, Mahardhika MR. The association of IL-1 Alpha level and TNF Alpha expressions on bone destruction in chronic suppurative otitis media and cholesteatoma. Indian J Otolaryngol Head Neck Surg. 2020;72:1–7. https://doi.org/10.1007/s12070-019-01704-z.
112. Kuczkowski J, Sakowicz-Burkiewicz M, Izycka-Swieszewska E, Mikaszewski B, Pawelczyk T. Expression of tumor necrosis factor-alpha, interleukin-1alpha, interleukin-6 and interleukin-10 in chronic otitis media with bone osteolysis. J Oto-Rhino-Laryngol Rel Spec. 2011;73:93–9. https://doi.org/10.1159/000323831.
113. Vitale RF, Ribeiro FDAQ. O papel do Fator de Necrose Tumoral Alfa (TNF-alfa) no processo de erosão óssea presente no colesteatoma adquirido da orelha média. Rev Bras Otorrinolaringol. 2007;73:123–7.
114. Kato A, et al. Interleukin-6 and tumour necrosis factor alpha synthesized by cholesteatoma cells affect mucociliary function in the eustachian tube. Acta Otolaryngol Suppl. 1998;538:90–7. https://doi.org/10.1080/00016489850182792.
115. Vitale RF, Pereira CSB, Alves AL, Fregnani J, Ribeiro FQ. TNF-R2 expression in acquired middle ear cholesteatoma. Braz J

Otorhinolaryngol. 2011;77:531–6. https://doi.org/10.1590/S1808-86942011000400020.
116. Sudhoff H, Borkowski G, Bujia J, Hildmann H, Fisseler-Eckhoff A. Immunohistochemical studies with middle ear mucosal remnants in cholesteatoma. HNO. 1997;45:630–5. https://doi.org/10.1007/s001060050138.
117. Bujia J, et al. Interleukin 1 (IL-1) and IL-1-receptor antagonist (IL-1-RA) in middle ear cholesteatoma: an analysis of protein production and biological activity. Eur Arch Otorhinolaryngol. 1996;253:252–5. https://doi.org/10.1007/BF00171137.
118. Schilling V, Negri B, Bujia J, Schulz P, Kastenbauer E. Possible role of interleukin 1 alpha and interleukin 1 beta in the pathogenesis of cholesteatoma of the middle ear. Am J Otol. 1992;13:350–5.
119. Chung JW, Yoon TH. Different production of interleukin-1alpha, interleukin-1beta and interleukin-8 from cholesteatomatous and normal epithelium. Acta Otolaryngol. 1998;118:386–91. https://doi.org/10.1080/00016489850183485.
120. Bujia J, Kim C, Ostos-Aumente P, Lopez-Villarejo J, Kastenbauer E. Enhanced epithelial proliferation due to elevated levels of interleukin-1 receptors in middle ear cholesteatomas. Eur Arch Otorhinolaryngol. 1997;254:6–8. https://doi.org/10.1007/BF02630748.
121. Ren X, Chen W, Cui P, Zhang QA. The expression of interleukin-1α in middle ear cholesteatoma [J]. Chinese Arch Otolaryngol Head Neck Surg. 2005;6
122. Aumente PO, Bujia J, Kim C, Jimenez Gimenez J, Lopez Villarejo P. A quantitative study of the presence of interleukin-1 and interleukin-6 in cholesteatoma of the middle ear. Acta Otorrinolaringol Espanola. 1996;47:259–62.
123. Sato N, Matsumoto H, Akimoto Y, Fujii A. The effect of IL-1alpha and nifedipine on cell proliferation and DNA synthesis in cultured human gingival fibroblasts. J Oral Sci. 2005;47:105–10. https://doi.org/10.2334/josnusd.47.105.
124. Sauder DN, Stanulis-Praeger BM, Gilchrest BA. Autocrine growth stimulation of human keratinocytes by epidermal cell-derived thymocyte-activating factor: implications for skin aging. Arch Dermatol Res. 1988;280:71–6. https://doi.org/10.1007/BF00417707.
125. Helgaland T, Engelen B, Olsnes C, Aarstad HJ, Vassbotn FS. In vitro cholesteatoma growth and secretion of cytokines. Acta Otolaryngol. 2010;130:815–9.
126. Hozawa K, Adachi M, Shiga N, Takasaka T. Pathogenesis of attic cholesteatoma. Otol Japan. 1999;9:197–201.
127. Fanglei Y, et al. The Expression of STAT3 and SOCS3 Protein in the Middle Ear Cholesteatoma. J Audiol Speech Pathol. 2016;24:265–8.
128. Wu Y, Tang X, Shao W, Lu Y. Effect of CT manifestations of cholesteatoma on MMP-2, MMP-9 and IL-6 in the serum of patients. Exp Ther Med. 2019;17:4441–6. https://doi.org/10.3892/etm.2019.7484.
129. Liu W, et al. Activation of the IL-6/JAK/STAT3 signaling pathway in human middle ear cholesteatoma epithelium. Int J Clin Exp Pathol. 2014;7:709–15.
130. Kim CS, Lee CH, Chung JW, Kim CD. Interleukin-1 alpha, interleukin-1 beta and interleukin-8 gene expression in human aural cholesteatomas. Acta Otolaryngol. 1986;116:302–6. https://doi.org/10.3109/00016489609137846.
131. Hongwei Z, Qianmei C, Huiping Y. Expression of Interleukin-8 and Interleukin-6 in the middle ear cholesteatoma epithelial [J]. J Audiol Speech Pathol. 2005;5
132. Song H-I, Xue Q-H, Zhu H-B. The expression of GM-CSF and the action of GM-CSF in cholesteatoma. 武汉冶金科技大学学报 (自然科学版). 1999;4
133. Huang T, Yan S-D, Huang C-C. Colony-stimulating factor in middle ear cholesteatoma. Am J Otolaryngol. 1989;10:393–8.
134. Yoshikawa M, et al. Identification of specific gene expression profiles in fibroblasts derived from middle ear cholesteatoma. Arch Otolaryngol Head Neck Surg. 2006;132:734–42. https://doi.org/10.1001/archotol.132.7.734.
135. Hamzei M, et al. Osteoclast stimulating and differentiating factors in human cholesteatoma. Laryngoscope. 2003;113:436–42. https://doi.org/10.1097/00005537-200303000-00009.
136. Hattersley G, Owens J, Flanagan A, Chambers T. Macrophage colony stimulating factor (M-CSF) is essential for osteoclast formation in vitro. Biochem Biophys Res Commun. 1991;177:526–31.
137. Shirakata Y, et al. Heparin-binding EGF-like growth factor accelerates keratinocyte migration and skin wound healing. J Cell Sci. 2005;118:2363–70. https://doi.org/10.1242/jcs.02346.
138. Xie S, et al. HB-EGF expression as a potential biomarker of acquired middle ear cholesteatoma. Acta Otolaryngol. 2017;137:797–802. https://doi.org/10.1080/00016489.2017.1284343.
139. Kuczkowski J, Sakowicz-Burkiewicz M, Izycka-Swieszewska E. Expression of the receptor activator for nuclear factor-kappaB ligand and osteoprotegerin in chronic otitis media. Am J Otolaryngol. 2010;31:404–9. https://doi.org/10.1016/j.amjoto.2009.06.004.
140. Kuczkowski J, et al. Molecular control of bone resorption in chronic otitis media with cholesteatoma. Pol Otolaryngol. 2010;64:219–24. https://doi.org/10.1016/S0030-6657(10)70019-6.
141. Jeong JH, et al. Expression of RANKL and OPG in middle ear cholesteatoma tissue. Laryngoscope. 2006;116:1180–4. https://doi.org/10.1097/01.mlg.0000224345.59291.da.
142. Ma Y, Ye S. The expression of receptor activator nuclear factor-kappaB ligand and osteoprotegerin in cholesteatoma. J Clin Otorhinolaryngol Head Neck Surg. 2008;22:293–5.
143. Xie S, Pan Z, Yin T, Ren J, Liu W. Expression of PTHrP and RANKL in acquired middle ear cholesteatoma epithelium. Acta Otolaryngol. 2020;140:351–5. https://doi.org/10.1080/00016489.2020.1717609.
144. Haruyama T, Furukawa M, Kusunoki T, Onoda J, Ikeda K. Expression of IL-17 and its role in bone destruction in human middle ear cholesteatoma. ORL J Otorhinolaryngol Relat Spec. 2010;72:325–31. https://doi.org/10.1159/000319897.
145. Chen AP, et al. Expression levels of receptor activator of nuclear factor-kappaB ligand and osteoprotegerin are associated with middle ear cholesteatoma risk. Acta Otolaryngol. 2015;135:655–66. https://doi.org/10.3109/00016489.2015.1011789.
146. Miyasato M, Takeno S, Hirakawa K. Expression of RANKL and proliferation abilities of cultured human middle ear cholesteatoma epithelial cells. Hiroshima J Med Sci. 2013;62:1–6.
147. Likus W, et al. Bacterial infections and osteoclastogenesis regulators in men and women with cholesteatoma. Arch Immunol Ther Exp. 2016;64:241–7. https://doi.org/10.1007/s00005-015-0373-7.
148. Gong N, et al. Keratinocytes-derived exosomal miRNA regulates osteoclast differentiation in middle ear cholesteatoma. Biochem Biophys Res Commun. 2020;525:341–7. https://doi.org/10.1016/j.bbrc.2020.02.058.
149. Park CW, Jang YH, Tae K, Kim SK, Lee KC. Experimental study on TGF-beta1 gene expression in cholesteatoma. Korean J Otolaryngol Head Neck Surg. 1997;40:69–75.
150. Lang S, Schilling V, Wollenberg B, Mack B, Nerlich A. Localization of transforming growth factor-beta-expressing cells and comparison with major extracellular components in aural cholesteatoma. Ann Otol Rhinol Laryngol. 1997;106:669–73. https://doi.org/10.1177/000348949710600810.
151. Huisman MA, de Heer E, Ten Dijke P, Grote JJ. Transforming growth factor beta and wound healing in human cholesteatoma. Laryngoscope. 2008;118:94–8. https://doi.org/10.1097/MLG.0b013e31814faafa.

152. Huisman MA, de Heer E, Dijke PT, Grote JJ. Transforming growth factor β and wound healing in human cholesteatoma. Laryngoscope. 2008;118:94–8.
153. Andrew L, Abraham D. TGF-β-signaling and the fibrotic response. FASEB J. 2004;18:816.
154. Sandig H, et al. Fibronectin is a TH1-specific molecule in human subjects. J Allergy Clin Immunol. 2009;124:528–35. https://doi.org/10.1016/j.jaci.2009.04.036.
155. Yang X, et al. Expression of transforming growth factor-beta 1 matrix metalloproteinase-1 and its inhibitor in human middle ear cholesteatoma. Zhonghua Er Bi Yan Hou Ke Za Zhi. 2002;37:121–3.
156. Schmidt M, Grunsfelder P, Hoppe F. Induction of matrix metalloproteinases in keratinocytes by cholesteatoma debris and granulation tissue extracts. Eur Arch Otorhinolaryngol. 2000;257:425–9. https://doi.org/10.1007/s004050000249.
157. Schmidt M, Grunsfelder P, Hoppe F. Up-regulation of matrix metalloprotease-9 in middle ear cholesteatoma—correlations with growth factor expression in vivo? Eur Arch Otorhinolaryngol. 2001;258:472–6. https://doi.org/10.1007/s004050100359.
158. Yang Y, Bazhin AV, Werner J, Karakhanova S. Reactive oxygen species in the immune system. Int Rev Immunol. 2013;32:249–70.
159. Knight JA. Review: free radicals, antioxidants, and the immune system. Ann Clin Lab Sci. 2000;30:145–58.
160. Baysal E, et al. Oxidative stress in chronic otitis media. Eur Arch Otorhinolaryngol. 2013;270:1203–8. https://doi.org/10.1007/s00405-012-2070-z.
161. Celebi Erdivanli O, Sanli A. Is there a relationship between myeloperoxidase activity and conductive hearing loss in chronic otitis media complicated by cholesteatoma? Ear Nose Throat J. 2015;94:166–92.
162. Garrett IR, et al. Oxygen-derived free radicals stimulate osteoclastic bone resorption in rodent bone in vitro and in vivo. J Clin Investig. 1990;85:632–9. https://doi.org/10.1172/JCI114485.
163. Eskiizmir G, Yuceturk AV, Onur E, Var A, Temiz P. The imbalance of enzymatic antioxidants in cholesteatoma. Acta Otolaryngol. 2009;129:1187–91. https://doi.org/10.3109/00016480802593489.
164. Bujia J, et al. Antibodies to the minor cartilage collagen type IX in otosclerosis. Am J Otol. 1994;15:222–4.
165. Shinoda H, Huang CC. Localization of intercellular adhesion molecule-1 in middle ear cholesteatoma. Eur Arch Otorhinolaryngol. 1995;252:385–90. https://doi.org/10.1007/BF00167306.
166. Schilling V, Bujía J, Negri B, Schulz P, Kastenbauer E. Immunologically activated cells in aural cholesteatoma. Am J Otolaryngol. 1991;12:249–53.
167. Kuczkowski J, Bakowska A, Mikaszewski B. Immunomorphological evaluation of cholesteatoma. Otolaryngol Polska (Pol Otolaryngol). 2004;58:289–95.
168. Aberg B, Jontell M, Edstrom S. Analysis of class II antigen expressing cells in cholesteatoma epithelium. Acta Otolaryngol. 1998;106:186–91. https://doi.org/10.3109/00016488809106424.
169. Negri R, Schilling V, Bujia J, Kastenbauer E. Immunohistochemical identification of cholesteatoma-associated macrophage populations. Laryngo Rhino Otol. 1992;71:168–73. https://doi.org/10.1055/s-2007-997270.
170. Prinsley P, Jennings B, Philpott C, Bhutta M. Genetics of cholesteatoma project: presenting author: Peter Prinsley. J Laryngol Otol. 2016;130:S113–4.
171. Jennings BA, Prinsley P, Philpott C, Willis G, Bhutta MF. The genetics of cholesteatoma. A systematic review using narrative synthesis. Clin Otolaryngol. 2018;43:55–67. https://doi.org/10.1111/coa.12900.
172. Desloge RB, et al. DNA analysis of human cholesteatomas. Am J Otol. 1997;18:155–9.
173. Welkoborsky HJ, Jacob RS, Hinni ML. Comparative analysis of the epithelium stroma interaction of acquired middle ear cholesteatoma in children and adults. Eur Arch Otorhinolaryngol. 2007;264:841–8. https://doi.org/10.1007/s00405-007-0328-7.
174. Ecsedi S, et al. Chromosomal imbalances are associated with increased proliferation and might contribute to bone destruction in cholesteatoma. Otolaryngol Head Neck Surg. 2008;139:635–40. https://doi.org/10.1016/j.otohns.2008.07.019.
175. Kojima H, Miyazaki H, Shiwa M, Tanaka Y, Moriyama H. Molecular biological diagnosis of congenital and acquired cholesteatoma on the basis of differences in telomere length. Laryngoscope. 2001;111:867–73. https://doi.org/10.1097/00005537-200105000-00021.
176. Jotic A, et al. Polymorphisms in Toll-like receptors 2 and 4 genes and their expression in chronic suppurative otitis media. Auris Nasus Larynx. 2015;42:431–7. https://doi.org/10.1016/j.anl.2015.04.010.
177. Sangal N, et al. Association of CARD8 activating polymorphism with bone erosion in cholesteatoma patients. Laryngoscope. 2021;131:E605–11. https://doi.org/10.1002/lary.28741.
178. Zivkovic M, Kolic I, Jesic S, Jotic A, Stankovic A. The Allele 2 of the VNTR polymorphism in the gene that encodes a natural inhibitor of IL-1beta, IL-1RA Is favorably associated with chronic otitis media. Clin Exp Otorhinolaryngol. 2018;11:118–23. https://doi.org/10.21053/ceo.2017.01060.
179. Prinsley P, et al. The genetics of cholesteatoma study. Loss-of-function variants in an affected family. Clin Otolaryngol. 2019;44:826–30. https://doi.org/10.1111/coa.13365.
180. Barnes PJ. Targeting the epigenome in the treatment of asthma and chronic obstructive pulmonary disease. Proc Am Thorac Soc. 2009;6:693–6. https://doi.org/10.1513/pats.200907-071DP.
181. Shanmugam MK, Sethi G. Role of epigenetics in inflammation-associated diseases. Sub-Cellular Biochem. 2013;61:627–57. https://doi.org/10.1007/978-94-007-4525-4_27.
182. Agrawal A, Tay J, Yang GE, Agrawal S, Gupta S. Age-associated epigenetic modifications in human DNA increase its immunogenicity. Aging. 2010;2:93–100. https://doi.org/10.18632/aging.100121.
183. Villagra A, Sotomayor EM, Seto E. Histone deacetylases and the immunological network: implications in cancer and inflammation. Oncogene. 2010;29:157–73. https://doi.org/10.1038/onc.2009.334.
184. Naik S, et al. Inflammatory memory sensitizes skin epithelial stem cells to tissue damage. Nature. 2017;550:475–80. https://doi.org/10.1038/nature24271.
185. Albino AP, et al. Expression of p53 protein in human middle ear cholesteatomas: pathogenetic implications. Am J Otol. 1998;19:30–6.
186. Palko E, et al. The c-MYC protooncogene expression in cholesteatoma. Biomed Res Int. 2014;2014:639896. https://doi.org/10.1155/2014/639896.
187. Ozturk K, Yildirim MS, Acar H, Cenik Z, Keles B. Evaluation of c-MYC status in primary acquired cholesteatoma by using fluorescence in situ hybridization technique. Otol Neurotol. 2006;27:588–91. https://doi.org/10.1097/01.mao.0000226290.04048.d9.
188. Holly A, Sittinger M, Bujia J. Immunohistochemical demonstration of c-myc oncogene product in middle ear cholesteatoma. Eur Arch Otorhinolaryngol. 1995;252:366–9. https://doi.org/10.1007/BF00178279.
189. Bayazit YA, Karakok M, Ucak R, Kanlikama M. Cycline-dependent kinase inhibitor, p27 (KIP1), is associated with cholesteatoma. Laryngoscope. 2001;111:1037–41. https://doi.org/10.1097/00005537-200106000-00019.
190. Yamamoto-Fukuda T, Akiyama N. Keratinocyte growth factor signaling promotes stem/progenitor cell proliferation under p63 expression during middle ear cholesteatoma formation. Curr Opin Otolaryngol Head Neck Surg. 2020;28:291–5. https://doi.org/10.1097/MOO.0000000000000655.

191. Friedland DR, Eernisse R, Erbe C, Gupta N, Cioffi JA. Cholesteatoma growth and proliferation: posttranscriptional regulation by microRNA-21. Otol Neurotol. 2009;30:998–1005. https://doi.org/10.1097/MAO.0b013e3181b4e91f.
192. Zhang W, Chen X, Qin Z. MicroRNA let-7a suppresses the growth and invasion of cholesteatoma keratinocytes. Mol Med Rep. 2015;11:2097–103. https://doi.org/10.3892/mmr.2014.2971.
193. Li N, Qin ZB. Inflammation-induced miR-802 promotes cell proliferation in cholesteatoma. Biotechnol Lett. 2014;36:1753–9. https://doi.org/10.1007/s10529-014-1545-y.
194. Mishiro Y, Sakagami M, Kitahara T, Kondoh K, Okumura S. The investigation of the recurrence rate of cholesteatoma using Kaplan-Meier survival analysis. Otol Neurotol. 2008;29:803–6. https://doi.org/10.1097/MAO.0b013e318181337f.
195. Mustafa A, Heta A, Kastrati B, Dreshaj S. Complications of chronic otitis media with cholesteatoma during a 10-year period in Kosovo. Eur Arch Otorhinolaryngol. 2008;265:1477–82. https://doi.org/10.1007/s00405-008-0707-8.
196. Kaya E, et al. Investigation of the presence of biofilms in chronic suppurative otitis media, nonsuppurative otitis media, and chronic otitis media with cholesteatoma by scanning electron microscopy. ScientificWorldJournal. 2013;2013:638715. https://doi.org/10.1155/2013/638715.
197. Chole RA, Faddis BT. Evidence for microbial biofilms in cholesteatomas. Arch Otolaryngol Head Neck Surg. 2002;128:1129–33. https://doi.org/10.1001/archotol.128.10.1129.
198. Hudson BI, Lippman ME. Targeting RAGE signaling in inflammatory disease. Ann Rev Med. 2018;69:349–64. https://doi.org/10.1146/annurev-med-041316-085215.
199. Opal SM, et al. Effect of eritoran, an antagonist of MD2-TLR4, on mortality in patients with severe sepsis: the ACCESS randomized trial. JAMA. 2013;309:1154–62. https://doi.org/10.1001/jama.2013.2194.
200. Rice TW, et al. A randomized, double-blind, placebo-controlled trial of TAK-242 for the treatment of severe sepsis. Crit Care Med. 2010;38:1685–94. https://doi.org/10.1097/CCM.0b013e3181e7c5c9.
201. Liao J, Wu F, Lin W, Huang Z. Taraxerol exerts potent anticancer effects via induction of apoptosis and inhibition of Nf-kB signalling pathway in human middle ear epithelial cholesteatoma cells. Trop J Pharm Res. 2018;17:1011–7.
202. Kara A, et al. Evaluation of the effect of diclofenac sodium and 5-fluourasil in a 3D cholesteatoma cell culture model. Otol Neurotol. 2019;40:1018–25. https://doi.org/10.1097/MAO.0000000000002297.

Advanced Hearing and Balance Evaluation in Otitis Media

44

Rafael da Costa Monsanto, Leandro Guena de Castro, Matheus Saito, José Carlos Convento Junior, and Norma de Oliveira Penido

Introduction

Otitis media, defined as the presence of middle ear inflammation or infection, is a highly burdening disease [1]. The high burden of otitis media is aggravated by its high worldwide incidence: acute otitis media (AOM) affects ~709 million people yearly, and it was estimated that over 31 million new cases of chronic otitis media (COM) are diagnosed worldwide [1, 2]. The World Health Organization (WHO) estimated that complications of otitis media are responsible for 28,000 deaths every year. These complications include (but are not limited to) intratemporal (acute mastoiditis, labyrinthitis, labyrinthine fistula and petrous apicitis, for example) and intracranial complications (sigmoid sinus thrombosis, intracranial abscess, and meningitis) [2].

The association of otitis media and inner ear lesions has been extensively studied in the past 4 decades. Adam Politzer, in 1894, was the first to hypothesize that patients with otitis media might be at risk of developing hearing loss [3]. Many experimental studies then dedicated to understanding the pathophysiological mechanisms involved with auditory sequela secondary to otitis media. However, it was only in 1972 that Paparella et al. [4] published a pioneer translational study corroborating the presence of sensorineural hearing loss, also demonstrating its otopathological correlates. The authors showed high-frequency hearing loss in patients with COM, which correlated otopathologically with loss of cochlear hair cells in the basal turn of the cochlea. These findings were later corroborated by many experimental and clinical studies. More recently, the WHO [5] demonstrated that otitis media is the third leading cause of hearing impairment, and Cordeiro et al. [6] revealed that a single episode of uncomplicated AOM may result in permanent hearing loss. Tinnitus is also a frequent complaint in patients with otitis media: a cohort study of 30 years including over 2000 participants revealed that children who had recurrent AOM or chronic otitis media with effusion (OME) had worse hearing and a higher prevalence of tinnitus in adulthood as compared with controls [7].

Based on the observations of cochlear/auditory sequela of otitis media, the presence of an associated peripheral vestibular lesion was also hypothesized. As vestibular problems are not major complaints of most patients with otitis media, this hypothesis has not been explored in depth [8] Many authors associated dizziness or vertigo in otitis media patients with the presence of perilymphatic fistula, variation in the middle ear pressure, or other associated clinical problems (such as metabolic diseases and benign paroxysmal postural vertigo) Nonetheless, clinical and experimental evidence demonstrated that otitis media can independently result in vestibular damage [9]. Histopathological studies in human temporal bones demonstrated loss of vestibular hair cells in the saccular and utricular macula of temporal bones with COM [10]. A cohort study showed that adults with a history of recurrent AOM or COM in childhood had a much higher prevalence of self-reported dizziness as compared with ones without a history of otitis media [11]. Thus, it seems that although the vestibular sequela of otitis media may be less burdening than auditory symptoms, these should be assessed to allow prevention and assertive treatment as required [12].

R. da Costa Monsanto (✉)
Department of Otolaryngology, Head & Neck Surgery, Banco de Olhos de Sorocaba Hospital, Sorocaba, SP, Brazil

Department of Otolaryngology, Head & Neck Surgery, Universidade Federal de São Paulo/Escola Paulista de Medicina (UNIFESP/EPM), São Paulo, SP, Brazil

Department of Otolaryngology, Head & Neck Surgery, University of Minnesota, Minneapolis, MN, USA
e-mail: rdacosta@umn.edu

L. G. de Castro · M. Saito · J. C. C. Junior
Department of Otolaryngology, Head & Neck Surgery, Banco de Olhos de Sorocaba Hospital, Sorocaba, SP, Brazil

N. de Oliveira Penido
Department of Otolaryngology, Head & Neck Surgery, Universidade Federal de São Paulo/Escola Paulista de Medicina (UNIFESP/EPM), São Paulo, SP, Brazil

M. V. Goycoolea et al. (eds.), *Textbook of Otitis Media*, https://doi.org/10.1007/978-3-031-40949-3_44

However, assessing vestibular function in patients with otitis media is challenging: the results of several vestibular function tests (such as caloric test, and Vestibular Evoked Myogenic Potential—VEMPs) are negatively influenced by the presence of the middle ear abnormalities (tympanic membrane perforation, fibrosis, effusion, and cholesteatoma) and the presence of conductive hearing loss [8]. Therefore, it is arguable whether the findings demonstrate the presence of vestibular deficiency or are the result of these technical artifacts. Other vestibular tests that are not influenced by these limitations (e.g., rotatory chair, video-head impulse test, and posturography) are expensive and unavailable in some locations [10].

The inner ear sequelae of otitis media may result in varying degrees of hearing and vestibular problems. The high-frequency hearing loss, which is commonly observed in patients with otitis media, may result in deterioration in music perception, sound localization and speech perception problems (especially in noisy environments), and tinnitus [6]. The hearing loss associated with unaddressed otitis media also results in language and development delays and may lead over time to academic underachievement, higher rates of unemployment, lower salary, and even increase the risks of neurodegenerative diseases, including Alzheimer and dementia [13, 14]. The impact of vestibular impairment secondary to otitis media has been less explored in the literature; however, children with otitis media are reported as "clumsy" and tend to fall more often than controls. Additionally, the development of gross and fine motor skills is delayed, and the posturography results are much worse in children with otitis media [15]. In adults, COM leads to a high prevalence of vestibular symptoms (40-60%), abnormal caloric and cervical vestibular-evoked myogenical potentials (cVEMP) tests, lower limit of stability and increased sway in posturographic evaluation [12].

In this chapter, we will explore in detail the auditory and vestibular function tests that are available in the clinical practice to evaluate patients with otitis media.

Anamnesis and Physical Examination

Anamnesis

The most frequent symptoms of acute otitis media (AOM) are otalgia and fever, followed by the presence of otorrhea. Adequate treatment results in resolution of the infection without any further complications. Potential sequelae of AOM include chronic perforation of the tympanic membrane, hearing loss, tinnitus, and vestibular symptoms. The presence of a chronic eardrum perforation is a frequent cause of recurrent otorrhea and middle ear infections, requiring surgical treatment over time. AOM may also result in intracranial and intratemporal complications such as mastoiditis, labyrinthitis, petrositis, meningitis, cerebellar abscess, and sigmoid sinus thrombosis. In AOM patients presenting with severe vestibular symptoms, diplopia, facial paralysis, severe headache, high fever, lethargy, vomiting, or neck stiffness should be thoroughly investigated for the presence of intratemporal or intracranial complications (Fig. 44.1).

Otitis media with effusion (OME) results from the presence of middle ear fluid for more than 3 months. The accumulation of middle ear effusion may occur for several reasons, the most frequent being Eustachian tube dysfunction. OME has a peak incidence in children, as the Eustachian tube in this population is shorter, more horizontal, and has a smaller lumen as compared with adults – it was observed that virtually 100% of preschool children will experience at least one transitory episode of OME [16]. As in most cases, the middle ear effusion is sterile, the presence of symptoms related with an acute infection are infrequent in OME. However, the accumulation of fluid may result in increased susceptibility for developing AOM through the course of the disease. Adults with OME frequently present with aural fullness, and less frequently with tinnitus and vestibular symptoms. In children, the symptoms may be less specific than in adults. Most frequently, OME is suspected in children with difficulties in speech and reading, delayed

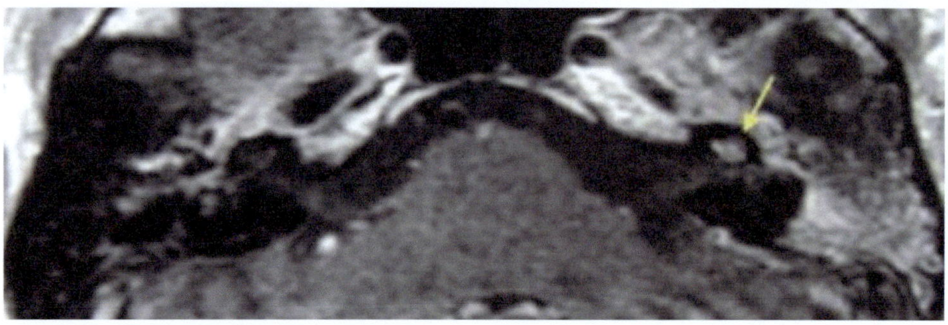

Fig. 44.1 Magnetic resonance imaging of a 23-year-old female patient with acute otitis media (AOM) who presented with a severe hearing loss in the left ear and vertigo. In hear physical examination, otoscopy revealed the presence of intense erythema and bulging of the left ear. Clinical vestibular examination revealed the presence of left-beating nystagmus, and Romberg test revealed a tendency fall to her left side. T1- weighted MRI with contrast showed intense enhancement of the cochlea (yellow arrow), suggesting acute labyrinthitis.

response to auditory input, limited vocabulary, and disturbances in attention. It was observed that the most frequent symptoms reported by the caregivers of children with OME are otalgia (76%), sleep disruption (64%), behavioral problems (49%), speech or hearing impairment (33-62%), and disequilibrium (15%) [16].

Chronic otitis media (COM), defined as the presence of chronic (>3 months) inflammation of the middle ear, may result in a myriad of clinical symptoms. Several authors have attempted to categorize COM to facilitate development of pathology-oriented diagnosis and treatment algorithms. Most frequently, studies report COM as either (1) nonsuppurative COM, defined as cases with a chronic perforation of the tympanic membrane secondary to otitis media with infrequent otorrhea; (2) chronic suppurative otitis media (CSOM), encompassing cases with frequent or intractable otorrhea; and (3) COM with cholesteatoma, defined as cases presenting with cholesteatoma identified in the middle ear or mastoid [17]. Paparella [18], also introduced the concept of "silent otitis media,", comprising patients who have tissue abnormalities in the middle ear cleft and mastoid (such as fibrosis, cholesterol granuloma, ossicular chain erosion, granulation tissue, or cholesteatoma) behind an intact eardrum. Considering the numerous potential sites of middle ear lesion secondary to otitis media, the clinical presentation of COM may significantly vary among patients. The most frequent clinical symptom described by patients with COM is hearing loss, affecting over 95% of the patients [12]. Other frequent symptoms are tinnitus, otorrhea, otalgia, dizziness, or vertigo. Less frequently, COM may result in deafness and facial nerve paralysis. COM also associates with intracranial and intratemporal complications, being more frequent (80%) than AOM-associated (20%) complications [19]. de Oliveira Penido et al. [2] estimated the incidence of intracranial complications of COM at 0.8%. Therefore, symptoms that may indicate an intracranial complication (such as the onset of profound hearing loss, severe vestibular symptoms, facial or abducens nerve paralysis, and other neurological symptoms) should be thoroughly investigated (Fig. 44.2).

Although vestibular symptoms are less frequent complaints as compared with hearing impairment in otitis media,

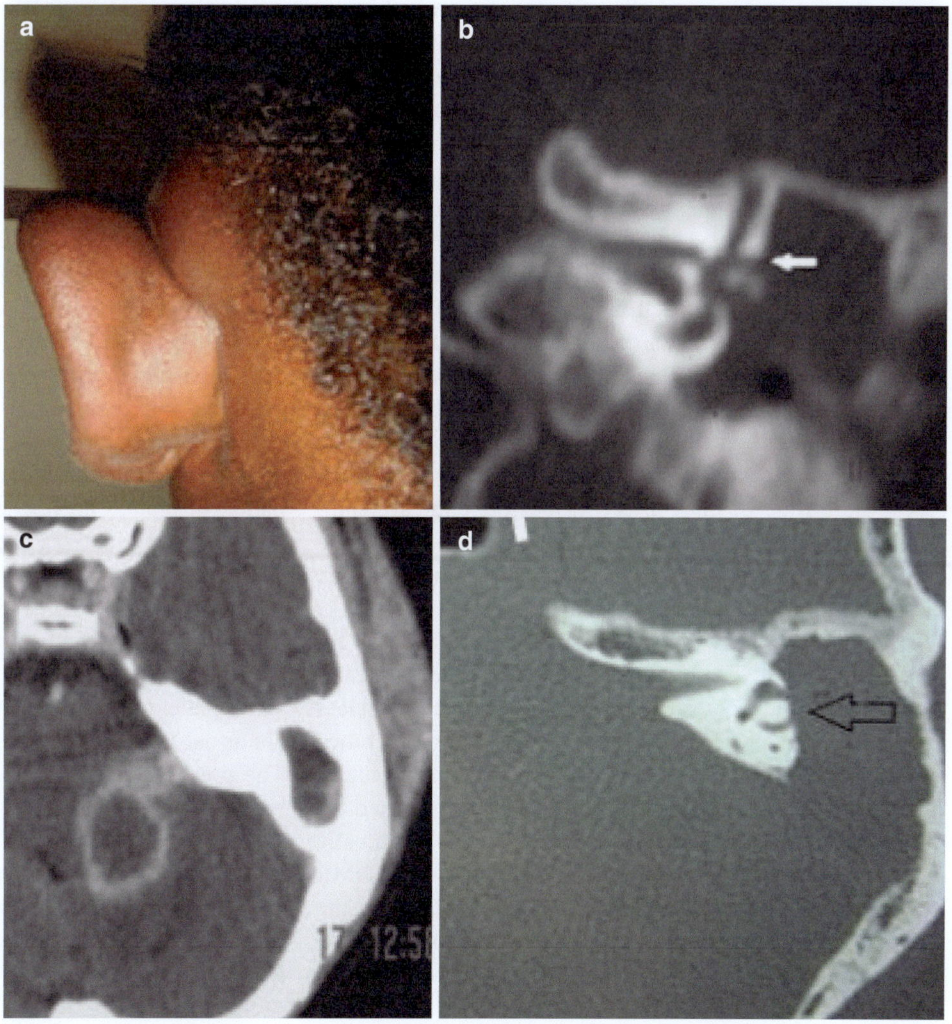

Fig. 44.2 A 13-year-old with chronic otitis media presented with a retroauricular edema in the left ear (**a**), associated with a profound hearing loss in the left ear and intense disequilibrium. Computed tomography (CT) revealed soft tissue filling the middle ear and mastoid, with an associated erosion of the left semicircular canal (white arrow, **b**) and a large opening of the mastoid with the posterior cranial fossa (black arrow, **d**). Contrast-enhanced CT revealed a subperiosteal and cranial abscess (**c**)

it has been demonstrated that over 50% of patients with AOM and COM report symptoms that are attributable to vestibular dysfunction [12]. Therefore, it is critical that the presence and characteristic of these symptoms are objectively assessed through structured anamnesis. Most patients with COM refer to the vestibular symptoms as disequilibrium, which is frequently triggered or worsened by the presence of otorrhea. In patients with AOM or COM exacerbations, patients may present vertigo and nystagmus, suggesting an acute vestibular lesion and the presence of labyrinthine fistula, especially in cases of cholesteatomatous COM (Fig. 44.2). In children, assessing vestibular symptoms can be challenging, as these are rarely reported by the patients and may not be perceived by the caregivers [20]. Children with OME or COM are more prone to falling and have delayed fine and gross motor development as compared with children without otitis media.

Physical Examination

The physical examination is critical to the diagnosis of otitis media. A precise diagnosis allows for timely and adequate treatment, in addition to prevention of sequelae and complications. The hearing evaluation in patients with otitis media initiates with an adequate otoscopy. As otitis media may result in hearing loss through a variety of pathophysiological mechanisms, these must be carefully examined to increase the chances of an adequate diagnosis and indicate potential treatment and prevention strategies.

The tympanic membrane (TM) should be examined thoroughly. The TM is abnormal in virtually 100% of patients with otitis media. However, the presence of a near-normal tympanic membrane may not indicate the absence of an underlying disease: patients with Eustachian tube dysfunction and chronic middle ear inflammation may present with only mild opacity and retraction of the eardrum. In these cases, the physician must also consider the clinical symptoms in the equation, in addition to audiometric results and imaging tests (when required). The otoscopy may indicate the type of otitis media and the adequate treatment. AOM is suspected in patients with erythema and bulging of the TM, in association with the presence of clinical symptoms such as otalgia, fever and/or otorrhea. In patients with aural fulness and hearing loss presenting with chronic (>3 months) retrotympanic middle ear effusion, in association with bulging or retraction of the tympanic membrane, must be screened for otitis media with effusion or silent otitis media. Pneumatic otoscopy is an important adjuvant in the diagnosis of OME in children, as a recent clinical practice guideline from the AAO [16] has demonstrated its efficacy in comparison to other diagnostic tools.

Cases presenting with a chronic tympanic membrane perforation with persistent or intractable suppuration are indicative of CSOM. Cholesteatoma can be in the otoscopic examination, and it may associate with the findings of middle ear inflammation and erosion of the scutum and ossicular chain. The absence of a TM perforation does not exclude the possibility of COM: Paparella et al. [18, 21] have demonstrated, through histological temporal bone and clinical studies, the presence of tissue changes that indicate chronic otitis media (fibrosis, granulation tissue, bone erosion, cholesterol granuloma, and cholesteatoma) in patients with an intact membrane. Also, the otoscopy may indicate potential abnormalities resulting in conductive hearing loss and indicate potential strategies for hearing restoration. The extension of the bony erosion and ossicular chain abnormalities secondary to otitis media may indicate the need for ossicular reconstruction or the use of prosthesis to allow optimal hearing restoration in cases where otologic surgery is warranted.

A thorough neurotologic examination is critical to evaluate potential vestibular impairment secondary to otitis media. Although many tools and devices are available in the clinical practice to evaluate vestibular function, the presence of conductive hearing loss and the middle ear abnormalities that are frequent in otitis media has a negative impact in some of these tests (such as caloric tests and VEMPs). Thus, the vestibular evaluation should be performed with tests that are not influenced significatively by the presence of these abnormalities. In this regard, clinical vestibular tests are essential to the diagnosis of vestibular impairment in patients with otitis media, as they may indicate the presence of vestibular dysfunction with minimal influence of the middle ear status. Among the tests used are the static (Romberg test) and dynamic (gait and Fukuda stepping tests) equilibrium tests, cerebellar function tests (index-index, index-nose, and diadochokinesis), assessment of the presence of nystagmus (spontaneous with and without visual fixation), head impulse and head-shaking tests, muscular tone and strength, examination of cranial nerves, and positional tests (Dix-Hallpike and head roll). In cases of noncomplicated AOM, OME, and COM, the clinical vestibular function tests frequently yield normal results; in some cases, patients may present mild instability in the Romberg test or lateral shifts in the Fukuda stepping test. In cases of more severe AOM and CSOM, some patients may present spontaneous nystagmus and an abnormal head impulse test in the side of the affected ear. The presence of spontaneous nystagmus and an abnormal head impulse test, in association with severe vestibular symptoms (including vertigo or postural instability) may indicate an increased risk of labyrinthitis, labyrinths fistula, an intracranial complication. Thus, these patients should be monitored closely to allow timely treatment if an intracranial complication is detected.

Hearing Evaluation

The gold-standard test to assess hearing in patients with otitis media is the pure-tone audiometry and speech tests. The tuning fork tests can be used to evaluate the type of hearing loss in the affected ears, being are especially useful in cases where an inner ear complication is suspected or in cases where a pure-tone audiometry is not readily available. Otitis media result in hearing loss in virtually 100% of the cases, with the most frequent type of hearing deficit being conductive, present in almost all forms of otitis media. However, it has been extensively demonstrated that some patients with otitis media develop sensorineural hearing loss, being most frequent in patients with CSOM.

Tonal Audiometry

The pure-tone audiometry is the most frequently used test for evaluating hearing thresholds, and it could be tested through air and bone conduction. Hearing thresholds are defined, as per the "American National Standards Institute" (2004) as "the minimum effective sound pressure level of an acoustic signal producing an auditory sensation in a specified fraction of the trials. The most accepted classification of the severity of hearing loss is: (1) mild (thresholds ranging from 26 to 40 dBHL); (2) moderate (41–55 dBHL); (3) moderately severe (56–70 dBHL); severe (71–90 dBHL); and profound (thresholds exceeding 90 dBHL).

Pure-Tone Air-Conduction Testing

The air-conduction testing measures the function of the external, middle, and inner ears. The pure tones are tested in the frequencies of 250–8000 Hz, in octave spacings. Although the pure-tone air conduction testing is potentially the most valuable hearing test, it does not provide specific information regarding the etiology of the auditory pathology when used in isolation. Thus, in the event of the air-conduction testing reveals thresholds exceeding 25 (adults) or 15 (children) dBHL, the test must be complemented by the bone-conduction testing.

Pure-Tone Bone-Conduction Testing

The bone-conducted stimulus reaches the cochlea directly, without going through the external and middle ears, through the skull bones, as the signal of a pure tone is presented to the patient through a bone vibrator that is placed on the mastoid to obtain hearing thresholds. Thus, the bone-conduction audiometry is remarkably useful in patients with a suspected conductive or mixed hearing loss. When the bone-and air-conduction audiometry is performed in association, a difference between the measured thresholds exceed 10 dBHL indicates the presence of a conductive hearing loss, which may or may not associate with a sensorineural hearing loss.

Speech Testing

Speech testing ("vocal audiometry") aims to assess the ability to perceive and recognize speech. A basic audiometric evaluation should routinely include speech testing. Among the tests used are the speech detection thresholds (SDT), speech reception thresholds (SRT), and speech discrimination scores. Both the SDT and SRT can be obtained using either air- or bone-conduction.

- Speech detective threshold (SDT): Measures the lowest sound intensity that the patient can detect the presence of 50% of the speech signals that are presented through the headphone. This test does not evaluate the recognition of speech, but the sound intensity that the patient acknowledges that he is listening to the speech signal. The SDT usually coincides with the pure-tone average, which is the average of the thresholds obtained with the pure-tone audiometry in the frequencies of 500, 1000, and 2000 Hz.
- Speech reception threshold (SRT): Corresponds to the lowest intensity that the patient can repeat 50% of the speech material. The SRT is usually 8–9 dB higher than the SDT.
- Speech discrimination: Determination of the speech discrimination is a more complex task as it evaluates the listener's ability to recognize speech. In conjunction with the pure-tone audiometry, it can help determine the differential diagnosis of hearing loss, provide information regarding the ability to communicate effectively, provide information regarding central auditory function, and provide insights about effectiveness of certain hearing rehabilitation strategies. The most frequent test used to evaluate discrimination is to present monosyllabic words in an open-set format. Patients with a pure conductive hearing loss frequently achieve optimal speech discrimination scores when the test is conducted using an adequate sound intensity. In patients with sensorineural hearing loss, the results may vary significantly among patients: patients with loss of sensorial cochlear cells frequently have lower discrimination scores as compared with nondiseased peers. In patients with lesions affecting the vestibulocochlear nerve, central auditory pathway, or even the auditory cortex, the discrimination scores are even lower, and this phenomenon can be seen even in patients with a normal or mild-to-moderate hearing loss in the pure-tone audiometry. In patients with otitis media, it has been demonstrated that their neural apparatus is frequently spared from the lesion secondary to the middle-ear inflammation. Therefore, even in patients with more severe degrees of mixed hearing loss, the discrimination

scores are within normal range or mildly abnormal. However, cases who had suffered an otitis media-related inner ear complication may present with very low discrimination scores.

Extended High-Frequency Audiometry

The extended high-frequency audiometry is performed in an acoustic booth using earphones that are calibrated to emit sounds at frequencies ranging from 8000 to 16,000 Hz. Theoretically, the extended high-frequency audiometry might constitute an ideal exam to evaluate initial hearing loss secondary to otitis media, as it has been demonstrated that the hook of the cochlea, which is adjacent to the round window membrane, is the primary lesion site secondary to otitis media [22]. However, the extended high-frequency audiometry is not yet validated for clinical use, as there are no normality values defined for these frequencies, and a wide variation in their results is seen in the normal population [6].

Despite these limitations, some authors dedicated to testing potential hearing losses affecting the extended high frequencies in patients with otitis media. Kasemodel et al. [22] revealed that patients with acute otitis media present with sensorineural hearing loss affecting the extended high frequencies in the first seven days from the onset of the disease. Cordeiro et al. [6] further revealed that a single episode of acute otitis media causes a significant and permanent elevation of hearing thresholds in the extended high frequencies (8–16 kHz) as compared with the non-diseased contralateral side.

Acoustic Immittance

The acoustic immittance aims to perform an objective measurement of the functional integrity of the tympanic-ossicular ensemble. The screening test named "acoustic immittance" test was based on the phenomena of "acoustic admittance," which is the amount of energy flowing through a system, and "acoustic impedance,", which is an opposition to the flow of sound energy. Measuring the acoustic immittance allows for identification and classification of peripheral (middle ear) and central auditory disorders. The most frequently used tests to evaluate acoustic immittance are the tympanometry and stapedial reflex measures.

Tympanometry

The tympanometry test was developed based on the observation that in cases where the middle ear and eustachian tube are normal, the best complacency of the tympanic membrane/ossicular chain system will occur when the pressure within the external auditory canal tends to equal the atmospheric pressure. Thus, in this test, an air-tight sealed probe is inserted into the ear canal, and it provides both positive and negative pressures onto the eardrum. Then, the probe measures the amount of acoustic energy reflected from the eardrum, providing information regarding transmission characteristics of the middle ear.

The result obtained with the tympanometry test is a direct estimate of the magnitude of the reflected acoustic energy. In a normal ear, the acoustic admittance is maximal when the pressure in the external auditory canal is equal to the atmospheric pressure. In cases presenting with an abnormal middle ear pressure, Eustachian tube dysfunction, ossicular chain abnormalities, or presence of middle ear effusion, the acoustic impedance increases, and the admittance decreases. To provide a more visual and intelligible demonstration of the results, Jerger [23] classified the potential results in a graphic representation. The types of tympanograms were classified as follows:

- Type A: Indicates a normal middle-ear pressure, in cases where the peak is at 0daPa. There are two sub-categories of A-type curves: As, which indicates a pressure peak at 0 that is reduced in amplitude, suggestive of ossicular chain fixation; and Ad, which indicates an unusually high-pressure peak at 0, suggesting ossicular chain discontinuity.
- Type B: Constitutes a "flat line" tympanogram, which indicates no point of maximum compliance. It indicates a mass-pressure effect behind the eardrum, which is seen in cases of serous or mucoid otitis media, space-occupying lesions of the middle ear (such as cholesteatoma or tumors), or a perforation of the tympanic membrane with a sealed Eustachian tube.
- Type C: Is graphically represented by the peak of compliance located in a negative pressure area, suggestive of the presence of negative middle ear pressure. It is frequently seen in early stages of otitis media without a significant amount of effusion.

The tympanometry is extremely useful in cases of otitis media with effusion and silent otitis media, as it reveals the presence of middle ear effusion and negative pressure in the middle ear, as well as the presence of tissue abnormalities in the middle ear. In cases of acute otitis media, as the tympanometry is not essential as a diagnostic tool, it is not recommended as it could result in worsening of the otalgia and discomfort of the patient. In patients with chronic otitis media presenting with a tympanic membrane perforation, the tympanometry offers a very limited benefit, being used in selected cases to evaluate the function of the Eustachian tube.

Stapedial Reflexes

The stapedial reflex is a protective mechanism dedicated to lower the sound intensity in cases of exposure to loud sounds. When the reflex pathway is activated, the stapedius muscle in both ears' contracts, stiffening the ossicular chain, resulting in a change in immittance. This pathway is composed of the cochlea, the VIII nerve, the ventral cochlear nucleus, the superior olive complex, the facial motor nucleus, and the facial nerve motor branch. Stapedial reflexes are useful in the differential diagnosis of hearing loss as they suggest the location of the injury.

Although testing the stapedial reflexes is useful for a complete audiologic diagnosis, it offers limited benefits in cases of otitis media. The test of the stapedial reflex is negatively influenced by the presence of middle ear disorders, as they prevent the tympanic membrane from showing a change in compliance when the stapedial muscle is contracted. Therefore, both ipsilateral and contralateral reflexes are bilaterally absent when the patient has a conductive hearing loss in the tested ear.

Otoacoustic Emissions

The active motility of outer hair cells serves as an amplifier of the displacement of the cochlear partition, which results in sound waves (termed "cochlear echoes") that are detectable at low intensities. These emissions may be detected spontaneously, or with a higher intensity following a sound stimulus, which is the "evoked otoacoustic emission". As spontaneous emissions may be absent in some patients, the evoked otoacoustic emissions are consistently detected in patients who have intact cochlear and middle ear apparatus. The evoked emissions can be tested using a transient, brief stimulus (such as a click or a brief tone burst (transient evoked otoacoustic emissions—TEOE) or using pure-tones separated by a specific frequency difference (distortion-product otoacoustic emissions—DPOE).

Testing the otoacoustic emissions is critical for an adequate audiological diagnosis in the present days. However, it offers very limited benefits when applied to patients with otitis media, as the presence of middle ear effusion, ossicular chain erosion or fixation, middle-ear tissue pathology, and tympanic membrane abnormalities do not allow for adequate detection of the otoacoustic emissions.

Auditory Brainstem Responses

The auditory brainstem response (ABR) represents the electric activity of the distal portion of the auditory pathway. The electrical impulses are recorded with surface electrodes, and they are represented graphically as "waves" as the impulses are transmitted through central auditory pathway landmarks. The ABR might be recorded using standard or disposable surface electrodes positioned on the forehead or at the vertex, on the medial surface of the ipsilateral or contralateral earlobe; the ground electrode is placed on the center of the forehead.

A normal ABR is comprised of 5–7 peaks that occur within a time frame of less than 10ms; however, only the first 5 peaks are considered within the test. The waves are elicited as they are captured in central auditory landmarks: wave I is originated at the level of the distal cochlear nerve, and the wave V at the level of lateral lemniscus in the midbrain. In a normal person, the latency of the waves I, III, and V (which are the most consistently identified waves) is consistent and can be used for evaluating normality of the electrical conduction of the stimuli. Abnormal values might occur when there is presence of middle ear pathology interfering with the conduction of the sound wave (occasion where the latency of the wave I is prolonged, but the interpeak interval between waves I–III–V are normal), or when a neural abnormality is present (resulting in complete absence of ABR waves, increased interpeak intervals and/or latency between waves I–III–V, or absence of one or more waves). It is also possible to evaluate the hearing thresholds at the tested frequencies, being considered as hearing thresholds the minimum sound intensity where the wave V is still detected in the ABR.

Considering patients with otitis media, the ABR is extremely useful to evaluate and diagnose children with otitis media with effusion or chronic otitis media who cannot perform the audiogram adequately. In these cases, the ABR can provide an adequate differential diagnosis between the presence of other potential causes of hearing loss (cochlear and central) from a pure conductive deficit caused by middle ear pathology. It can also indicate the best hearing rehabilitation strategy in cases presenting with a more intense hearing loss, being extremely useful in cases where a cochlear implant may be indicated. In older patients with otitis media, the ABR might be used only in selected cases, as the pure-tone audiometry is frequently sufficient to provide optimal evaluation of hearing.

Vestibular Function Tests

Caloric Tests

Caloric tests have been widely used in the study of vestibular function. However, the use of the caloric tests in patients with otitis media has not been extensively used for several reasons. First, the initially proposed caloric tests using water stimulation was not adequate to patients with otitis media, as it was not well tolerated by young children, and the application of water in patients with ventilation tubes, tympanic membrane perforations, and open mastoid cavities could result in extreme discomfort and infection. Paparella et al. [24] were the first authors to propose the use of air caloric tests to evaluating vestibular function in patients with otitis media. In their preliminary study, the authors observed that (1) patients with ventilation tubes and small perforations of the tympanic membrane had similar caloric test results as compared with the contralateral, nondiseased ear; (2) patients with large tympanic membrane perforations showed hyperactive responses, including shorter latency, increased amplitude, and higher frequency of nystagmus; and (3) in patients who had large perforations and moist ear, an inverted or contralateral nystagmus was observed. The authors conclude that the air caloric test can be safely used in patients with otitis media. Recent studies have also shown the high prevalence of caloric test abnormalities in patients with CSOM. The results of air caloric tests in patients Siampara et al. [25] observed the prevalence of canal paresis at 5.3% in patients with chronic suppurative otitis media. In the studies of Mostafa et al. [26] and Gianoli and Soileau [27], however, the prevalence of canal paresis was much higher (61.6% and 72%, respectively).

Some considerations must be made regarding the use of caloric test to evaluate peripheral vestibular function in patients with otitis media. As otitis media may result in a variety of abnormalities affecting the middle ear structures, the results of the caloric test might not fully represent the vestibular function. Furthermore, the results of the caloric tests in patients with middle ear pathology have not yet been validated, and therefore it is not possible to affirm whether an "abnormal" result is indicative of vestibular dysfunction or the result of a hyper- or hypo- stimulation of the labyrinth due to the middle ear abnormalities [8, 12]. However, it has been suggested that caloric tests can be used to evaluate the presence and progression of inner ear complications of otitis media such as suppurative labyrinthitis: in an initial phase, inflammation of the labyrinthine structures result in hyperexcitation, progressing over time to an absolute hypofunction (more frequent). Even in these cases, however, the presence of middle ear effusion can attenuate the caloric response, causing a false-positive result. In conclusion, it seems that although caloric tests can be used in patients with otitis media, their results must be interpreted with caution and correlated with clinical data.

Rotatory Chair Testing

The rotatory chair testing is one of the potential vestibular function tests that may be used in patients with otitis media, as the presence of middle ear abnormalities and sound conduction deficits do not influence significantly in their results. Additionally, the rotational testing is less bothersome to the patients than caloric testing. However, unlike caloric tests, both ears are stimulated simultaneously. In this test, a high-torque motor-driven chair and a specific software to analyze the results are needed.

In this test, the patient is placed in a dark environment, and is subjected to 10 cycles of sinusoidal head-velocity stimulus for each tested frequency, typically ranging from 0.01 to 0.7Hz. Then, the eye movements through the exam are recorded using video-oculography goggles. The results are averaged over successive cycles, and gain, phase, asymmetry, and bias velocity are calculated. While phase refers to the temporal shift in eye velocity relative to head velocity, the gain is the amplitude of the maximum slow-phase eye velocity divided by amplitude of the maximum stimulus velocity. Directionally dependent asymmetries can indicate relative weakness of function in one of the labyrinths in relation with the other.

In patients with otitis media, the rotatory chair test can be an alternative to the caloric tests to evaluating peripheral vestibular abnormalities, especially in patients with unilateral disease. Nonetheless, a few critical aspects must be taken into consideration. First, both labyrinths are stimulated simultaneously, and therefore it is not possible to study each ear separately. Second, patients with chronic, compensated vestibular losses (which seems to be the case of most patients with otitis media) [12], patients may exhibit minimal asymmetries, having normal gain and phase. And last, the rotatory chair is an expensive device, being unavailable in some locations. On the other hand, the rotatory chair test can be used to corroborate an abnormal caloric test result in a patient with otitis media. Moreover, it evaluates the vestibuloocular reflex in a different test frequency as compared with the caloric test, providing a more comprehensive evaluation of the function of the semicircular canals as compared with each test in isolation.

A recent systematic review [8] has indicated only two studies involving rotatory chair testing in patients with otitis media. Ben-David et al. [28] evaluated 50 children with OME: in their study, no significant differences in the rotatory chair test was found as compared with healthy children. Mostafa et al. [26] and Gianoli and Soileau [27] evaluated patients with CSOM: in both studies, the authors estimated the prevalence of rotatory chair abnormalities at 70% and 72%, respectively. Interestingly, both studies showed that there was a significative correlation between the presence of phase defects in the rotatory chair with the presence of caloric weakness, suggesting that these results are indicative of peripheral vestibular dysfunction secondary to chronic suppurative otitis media.

Electrooculography (EOG) and Videooculography (VOG)

A device can be used to detect and measure eye movements using a variety of stimuli, providing important information regarding vestibular function. The EOG device was the most used for many years, being still used in some centers. In this test, the eye acts as an electric dipole oriented along its long axis, and movements of the dipole in relation to the surface electrodes produce an electric signal that correspond to eye position [29]. It is possible to detect and record horizontal and vertical eye movements; the vertically aligned electrodes, however, sense voltage associated with eye and lid movement, limiting the use of the device in assessing vertical eye movement. One limitation of the EOG is that it cannot measure torsional eye movements, and therefore these should be evaluated directly by the examiner or using Frenzel lenses [30]. Although the ENG is a simple, noninvasive, and reasonably accurate procedure for routine vestibular assessment, it has some disadvantages, such as interference from muscle electrical activity and ambient electric noise [29]. The VOG has become widely used in recent years, as it provides a three-dimension recording of eye movements by using infrared cameras. It has the advantage of being noninvasive, easy to position, and do not associate with the position drifts seen with the EOG.

The use of EOG/VOG to evaluate vestibular function in patients with otitis media has been reported in the past. A systematic review of the literature demonstrated that—in patients with OME—there was a significantly higher prevalence of abnormal EOG results as compared with controls: from the EOG tests on 334 children with OME, abnormal findings were reported in 120 (25.9%) [8]. In patients with AOM, the prevalence of abnormal EOG results was much higher: abnormalities were demonstrated in 93% of the patients in the acute phase of AOM, all suggestive of peripheral pathology. Most patients with spontaneous nystagmus (92.8%) had irritative-type nystagmus beating toward the affected ear; only one patient had paretic type nystagmus beating toward the contralateral ear. In patients with CSOM, the same systematic review revealed that 56% of 175 patients had spontaneous nystagmus identified in their EOG. The abnormal ENG results in patients with AOM and CSOM possibly reflect the presence of labyrinthine dysfunction secondary to passage of inflammatory mediators from the middle to the inner ear [4, 9, 10, 18, 21, 31].

Subjective Vertical Visual Test

The subjective vertical visual (SVV) is one of the vestibular function tests that is not influenced by the presence of conductive hearing loss. This test was conceived based on the premise that a normal person can maintain the sense of verticality even without visual cues. The subjective vertical visual is a promising test aimed to evaluating vestibular dysfunction secondary to otitis media for several reasons. Histopathological and clinical studies demonstrated that the otolithic organs are the most frequent lesion sites secondary to otitis media [10], while semicircular canals are spared until more advanced stages of disease [10, 32]. Thus, the SVV comprises a test dedicated to evaluating otolithic function that is not significantly influenced by the presence of middle ear pathology and conductive deficits, which is the case of vestibular evoked myogenic potentials (VEMPs), for example. Although initially proposed SVV tests evaluated both labyrinths simultaneously, dynamic protocols (such as the off-vertical axis rotation) can differentiate the laterality of the lesion.

It has been suggested that the SVV test should be used in the following situations [33]: (1) In all patients presenting with acute vertigo, as a pathologic SVV deviation is a highly sensitive indicator of acute damage of the peripheral or central graviceptive pathways and (2) in all cases in which acute brainstem infarction is suspected, even in the absence of perceptual or postural symptoms. SVV tilts due to unilateral brain stem lesions are of topographic value for they indicate the level or the side of the lesion; (3) in patients with ocular motor symptoms, as testing for monocular and binocular SVV can help to differentiate between a peripheral and a central origin of the symptoms. Apart from its clinical use in the differentiation of central vestibular disorders, the SVV results is a strong indicator of the function of otolithic organs in cases where a peripheral vestibular lesion is suspected, which seems to be the case of otitis media.

Although the SVV test might constitute a reliable method to assessing peripheral vestibular function in patients with otitis media, this has not yet been studied in depth. Lee et al. [34] used a computer software to show a vertical line that patients with CSOM should put into the vertical position using a remote control. The authors observed abnormal SVV results in 20% of the patients with CSOM. More recently, Monsanto et al. [12] observed an abnormal tilting of the SVV (>2.0°) in 68.6% of the 51 patients with CSOM, and the mean deviation of the true vertical was also higher in patients with CSOM as compared with controls (CSOM, 3.66°; controls, 0.76°). Additionally, the authors observed a significant correlation between the presence of abnormal SVV results with the presence of vestibular symptoms. Assuming (based on previous clinical observation and results of histopathological studies) that otitis media result in a peripheral vestibular lesion, these results seem to indicate otolithic dysfunction. However, these results must be interpreted with caution, as 1) the SVV test does not evaluate peripheral vestibular function in isolation and 2) it has limitations in assessing peripheral vestibular function in patients with chronic vestibular symptoms. Different SVV testing methods have been proposed:

Off-vertical Axis Rotation (OVAR)

In the OVAR test, deviations of the true vertical are determined using static or dynamic protocols. A device is used to present a luminous line in a dark environment – then, the patient is asked to rotate the luminous line at the point they perceive that is aligned with the vertical axis.

In the dynamic protocol, the patient subjected to a rotation of 300 deg/sec [35]. Once the patient has been rotating at a constant velocity for approximately one minute and the per-rotary nystagmus has subsided, the patient is asked to manipulate a laser line on the wall (using a handheld remote) until it is perceived in the true vertical position. The most critical advantage of this method is that it allows testing of each utricle independently, as the centripetal acceleration applied to either the right or left labyrinth allows for independent utricular evaluation without influence from the other ear [36].

In the static protocol, the test is performed similarly but without spinning the patient off axis. Although this test may be technically easier to perform and more comfortable to the patient, it has been shown that the static SVV protocol may result in simultaneous stimulation of both otolithic organs.

Virtual Reality Goggles

Many manufacturers have developed virtual reality goggles that aims to digitally determine the subjective vertical visual. In all these devices, the patient is placed in a dark environment, and the virtual reality goggles are placed in position. The patients are then asked to move a fluorescent line using a remote control until the position that it is perceived at the vertical position.

Hemispheric Dome Method

In this test, [33] patients sit with their chin resting on a fixed pad and are instructed to look at a horizontal line placed in a hemispheric dome, 60 cm in diameter, which is rotated around their line of sight. To avoid influence of external orientation references, the dome covers the entire visual field of the patients and is covered with a random pattern of colored dots. A rotating linear target is then placed 30 cm in front of the patient—the target and dome are then rotated to a randomized offset position, and the patients are instructed to align the target in the vertical position using a remote control. The angle between the adjusted orientation and the true spatial vertical is then determined by a computer software.

Bucket Test

The bucket test [33] is a simple and inexpensive method to assess the SVV. In this test, a bucket is modified to measure deviations of the true vertical. The bucket test has been shown to be a reliable method for assessing the presence of central or peripheral vestibular lesions, with more than 90% intratest and intertest reliability [33, 37]. In this method, the authors used a 15.0-L bucket (rim diameter = 35.5 cm; depth = 33.0 cm; bottom diameter = 31.5 cm). A fluorescent tape was used to draw a vertical line in its internal base, and in the outer base of the bucket, a string with a small weight was pinned to the center. In the rim of the external base of the bucket, a protractor scale was taped, in which 0° coincided with the straight line drawn inside of the bucket; the 0° position was defined as the true vertical (Fig. 44.1b). As the bucket was rotated, the straight line was pulled down by the weight, which indicated the angle of deviation (in degrees) from the true vertical. The examiner rotates the bucket in a clockwise or counterclockwise direction until the string pointed to a deviation of ±20°, and then the bucket was slowly rotated back toward the 0° position. Patients are instructed to verbalize "stop" in the moment the internal line reaches the true vertical position. The angular deviations of the true vertical were measured in degrees (clockwise direction was labeled with a "positive" sign and deviations in the counterclockwise directions as "negative")

The main advantages of the bucket method [33] in assessing the SVV are (1) the tool uses inexpensive material and easy to assemble; (2) it does not require extensive training; (3) the results are easy to interpret; (4) the test is easy to perform, and the results have been validated; and (4) it could be used in virtually all types of vestibular problems.

Posturography

The posturography provides a quantitative measurement of the integration of vestibular, visual, and proprioceptive inputs that maintain postural balance control. The posturography may be performed either using dynamic or static platforms. The most widely used device is the computerized dynamic posturography named Equitest®. In this test, the patient stands on a movable platform and is subjected to a movable visual surround. The center of pressure position is recorded by pressure-sensitive gauges located in the platform, which is also used to evaluate the postural sway. Static posturography tests are less commonly reported in the literature. The most frequently used static posturography device is the Balance Rehabilitation Unit® (BRU) [38]. The BRU has a force platform that measures displacement of the center of pressure, while patients are exposed to somatosensorial (eyes closed, standing on a medium density foam mattress with eyes closed), vestibular and visual (saccadic, optokinetic) stimuli through virtual reality goggles. The postural control is analyzed under 3 parameters: (1) limit of stability (LOS) = area in which the volunteers can intentionally dislocate their center of pressure (cm^2); (2) sway area = area comprising 95% of the dislocations of the center of pressure in each specific test (cm^2); and (3) sway velocity = total distance of dislocation divided by the duration of the test (cm/s).

The posturography is useful in several situations, especially those involving unilateral or bilateral vestibular hypofunction, brainstem stroke, cerebellar ataxia, extrapyramidal disorders, and cerebellopontine angle neoplasms. The results reveal specific aspects that could result in a tailored vestibular rehabilitation strategy. In this regard, although posturography test does not evaluate peripheral vestibular function in isolation and does not directly provide identification of the specific site of lesion, it has been hypothesized that the specific tests that deprives the patients from visual cues and proprioception (such as the sensory organization test of the Equitest device) might reflect utricular function [39]. Liu et al. [39] observed a significant positive correlation between the results of the sensory organization test with the ocular VEMP, a finding that seems to support this hypothesis.

As the results of the posturography are not influenced by the presence of middle ear pathology or conduction deficits, many authors have used the posturography to evaluate equilibrium in patients with otitis media. In children with OME, posturography results revealed higher mean velocity, more falls during the exams, and increased sway amplitude during high-frequency stimuli as compared with healthy children (24, 36). In most of these studies, the posturography abnormalities seemed to complete subside after insertion of ventilation tubes. Gawron et al. [40], however, showed that where despite improvements, OME subjects still performed worse than controls after 4 weeks of grommet insertion.

In patients with CSOM, Mostafa et al. [26] did not observe significant abnormalities in the posturography test. The authors, however, did not include a control group for comparison purposes. Monsanto et al. [12], in a controlled study including 126 patients with CSOM, observed that patients had worse limit of stability and increased sway as compared with controls. The authors also observed a significant correlation between the abnormal posturography results with the presence of vestibular symptoms, abnormal clinical vestibular function tests, and increased deviations in the SVV test ($P < 0.05$).

Video Head Impulse Test: Video-HIT

The video-HIT is a bedside test used to evaluate function of the semicircular canals, providing objective measures of the gain of the vestibuloocular reflex (VOR) for each canal separately [41]. The quantitative testing allows recording of short-latency eye movements that may be missed under bedside conditions. In comparison with the caloric and rotatory chair tests, it evaluates movements that are much faster, which makes the video-HIT a great addition to the matter of vestibular function testing. The video-HIT test requires goggles with a high-resolution video camera that will capture the movement of the eyes during the head tilt. The examiner proceeds with the head movements toward the direction of each specific semicircular canals. The movements of the eyes and head are recorded graphically in a computer software, and individual impulses with artifacts can be excluded to ensure consistency of the results. The software evaluates the presence of corrective saccades and calculates the VOR gain by providing the ratio of the amplitude of the eye movements by the amplitude of the head movement.

Testing the vestibular function in patients with otitis media is challenging, as many of the tests that are available in the daily practice (such as VEMPs and caloric tests) do not have their results validated for the use in patients with middle ear pathology and conductive deficits. As the video-HIT does not suffer the influence of the middle ear pathology and allows for testing each semicircular canal individually, the video-HIT constitutes a remarkable asset in objectively evaluating the VOR.

As the video-HIT test has only become widely available more recently, not many studies dedicated to using this diagnostic tool in patients with otitis media. Tomaz et al. [42] observed a higher prevalence of corrective saccades in patients with chronic suppurative otitis media with and without cholesteatoma as compared with controls. The authors also demonstrated a significantly lower gain of the anterior semicircular canal of the affected ear of patients with cholesteatoma as compared with controls ($P < 0.001$), but no significant differences were observed in the gain of the lateral and posterior canals between patients with chronic otitis media and controls ($P > 0.05$). D'Albora et al. [43] described video-HIT test results in two patients with a cholesteatoma-induced lateral semicircular canal erosion, revealing an abnormally low vestibuloocular reflex gain and the presence of corrective saccades in both patients. Covelli et al. [44] also suggested that the video-HIT test could constitute a useful tool to evaluate residual vestibular function in patients with labyrinthine fistula caused by CSOM that will be later operated.

Although the video-HIT is a promising tool in the evaluation of peripheral vestibular function in patients with otitis media, some limitations that are inherent to the test should be highlighted [12]: (1) the sensitivity of video-HIT may not allow accurate detection of chronic, compensated abnormalities affecting the semicircular canals, [45]; (2)

because VHIT measures the VOR at high frequency, it is possible that abnormalities affecting the semicircular canal function in the lower frequencies could have been missed [46]; and (3) semicircular canals seem to be less affected by the inflammatory damages caused by COM than the otolithic organs, as suggested by histopathological evidence [12, 32, 47]

Vestibular-Evoked Myogenic Potentials (VEMP)

VEMPs are electromyographic responses derived from the vestibular labyrinth evoked by sound, vibration, or electrical stimulation [48]. In healthy subjects, auditory stimulation results in a relaxation of the ipsilateral sternocleidomastoid muscle. These cervical VEMP (cVEMP) responses occur at a short latency (12 ms) in reaction to the click stimulus. After the c-VEMP was proposed, it was observed the extraocular musculature also respond to vestibular stimulation through bone-conducted stimuli – this test modification was named ocular VEMP (oVEMP) [49]. While the cVEMP responses are result of selective activation of the sacculus, the oVEMP corresponds to the utricular function [48, 50].

The VEMP tests have become cornerstones of laboratory diagnosis of vestibular problems. It has been widely used to diagnose Meniere's disease, vestibular Migraine, and superior semicircular canal dehiscence. In the specific case of otitis media, as it has been observed that the otolithic organs are the most critical lesion sites secondary to otitis media, many authors have dedicated to study the use of VEMPs as a diagnostic tool to evaluate vestibular function. A systematic review [8] identified a total of 10 studies that evaluated the VEMP results in patients with otitis media with effusion (3 studies) and chronic suppurative otitis media (7 studies). In the studies involving patients with OME, a total of 101 children were included: VEMP tests using air-conducted stimuli did not elicit detectable responses in most patients with OME, and bone-conducted stimuli VEMP results varied greatly among studies (2–30% of absence of responses). Critical analysis of the amplitude and latency of p13 and n26 waves was very inconsistent among these studies using bone-conduction stimuli, varying from no significant differences in both latencies or in amplitude to delayed latencies and significantly smaller amplitudes as compared with controls. The studies including patients with chronic suppurative otitis media comprised a total of 277 patients (317 ears), most of which used cVEMPs (217 patients and 257 ears) in isolation, and 1 study (85 patients, 117 ears) tested both cVEMPs and oVEMPs. Assuming abnormal VEMPs as the absence of response or delayed latency/decreased amplitude of the waves p13-n26, the oVEMP was abnormal in 72 of 106 ears (68%). The cVEMP test yielded abnormal results in 160 of 317 ears (50.4%). There was also a great controversy regarding the association between abnormal VEMP results with the presence of vestibular symptoms, with some authors observing a significant positive correlation between these two variables while others did not.

Although a vestibular testing that would allow evaluation of the function of otolithic organs would be critical in patients with otitis media, the VEMPs should be used with caution. The VEMP results suffer a great negative influence of conductive hearing deficits that are hallmarks of otitis media, as the standard test battery includes air-conducted vestibular stimuli. An alternative that was proposed was the use of bone-conduction stimuli, which could potentially circumvent the negative influence of the conductive hearing loss. However, it has been observed that the use of bone-conductive stimuli seems to stimulate both labyrinths simultaneously, which can compromise the validity of the results. Therefore, it seems that the VEMP might be used only in selected cases, and their results should be interpreted in association with the clinical symptoms and results of other vestibular tests in conjunction.

Imaging Evaluation of the Cochlea and Peripheral Vestibular System

Imaging tests are rarely necessary to the diagnosis of uncomplicated otitis media, as a positive clinical history, in association with the physical examination findings, are sufficient to seal the diagnosis in most cases. However, some situations require the use of imaging tests, especially cases requiring surgical treatment or those in which a complication of otitis media is suspected.

Cases of AOM and COM may associate with a variety of inner ear complications. These are suspected in cases presenting with persistent fever, significant or abrupt hearing loss, intense tinnitus, vestibular symptoms, facial paralysis, and/or signs of increased intracranial pressure or altered mental state. A cohort [19] showed that intracranial complications are much more frequent in patients with COM (80%) as compared with AOM (20%). The bone erosion resulting from chronic middle ear inflammation and the presence of cholesteatoma seems to be the cause for such higher incidence of complications in patients with COM (Fig. 44.3). Nonetheless, otitis media may cause auditory and vestibular symptoms even in the absence of a clear erosion of the bony labyrinth due to passage of inflammation products through the round window membrane [51, 52].

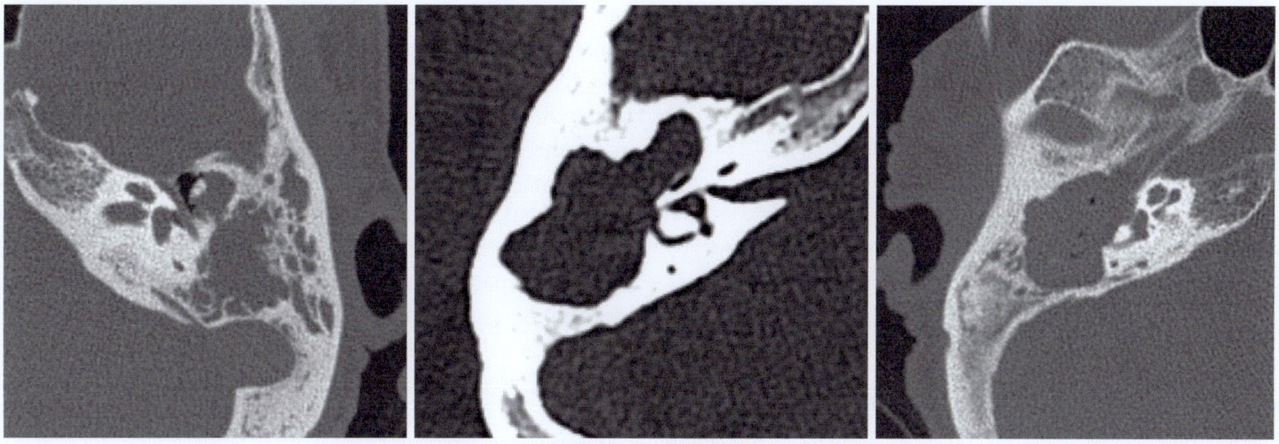

Fig. 44.3 Three computed tomography scans of the temporal bone from three different patients with cholesteatoma showing erosion of the middle ear and mastoid. The first image shows a bony erosion restricted to the scutum and mastoid antrum. The second image shows intense erosion of the temporal bone with a small communication between the membranous portion of the lateral semicircular canal and the mastoid. The last picture shows the presence of a large erosion of the lateral semicircular canal

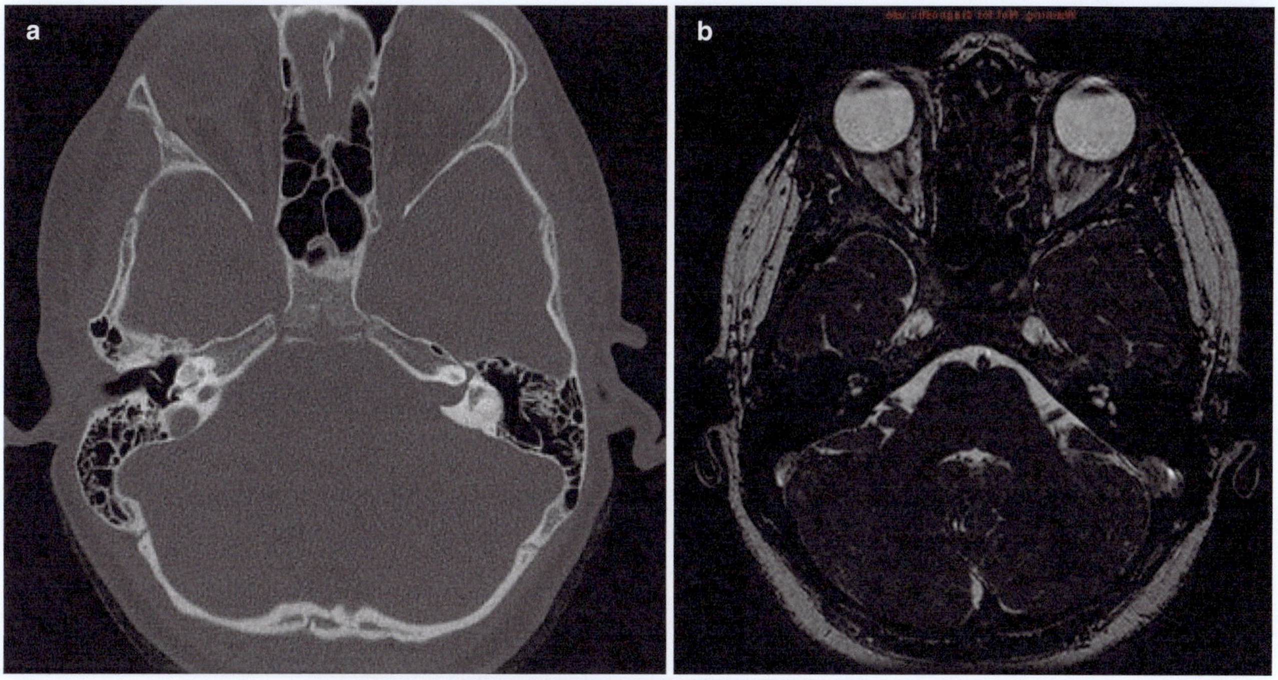

Fig. 44.4 (**a**) A computed tomography scan of a patient with cochlear ossification as consequence of otitis media-associated labyrinthitis ossificans in the right ear. (**b**) T2WI MRI scan of the same patient, revealing a decreased T2 signal in the cochlea

The presence of acute auditory and vestibular symptoms in patients with otitis media must be thoroughly assessed for the presence of an intratemporal or intracranial complication. If these complications are suspected, the MRI is preferred to the CT scan. However, the use of CT scans may be useful to evaluate the presence of cochlear or vestibular ossification in cases of labyrinthitis ossificans and meningitis (Fig. 44.4), and contrasted CTs can identify an intracranial abscess (Fig. 44.2) if an MRI is not readily available.

The MRI scans are particularly useful in the evaluation of labyrinthitis secondary to otitis media: in patients with labyrinthitis, gadolinium T1-weighted images (T1WI) show cochlear and vestibular enhancement, and a cochlear hyperintensity is also observed in the T2-flair (Fig. 44.5).

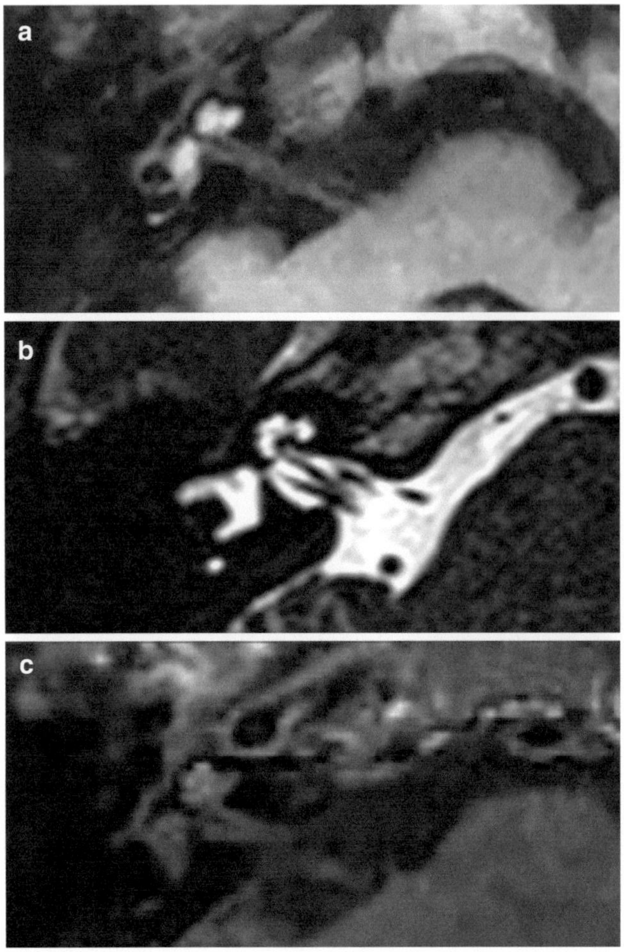

Fig. 44.5 Three coplanar magnetic resonance imaging pictures of a patient with acute otitis media presenting with vertigo and profound hearing loss. (**a**) A T1WI with fat suppression and gadolinium MRI showing a cochlear and vestibular enhancement. (**b**) T2WI showing an isointense signal of the cochlea and vestibule in relation to the cerebrospinal fluid. (**c**) T2-flair imaging showing increased cochlear signal, suggestive of acute labyrinthitis

Conclusions

As it has been extensively demonstrated that otitis media can result in significant hearing loss and abnormal peripheral vestibular function, it is critical that patients with different forms of otitis media are subjected to a comprehensive study of the hearing and vestibular function. Although hearing can be easily assessed using standard pure-tone audiometry and speech tests, evaluating the vestibular symptoms is challenging for several reasons. Some vestibular function tests are negatively influenced by the presence of conductive hearing loss and middle ear pathology (VEMPs and caloric tests), some stimulate both labyrinths simultaneously (rotatory chair, SVV, and bone-conducted VEMPs), some do not evaluate vestibular function in isolation (posturography), and others are expensive and unavailable in some centers (rotatory chair, posturography, and video-HIT). Despite these many difficulties, the results of these vestibular tests complement the anamnesis and physical examination and can provide remarkable clues toward the magnitude of the vestibular impairment. These tests also might indicate the presence of an inner ear complication secondary to otitis media and provide information that can result in a pathology-oriented development of rehabilitation strategies. Imaging tests such as CT scans and MRIs may be used in the evaluation of potential labyrinthine and intracranial complications of otitis media.

References

1. Monasta L, Ronfani L, Marchetti F, Montico M, Brumatti LV, Bavcar A, Grasso D, Barbiero C, Tamburlini G. Burden of disease caused by otitis media: systematic review and global estimates. PLoS One. 2012;7:e36226. https://doi.org/10.1371/journal.pone.0036226.
2. de Oliveira Penido N, Chandrasekhar SS, Borin A, de Albuquerque Maranhão AS, Testa JRG. Complications of otitis media—a potentially lethal problem still present. Braz J Otorhinolaryngol. 2016;82:253–62. https://doi.org/10.1016/j.bjorl.2015.04.007.
3. Politzer A, Ballin MJ. Politzer's text-book of the diseases of the ear for students and practitioners. Ind Med Gaz. 1927;62:410–1.
4. Paparella MM, Oda M, Hiraide F, Brady D. Pathology of sensorineural hearing loss in otitis media. Ann Otol Rhinol Laryngol. 1972;81:632–47. https://doi.org/10.1177/000348947208100503.
5. World Health Organization. (2018). Addressing the rising prevalence of hearing loss.
6. Cordeiro FP, da Costa Monsanto R, Kasemodel ALP, de Almeida Gondra L, de Oliveira Penido N. Extended high-frequency hearing loss following the first episode of otitis media. Laryngoscope. 2018;128:2879–84. https://doi.org/10.1002/lary.27309.
7. Aarhus L, Tambs K, Kvestad E, Engdahl B. Childhood otitis media: a cohort study with 30-year follow-up of hearing (The HUNT Study). Ear Hear. 2015;36:302–8. https://doi.org/10.1097/AUD.0000000000000118.
8. Monsanto RDC, Kasemodel ALP, Tomaz A, Paparella MM, Penido NDO. Current evidence of peripheral vestibular symptoms secondary to otitis media. Ann Med. 2018;50:391–401. https://doi.org/10.1080/07853890.2018.1470665.
9. da Costa Monsanto R, Erdil M, Pauna HF, Kwon G, Schachern PA, Tsuprun V, Paparella MM, Cureoglu S. Pathologic changes of the peripheral vestibular system secondary to chronic otitis media. Otolaryngol Head Neck Surg. 2016;155:494–500. https://doi.org/10.1177/0194599816646359.
10. da Costa Monsanto R, Schachern P, Paparella MM, Cureoglu S, de Oliveira Penido N. Progression of changes in the sensorial elements of the cochlear and peripheral vestibular systems: the otitis media continuum. Hear Res. 2017;351:2–10. https://doi.org/10.1016/j.heares.2017.05.003.
11. Aarhus L, Tambs K, Hoffman HJ, Engdahl B. Childhood otitis media is associated with dizziness in adulthood: the HUNT cohort study. Eur Arch Otorhinolaryngol. 2016;273:2047–54. https://doi.org/10.1007/s00405-015-3764-9.

12. Monsanto RDC, Kasemodel ALP, Tomaz A, Abrahão Elias TG, Paparella MM, de Oliveira Penido N. Evaluation of vestibular symptoms and postural balance control in patients with chronic otitis media. J Vestib Res. 2020; https://doi.org/10.3233/VES-200691.
13. Lin FR, Metter EJ, O'Brien RJ, Resnick SM, Zonderman AB, Ferrucci L. Hearing loss and incident dementia. Arch Neurol. 2011;68:214–20. https://doi.org/10.1001/archneurol.2010.362.
14. Livingston G, Sommerlad A, Orgeta V, Costafreda SG, Huntley J, Ames D, Ballard C, Banerjee S, Burns A, Cohen-Mansfield J, Cooper C, Fox N, Gitlin LN, Howard R, Kales HC, Larson EB, Ritchie K, Rockwood K, Sampson EL, Samus Q, Schneider LS, Selbæk G, Teri L, Mukadam N. Dementia prevention, intervention, and care. Lancet. 2017;390:2673–734. https://doi.org/10.1016/S0140-6736(17)31363-6.
15. Casselbrant ML, Furman JM, Rubenstein E, Mandel EM. Effect of otitis media on the vestibular system in children. Ann Otol Rhinol Laryngol. 1995;104:620–4. https://doi.org/10.1177/000348949510400806.
16. Rosenfeld RM, Shin JJ, Schwartz SR, Coggins R, Gagnon L, Hackell JM, Hoelting D, Hunter LL, Kummer AW, Payne SC, Poe DS, Veling M, Vila PM, Walsh SA, Corrigan MD. Clinical practice guideline: otitis media with effusion (update). Otolaryngol Head Neck Surg. 2016;154:S1–S41. https://doi.org/10.1177/0194599815623467.
17. Bluestone CD, Gates GA, Klein JO, Lim DJ, Mogi G, Ogra PL, Paparella MM, Paradise JL, Tos M. 1. Definitions, terminology, and classification of otitis media. Ann Otol Rhinol Laryngol. 2002;111:8–18. https://doi.org/10.1177/00034894021110S304.
18. Paparella MM, Shea D, Meyerhoff WL, Goycoolea MV. Silent otitis media. Laryngoscope. 1980;90:1089–98. https://doi.org/10.1288/00005537-198007000-00003.
19. Penido ND, Borin A, Iha LCN, Suguri VM, Onishi E, Fukuda Y, Cruz OLM. Intracranial complications of otitis media: 15 years of experience in 33 patients. Otolaryngol Head Neck Surg. 2005;132:37–42. https://doi.org/10.1016/j.otohns.2004.08.007.
20. Casselbrant ML, Villardo RJM, Mandel EM. Balance and otitis media with effusion. Int J Audiol. 2008;47:584–9. https://doi.org/10.1080/14992020802331230.
21. Paparella MM, Schachern PA, Cureoglu S. Chronic silent otitis media. Orl-J Oto-Rhino-Laryngol Rel Specialties. 2002;64:65–72. https://doi.org/10.1159/000057783.
22. Kasemodel ALP, Costa LEM, Monsanto RDA, Penido NDO. Sensorineural hearing loss in the acute phase of a single episode of acute otitis media. Braz J Otorhinolaryngol. 2020;86(6):767–73. https://doi.org/10.1016/j.bjorl.2019.06.001.
23. Jerger J, Speaks C, Trammell JL. A new approach to speech audiometry. J Speech Hear Disord. 1968;33:318–28. https://doi.org/10.1044/jshd.3304.318.
24. Paparella MM, Rybak L, Meyerhoff WL. Air caloric testing in otitis media. (preliminary studies). Laryngoscope. 1979;89:708–14.
25. Siampara L, Mann SBS, Panda NK, Mehra YN. Audiovestibular profile in unilateral chronic suppurative otitis media. Indian J Otolaryngol Head Neck Surg. 1997;49:107–11. https://doi.org/10.1007/BF03023784.
26. Mostafa BE, Shafik AG, El Makhzangy AMN, Taha H, Abdel Mageed HM. Evaluation of vestibular function in patients with chronic suppurative otitis media. ORL J Otorhinolaryngol Relat Spec. 2013;75:357–60. https://doi.org/10.1159/000357475.
27. Gianoli GJ, Soileau JS. Chronic suppurative otitis media, caloric testing, and rotational chair testing. Otol Neurotol. 2008;29:13–5. https://doi.org/10.1097/mao.0b013e31815c2589.
28. Ben-David J, Podoshin L, Fradis M, Faraggi D. Is the vestibular system affected by middle ear effusion? Otolaryngol Head Neck Surg. 1993;109:421–6. https://doi.org/10.1177/019459989310900306.
29. Blakley BW, Chan L. Methods considerations for nystagmography. J Otolaryngol Head Neck Surg. 2015;44:25. https://doi.org/10.1186/s40463-015-0078-2.
30. Ben-David Y, Hafner H, Fradis M, Krasnitz G, Podoshin L. Do Frenzel glasses have a place in the modern electronystagmography laboratory. Am J Otol. 1996;17:89–92.
31. Paparella MM. Interactive inner-ear/middle-ear disease, including perilymphatic fistula. Acta Otolaryngol Suppl. 1991;485:36–45.
32. Chang C-W, Cheng P-W, Young Y-H. Inner ear deficits after chronic otitis media. Eur Arch Otorhinolaryngol. 2014;271:2165–70. https://doi.org/10.1007/s00405-013-2714-7.
33. Zwergal A, Rettinger N, Frenzel C, Dieterich M, Brandt T, Strupp M. A bucket of static vestibular function. Neurology. 2009;72:1689–92. https://doi.org/10.1212/WNL.0b013e3181a55ecf.
34. Lee D-H. How to improve the accuracy of diagnosing otitis media with effusion in a pediatric population. Int J Pediatr Otorhinolaryngol. 2010;74:151–3. https://doi.org/10.1016/j.ijporl.2009.10.029.
35. Akin FW, Murnane OD. Subjective visual vertical test. Semin Hear. 2009;30:281–6. https://doi.org/10.1055/s-0029-1241128.
36. Clarke AH, Schönfeld U, Hamann C, Scherer H. Measuring unilateral otolith function via the otolith-ocular response and the subjective visual vertical. Acta Otolaryngol Suppl. 2001;545:84–7. https://doi.org/10.1080/000164801750388180.
37. Böhmer A, Rickenmann J. The subjective visual vertical as a clinical parameter of vestibular function in peripheral vestibular diseases. J Vestib Res. 1995;5:35–45.
38. Cusin FS, Ganança MM, Ganança FF, Ganança CF, Caovilla HH. Balance Rehabilitation Unit (BRUTM) posturography in Menière's disease. Braz J Otorhinolaryngol. 2010;76:611–7. https://doi.org/10.1590/S1808-86942010000500013.
39. Liu J, Zhou R, Liu B, Leng Y, Liu J, Liu D, Zhang SL, Kong WJ. Sensory organization test principally reflects utricular function. Acta Otolaryngol. 2017;137:1143–8. https://doi.org/10.1080/00016489.2017.1342143.
40. Gawron W, Pośpiech L, Orendorz-Fraczkowska K. An evaluation of postural stability and the effects of middle-ear drainage on vestibulo-spinal reflexes of children with chronic otitis media with effusion. Int J Pediatr Otorhinolaryngol. 2004;68:1175–9. https://doi.org/10.1016/j.ijporl.2004.03.017.
41. MacDougall HG, Weber KP, McGarvie LA, Halmagyi GM, Curthoys IS. The video head impulse test. Neurology. 2009;73:1134–41. https://doi.org/10.1212/WNL.0b013e3181bacf85.
42. Tomaz A, Monsanto RDC, Cusin FS, Kasemodel ALP, Penido NDO. Evaluation of the vestibulo-ocular reflex in patients with chronic otitis media. Braz J Otorhinolaryngol. 2022;88(5):675–82. https://doi.org/10.1016/j.bjorl.2020.09.006.
43. D'Albora R, Silveira L, Carmona S, Perez-Fernandez N. Diagnostic bedside vestibuloocular reflex evaluation in the setting of a false negative fistula test in cholesteatoma of the middle ear. Case Rep Otolaryngol. 2017;2017:2919463. https://doi.org/10.1155/2017/2919463.
44. Covelli E, Talamonti R, Benincasa AT, Filippi C, Marrone V, Tarentini S, Monini S, Barbara M. Video head impulse test in labyrinthine fistula due to middle ear cholesteatoma. J Int Adv Otol. 2019;15:283–8. https://doi.org/10.5152/iao.2019.5678.
45. Mezzalira R, Bittar RSM, do Carmo Bilécki-Stipsky MM, Brugnera C, Grasel SS. Sensitivity of caloric test and video head impulse as screening test for chronic vestibular complaints. Clinics (Sao Paulo). 2017;72:469–73. https://doi.org/10.6061/clinics/2017(08)03.
46. Ramos BF, Cal R, Carmona S, Maia FZE. VVOR and VORS testing as a tool in the diagnosis of unilateral and bilateral vestibular hypofunction. Rev ORL. 2018;9:1–2. https://doi.org/10.14201/orl.18856.
47. Kodama A, Ishii T, Oka Y, Uebo K. Inner ear histopathology of human temporal bone with chronic otitis media. Equilibrium Res. 1988;47(Suppl. 4):94–100. https://doi.org/10.3757/jser.47.Suppl-4_94.

48. Murofushi T, Kaga K. Recording and assessing VEMPs. In: Vestibular evoked myogenic potential: its basics and clinical applications. Tokyo: Springer Japan; 2009. p. 25–33. https://doi.org/10.1007/978-4-431-85908-6_4.
49. Chihara Y, Iwasaki S, Ushio M, Murofushi T. Vestibular-evoked extraocular potentials by air-conducted sound: another clinical test for vestibular function. Clin Neurophysiol. 2007;118:2745–51. https://doi.org/10.1016/j.clinph.2007.08.005.
50. Colebatch JG, Halmagyi GM, Skuse NF. Myogenic potentials generated by a click-evoked vestibulocollic reflex. J Neurol Neurosurg Psychiatry. 1994;57:190–7.
51. Goycoolea MV. Clinical aspects of round window membrane permeability under normal and pathological conditions. Acta Otolaryngol. 2001;121:437–47.
52. Goycoolea MV, Paparella MM, Goldberg B, Carpenter AM. Permeability of the round window membrane in otitis media. Arch Otolaryngol. 1980;106:430–3.

Radiological Evaluation of the Temporal Bone in Chronic Otitis Media

45

Mauricio Noschang Lopes da Silva,
Marcela Lehmkuhl Damiani, and Sady Selaimen da Costa

Introduction

The temporal bone has a complex anatomy, and radiology helps to understand it. Mastoid radiography can provide data such as temporal bone pneumatization, *tegmen,* and lateral sinus position. However, computed tomography (CT) is the best diagnostic test for involvement of temporal bone structures resulting from chronic inflammation, and the use of contrast is not routinely necessary in cases of chronic otitis media (COM). The indications for performing CT in the context of chronic otitis media are presence of cholesteatoma in physical examination; history of persistent otologic suppurations; and pronounced hearing loss, sometimes incompatible with otoscopy.

COM patients with symptoms neurological must undergo magnetic resonance imaging (MRI) to exclude abscesses and sinus thrombosis sigmoid. MRI can also be useful to assess possible intracranial extension of cholesteatoma or to differentiate it from cholesterol granulomas and granulation tissue. Moreover, this test is important in diagnosis of recidivism in closed cavity tympanomastoidectomy or subtotal petrosectomy.

History of Imaging Exams

The beginning of radiology in the head and neck was through conventional radiographs. They were performed mainly for fractures and to locate foreign bodies. Some researchers have fervently sought other applications. Eugene W. Caldwell (1870–1918) became fascinated by X-rays just 2 years after Roentgen's discovery [1]. He was an electrical engineer, but studied medicine and graduated in 1902. He dedicated his research work to the sinuses and played a key role in the development of sinusitis diagnosis. He died at the age of 48 from radiation-induced metastatic skin cancer.

The temporal bone has more complex anatomy and special views had to be developed to depict its compartments. Particularly, the middle ear and mastoid were given special attention for the evaluation of infection and cholesteatoma. In 1906, Dr. Arthur Schüller (1874–1957), an Austrian neuroradiologist considered one of the founders of this subspecialty, described an oblique view of the mastoid (tube at an angle of 25° caudally), through plain radiography, aiding in the evaluation of trauma and pneumatization of the temporal bones (Fig. 45.1).

Conventional radiographs have evolved, but they were still precarious in the detailed assessment of head and neck anatomy. In 1931, there was the second major milestone in radiology: the introduction of linear tomography by Dr. Ziedses des Plantes from the Netherlands. Using this technique, tissue planes of varying thickness were visualized in detail, excluding anatomical structures above and below the selected plane. The technique was based on linear movements in opposite directions, between the movement of the tube and the cassette containing the film.

From there, polytomography emerged with a pluridirectional and hypocycloidal unit. Galdino Valvassori, a member of the University of Chicago team from 1960 onward, worked with this new unit on research carried out on a large human temporal bones (HTB) from Dr. Lindsey, chairman of otolaryngology at the University of Chicago. These studies have led to important publications on conditions such as cholesteatoma, pathology of the internal auditory canal, otosclerosis, and diseases of the posterior

M. N. L. da Silva (✉) · M. L. Damiani
Hospital de Clínicas de Porto Alegre, Universidade Federal do Rio Grande do Sul, Porto Alegre, Brazil

S. S. da Costa
Universidade Federal do Rio Grande do Sul, Porto Alegre, Rio Grande do Sul, Brazil

M. V. Goycoolea et al. (eds.), *Textbook of Otitis Media*, https://doi.org/10.1007/978-3-031-40949-3_45

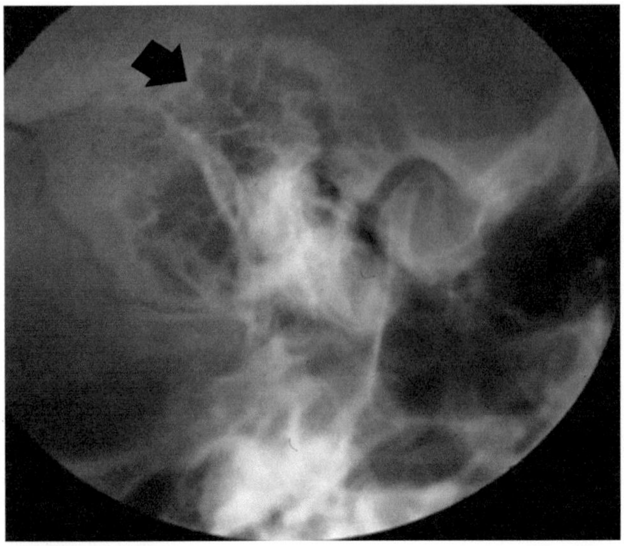

Fig. 45.1 Normally pneumatized mastoid—conventional radiography—Schüller [1] view

fossa. Their experiences were summarized and published in 1966 in a book on temporal bone tomography and in 1973 in an atlas [2].

An important historic achievement came in 1972 with the introduction of CT by Godfrey Hounsfield of Great Britain, who was a computer specialist. The foundation of CT was based on mathematical equations that had been formulated in 1963 and 1964 by AM Cormack, a professor of physics at Tufts University in Boston. In 1979, both researchers were awarded the Nobel Prize in Medicine for this remarkable discovery. CT has allowed the differentiation of normal and abnormal soft tissues and bone structures and its development in recent years, through helicoidal CT, has allowed rapid examinations and thinner cuts, with the ability to reconstruct three-dimensionally.

A third important milestone in radiology occurred with the introduction of MRI. The principles of this examination are based on the theory of spin and were first demonstrated by Isidor Rabi in 1938 [3, 4], who tested the emission of a particle beam through a magnetic field and showed that it can emit waves at dependent frequencies and the charge of the particles and the strength of the magnetic field. In 1946, Bloch and Purcell [3, 5–7] demonstrated the same principles applied to liquids and solids and, in 1978, Young and Clow [3, 8] obtained the first magnetic resonance imaging of the brain, enabling the development of neuroanatomical studies in a unique way.

Computed Tomography of Temporal Bones

CT is an excellent exam to evaluate the structures of the temporal bone [9], as well as the changes caused by otitis media. The cuts must be 1–2 mm thick and the images presented in the axial, sagital, and coronal planes, being the images carefully evaluated in windows for bone, soft tissue and liquid. Its use is becoming more and more indicated, especially in surgical cases, because through it, the diagnosis can be confirmed, the involvement of the ear by the disease can be accurately measured and the surgical team prepared for possible anatomical variations capable of complicating a surgery.

The COM presents alterations well described in the tomographic studies. It is possible to visualize the presence of effusion in the middle ear and mastoid, bone erosions, degree of pneumatization mastoid, position of the lateral sinus and the relationship between the temporal bone and the great vessels [10]. In addition, modern helicoidal image acquisition techniques and high-resolution slices allow the evaluation of smaller structures more accurately. The state of the tympanic membrane, the ossicular chain, and the entire course of the facial nerve can be estimated. However, often some structures are not carefully observed through this exam, mainly due to the lack of standardized routine of analysis. Thus, the systematic use of this test in the evaluation of patients with cholesteatoma is essential.

Currently, there are no reasons to dismiss CT. It has a much lower cost than in the past, rapid performance and minimal morbidity. The minimum assessment includes mastoid pneumatization, opacifications, facial nerve path, *tegmen* position, bone erosions, ossicular chain, relationship of the great vessels and sigmoid sinus, aeration of the protympanum, bone spur of Chaussé, and anatomical variations [11, 12]. It is important to standardize a *"check list"* (Figs. 45.2 and 45.3) so that there is no risk of neglecting any structure or compartment, avoiding surprises during the operation.

The figures presented show the characteristics considered the most important in the radiological analysis in the axial and coronal planes of temporal bones [12]. The structures and form of evaluation are described in Tables 45.1, 45.2, 45.3, and 45.4.

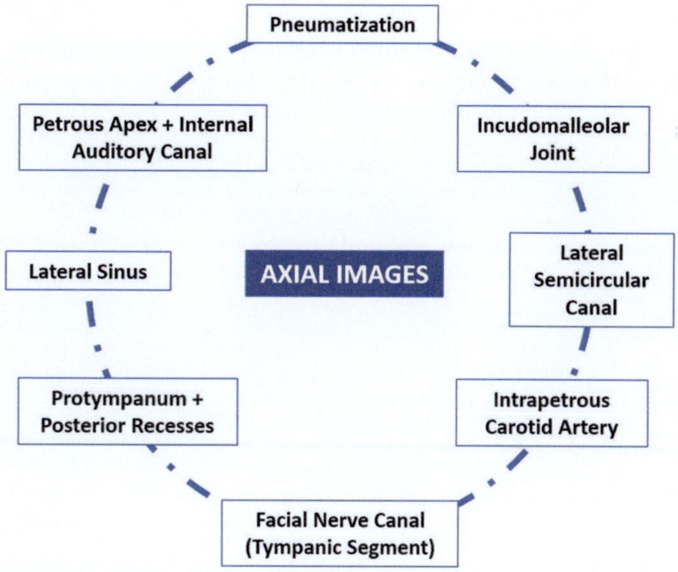

Fig. 45.2 List of structures seen in the axial plane

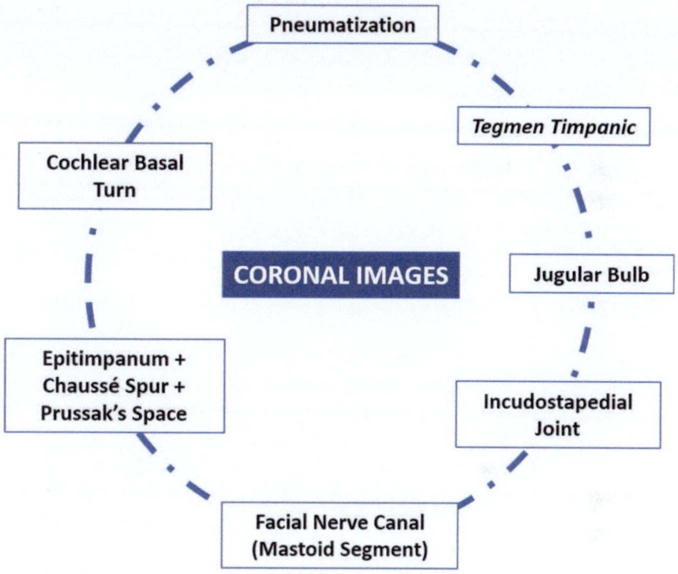

Fig. 45.3 List of structures seen in the coronal plane

Table 45.1 Radiological interpretation of structures

	Coronal plane	Axial plane	Evaluation
External auditory canal	At the level of the basal turn of the cochlea and the IAC—Fig. 45.4	At the level of the basal turn of the cochlea, the TMJ (anterior) and the mastoid cells (posterior) are visualized—Fig. 45.5	Normal, eroded, or filled with material (soft tissue or bone)
Tympanic membrane	At the same level as the EAC, head, neck, and proximal part of the malleus manubrium—Fig. 45.4	At the same level as the EAC, sections showing the posterior recesses—Fig. 45.5	Normal, retracted, perforated, thickened or with tympanosclerosis— Fig. 45.4
Mesotympanum	Sections between the cochlea (anterior) and the IAC (posterior)	Level between the basal turn of the cochlea (lower) to the appearance of all the turns (upper) —Fig. 45.6	Aeration or filled
Protympanum	–	At the level of the basal turn of the cochlea. Previous: TMJ. Posterior: carotid canal and anterior portion of the otic capsule—Fig. 45.7	Aeration or filled
Retrotympanum	–	On the same level as the pro-tympanum. Facial nerve in second genu (between tympanic and mastoid segments) divides posterior recesses into sinus tympani (medial) and facial nerve recess (lateral) – Fig. 45.7	Aeration or filled
Epitympanum	Sections between the cochlear turns and the facial nerve section at the second genu (anterior) up to the SSCC view (posterior) – Fig. 45.8	showing the incudomalleolar joint—Fig. 45.9	Aeration or filled
Bone spur of Chaussé and prussak space	Level of the cochlear turns, in the transition to the labyrinth, with observation of the malleus head and neck—Figs. 45.8 and 45.10	–	Bone Spur of Chaussé: Intact or eroded . Prussak space: compartment between Chaussé and the malleus head. Aerated or veiled.
Lateral semicircular canal (LSC) and superior semicircular canal (SSC)	Between the levels of the epitympanum (anterior) to the mastoid antrum (posterior)—Fig. 45.11	The LSC can be visualized in the section that shows the cochlea and the modiolus, in addition to the incudomalleolar joint—Fig. 45.12	Integrity or presence of labyrinthine fistulas.
Tympanic tegmen	Along the entire length of the middle ear and mastoid. From the beginning of the cochlea (anterior) to the most posterior regions of the mastoid—Figs. 45.13 and 45.14	–	Integrity and position
Intrapetrosal carotid artery	–	From its vertical (lower) portion and its relations with the hypotympanum and jugular foramen, to its horizontal (upper) portion and its interaction with Eustachian tube—Fig. 45.15	Normal, dehiscent or salient.
Jugular bulb	Inferior to the cochlea and labyrinth—Figs. 45.16 and 45.17	Posterior to the carotid artery, at lower levels	Normal, dehiscent, or salient
Cortical bone of the posterior fossa	–	At the level of the lateral sinus cut—Fig. 45.18	Integrity
Sigmoid sinus	–	At the mastoid and posterior fossa levels—Fig. 45.18	Normal, dehiscent, or salient
Petrous apex	–	At the Internal Auditory Canal level—Fig. 45.19	Pneumatized or not. Evaluate pathologies such as effusion, destruction of septa or tumors
Cochlea	–	Figure 45.20a	Malformations, erosions, or calcifications
Internal Auditory Canal (IAC)	–	Figure 45.20b	Sign of enlargement, possible invasion by cholesteatoma or tumors.

Table 45.2 Radiological interpretation of the ossicular chain: malleus, incus, and stapes

Ossicular chain	
Malleus	
Head (Fig. 45.21a, b)	Coronal plane (Fig. 45.21a): at the level of Prussak's space. Axial plane (Fig. 45.21b): in the region of the epitympanum, at the level of the horizontal segment of the facial nerve, the IAC and the LSC
Neck (Fig. 45.22a, b)	Coronal plane (Fig. 45.22a): at the level of bone spur of Chaussé. Axial plane (Fig. 45.22b): section showing the cochlea with the modiolus
Handle (Fig. 45.23)	Coronal plane: section where the TM, the cochlea and the transversal section of the facial nerve (labyrinthine and tympanic segments) can be observed
Evaluation	Normal, eroded, absent or involved by tympanosclerosis (Fig. 45.24)
INCUS	
Body (Fig. 45.25)	Axial plane: intermediate level between the head and neck of the malleus, in the section where the cochlea and LSC can be seen. It is possible see the short process
Long process and incudostapedial joint (Figs. 45.26 and 45.27)	Viewed with the stapes
Evaluation	Normal, eroded, absent, or involved by tympanosclerosis
Stapes	
Coronal plane (Fig. 45.27)	Level where the vestibule, basal turn of the cochlea, LSC and SSC are observed
Axial plane (Fig. 45.26)	Level where the cochlea, vestibule, IAC, and petrous apex are observed
Evaluation	Normal, eroded, absent, or involved by tympanosclerosis

Table 45.3 Radiological interpretation of the mastoid

Mastoid	
Coronal plane (Fig. 45.27)	Level where the vestibule, basal turn of the cochlea, LSC and SSC are observed
Axial plane (Fig. 45.26)	Level where the cochlea, vestibule, IAC, and petrous apex are observed
Evaluation	It is classified as sclerotic, diploic, or pneumatized (Figs. 45.28, 45.24, 45.29, 45.30). Sclerosis: absence of pneumatization. Diploic: 10 or fewer cells between 2 and 5 mm in size, plus a pneumatized antrum. Mastoids with partial pneumatization . Pneumatized: completely aerated, with more than 10 cells of the size mentioned above, in addition to a pneumatized antrum. Then it is divided into 3 spaces: antrum, tip, and "mid" . mastoid" (intermediate region). Presence or not of veiling in each space (Fig. 45.31)

Table 45.4 Radiological interpretation of the facial nerve

Facial nerve	
Tympanic segment (Figs. 45.32 and 45.33)	Axial plane: the entire course, including the first genu, at the level of the incudomalleolar joint. Coronal plane: cross section under the LSC.
Mastoid segment (Fig. 45.32)	Coronal plane: at the level of the stylomastoid foramen, inferior to the LSC.
Evaluation	Normal or eroded bone canal, dehiscent nerve or not.

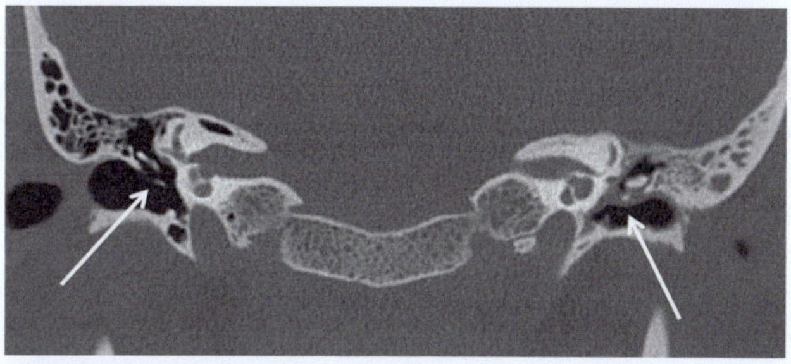

Fig. 45.4 Coronal plane. Comparison between the two ears. Right ear with normal TM and external auditory canal without alterations (left side arrow). Left ear with perforated TM and presence of soft tissue material in the external auditory canal (right side arrow)

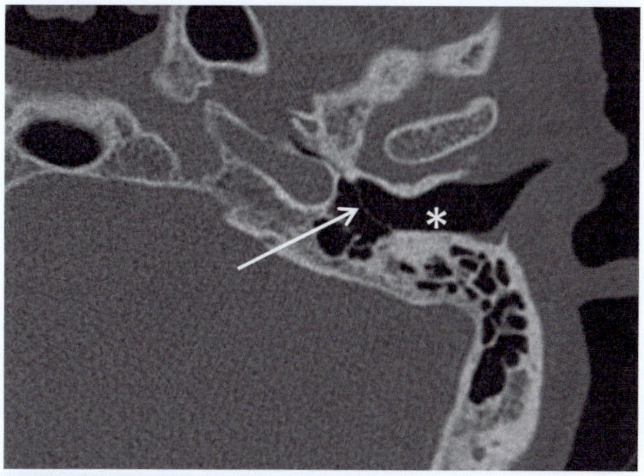

Fig. 45.5 Left ear axial plane. Tympanic membrane (arrow) and EAC (asterisk)

Based on this suggested systematization (Figs. 45.34, 45.35, 45.36, and 45.37) and examples of pathological temporal bones, it becomes easier to assess the presence of disease, stage the involvement of the middle ear and mastoid, and safely propose surgeries through CT of the temporal bones.

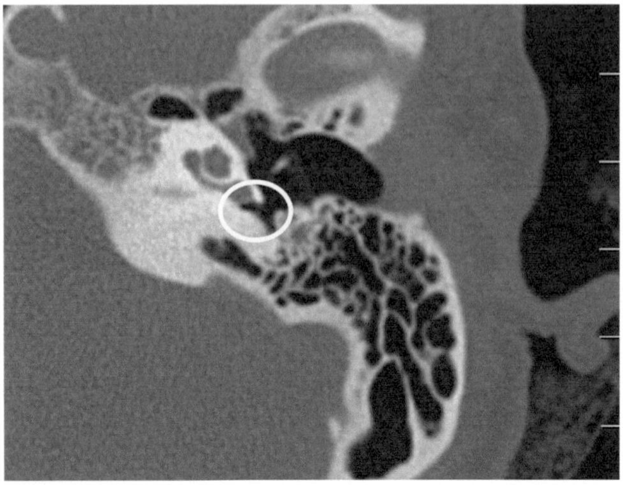

Fig. 45.6 Left ear axial plane. Round window niche (ellipse)

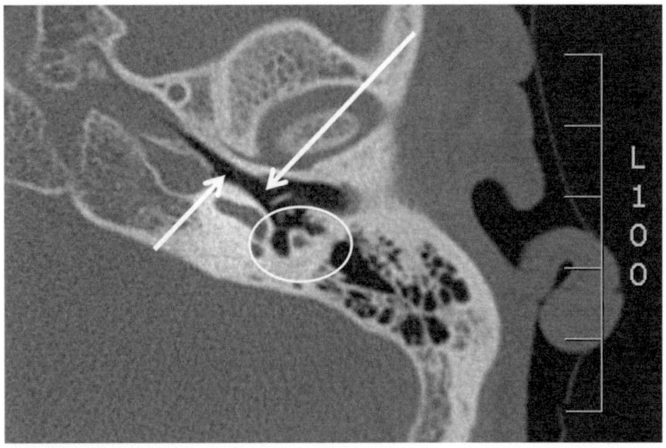

Fig. 45.7 Left ear axial plane. Aerated protympanum (short arrow), aerated mesotympanum (long arrow), and posterior recesses (ellipse). Note the facial nerve in the center of the ellipse dividing the sinus tympani (more medial) from the facial recess (more lateral)

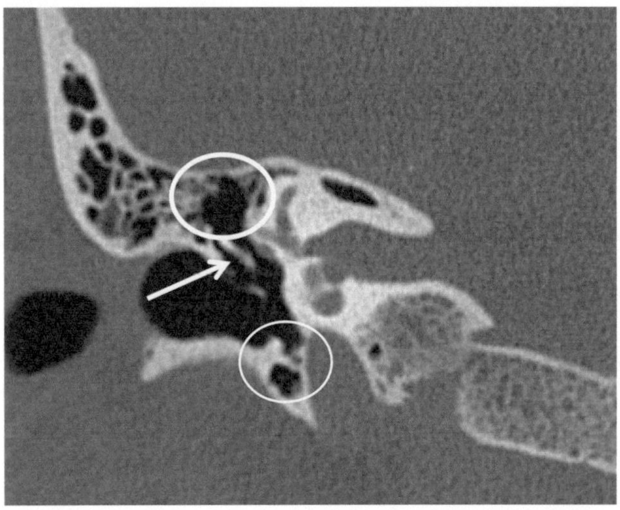

Fig. 45.8 Right ear coronal plane. Aerated epitympanum (upper ellipse); free Prussak space, between the lateral wall of the attic and the ossicular chain (arrow); free hypotympanic cells (lower ellipse)

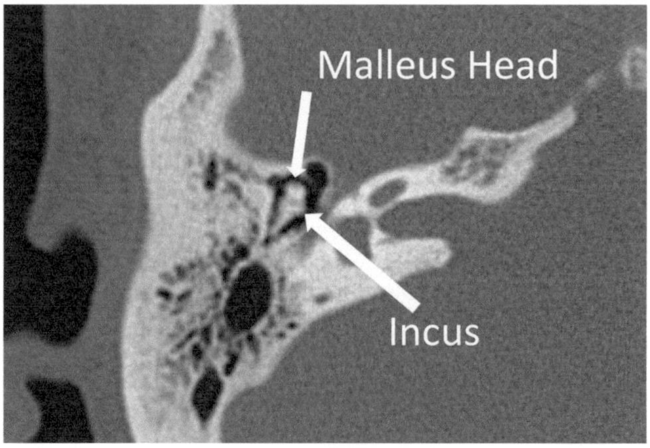

Fig. 45.9 Right ear axial plane: visualization of the incudomalleolar joint in the epitympanum

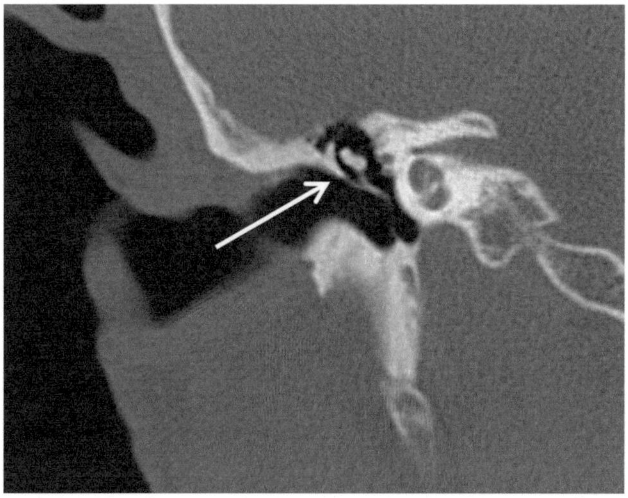

Fig. 45.10 Right ear coronal plane. Bone Spur of Chaussé (arrow)

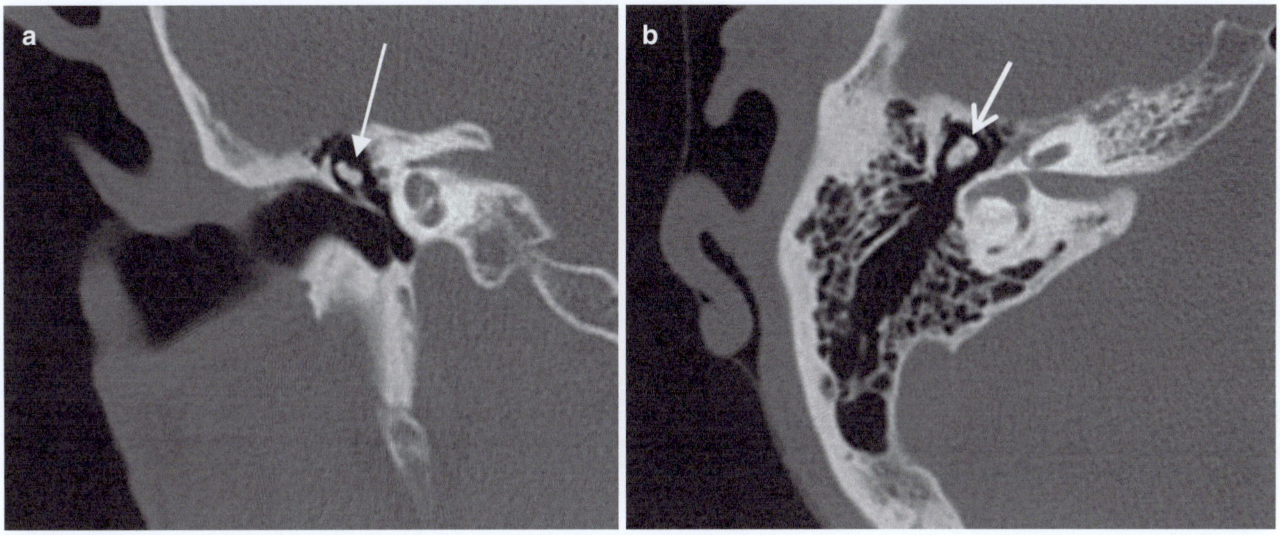

Fig. 45.11 Malleus head (arrows). In (**a**), right ear coronal plane. In (**b**), the same ear in the axial plane

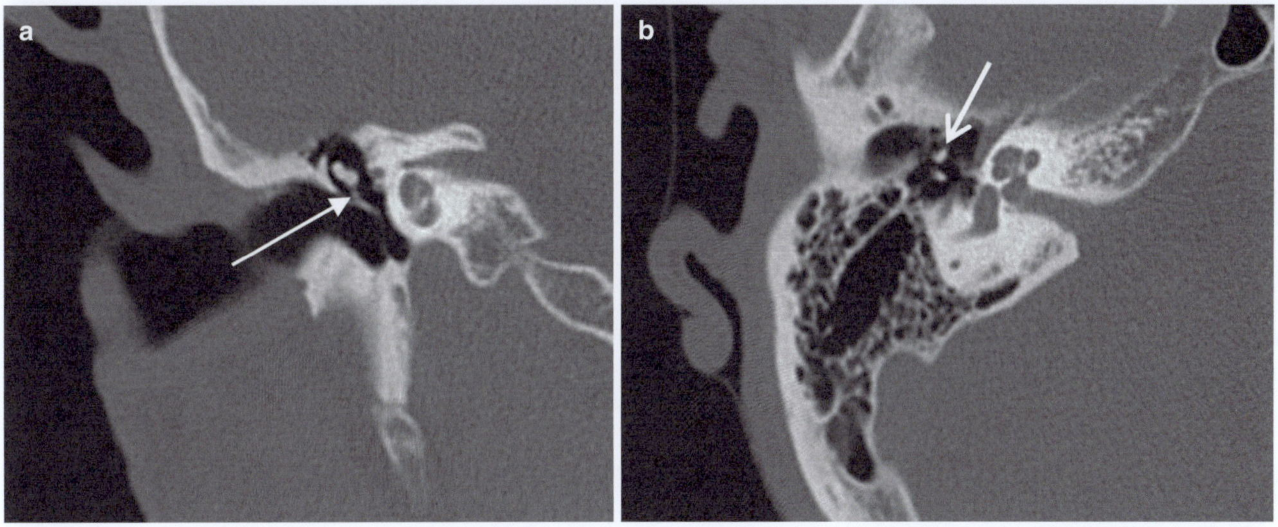

Fig. 45.12 Malleus neck (arrows). In (**a**), right ear coronal plane. In (**b**), the same ear in the axial plane

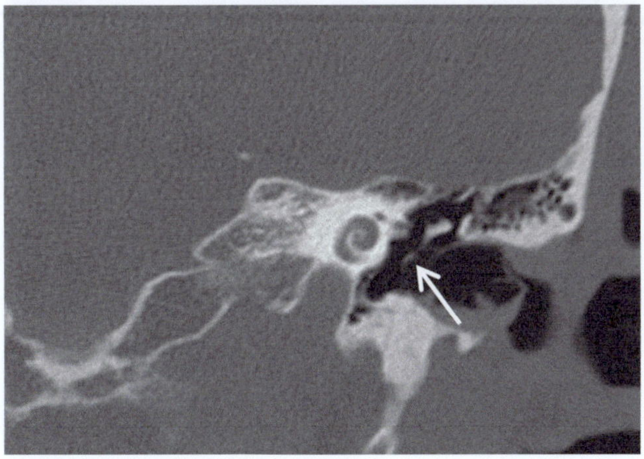

Fig. 45.13 Malleus handle (arrow)

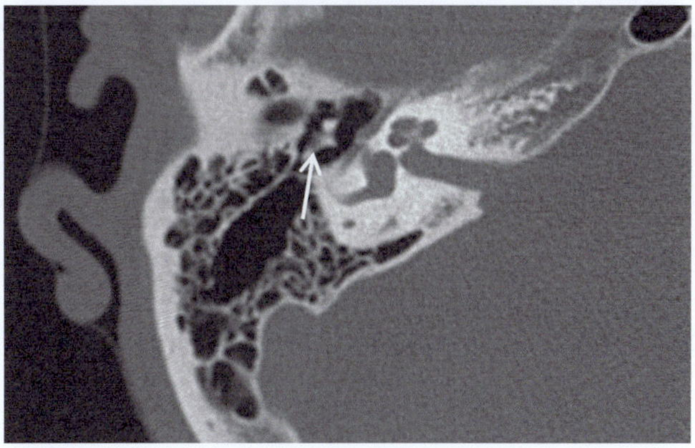

Fig. 45.14 Incus body with a short process (arrow)

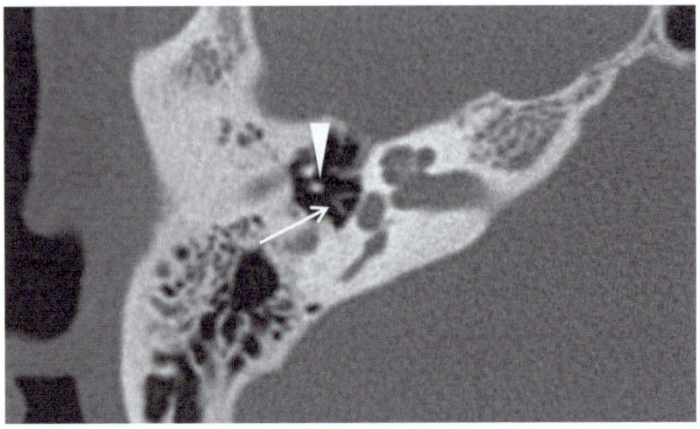

Fig. 45.15 Axial plane of the right ear: visualization of the long process of the incus (arrowhead), stapes (arrow), footplate, and vestibule. Normal ossicular chain

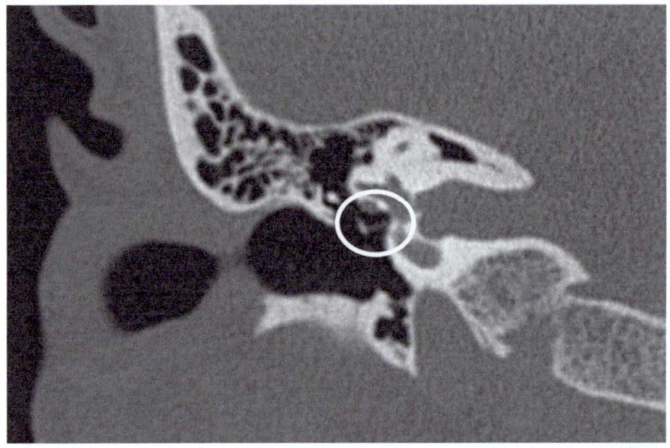

Fig. 45.16 Right ear coronal plane. Incudostapedial joint with visualization of the oval window (ellipse) in the mesotympanum

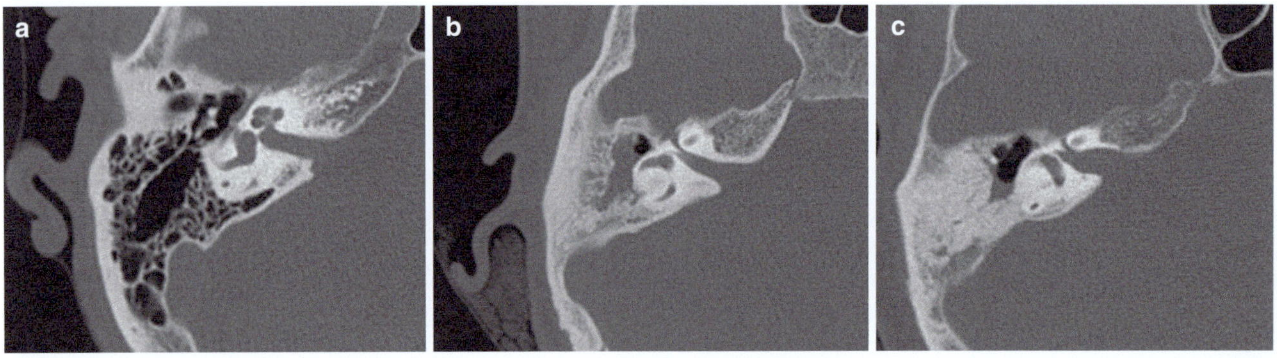

Fig. 45.17 Axial plane of the right ear of 3 patients: pneumatized mastoid in (**a**), diploic in (**b**) and sclerotic in (**c**)

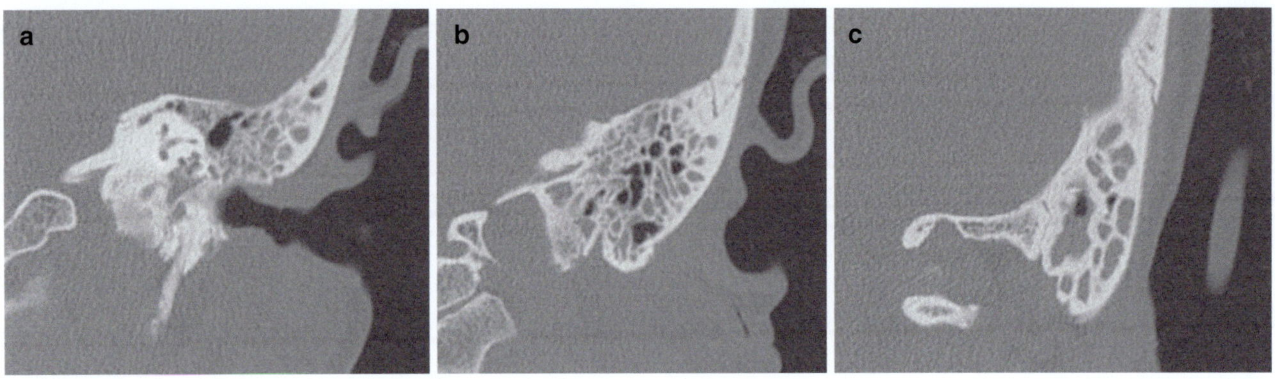

Fig. 45.18 Left ear coronal plane: pneumatized and veiled mastoid compartments. (**a**) Antrum. (**b**) Mid mastoid. (**c**) Mastoid tip

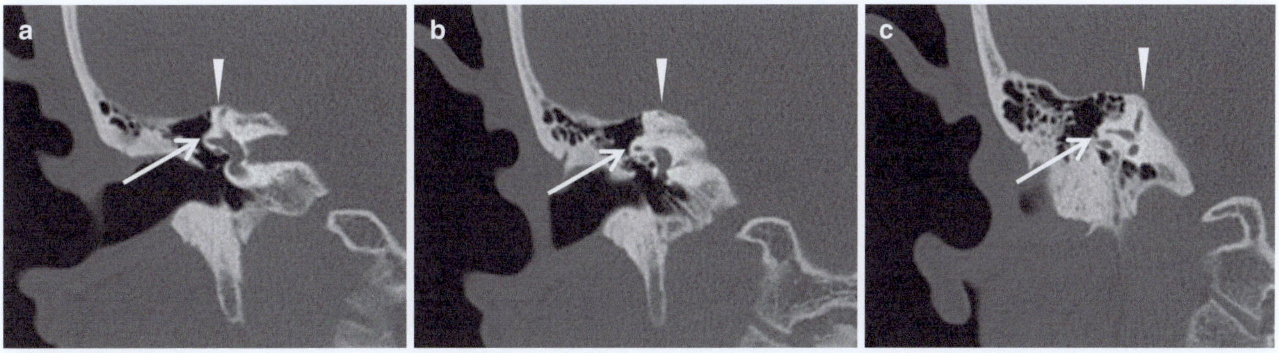

Fig. 45.19 Coronal plane of the right ear: LSC (arrow) and SSC (arrowhead) in view at the level of the epitympanum in (**a**), the aditus in (**b**) and the antrum in (**c**)

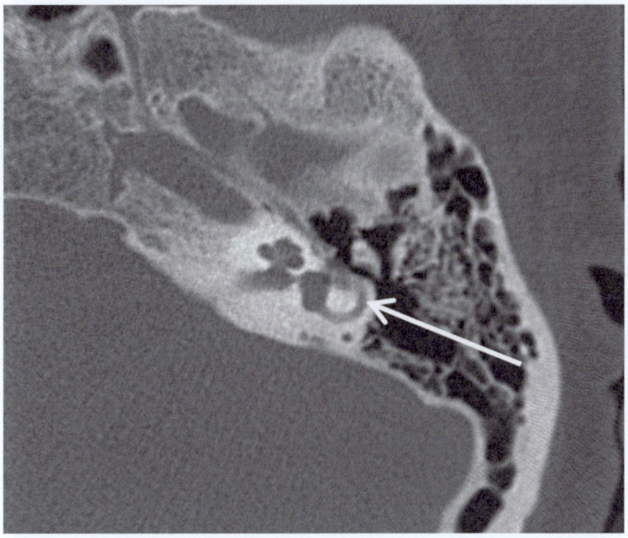

Fig. 45.20 Left ear axial plane: LSC (arrow)

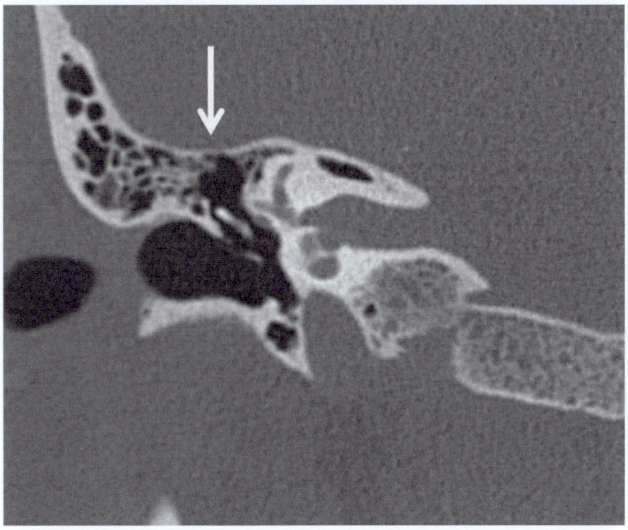

Fig. 45.21 Right ear coronal plane. *Tegmen timpani* (arrow)

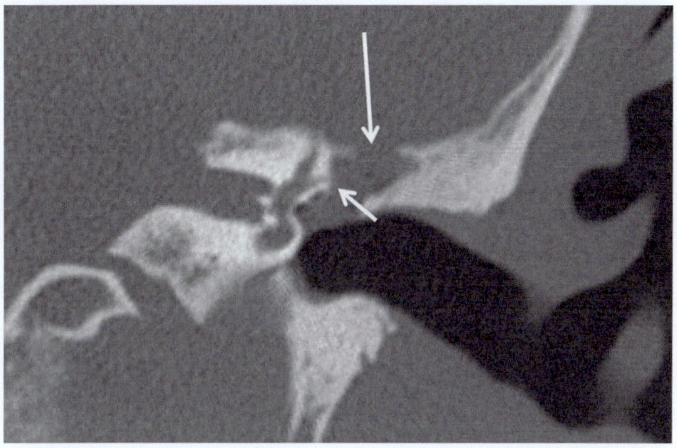

Fig. 45.22 Coronal plane—left ear. Tegmen's erosion (long arrow) and LSC fistula (short arrow). Veiling of the tympanic cavity in the region of the oval window and epitympanum suggesting cholesteatoma

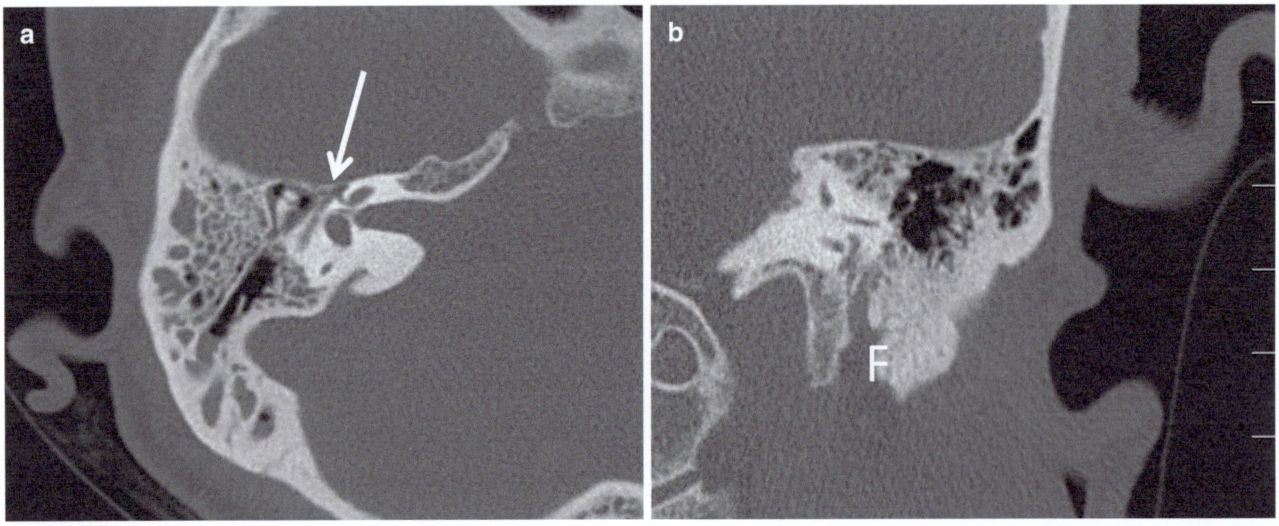

Fig. 45.23 Visualization of the facial nerve path. (**a**) Axial plane, right ear: tympanic segment of the facial nerve and first genu (arrow). (**b**) Coronal plane, left ear: mastoid segment of the facial nerve (F)

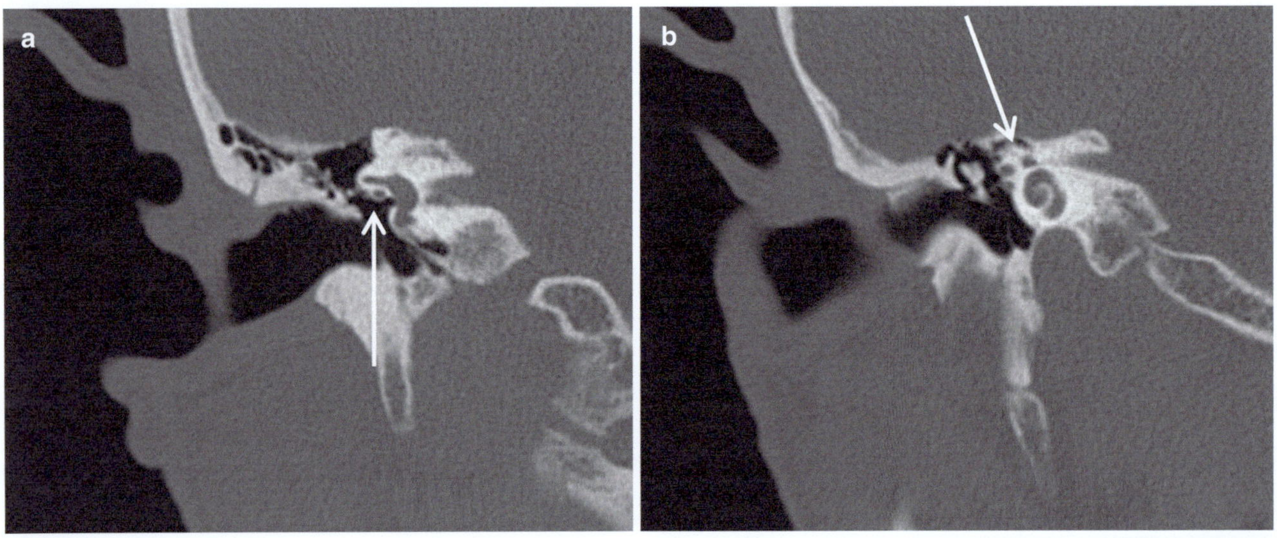

Fig. 45.24 Visualization of the facial nerve path (arrows)—right ear coronal plane. (**a**) Cross section of the tympanic segment of the facial nerve. (**b**) Cross-section of the labyrinthine (more medial) and tympanic (more lateral) segments

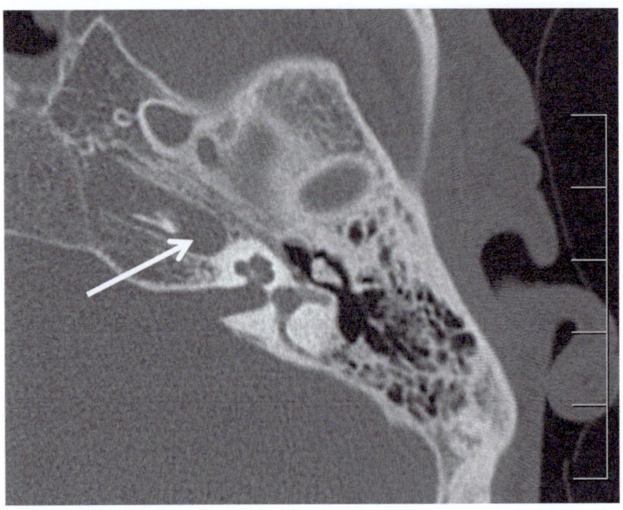

Fig. 45.25 Intrapetrous carotid artery (arrow)

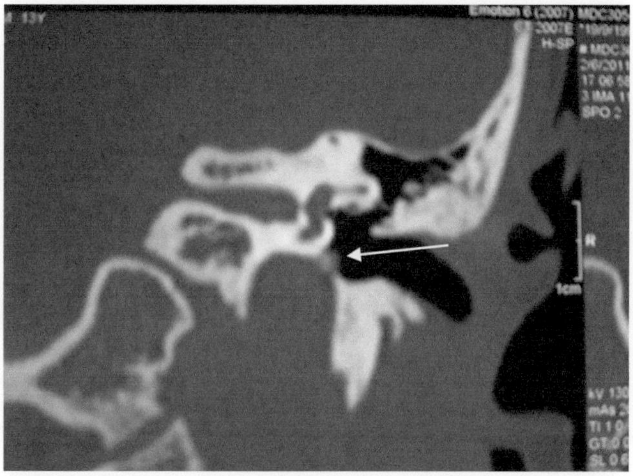

Fig. 45.26 Left ear coronal plane: dehiscent jugular bulb (arrow)

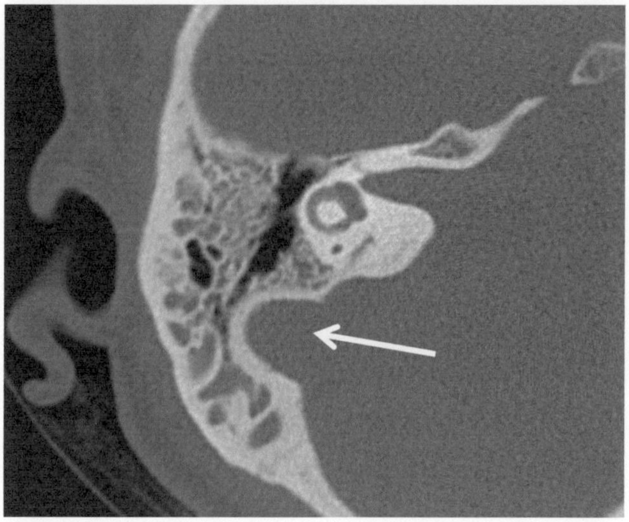

Fig. 45.27 Right ear axial plane: prominent sigmoid sinus, but with integrity of the posterior fossa cortex (arrow)

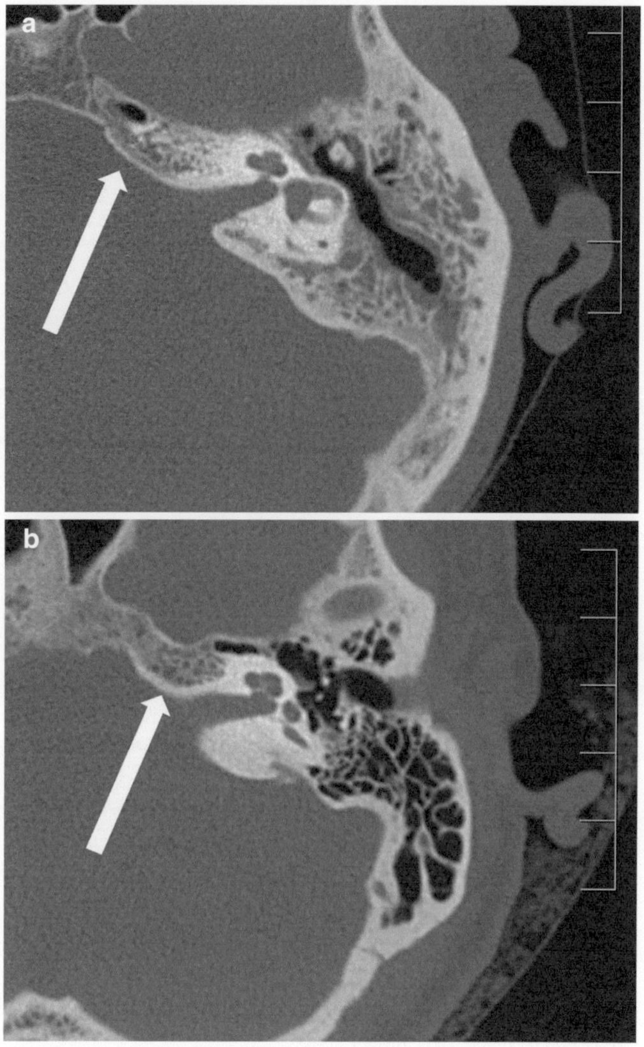

Fig. 45.28 Axial plane left ear of different patients. View of the petrous apex (arrows). In (**a**), cell pneumatization next to the clivus. In (**b**), pneumatization of supracochlear cells

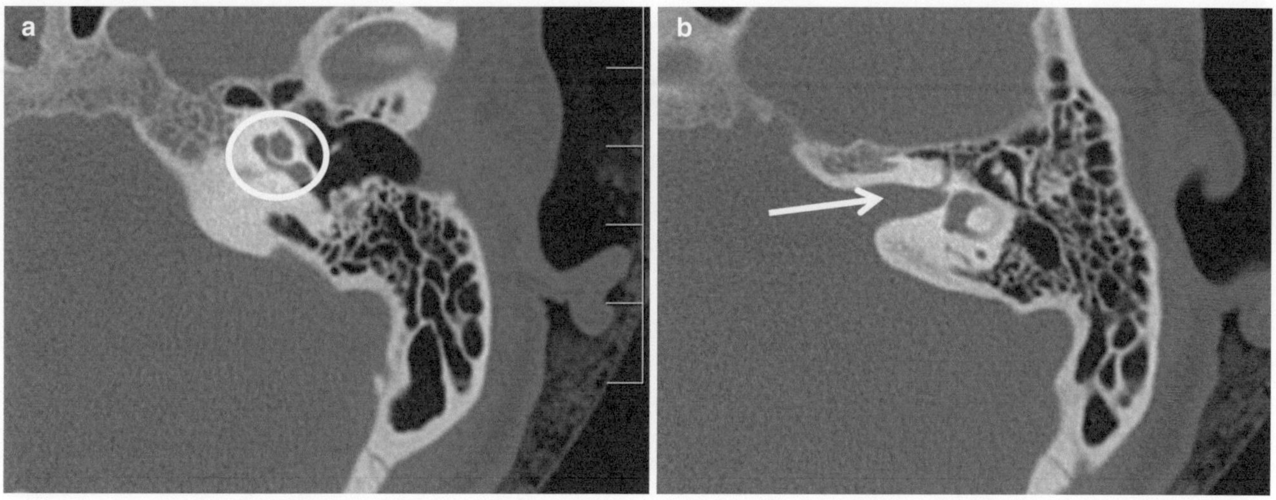

Fig. 45.29 Left ear axial plane. (**a**) Visualization of normal cochlear turns (ellipse). (**b**) Normal internal auditory canal (arrow)

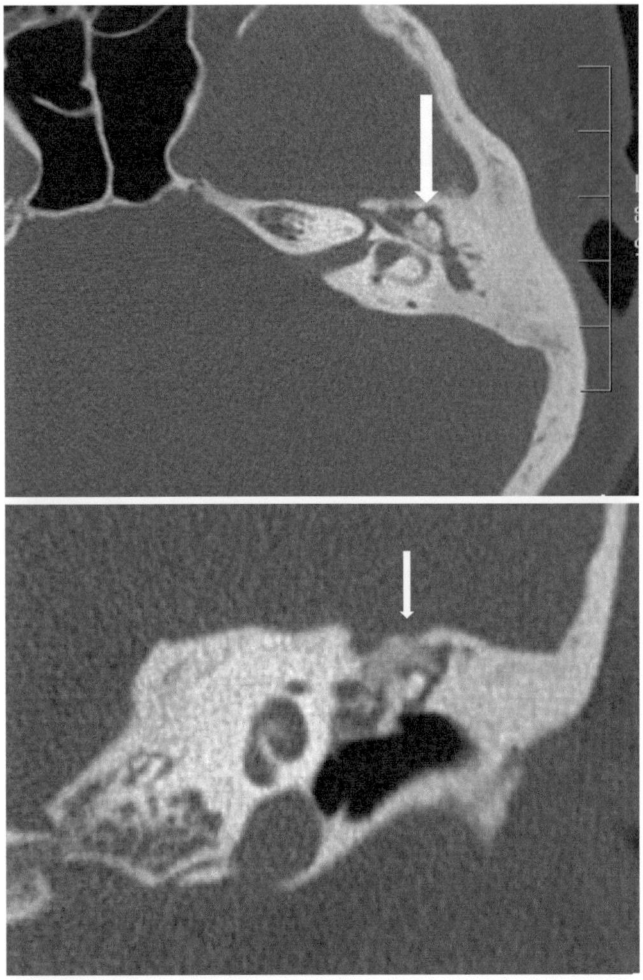

Fig. 45.30 Tympanosclerosis involving the ossicular chain of the left ear. (**a**) Axial plane. (**b**) Coronal plane

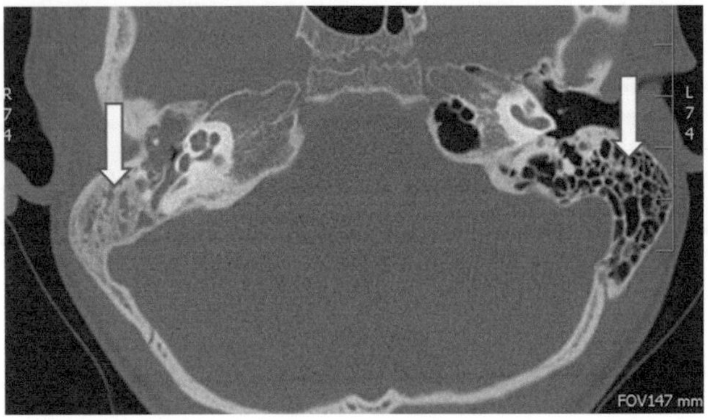

Fig. 45.31 Right ear axial plane: reduction of mastoid pneumatization and opacification. Left ear pneumatized mastoid

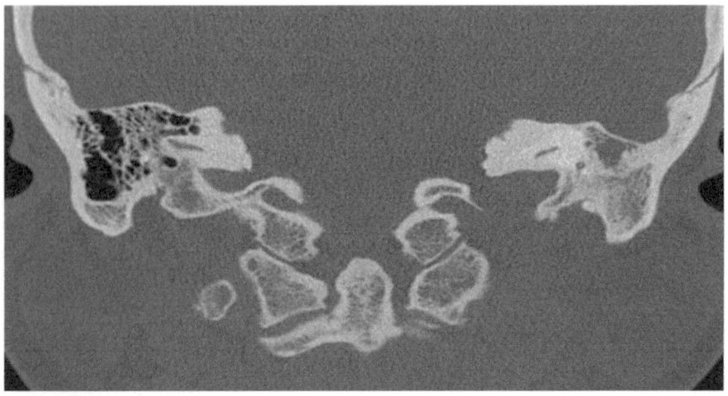

Fig. 45.32 Coronal plane—Right ear: Pneumatized mastoid. Left ear: sclerotic and with a veiled antrum

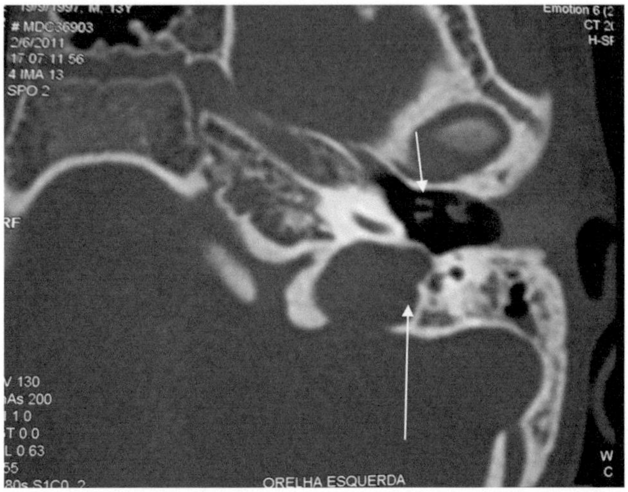

Fig. 45.33 xial plane—left ear. Protruding jugular bulb in the tympanic cavity (long arrow) and presence of ventilation tube in the tympanic membrane (short arrow)

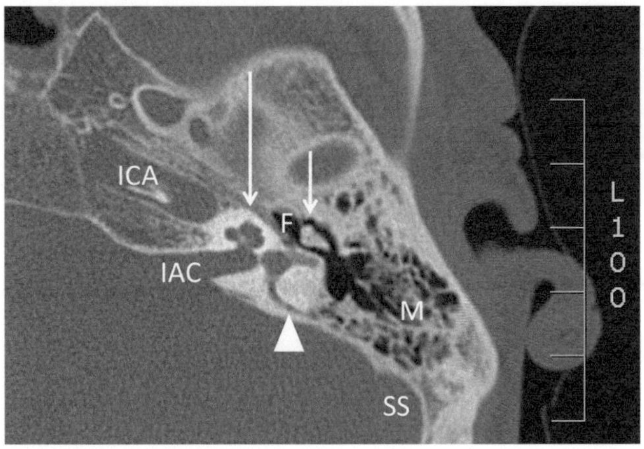

Fig. 45.34 Structures seen in an upper axial plane section of the left ear: intrapetrous carotid artery (ICA), internal auditory canal (IAC), cochlear turns (long arrow), facial nerve (F), incudomalleolar joint (short arrow), lateral semicircular canal (arrowhead), mastoid cells (M), and sigmoid sinus (SS)

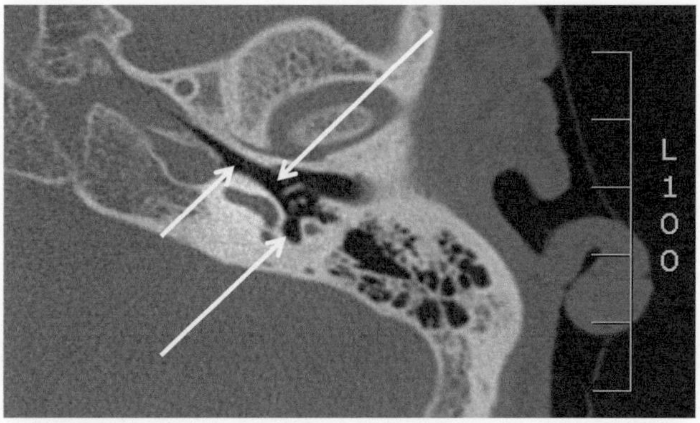

Fig. 45.35 Tympanic compartment seen in the down axial plane of the left ear: protympanum (short arrow), mesotympanum (long arrow), and retrotympanum (middle arrow)

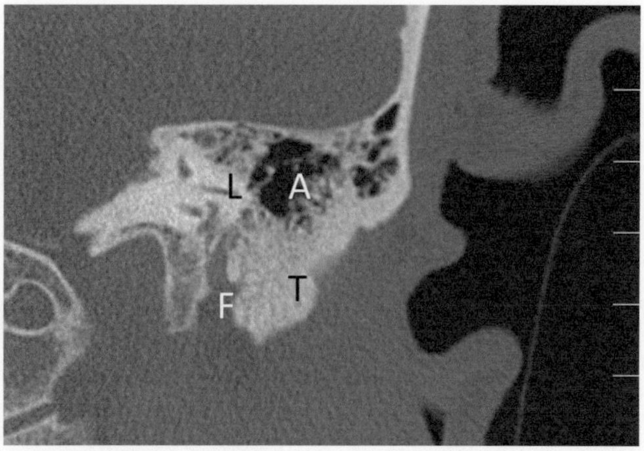

Fig. 45.37 Mastoid compartments seen in the coronal plane—left ear: antrum (A), mastoid tip (T), vertical segment of the facial nerve (F), lateral semicircular canal (L)

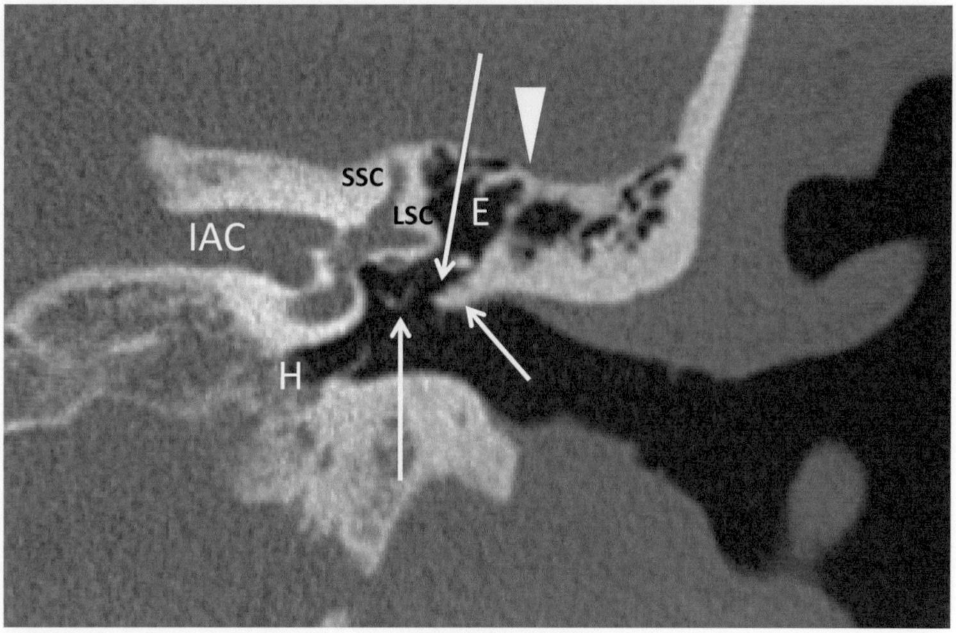

Fig. 45.36 Structures seen in the coronal plane—left ear: epitympanum (E), Prussak's space (long arrow), Bone Spur of Chaussé (short arrow), tegmen (arrowhead), hypotympanum (H), incudostapedial joint with visualization of the stapes in the oval window (middle arrow), superior semicircular canal (SSC), lateral semicircular canal (LSC), and internal auditory canal (IAC)

Magnetic Resonance Imaging

MRI has gained space in medical practice due to its great benefit of better characterization of soft tissues. It is a noninvasive test that is based on the use of nonionizing electromagnetic radiation, where atomic nuclei are exposed to a large magnetic field, absorbing and re-emitting electromagnetic waves at specific frequencies. This wealth of emitted signals generates a lot of information, depending on the sequence used. In the context of intracranial images, radiofrequency waves stimulate hydrogen ions due to their high concentration in biological tissue. The signal is predominantly derived from fat and water, with the fat becoming hyperintense on the T1 sequence and the water on the T2 sequence. Structures that contain calcium or have air inside are hypointense in both T1 and T2 [13–17].

Regarding otitis media, the use of MRI has some more specific indications: neurological symptoms in cases with acute or chronic otitis media, to investigate possible intracranial complications; rule out meningocele when *tegmen timpani* is found with discontinuity on CT; involvement of the petrous apex on CT, allowing differentiation of lesions; and for differential diagnosis with neoplasms, when there is suspicion.

Another very important use of MRI is in cholestetaoma evaluation, specifically in the *non-echoplanar diffusion weighted* (DWI). Temporal bone CT is limited in the evaluation of recidivism in patients undergoing Wall-up tympanomastoidectomy or petrosectomy, and the use of MRI-DWI makes it possible. For this assessment, the test has a sensitivity of 90%, specificity of 100%, positive predictive value of 100%, and negative predictive value of 96%. DWI is based on the rate of water movement in tissue and, in pathological cases, is restricted. Thus, cholesteatoma presents with water restriction in the MRI-DWI [14–17].

It is important to keep in mind how the temporal bone appears on an MRI and to know how to interpret the changes when they are present. Findings should be consistent with the patient's clinic and previous CT scan. Figures 45.38, 45.39, 45.40, 45.41, 45.42, 45.43, 45.44, 45.45, and 45.46 show some findings in MRI. Table 45.5 summarizes MRI findings in chronic otitis media.

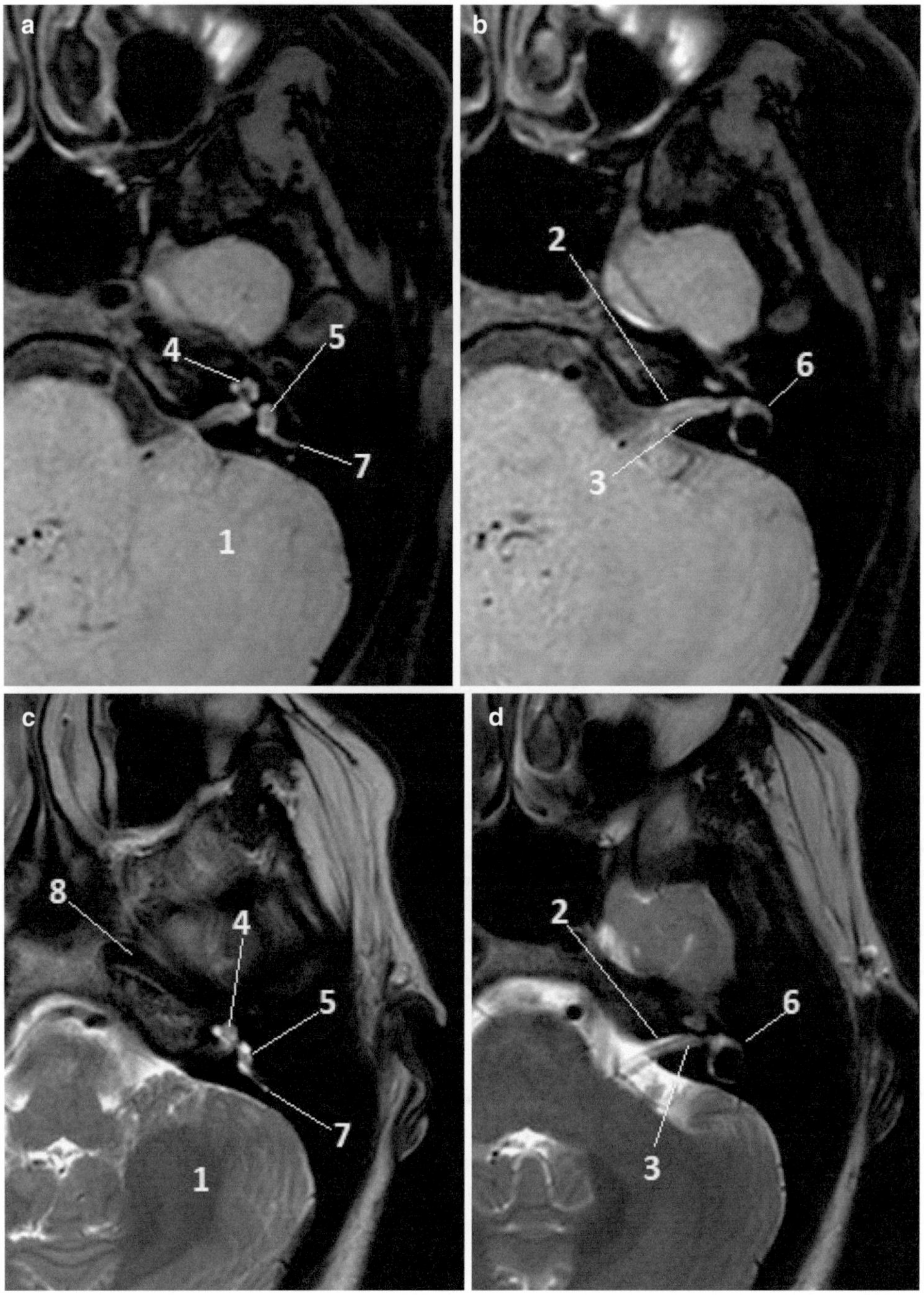

Fig. 45.38 Axial MRI (left ear) without alterations. AB: T1 sequence without contrast. CD: T2 sequence. 1—Cerebellum, 2—cochlear nerve, 3—inferior vestibular nerve, 4—cochlea, 5—vestibule, 6—LSC, 7—PSC and 8—ICA

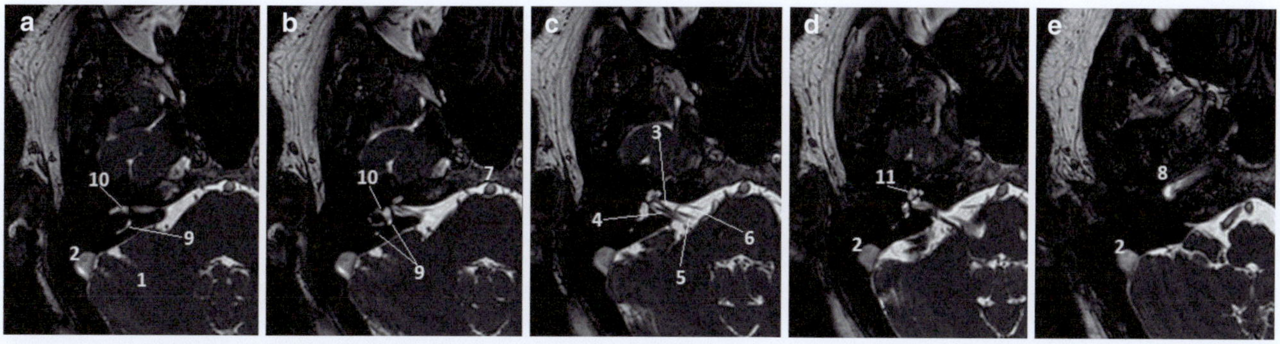

Fig. 45.39 Axial MRI (right ear) without alterations, T2 sequence. 1—Cerebellum, 2—sigmoid sinus, 3—cochlear nerve, 4—inferior vestibular nerve, 5—facial nerve, 6—anteroinferior cerebellar artery (AICA), 7—basilar artery, 8—ICA, 9—PSC, 10—LSC and vestibule, 11—cochlear

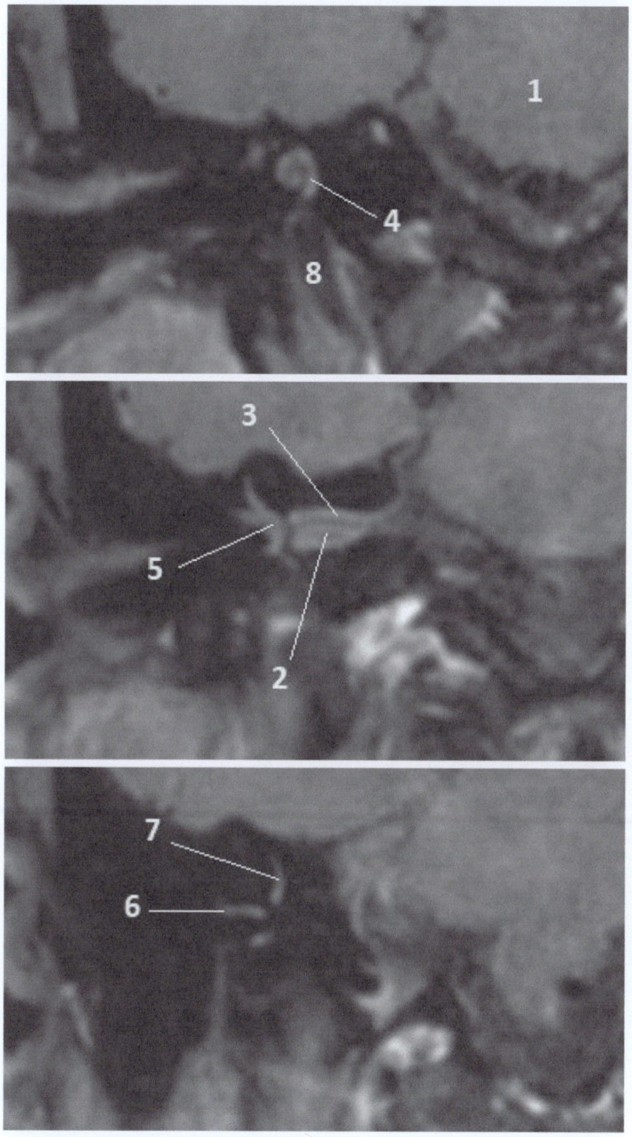

Fig. 45.40 Coronal MRI (normal right ear), T1 sequence without contrast. 1—Brainstem, 2—inferior vestibular nerve, 3—superior vestibular nerve, 4—cochlea, 5—vestibule, 6—LSC, 7—SSC, 8—ICA

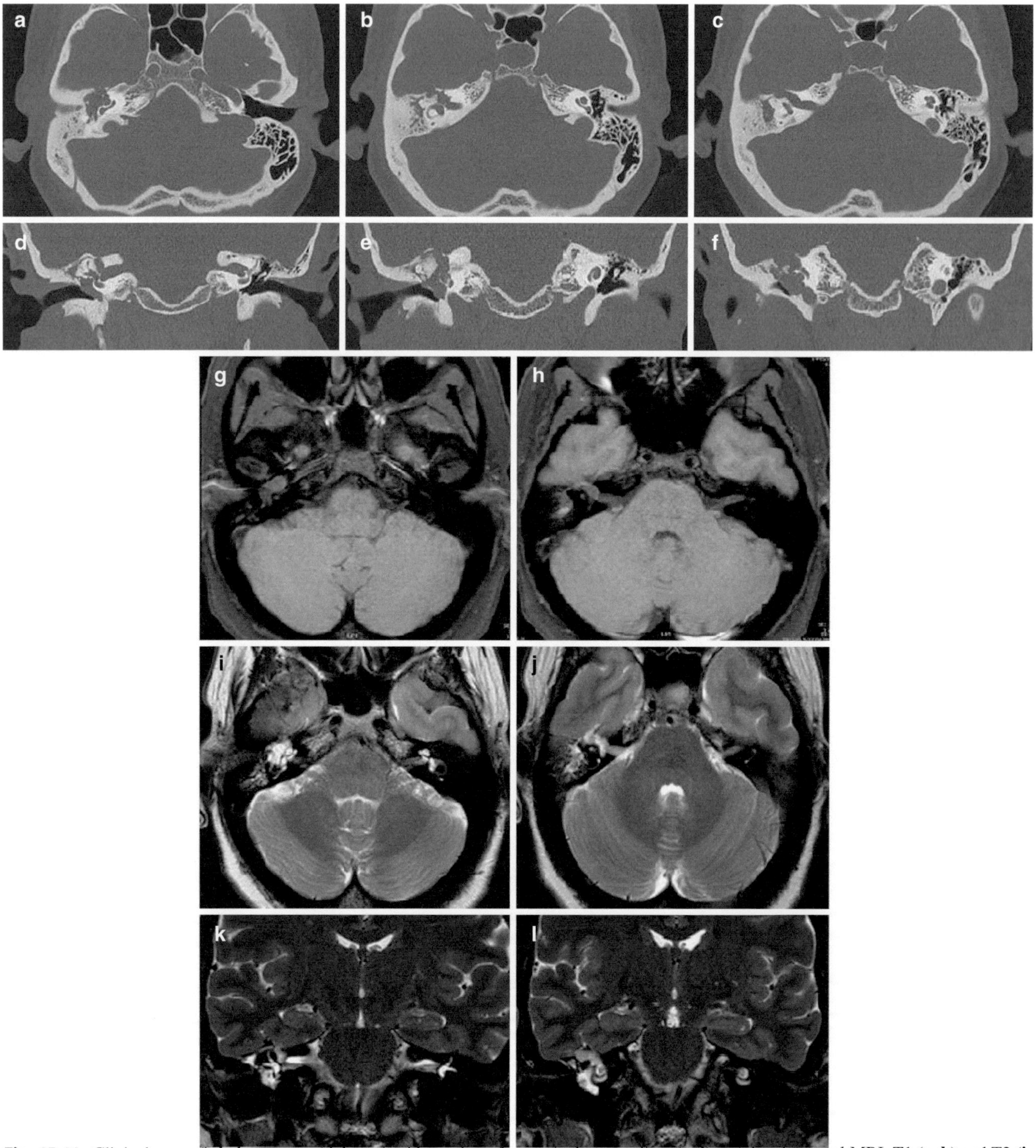

Fig. 45.41 Clinical case of cholesteatoma (right ear) with erosion of the *tegmen timpani*, cochlear fistula, and invasion of the geniculate ganglion. (**a**–**f**): axial and coronal CT sections of the temporal bones, noting cortical bone erosion of the middle fossa, cochlear turns and geniculate ganglion. (**g**, **l**): axial and coronal MRI, T1 (**g**, **h**) and T2 (**i**, **j**, **k**, **l**) sequences, suggesting cholesteatoma (hyposignal on T1 and hypersignal on T2)

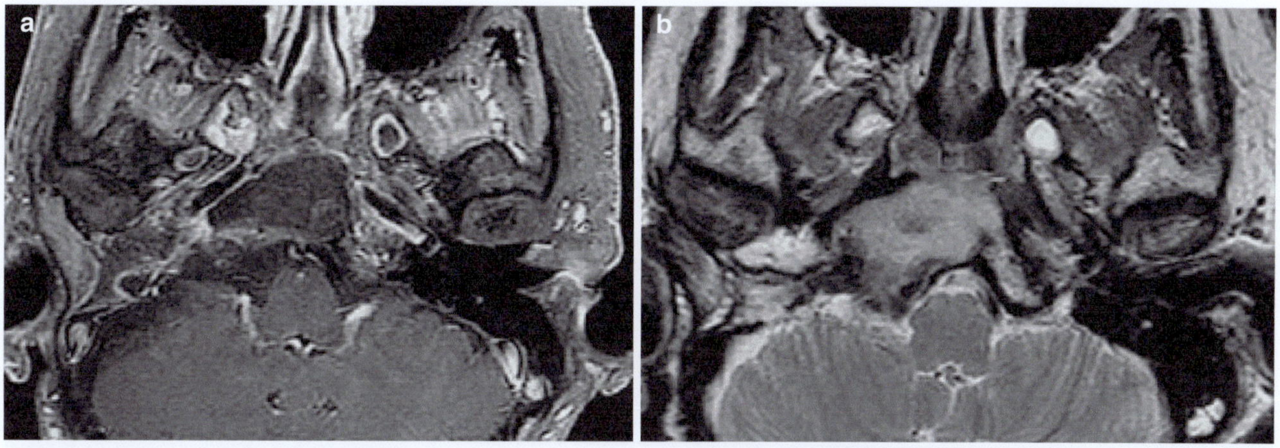

Fig. 45.42 (**a**, **b**) Cholesteatoma in the petrous apex and clivus on the right ear. (**a**) T1 sequence, lesion with hyposignal; (**b**) T2 sequence, lesion with hypersignal

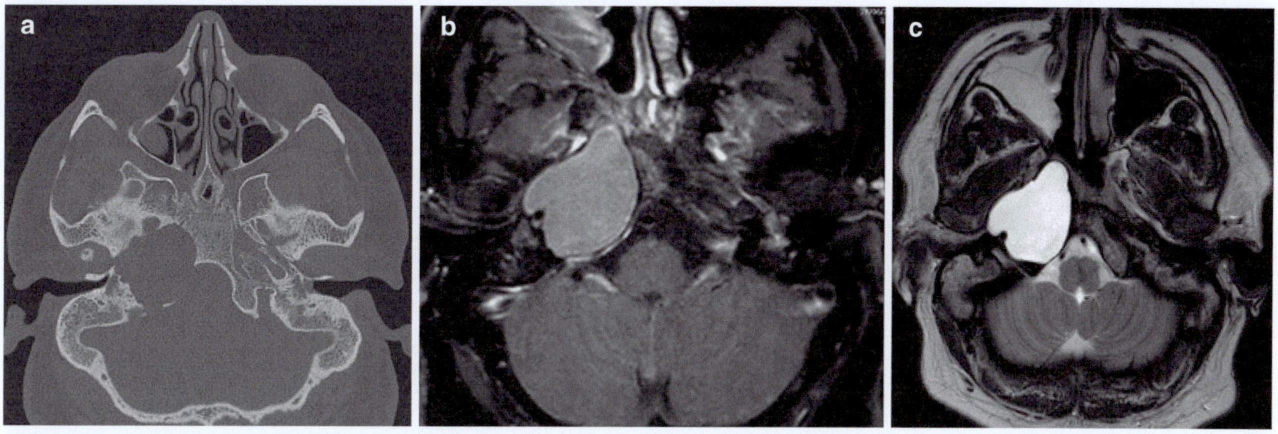

Fig. 45.43 (**a**–**c**) Cholesterol granuloma in the petrous apex on the right extending into the parapharyngeal and retropharyngeal spaces. (**a**) CT temporal bones, axial section. (**b**) Axial MRI, T1-enhanced sequence, with a hyperintense lesion without contrast enhancement. (**b**)—Axial MRI, T2 sequence, hyperintense signal

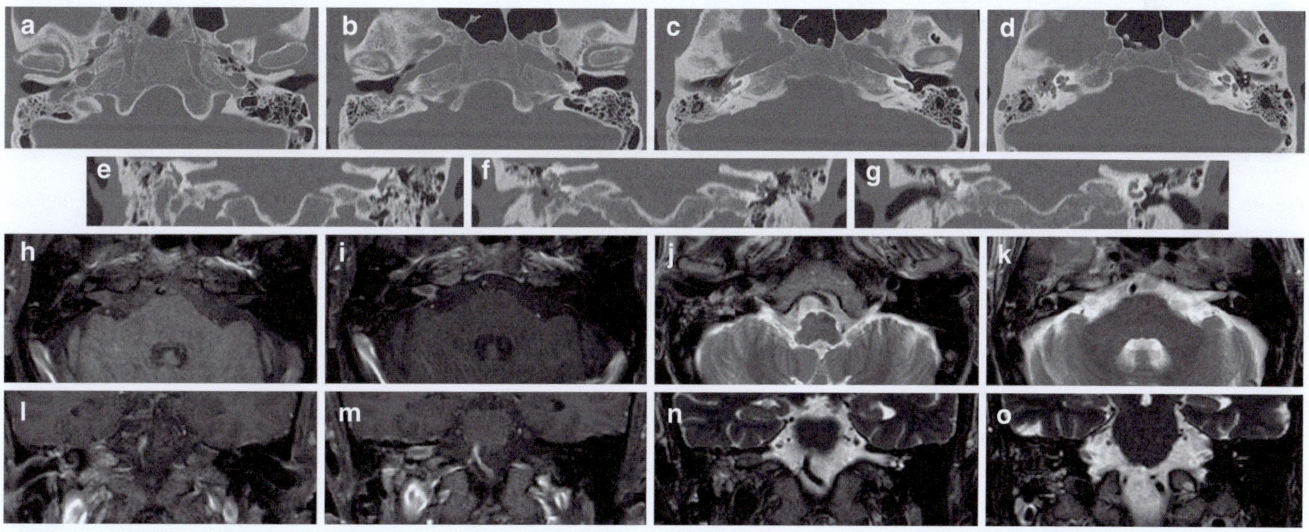

Fig. 45.44 (**a**–**o**) Clinical case of right petrositis due to otitis media complication. (**a**–**g**) CT of temporal bones, axial and coronal sections, there is opacification of the middle ear and petrous apex, in addition to erosion of mastoid cells and the facial canal in its mastoid portion. There is erosion of vestibule, basal turn of the cochlea and in the lateral portion of the ICA. (**h**–**o**) MRI in axial and coronal sections, T1 sequences with contrast (**h**, **i**, **l**, **m**) and T2 (**j**, **k**, **n**, **o**), there are signs of disease extension also to the internal auditory canal

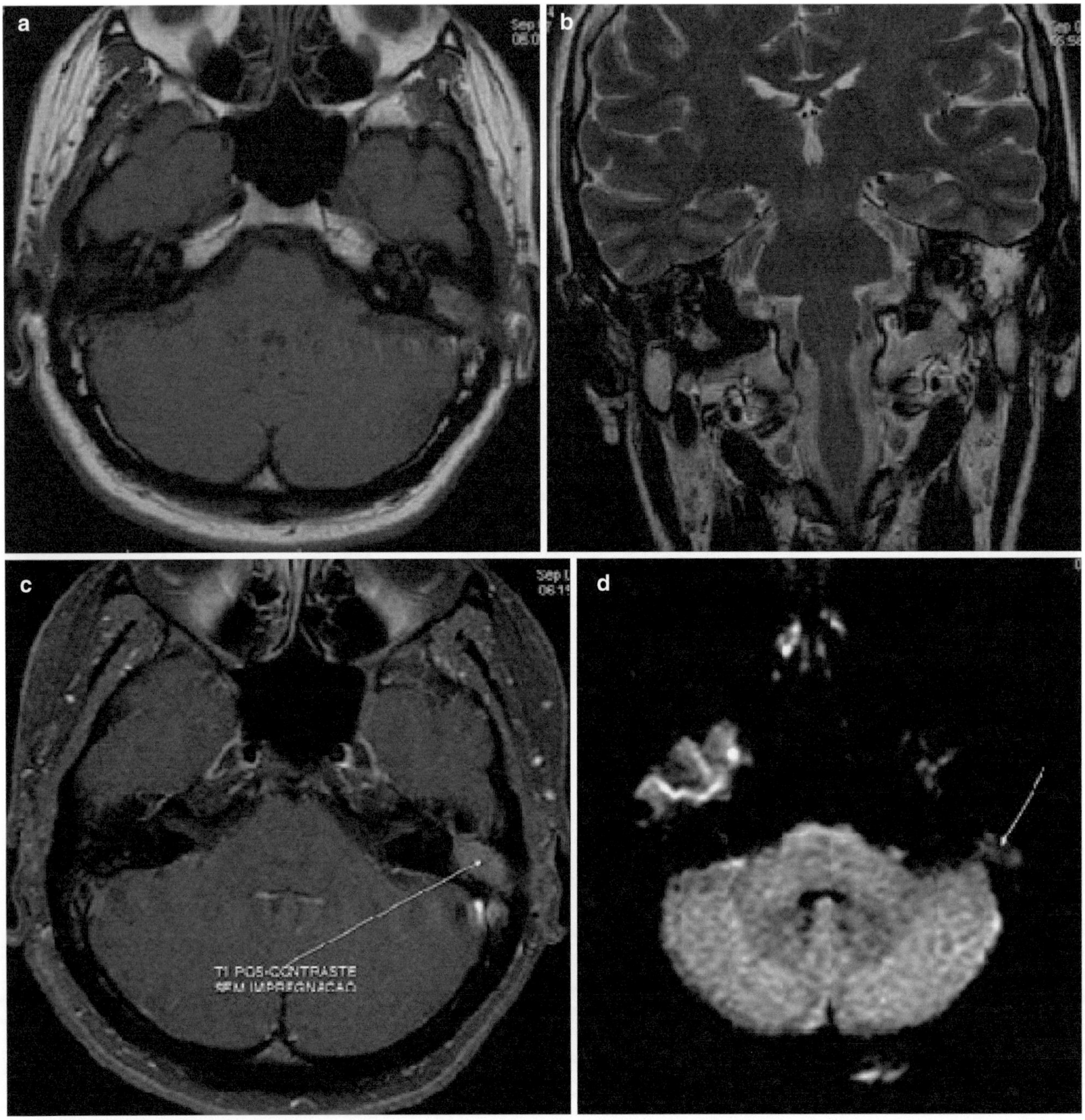

Fig. 45.45 (**a**–**d**) MRI in axial sections, evaluation of residual cholesteatoma after closed left tympanomastoidectomy surgery. (**a**) T1 sequence, hyposignal. (**b**) T2 sequence, hypersignal. (**c**) T1 sequence with contrast, without enhancement. (**d**) Diffusion restriction, indicative of disease recurrence

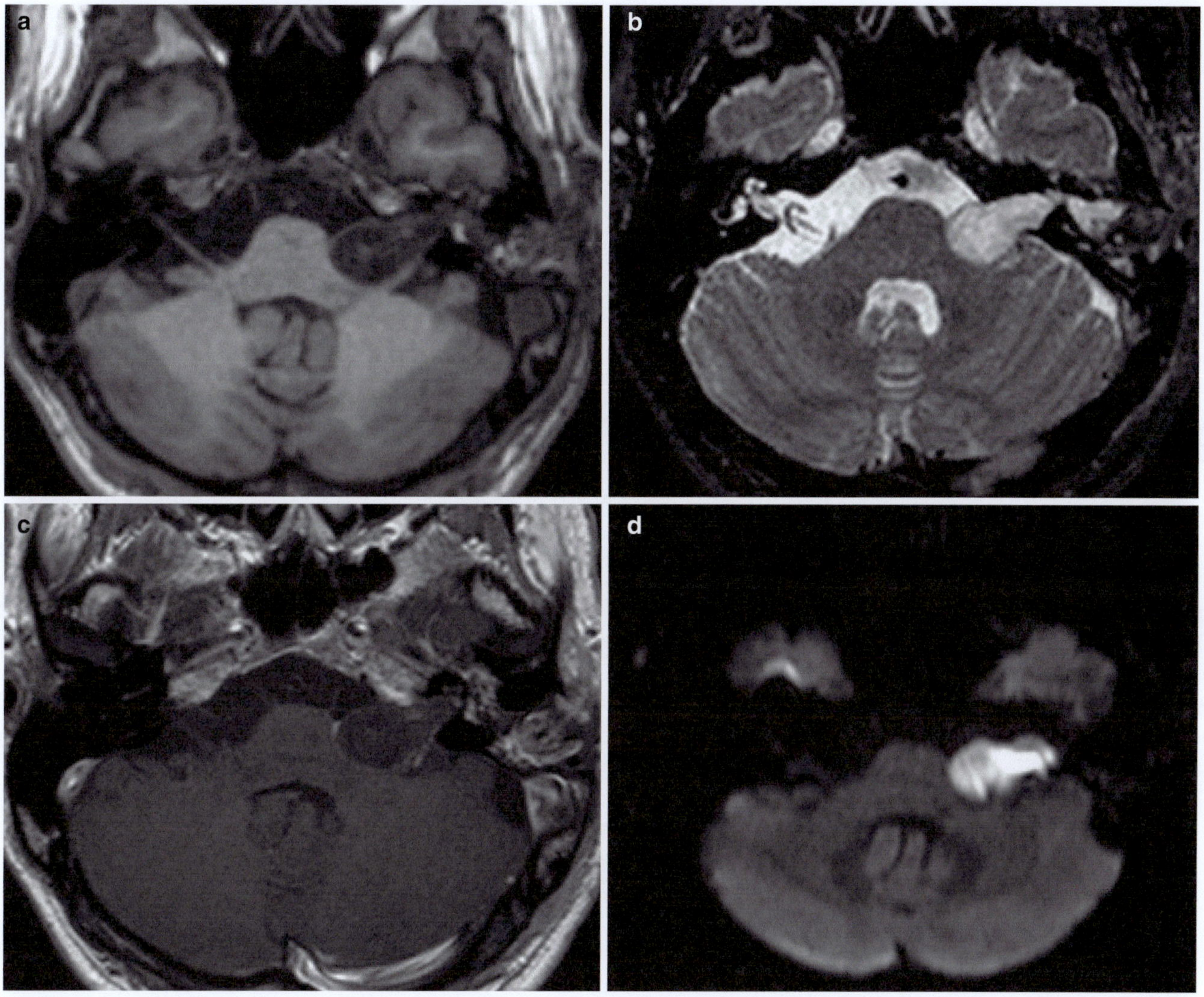

Fig. 45.46 (**a–d**) MRI in axial sections, evaluation of lesion found on CT of temporal bones for differential diagnosis. (**a**) T1 weighted, hyposignal. (**b**) T2 weighted, hypersignal. (**c**) T1 with gd, mild capsule enhancement. (**d**) Diffusion restriction, indicative of cholesteatoma

Table 45.5 Radiologic interpretation on MRI within the spectrum of chronic otitis media

	T1	T2	Post-gadolinium T1	DWI
Cholesteatoma	Hyposignal	Hypersignal	No enhancement	Diffusion restriction
Cholesterol granuloma	Hypersignal	Hypersignal	No enhancement	Without restriction
Effusion	Hyposignal	Hypersignal	No enhancement	Without restriction

Clinical–Radiological Correlation

Medical practice must, imperatively, be guided by a properly collected clinical history and a complete physical examination. The request for additional exams, regardless of whether CT or MRI, should always be guided by prior clinical reasoning, in addition to having the objective of promoting the diagnostic hypothesis. The isolated interpretation of the exam is not advised.

Below, we will present some cases to better elucidate this important correlation in daily practice.

Clinical Case 1

Female patient, 17 years old, with a history of frequent otitis in the left ear for 18 months, in addition to progressive ipsilateral hearing loss. Otoscopy showed marginal tympanic perforation in posterior quadrants with signs suggestive of previous retraction (erosion of the long process of the incus, timpanoestapedopexy (Fig. 45.47a, b), tympanic remnants under the promontory) and normal middle ear mucosa on the left. The tuning fork tests showed Weber lateralizing to the left and Rinne negative to the left. Examination of the right ear showed no particularities. Audiometry showing moderate conductive hearing loss on the left ear (Fig. 45.47c). CT scan of the temporal bones presented a hypopneumatized mastoid, but without opacifications (Fig. 45.47d–i). Besides, it was observed incudostapedial disarticulation and ankylosis of the malleus head.

Clinical Case 2

Male patient, 17 years old, had otorrhea in the right ear for more than 5 years, in addition to progressive ipsilateral hearing loss and tinnitus. The otoscopy showed a cholesteatoma, and it was no longer possible to visualize the ossicular chain. On the left, intact eardrum with retraction in the posterosuperior quadrant (Fig. 45.48a). The tunning fork tests showed Weber lateralizing to the right and Rinne was negative in both ears. Audiometry showed moderate conductive loss on the right and mild on the left (Fig. 45.48c). Temporal bone CT shows a clear difference between the ears (Fig. 45.48d–g). On the right, a hypopneumatized mastoid can be seen, filled with soft tissue content, in addition to extensive erosion of the bone spur of Chaussé and the ossicular chain. On the left, the mastoid is pneumatized and, in the middle ear, a small concentration of soft tissue tissue, associated with a thickened tympanic membrane, is visualized in the topography of the incudostapedial joint.

Clinical Case 3

Male patient, 63 years old reported progressive hearing loss and bilateral tinnitus. Worked for many years in noisy environments without using protective equipment. One year ago, he had a traumatic perforation of the right tympanic membrane. At otoscopy, a wide tympanic perforation in the right ear with clear identification of the ossicular chain, tympanic ostium of the Eustachian tube and round window (Fig. 45.49a, b). On the left, there were no significant changes. Tuning fork tests Weber lateralizing to the right and Rinne was positive in both ears. Audiometry showed moderate mixed hearing loss on the right and a sensorioneural deafness in

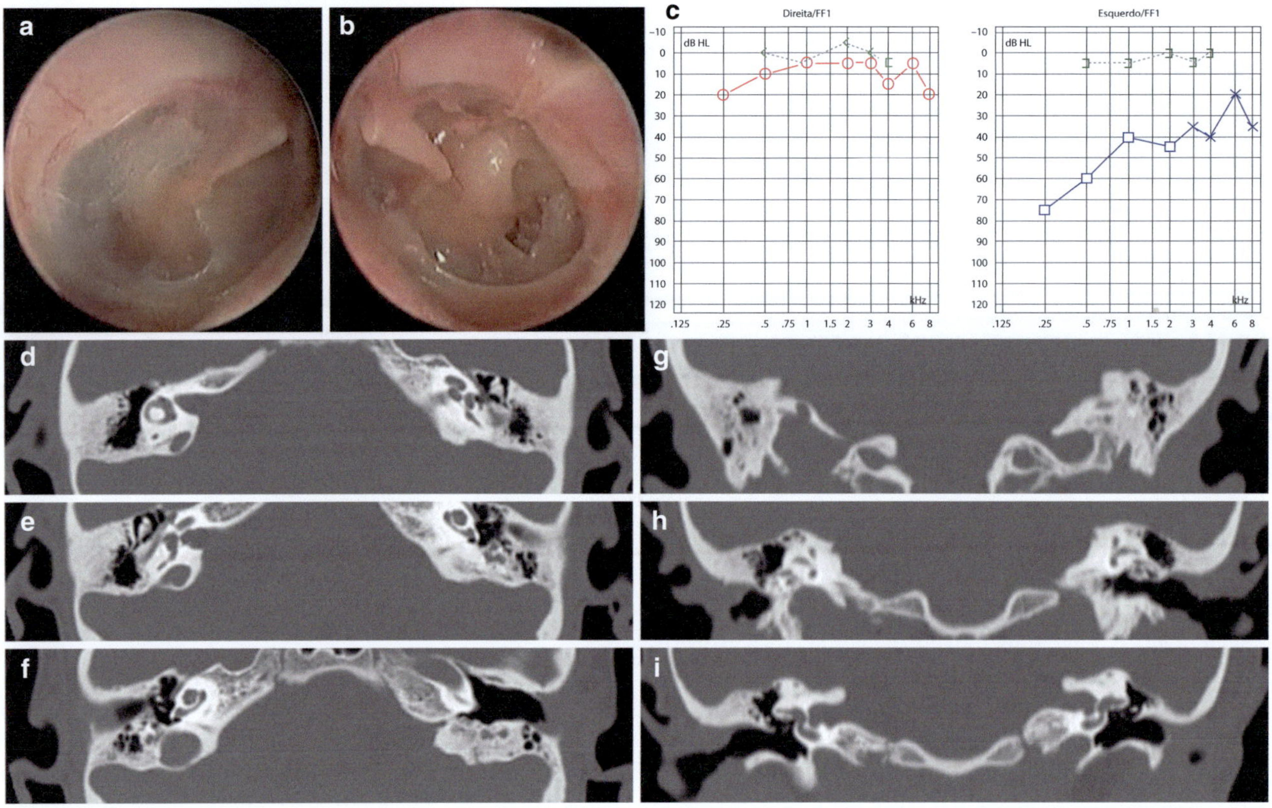

Fig. 45.47 AI: Clinical case 1. (**a**, **b**) otoscopy. (**c**) audiometric exam. (**d**–**f**) CT of temporal bones, axial slices. (**g**–**i**) CT of temporal bones, coronal slices. Ossicular chain discontinuity can be seen in (**e**) and (**i**). Malleus head ankylosis in D

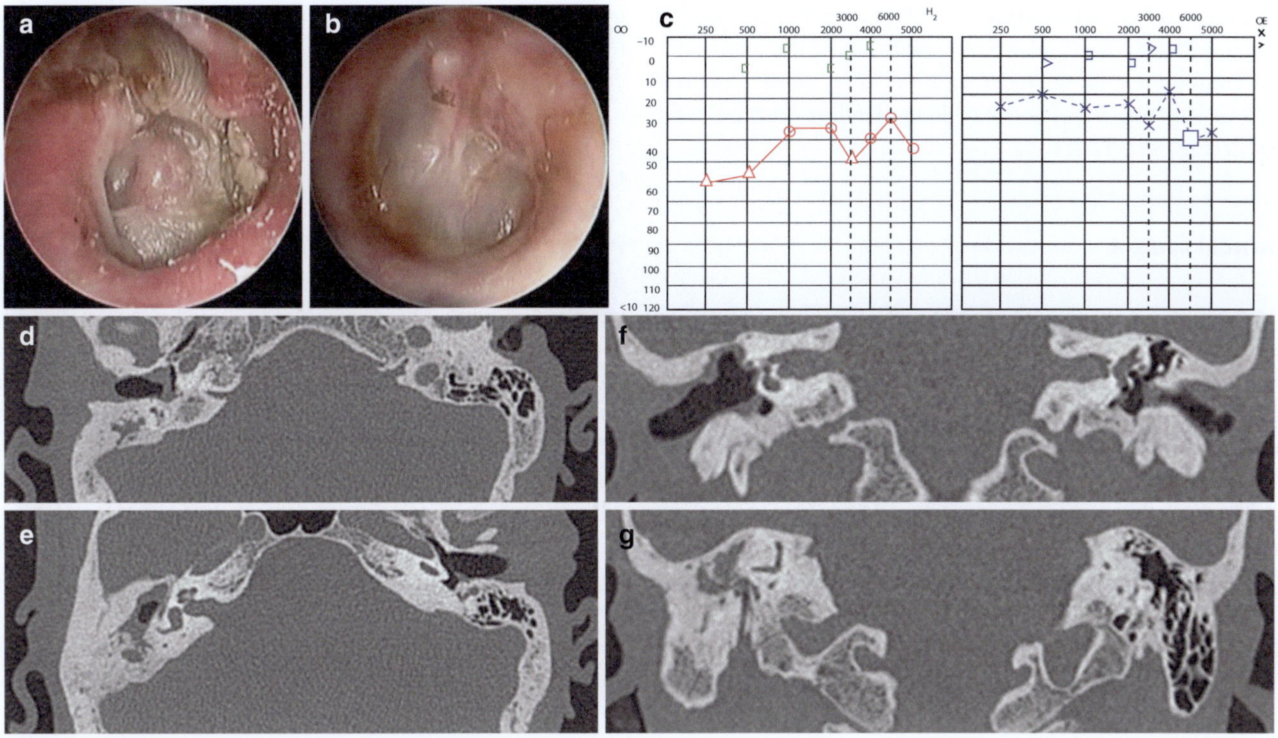

Fig. 45.48 (a–i) Clinical case 2. (a, b) Otoscopy. (c) Audiometric exam. (d, e) CT of temporal bones, axial slices. (f, g) CT of temporal bones, coronal slices. Notably, there is a different pattern of pneumatization between the both mastoids

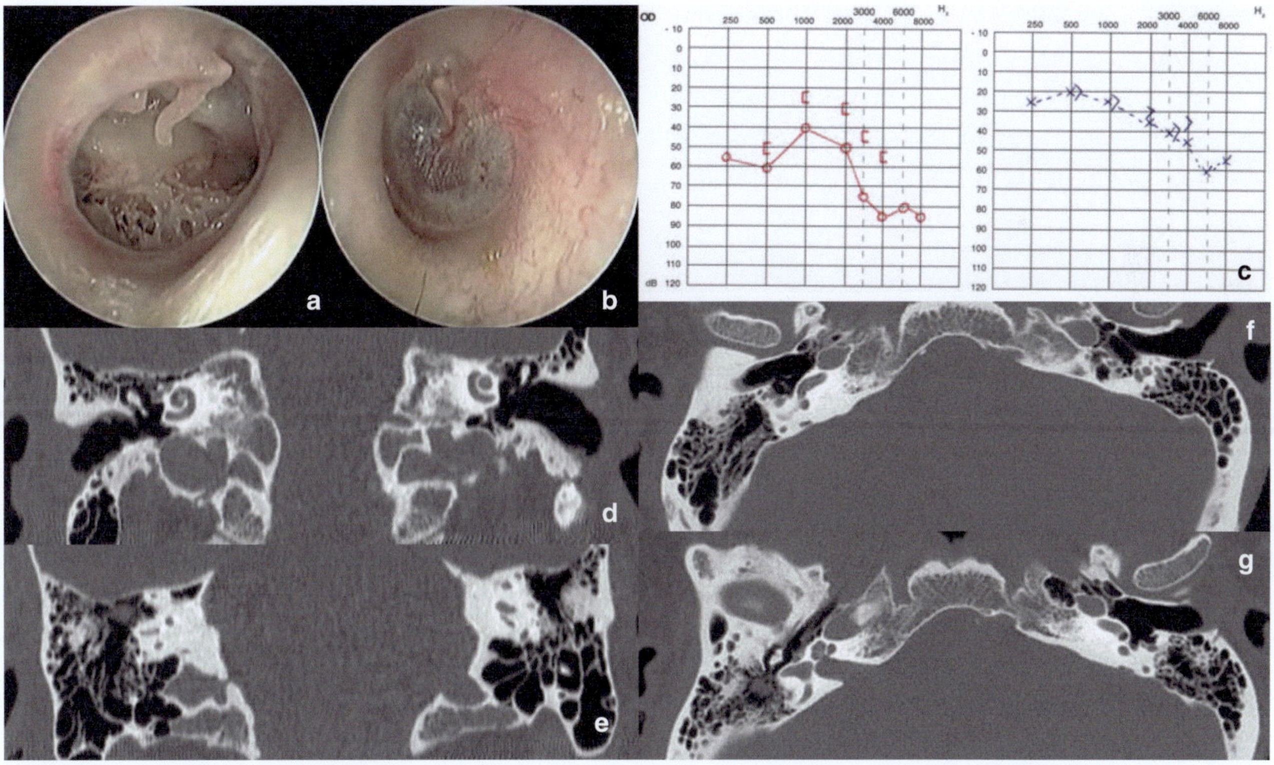

Fig. 45.49 (a–g) Clinical case 3. (a, b) Otoscopy. (c) Audiometric exam. (d, e) CT of temporal bones, coronal slices. (f, g) CT of temporal bones, axial slices. We visualized adequate aeration of the mastoid and middle ear bilaterally, in addition to a preserved ossicular chain

high frequencies on the left (Fig. 45.49c). Temporal bone CT shows adequate mastoid development bilaterally with adequate middle ear aeration, in addition to an intact ossicular chain, indicating the absence of long-standing chronic otitis media (Fig. 45.49d–g).

Clinical Case 4

Male patient, 55 years old, with progressive bilateral hearing loss for more than 20 years, user of individual hearing aid (HA) for 10 years. He reported intermittent otorrhea in both ears, 3–4 episodes a year. The otoscopic examination of the right ear showed significant retraction of the *pars tensa* and medialization of the malleus handle, without attical retraction or epithelial accumulation (Fig. 45.50a, b). On the left, eardrum perforation in the anterior quadrants and amputation of the malleus handle, in addition to slight attical retraction. Audiometry showed bilateral severe mixed hearing loss. CT showed hypopneumatization of the mastoids, in addition to opacification of the mastoids cells and epitympanum, and clear visualization of retractions of the pars tensa in both ears (Fig. 45.50c). The image also suggests ossicular erosion on the left (Fig. 45.50d–i).

Clinical Case 5

Patient, 70 years old, hypertension, and insulin-dependent diabetes. He reported a history of bilateral progressive hearing loss for about 7 years and occasional otorrhea in the right ear during this period. Otoscopy of the right ear revealed an attical cholesteatoma and retraction in the posterosuperior quadrant (Fig. 45.51a, b). On the left, perforation in the posteroinferior quadrant with tympanic remnants on the promontory. Acumetry with tuning fork of 512 Hz, Weber test with sound lateralization to the left and negative Rinne bilaterally. Audiometry showed mild conductive loss on the right and moderate mixed loss on the left (Fig. 45.51c). CT showed mastoid hypopneumatization and opacification, in addition to erosion of the ipsilateral bone spur of Chaussé. On the left, the entire chain can be seen (Fig. 45.51d–g).

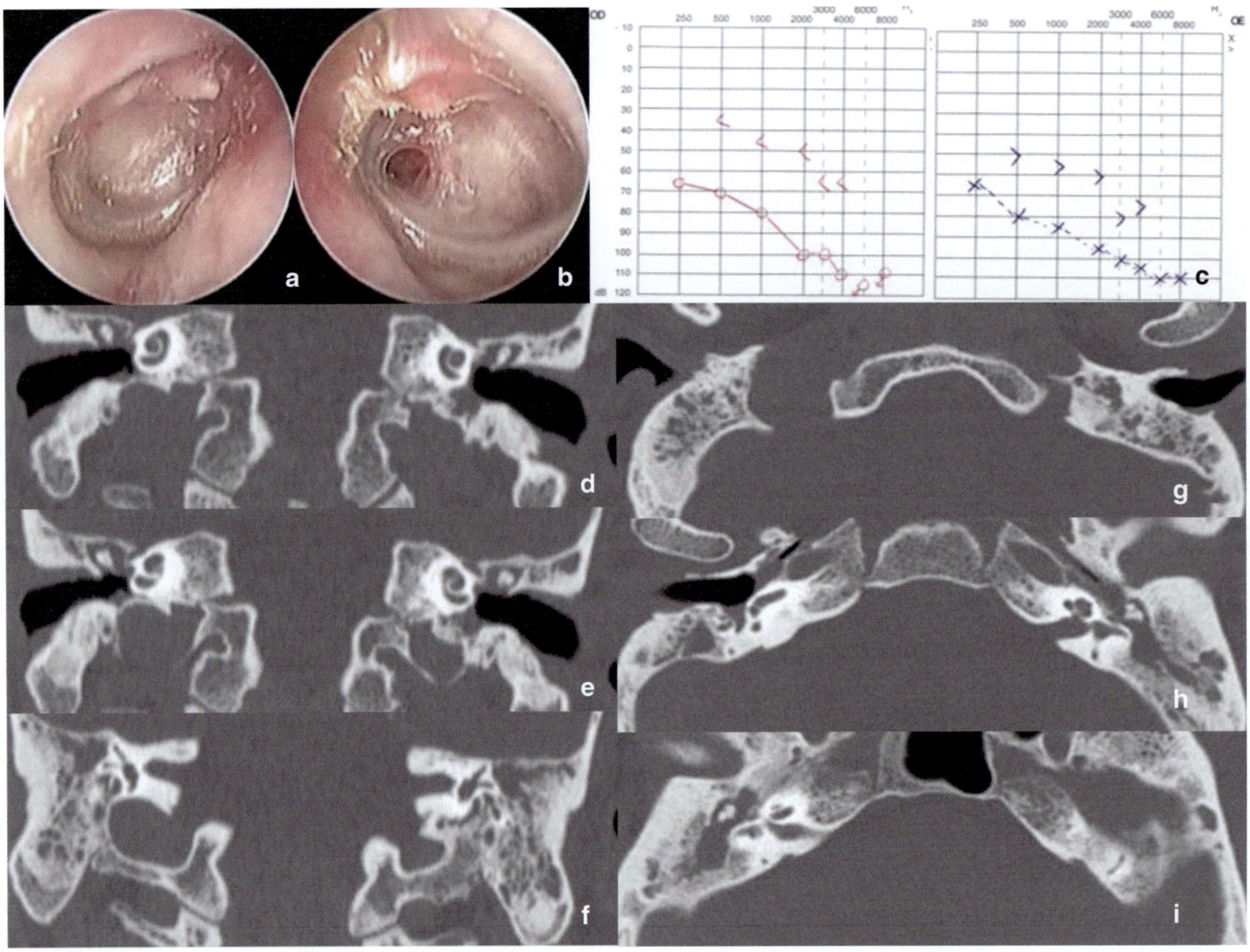

Fig. 45.50 (**a–i**) Clinical case 4. (**a**, **b**) otoscopy. (**c**) audiometric exam. (**d–f**) CT coronal plane. (**g–i**) CT axial plane

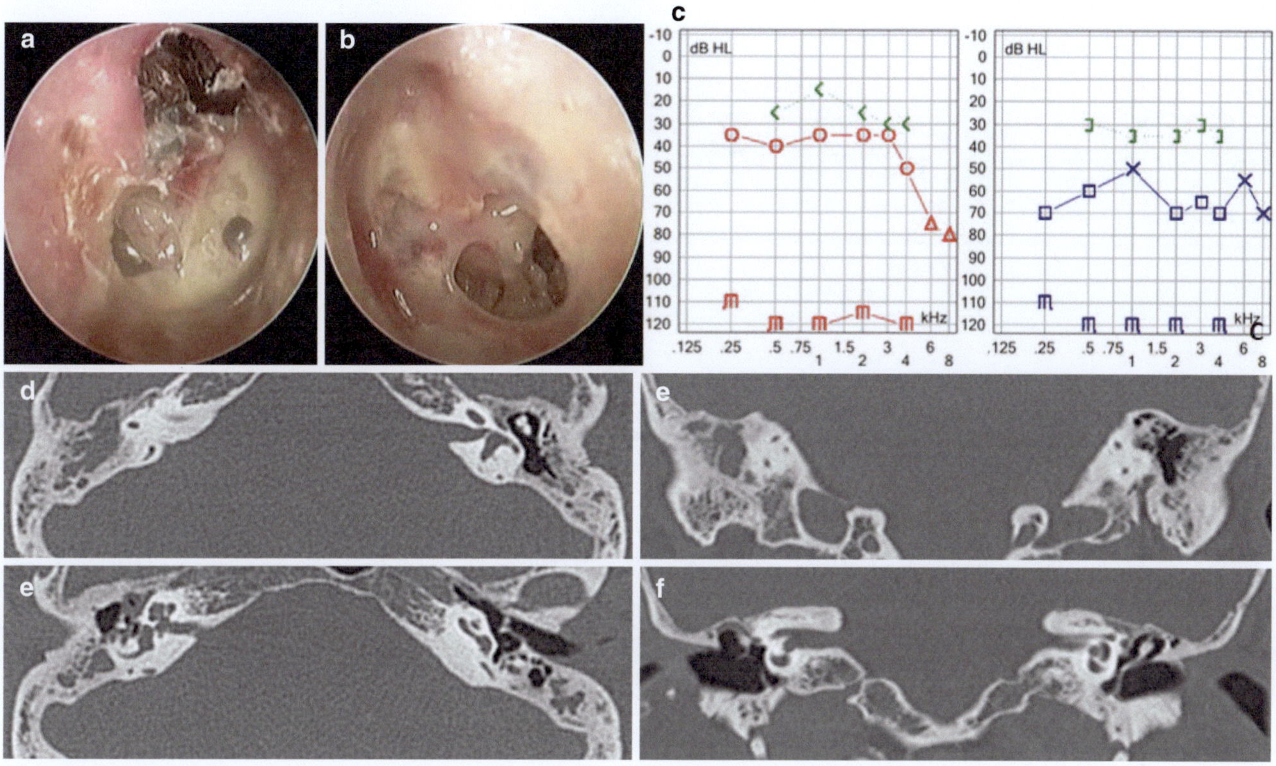

Fig. 45.51 (**a–g**) Clinical case 4. (**a**, **b**) Otoscopy. (**c**) Audiometric exam. (**d**, **e**) CT of temporal bones, axial slices. FG: CT of temporal bones, coronal slices. There is hypopneumatization of the mastoids, but there is a difference in the filling of the mastoid cells and the epitympanum on the right ear. On the left, observe medialization of the malleus handle with possible promontory touch

Final Considerations

Anamnesis and physical examination will always be the starting points in the evaluation of a patient with otitis media. Complementary imaging improves medical assessment and makes more accurate diagnoses. It is essential to have a schematized routine in the evaluation of these exams. In addition, the radiological tests provide more security in surgical approaches.

References

1. Weber AL. History of head and neck radiology: past, present, and future. Radiology. 2001;18:15–24.
2. Valvassori GE. Radiographic atlas of the temporal bone: book II. American Academy of Ophthalmology and Otolaryngology; 1964.
3. Viard A, Eustache F, Segobin S. History of magnetic resonance imaging: a trip down memory lane. Neuroscience. 2021;474:3–13.
4. Rabi II, Zacharias JR, Millman S, Kusch P. A new method of measuring nuclear magnetic moment. Phys Rev. 1938;53:318.
5. Bloch F. Nuclear induction. Phys Rev. 1946;70:460–74.
6. Bloch F, Hansen WW, Packard M. The nuclear induction experiment. Phys Rev. 1946;70:474–85.
7. Purcell EM, Torrey HC, Pound RV. Resonance absorption by nuclear magnetic moments in a solid. Phys Rev. 1946;69:37–8.
8. Young I, Clow H. Britain's brains produce first NMR scans. New Sci. 1978;80(588):b26.
9. Swartz JD, Daniels DL, Hamsberger HR, et al. The Temporal bone. Am J Neuro Radiol. 1996;17:201–4.
10. Lemmerling MM, De Foer B, VandeVyver V, et al. Imaging of the opacified middle ear. Eur Radiol. 2008;66:363–71.
11. Swartz JD. Current imaging approach to the temporal bone. Radiol. 1999;171:309–17.
12. Swartz JD, Harnsberger HR, Mukherji SK. The temporal bone: contemporary diagnostic dilemmas. Radiol Clin N Am. 1998;36:819–53.
13. Yousaf T, Dervenoulas G, Politis M. Advances in MRI methodology. Int Rev Neurobiol. 2018;141:31–76.
14. De Foer B, Vercruysse J-P, Bernaerts A, et al. Detection of postoperative residual cholesteatoma with non-echo-planar diffusion-weighted magnetic resonance imaging. Otol Neurotol. 2008;29(4):513–7.
15. Fruauff K, Coffey K, Chazen JL. Phillips CD Temporal bone imaging. Top Magnetic Resonance Imaging. 2015;24(1):39–55.
16. De Foer B, Vercruysse J-P, Bernaerts A, et al. Middle ear cholesteatoma: non-echo-planar diffusion-weighted MR imagins versus delayed gadolinium-enhanced T1-weighted MR imagins—value in detection. Radiology. 2010;255(3):866–72.
17. Moura MVT, Taranto DOL, Garcia MM. Cholesteatoma: utility of the diffusion sequence without planar echo. Radiol Bras. 2012;45(5):283–7.

Surgical Anatomy of the Middle Ear Cleft and Mastoid

46

Sady Selaimen da Costa, Douglas K. Reinhardt, and Marcela Lehmkuhl Damiani

Introduction

Middle ear surgery requires constant attention to details, as the boundaries between success and failure are delicate. The surgical outcome results from a series of steps to be aware of during the pre, intra, and postoperative periods. The operative technique does not represent any magical gift or a "congenital inheritance" in a talented surgeon, nevertheless, the result of a long and demanding period of theoretical and practical training.

Five basic principles guide the surgeon's operative improvement: (1) a solid theoretical basis of the pathology; (2) profound anatomical knowledge; (3) constant training in dissection laboratories; (4) close observation of more experienced surgeons; and (5) up-to-date and continuing medical education.

Middle Ear Surgery

The dimensions of the middle ear are inversely proportional to the delicacy of its structures (tympanic membrane, ossicular chain, windows, and facial nerve), as well as to the importance of the surrounding organs (labyrinth, internal carotid artery, lateral sinus, jugular gulf, and middle and posterior cerebral fossa). Thus, maximized attention to care in the operative field is imperative.

It is essential to obtain a wide operative field with excellent exposure. Therefore, the selection of an appropriate access route for the magnitude of the proposed procedure and the achievement of effective hemostasis are essential.

There are three main access routes to the middle ear: transcanal, endaural, and retroauricular. The option for one or the other will depend on the analysis of a whole set of characteristics related to the type, location, and extent of the pathological process and a series of particularities specific to the patient, surgeon, and the infrastructure of the place of care. In summary, the approach to the middle ear should always be individualized (Chart 46.1).

Chart 46.1 Determining the Surgical Technique

1. **Factors related to the pathological process**
   - Type, degree, and extent of the pathology
   - Hearing loss
   - Associated complications
2. **Patient-related factors**
   - Contralateral ear
   - General state
   - Age
   - Origin
   - Profession
3. **Factors related to surgery**
   - Surgeon's experience
   - Surgical center infrastructure and available materials

Furthermore, the postoperative result should also be guided by well-defined objectives, also individualized for each patient and sometimes evaluated intraoperatively: identification and treatment of the pathology, obtaining a dry and safe ear, and, if possible, auditory gain [1, 2].

It is clear that, in parallel with the traditional anatomical study, it is necessary for us to have well-established concepts in surgical and pathological anatomy, since the criteria for accessibility and resectability of a lesion come from the analysis of a whole set of characteristics specific to the disease itself, to the extent of their involvement and the general conditions of the patient [3–6]. In other words, the anatomical

S. S. da Costa (✉)
Department of Otolaryngology, Head & Neck Surgery, School of Medicine, Universidade Federal do Rio Grande do Sul, Porto Alegre, Brazil

D. K. Reinhardt
Hospital São Lucas da PUCRS, Porto Alegre, Brazil

M. L. Damiani
Hospital de Clínicas de Porto Alegre, Porto Alegre, Brazil

M. V. Goycoolea et al. (eds.), *Textbook of Otitis Media*, https://doi.org/10.1007/978-3-031-40949-3_46

study must be expanded and adapted to the surgeon's needs, clearly establishing the dividing marks between the feasible and the impossible [7, 8]. This pragmatic approach, characteristic of surgical anatomy, involves the elaboration of a rational operative strategy that will include the recognition of several anatomical repairs from the surface to the deepest planes [4, 9]. These structures, henceforth referred to as "landmarks," must be accessed and identified sequentially, indicating precisely and safely the paths to be followed until our main objective is achieved [3, 10].

Approaching the middle ear can be structured in different ways based on these landmarks, however, always attending common characteristics:

- Surgical accessibility;
- Easy identification;
- Sequential anatomical position: lateromedially in lateral accesses and craniocaudally in accesses via the middle fossa;
- Resistance to distortions caused by pathological processes;
- Location at different levels of the temporal bone.

The objective of this chapter is to describe the surgical anatomical landmarks in the middle ear and mastoid. Thus, in the following Tables 46.1, 46.2, 46.3, 46.4, 46.5, 46.6, 46.7, and 46.8 and Figs. 46.1, 46.2, 46.3, 46.4, 46.5, 46.6, 46.7, and 46.8, we will describe a set of references at different levels of the temporal region. Regardless of the access chosen, several of these landmarks, if not all, must be rigorously observed throughout the dissection, from the superficial to the deepest planes.

Table 46.1 Level I landmarks—superficial

Helix	• Posterior limit of type II Lempert incision • Provides the contour of the auricular pavilion and must not have its cartilage violated
External auditory meatus (EAM)	• EAC external opening whose diameter and malleability should be considered when choosing the access
Concha of auricle	• The only cartilage that can be violated in the endaural (Koerner flap) and retroauricular (meatoplasty) approaches • Its remodeling is mandatory in open mastoidectomy (meatoplasty)
Tragus	• Anterior limit of Lempert type II incision • Cartilage donor site for reconstructions
Anterior notch	• Groove between helix (posteriorly) and tragus (anteriorly) • Type II Lempert incision site • Reference for removal of fascia in endaural access
Ear lobe	• Useful for harvesting fat for window plugging
Retroauricular line	• Retroauricular incision site
Mastoid process	• Temporal bone inferior limit • Protects the facial nerve, medially • Underdeveloped in children: risk of facial nerve injury in the stylomastoid foramen
Hairline	• Superficial projection of linea temporalis and middle cranial fossa

Table 46.2 Level II landmarks—subcutaneous level

Posterior border of EAM	• Identification of the posterior border of the EAM in the retroauricular approach.
Mastoid periosteum	• Used as a pedicled flap in the obliteration of open cavities. • Used as free graft • Anchoring of self-static retractors
Temporalis muscle and fascia	• Temporal scale reference. • Site for graft harvesting
Linea temporalis	• Upper limit of the dissection indicating the position of the dura mater in the middle fossa.

Table 46.3 Level III landmarks—subperiosteal

Linea temporalis	• Upper limit of the dissection indicating the position of the dura mater in the middle fossa
Henle's spine	• Constant reference point in the retroauricular approach. • Classically used as a projection on the surface of the antrum
Cribriform area and Macewen's triangle	• Particularly in children, this set of small foramina can function as a drainage route for purulent secretions from the mastoid to the sub-periosteal space. • Lateral limit of the mastoid cavity
Posterior wall of external auditory canal (EAC)	• Anterior limit of closed mastoidectomy. • Also used as a projection of the position of the antrum on the surface
Mastoid process	• Insertion point of the sternocleidomastoid muscle. • Inferior reference of dissection during mastoidectomy
Mastoid foramen	• Vascular foramen through which the emissary vein travels to the lateral sinus and the mastoid branch of the occipital artery. • Bleeding site during wide exposure of the mastoid in otoneurological procedures

Table 46.4 Level IV landmarks—meatus

Tympanosquamous suture	• Between the tympanic bone and temporal squama. • Anterior limit of the vascular area • Area of difficult dissection of the flap
Tympanomastoid suture	• Between the tympanic bone and the mastoid around 1 o' clock. Posterior limit of the vascular area. • Area of difficult dissection of the flap • Serves as a channel for Arnold's nerve (branch of the vagus nerve) • Route of spread of infections from the external auditory canal to the base of the skull (malignant external otitis)
Vascular strip area	• Densest skin area of the EAC between 11 o' clock and 1 o' clock • Vascular supply of the EAM
Anterior EAC wall	• Frequent bony bulging and posterior limit of the temporomandibular joint
Tympanic annulus	• Point of insertion of the tympanic membrane into the tympanic sulcus. Absent between the 11 o' clock and 1 o' clock positions. • Its identification is fundamental in the elevation of the tympanomeatal flap, preserving the tympanic integrity
Tympanic membrane—*pars tensa*	• Middle ear window to the outside, laterally limiting the mesotympanic region. • Site of focal or diffuse retractions, central and marginal perforations (which may progress to secondary cholesteatomas). • Site of primary cholesteatomas (posterosuperior)
Tympanic membrane—*pars flaccida*	• Lateral limit of Prussak's space being a legitimate mirror of intratympanic pressure variations. • Site of primary (attic) cholesteatomas
Incisura rivini	• Also known as the *incisura tympanica*, it represents a natural dehiscence of the tympanic bone. • An important point of reference during elevation of the tympanomeatal flap, as in its posterior portion the tympanic ring can be easily identified leaving the tympanic sulcus

Table 46.5 Level V landmarks—superficial mastoid

Posterior wall of EAC	• Anterior limit of closed mastoidectomy
Tegmen tympani and dura mater of middle cranial fossa	• Upper limit of mastoidectomy • Frequent site of bone erosions
Lateral sinus	• Posterior limit of mastoidectomy • Important in otoneurological approaches
Citelli's angle	• Acute angle formed between the dura mater (superiorly) and the lateral sinus (posteriorly) • Key reference in translabyrinthine access to the internal auditory canal
Root of zygoma	• Anterior extension of tegmen tympani • Anterolateral boundary of the epitympanum
Koerner's septum	• Limit of mastoid pneumatization proceeding from the superior sac (squamous) and the middle sac (petrosa) • Also known as the petrosquamous lamina or false antrum. • Landmark on the posterior approach to the antrum
Mastoid process	• Insertion point of the sternocleidomastoid muscle. • Inferior pole of dissection during mastoidectomy

Table 46.6 Level VI landmarks—deep mastoid

Posterior wall of EAC	• Anterior limit of closed mastoidectomy frequent site of bone erosions
Tegmen timpani and dura mater of middle cranial fossa	• Upper limit of mastoidectomy • Frequent site of bone erosions
Lateral sinus	• Posterior limit of mastoidectomy • Important in otoneurological approaches
Citelli's angle	• Acute angle formed between the dura mater of the middle fossa (superiorly) and the lateral sinus (posteriorly) • Key reference in translabyrinthine access to the internal auditory canal
Mastoid antrum	• Large mastoid cell, the most constant and the only one present since birth. • Site of infection and abscess formation by direct contiguity in acute otitis media
Lateral semicircular canal	• Medial limit of mastoidectomy • Key structure for the location of the second genu of the facial nerve (inferomedially) and incudal fossa (anteriorly). • Frequent site of perilymphatic fistula due to bone erosion
Posterior semicircular canal	• Anteromedial limit of the lateral sinus • Reference in retrolabyrinthine approaches to the internal auditory canal • Reference to the endolymphatic sac • Next to the lateral channel, they make up the so-called solid angle
Trautmann's triangle	• Triangle bounded by posterior semicircular canal, tegmen tympani, and lateral sinus • Along with Donaldson's line (perpendicular to the posterior canal) they are fundamental in identifying the endolymphatic sac
Incudal fossa and incus short process	• Refer anteriorly to the epitympanum and incudo-malleolar joint • The short process of the incus points to the facial recess
Cog	• Bony spike extending from tegmen tympani anterior to malleus head. • Boundary between the anterior and posterior epitympanum. • Landmark in locating the most proximal portion of the tympanic segment of the facial nerve
Digastric ridge	• Origin of the digastric muscle • Internally in the mastoid, it presents its anterior limit in the stylomastoid foramen, being an extremely useful reference point in the most caudal location of the vertical facial segment

Table 46.7 Level VII landmarks—closed mastoidectomy (facial recess)

Posterior wall of EAC	• Lateral bony boundary of the facial recess
Lateral semicircular canal	• Posterosuperior reference of the second genu of the facial nerve
Facial nerve—mastoid (vertical) segment	• Medial limit of the facial recess
Chorda tympani nerve	• Along with the posterior wall of the EAC, it represents the lateral boundary of the facial recess. • Must be repaired during manipulation of the incudo-stapedial joint
Incudal fossa and incus short process	• Incudal fossa: between the end of the short process of the incus and lateral to the facial nerve • Upper limit of the facial recess
Piramidal eminence	• Stapedius muscle tendon emergence point. • Represents the floor of the facial recess and the roof of the tympanic sinus
Stapes	• Smallest and most delicate bone in the human body. • Housed in the niche of the oval window, it inferiorly limits the tympanic segment of the facial nerve, which may be dehiscent

Table 46.8 Level VIII landmarks—open mastoidectomy

Cochleariform process	• Constant anatomical reference located at the midpoint of the middle ear between the meso and epitympanum. • Anterior limit of the tympanic segment of the facial nerve
Facial nerve—tympanic (horizontal) segment	• Situated in an often dehiscent bony canal • Bordered anteriorly by the cochleariform process, posteroinferiorly by the stapes, and superiorly by the lateral semicircular canal
Aditus AD antrum	• Small triangular passageway between the attic anteriorly and the antrum posteriorly • Mastoid aeration channel whose patency is vital for the homeostasis of the cell complex
Mastoid antrum	• Large mastoid cell, more constant, and the only one present since birth. • Site of infection and abscess formation by contiguity in acute otitis media
Lateral semicircular canal	• Medial limit of mastoidectomy • Key structure for the location of the second genu of the facial nerve (inferomedially) and incudal fossa (anteriorly). • Frequent site of perilymphatic fistula due to bone erosion
Facial nerve—second genu	• Located inferior to the lateral canal • Transition between the tympanic (horizontal) and mastoid (vertical) segments of the facial nerve • Segment of the facial nerve most frequently injured in approaches to the middle ear
Facial nerve—mastoid (vertical) segment	• Segment extending superiorly from the knee to the stylomastoid foramen • Bounds in the open cavities the meso and hypotympanum (anteriorly) and the mastoid cavity (posteriorly) • It must be sufficiently recessed in open cavities, allowing perfect epithelialization and self-cleaning capacity of the cavity
Piramidal eminence and stapedius muscle	• Essential in locating the stapes and cleaning the facial recess region
Stapes and oval window	• Constant site of inflammatory pathologies that involve and destroy the stapes superstructure (cholesteatomas/ inflammatory tissue)
Round window	• Opening of the scala tympani in the middle ear • Main transfer route of inflammatory pathology between middle/inner ear compartments
Hipotympanum	• The lower floor of the middle ear, limited laterally by the tympanic bone and inferiorly by a thin, and sometimes dehiscent, bony lamina and by the jugular gulf
Protympanum and auditory tube opening	• Most anterior region of the mesotympanum and common site of obstruction to the auditory cleft aeration routes • Lateral relationship of the vertical segment of the bone canal (sometimes dehiscent) through which the intrapetrous carotid artery passes • Middle ear contamination channel from the rhinopharynx
Tensor tympani muscle semicanal	• Middle ear protrusion, anterior to the cochleariform process. Floor of the anterior epitympanum which is separated from the rest of the tympanic cavity by a fold of mucous in 90% of the time
Cog	• Bony spike extending from tegmen tympani anterior to malleus head. • Boundary between the anterior and posterior epitympanum. • Landmark in locating the most proximal portion of the tympanic segment of the facial nerve
Epitympanum (attical region)	• Upper floor of the middle ear bounded laterally by the scutum. • Houses the incudo-malleolar joint
Anterior epitympanum	• Anterior to the malleus head and cog and separated from the anterior mesotympanum by the fold of the tensor tympani muscle • Frequent site of residual cholesteatoma
Mastoid cavity	• Cell complex with an average volume of 12 cm^3. • It must be completely exantered in the presence of gross pathologies. • Usually poorly pneumatized (sclerotic) in chronically infected ears

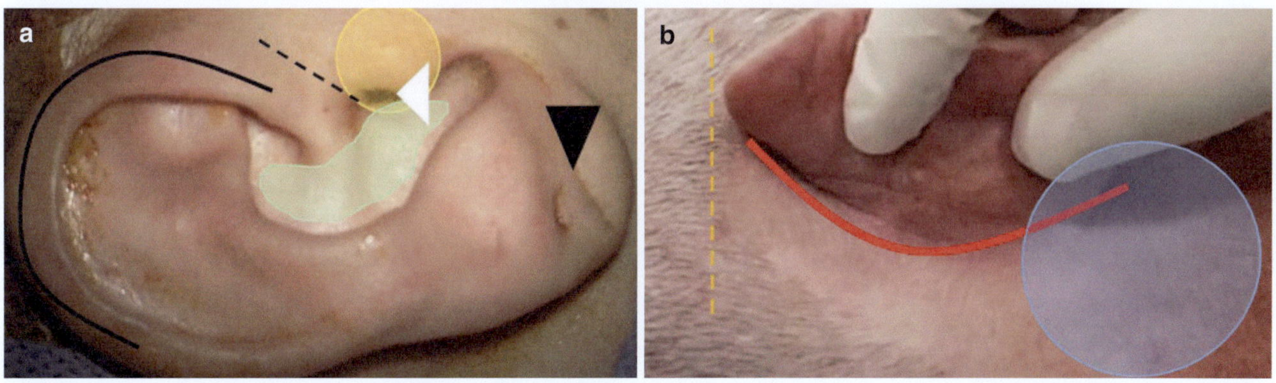

Fig. 46.1 Level I landmarks—superficial. (**a**) Helix (continuous black line); EAM (white arrowhead); concha (green hatching); tragus (yellow hatched); anterior notch (black dashed line); lobe (black arrowhead); (**b**) retroauricular notch (solid red line); mastoid process (blue dot); hairline (dashed orange line)

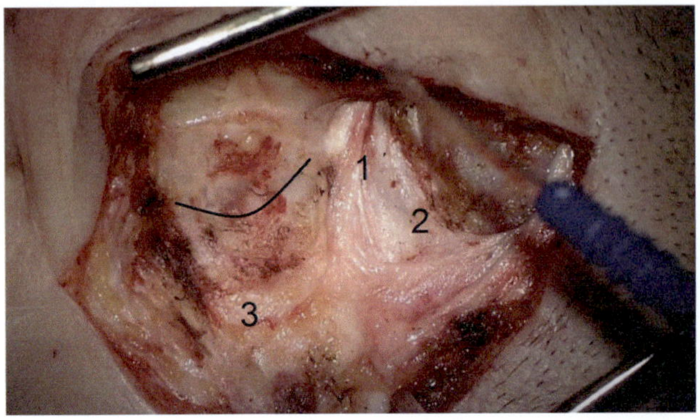

Fig. 46.2 Level II landmarks—subcutaneous level. Left ear: Posterior border of EAM (curved line); temporalis line (1), temporalis muscle and fascia—partially removed (2), mastoid periosteum (3)

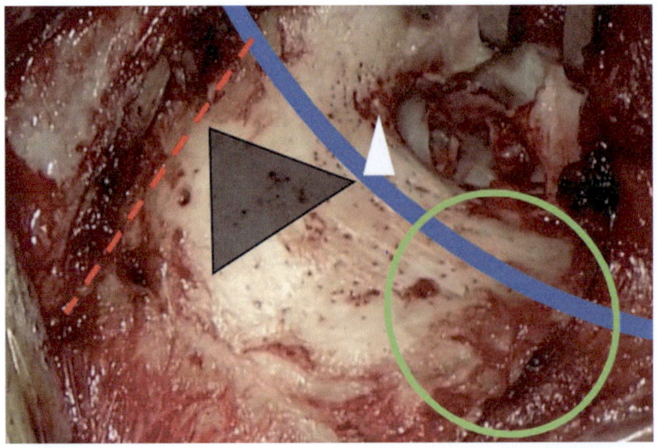

Fig. 46.3 Level III landmarks—subperiosteal. Temporalis line (red dashed line); Spine of Henle (white arrowhead); cribriform area and Macewen's triangle (black arrowhead); EAC posterior wall (solid blue line); mastoid process (green circle)

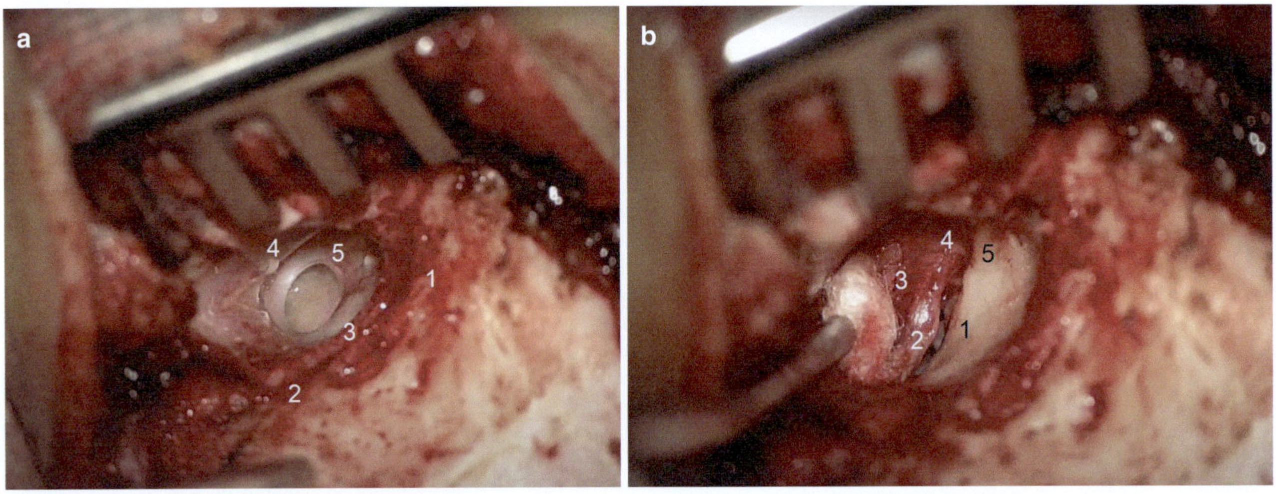

Fig. 46.4 (**a**) Level IV landmarks—meatus. Left ear: tympanosquamous suture (1); tympanic-mastoid suture (2), vascular band (3), anterior edge of EAC (4), perforated tympanic membrane (5). (**b**) Level IV landmarks—meatus. Left ear: tympanic ring (1); annular ligament (2), pars tensa (3), pars flaccida (4), Rivinus' notch (5)

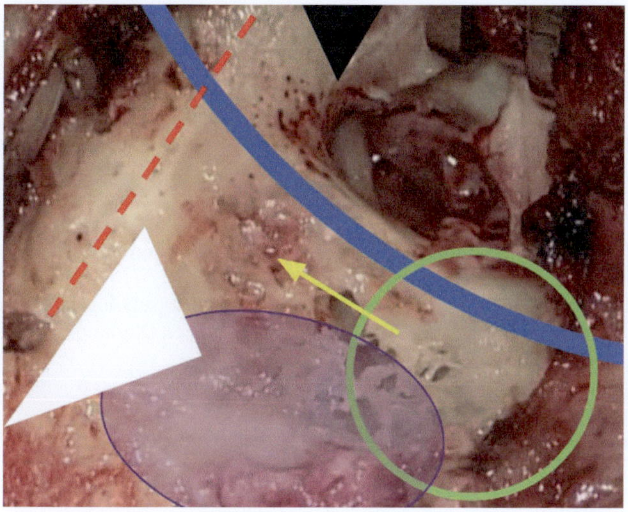

Fig. 46.5 Level V landmarks—superficial mastoid. EAC posterior wall (solid blue line); Tegmen timpani (red dashed line); lateral sinus (purple hatched); Citelli angle (white arrowhead); Zygoma root (black arrowhead); Koerner's septum (yellow arrow); mastoid process (green circle)

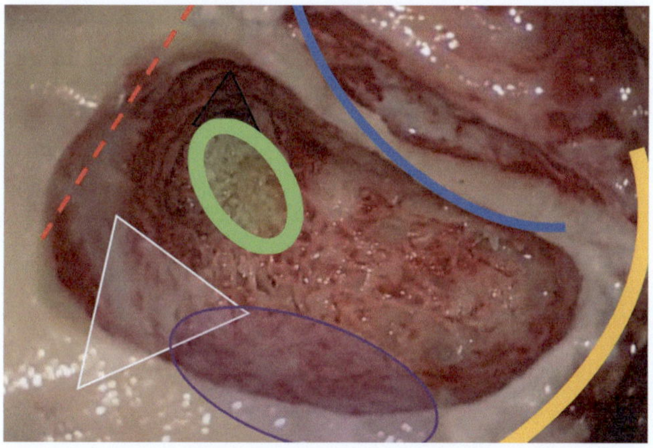

Fig. 46.6 Level VI landmarks—deep mastoid. EAC posterior wall (solid blue line); Tegmen timpani (red dashed line); lateral sinus (purple hatched); Citelli angle (white arrowhead); lateral semicircular canal (green hatched); incudal fossa and short process of the incus (black arrowhead); digastric groove (solid orange line)

Considering that the purpose of this chapter is to show the range of options present in the approach to chronic otitis media, we tried didactically to group landmarks at different levels of the temporal region. Regardless of the access chosen, several of these landmarks, if not all, must be rigorously observed throughout the dissection, from the superficial to the deepest planes.

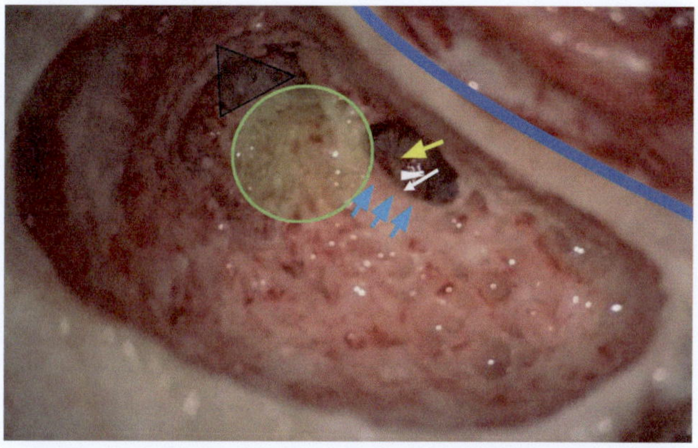

Fig. 46.7 Level VII landmarks—closed mastoidectomy (facial recess): EAC posterior wall (solid blue line); lateral semicircular canal (green hatched); vertical segment of the facial nerve (blue arrows); incudal fossa and short process of the incus (black arrowhead); pyramidal eminence (white arrowhead); stapes (yellow arrow)

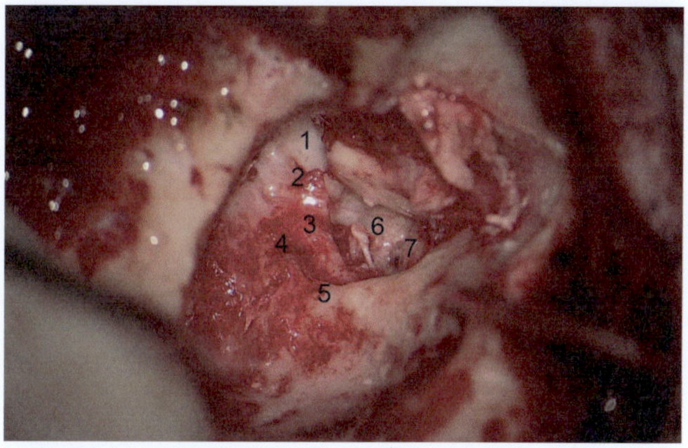

Fig. 46.8 Level VIII landmarks—open mastoidectomy, right ear: cog (1); cochleariformprocess(2); facial nerve—tympanic segment (3); lateral semicircular channel (4); facial nerve—mastoid segment (5); stapes over oval window (6)—note the absence of incus and malleus; round window (7). [11–14]

References

1. Luers JC, Hüttenbrink KB. Surgical anatomy and pathology of the middle ear. J Anat. 2016;228(2):338–53. https://doi.org/10.1111/joa.12389. Epub 2015 Oct 19.
2. Cruz OLM, Costa SS. Mastoidectomia. Otologia clínica e cirúrgica. Rio de Janeiro: Revinter; 2000. p. 271–87.
3. Costa SS, Colli BO, Fonseca N. Anatomia cirúrgica da artéria carótica interna intrapetrosa. J Bras Neurocir. 1996;7:30–43.

4. Goldenberg RA. Surgeon's view of the skull base from the lateral approach. Laryngoscope. 1984;94(suppl. 36):1–21.
5. Ogawa K, Inoue Y, Yamamoto M, Ikeda S, Kansaki J. Surgical anatomy for the extended cranial fossa approach. Acta Otolaryngol (Stockh). 1991;487:41–7.
6. Saleh E, Naguib, Cokkeser Y, Aristegui M, Sanna M. Lower skull base: anatomic study with surgical implications. Ann Otol Rhinol Laryngol. 1995;104:57–61.
7. Koriwchak M. Temporal bone cancer. Am J Otol. 1993;14: 623–6.
8. Piromchai P, Wijewickrema S, Smeds H, Kennedy G, O'Leary S. Correlations of external landmarks with internal structures of the temporal bone. Otol Neurotol. 2015;36(8):1366–73. https://doi.org/10.1097/MAO.0000000000000824.
9. Catalano PJ, Eden AR. An external reference to identify the internal auditory canal in middle fossa surgery. Arch Otolaryngol Head Neck Surg. 1993;108:111–6.
10. Goycoolea MV, Paparella MM, Nissen RL. Atlas of otologic surgery. Philadelphia: W. B. Saunders; 1989.
11. Arnoldner C, et al. Manual of otologic surgery. 1st ed. Springer; 2015.
12. Fisch U, et al. Tympanoplasty, mastoidectomy, and stapes surgery. 2nd ed. Thieme; 2011.
13. Francis HW, Niparko JK. Temporal bone dissection guide. 2nd ed. Thieme; 2016.
14. Mutlu C, Costa SS, Paparella MM. Clinical histopathological correlations of pitfalls in middle ear surgery. Eur Arch Otorhinolaryngol. 1998;255:189–94.

47 The Endoscopic Anatomy of Temporal Bone

Muaaz Tarabichi, Aneesa Ansar, Mustafa Kapadia, and Daniele Marchioni

Endoscopic Anatomy of the External Auditory Canal

It is important to inspect the anatomy of the external auditory canal (EAC), the tympanic membrane (TM), and the structures visible through the translucent TM. Understanding the anatomy of temporal bone from the CT scan sections prior to the surgery is of paramount importance. An axis drawn through the ear canal will be directing you to the attic. On removal of the scutum seen in between will give us a wide and open access to the attic, which forms the natural cul de sac of the external auditory canal (Fig. 47.1).

The blood vessels of the TM originate from the EAC. They supply in a lateral to medial direction. The skin of EAC and the epithelial layer of the TM form the bleeding elements of the external ear (Fig. 47.2). The friable skin and epithelium of the TM can be seen distinctly in the Fig. 47.3.

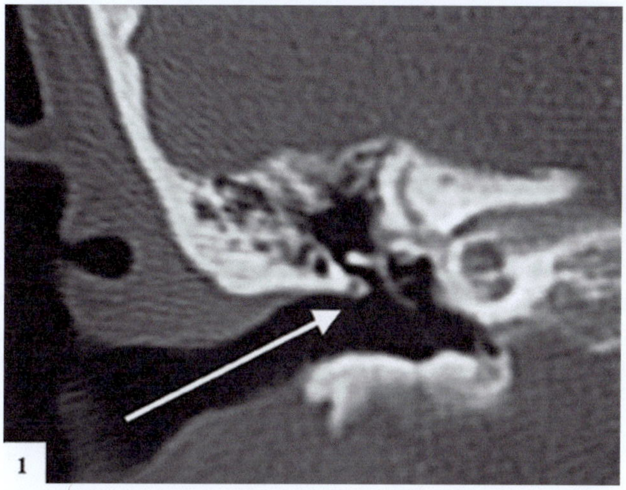

Fig. 47.1 Right ear: Coronal CT section through the external auditory canal (EAC) and middle ear. Note that the axis of the EAC slopes upward. The scutum represents the real "bottom of the EAC" rather than the mesotympanum. If the scutum is removed, this would allow direct access to the attic, the area frequently involved in cholesteatoma growth

Enlargement of the Ear Canal

The axis of the external auditory canal is directed superiorly and the scutum forms the medial end of the ear canal. It is also common to find bony over hangings in the EAC. The location and extent of it should be well noted (Figs. 47.1 and 47.4). Anterior or even an inferior overhang are commonly seen in many anatomical specimens. These can be curated out in all directions to achieve a panoramic view of the annulus using the 0° endoscope, keeping in mind the fact that the bony annulus is very variable in relation to the adjacent critical structures. Always consider the possibility of a high jugular bulb, anterior sigmoid sinus, a low lying dura, and the facial nerve (Figs. 47.5 and 47.6).

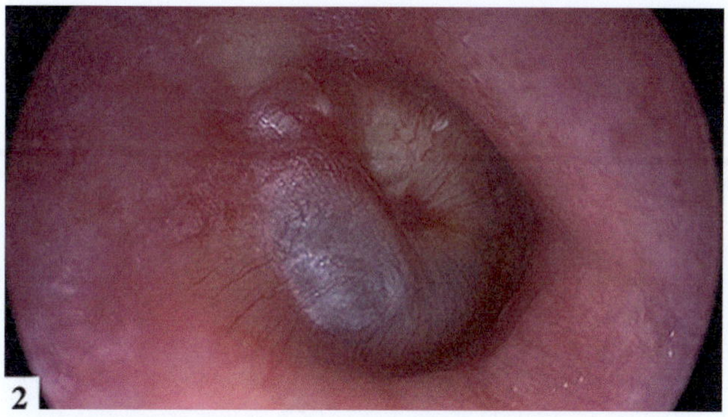

Fig. 47.2 Endoscopic view of the tympanic membrane (TM) in a right ear with cholesteatoma showing through. *Note the blood vessels arising from the EAC and supplying the TM*

M. Tarabichi · A. Ansar (✉) · M. Kapadia
Department of Otolaryngology, Tarabichi Stammberger Ear and Sinus Institute, Dubai, UAE
e-mail: aansar@tarabichi.org

D. Marchioni
Department of Otolaryngology, University of Modena, Modena, Italy

M. V. Goycoolea et al. (eds.), *Textbook of Otitis Media*, https://doi.org/10.1007/978-3-031-40949-3_47

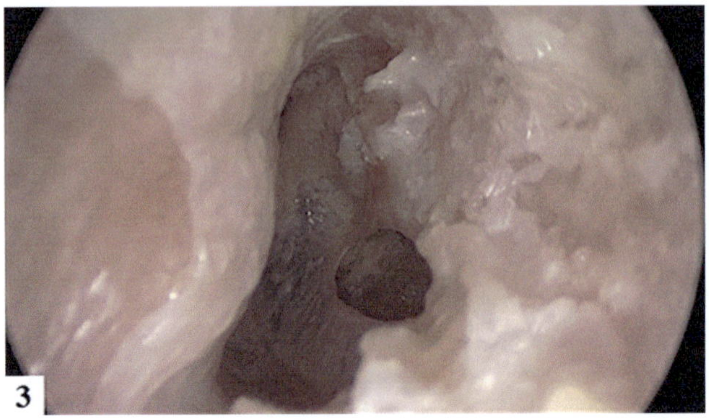

Fig. 47.3 Left ear: The skin of the canal has been removed along with the epithelial layer of the TM. The EAC has been enlarged. *Note the boundaries of the fibrous annulus (**white spots**); Chorda tympani (**Ct**); posterior mallear ligament (**Pml**)*

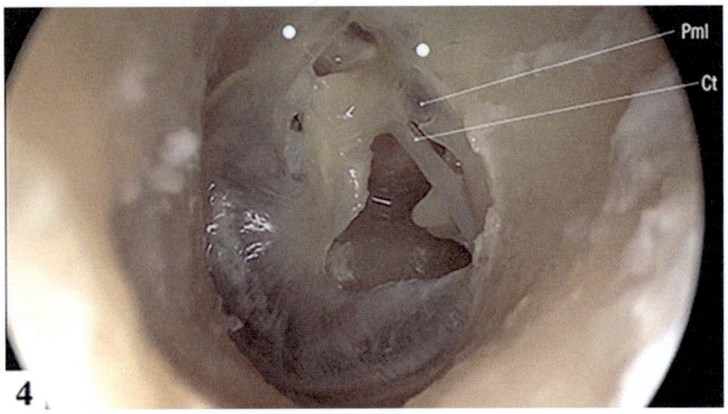

Fig. 47.4 Left ear: Endoscopic view of an anatomic specimen with a small perforation. *Note the size and location of the considerable anterior bony overhang in the external auditory canal*

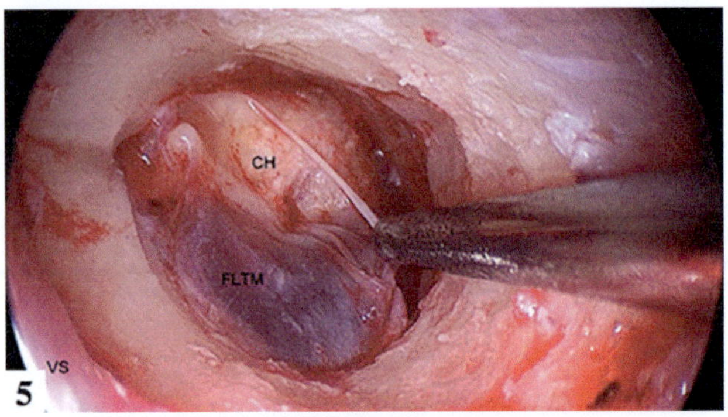

Fig. 47.5 Right ear: The canal wall is curetted to obtain a panoramic view of the tympanic ring using the 0° endoscope. *Vascular strip (**VS**); fibrous layer of tympanic membrane (**FLTM**); cholesteatoma (**CH**)*

Fibrous annulus—The glistening white fibrous annulus is anchored in a bony groove. It is incomplete in the upper posterior part of tympanic membrane. The fibrous annulus will be visible inferiorly and is incomplete at its upper end (Figs. 47.2 and 47.3). The annulus serves as a good landmark for the incision for the vascular strip.

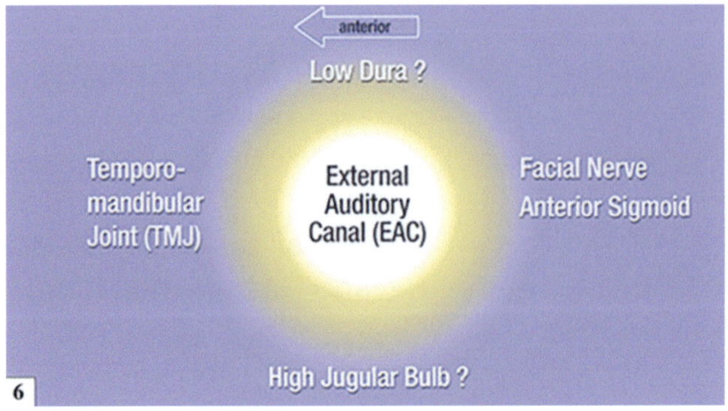

Fig. 47.6 Schematic anatomical representation of the left EAC with *surrounding structures* that need to be considered when enlarging the ear canal

Endoscopic Anatomy of the Middle Ear

After detaching the fibrous layer of the TM from the upper part of malleus handle and mobilizing from the bony sulcus, it is deflected inferiorly (Fig. 47.7). Separate the TM from the malleus handle starting from the lateral short process of the malleus and extending toward the umbo. The posterior malleolar ligament can be seen overlying the chorda tympani (Fig. 47.8).

Endoscopic Anatomy of the Retro Tympanum

On removing the bony annulus posteriorly gives a full access to the facial recess and sinus tympani. The posterior canal wall needs to be almost flushed with the pyramidal eminence. The pyramidal eminence accurately marks the level of the vertical segment of the facial nerve. It is safer to curette the bone superficial to that level. The facial recess present as a small depression on the posterior border of tympanic cavity (Fig. 47.9).

Figures 47.10 and 47.11 shows the retro tympanic anatomy. To see the retro tympanic anatomy clearly, the posterior aspect should face away from you and the axis of the scope's direction of viewpoints away from you. The presence of a sub pyramidal space and its entry point is to be noted.

The schematic diagram shows the drawing of the *sub pyramidal space (sps)* (Fig. 47.12) and the variable morphology of the *pyramidal eminence* (Fig. 47.13) and description.

The ⟹ refers to the communication of **sps**; facial nerve (**fn**); stapes (**s**); ponticulus (**p**); promontory (**pr**); round window (**rw**); subiculum (**su**).

The anatomy of the *sinus tympani* and *ponticulus promontorii* also varies with each individual. The variable morphology of the sinus tympani and ponticulus promontorii is described with the different types (Figs. 47.14, 47.15, 47.16,

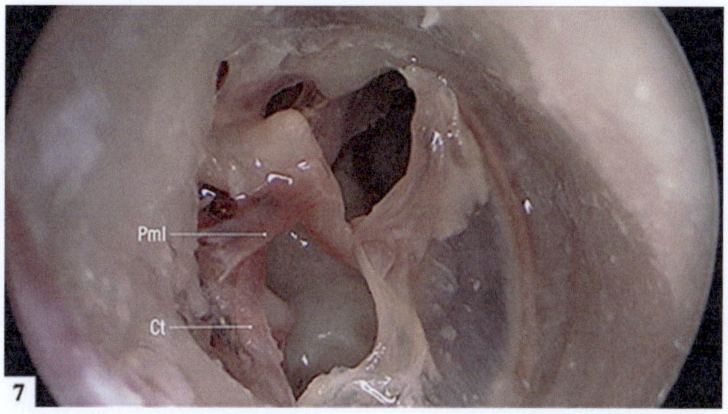

Fig. 47.7 Right ear: Fibrous layer of the TM is pulled down off the malleus handle revealing *the posterior mallear ligament (**Pml**) and the chorda tympani (**Ct**)*

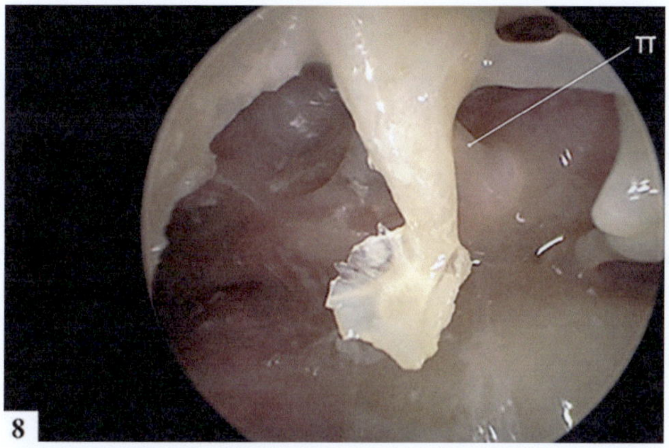

Fig. 47.8 Left ear: The fibrous layer of the TM along with the fibrous annulus has been removed and separated from the malleus handle. *The tendon of the tensor tympani (**TT**)*

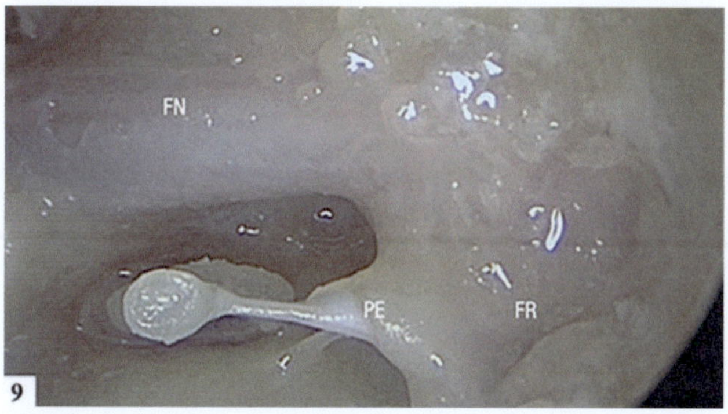

Fig. 47.9 Left ear. Endoscopic view through a transcanal endoscopic access after minor removal of bone*; the facial recess (**FR**) is very shallow and more of a flat depression, superficial to the pyramidal eminence (**PE**), and the vertical segment of facial nerve (**FN**).* Also note the horizontal segment of the facial nerve

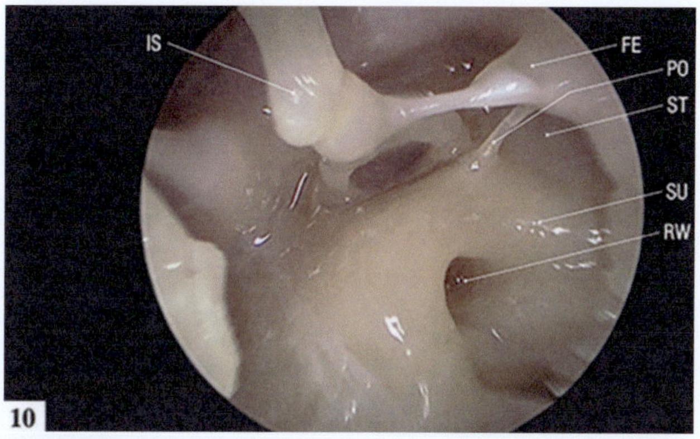

Fig. 47.10 Left ear: Endoscopic view of the retrotympanum. *Incudostapedial joint (**IS**); pyramidal eminence (**PE**); ponticulus (**PO**); sinus tympani (**ST**); subiculum (**SU**); round window (**RW**)*

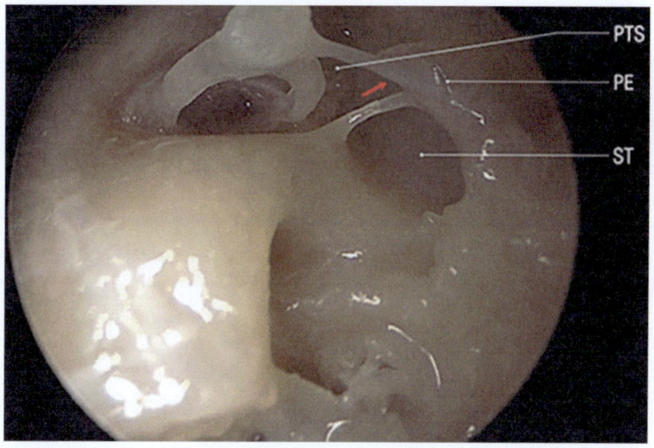

Fig. 47.11 Left ear. The entry points of the subpyramidal space (→) of this specimen are a specific feature of *'type A', connecting both the sinus tympani (**ST**) and posterior tympanic sinus (**PTS**). Pyramidal eminence (**PE**)*

and 47.17). The tegmen of the round window niche and anterior and posterior pillars are to be identified on identification of the round window niche (Fig. 47.18).

Endoscopic Anatomy of the Hypotympanum

In order to view the hypotympanum, a 30° endoscope is preferred with the removal of any inferior bony overhang and enlarging the access to the inferior and the posterior-inferior part of the retro tympanum. The subiculum separates inferior from superior retro tympanum. The subiculum also shows different variations in each specimen (Figs. 47.19, 47.20, and 47.21).

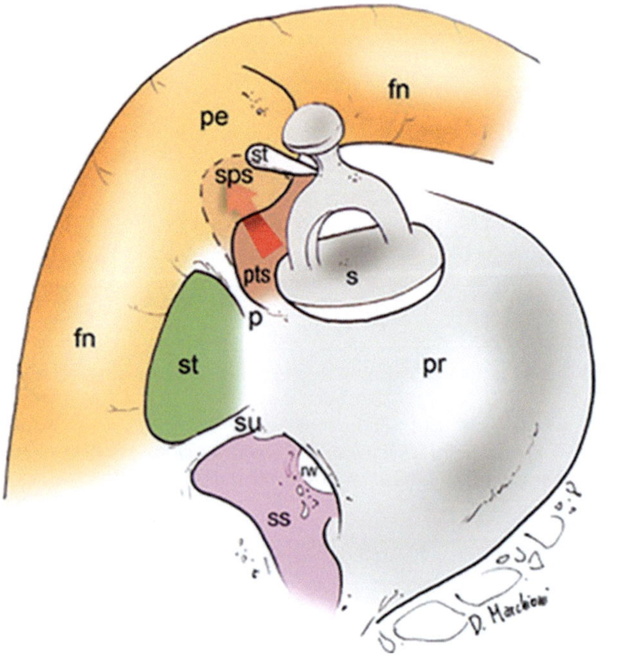

Fig. 47.12 Schematic drawing of subpyramidal space (sps) of a right ear. *Facial nerve (**fn**); pyramidal eminence (**pe**); stapes tendon (**st**); ponticulus (**p**); posterior sinus tympani (**pts**); stapes (**s**); sinus tympani (**st**); promontory (**pr**); round window (**rw**); subiculum (**su**); sinus subtympanicus (**ss**)*

Finiculus is a ridge of bone from the anterior and inferior slip of the round window separating the inferior retro tympanum from hypotympanum (Fig. 47.22). The styloid eminence, jugular bulb including the curvature of the basal turn of cochlea can be seen in a well pneumatised infracochlear space.

Endoscopic Anatomy of the Epitympanum

After a careful limited atticotomy meticulously, preserving the lateral incudo malleolar ligament and the lateral malleolar ligament on the medial aspect of the scutum. These are two friable ligaments along with the neck of malleus forms the roof and medial aspect of the Prussak's space Fig. 47.23).

These suspensory ligaments separates the area between scutum and ossicles by forming the lateral part of the epitympanic diaphragm. These ligaments act as the gateway for the spread of attic cholesteatoma (Fig. 47.24).

On extending the atticotomy, the anterior epitympanic space can be seen. The epitympanic space is separated from the supratubal space by the Sheehy's cog. The tensor fold is seen spreading across the cog and the tensor tympani (TT) (Figs. 47.25, 47.26, 47.27, 47.28, 47.29, and 47.30).

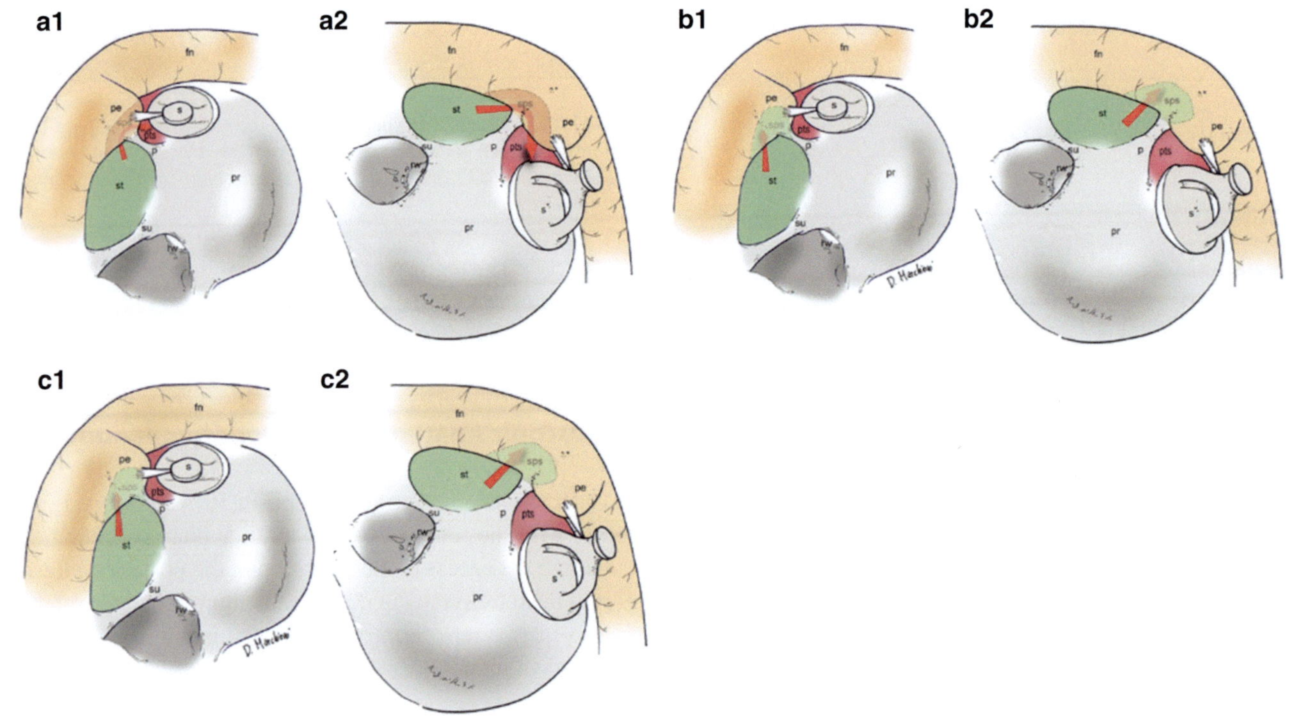

Fig. 47.13 Variable morphology of the **pyramidal eminence** (**pe**) in a right ear demonstrated by two types of perspectives: an anatomic view (**a1, b1, c1**) and a surgical endoscopic view (**a2, b2, c2**) through an angled-view scope while looking in the posterior direction. **a b c** Morphological variations of the **pe**, sinus tympani (**st**), and posterior sinus tympani (**pts**) communicating through the subpyramidal space (**sps**). Partial morphology of the **pe**. The subpyramidal space (**sps**) is communicating with the sinus tympani. Partial morphology of the **pe**. The subpyramidal space (**sps**) is communicating with the posterior sinus tympani (**pts**)

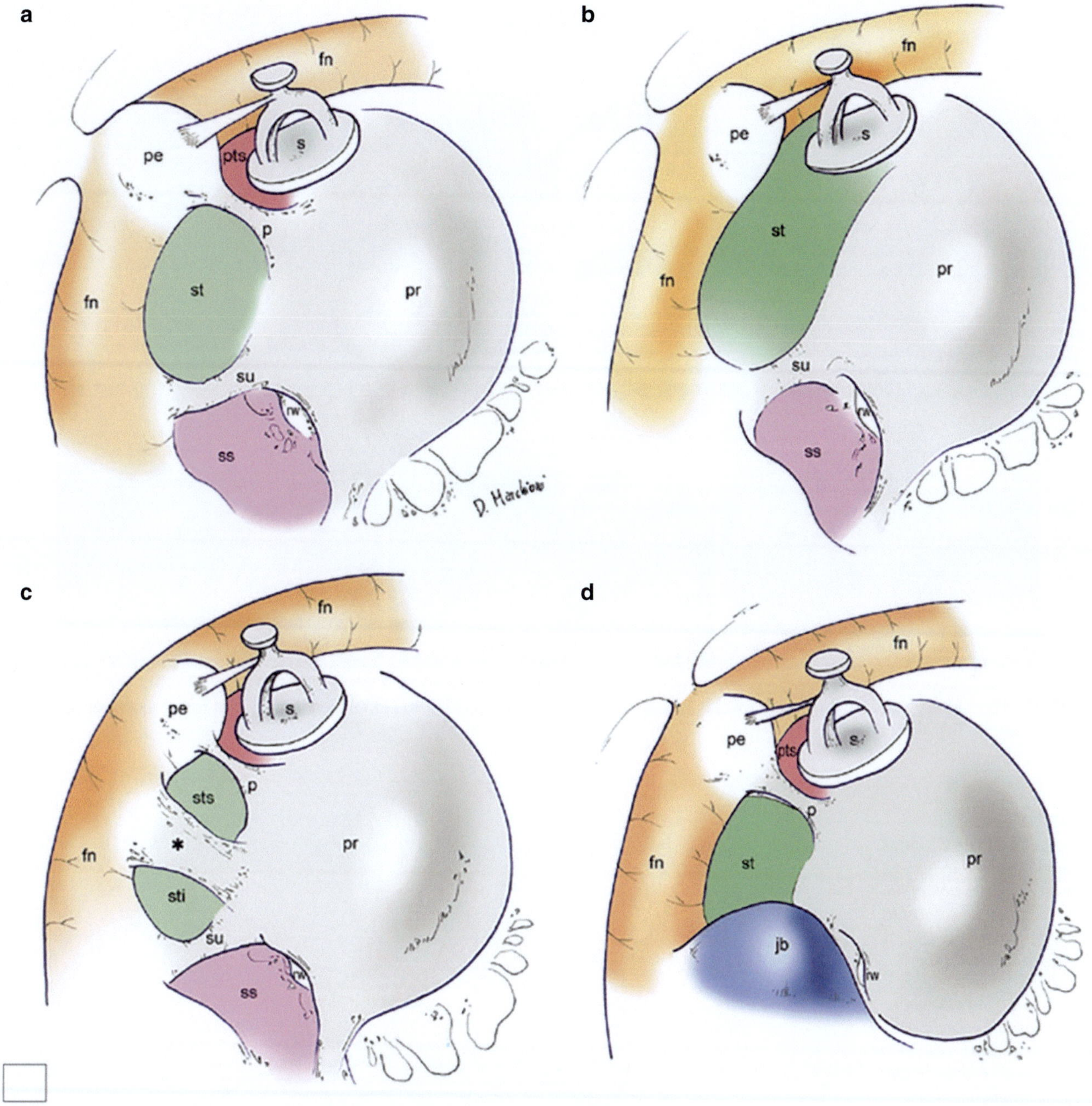

Fig. 47.14 The variable morphological appearance of the **sinus tympani**. *Facial nerve (**fn**); posterior sinus tympani (**pts**); pyramidal eminence (**pe**); promontory (**pr**); stapes (**s**); round window (**rw**); subiculum (**su**); jugular bulb (**jb**); sinus subtympanicus (**ss**); sinus tympani (**st**); ridge separating the sinus tympani into two parts (*); superior part of sinus tympani (**sts**); inferior part of sinus tympani (**sti**)*

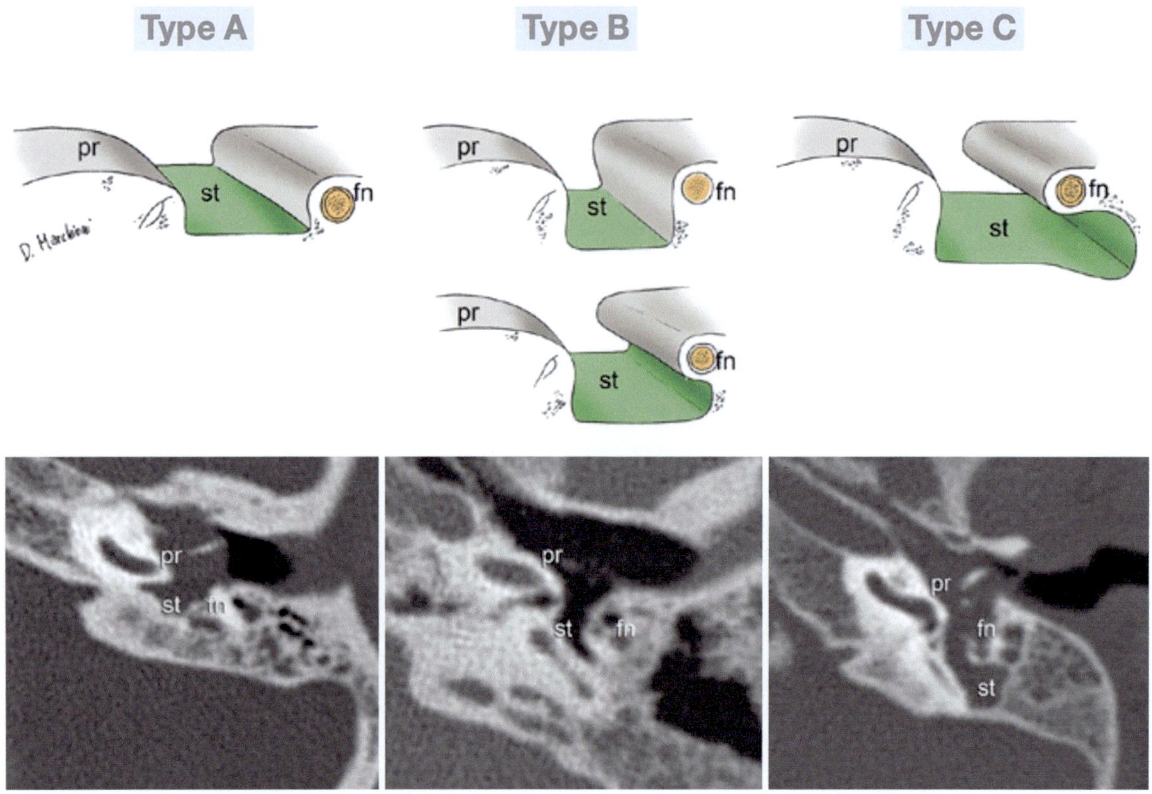

Fig. 47.15 The various types of **sinus tympani** classified according to depth and extension in relation to the facial nerve. Cochlear promontory (**pr**); facial nerve (**fn**); sinus tympani (**st**)

Fig. 47.16 Schematic drawing of a "**Type C**" **sinus tympani.** *The ⟹ indicates the posterior extension of the sinus tympani with respect to the third portion of the facial nerve (**fn**). Chordal ridge (**cr**); chorda tympani nerve (**ctn**); lateral tympanic sinus (**lts**); facial sinus (**fs**); incus (**in**); malleus (**ma**); ponticulus (**p**); pyramidal eminence (**pe**); cochlear promontory (**pr**); posterior sinus tympani (**pts**); stapedial tendon (**st**); stapes (**s**); subiculum (**su**); round window (**rw**)*

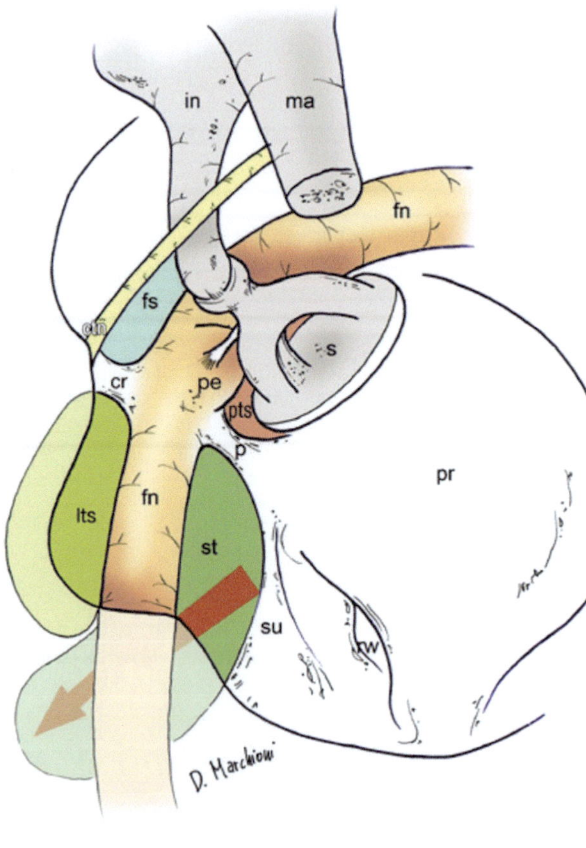

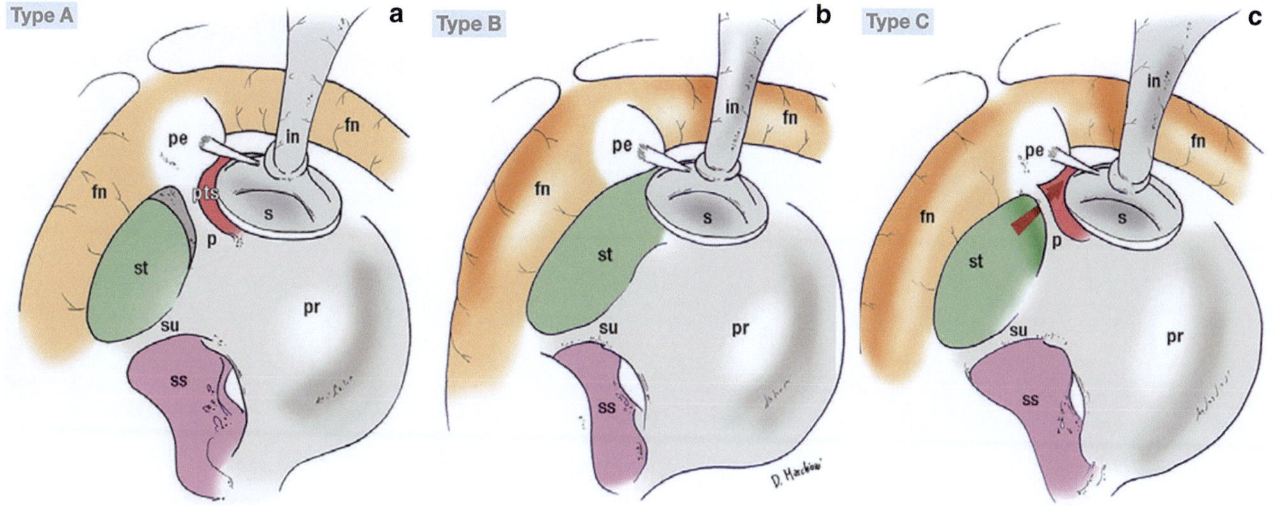

Fig 47.17 (**a–c**) The variable morphological appearance of the **ponticulus promontorii** (**p**). *Ridge ponticulus (**Type A**); incomplete ponticulus (**Type B**), bridge ponticulus (**Type C**). Facial nerve (**fn**); incus (**in**); ponticulus (**p**); pyramidal eminence (**pe**); posterior sinus tympani (**pts**); cochlear promontory (**pr**); stapedial tendon (**st**); stapes (**s**); subiculum (**su**); sinus subtympanicus (**ss**)*

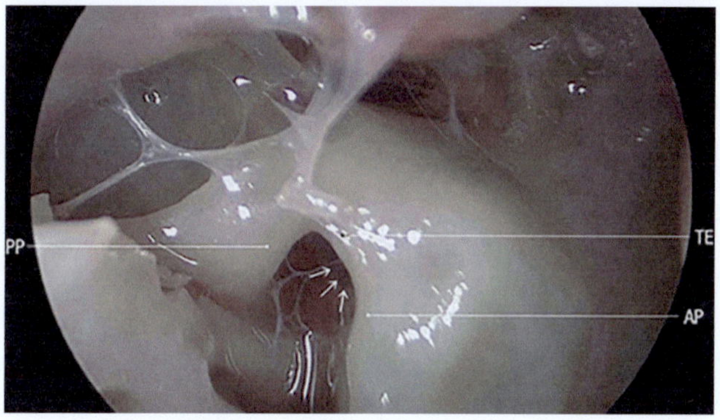

Fig. 47.18 Right ear. Endoscopic view of the round window niche. *Tegmen of the round window niche (**TE**); anterior pillar (**AP**); posterior pillar (**PP**); round window membrane (⟹)*

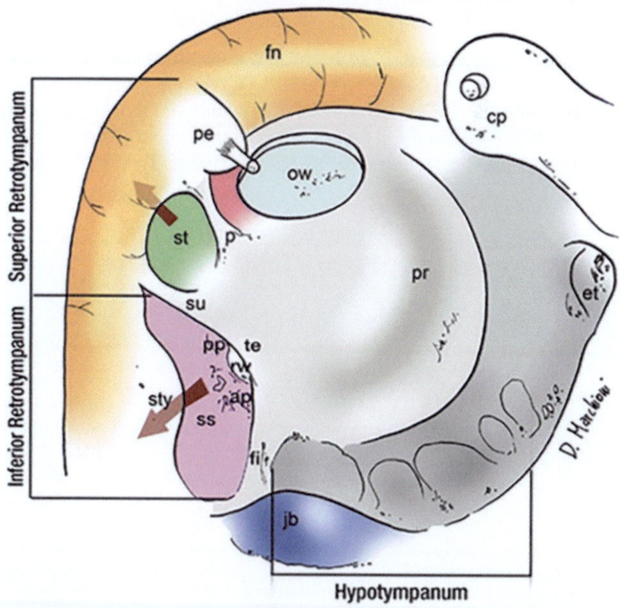

Fig. 47.19 Right ear. Schematic anatomical survey drawing of the **retrotympanum and hypotympanum.** *The finiculus (**fi**)* appears as a bony ridge which arises from the anterior and inferior lip of the round window and separates the inferior retrotympanum from the hypotympanum. *The subiculum (**su**)* marks the boundary between the superior and inferior retrotympanum. Right side. *Facial nerve (**fn**); pyramidal eminence (**pe**); oval window (**ow**); cochleariform process (**cp**); sinus tympani (**st**); ponticulus (**p**); subiculum (**su**); posterior pillar (**pp**); tegmen of round window niche (**te**); cochlear promontory (**pr**); Eustachian tube (**et**); round window (**rw**); styloid eminence (**sty**); sinus subtympanicus (**ss**); anterior pillar (**ap**); finiculus (**fi**); jugular bulb (**jb**)*

Endoscopic View down the Eustachian Tube

An angled endoscope is used to look further down into the eustachian tube. The relationship between the carotid artery and the bony canal for TT muscle (Fig. 47.29). The size and depth of the supra tubal recess vary considerably. On rotating further superiorly and posteriorly, the TT fold can be seen separating the supratubal recess from the anterior attic. The position and shape of the TT fold are also highly variable and are related to the size of the supra tubal recess (Fig. 47.30). The TT fold is almost a horizontal structure that closes the anterior attic and separates it from the eusta-

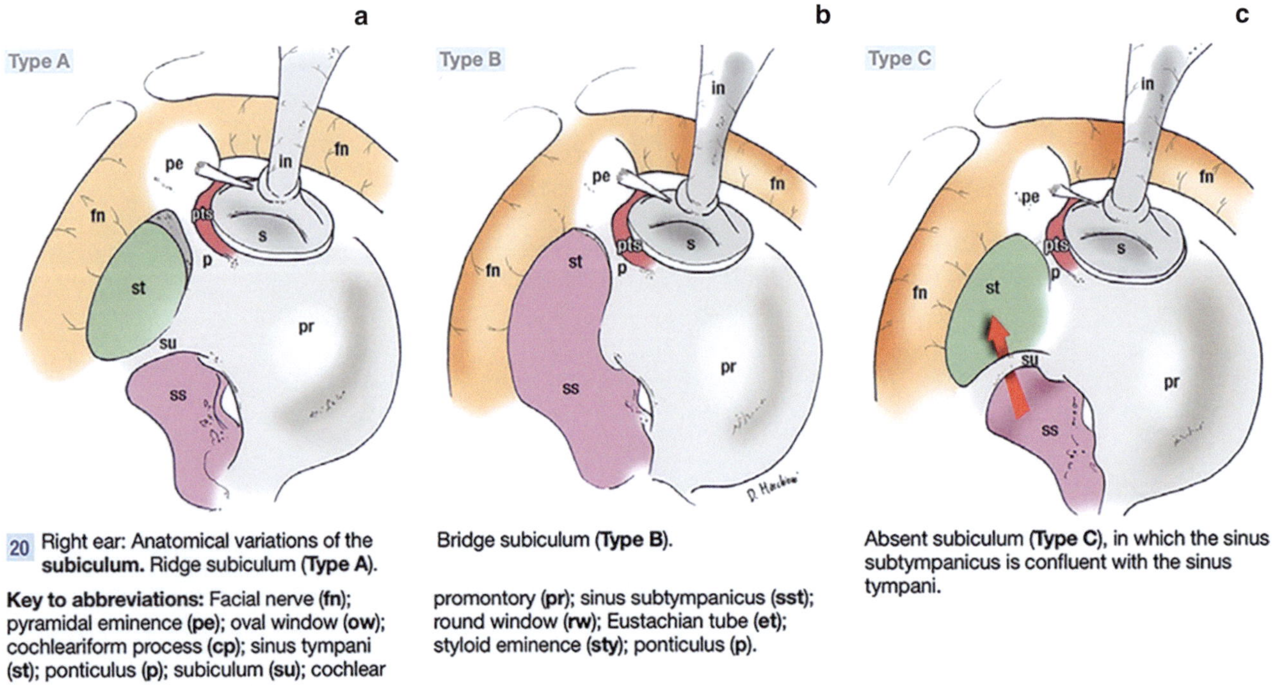

Fig. 47.20 (a–c) Right ear: Anatomic variations of the subiculum. *(A) **Ridge subiculum.** (B) **Bridge subiculum.** (C) **Absent subiculum***, **Key to abbreviations**: *Facial nerve (**fn**); pyramidal eminence (**pe**); oval window (**ow**); cochleariform process (**cp**); sinus tympani (**st**); ponticulus (**p**); subiculum (**su**); cochlear bridge subiculum (**Type B**). promontory (**pr**); sinus subtympanicus (**sst**); round window (**rw**); Eustachian tube (**et**); styloid eminence (**sty**); ponticulus (**p**). Absent subiculum (**Type C**), in which the sinus subtympanicus is confluent with the sinus tympani*

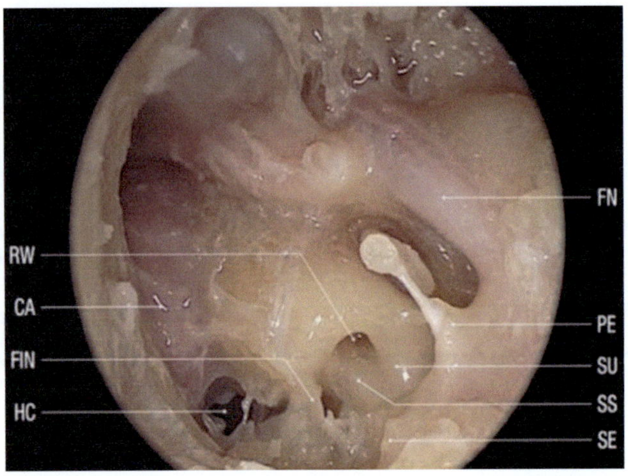

Fig. 47.21 Left ear: Endoscopic panoramic view of the tympanic cavity with special focus on the retrotympanum. *Facial nerve (**FN**); subiculum (**SU**); sinus subtympanicus (**SS**); styloid eminence (**SE**); round window (**RW**); finiculus (**FIN**); carotid artery (**CA**); hypotympanic air cell (**HC**)*

chian tube when the supratubal recess is poorly developed. It begins with the tendon of TT and inserts along a bony ridge formed by the encasement of the TT muscle and extends into the anterior epitympanic spine (Figs. 47.31, 47.32, and 47.33).

If the supratubal recess is well developed as in this specimen, the tensor tympani then holds two parts. The vertical part attaches to the cog and forms the wall separating the anterior attic from the supratubal recess. The horizontal segment attaches to the TT tendon and the most anterior part of the bony ridge which is formed by the bony canal for the TT muscle. The horizontal part of TT fold also contributes to the floor of the supratubal recess if it is well developed (Figs. 47.31, 47.32, 47.33, and 47.34).

The epitympanic ventilation is maintained through the tympanic isthmus formed between the incudo stapedial joint and the TT tendon. A complete TT fold and a closed lateral attic space prevents the ventilation through the anterior attic (Fig. 47.35).

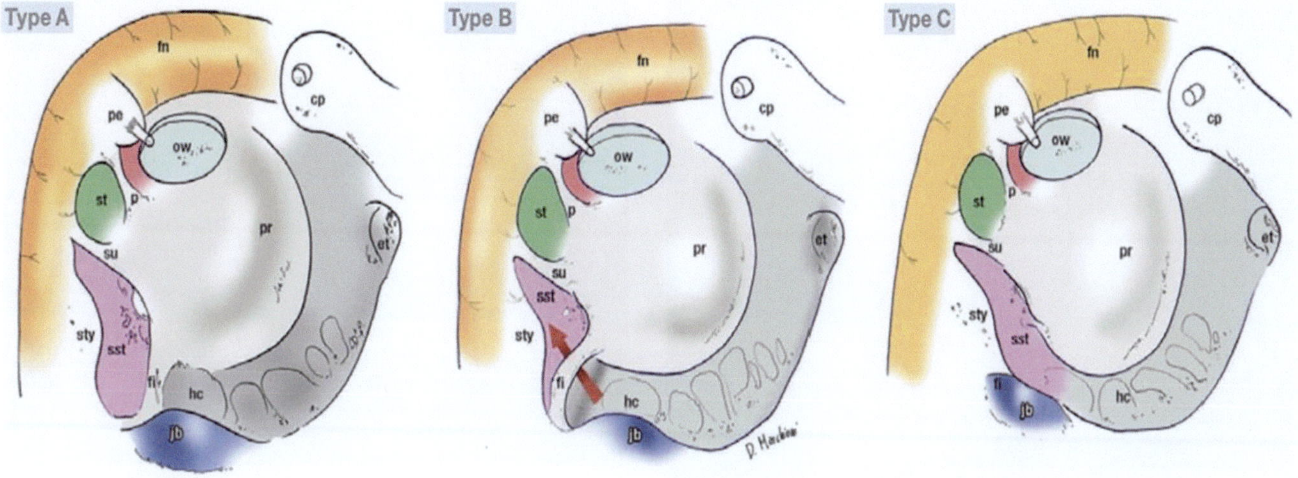

Fig. 47.22 Anatomical variations of the *finiculus (fi)*. Right side. *Ridge finiculus (**Type A**); Bridge finiculus (**Type B**). Absent finiculus (**Type C**). **Key to abbreviations:** facial nerve (**fn**); pyramidal eminence (**pe**); oval window (**ow**); cochleariform process (**cp**); sinus tympani (**st**); ponticulus (**p**); subiculum (**su**); round window (**r w**); cochlear promontory (**pr**); Eustachian tube (**et**); styloid eminence (**sty**); sinus subtympanicus (**sst**); finiculus (**fi**); jugular bulb (**jb**); styloid eminence (**sty**); ponticulus (**p**); hypotympanic air cell (**hc**)*

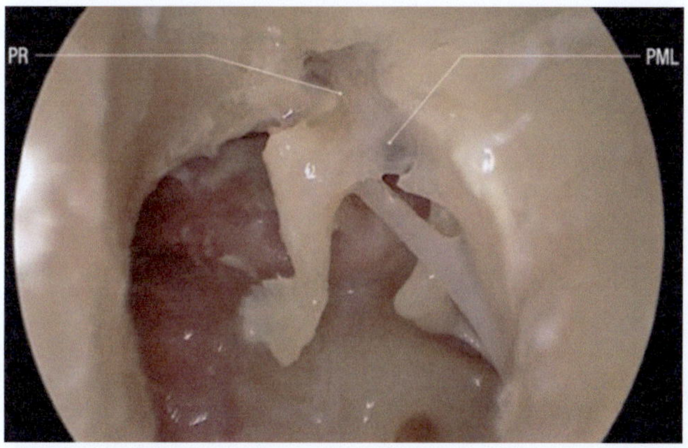

Fig. 47.23 Left ear: *Prussak's space (**PR**); posterior mallear ligament (**PML**)*

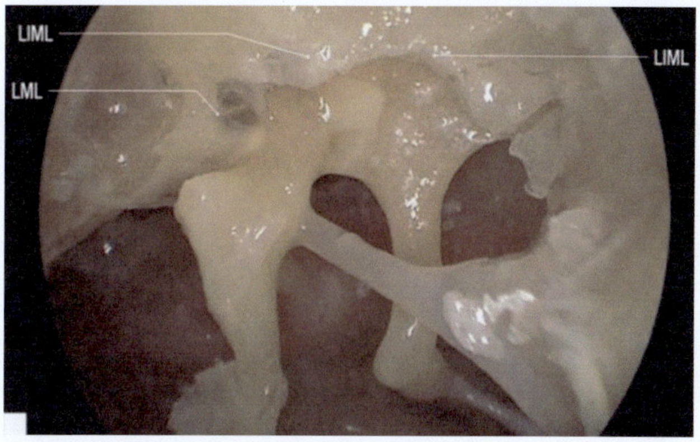

Fig. 47.24 Left ear: The relatively straight insertion line of the *lateral incudo-mallear ligament (**LIML**) and the downward sloping insertion line of the lateral mallear ligament (**LML**)*

The Incus is removed here to visualize the articular facet with malleus and stapes (Figs. 47.36 and 47.37). The horizontal segment of the facial nerve and the second genu, the lateral semi-circular canal, and remnant of the superior incudal ligament can be seen in the picture (Fig. 47.38).

The malleus is nipped above the neck at a superior level to preserve the anterior mallear ligament and the TT tendon. The TT tendon is seen attached to the handle and neck of the malleus (Fig. 47.39) The head of malleus is removed by preserving the suspensory ligaments and mobilizing the handle anteriorly. We can now observe the TT tendon attaching to the neck of malleus, course of chorda tympani (CT) nerve, anterior aperture of the bony canal into which the CT nerve runs into. Note the topographical relationship of the CT nerve to the AML, the anterior tympanic spine, and the attachment of the anterior mallear ligament (Fig. 47.40).

Upon transecting the TT tendon and the malleus handle, we can very well see the fibers of the horizontal segment of the facial nerve, its first genu after arising from the IAC, relationship of geniculate ganglion (GG), relation of the second genu, the lateral semi-circular canal, and the remnant of TT fold.

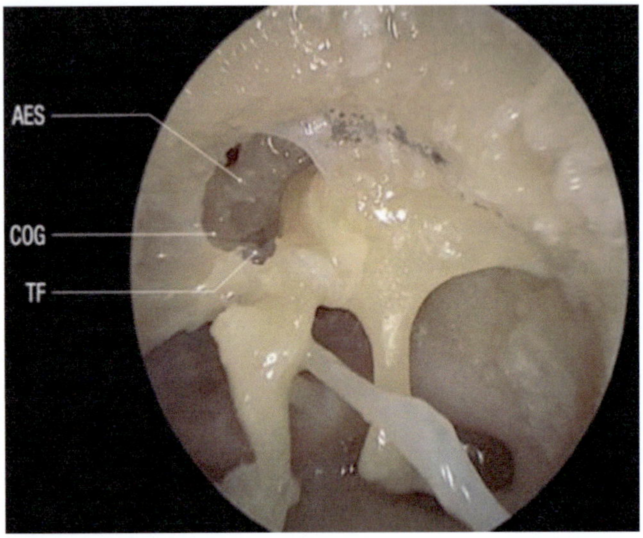

Fig. 47.25 Left ear: *Anterior epitympanic space (**AES**); Sheehy's cog (**COG**), separating the supra tubal recess from the anterior epitympanic space; tensor tympani folds (**TF**)*, partially visible and closing off the attic from direct ventilation of the supratubal recess and the Eustachian tube

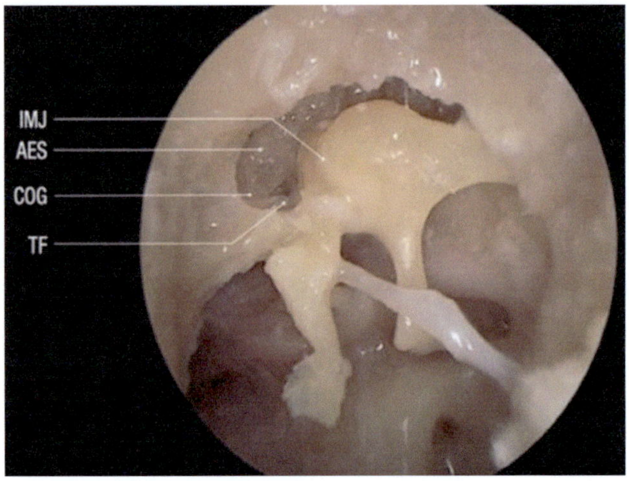

Fig. 47.27 Left ear: The ossicles have been fully exposed within the attic allowing to clearly visualize the incudo-mallear articulation line. *Incudo-mallear joint (**IMJ**); anterior epitympanic space (**AES**); Sheehy's cog (**COG**) separating the supratubal recess from the anterior epitympanic space; tensor tympani fold (**TF**)*, partially visible and preventing the attic from direct ventilation via the supratubal recess and the Eustachian tube

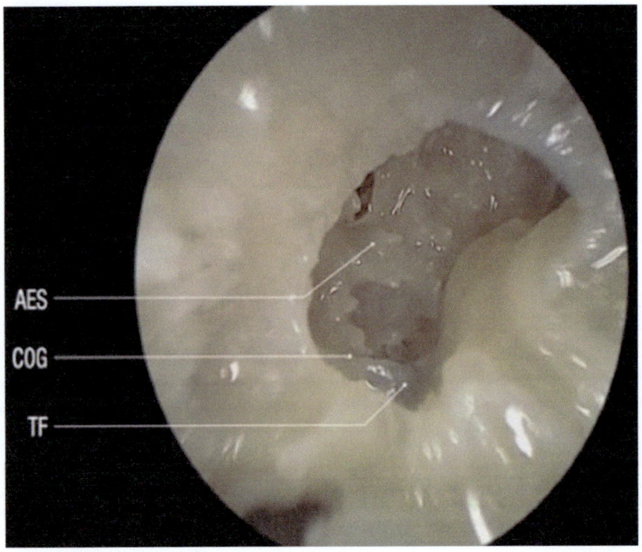

Fig. 47.26 Left ear: Close-up view of the *anterior epitympanic space (AES)*

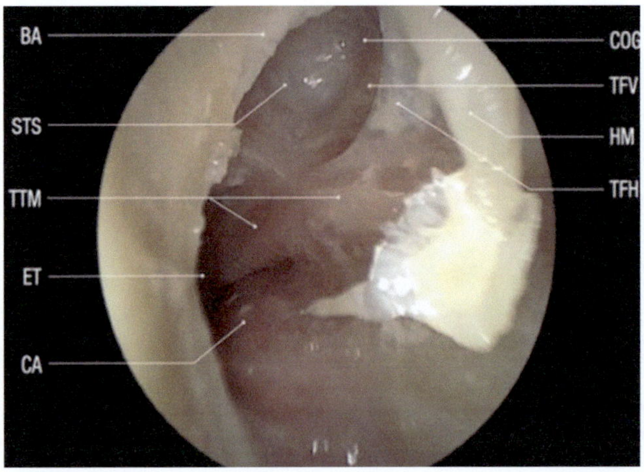

Fig. 47.28 Left ear: *handle of malleus (**HM**); supratubal recess (**STS**); anterior surface of Sheehy's cog (**COG**) separating the attic from the supra-tubal recess; vertical segment of the tensor tympani fold (**TFV**), which—given its entire integrity—closes off the attic from the Eustachian tube; horizontal segment of the tensor tympani fold (**TFH**) which* partially *contributes to the floor of the supratubal recess anteriorly; bony encasement of the tensor tympani muscles (**TTM**); bony annulus (**BA**); carotid artery (**CA**)*

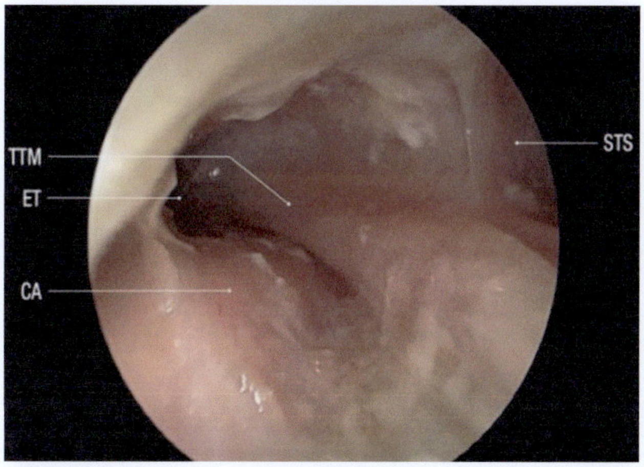

Fig. 47.29 Left ear: Endoscopic view down the *Eustachian tube (**ET**). Bony encasement of the tensor tympani muscle (**TTM**);bony annulus (**BA**); carotid artery (**CA**)*

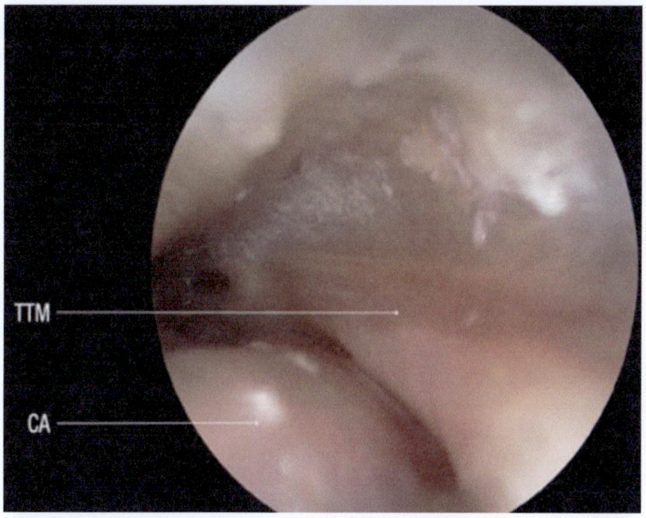

Fig. 47.30 Using a 45°-scope, it is occasionally possible to view the opening of the Eustachian tube to the nasopharynx. *Carotid artery (**CA**); tensor tympani muscle (**TTM**)*

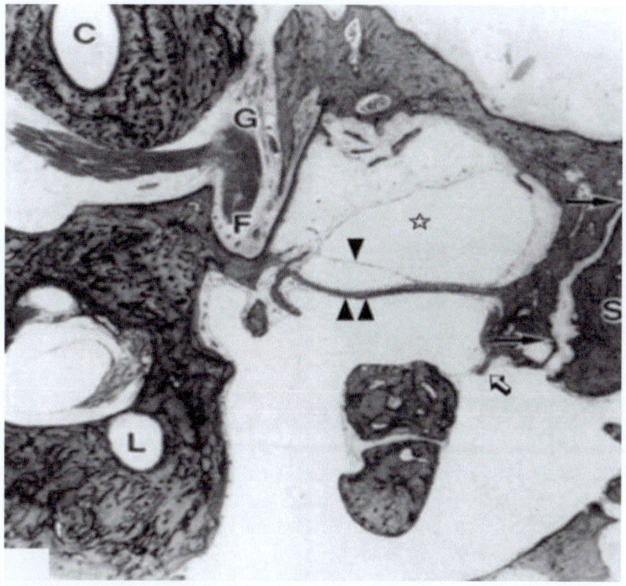

Fig. 47.31 Histologic section through a dome-shaped supratubal recess (☆). *The outermost plate (➡) of the petrosa; a spur (↖) projecting toward the mallear head, to which attaches a mucosal fold that stems from the anterior mallear ligament; sheehy's cog (▲▲); tensor tympani folds (▼); geniculate ganglion (**G**); cochlea (**C**); lateral semicircular canal (**L**)*

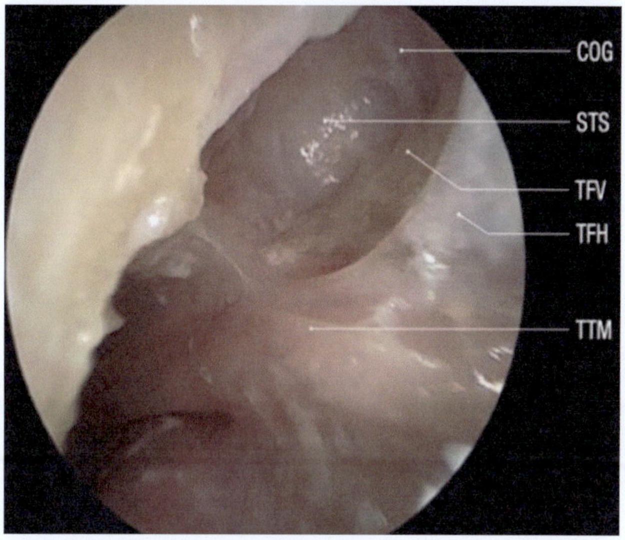

Fig. 47.32 Left ear: Endoscopic anatomy of the tensor tympani fold in a specimen with a well-developed *supratubal recess (**STS**). The tensor tympani folds are composed of two segments, a vertical part (**TFV**) that attaches to Sheehy's cog (**COG**), and a horizontal part (**TFH**) that partly contributes to the floor of the supratubal recess anteriorly; bony encasement of the tensor tympani muscle (**TTM**)*

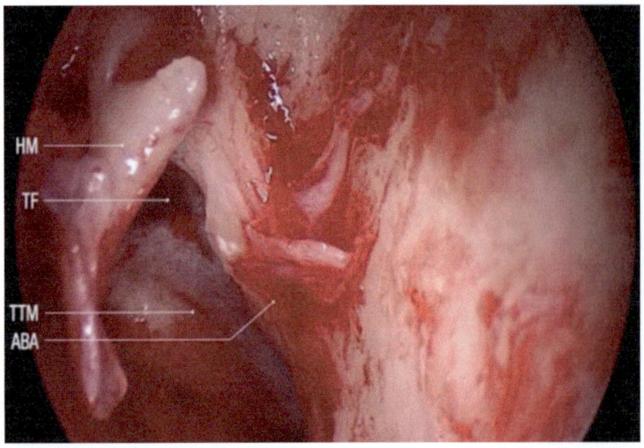

Fig. 47.33 Right ear: Unlike the anatomic specimen shown in Fig. 47.31, this is a poorly developed supratubal recess in a surgical case. View through a 70°-scope, upward and backward. *The tensor tympani fold (**TF**) here, different from the one shown in* Fig. 47.31, *is almost a horizontal structure. Handle of malleus (**HM**); tensor tympani muscle (**TTM**), anterior bony annulus (**ABA**)*

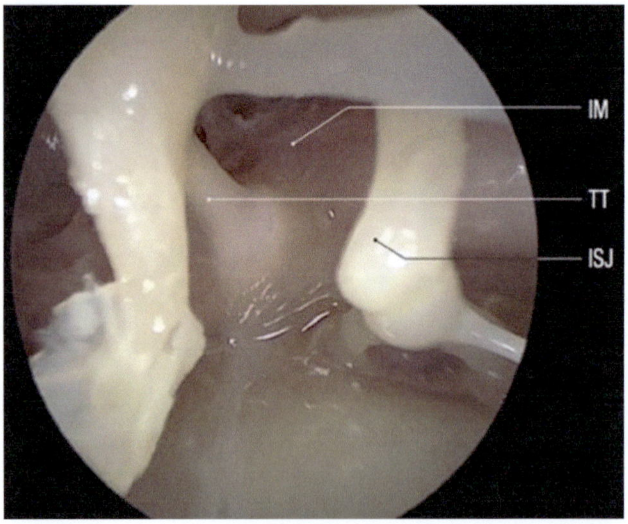

Fig. 47.35 Left ear: *tympanic isthmus (**IM**)* forms the only passageway for attic ventilation in the presence of complete tensor folds. *Tensor tympani tendon (**TT**); incudo-stapedial joint (**ISJ**)*

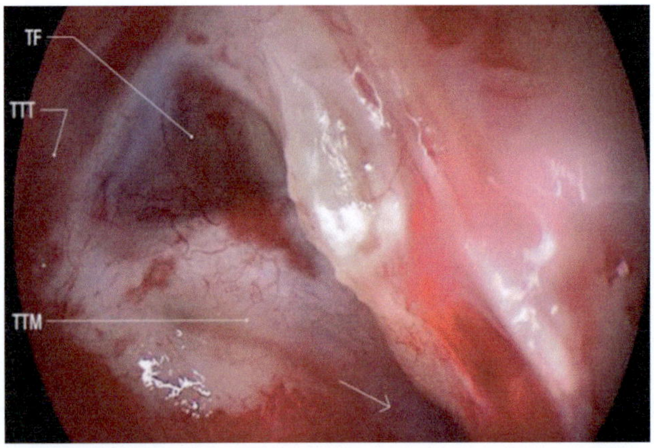

Fig. 47.34 Right ear: Endoscopic close-up view of the tensor tympani fold (**TF**) shown in Fig. 47.32. *Bony encasement of the tensor tympani muscle (**TTM**); tensor tympani tendon (**TTT**) inserting on the neck of the malleus. Funnel-shaped entrance to the Eustachian tube (—▷)*

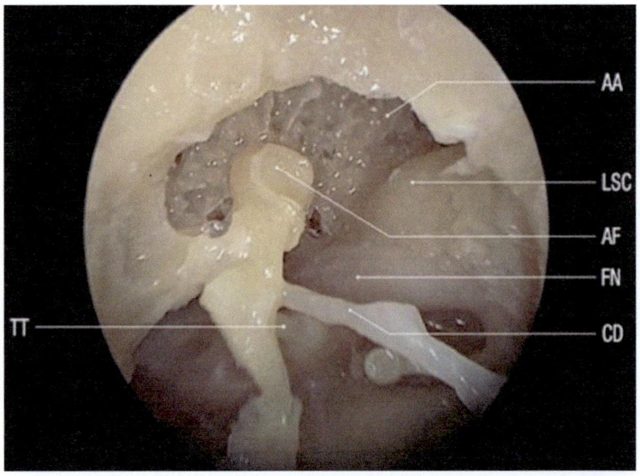

Fig. 47.36 Left ear: Endoscopic view after removal of the incus. *Articular facet of the head of malleus (**AS**); horizontal segment of the facial nerve (**FN**); lateral semicircular canal (**LSC**); Additus ad antrum (**AA**); chorda tympani (**CD**); tensor tympani tendon (**TT**)*

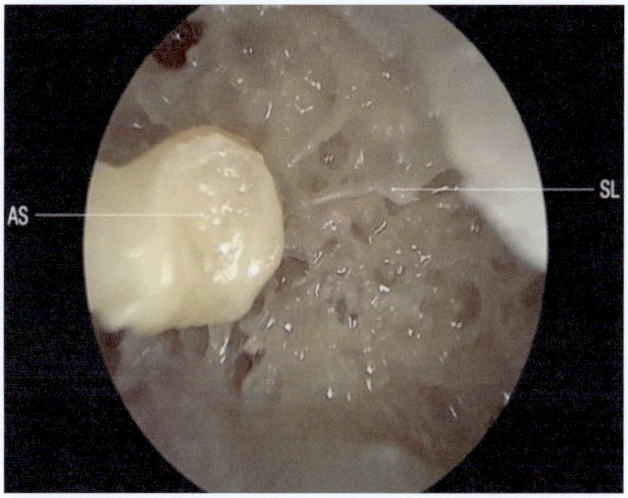

Fig. 47.37 Left ear: Endoscopic view of the attic after removal of the incus. *Articular surface of the head of malleus (**AS**); remnant of the superior ligament (**SL**) of the incus attaching to the tegmen tympani*

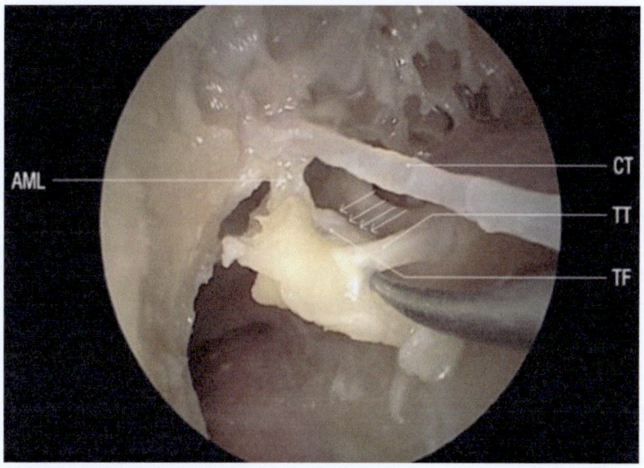

Fig. 47.39 Left ear: The handle of malleus has been mobilized anteriorly to expose the tensor tympani fold which is released from its attachments; the starting point of the white arrows indicate the original position of the fold and the tips show the current point following lateralization of the malleus handle. *Tensor tympani tendon (**TT**); chorda tympani (**CT**); tensor tympani fold (**TF**) after dislocation from its original position; anterior mallear ligament (**AML**)*

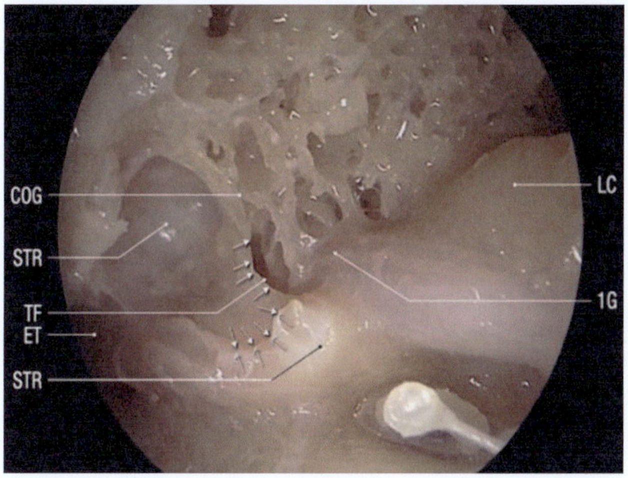

Fig. 47.38 Left ear: Endoscopic view after transection of the tensor tympani tendon and removal of the malleus handle, the anterior tympanic spine, anterior mallear ligament, and the chorda tympani. *Sheehy's cog (**COG**); remnant of the tensor tympani fold (**TM**); insertion point (⟹) of the partially removed vertical segment of the tensor tympani fold; insertion point (⟸) of the completely removed horizontal segment of the tensor tympani fold; supratubal recess (**STR**); Eustachian tube (**ET**); cochleariform process (**CP**); first genu (**1G**) of the facial nerve and neighbouring geniculate ganglion; lateral semicircular canal (**LC**)*

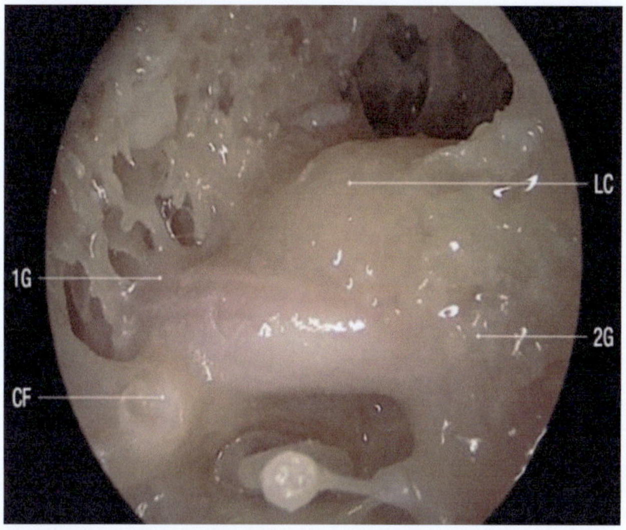

Fig. 47.40 Left ear: Endoscopic view of the horizontal segment of the facial nerve demonstrating its topographical relationship to the lateral semi-circular canal. *First genu (**1G**); second genu (**2G**); lateral canal (**LC**); cochleariform process (**CP**)*

References

1. Baki FA, El Dine MB, El Said L, et al. Sinus tympani endoscopic anatomy. Otolaryngol Head Neck Surg. 2002;127:158–62.
2. Thomassin JM, Korchia D, Doris JM. Endoscopic guided otosurgery in the prevention of residual cholesteatomas. Laryngoscope. 1993;103:939–43.
3. Badr-El-Dine M. Value of ear endoscopy in cholesteatoma surgery. Otol Neurotol. 2002;23:631–5.
4. Tarabichi M. Endoscopic management of acquired cholesteatoma. Am J Otol. 1997;18:544–9.
5. Tarabichi M. Endoscopic management of limited attic cholesteatoma. Laryngoscope. 2004;114:1157–62.
6. Bowdler DA, Walsh RM. Comparison of the otoendoscopic and microscopic anatomy of the middle ear cleft in canal wall-up and canal wall-down temporal bone dissections. Clin Otolaryngol Allied Sci. 1995;20:418–22.
7. Bottril ID, Poe DS. Endoscope-assisted ear surgery. Am J Otol. 1995;16:158–63.
8. Karhuketo TS, Puhakka HJ, Laippala PJ. Endoscopy of the middle ear structures. Acta Otolaryngol Suppl. 1997;529:34–9.

Surgical Treatment of Chronic Otitis Media: Menu of Solutions

48

Sady Selaimen da Costa, Fabio Andre Selaimen, Mauricio Noschang Lopes da Silva, and Douglas K. Reinhardt

Introduction

As can be seen from its definition, the inflammatory process always associated with otitis media can be found focally in some area of the middle ear (ME) or generalized, completely filling the ME/mastoid complex and, not infrequently, extrapolating the limits of the temporal bone causing serious and even fatal extratemporal complications.

An obvious therapeutic implication of this diversity of clinical forms is the absolute impossibility of, with a single procedure, being able to solve all the conditions potentially found there. Thus, throughout history, a constellation of surgeries and additional surgical steps have been designed focusing on the point-by-point resolution of a series of situations related to the inflammatory processes intrinsically related to otitis media.

The aim of this chapter is to briefly review the most common procedures that were dialectically designed for the surgical treatment of the various forms of presentation of this prevalent disease. Our idea here is simply to present an overview of this immense arsenal. Of course, we do not intend to exhaust the subject. For more details, the reader can refer to the specific chapters (tympanoplasty, tympanomastoidectomy, and petrosectomy). We will begin by describing the most used access routes and, later, the accesses that involve bone removal.

S. S. da Costa (✉)
Department of Otolaryngology, Head & Neck Surgery, School of Medicine, Universidade Federal do Rio Grande do Sul, Porto Alegre, Brazil

F. A. Selaimen · M. N. L. da Silva
Hospital de Clínicas de Porto Alegre, Porto Alegre, Brazil

D. K. Reinhardt
Hospital São Lucas da PUCRS, Porto Alegre, Brazil

Transchanal Approach

Indications: Pros and Cons

Originally, the transcanal access was developed by Lempert in the 30s in order to section the sympathetic tympanic plexus located on the promontory, which was believed to be responsible for the origin of tinnitus [1]. Afterward, this approach was adapted by Rosen for mobilization of the stapes in cases of otosclerosis and then improved by Shea in stapedectomy procedures.

This access should be reserved for situations where exploration is limited to the tympanic membrane, mesotympanum and/or hypotympanum, never being indicated when manipulation of the epitympanum and/or mastoid is anticipated [2]. We list below (Table 48.1) some procedures that can be satisfactorily performed by this route with the aid of a posterior tympanomeatal flap [2–7].

Basic Technique

We use a local anesthetic with a vasoconstrictor, usually 2% lidocaine with 1:100,000 epinephrine, under an insulin syringe that allows for easy injections. A nasal or Lempert

Table 48.1 Transcanal access applications

1.	Stapedectomy
2.	Trans-canal labyrinthectomy
3.	Myringotomy
4.	Myringoplasty
5.	Tympanoplasty
6.	Closure of perilymphatic fistulas
7.	Tumor biopsy
8.	Posterior ampullary nerve section
9.	Ossiculoplasty
10.	Tympanic glomus tumor removal
11.	Jacobson nerve section
12.	Section of the tendon of the tensor tympani muscle
13.	Exploratory tympanotomy

M. V. Goycoolea et al. (eds.), *Textbook of Otitis Media*, https://doi.org/10.1007/978-3-031-40949-3_48

speculum is used for the initial injections in the inferior, superior, and posterior quadrants of the external auditory canal (EAC), which can be modified depending on the flap to be used. The infiltration must be slow to avoid the formation of bubbles and maceration of the canal skin. When the anesthetic infiltration is adequate, it is possible to visualize the skin dissection of the external auditory canal from the injection point to the tympanic annulus.

The choice of a speculum with adequate size is essential, as it allows a satisfactory surgical visualization and the possibility of bimanual work [8]. A sickle scalpel is used for the first vertical incision at the 12 o'clock position, in a straight line toward the surgeon. A second vertical incision is made at the 6 o'clock position, curving toward the first vertical incision. A third incision—horizontal—can be made with Rosen's scalpel on the edge of the speculum, connecting the first and second vertical incisions [2]. While making the incisions, the underlying bone must be "felt" with the instrument, even to the point of producing noise, thus confirming the complete section of the skin.

The junction of the skin with the tympanic annulus at the 12 o'clock position corresponds to the so-called vascular strip being generally thicker and richer in vessels and connective tissue [8]. The complete section of this area is of utmost importance, and Bellucci scissors are very useful in this step. One should not try to mobilize the flaps or enter the middle ear until there is complete release of the skin flaps [8].

After releasing the cutaneous margins, the surgeon uses a duckbill elevator or Rosen's knife to start the dissection, which must be performed slowly and carefully in order to keep the tympanomeatal flap intact, since this is responsible for the blood supply and healing will depend on this. The tip of the suction tip (keeping the flow port uncovered) should be used against the elevator blade to keep the flap dry. During detachment, special attention is given to the region corresponding to the tympanomastoid suture line, since it is often prominent, creating a legitimate groove where the skin of the auditory canal penetrates and is firmly inserted. This anatomical accident can be circumvented by visualizing the soft tissue penetrating the bone trough, allowing its fibers to be dissected over the suture or simply sectioned.

The skin is elevated evenly, avoiding aspiration of the flap and tunneling, until reaching the tympanic annulus which is easily identified at the node of Rivinus (at the posterior boundary between the tensa and flaccida segments of the tympanic membrane—TM). After identification, it is gently lifted, taking care to work with the lift pressed against the bone.

After elevating and moving away the tympanic annulus, a needle or a curved sickle knife can be used to break the mucosa, accessing the middle ear always below the annulus and, if possible, inferiorly toward the round window. At this point, the duckbill must be introduced through the initial orifice and compressed against the tympanic sulcus, mobilizing it inferiorly to completely release the posterior–inferior tympanic membrane. Superiorly, a sickle knife or a needle can be used to release the posterosuperior tympanic membrane, taking care not to injure the ossicles during this step. The chorda tympani nerve must be identified and carefully removed from the field of work. If this maneuver causes it to stretch, it is best to simply section it with Bellucci scissors. This nerve must not be pinched and pulled in an inferior–superior direction, under the risk of producing an injury to the vertical segment of the facial nerve.

In the presence of an anterior bulging of the EAC, incisions at 12 and 6 o'clock can be joined through a curvilinear incision a few millimeters from the tympanic annulus. A laterally pedicled flap can be developed and the bone canal rectified with the aid of curettes and a drill, allowing better exposure of the anterior mesotympanum. During this step, the bony boundary over the temporomandibular joint capsule should be observed due to the possibility of its being violated.

After the objective of the surgical act is achieved, the flap is then replaced in its original position and the EAC is patched with compressed sponges or with antibiotic ointments. The external auditory meatus is covered with a sterile cotton.

Retroauricular Approach

Indications: Pros and Cons

The retroauricular approach is credited to Galen, who approximately 1800 years ago already used it in order to remove "rotten bone" from diseased mastoids (*apud* [2]). More modernly, this access was reintroduced into clinical practice in 1853 by Sir William Wilde, who recommended it in the treatment of suppurative mastoiditis as a complication of otitis media (*apud* [2]).

According to the classic textbook on otological surgery by Nadol and Schuknecht [9], the retroauricular access quickly became the legitimate "workhorse" of the modern otologist due to the wide exposure of the mastoid that it offers, combined with its incomparable versatility and flexibility. This approach, with the addition of small variations, can be adapted for most otological procedures (Table 48.2). The wide exposure offered by it facilitates the identification of key anatomical references in the lateral temporal approaches, thus minimizing the risks of inadvertent injuries to noble structures. Other advantages of the retroauricular approach consist of the practicality offered in the creation of superior or inferior pedicled musculo-periosteal flaps (used to obliterate open cavities) and the ease in obtaining hemostasis. In contrast to the endaural approach (which allows a

Table 48.2 Retroauricular access applications

1.	**Simple mastoidectomy**
	(a) Acute mastoiditis
	(b) Endolymphatic sac surgery
	(c) Translabyrinthine labyrinthectomy
2.	**Closed tympanomastoidectomy (Wall *up canal)***
	(a) Non-cholesteatomatous chronic otitis media
	(b) Cochlear implant
	(c) Facial nerve decompression
3.	**Open tympanomastoidectomy (Wall *down canal)***
	(a) Chronic cholesteatomatous otitis media
	(b) Tumors
4.	**Management of congenital aural atresia**
5.	**Exposure of the hypotympanum**
	(a) Glomus tumor
	(b) Posterior ampullary nerve section
6.	**Access to the lateral base of the skull**

direct view of the membrane and tympanic cavity), the retroauricular approach offers the surgeon an "acute angle" approach to these structures. This "beveled" view minimizes interference caused by convexities of the anterior wall of the auditory canal, offering an excellent exposure of the anterior half of the tympanic membrane, the protympanum, and the tympanic orifice of the Eustachian tube.

Alongside these advantages, the cosmetic results of the incision are acceptable, as it can be hidden in the retroauricular fold or later in the hairline.

The possibility of employing this incision in the treatment of virtually all temporal surgical conditions creates the added advantage of familiarity through repetition. In this sense, the speed, exposure, and, above all, the flexibility offered by this access route cannot be emphasized enough.

Thus, the retroauricular approach may be indicated as the first step in several procedures, such as simple mastoidectomy, closed or open tympanomastoidectomy, resection of some tumors, and for better hypotympanic exposure. A modification of the incision so that it is located more posterior to the retroauricular sulcus allows exposure of the cerebellopontine angle in surgery for vestibular schwannomas and facilitates the transcochlear approach to the petrous apex and the retrolabyrinthine/retrosigmoid sections of the vestibular nerve. The length of the incision to the neck allows sufficient exposure for removal of jugular glomus tumors through the infratemporal fossa. The addition of an extension of the incision anteriorly to the pinna (forming a kind of Y), provides the necessary exposure for lateral accesses to the skull base, including the resection of the temporal bone.

Basic Technique

Whenever we decide for the retroauricular approach, we prefer general anesthesia with orotracheal intubation, as the magnitude of the procedure usually requires it. The patient's head should be as close as possible to the surgeon, taking care not to project the shoulder superiorly in such a way as to hinder its movements. The head should be positioned in extension, resting on a small "crown" or using a fixator specially developed for otological surgeries. The table is usually placed a few degrees in the inverted Trendelenburg position and shifted slightly toward the surgeon [10].

Hair must be shaved to three centimeters above and behind the ear, sparing the whiskers. With the help of nurses, a cap is made and must be firmly attached to the head with adhesive tape and micropore. In our routine, prior to the surgeon's brushing, we perform infiltrations. We used a local anesthetic with a vasoconstrictor (2% lidocaine with 1:100,000 epinephrine) under a 3 mL disposable syringe coupled to an abocath 22 needle and the aid of a nasal or Lempert speculum, in order to obtain hemostasis and facilitate the elevation of the skin flaps. The infiltration must be done slowly to avoid the formation of bubbles and maceration of the skin in the canal, as previously mentioned in the transcanal technique. Soon after, an additional injection must be made along the retro-auricular sulcus, avoiding injecting anteriorly to the tragus or deep to the mastoid tip (mainly in children), preventing an undesirable anesthesia of the facial nerve, respectively, close to the parotid or the foramen stylomastoid. The fact that we perform the infiltration at this moment speeds up the beginning of the procedure and, obviously, increases the effectiveness of the vasoconstriction.

After dressing, antisepsis of the surgical field (aqueous iodophor) and delimitation of the surgical area, an incision is made next to the retroauricular sulcus, slightly posterior to the insertion angle of the auricular pavilion in the temporal bone in order to avoid postoperative scar retractions. The scalpel is handled with the dominant hand while the other pulls the pinna anteriorly to expose the operative field (a task that can also be performed by an assistant). The first incision extends curvilinearly from the tip of the mastoid to a point roughly located on the temporal line and still hidden behind the most cranial portion of the pinna. Deep down, it involves the skin and subcutaneous cellular tissue. The rudimentary retroauricular muscle plane is next to be incised, and small blood vessels can be electrocoagulated directly and without wasting time. Once in the musculo-periosteal plane, the dissection progresses anteriorly until the posterior semicircle of the EAC is completely delineated, inferiorly with exposure of the mastoid tip periosteum, and superiorly until revealing the temporal muscle line. Posteriorly, the dissection proceeds over the periosteum for a variable distance that will be directly related to the extent of the procedure. In this step, we identify the periosteal plane by elevating the soft tissues with a Sehn–Müller retractor. Even in tympanoplasties, we develop, at the very least, a pocket of periosteum that will serve as a fibrous band supporting the posterior arm of the self-retaining retractor.

At the upper pole of the incision, a three-prong retractor is positioned, and the deeper tissues are divulsed with the aid of Metzembaum scissors, quickly exposing the fascia of the temporal muscle, easily recognized by its characteristic color and shine. With a scalpel (blade 15), a roughly circular incision is made over the fascia, and using or not using hydrodissection, it is separated from the adjacent muscle and conventionally prepared.

After obtaining and treating the temporal fascia, attention is redirected to the operative field where we identify the posterior semicircle of the auditory canal, mastoid periosteum, temporal line, temporal muscle, and mastoid tip. The next step is performed with the electric scalpel, and a septum dissector involves creating a periosteal flap. This flap may have a roughly triangular configuration (anteriorly pedicled or type 1), cylindrical (inferiorly pedicled or type 2) or quadrangular (superiorly pedicled or type 3). The option for one or the other varies from surgeon to surgeon and, in our opinion, will depend on surgical planning and anticipation of subsequent steps. Thus, in conventional, flexible tympanoplasties, and ossiculoplasties, we prefer the type 1 flap, as during its detachment we sequentially identify key landmarks and the flap itself, due to its resistance, is used in the anterior anchoring of the retractors. In open mastoidectomies, we developed inferiorly pedicled flaps (type 2), as in these occasions they present themselves as an unmatched option in the obliteration of cavities of exaggerated dimensions. In closed mastoidectomy, however, we used the type 3 flap, since at the end of the procedure it can be more easily repositioned and sutured to its original position. This maneuver makes it possible to close the retroauricular incision in two planes (periosteal and cutaneous), significantly improving the cosmetic result by positioning the external ear in a more anatomical position and minimizing skin retraction into the mastoidectomy cavity. Making the flap depends on the individual preference of each surgeon, and we emphasize its importance by emphasizing its almost "a thousand and one uses" (Table 48.3).

After creating the flap, it is folded back and kept eccentric to the operative field with the help of retractors. This maneuver takes us directly to the following landmarks: posterior wall and skin of the EAC, temporal line, spine of Henle, cribriform area/triangle of Macewen, and mastoid process.

Table 48.3 Uses of the periosteal flap

(a) Tympanic graft
(b) Graft for TORP™ and PORP™
(c) Graft for windows
(d) Canal wall reconstruction
(e) Anchoring of retractors in the transposition of the pinna
(f) Tubal orifice obstruction in the open technique
(g) Consistency of the suture line in the closed technique
(h) Reinforcement of atrophic TM

Once the skin on the posterior wall of the EAC is clearly identified, we make a horizontal incision. For this purpose, we used a scalpel (blade 15) sectioning the skin in the posterior 180° of the junction between the bony and cartilaginous canal. Additionally, two relief incisions are made at 6 and 12 o'clock directed laterally to the concha, thus delimiting a Koerner's flap. This flap, after being completely released, is inverted, added to the pinna and fixed anteriorly with the retractors, exposing the 360° of the EAC and the next references: tympanic-mastoid suture, tympanic-squamous suture, anterior wall of the canal, and tympanic membrane.

With the lenticular or sickle knife or even with the scalpel blade 15, two vertical incisions are created at 11 and 7 o'clock from the annulus to the side of the horizontal incision, defining a wide tympanomeatal flap.

After elevation of the posterior flap, the canal can be resized in order to maximize exposure of the middle ear contents. When there is an anterior bulging, the 11 and 7 o'clock positions can be joined through a curved incision a few millimeters from the annulus. A laterally pedicled flap is created with the aid of the 90° Rosen, and the anterior bony canal can be straightened with cutting and diamond burs. During this step, care must be taken to avoid exposure of the temporomandibular joint (TMJ) capsule. Drilling proceeds superiorly–inferiorly and from lateral to medial, until adequate exposure of the EAC, tympanic remnants, anterior edge, and protympanum is achieved. In the case of a posterior canalplasty is necessary, as we progress medially and inferiorly, the presence of a facial nerve should be anticipated in its mastoid segment, more laterally and anteriorly projected.

At the end of the previously proposed procedure, the middle ear must again be exuberantly irrigated and debris suctioned, returning the tympanomeatal flap to its original position. The external auditory canal is completely and firmly filled with pieces of sponge, the first of which must be molded into a cylindrical shape and firmly positioned in the anterior tympanic sulcus in order to press the flap anteroinferiorly against the bone wall. This maneuver is essential to ensure the so-called control of the anterior edge—a key element in the functional success of any tympanoplasty. After this step, the canal is completely filled with sponges up to the height of the incisions. The retractors are relieved and removed and the incisions sutured in one or two planes.

In situations where an open cavity is created, a proportional meatoplasty is mandatory. The external auditory meatus is sealed with hydrophilic gauze soaked in antibiotic ointment, and the external dressing is made according to the magnitude of the procedure. Whenever we use the retroarticular approach, at the end of the procedure, we personally coordinate the performance of this dressing, since all care must be observed in the manipulation of the patient's head, which, at this moment, may still be intubated. We use a filling of the concha with sterile cotton and several layers of gauze that are positioned over and under the auricle. A bandage with 12 cm bandages and adhesive tape is firmly applied, taking care to leave the eyes and the contralateral ear exposed.

In Sheehy's classic lateral tympanoplasty technique (*onlay*), the incisions differ from those described above, since both the making of the so-called vascular strip and the circular incision 7external to it are performed initially and transcanally. Only after completing these incisions and retrogradely elevating the vascular strip will the surgeon's attention turn to the retroauricular incision.

Endaural Approach

Indications: Pros and Cons

Endaural approach was performed for the first time at the end of the nineteenth century, being credited to Kessel (*apud* [11]). However, the first attempts to use the cartilaginous incision were abandoned due to the problem of postoperative perichondritis. In 1930, Heermann developed the extra cartilaginous extension of the endaural incision, a technique known to us today [2]. Eight years later, Lempert combined Sourdille's tympanomeatal flap with Heermann's extra cartilaginous incision in a single-step procedure [12]. Lempert's surgical approach involved three incisions, all extra cartilaginous and with excision of a triangle of skin, fibrous tissue, and periosteum of the posterosuperior portion of the external auditory canal. This approach was widely used by Lempert and subsequently by several generations of otologists, with some modifications, as the primary tympanomeatal approach route. Nowadays, although the popularity of the retroauricular approach has somewhat obscured the endaural approach, it remains an excellent access route to the temporal bone in certain circumstances [2].

The endaural access is excellent in cases where a meatoplasty and/or canaloplasty is necessary, and in those situations where a straight-line view of the auditory canal is important (large osteomas and exostoses). In large perforations and anterior perforations—especially if associated with convexity of the anterior canal—the endaural access combined with canaloplasty provides us with excellent exposure. This access route also promotes adequate visualization of the attic region, facilitating the removal of attic cholesteatomas and possibly those with a small extension to the mastoid antrum (Table 48.4).

On the other hand, as additional advantages, compared to the retroauricular route, intraoperative trauma and bleeding are less and the postoperative anatomical relationships with the pinna are more reliable. There are divergent opinions about when the endaural access, compared to the retroauricular one, provides a better or worse exposure of the tympanic sinus. In most cases, endaural approach should include a small meatoplasty in order to facilitate postoperative care and avoid the risk of fibrocartilaginous stenosis of the auditory canal opening.

Table 48.4 Applications of endaural access

1.	Need for canaloplasty or meatoplasty
2.	Large tympanic membrane perforations
3.	Previous perforations
4.	Attic cholesteatomas
5.	Cholesteatomas with small extension to the antrum

Basic Technique

In order to obtain a better exposure, it is recommended to use a nasal speculum to perform the anesthetic infiltrations as already described in the retroauricular access, adding an extra injection in the region of the notch. The anatomical references used are: external auditory canal and meatus; tragus; concha; helix; crus of helix; anterior notch; and lobule.

In the traditional Lempert technique, initially, a Koerner flap is made through two vertical incisions in the external auditory canal located at 12 and 6 o'clock. These incisions are made with a #15 scalpel blade and extend from a few millimeters from the tympanic annulus, progressing laterally to the osteocartilaginous junction of the canal. A third incision—horizontal—connects the two vertical incisions, medially delimiting a cutaneous flap that is elevated in a retrograde manner. The vertical incisions are enlarged with the scalpel until slightly penetrating the conchal cartilage. The Lempert elevator is then used to elevate the Koerner flap and partially expose the mastoid cortex. The vertical incision located at 12 o'clock can be enlarged over the notch to expose the fascia of the temporalis muscle. At this moment, a meatoplasty can be easily performed by everting the Koerner flap and dissecting the fibrous tissue that leads us to the anterior margin of the conchal cartilage. Keeping the skin of the flap intact, this cartilage is isolated by removing a slice as generous as needed with the scalpel.

The traditional Lempert incisions (types I, II, and III) can also be modified in three ways. A reduced endaural approach involves a Lempert type I incision combined with a small pic made over the notch region to facilitate placement of a small self-retaining retractor that allows for bimanual surgery [13, 14]. A median approach includes the Lempert II incision more superiorly, as well as the Lempert III incision, in order to allow adequate retraction of the posterior flap and expose part of the mastoid cortex adjacent to the posterior canal. The enlarged version of the endaural incision includes the Lempert type II incision extending into the *temporalis fascia region* and the Lempert III incision inferiorly to allow soft tissue retraction and exposure of the cortex and mastoid tip in its entirety.

In this modified Lempert technique, the first incision (Lempert I) is made semi-circumferentially between 6 and 12 o'clock in the posterior wall of the canal at the osteocartilaginous junction. This incision should completely transfix the soft tissues reaching the bone. The second incision (Lempert II) is made between the tragus, helix crus, and anterior notch, taking care not to expose or damage the helix cartilage during this maneuver. The length of this incision is related to the degree of exposure required for the procedure, ranging from a few millimeters (exploratory tympanotomy) to a few centimeters (mastoidectomy). The Lempert type II incision can be deepened in order to expose the plane of the temporal fascia in cases where the need for a graft is anticipated. The areolar tissue is then separated from the true fascia by means of dissection, and local anesthetic is injected under the fascia to separate it from the muscle. Completely section the fascia with the scalpel and remove the fascia (in an ovoid shape). After this, the fascia is placed on a silicone block, with the bottom facing upwards, and all the muscle fibers still adherent are resected. The silicone block is placed under an electric lamp, and in about 10 min, the fascia will be dry.

Care must be taken not to deepen the incision immediately after the subcutaneous plane during this step, since branches of the artery and superficial temporal vein are found in this topography. The residual skin of the auditory canal (cartilaginous portion) is preserved and elevated completely exposing the posterior wall of the external auditory canal. Two-prong self-retaining retractors are positioned at right angles to stabilize the flaps and facilitate exposure. With attention again focused on the external auditory canal, a curved scalpel is used to make the first vertical incision at 11 o'clock, from the annulus toward the Lempert type I incision (#1). A second vertical incision (#2) is made at 7 o'clock, curving towards incision #1. Such incisions and Lempert type I define a broad superior–posterior–inferior tympanomeatal flap. The length and width of this flap may vary according to anticipated pathological conditions. In a routine type I tympanoplasty, a 6 mm flap should be sufficient, and the vertical incisions can be located at 12 and 6 o'clock, while in a more extensive exploration with a small aticotomy, or in cases where it is removed the bony canal, an 8 mm flap should be required. After releasing the skin edges, the surgeon uses a duckbill elevator or even a Rosen knife to slowly and carefully separate the skin flap from the underlying bone in order to preserve the flap intact. The suction can be used with the tip applied against the elevator blade in order to keep the field bloodless. The skin is evenly lifted until it reaches the tympanic annulus. Sometimes dissection is made impossible due to a very narrow or tortuous external auditory canal. Regardless of the cause of the narrowing, the canal must be surgically straightened to facilitate access to the middle ear. When opting for a canalplasty, we prefer to carry out the same before penetrating the interior of the middle ear cleft.

At the end of the procedure, the tympanic-meatal flap is carefully repositioned to its original position, the external auditory canal is completely and firmly filled with pieces of sponge, slightly moistened up to the height of the incisions. The retractors are relieved and removed and the incisions sutured in one or two planes. As in the retroauricular access, the external auditory meatus is sealed with hydrophilic gauze soaked in antibiotic ointment and the external dressing is made according to the magnitude of the procedure.

Transcanal Endoscopic Approach

The established use of the microscope in the field of ear surgeries is undeniable, presenting different exposures according to the approaches previously described. However, its "straight line" visual field makes it impossible to fully see certain areas of the middle ear and, therefore, the use of the endoscope has gained great space in surgical complementation through its angular view. The endoscope was introduced as an auxiliary method in microscopic surgeries, notably in wall-up tympanomastoidectomy and, over the years, it has become a valid option in middle ear surgeries by providing increasingly less invasive procedures with its isolated use.

Its main objective is the direct visualization of certain recesses of the middle ear cleft, thus reducing the need for larger resections of bones and soft tissues. The highest rates of residual disease in wall-up cholesteatoma surgery occur in the anterior epitympanum, facial recess and tympanic sinus, reaching 40% of cases. The use of angled endoscopes directly aids in examining these regions during surgery. A randomized clinical trial with 57 patients concluded that the application of the endoscope to review the posterior recesses at the end of the wall-up tympanomastoidectomy actually decreased the rate of residual disease and recurrence in pars tensa cholesteatomas.

One year after the first surgery, the second look of the cholesteatoma can be performed only with the endoscopic examination of the auditory cleft, to the detriment of the surgical opening traditionally performed. In addition to visualizing areas of possible residual disease, the endoscope can assess the permeability of the tympanic diaphragm—markedly, in the tympanic tensor fold, being a valuable tool in the assessment of the etiopathogenesis of chronic otitis media.

The use of the endoscope alone has been shown to be feasible and even comparable to the microscopic technique in tympanoplasty, ossiculoplasty, and stapedotomies surgeries.

When performing transcanal endoscopic surgery, the need for canaloplasty is reduced, and the retroauricular approach is avoided, resulting in a less invasive procedure. Training in the technique in a dissection laboratory prior to its surgical use is recommended.

Disadvantages of the endoscope over the microscope include

- Use of one hand exclusively for holding the device
- Loss of depth perception
- Need for frequent cleaning of the device lens
- Competition for space with instruments
- Difficulty in field hemostasis

Basic Technique

For the application of the endoscope in middle ear surgery, it is necessary to set up the operating room before starting the procedure. The video tower should be ideally positioned in front of the surgeon and at eye level, in order to cause as little neck discomfort as possible during the procedure. The surgical team should position themselves on the opposite side of the surgeon and the microscope should be close, allowing easy access when and if necessary. In case of difficulty in hemostasis, consideration should be given to converting the procedure to the microscope. Alternatively, the surgeon may choose to perform the endoscopic procedure standing up, similarly to nasosinusal endoscopic surgeries, or sitting down.

Similar to the microscopic technique, both arms must be supported during the procedure. The camera should be held firmly, with the endoscope shaft resting gently over the cartilaginous external meatus. The dominant hand should be used for instrumentation.

It is recommended to perform a trichotomy of the external acoustic meatus to avoid soiling the endoscope lens. When the camera is introduced, there may be compression of the external canal walls over its fiber, which must be avoided. Optical compression leads to image distortion during the procedure and possible equipment damage. It is recommended to place a container with *defoger substance* close to the surgical field, in order to reduce the time required for cleaning the optics.

Care with hemostasis does not differ from the microscopic technique: reverse Trendelenburg decubitus, infiltration with lidocaine + epinephrine 1: 100,000 and/or use of cotton soaked in epinephrine for local hemostasis. Infiltration, when performed, should be performed slowly in the posterior–superior portion of the canal due to the richer vascular anatomy in this location.

The heat dissipation of the endoscope over the surgical field is potentially harmful. Light intensity should be maintained at less than 50% and a minimum distance of 5 mm between the endoscope tip and noble structures, such as the facial nerve and oval and round windows. Frequent saline instillations help to reduce the temperature in the field. In order to reduce the risk of trauma to the middle ear structures with the endoscope tip, it is recommended to always keep it lateral to the tympanic annulus.

Initially, the right-handed surgeon may feel more comfortable operating on the left ear. This is due to less compression due to the anterior angulation of the external meatus and the entrance of the camera more directly to the posterior recesses and ossicular chain.

The use of microscope instruments is often sufficient for endoscopic instrumentation. However, the adoption of angled instruments favors the manipulation of the surgical field, and many times it is necessary to acquire new materials for the full performance of the endoscopic surgery of the middle ear.

The making of the tympanomeatal flap must be adapted to the proposed surgery, varying the positions of the incisions and their extension, and their detachment performed uniformly and without tunneling. Fascia grafts can be harvested through an external incision or one can choose to extend the tympanic-meatal flap incision to the end of the bone canal, similarly to the Lempert incision. The skin flap is then elevated, accessing the temporal fascia through the same incision as the meatal flap and avoiding a more external incision.

At the end of the procedure, the tympanic-meatal flap is carefully repositioned to its original position, the external auditory canal is completely and firmly filled with pieces of surgical sponge, slightly moistened up to the height of the incisions. The external auditory meatus is sealed with hydrophilic gauze soaked in antibiotic ointment and the external dressing made locally.

Principles of Tympanoplasty

Over the years, definitions and classifications of tympanoplasty have been proposed by various authors but still today the one presented by Wüllstein is used by most otologic surgeons:

Myringoplasty: Refers to a procedure in which a tissue graft is used to close a perforation of the tympanic membrane. The most commonly used tissue grafts are temporalis fascia, vein, ear lobe adipose tissue, and subcutaneous connective tissue. Some authors define myringoplasty as a surgery confined to the drumhead itself, with no instrumentation of the middle ear and without lifting the membrane from its original position.

Tympanoplasty: Includes all procedures when the drum is lifted from its position in the ear canal and there is instrumentation of the middle ear cleft. According to the magnitude of the procedure, it can be divided into five subgroups:

Type I Tympanoplasty: Is usually performed by an approach through the external auditory canal and consists of exploration of the middle ear, the inspection of the ossicular chain and possible removal of minor disorders. The drumhead is repaired with an autogenous tissue graft.

Type II Tympanoplasty: Implies a surgical operation to remove the disease, followed by a reconstructive procedure to re-establish the lever mechanism of the ossicular system. It is usually performed through the external auditory canal and includes the removal of the posterosuperior bony meatal rim as well as repair of the tympanic membrane defect. The most common ossicular reconstruction is the introduction of a bone or cartilage graft between an eroded incus and the head of the stapes.

Type III Tympanoplasty: Is performed when the disease precludes a re-establishment of a normal sound-conducting system. It implies removal of the diseased tissue from the middle ear cleft and mastoid and preparation of the ear for either advancement of the tympanic membrane to the head of the stapes or placement of a tissue graft on the head of the stapes.

Type IV Tympanoplasty: Is performed when ossicular disease is extensive, including absence of the supra-structure of the stapes. Here the tympanic membrane or a tissue graft bridges the hypotympanic cavity and exteriorizes the oval window niche. The sound waves pass directly to through the footplate while the round window membrane remains protected in an air-containing pocket ventilated by the Eustachian tube.

Type V Tympanoplasty: It can be performed in a special situation when a type III or IV tympanoplasty succeeds in eliminating the disease process and a protected aerated hypotympanum has been established but hearing has not improved because of fixation of the footplate. A second procedure is performed as an attempt to create a fistula on the lateral semicircular canal or removing the footplate and sealing the vestibule with an autologous tissue. Both type IV and V tympanoplasty are rarely performed nowadays.

Tympanoplasty: Traditional Guidelines

Modern practice dictates grafting the tympanic membrane defect with connective tissue, most commonly with temporalis fascia. This fascia acts as a scaffolding to support regenerating mucosa on the medial aspect of the drum or squamous epithelium on the lateral side of the drum. Consequently, the fascia may be inserted below the drum remnant (underlay technique) or above the drum remnant (overlay technique). Both techniques show similar healing and hearing results and both have pros and cons. As we said before capable otologists who are advocates of either technique appear to obtain almost identical results.

In our group, we have employed both techniques. The choice of one or another is dependent on the patient's characteristics.

Underlay

This technique was originally described by Shea and Austin and Shea subsequently made further refinements. We preferably use the underlay technique in the first surgery of a central dry perforation. Regarding the approach, we employ the transcanal approach when the case fulfils the following conditions: (1) first surgery; (2) large external auditory meatus; (3) simple chronic otitis media; (4) central perforation; (5) air-bone gap less than 25 dB; and (6) all the margins are visible. The retroauricular approach is preferred whenever (1) revision surgery; (2) narrow external auditory meatus; (3) cholesteatoma or granulation tissue—mastoid instrumentation is anticipated-; (4) marginal perforation; (5) air–bone gap greater than 25 dB; and (6) anterior margin is not visible.

The surgical technique of the underlay tympanoplasty is briefly summarized in Table 48.5.

The advantages of this technique are its simplicity, previous margin blunting and graft lateralization are avoided, and the drum stays at the correct level relative to the annulus and ossicles. The disadvantages include limited exposure of the middle ear contents, increased failure rates due to limited bed size for the graft, reduced middle ear space, and facilitating intratympanic adhesions.

Table 48.5 Transcanal Underlay Tympanoplasty: Step by step technique

OTOLOGIC SURGERY
Surgical Technique

Transcanal Underlay Tympanoplasty

1. **Canal incisions at 6 and 12 h**
2. **Elevation of the tympanomeatal flap**
3. **Freshen the margins of the perforation**
4. **Exploratory tympanotomy**
5. **Fascia graft placement under the drum remnant**
6. **Gelfoam packing**
7. **Return the fascia and the tympanomeatal flap to position**
8. **Packing the external auditory canal**

Overlay

The modern overlay tympanoplasty is credited to Sheehy and Glasscock (apud [8]). We generally employ this technique in multiple interventions and marginal perforations. We always use the behind the ear approach in this situation.

The surgical technique of the overlay tympanoplasty is briefly summarized in Tables 48.6 and 48.7.

The advantages of this technique are the excellent visualization of the anterior meatal recess, higher success rates because the drum is replaced almost "in toto" and the middle ear space is not reduced. The disadvantages are well known and include the blunting of the anterior meatal recess, the lateralization of the graft, thickening of the neotympanum, squamous cyst formation if the drum is not completely denuded, and the technique is too laborious for small central perforations.

Table 48.6 Postauricular Overlay Tympanoplasty: Step by step technique

OTOLOGIC SURGERY
Surgical Technique

Postauricular Overlay Tympanoplasty

1.Verical canal incisions at 11 and 01 h
2.Horizontal incision close to the annulus between 11 and 1 h
3.Retrograde elevation of the vascular strip
4.Horizontal incision at the border of the speculum from 1 to 11 h
5.Postauricular incision
6.Temporalis fascia harvest
7.Anterior transposition of the pinna and the vascular strip
8.Dissection of the canal wall skin
9.Dissection of the skin from the annulus

Table 48.7 Postauricular Overlay Tympanoplasty: Step by step technique (cont.)

OTOLOGIC SURGERY
Surgical Technique

Postauricular Overlay Tympanoplasty

10.Anterior and posterior canaloplasty
11.Cleaning of the tympanic membrane remnants
12.Exploratory tympanotomy and ossiculoplasty
13.Trimming the fascia and the canal skin
14.Positioning the fascia and the canal skin
15.Packing the anterior angle and the external canal
16.Suturing the postauricular wound
17.Applying the dressings

Surgical Approaches Involving Bone Removal

Knowledge and mastery of the surgical approaches (together with their adaptations) discussed in this chapter are basic for performing any surgical procedure on the temporal bone. A correctly chosen approach makes possible a series of possibilities or additional steps that will be guided primarily and exclusively by the underlying disease and the transoperative findings. Even though the description of these steps goes beyond the objectives of this chapter, we will briefly review the main bony approaches to the middle ear/mastoid complex. For more details, the reader should consult specific chapters in this book.

Simple Mastoidectomy

This surgery was first described by Riolanus in 1649, and Petit in 1736 was the first to successfully perform it [15]. Surgery fell into ostracism until 1873 for having caused the death of the royal physician of Denmark, operated under inappropriate conditions [16]. Schwartze, in 1873, was the first to systematize this procedure, detailing its technique and indications [17]. In the late nineteenth century, pre-antibiotic times, surgery enjoyed general acceptance and was proclaimed an unsurpassed measure in saving lives.

Simple mastoidectomy involves total exenteration of the mastoid cell system, without interfering with the middle ear content and preserving the posterior wall of the external auditory canal. Its main indications are coalescent mastoiditis, exposure of the endolymphatic sac, trans-labyrinthine, and perilabyrinthine procedures.

Radical Mastoidectomy

In 1873, Von Tröltsch introduced a modification of Schwartze's simple mastoidectomy with the aim of preventing persistent postoperative otorrhea resulting from the presence of residual pathology in the mastoid [18]. The term "radical" was later coined by Von Bergmann for those cases in which the posterior and superior walls of the external auditory canal were removed [19]. In 1889, Cluster described this surgery as it is known today (apud [11]).

This procedure allows the complete exenteration of the pathology located in the tympanic cavity, antrum, and mastoid with the consequent creation of a cavity where the middle ear and external auditory canal merge into a single structure with regular edges and surfaces, exteriorized through the external acoustic meatus which is surgically enlarged (meatoplasty).

The surgery is performed after a retroauricular incision. Bone removal can be done by two different routes: from the outside to the inside (*outside-in,* when the antrum is explored through the mastoid fossa, like a simple mastoidectomy) or from the inside to the outside (*inside-out,* when the external auditory canal, it is widened by drilling the posterior wall, followed by an atticotomy and exposure of the antrum via an aditus). This technique exposes several important structures such as the stapes, the facial nerve, and the lateral semicircular canal, ensuring their protection from inadvertent injuries. The posterior wall is lowered almost to the level of the facial nerve canal and the diseased mastoid cells are completely removed. After this step has been completed, the remains of the eardrum are removed along with the ossicles (with the exception of the stapes), the middle ear mucosa, and the tensor tympani. The Eustachian tube opening is obstructed, and a generous meatoplasty is performed.

This technique is indicated in extensive or recurrent tympanic-mastoid pathologies associated with intracranial complications or in which restoration of auditory function, even partially, is not feasible. Also done in some procedures for resection of temporal bone tumors.

Modified Radical Mastoidectomy

This procedure had its technical development from radical mastoidectomies through surgical variants that aimed at preserving hearing. Some authors such as Jansen and Körner suggested the preservation of ossicles and tympanic membrane in certain radical surgeries, but it was Bondy in 1910 who originally described the modified radical mastoidectomy [20, 21].

Bondy's technique has common aspects with radical surgery, but the middle ear content is preserved intact. Access can be retroauricular or endaural. An extensive tympanomeatal flap is made with two vertical incisions, respectively, at **6 and 9 o'clock,** which are extended to the tympanic annulus. This flap is raised, the upper wall of the canal is removed, and the posterior wall is lowered to the level of the facial nerve canal. Next, the cholesteatoma is removed from the attic and, subsequently, from the antrum, allowing its matrix to be preserved. The skin flap is then rotated to cover the attic and mastoid region. Years later, meatoplasty was incorporated into this procedure.

Modified radical mastoidectomy is indicated exclusively for attic-antral cholesteatoma with normal mesotympanum, *pars flaccida perforations,* and hearing within normal limits.

Open Tympanomastoidectomy (Wall Down)

The development of surgical otomicroscopy enabled the creation and incorporation of several tympanoplasty techniques to Bondy's modified radical mastoidectomy. Open tympanomastoidectomy is nothing more than a refinement of Bondy's technique, associated with surgical instrumentation of the middle ear for the removal of pathological processes with modern tympanoplasty techniques.

We indicate this technique in cholesteatoma recurrences after initial use of the closed technique, in large cholesteatomas with destruction of the posterior wall, in dehiscence of the middle fossa floor and in cases of natural lateral sinus that preclude adequate access to the antrum. We also employ this technique in some special syndromic populations.

Closed or Combined Tympanomastoidectomy (or Wall Up)

In 1958, Jansen described posterior tympanotomy [22]. Other ear surgeons have also described it in detail, including Sheehy & Patterson [23] and Glasscock III and Miller [24]. This technique, in addition to preserving the anatomical configuration of the ear, launched the pillars for the appearance of the so-called combined tympanomastoidectomy or canal wall-up tympanomastoidectom.

In this procedure, the posterior wall of the external auditory canal is kept intact, and the pathology of the middle ear is exposed through the opening of the facial nerve recess.

Initially, a simple mastoidectomy is performed and, after identifying the fossa incudis, a triangular area limited superiorly by the bone of the incudal fossa (incus buttress), medially by the superior mastoid segment of the facial nerve and laterally by the chorda tympani nerve is identified and the bone is initially removed with a large cutting bur, which is gradually replaced by smaller diamond burs until the facial recess is opened and enlarged, allowing the visualization of the pyramidal eminence, the oval and round windows, the tympanic segment of the facial nerve, the cochleariform process, and the ET ostium. After complete removal of the pathological tissues, the ear is reconstructed and the eardrum grafted with a fascia, perichondrium, or periosteum.

This technique is indicated in cases of middle ear cholesteatomata, chronic otitis media with granulation tissue, facial nerve decompression, tympanic glomus, and cochlear implants.

Anteroposterior Mastoidectomy

Farrior, in 1968, described and advocated the performance of a simple mastoidectomy associated with an anterior atticotomy, hypotympanectomy, and tympanoplasty [25]. This access offers flexibility in viewing and removing pathologies located in the mesotympanum, epitympanum, and mastoid.

Its approach is similar to the combined tympanomastoidectomy, with the difference that, in anteroposterior mastoidectomy, performing an atticotomy increases the exposure of the middle ear by removing the bone from the upper wall of the EAC and *scutum*. A 2 mm bone bridge is maintained between the *tegmen* and the most posterior portion of the EAC, separating the atticotomy anteriorly and the mastoid cavity posteriorly. Before middle ear reconstruction, the aditus is obliterated with muscle, cartilage, or bone pate in order to avoid the formation of a secondary retraction pocket.

This approach is indicated in cases of primary cholesteatomas involving the *scutum* or extending posteriorly to the stapes in patients with well-pneumatized temporal bones.

Osteoplastic Epitimpanotomy

This surgery developed by Sabrina Wullstein combines wide exposure of attico-antral cholesteatomas with maintenance of the EAC superior wall with a normal configuration [26].

After removing the bony surface above and behind the EAC, the meatal skin on the superior and posterior walls is elevated to the node of Rivinus. These walls are thinned at the same time that the EAC is enlarged without, however, penetrating the antral and attic cells. A bony lip to be removed is demarcated with the aid of a diamond bur and deepened enough until it can be broken and removed with a dissector. Thus, a wide attic-antral exposure is obtained.

The cholesteatoma is removed, the middle ear is reconstructed, the cortical bony lamina is replaced, and the tympanic graft is positioned. This technique is indicated for cholesteatomas confined to the attic-antral region.

Intact Bridge Tympanomastoidectomy (IBM)

Open-cavity mastoidectomy is usually relatively successful in removing mastoid and middle ear disease. However, it has well-known drawbacks, namely, a life-long cavity and poor hearing results in most cases. The closed-cavity technique, on the other hand, has better preservation of function, but traditionally a higher failure rate in eradicating disease and more challenging surgical steps. In the early eighties, Paparella developed the IBM with the objective of minimizing the undesirable complications of open cavities, and at the same time, eradicating the disease and reconstructing the middle ear in a single surgical step [27]. He proclaimed that, with this procedure, it was possible to combine the positive aspects of both open and closed techniques, with low recurrence rates associated with considerable auditory gains. The IBM is indicated for patients with chronic otitis media and mastoiditis, intractable cholesteatoma, cholesterol granuloma, or granulation tissue in the mastoid, middle ear, or attic, either as a first operation or, if there has been prior surgery, to revise where the earlier procedure has left an intact posterior canal wall or bridge. Because most patients with chronic otitis media and mastoiditis do have small, sclerotic, hypocellular mastoids, they are ideal candidates for the IBM.

Both the endaural or retroauricular approaches may be employed. The fascia of the temporal muscle is removed, followed by elevation of a large tympanomeatal flap and complete exposure of the mastoid cortex. In the next step, the walls of the EAC are drilled as much as possible, performing a plastic surgery of this canal that allows a 360° visualization of the eardrum or its remnants. When indicated, a thorough open mastoidectomy is done, preserving the bridge. The height and sculpturing of the bridge will depend upon the presence of disease in the region. The height of the bridge should be enough to provide an increase of the posterior mesotympanic space and allowing adequate removal of pathologic tissue in the mastoid. The aditus is also enlarged to remove diseased tissue in the epitympanic space. In cases presenting with extensive disease affecting the attic, an atticotomy should be added to the procedure. The facial or suprapyramidal recess is cleaned but not drilled open. The mastoidectomy should extend to the point where all pathologic tissue is removed, and the bony walls seen are free from disease. Through this technique, the middle ear is enlarged in depths and diameter, which facilitates tympanoplasty and ossiculoplasty, as well as removal of pathology. The Atticus and the shape and location of the bridge are important to accomplish the goal through improved visualization. After the necessary instrumentation of the middle ear is completed a wide meatoplasty is performed, which accommodates the introduction of the surgeon's index finger. Obliteration of the mastoid, as well as the use of a free skin graft, are optional.

Soft Tissue Complementary Steps

Meatoplasty

Meatoplasty is a surgical procedure that aims to enlarge the opening of the external ear and create a skin flap that will serve as a matrix in the epithelialization of the neocavity. In 1893, Stacke described for the first time the external acoustic meatus skin flap as a complement to the radical mastoidectomy described by Zaufal in 1890 [28].

Meatoplasty has become an essential complementary surgical procedure in open cavity tympanomastoidectomy and in surgeries of the stenosed external auditory canal. It may also be employed as a complementary surgical step in canaloplasty, tympanoplasty, closed cavity tympanomastoidectomy, and in some otoneurological procedures [29]. Also, in cases of congenital or acquired stenosis (refractory external otitis, trauma, neoplasms, and iatrogenesis) of the external auditory canal, performing a meatoplasty is fundamental. The new meatus will be defined by the remodeling of four types of tissues: skin, cartilage, subcutaneous tissue, and bone. Which of these planes will be manipulated will depend on the pathology in question, the main surgical procedure performed and the size of the desired opening [30].

An adequate meatal opening allows us easy access to the auditory canal, tympanic membrane, and open neocavities, providing the handling of these regions for proper postoperative *toilet* [31].

Accompanying the main surgical procedure, the meatoplasty can be performed through endaural or retroauricular approaches. We opted for the second one for being more practical since we will have a direct view of all manipulated structures.

Although the meatoplasty is commonly the last surgical step in the main procedure, it should be remembered that the first incisions in the skin of the canal coincide with the first steps of meatoplasty.

The surgical technique involves two vertical incisions made at 1 and 5 o'clock, extending superiorly into the canal and joining inferiorly 5 mm from the tympanic annulus. These incisions will delimit the caudal portion of the Köerner flap [32]. After completing the work done on the mastoid and middle ear, we removed the self-retaining retractors, control any residual bleeding, and proceed with the meatoplasty.

For such the surgeons holds the ear with the index finger and thumb in tweezers, pushing the concha backwards with the middle finger, which will have the function of support and guide for tissue dissection. As we dissect the subcutaneous tissue, we pinch it and pull it upwards. The excess of this tissue can be removed and discarded.

We identified and released the conchae cartilage from the skin anteriorly. Its free edge is then resected in an ellipse, without approaching its upper portion. At this moment, the sensitivity of the pulp of the middle finger and the constant visualization of the concha anteriorly will prevent trauma to the skin in this region. The next step will be the lengthening of the vertical canal incisions. The higher they extend toward the free skin of the concha, the greater the amplitude of the meatus. A good parameter is when the meatus freely accepts the index finger. A generous skin flap is thus created, the Köerner flap, which should be as wide as possible, intact, neither thick nor thin.

After making the flap, we apply one or two 3-zero vicryl sutures, close to its base to the neighboring subcutaneous tissue superiorly, with the aim of pulling it backward, which will promote healing tension, forcing the flap against the bone wall of the neocavity.

Finally, we filled the newly created cavity with cardiac tape with antibiotic ointment. This plug will be removed in 2 weeks, during which time systemic antibiotic coverage may be extended. At the end of 45 days, depending on the level of granulation observed, the cavity, if not properly and completely healed may be covered with thin free skin flaps taken from the medial region of the arm (Thiersch Graft). This procedure, however, is rarely necessary.

References

1. Lempert J. Tympanosympathectomy: a surgical technic for the relift of tinnitus aurium. Arch Otolaryngol. 1946;43:199–212.
2. Gulya AJ. Soft tissue incisions and approaches. In: Nadol JB, Schuknecht HF, editors. Surgery of the ear and temporal bone. New York: Raven Press; 1993.
3. Epley JM. Reflexogenic vertigo treated by tensor tympanic transection. Otolaryngol Head Neck Surg. 1981;89:849–53.
4. Gacek RR. Transection of the posterior ampullary nerve for the relief of benign paroxysmal positional vertigo. Ann Othol Rhinol Laryngol. 1974;83:596–605.
5. Glasscock ME III, Harris PE, Newsome G. Glomus tumors: diagnosis and treatment. Laryngoscope. 1974;84:2006–32.
6. Schuknecht HF. Myringoplasty. Clin Otolaryngol. 1976;1:53–65.
7. Hammerschlag PE, Schuknecht HF. Transcanal labyrinthectomy for intractable vertigo. Arch Otolaryngol. 1981;107:152–6.
8. Glasscock ME III, Shambaugh GE. Surgery of the ear. Philadelphia: WB Sauders Company; 1999.
9. Nadol JB, Schuknecht HF, editors. Surgery of the ear and temporal bone. New York: Raven Press; 1993.
10. Goycoolea MV, Paparella MM, Nissen RL. Atlas of otologic surgery. Philadelphia: WB Saunders; 1989.
11. Miglets A, Paparella MM, Saunders WH. Atlas of ear surgery. 4th ed. Saint Louis: Mosby Company; 1986.
12. Lempert J. Improvement of hearing in cases of otosclerosis. Arch Otolaryngol. 1938;28:42–97.
13. Alleva M, Paparella MM, Morris MS, da Costa SS. The flexible/intact brigde tympanomastoidectomy technique. Otolaryngol Clin North Am. 1989;2:41–50.
14. Shupak A, Doweck I, Greenberg E. Diving related inner ear injuries. Laryngoscope. 1991;101:173–9.
15. Petit JL. Trailé des maladies chirugicales. Paris; 1774.
16. Ballance CA. Essays on the surgery of temporal bone. London: Mc Millan; 1919.
17. Scwartze HH, Eysell CG. Uber die Kunstliche Eröffnung des Warzenfortsatzes. Arch Ohrenh. 1983;7:156.
18. Von Trölsch AF. Lehrbuch der ohrenheilkunde mit einschluss der anatomie des ohres. Leipzig: Fogel; 1873.
19. Von Bergmann E. Die chirurgische behandlung von himkrankheiten. Berlin; 1889.
20. Bondy G. Totalaufmeisselun mit erhaltung von trommelfell und gehörknöchelchen. Dermatol Monatsschr. 1910;44:15.
21. Körner O. Die eitrigen erkrakungen des schläfenbeins. Wiesbaden: Bergmann; 1899.
22. Jansen C. Über radikaloperation und tympanoplastik. Sitz ber Fortbild Arztekann Ob. 1958;18:2–7.

23. Sheehy JL, Patterson ME. Intact canal wall tympanoplasty with mastoidectomy. Laryngoscope. 1967;77:1502.
24. Glasscock ME III, Miller GW. Intact canal wall tympanoplasty in the Management of Cholesteatoma. Laryngoscope. 1976;86:1639.
25. Farrior JB. Tympanoplasty in 3D. Rochester, MN: American Academy of Ophthalmology and Otolaryngology; 1968.
26. Wüllstein SR. Osteoplastic epytympanotomy. Ann Othol Rhinol Laryngol. 1974;83:663.
27. Paparella MM, Jung TTK. Intact brigde tympanomastoidectomy (IBM): combined essentials feature of open vs. closed procedures. J Laryngol Otol. 1983;97:575–85.
28. Shambaugh GE, Glasscock ME. Tympanoplasty. In: Surgery of the ear. 3rd ed. Philadelphia: Saunders; 1980.
29. Meyerhoff WL, Pollock KJ, Roland PS, Mickey B. Modified Rambo meatoplasty in translabyrinthine tumor removal. Otolaryngol Head Neck Surg. 1991;104:100–2.
30. Portman M, Guerrier Y. Traité de technique chirurgicale ORL et cervico-faciale. Take 1. Masson Cic; 1975.
31. Osborne JE, Terryrm, Gandhi AG. Large meatoplasty technique for mastoid cavities. Clin Otolaryngol North Am. 1985;10:357–60.
32. Blake P, Morrissey G. Canal wall down techiques for managing cholesteatoma. Aust NZJ Surg. 1991;61:914–8.

Tympanoplasty: Underlay Technique Step by Step and the Complex Tympanoplasty

49

Fábio André Selaimen, Mauricio Noschang Lopes da Silva, and Sady Selaimen da Costa

Introduction

Current tympanoplasty techniques involve repairing the tympanic membrane defect by placing a graft over or under the borders of the perforation. The graft works as a bridge, allowing regeneration of the squamous epithelium of the external ear, on its lateral side, and of the middle ear mucosa, on its medial side. The surgical technique may vary depending on the access, the position of the graft, and the reconstruction (or not) of the ossicular chain.

Regarding the surgical approaches, there are four described techniques:

- Transcanal: the surgeon works through the ear specula, which can be affixed to the table using a specific device (holder), or by the surgeon's nondominant hand.
- Endoscopic: with the advent of endoscopic ear surgery, the transcanal approach is being redefined, with a broader view and novel possibilities.
- Endaural: through the Lempert I, II, and III incisions and positioning of the autostatic retractors.
- Retroauricular: described subsequently in this chapter.

The four approaches are debated in a specific chapter in this book, with a step-by-step descriptions, indications, and illustrations. We suggest reading the specific chapter. In our group, we prefer the retroauricular, as it provides greater exposure and, therefore, the greater possibility of managing unforeseen intraoperative events. Below we list the criteria needed to use the transcanal or endaural approach:

F. A. Selaimen (✉) · M. N. L. da Silva
Hospital de Clínicas de Porto Alegre, Porto Alegre, Brazil

Instituto Gaúcho de Otorrinolaringologia, Porto Alegre, Brazil

S. S. da Costa
Hospital de Clínicas de Porto Alegre, Porto Alegre, Brazil

Universidade Federal do Rio Grande do Sul, Porto Alegre, Brazil

Instituto Gaúcho de Otorrinolaringologia, Porto Alegre, Brazil

- First surgery.
- Favorable external auditory canal (EAC).
- Absence of cholesteatoma.
- Tympanic perforation in the posterior quadrants.
- Air–bone gap less than 25 dB.
- All visible borders of the perforation.

When the above criteria are not met, which occurs in most patients who come to our offices, the retroauricular approach will be preferred.

Regarding the graft position, the two surgical techniques traditionally used are the underlay, which places the graft under the tympanic remnant (Austin's medial technique), and the overlay, which places the graft over the remnant (Sheehy's lateral technique). Experienced otologists obtain almost identical results with the chosen technique. Also, in smaller perforations, it is possible to use the inlay technique when the graft is positioned in the same plane as the tympanic membrane.

In our group, we preferentially use the underlay technique, which will be detailed subsequently. The advantages of this surgical technique of tympanoplasty consist in its simplicity, in the ability to avoid deletion of the angle between the tympanic membrane and the EAC (blunting) or lateralization of the graft.

Pathogenesis-Oriented Surgery

As discussed in the chapter "Tympanic Membrane Perforations and Tympanoplasty: New Profiles, New Strategies" we are critical of the traditional classification of tympanic perforations as central or marginal. We strongly recommend reading the specific chapter, as the management described in the following paragraphs will be significantly influenced by the kind of perforation. The reason for our disagreement with the classification is that it expresses little about the probable pathogenesis of the perforation and also does not bring any specific changes in surgical management.

M. V. Goycoolea et al. (eds.), *Textbook of Otitis Media*, https://doi.org/10.1007/978-3-031-40949-3_49

On the other hand, the classification as *inside-out* or *outside-in*, based on signs of previous retraction, allows us to infer the pathogenesis of the perforation. In summary, it attempts to differentiate a previously healthy ear from a chronically dysfunctional one.

In line with this reasoning, the treatment guided by the pathogenesis will be very differentiated according to the type of perforation. In the group of *inside–out* perforations, the proposed pathogenesis translates to a healthy middle ear, which suffered punctual aggression in time that led to the perforation. Thus, the surgical treatment only aims to "close the hole."

The *outside–in* perforations translate to the end of a chronic dysfunctional middle ear, with deaeration, probably originating from the Eustachian tube dysfunction. This chronic negative pressure in the middle ear will develop a progressive retraction of the tympanic membrane until its segmental necrosis due to ischemia, thus generating the perforation. This journey of the normal until the perforated tympanic membrane leaves marks in its path: the four described signs of retraction associated with the perforation. Thus, in addition to just "closing the hole" (as in the *inside-out* perforation), more steps will be needed to reestablish the physiology of the middle ear in the outside–in. We can list the additional steps that may be required according to each case:

- The use of more resistant grafts, such as cartilage associated with the temporal fascia (double graft), thus preventing future retraction.
- The insertion of a concomitant ventilation tube, thus ensuring adequate ventilation in the immediate- and midterm postoperative periods, mainly if the Eustachian tube function cannot be restored.
- Lateralization of the malleus (including sectioning the tendon of the tensor tympani), thus allowing air circulation from the Eustachian tube throughout the entire middle ear.
- Cleaning of epithelium adhered to the promontory (and often occupying posterior recesses), thus preventing the formation of a cholesteatoma in the future.
- The use of angled optics to inspect posterior recesses, hypotympanum and supratubal recesses.
- Ossicular chain reconstruction since ossicular erosion is more frequent in this group of perforations.
- Procedures aimed at improving Eustachian tube function.

The Simple Tympanoplasty

The term "simple tympanoplasty" traditionally refers only to the instrumentation of the middle ear. It receives this nomenclature because it is not associated with mastoidectomy, which would characterize tympanomastoidectomy. However, based on the study and reclassification of tympanic membrane perforations, we agreed to rename "simple" tympanoplasty the technique limited to the closure of the perforation. In other words, when additional procedures are not necessary to restore the physiology of the middle ear, tympanoplasty will receive the name "simple." It can be performed through any access route and following any graft positioning. We recommend it to be performed in patients with *inside-out* perforations since those are the perforations with a healthy middle ear in the background. The terminology contrasts the "complex tympanoplasty," recommended for *outside-in* perforations and in which additional procedures will be required, on demand, according to each patient, to reestablish normal physiology in the middle ear.

Surgery Description: Step by Step

Next, we will describe in detail and illustrate step-by-step, our preferred surgical technique: retroauricular approach, with the placement of the graft under the borders of the tympanic remnant (underlay). The standard technique of simple tympanoplasty for *inside-out* perforation will be initially described. Later in the chapter, we will describe the additional steps required in the *outside-in*.

Step 1: Preparation of the Surgical Field and Infiltration

After a small trichotomy of the retroauricular region, antisepsis of the operative field is performed. Subsequently, the surgical field is delimited with the placement of plastic or fabric drapes. The use of adhesive plastic drapes (Fig. 49.1) is very helpful, as it keeps the surgical drapes dry, even when there is a need for irrigation for mastoidectomy.

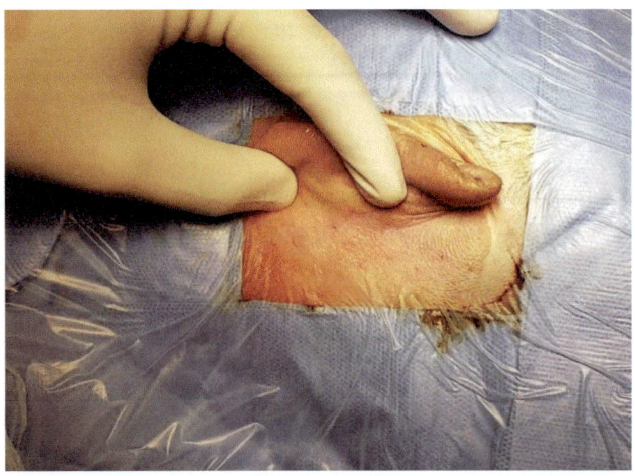

Fig. 49.1 Completion of preparation of the surgical field, delimited by plastic adhesive fields—left ear

Once the field is prepared, local infiltration is performed with a 2% xylocaine solution with adrenaline (1:1,000,000), waiting at least 5 min for the incision so that the rebound effect of adrenaline does not cause more bleeding than expected.

Step 2: Obtaining the Cartilage Graft (When Necessary)

When the surgeon chooses to perform a cartilage graft, we prefer cartilage from the tragus. In addition to minimal aesthetic and functional alteration with the incisions made, the tragus cartilage has, in most cases, the ideal thickness and shape for tympanoplasty. In addition, its slight concavity allows the edges of the cartilage to fit perfectly under the edges of the tympanic remnant.

Initially, an incision is performed in the tragus on the face of the EAC (Fig. 49.2a), using the entire length available (Fig. 49.2b). Afterward, the skin is detached from the perichondrium using delicate scissors with a curved tip. Once the entire posterior face of the cartilage is free (Fig. 49.2c), an incision is performed in the cartilage itself, transfixing it. In this incision, it is necessary to observe the preservation of the cartilage domus, maintaining at least 2 mm superiorly to prevent the tragus from collapsing and thus resulting in a very unpleasant esthetic defect.

With the use of tissue forceps, the cartilage is pulled posteriorly, and anterior detachment is performed, maintaining the perichondrium (Fig. 49.2d). Once the cartilage is free anteriorly and posteriorly, we make straight upper and lower incisions. Finally, an incision is made medially in the carti-

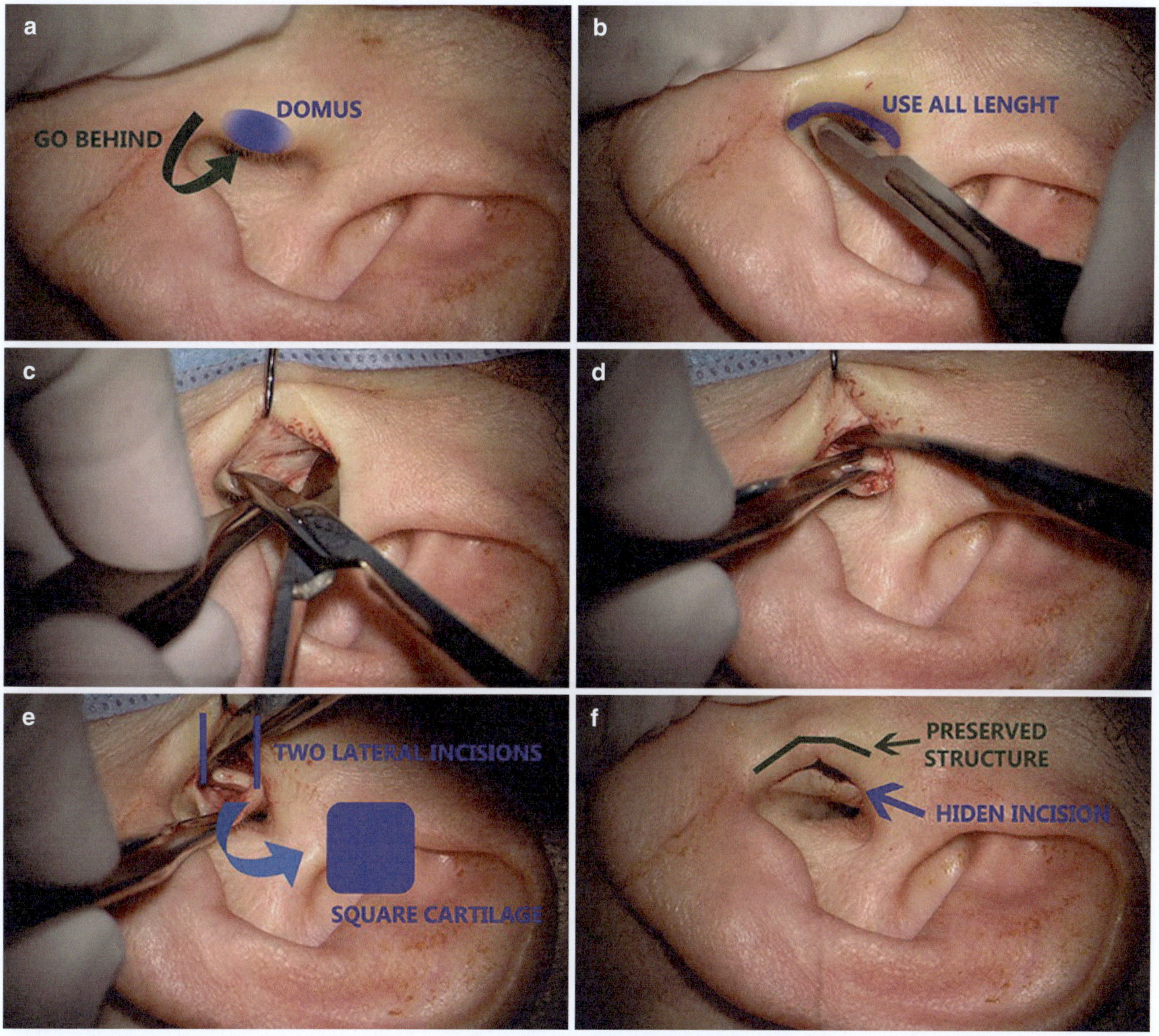

Fig. 49.2 Tragus cartilage removal, step by step. (**a**) Exposure of the EAC face of the tragus cartilage; (**b**) Demonstration of the skin incision (position and length); (**c**) Detachment of the skin and subcutaneous tissue, maintaining the cartilage perichondrium; (**d**) Incision of the anterior surface of the tragus cartilage; (**e**) Removal of cartilage in a square format; (**f**) Final appearance, with preserved structure (due to the preservation of the cartilage domus) and minimal aesthetic defect

lage, which will unify the previous incisions, resulting in a square cartilage, with the perichondrium preserved on both sides (Fig. 49.2e).

Finally, careful hemostasis is performed since exaggerated cauterization (even with bipolar cautery) can lead to necrosis of the thin skin of the tragus. The skin can be closed using a monofilament thread, absorbable or not. The 4-0 mononylon is preferred, as it generates less crust formation.

Step 3: Retroauricular Approach

The incision is performed approximately 1 cm behind the retroauricular sulcus (Fig. 49.3). Thus, it avoids lateral displacement of the pavilion in the immediate and late postoperative period, which can occur when the incision is made directly in the sulcus. In addition, it allows the creation of muscle-periosteal flaps suitable for wide exposure of the mastoid.

The dissection in the plane of the superficial fascia must continue until the contour of the membranous EAC portion is exposed in the region corresponding to the beginning of the zygomatic process above and the tip of the mastoid below.

Then, the temporal fascia must be obtained for the reconstruction of the tympanic membrane. With the autostatic retractor, the fascia of the pre-zygomatic region is exposed. Next, we perform a slight infiltration of 2% xylocaine solution in the plane between the fascia and the muscle, allowing an initial dissection and reduced bleeding (Fig. 49.4). After removing the fascia, it must be placed to dry on a sterile surface exposed to the environment. We do not recommend using a hot air source.

Back to the surgical field, an incision creates the muscle-periosteal flap. We usually make two incisions, one above and the other below the EAC, joined posteriorly by a vertical incision so that a quadrangular flap is designed, pedicled at the top, in continuity with the membranous portion of the EAC. The detachment is performed in a subperiosteal plane. Once the muscle-periosteal flap is completed (Fig. 49.5), the cribriform region, the Henle suprameatal spine, and the entire contour of the bony EAC are exposed, indicating the place where the detachment of the skin from the EAC will begin.

Step 4: EAC Incision and Skin Flaps

The next step is an incision in the skin of the EAC, in its posterior portion, performed after making the muscle-periosteal flap and consequent exposure of the lateral third. Thus, with a No. 15 scalpel blade, the skin is incised with penetration into the lumen of the canal via the posterior path. The incision should be made around 2–3 mm below the bone edge of the external acoustic meatus, thus preventing the tympanomeatal flap from becoming too thick. Figure 49.6 shows the EAC incision.

After the skin incision, allowing adequate exposure of the entire surgical field, the need for canaloplasty is evaluated. Before starting the detachment of the tympanomeatal flap, obtaining a 360° visualization of the tympanic membrane in the surgical field (without repositioning the microscope) is essential. Figure 49.7 illustrates a left ear where canaloplasty is required.

Step 5: Anterior Canaloplasty

After incision of the posterior flap and exposure of the EAC, if the TM cannot be entirely visualized (360°), canaloplasty is required (Fig. 49.8).

Using a 90° round knife, an incision is made in the anterior skin of the EAC immediately lateral to the tympanic ring

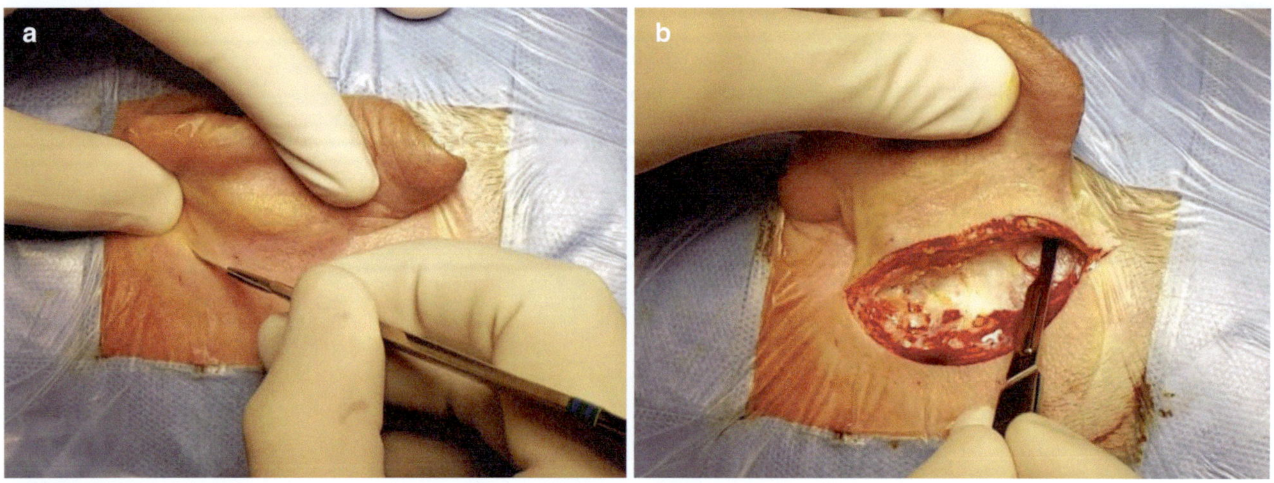

Fig. 49.3 Retroauricular incision—left ear. (**a**) Note that the surgeon's thumb demarcates the tip of the mastoid, preventing the incision from extending posteriorly and reducing the risk of injury to the facial nerve. (**b**) End of incision and beginning of detachment by planes

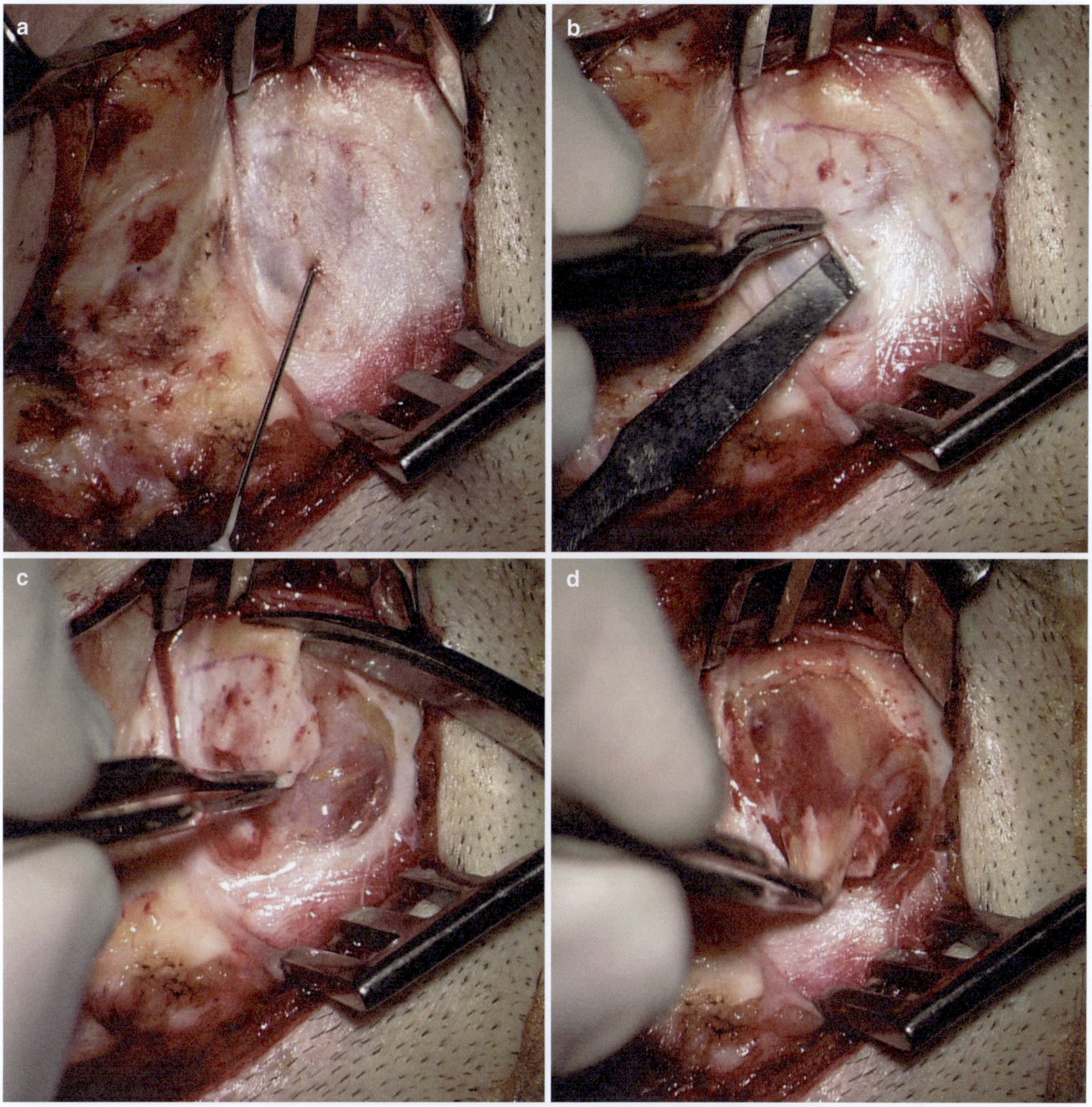

Fig. 49.4 Obtaining the temporal fascia—left ear. (**a**) Solution infiltration. (**b**) Detachment through a small incision. (**c**) Delimitation of the fascia. (**d**) Removal of the fascia by detachment

(Fig. 49.8a), pushing it laterally to create an anterior flap. Thus, the anterior bone canal can be smoothed with diamond burs until a complete 360° exposure of the TM is achieved.

At this stage, special care must be taken to prevent the temporomandibular joint capsule from being violated or jeopardizing the flaps with the drill.

Step 6: Revival of the Perforation Borders

After completing the access to the EAC and complete exposure of the TM with canaloplasty and before starting the detachment of the tympanomeatal flap, we proceeded to revive the perforation borders (Fig. 49.9). This step consists of the complete removal of the fibrous ring that encircles it, and the removal of small tympanosclerosis plaques that could affect the blood supply to the graft. This step can be performed with an ear needle or a sickle knife.

Step 7: Incisions of the EAC

A tympanomeatal flap is performed through skin incisions and detachment from the tympanic bone. First, two incisions

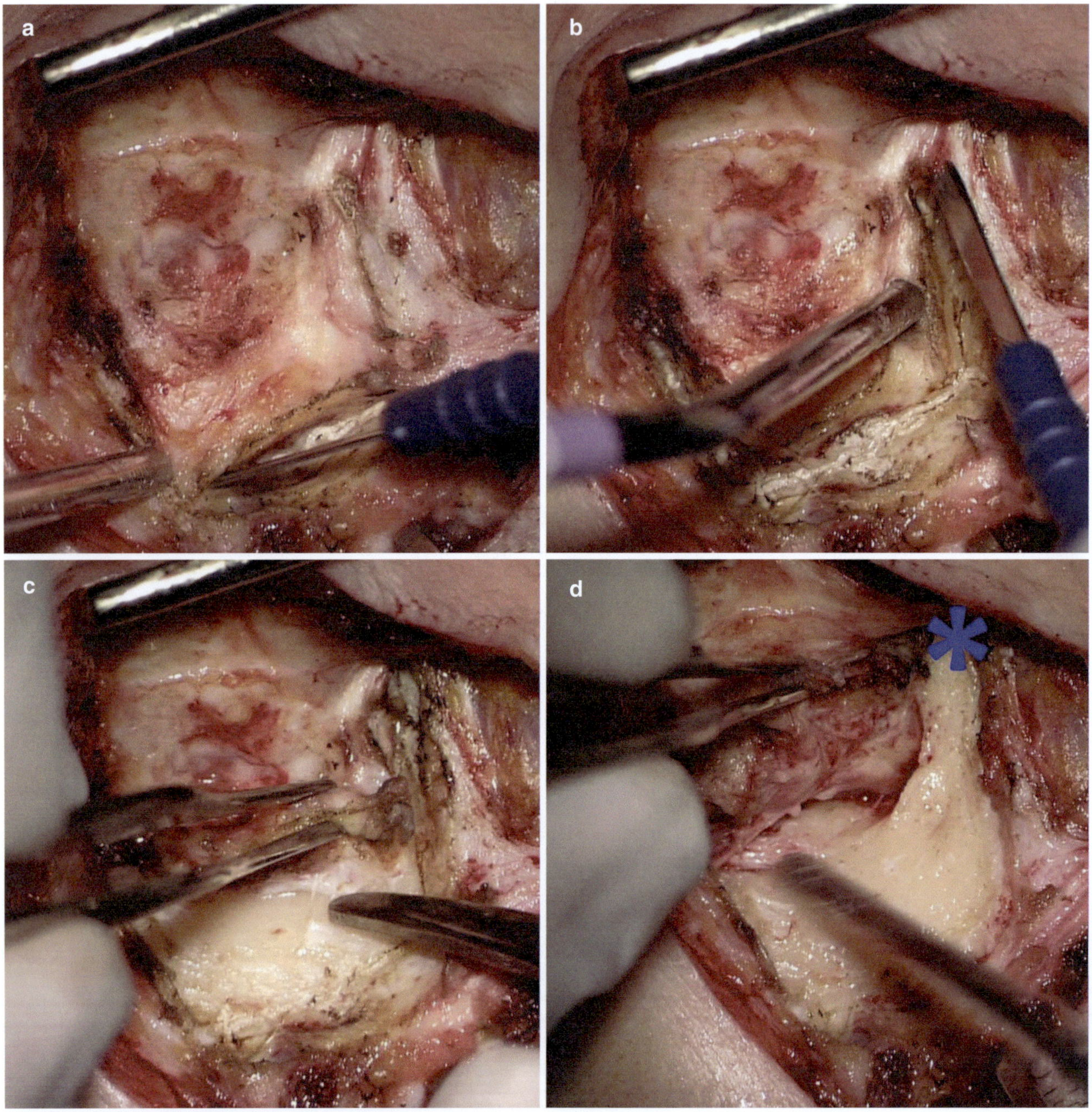

Fig. 49.5 Preparation of the muscle-periosteal flap—left ear. (**a**) Posterior incision. (**b**) Upper incision, parallel to the lower one, delimiting a quadrangular and anteriorly pedicled flap. (**c**) Detachment in the subperiosteal plane. (**d**) End of making the flap, delimiting the posterior wall of the EAC, and exposing the zygoma (blue asterisk)

are made, from medial to lateral, starting at the TM. Then, both incisions will be extended in the lateral direction until they meet the posterior EAC incision (which was made during the retroauricular approach). The upper incision begins lateral to and slightly posterior to the lateral process of the malleus (lateral to the sulcus of Rivinus). As a reference, we use the figure of an imaginary clock, whose 12 h are on the lateral process of the malleus. Therefore, the upper incision would correspond to 12 o'clock. The lower incision starts inferiorly, corresponding to 6 o'clock, and extends laterally to the end of the flap. Figure 49.10 illustrates those steps.

Step 8: Elevation of the Tympanomeatal Flap

Flap elevation must be performed with care and delicacy once the flap will partially provide the blood supply for tympanic healing; therefore, the less traumatic the dissection, the better the vascularization and, consequently, the healing. It can be done with a round knife (Fig. 49.11) or a flap elevator

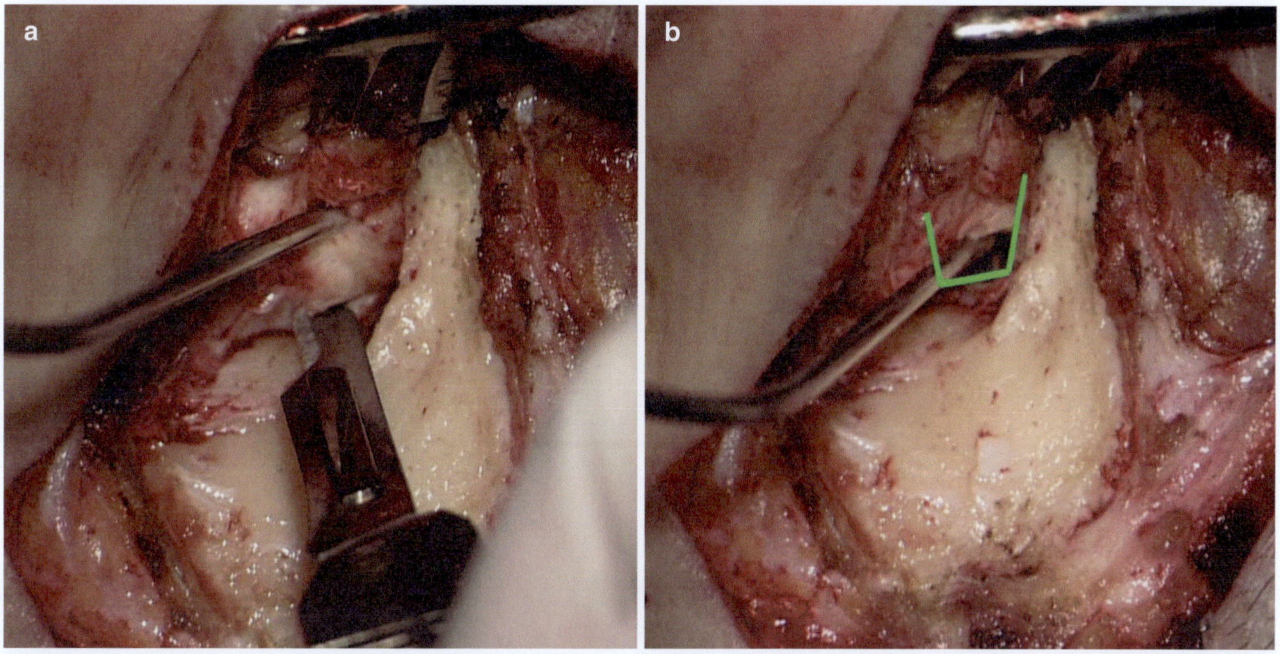

Fig. 49.6 EAC skin incision, posterior approach—left ear. (**a**) The skin is incised with a scalpel. (**b**) Rectangular incision, delimited superiorly and inferiorly, avoiding maceration of the EAC skin during ear traction

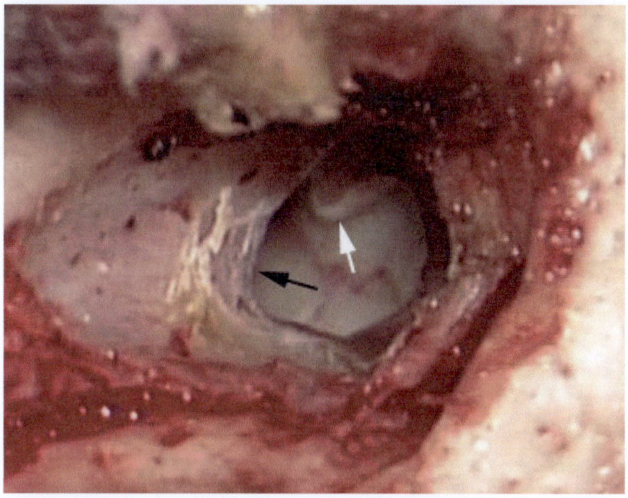

Fig. 49.7 Need for the canaloplasty—left ear. Note that we cannot see the anterior and inferior edges of the TM. Note the short distance between the anterior limit of the ECA (black arrow) and the malleus (white arrow), inferring that the EAC hides the anterior quadrants

(Rosen, Beales, or Hughes). Often, the use of cotton soaked in adrenaline can help in hemostasis, while it helps in the detachment of the skin.

Step 9: Middle Ear Access and Inspection

Once the flap has been detached medially to the level of the tympanic ring, we can identify the region where the tympanic ring is less firmly attached to the tympanic sulcus, that is, the posterosuperior quadrant (see chapter Tympanoplasty: From Basics to Beyond). Thus, an incision is performed between the EAC posterior bony wall and the tympanic annulus (Fig. 49.12) with a delicate instrument (needle or sickle scalpel). The chorda tympani nerve will sometimes be visible before the bony posterior wall. Thus, we make the incision between the annulus and the chorda tympani nerve. Next, this incision is enlarged superiorly to the lateral process of the malleus (12 o'clock) and inferiorly until the cells of the infracochlear tract of the mastoid are exposed (6 o'clock). In this way, we have an extensive exposure of the middle ear so that we proceed to inspect all structures to confirm (or eventually change, in case of findings not seen in the preoperative evaluation) the initial surgical plan.

The presence of tympanic remnants over the ossicular chain (except malleus) or adhered to the promontory should be considered signs of retraction associated with the perforation, characterizing it as an *outside-in* perforation. In those cases, additional steps may be necessary, not simply "closing the hole." Thus, we agreed to call surgery with additional steps "complex tympanoplasty," which will be addressed later in this chapter.

A perforation will be classified as *inside-out* if it does not show signs of retraction. We remind the reader that, at this moment, we describe "simple tympanoplasty." This procedure consists of the simple closure of the tympanic perforation, either with fascia graft, cartilage graft, or double graft (cartilage plus fascia), the latter being our preferred choice.

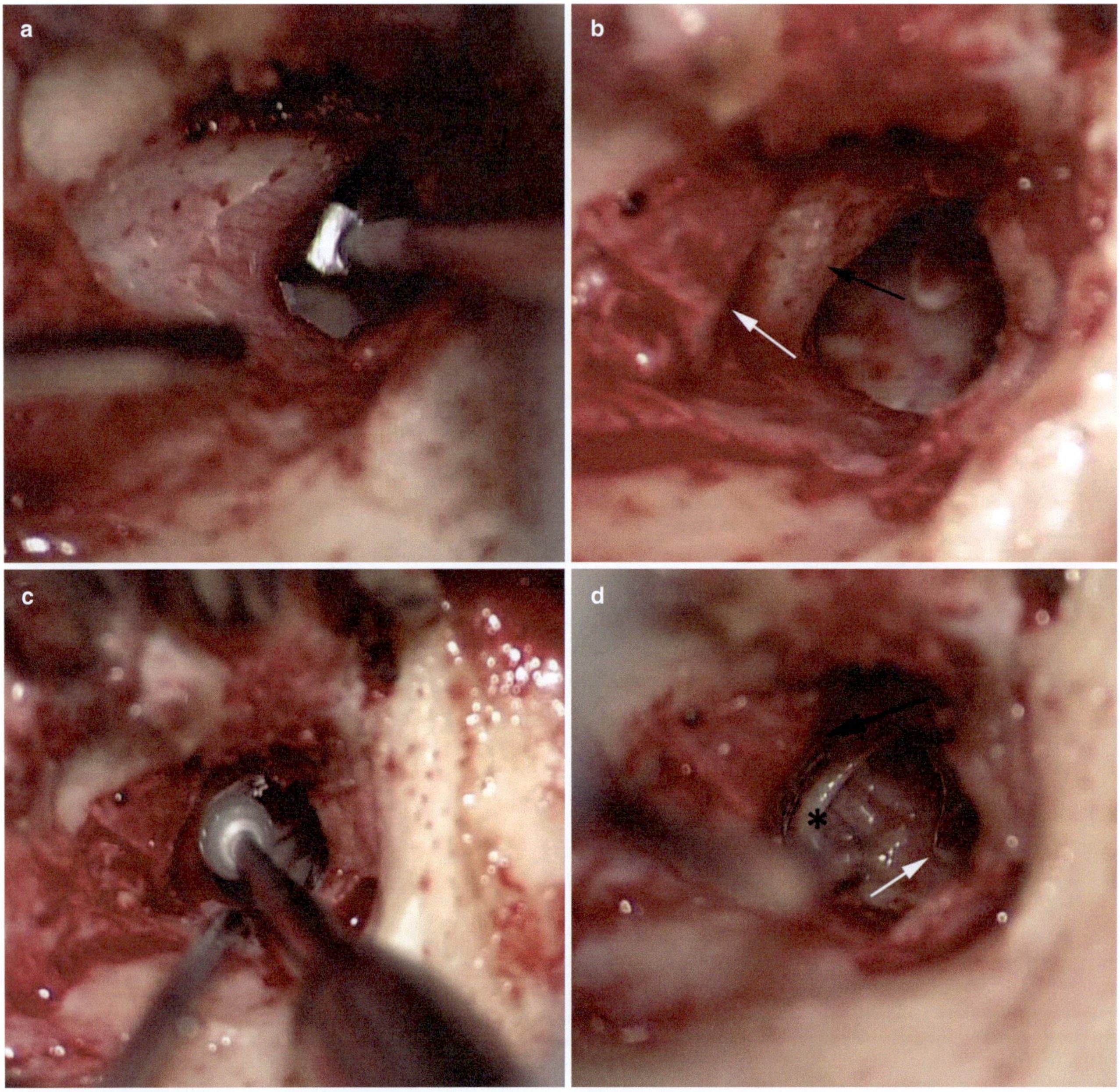

Fig. 49.8 Performing anterior canaloplasty—left ear. (**a**) Retrograde incision and detachment of the anterior skin flap with 90° round knife. (**b**) Bone exposure of the anterior EAC (black arrow), with skin flap preserved and flexed upward (white arrow). (**c**) Rectification of the bone wall with a diamond bur, (**d**) end of canaloplasty. Note the anterior tympanic border, which was not seen before (black asterisk). Note also the greater distance between the anterior bony limit of the EAC (black arrow) and the malleus (white arrow), especially in comparison to Fig. 49.7 before canaloplasty

Step 10: Placement of the Fascia Graft

Temporal muscle fascia is our material of choice for those cases, as it is easy to obtain and is removed during the retroauricular approach. With the aid of ear forceps (Hartmann or similar), the graft is placed under the remaining tympanic membrane as anteriorly as possible and extended over the promontory. The graft is then bent posteriorly to rest on the medial surface of the flap (a maneuver we call "pullback"). Figure 49.13 shows those maneuvers, as described below. The tympanomeatal flap is reflected anteriorly (Fig. 49.13a, black arrow shows the flap). Next, the fascia graft (Fig. 49.13b, black arrow) is taken over the promontory. Once the flap is posteriorly folded, the anterior extremity of the fascia is pinched and reflected posteriorly (Fig. 49.13c,

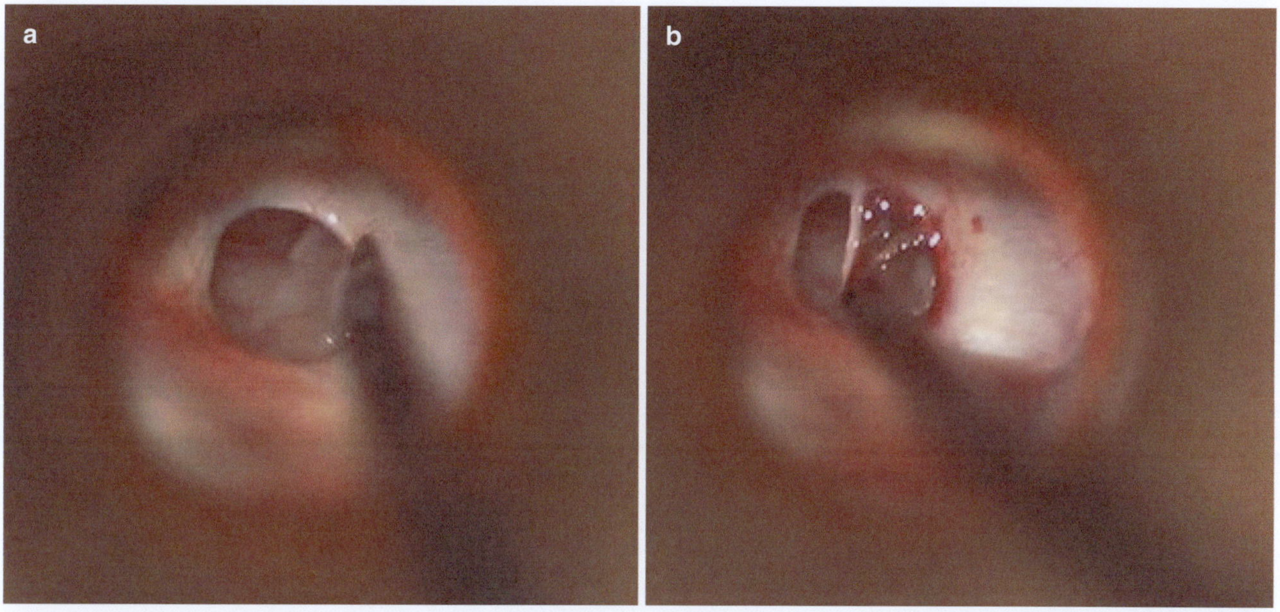

Fig. 49.9 Revival of the perforation borders—left ear, in transcanal approach. (**a**) A needle is used to incise behind the fibrous annulus. (**b**) Removal of the fibrous annulus around 360° of the perforation

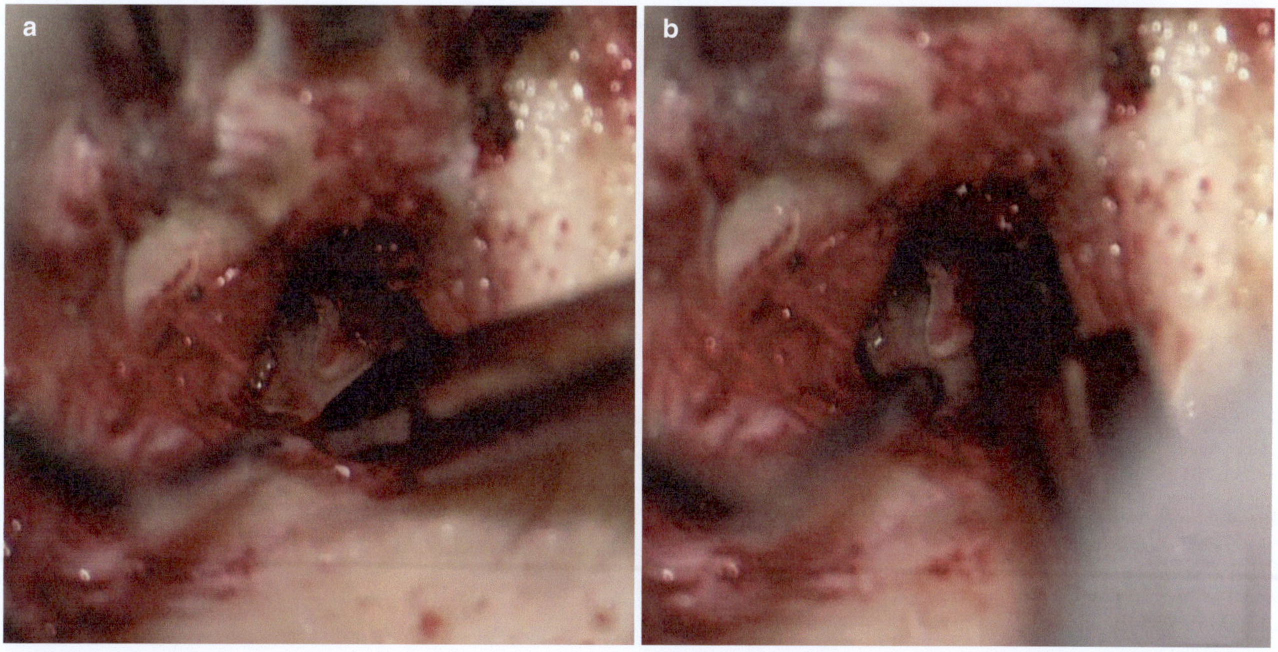

Fig. 49.10 EAC incisions—left ear. (**a**) Lower, or 6 h. (**b**) Superior, or 12 h, taking the lateral process of the malleus as a reference

black arrow). Finally, the fascia rests on the tympanomeatal flap (Fig. 49.13d, black arrow), exposing the middle ear again (but now through the perforation).

If the surgeon chooses only the fascia, proceed with the placement of a hemostatic sponge (Gelfoam®, Spongostan®, among others) filling the middle ear, from the promontory to the level of the tympanic remnants (Fig. 49.13e). The function of this layer is to maintain the fascia in place since the fascia will be positioned under the edges of the perforation. Also, it presses the fascia against the tympanic borders, thus facilitating adhesion and consequent epithelialization and closure of the perforation. Figure 49.13f demonstrates the fascia being detached from the tympanomeatal flap where it was at rest and positioned under the edges of the perforation.

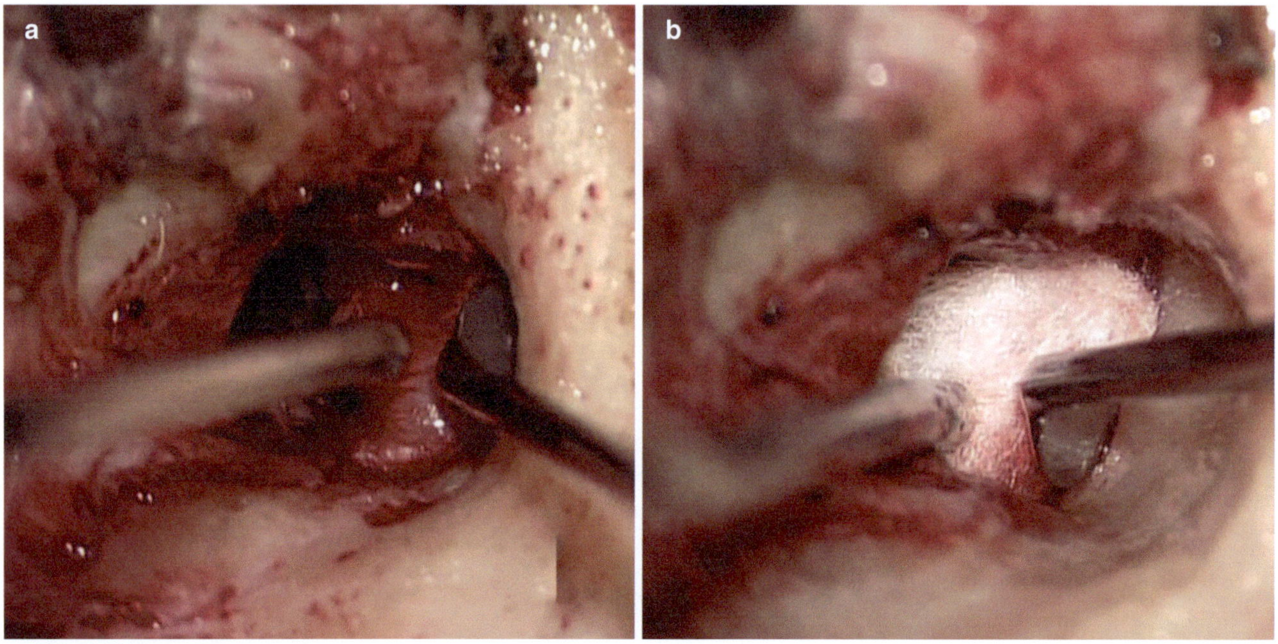

Fig. 49.11 Elevation of the tympanomeatal flap—left ear. (**a**) Using a 45° round knife, the skin is detached from the bone with extreme delicacy. (**b**) We can use cotton soaked in adrenaline to reduce bleeding and facilitate visualization of the tympanic ring

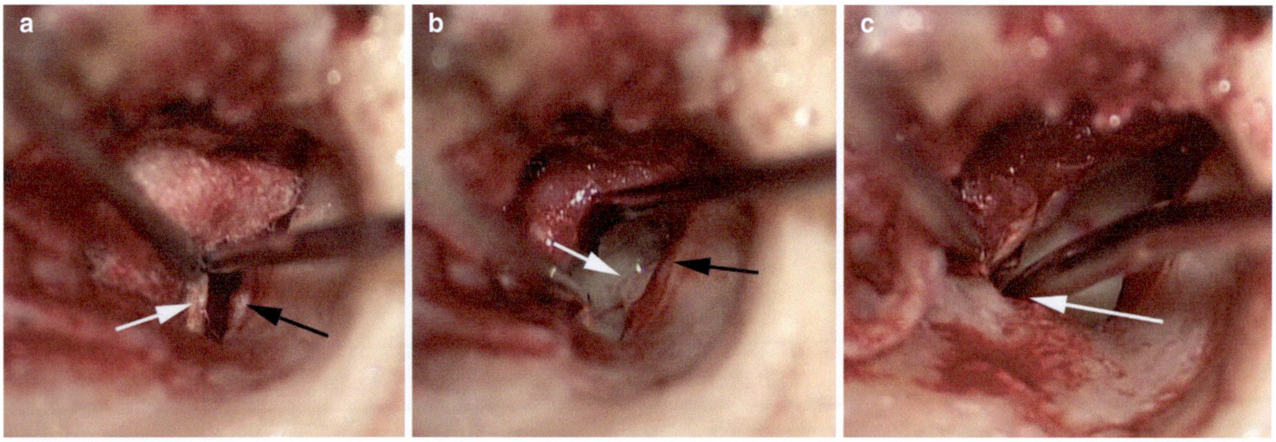

Fig. 49.12 Access to the left middle ear. (**a**) With a delicate instrument (sickle scalpel or needle), we separate the tympanic ring (white arrow) from the chorda tympani nerve (black arrow) and the posterior bone wall. The posterosuperior quadrant is where the tympanic ring is less adhered to the bone sulcus, being the preferential access site (taking care of the ossicular chain medially). (**b**) Exposure of the ossicular chain (white arrow) and chorda tympani in position (black arrow). (**c**) Inferior detachment (direction of the white arrow) of the tympanic ring, with a blunt instrument (Beales or Hughes elevator) to prevent its rupture

Step 11: Placement of the Cartilage Graft

In most surgeries, we choose to reinforce the graft with cartilage, as we believe this will increase the success rate of graft healing. Therefore, in our group, only a small group of perforations do not receive cartilage reinforcement. Those are small perforations (less than 25% of the tympanic area), without associated signs of retraction, with normal middle ear mucosa, and with generous tympanic borders around the entire perforation.

The choice of graft is the surgeon's choice, according to his skills and experience. However, although we strongly recommend the use of the double graft, we present below the criteria which, if present, we consider vital to use the double graft:

- Large perforations, since in those cases, the failure rate of tympanoplasty with fascia only is known to be higher.
- Narrow borders, especially anteriorly and inferiorly, as anchoring the fascia will be more difficult and, consequently, more likely to dislocation.
- Exuberant tympanosclerosis, since the tympanic remnant vascular supply will be poorer.

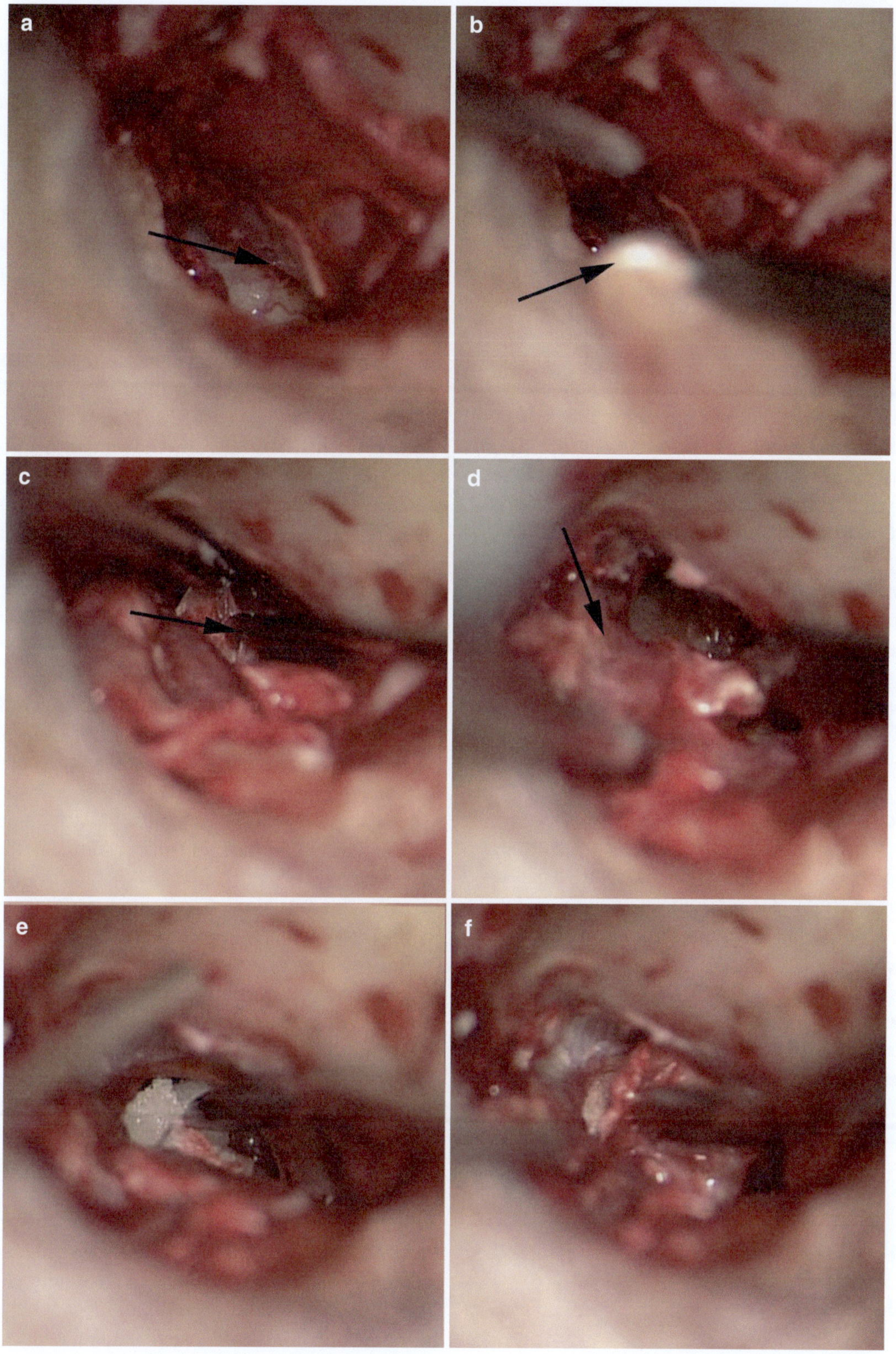

Fig. 49.13 Positioning of the fascia (as a single graft). (**a**) Elevated and anteriorly displaced tympanomeatal flap (black arrow), exposing the middle ear; (**b**) Temporal fascia flap (black arrow) being taken to the promontory; (**c**) Tympanomeatal flap returned to its place, with the fascia seen through the tympanic perforation in its original position (black arrow shows the end of the fascia); (**d**) Temporal fascia (black arrow) being reflected posteriorly to expose the middle ear, allowing the placement of the hemostatic sponge; (**e**) Hemostatic sponge being placed in the middle ear through the perforation; (**f**) Fascia is detached from the tympanomeatal flap again, so it is placed under the edges of the tympanic perforation

- Significant erosion of the incus long crus, where the thickness of the cartilage will facilitate a type 3 tympanoplasty (positioning the cartilage in direct contact with the head of the stapes).
- Failure in previous surgery that was performed only with fascia.

Step 12: Filling the Tympanic Cavity

At this step, we complete the filling of the middle ear with hemostatic sponge cubes Gelfoam®, Spongostan®, among others) up to the level of the tympanic ring. This is an additional effort to support the graft and avoid dislocation. Special attention is needed to the anterior quadrants since the malleus can be a barrier to the passage of the cubes. In addition, proximity to the Eustachian tube can cause early dissolution and leakage of the middle ear sponge. Enough amount of sponge cubes should be placed to push the graft against the perforation and lift it slightly.

Step 13: Repositioning the Tympanomeatal Flap

The tympanomeatal flap is returned to its original position, and every precaution must be taken to check whether it covers the fascia. Often at this point, the fascia is pushed under the flap, like "tightening a shirt at the waist." After this final check, the EAC is wholly filled with hemostatic sponge cubes.

Step 14: Closure of the Retroauricular Access

With the ear back in the anatomical position, hemostasis is performed. Subsequently, the retroauricular incision is sutured in layers, with particular attention to the muscular planes, thus avoiding the development of a protruding ear postoperatively.

Step 15: Bandage

Due to the execution of a retroauricular incision, some postoperative bleeding is expected. Therefore, we suggest making a dressing using molded gauze medial and lateral to the auricle. It will be held in position with a 10- or 12-cm circular bandage.

The Complex Tympanoplasty

Additional Steps

As mentioned above, in this type of perforation, there is a need for additional steps in an attempt to restore middle ear physiology. Thus, after step 9 and before step 10 described above, we will now describe the additional procedures in the perforations associated with retractions (*outside-in* perforations).

Malleus Lateralization

In the *outside-in* perforations, often the malleus is medialized, sometimes touching the promontory. This situation creates compartmentalization in the middle ear, isolating the posterior portion (posterior mesotympanum and the retrotympanum) from the anterior portion (anterior mesotympanum, supratubal recess, and Eustachian tube), as shown in Fig. 49.14. Consequently, the gas coming from the Eustachian tube will not reach the posterior portions. If not corrected, this lack of ventilation will be a relevant motive for tympanoplasty failure.

Therefore, it is necessary to lateralize the malleus and re-establish this aeration path. If the ossicular chain is intact and mobile, lateralization of the malleus must be done with extreme delicacy. The that will occur when pulling the malleus laterally movement (analog to a lever) can disarticulate the long incus crus from the head of the stapes. However, if an incudostapedial disarticulation already exists, the movement may be broader and possibly more effective. Also, in this step, it may be necessary to section the tendon of the tensor tympani muscle, facilitating lateralization of the manubrium of the malleus (Fig. 49.15).

Inspection of the Ostium of the Eustachian Tube

Despite going beyond the scope of this chapter, the mechanisms to restore the physiology of the Eustachian tube are an essential point in the management of *outside-in* perforations. Therefore, here we will limit ourselves to commenting on the need to visualize the tympanic ostium of the Eustachian tube.

After lateralization of the malleus, often with the section of the tensor tympani tendon, we will be able to visualize the region of the protympanum and the supratubal recess, as well as the middle ear opening of the Eustachian tube. Often, it will be covered by mucous strands or adhesions, which must be removed until the region is entirely free. It may be necessary to use an endoscope with angled optics for this step (see below in "systematization of the use of the endoscope").

Cleaning the Epithelium Adhered to Middle Ear Structures

Often, the retraction associated with the perforation will be very pronounced, going so far that the epithelium of the lateral layer of the TM will meet the ossicular chain, promontory, and even posterior recesses. If not removed, it can subsequently proliferate and generate a middle ear cholesteatoma (implantation theory).

The epithelium must be entirely removed from these regions using instruments such as retractors, micro forceps, sickle scalpels, and round knives. Using an endoscope is also critical to check the facial recess and sinus before closing the perforation.

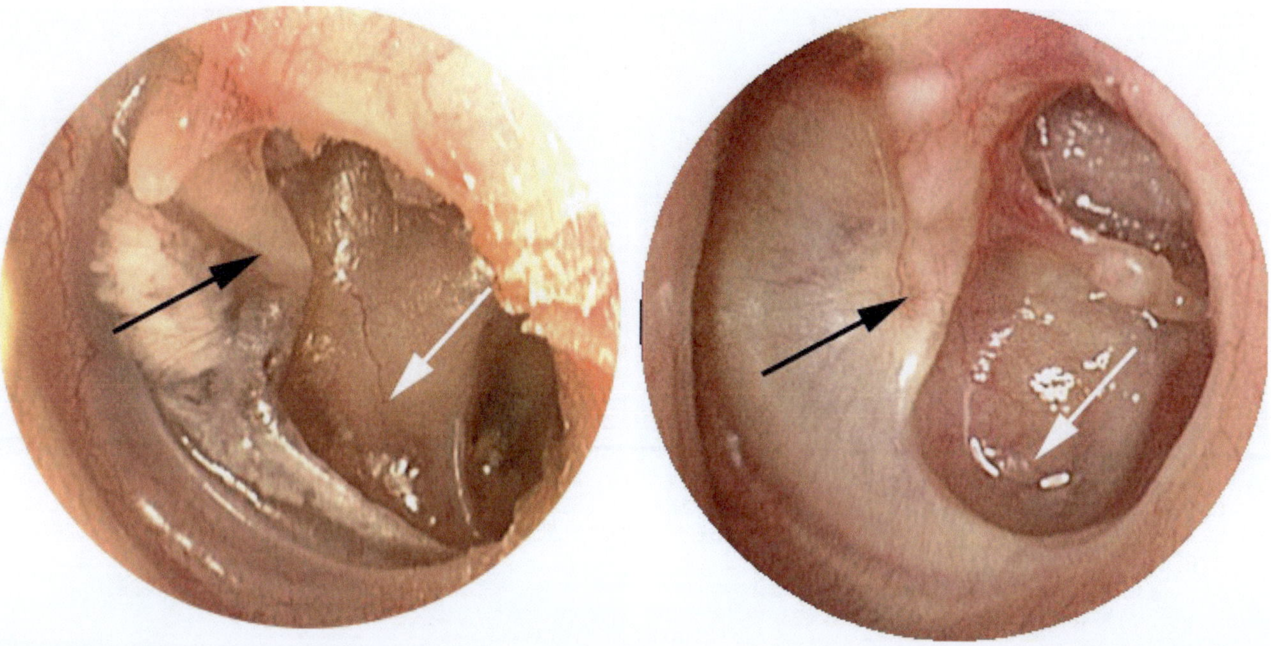

Fig. 49.14 Illustration of selective lack of ventilation of the posterior mesotympanum and retrotympanum, both in the left ear. Note that the medialized malleus (black arrows) brings the TM into contact with the promontory subiculum (white arrows), separating the anterior and posterior quadrants. As a result, the Eustachian tube cannot ventilate the posterior quadrants

Systematizing the Endoscope Usage

The endoscope with optics at an angle of 30 or 45° is of fundamental importance in *outside-in* perforation surgery. Including the steps already described above, the surgeon must have a systematic routine for using the endoscope (Fig. 49.16) to visualize all regions of the middle ear before closing the perforation.

We recommend performing a 360° turn of the middle ear, analyzing the following regions:

- Anterior and posterior epitympanum, in addition to the tympanic diaphragm.
- Supratubal recess, protympanum, and Eustachian tube.
- Hypotympanum mastoid cells.
- Round and oval windows.
- Retrotympanum and posterior recesses: tympanic sinus and facial recess.
- Aditus ad antrum: reopening, if closed.

Ossicular Chain Reconstruction

Once the inspection of the middle ear with the endoscope is finished, we will proceed with the reconstructive steps. First, the ossicular chain, if not intact, must be repaired. In *outside-in* perforations, the most frequently found damage is the erosion of incus long crus, often without contact with the stapes head. The primary reconstructions, in this case, will depend on the distance between the remnant of the long crus and the stapes and can be systematized as follows:

- Small distance between the long crus and the stapes: we can insert a bony or cartilaginous disc between them to restore the mobility of the ossicular chain. Also, bone cement is an excellent alternative to restoring mobility in these cases.
- Long distance between the long incus crus and the stapes (or incus absence): we can perform a type 3 tympanoplasty using the cartilage graft itself. The tragus cartilage is especially useful in these situations since it can be sculpted and positioned to occlude the tympanic perforation. At the same time, its thickness will allow a direct touch of the stapes head, configuring a type 3 reconstruction (Fig. 49.17).
- Although it is less frequent, in case of partial erosion or absence of the stapes superstructure, we recommend ossicular reconstruction to be performed in a second surgical stage. TORP-type prostheses can be inserted between the stapes footplate and the previously reconstructed tympanic membrane. However, it is essential that the otologist is sure of the physiological functioning of the middle ear, which is initially impossible at this first surgical stage. So, after repairing the defect in the tympanic membrane, we wait a period that can vary from 6 to 12 months. We can only perform the second surgical time later, with ossicular reconstruction with TORP.

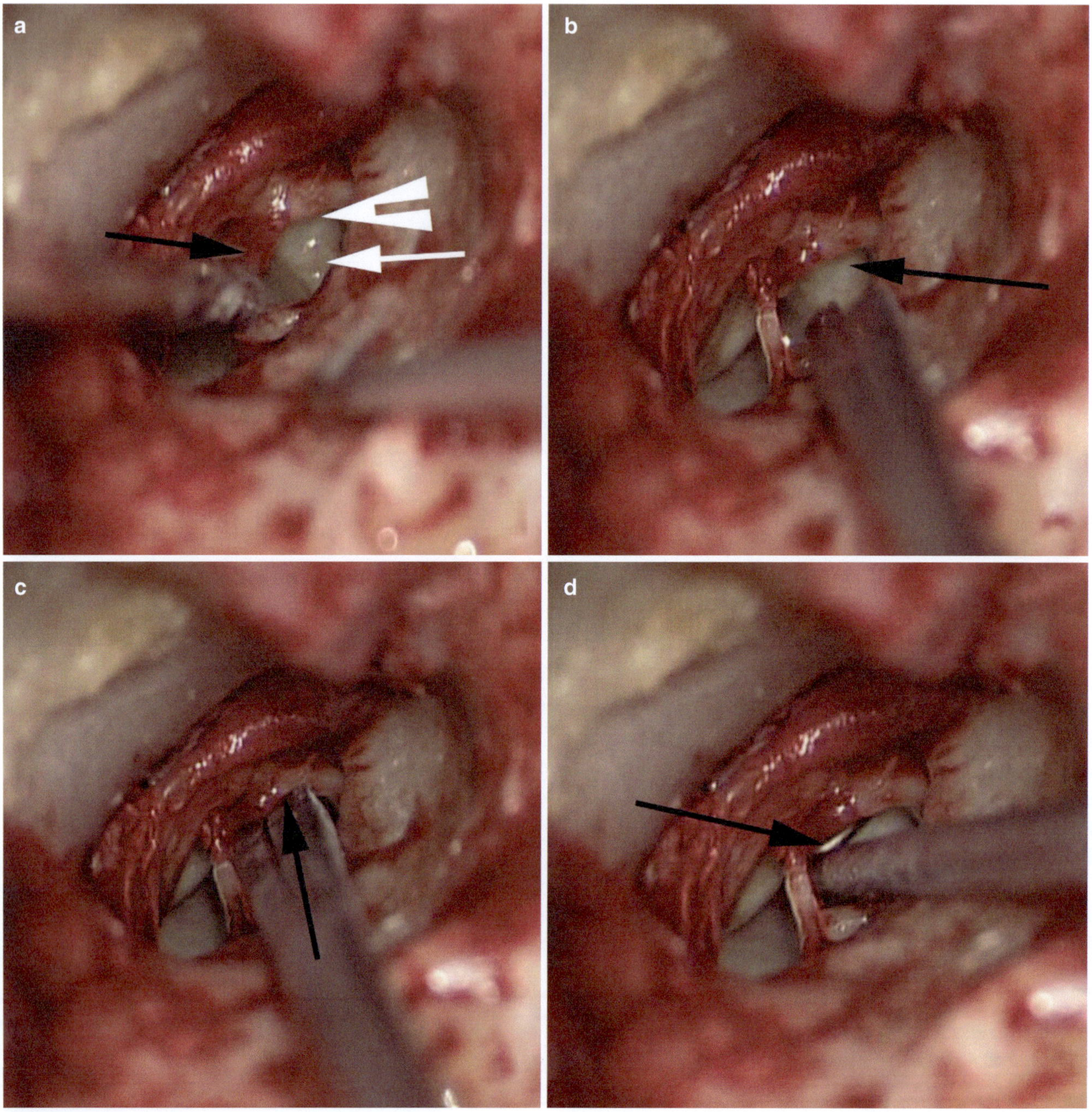

Fig. 49.15 Section of the tendon of the tensor tympani muscle in the left ear. (**a**) Identification of the facial nerve (white arrow) and cochleariform process (white arrowhead), possible after gentle lateral traction of the malleus manubrium (black arrow). (**b**) Identification of the tendon (black arrow) from the cochleariform process. (**c**) Cutting the tendon with micro-scissors that exert lateral tension on the malleus (direction of the black arrow), ensuring distance from the facial nerve and adequate traction for the cut. (**d**) Lateralization of the malleus, using a delicate hook (black arrow)

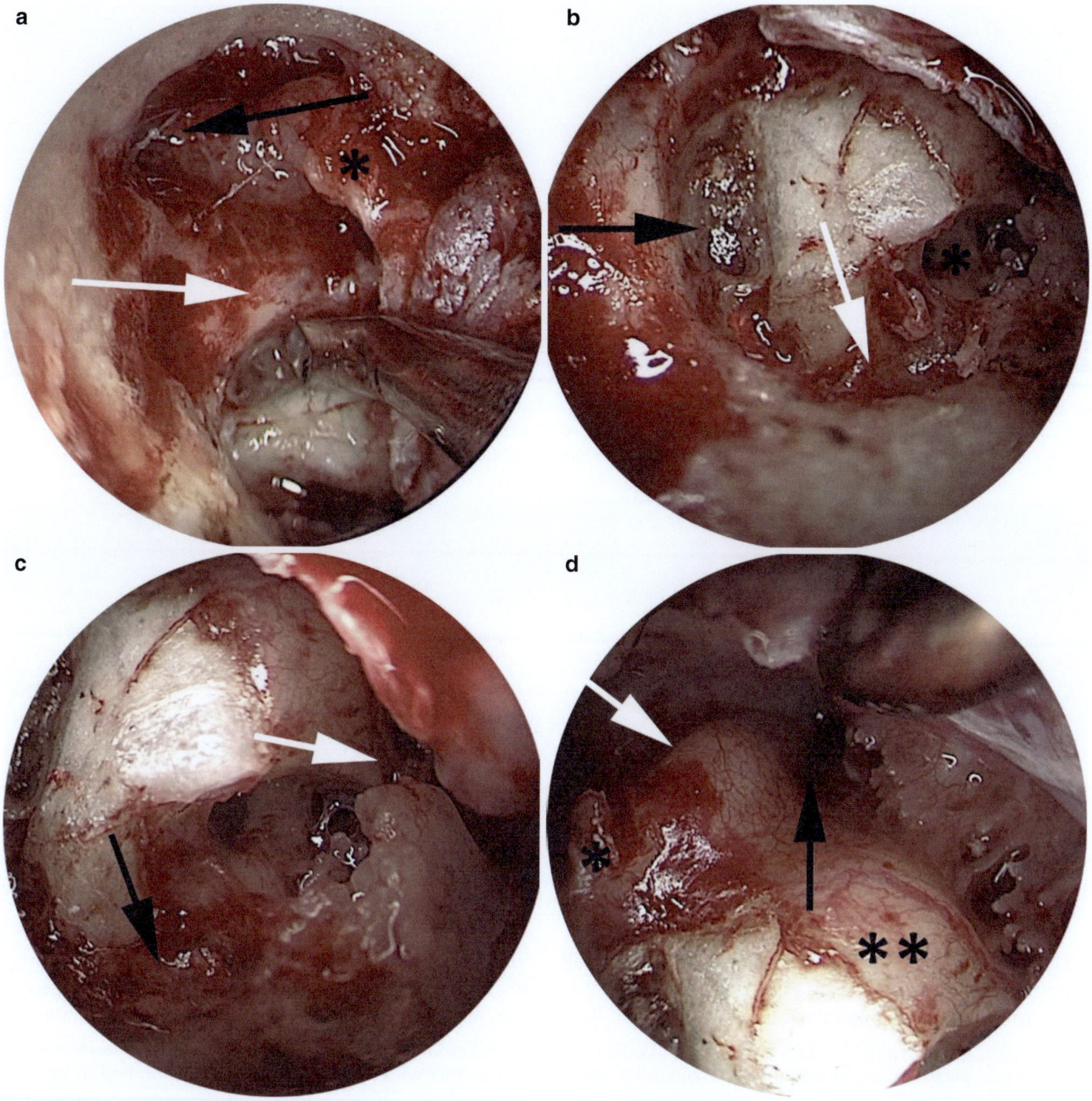

Fig. 49.16 Endoscopic revision of the middle ear. (**a**) Upper region, showing aditus ad antrum (black arrow), facial nerve (white arrow), and head of malleus (black asterisk). (**b**) Posterior region, showing the stapes footplate (black arrow), posterior recesses (white arrow), and round window (asterisk). (**c**) Lower region, with visualization of the posterior recesses (black arrow) and the cellular tract of the hypotympanum (white arrow). (**d**) Anterior region, with visualization of the Eustachian tube (black arrow), tensor tympani semicanalis (white arrow), cochleariform process (single asterisk), and cochlear promontory (two asterisks)

Use of More Resistant Grafts

Unlike the technique for *inside-out* perforation, in which the surgeon can use the graft of his choice, we recommend using more resistant grafts for *outside-in* perforations. Tragus cartilage is especially interesting in these situations. In addition to the adequate thickness in most cases, it has a slight curvature that will facilitate adherence to the tympanic remnant without gaps or unevenness (Fig. 49.18).

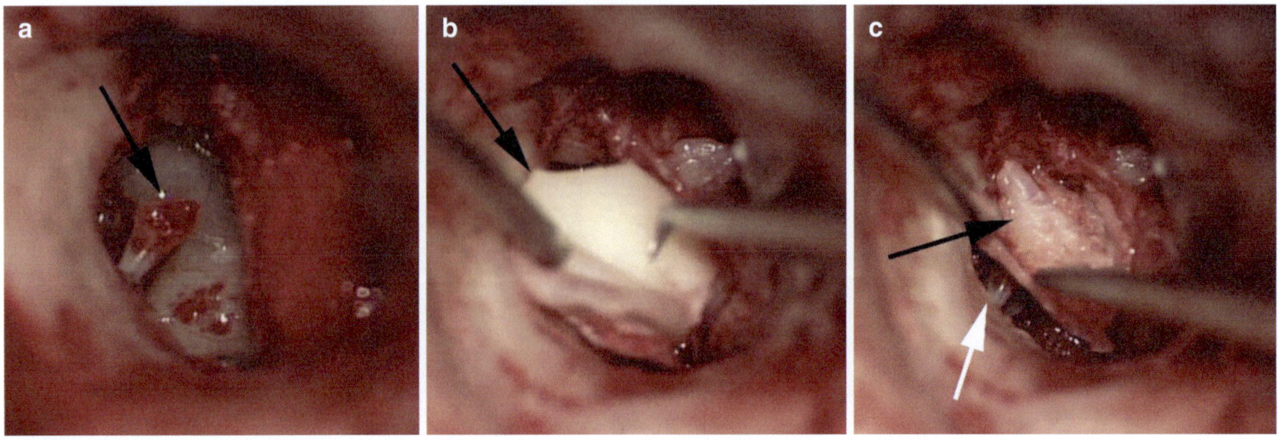

Fig. 49.17 Type 3 tympanoplasty with cartilage. (**a**) Identify the stapes head (black arrow) without the incus long crus. (**b**) Positioning of the cartilage over the stapes. (**c**) Visualization of the stapes head (white arrow) in direct contact with the cartilage. The thickness of the cartilage (black arrow) guarantees that there will be no gap between the tympanic membrane and the stapes head

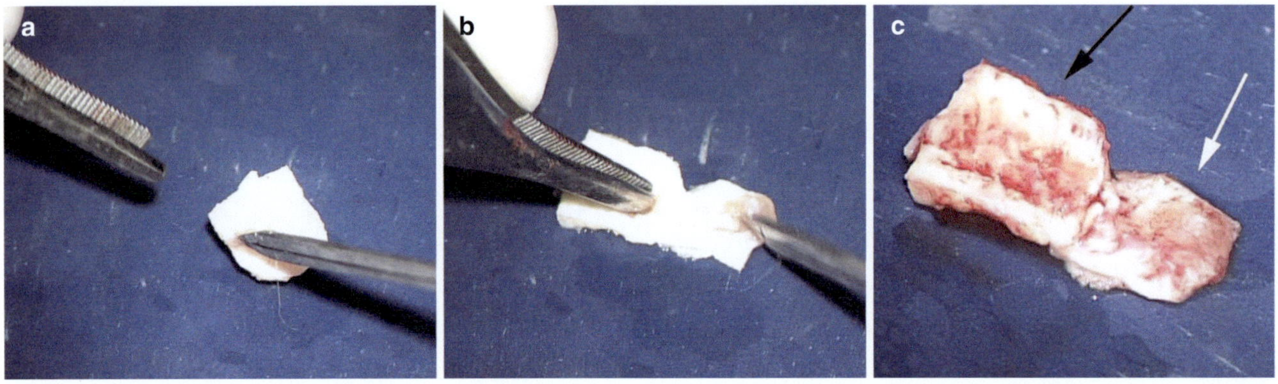

Fig. 49.18 Preparation of the cartilage that was extracted from the tragus. (**a**) Cartilage with the perichondrium. (**b**) Traction of the perichondrium on one side. (**c**) End of work with the cartilage, showing the concavity upward (black arrow) and the perichondrium almost completely detached (white arrow) but still connected to the cartilage

The temporal fascia will also be used to help finish and fill the borders. Thus, characterizing a double graft (fascia + cartilage), which will not only increase closure rates in the short term but also prevent progressive retraction and recurrence of *outside-in* perforations in the medium and long term. Following, we present step by step the cartilage positioning (Fig. 49.19).

Ventilation Tube Insertion

As paradoxical as this situation may seem, inserting a ventilation tube at the same time as the closure of perforation may often be indicated. While in *inside-out* perforations, in fact, this indication does not make sense, in *outside-in* perforations, the assurance of adequate ventilation is of vital importance, especially in the immediate postoperative period.

We start with the 1021 grommet, positioned in the anterior quadrants. Many patients will be stable in the medium and long term (even after the grommet extrusion and the TM's healing). However, a considerable number of patients will present retraction recurrence. We will indicate a new procedure with long-lasting grommet insertion in these cases.

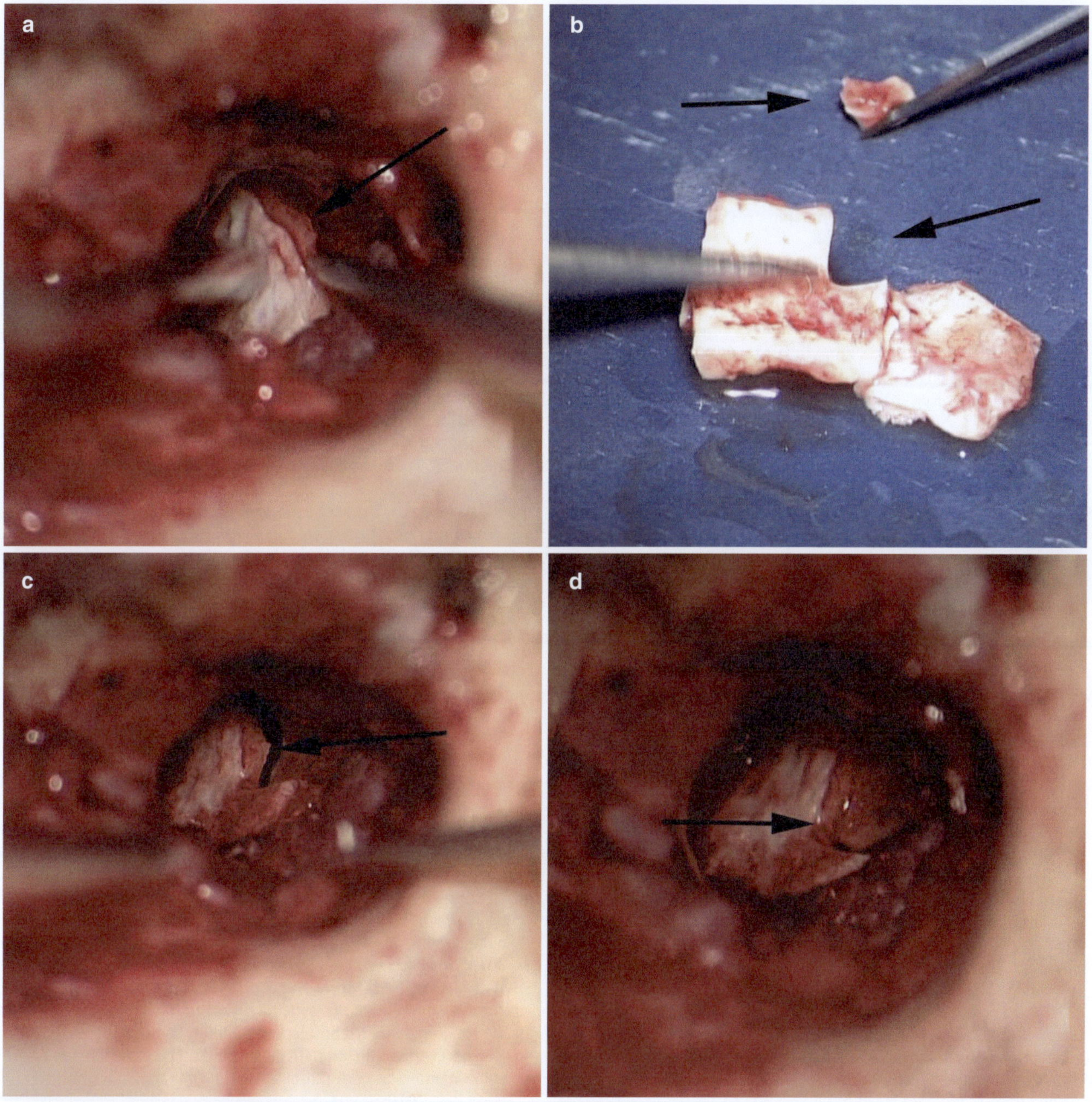

Fig. 49.19 Placement of cartilage graft in the left ear. (**a**) First placement, showing that the contact with the malleus projects the cartilage out of the middle ear (black arrow). (**b**) Removing part of the cartilage, making a housing for the malleus. (**c**) The black arrow points to the cleft made in the cartilage for fitting the malleus. (**d**) The black arrow points to the final position of the cartilage, integrated into the malleus and without irregularities (continuous surface)

Bibliography

Alleva M, Paparella MM, Morris MS, et al. The flexible/intact bridge tympanomastoidectomy technique. Otolaryngol Clin N Am. 1989;2:41–50.

Ars B, Decraemer W, Ars-Piret N. Lamina propria and tympanic retractions—morphological and physical details. Les Cah d'ORL. 1986:4.

Berger GB. Nature of spontaneous tympanic membrane perforation in acute otitis media in children. J Laryngol Otol. 1989;103(12):1150–3.

Bezold F. Cholesteatom, Perforation der Membrana flaccida und Tubenverschluß. Z Hals Nasen Ohrenheilk. 1890;20:5–29.

Bhattacharya S, Pal S, Saha S, Gure P, Roy A. Comparison of a microsliced modified chondroperichondrium shield graft and a temporalis fascia graft in primary type I tympanoplasty: a prospective randomized controlled trial. Ear Nose Throat J. 2016;95(7):274–83.

Celik O, Eskiizmir G, Ulkumen B, Karaca G. Impact of graft type on anatomical and functional outcome in type-I tympanoplasty. B-ENT. 2018;15:169–77.

Ciğer E, Balcı MK, İşlek A, Önal K. The wheel-shaped composite cartilage graft (WsCCG) and temporalis fascia for type 1 tympanoplasty: a prospective, randomized study. Eur Arch Otorhinolaryngol. 2018;275(12):2975–81. https://doi.org/10.1007/s00405-018-5171-5.

da Costa SS, Cruz OLM. Exploratory tympanotomy. Oper Tech Otolaryngol Head Neck Surg. 1996;7(1):20–6.

da Costa SS, de Dornelles C. Otite Média Crônica não-colesteatomatosa. In: da Costa SS, Cruz OLM, de Oliveira JAA, editors. Otorrinolaringologia: Princípios e Prática. 2nd ed. Porto Alegre: Artmed; 2006. p. 289–308.

da Costa SS, Rosito LPS, de Dornelles C, Sperling N. The contralateral ear in chronic otitis media. Arch Otolaryngol Head Neck Surg. 2008;134(3):290–3.

Gaihede M, Padurariu S, Jacobsen H, de Greef D, Dirckx JJJ. Eustachian tube pressure equilibration. Temporal analysis of pressure changes based on direct physiological recordings with an intact tympanic membrane. Hear Res. 2013;301:53–9.

Gyanwali B, Li H, Xie L, Zhu M, Wu Z. The role of tensor veli platini muscle (TVP) and levetor veli platini muscle (LVP) in the opening and closing of pharyngeal orifice of Eustachian tube. Acta Otolaryngol. 2015;136(3):249–55.

Hardman J, Muzaffar J, Nankivell P, Coulson C. Tympanoplasty for chronic tympanic membrane perforation in children: systematic review and meta-analysis. Otol Neurotol. 2015;36(5):796–804.

Jackler RK, Maria PLS, Varsak YK, Nguyen A, Blevins NH. A new theory on the pathogenesis of acquired cholesteatoma: mucosal traction. Laryngoscope. 2015;125(Suppl 4):1–14.

Juhn SK, Paparella MM, Goycoolea M, Kim CS, Giebink S. Pathogenesis of otitis media. Ann Otol Rhinol Laryngol. 1977;86(4):481–92.

Jumaily M, Franco J, Gallogly J, Hentzelman JL, Costa DJ, Wild APK, et al. Butterfly cartilage tympanoplasty outcomes: a single-institution experience and literature review. Am J Otol. 2018;39(4):396–400. https://doi.org/10.1016/j.amjoto.2018.03.029.

Knapik M, Saliba I. Pediatric myringoplasty: a study of factors affecting outcome. Int J Pediatr Otorhinolaryngol. 2011;75(6):818–23.

Levine S, Daly K, Giebink GS. Tympanic membrane perforations and tympanostomy tubes. Ann Otol Rhinol Laryngol. 1994;103:27–30.

Liese JG, Silfverdal SA, Giaquinto C, Carmona A, Larcombe JH, Garcia-Sicilia J, et al. Incidence and clinical presentation of acute otitis media in children aged <6 years in European medical practices. Epidemiol Infect. 2014;142(8):1778–88.

Malafronte G, Filosa B. One hundred twenty-five fat myringoplasties: does marginal perforation matter? Clin Otolaryngol. 2018;43(1):362–5.

Mansour S, Magnan J, Haidar H, Nicolas K. Tympanic membrane retraction pocket. Springer; 2015.

Martin C, Karkas A, Prades J. Tubotympanic system functioning. Eur Ann Otorhinolaryngol Head Neck Dis. 2017;134(3):177–84.

Mcdonald MH, Hoffman MR, Gentry LR, Jiang JJ. New insights into mechanism of Eustachian tube ventilation based on cine computed tomography images. Eur Arch Oto-Rhino-Laryngol. 2012;269(8):1901–7.

Meyerhoff WL, Kim CS, Paparella MM. Pathology of chronic otitis media. Ann Otol Rhinol Laryngol. 1978;87(6 pt 1):749–60.

Monasta L, Ronfani L, Marchetti F, Montico M, Brumatti L, Bavcar A, et al. Burden of disease caused by otitis media: systematic review and global estimates. PLoS One. 2012;7(4):e36226.

Neely JG. Tympanoplasty. In: Pillsbury III HC, Goldsmith III MM, editors. Operative challenges in otolaryngology head & neck surgery. Chicago: Year Book Medical Publisher; 1990. p. 24–32.

Onal K, Uguz M, Kazikdas K, Gursoy S, Gokce H. A multivariate analysis of otological, surgical and patient-related factors in determining success in myringoplasty. Clin Otolaryngol Off J ENT-UK. 2005;30(2):115–20.

Paço J, Branco C, Estibeiro H. The posterosuperior quadrant of the tympanic. Otolaryngol Head Neck Surg. 2009;140(6):884–8.

Principi N, Marchisio P, Rosazza C, Sciarrabba CS, Esposito S. Acute otitis media with spontaneous tympanic membrane perforation. Eur J Clin Microbiol Infect Dis. 2017;36(1):11–8. https://doi.org/10.1007/s10096-016-2783-9.

Rosito LPS, Canali I, Selaimen FA, Jung YP, Pauletti MGT, Deutsch KM, et al. Análise descritiva dos achados otoscópicos em perfurações marginais da membrana timpânica. Braz J Otorhinolaryngol. 2013;79(6 s1):2.

Rosito LPS, Costa SS, Schachern PA, Dornelles C, Cureoglu S, Paparella MM. Contralateral ear in chronic otitis media: a histologic study. Laryngoscope. 2007;117(10):1809–14.

Rosito LPS, Silveira Netto LF, Teixeira AR, da Costa SS. Classification of cholesteatoma according to growth patterns. JAMA Otolaryngol Head Neck Surg. 2016;142(2):168–72.

Rosito LPS, Sperling N, Teixeira AR, Selaimen FA, da Costa SS. The role of tympanic membrane retractions in cholesteatoma pathogenesis. Biomed Res Int. 2018;2018:1.

Ryan MA, Kaylie DM. What is the optimal age to repair tympanic membrane perforations in pediatric patients ? Laryngoscope. 2016;126(10):2201–2.

Sadé J, Avraham S, Brown M. Atelectasis. Retraction pockets and cholesteatoma. Acta Otolaryngol. 1981;92(5–6):501–12.

Schmiemann G, Kruschinksi C. Complication rate of out-patient removal of ear wax: systematic review of the literature. HNO. 2009;57(7):713–8.

Schuknecht HF. Surgical pathology. In: Pathology of the ear. Cambridge: Harvard University; 1974.

Selaimen FA, Rosito LPS, Silva MNL, Silva AL, Stanham VS, Costa SS. Central versus marginal tympanic membrane perforations: does it matter? An analysis of 792 patients. Acta Otolaryngol. 2021;141(2):122–8. https://doi.org/10.1080/00016489.2020.1831698. Epub 2020 Oct 29.

Selaimen FA, Rosito LPS, da Silva MNL, Stanham VS, Sperling N, da Costa SS. Tympanic membrane perforations: a critical analysis of 1003 ears and proposal of a new classification based on pathogenesis. Eur Arch Otorhinolaryngol. 2022;279(3):1277–83. https://doi.org/10.1007/s00405-021-06776-8. Epub 2021 Mar 27.

da Silva MNL, dos Muller J, Selaimen FA, Oliveira DS, Rosito LPS, da Costa SS. Tomographic evaluation of the contralateral ear in patients with severe chronic otitis media. Braz J Otorhinolaryngol. 2013;79(4):475–9.

Silveira Netto LF, da Costa SS, Sleifer P, Braga ME. The impact of chronic suppurative otitis media on children's and teenagers' hearing. Int J Pediatr Otorhinolaryngol. 2009;73(12):1751–6.

Stomackin G, Kidd S, Jung TT, Martin GK, Dong W. Effects of tympanic membrane perforation on middle ear transmission in gerbil. Hear Res. 2019;373:48–58.

Tong M, Yue V, Ku P, van Hasselt C. Preoperative topical ofloxacin solution for tympanoplasty: a randomized, controlled study. Otol Neurotol. 2002;23(1):18–20.

Tseng CC, Lai MT, Wu CC, Yuan SP, Ding Y. Comparison of the efficacy of endoscopic Tympanoplasty and microscopic Tympanoplasty: a systematic review and meta-analysis. Laryngoscope. 2017;127(8):1890–6.

World Health Organization. Chronic suppurative otitis media: burden of illness and management options. 2004.

Wullstein H. Funktionelle Operationen im Mittelohr mit Hilfe des freien Spaltlappen-Transplantates. Arch für Ohren Nasen Kehlkopfheilkd. 1952;161(2–6):422–35.

Zorzetto NL. Anatomia da orelha. In: da Costa SS, Cruz OLM, de Oliveira JAA, editors. Otorrinolaringologia: Princípios e Prática. 2nd ed. Porto Alegre: Artmed; 2006. p. 23–60.

Tympanoplasty: The Overlay Technique Step by Step

50

Fábio André Selaimen, Mauricio Noschang Lopes da Silva, and Sady Selaimen da Costa

Introduction

Tympanoplasty techniques currently employed involve repairing the tympanic membrane defect by positioning a tissue graft (most commonly the temporalis muscle fascia). These grafts act as a bridge allowing regeneration of the squamous epithelium of the external ear (on its lateral side) and the middle ear mucosa (on its medial side).

For this purpose, two surgical techniques have been traditionally used: the one that positions the graft below the tympanic remnant (medial technique, Austin or *underlay*) or above the remnant (lateral technique, Sheehy, or *overlay*). In experienced hands, both techniques present comparable results regarding tympanic membrane healing rates and restoration of auditory function.

According to Sheehy, an otological surgeon with little experience may have difficulty with any techniques, but these problems will differ depending on the technique used. In our group, we have preferably used Austin's technique, reserving Sheehy's for exceptional situations.

The previous chapters of this book explored in detail all aspects related to tympanoplasty, such as anatomical and physiological aspects and preoperative planning, as well as other surgical techniques and postoperative care. The purpose of this chapter is to present, step-by-step, the surgical technique for *overlay* tympanoplasty.

F. A. Selaimen (✉) · M. N. L. da Silva
Hospital de Clínicas de Porto Alegre, Porto Alegre, Brazil

Instituto Gaúcho de Otorrinolaringologia, Porto Alegre, Brazil

S. S. da Costa
Hospital de Clínicas de Porto Alegre, Porto Alegre, Brazil

Universidade Federal do Rio Grande do Sul, Porto Alegre, Brazil

Instituto Gaúcho de Otorrinolaringologia, Porto Alegre, Brazil

Indications and Contraindications

Tympanoplasty is a relatively safe procedure in experienced hands and should be indicated to eliminate a middle ear infection or restore the sound conduction mechanism in any healthy patient. It is clear that surgery loses its purpose in a functionally "dead" ear or with only residual cochlear function unless the suppurative component of the disease interferes with the patient's quality of life. It is also contraindicated in malignant neoplasms of the temporal bone or invasive and potentially lethal infections of the ear and adjacent tissues. Other contraindications depend on multiple conditions, and the decision process, where and when to operate, must be highly individualized. For example, the single or dominant ear should only be observed unless the infectious process is clinically uncontrollable, thus risking the integrity of the inner ear. In these situations, the authors agree that conservative procedures should be performed in an attempt to minimize additional cochlear damage. One should also not intervene in cases of repeated surgical failures in experienced hands, in ears with irreversible tubal dysfunctions, or in rare occasions of recurrent prosthesis extrusions.

We usually employ the *overlay* technique in multiple interventions and total (or subtotal) perforations. On these occasions, we always use the retroauricular approach. The advantages of this technique are the excellent visualization of the anterior meatal recess and the high success rates since the eardrum is replaced with almost its total area, and the middle ear space is not reduced. The graft will be placed over the mucosal and fibrous layers of the tympanic membrane (after the removal of the lateral layer), like shown in Fig. 50.1.

However, disadvantages are well known and include erasure of the anterior border (Fig. 50.2, known as "blunting"), graft lateralization (Fig. 50.3), thickening of the neotympanum, and formation of epidermoid cysts if the eardrum is not completely denuded. In addition to these disadvantages, we consider the lateral technique too laborious to be used in small central perforations.

M. V. Goycoolea et al. (eds.), *Textbook of Otitis Media*, https://doi.org/10.1007/978-3-031-40949-3_50

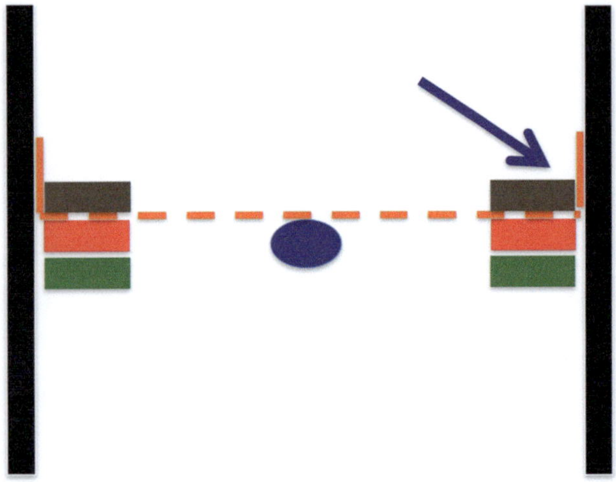

Fig. 50.1 Placement of the graft (orange dotted line), over the mucosal (green) and fibrous (red) layers of the tympanic membrane. In black, is represented the external auditory canal and, in gray, the lateral layer of the tympanic membrane (that will be removed). In blue, a section of the malleus

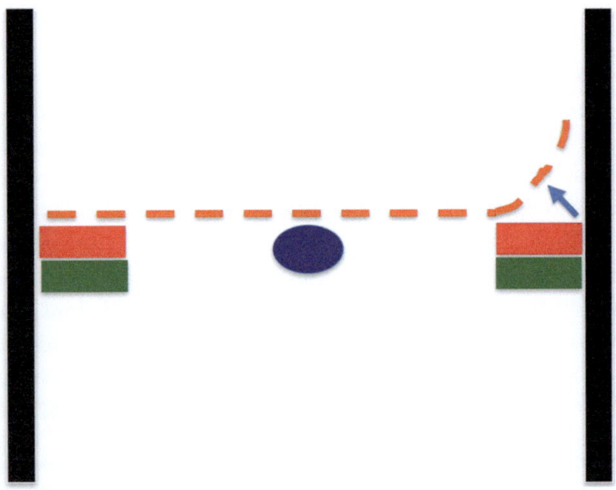

Fig. 50.2 Blunting of the tympanic membrane. Blunting occurs when there is loss of the normally acute (45–50°) anterior tympanomeatal angle, at the junction between the TM and external auditory canal

Most of these disadvantages are due to the lack of support provided by the tympanic remnant, especially in the anterior region. In underlay tympanoplasty, the graft is pressed by the hemostatic sponge lining against the tympanic remnant in the direction from the middle ear towards the external auditory canal. The graft is barred from lateralizing due to the annulus firmly adhering to the tympanic sulcus and maintaining tension on the remnant (Fig. 50.4).

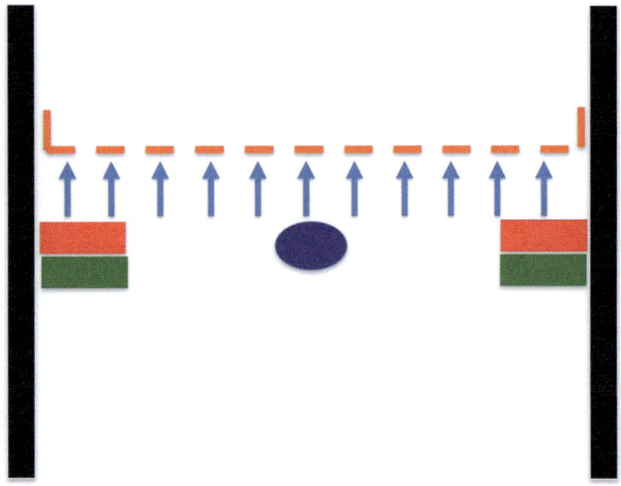

Fig. 50.3 Lateralization of the TM graft

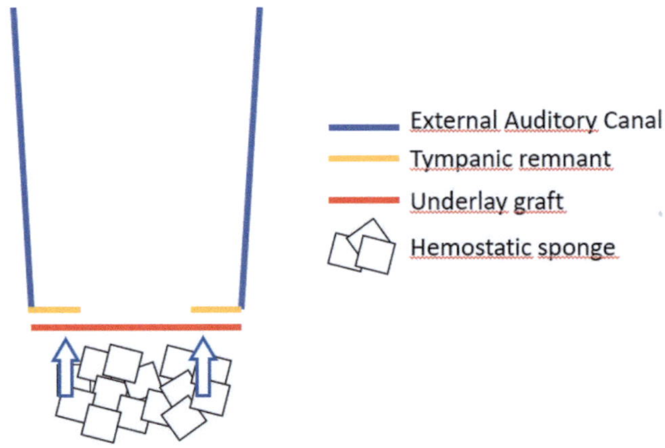

Fig. 50.4 Underlay tympanoplasty. Blue arrows represent the tension of the graft against the tympanic remnant

However, in overlay tympanoplasty, the graft is already lateral to the tympanic remnant. Thus, there is no way to use the stability of the tympanic annulus to stabilize the graft. The risk of graft lateralization in this technique is greater (Fig. 50.5).

The two situations described above will differ regarding the auditory results within the lateralized graft. In the case of the deletion of the anterior angle (blunting), the auditory result will be less impaired than in the complete lateralization of the graft. However, in the latter case, the auditory result will be terrible since the lateralized TM will not only be able to vibrate the ossicular chain but also act as a barrier to airway conduction for the middle ear. Figure 50.6 shows an otoendoscopy of an ear with graft lateralization.

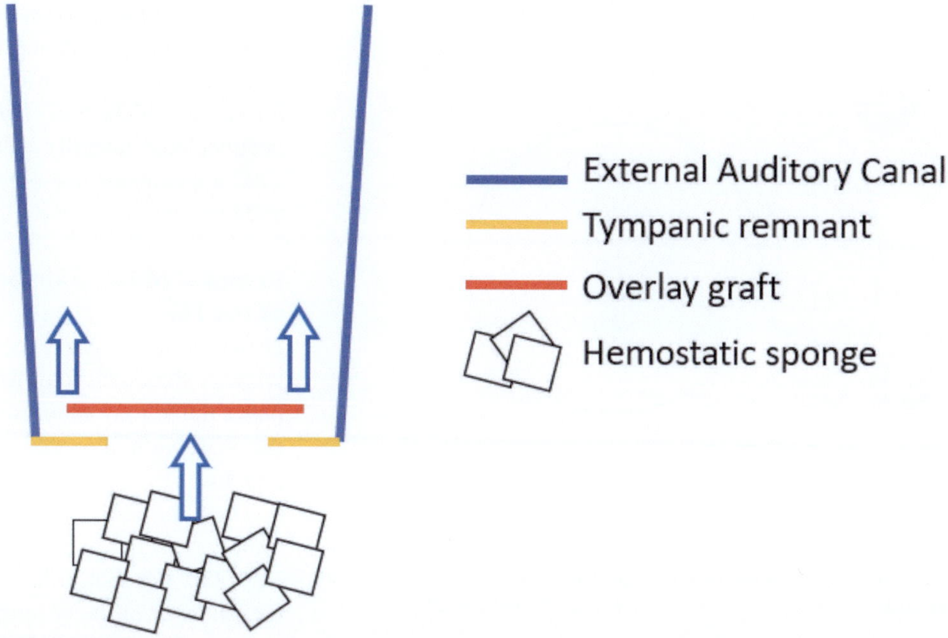

Fig. 50.5 Overlay tympanoplasty. Blue arrows represent the hemostatic sponge pressing the graft, which has not a firm surface to stabilize it

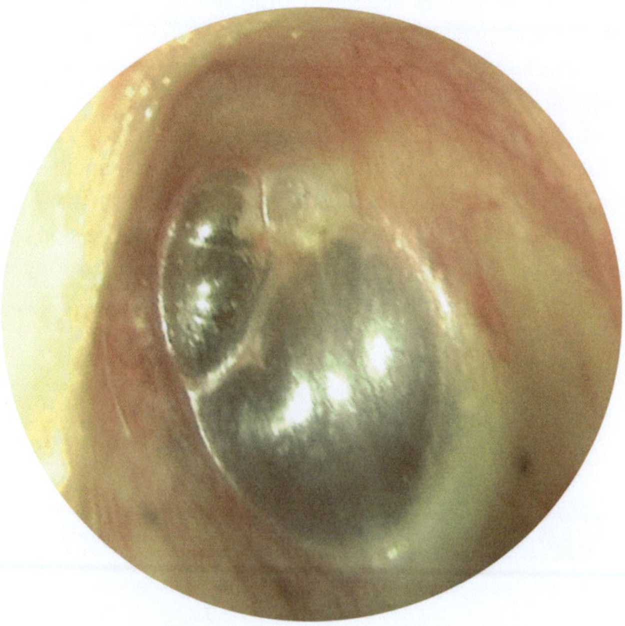

Fig. 50.6 Left ear, lateralized graft

Surgical Technique

Approaches

Optimal surgical exposure is a critical factor in the success of any surgery. The importance of the exposure cannot be attenuated, either if microscopic or endoscopic surgery is being considered. Traditionally, three different approaches were described in tympanoplasty: transcanal, endaural, and retroauricular. More recently, the endoscopic approach has been consolidated into surgical options. All the approaches are described in this book, we suggest the reader refer to the specific chapter.

The retroauricular approach is the "warhorse" of surgical otology and, with few modifications, can fit almost all temporal bone procedures. The wide exposure of the 360° of the external auditory canal (EAC) can be further improved through anterior and posterior canaloplasty. We have routinely employed this approach for narrow or sinuous canals, revision cases, large perforations, poor control of the anterior margin of the perforation, and when concomitant mastoidectomy is possible. Once the indications for overlay tympanoplasty mainly include the total (or subtotal) perforations, we elected the retroauricular approach as the preferred in those cases.

Overlay Technique Step by Step

External Auditory Canal Incisions (Transmeatal)

In order to delineate the vascular strip, we perform the first two incisions along the two suture lines at 1 and 11 o'clock (considering the malleus lateral process as 12 o'clock), as shown in Fig. 50.7. These incisions are oriented medially laterally, starting 2 mm from the tympanic annulus and extending beyond the osseocartilaginous junction. They are linked to each other through a third incision next to the annulus, thus creating a laterally pedicled flap. This flap, or vascular strip, contains the largest vascular contingent of the EAC and is then retrogradely elevated (from medial to lateral) with a Rosen knife.

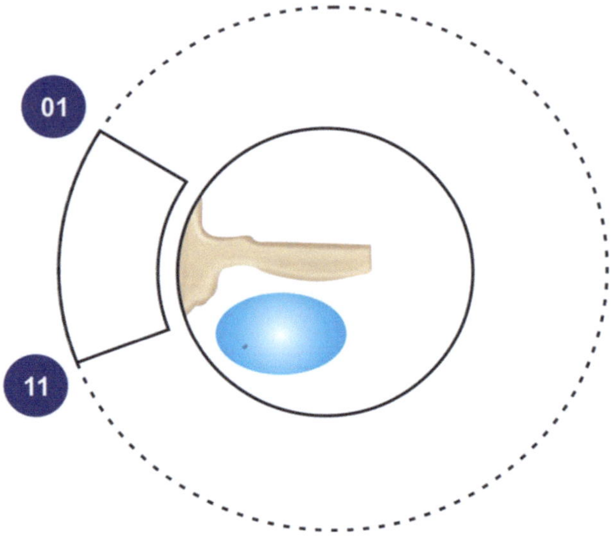

Fig. 50.7 Transmeatal incisions on overlay technique at 1 and 11 o'clock

Retroauricular Approach and Taking the Fascia

The retroauricular incision is made approximately 1 cm behind the pinna. It is performed this way, rather than in the retroauricular sulcus, as it does not cause postoperative discomfort for the patient, such as the use of glasses, and because it improves the approximation of the skin to the surgical wound. The incision reaches the temporalis muscle's fascia and the mastoid's periosteum. The ear is reflected anteriorly, and the plane of loose areolar tissue is traced anteriorly until the ear canal can be felt by palpation. The autostatic retractors are positioned at this time.

After controlling the bleeding with the cautery, the connective areolar tissue is set apart from the true temporalis fascia through sharp and blunt dissection. Then, a 3 × 2 cm piece of fascia is removed and spread on a plane surface (Teflon block, round tub, or other).

External Auditory Canal Exposure

After removing the fascia, the retroauricular incision is completed, and a periosteal flap is created. This flap is dissected anteriorly with a septal detacher. In this step, the lateral reference points are recognized sequentially: mastoid cortex, cribriform area, and Henle's spine. At this time, a semi-circular depression indicates that the CAE has been reached.

The microscope assists in further dissection until the EAC skin and the posterior margin of the vascular strip are both identified. With a scalpel blade #11, the EAC skin is incised at the osseocartilaginous junction. This incision starts from the posterior and most lateral edges of the vascular strip in an inferior direction. Then it ascends along the EAC's anterior wall until the vascular strip's anterior edge is reached.

Thus, the bony and cartilaginous portions of the EAC are almost entirely separated, facilitating anterior transposition of the external ear. During this maneuver, the vascular band is entirely detached from its bone bed and remains pedunculated laterally to the pinna. When the 360° of the EAC are exposed, the pinna and the vascular band are fixed and kept in position with autostatic retractors.

Removal of EAC Skin and the Lateral Surface of the TM

Using the microscope, the remaining canal skin is dissected with the Rosen elevator until the annulus is reached. At this point, the fibrous annulus is kept in its original position, and the dissection direction changes parallel and around the annulus.

Once the EAC skin is thoroughly dissected, it must be removed with the lateral layer of the TM, as shown in Fig. 50.8. For that, it has to be carefully separated from the medial layer of the tympanic remnant and, mainly, from the annulus. The annulus must be kept inserted in its bone groove in order to serve as a support for the graft. To perform this removal, the skin is separated from the ring superiorly or inferiorly, depending on the surgeon's viewing angle. Using a Rosen elevator, the surgeon tries to find a plane of dissection between these two structures. Once this plane is found, it must be followed circumferentially until the tympanic epidermal layer is completely removed. This maneuver, if appropriately done, separates the remaining skin from the canal precisely at the level of the tympanic ring. The skin can be kept in saline solution on the auxiliary table for as long as necessary.

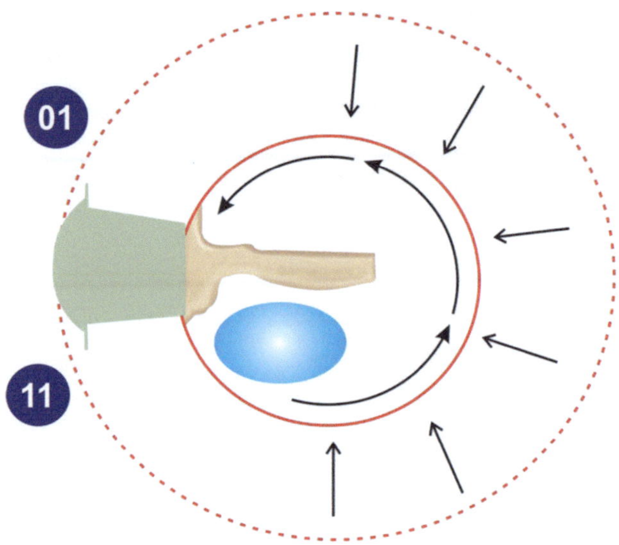

Fig. 50.8 Skin and epithelial layer of TM removal

Enlarging the Ear Canal

An ample canaloplasty is a crucial feature of the lateral *overlay* technique. Initially, the drill is used, and later, close to the annulus, the curette is used to remove residual small bony overhangs and epithelial remnants. Enlarging the anterior sulcus's exposure for perfect graft placement is imperative. After concluding this step and with a 360° vision of the ear canal, attention is directed to ensure that all epithelial remnants were removed either from the canal or the TM. Any residual niches of skin left behind may generate epithelial cysts in the postoperative period.

Exploratory Tympanotomy and Ossiculoplasty

Before grafting the TM, attention is directed to the middle ear contents. A methodical analysis is carried out emphasizing key anatomical landmarks checking the patency of the middle ear aeration channels: Eustachian tube opening, protympanum, the position of the malleus handle (which often will be found medialized), and the anterior and posterior tympanic isthmus. Next, the posterior recesses (round window niche, sinus tympani, and facial recess) are sequentially checked for hidden pathology (granulation tissue, cholesterol granuloma, or small epithelial cysts). Finally, the integrity of the ossicular chain is fully inspected, and its mobility is tested. Partial or total ossicular erosion or fixation is identified at this stage and managed if possible. When the middle ear's general conditions are far from ideal (thick mucosa, keratin islands over the promontory, gross ossicular destruction), the surgery should be staged, and ossicular reconstruction carried out in a second stage.

Packing the Middle Ear and Preparing the Fascia

Hemostatic sponge (Gelfoam, Spongostam) is prepared in various sizes and formats. We use medium size sponge blocks soaked in the physiologic solution to fill the middle ear up to the level of the annulus ring.

The fascia must be removed from the surface where it was placed and prepared with delicate scissors until a final circular product is obtained. The dimensions of this molded fascia must have the exact dimensions of the absent TM. The anterior edge of the fascia must be rounded to fit the annular sulcus, and an S-shaped incision is made in its medial portion creating a small slit to accommodate the malleus handle. Its length must be adjusted to allow part of the fascia to rest on the posterior wall of the EAC.

Preparing the EAC Skin

The conduit skin is prepared by cutting the irregular edges created in the initial dissection. Any excess skin must be removed. The piece of skin is accommodated in the silicone block with its periosteal face upward and the lateral margin closest to the surgeon. The skin is kept wet throughout the procedure. In order to avoid trapping air bubbles under this skin, we usually make small incisions of 1–2 mm parallel to its longest axis with a scalpel.

Placing the Fascia

Once the fascia is prepared, it is suspended by its anterior edge with delicate ear forceps ("alligator forceps") and immersed in saline solution to facilitate its manipulation. The graft is taken into the canal, and its anterior edge is placed over the tympanic annulus in the anterior sulcus. The slit created in the graft is placed under the malleus and pulled superiorly to the neck. The anterior half of the slit is then pulled over the *pars flaccida* to cover the region superior to the lateral process of the malleus. The graft must be placed over the tympanic ring at this point, as shown in Fig. 50.9, limited in the annular sulcus anteriorly and inferiorly. Superiorly, the posterior half of the graft should be accommodated below the TM *umbus* and malleus handle. As mentioned, the anterior half of the graft must cover the pars flaccida region, slightly overlapping the posterior half (at its upper pole) and extending to the superior wall of the EAC. The graft must also cover part of the posterior wall of the EAC, allowing the band to vascular rest on it.

Placing the EAC Skin

Once prepared as described above, the skin is grabbed with forceps at the lateral edge and placed into the EAC (Fig. 50.10). It is easier to position the skin if the medial edge touches the grafted fascia and is thus drawn into position, allowing surface tension to push the edge of the tissue into the anterior angle. This should result in a sharp angle between the fascia and the opposing skin. None should overlap the other; both are just touching at the junction between the annulus and the bony part of the canal.

The packing starts with strips of hemostatic sponge tightly compressed against the anterior sulcus. The rest of the canal is packed tightly with blocs of sponge, leaving a corresponding free space in the vascular strip. As pointed out by Sheehy, the canal skin should cover the bone from which it was removed and positioned slightly more medially and overlapping the fascia by a millimeter. Besides accelerating epithelization, it helps to prevent possible blunting.

Filling the Anterior Angle

Small strips or "rails" of hemostatic sponge soaked in the physiologic solution are positioned under pressure along the entire tympanic sulcus, ensuring the acute angle created between the graft and the EAC skin is maintained. This filling continues in layers until the medial half of the EAC and the anterior half of the TM are positioned in place.

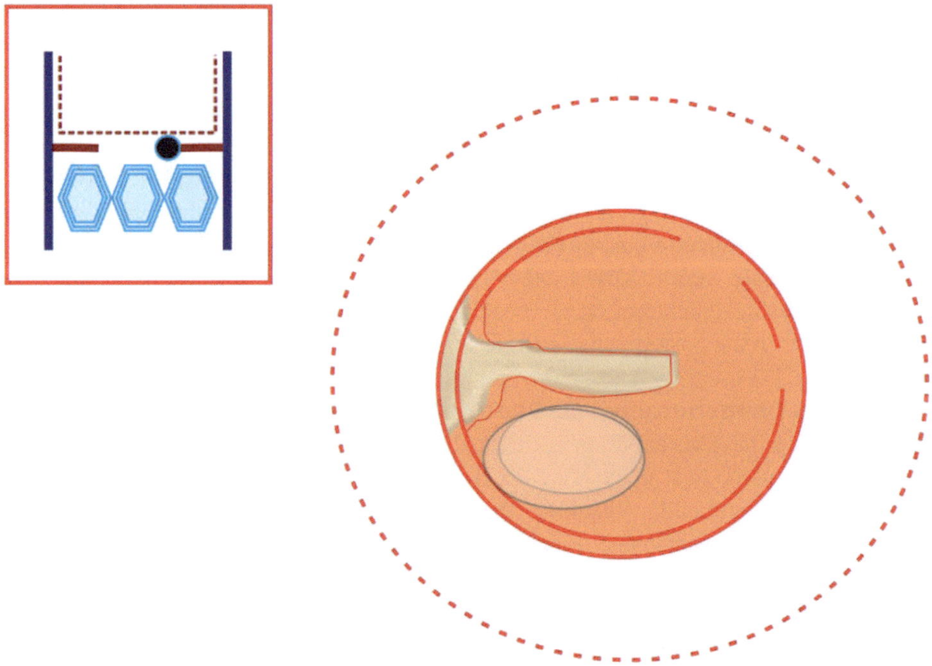

Fig. 50.9 Placement of fascia

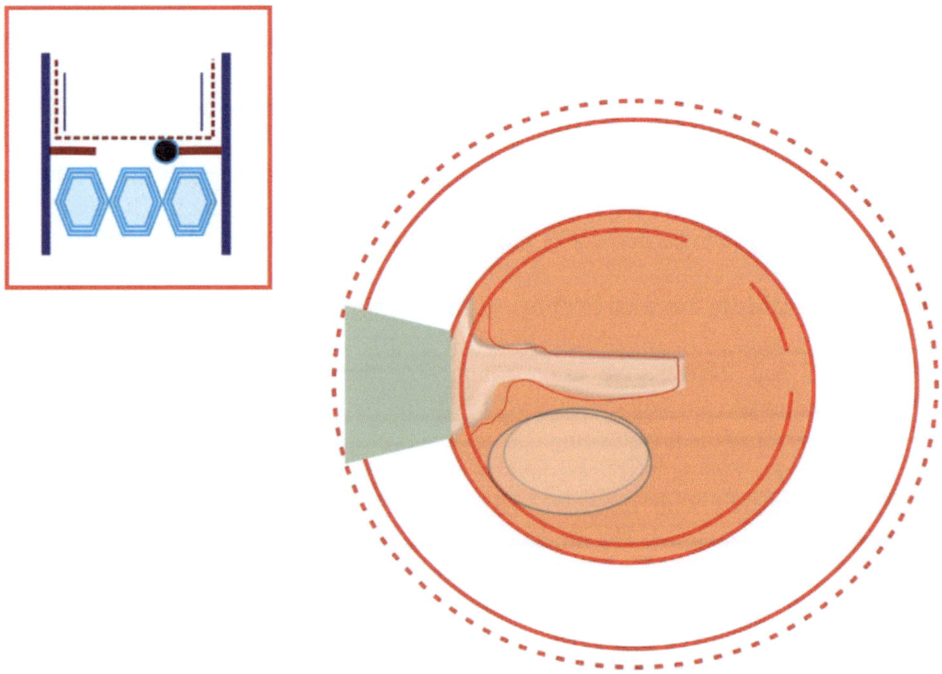

Fig. 50.10 Replacement of the canal skin

Once the above procedure is complete in the anterior part, the graft should be stable in the ear. We can work again through the transcanal approach by releasing the retractors and pulling the external ear to its original position. At this moment, the vascular stripe is released and positioned, overlapping the posterior portion of the graft. This maneuver is essential for accelerating healing and preventing postoperative infections. Additional hemostatic sponge cubes complete the filling of the EAC.

Closure of the Retroauricular Access

With the ear back in the anatomical position, hemostasis is performed. Subsequently, the retroauricular incision is sutured in layers, with particular attention to the muscular planes, thus avoiding the development of a protruding ear postoperatively.

Bibliography

Austin DF, Shea JJ Jr. A new system of tympanoplasty using vein graft. Laryngoscope. 1961;71:596–611.

Costa SS, Souza LCA, Piza MRT. The flexible endaural tympanoplasty. Otolaryngol Clin N Am. 1999;32:41340.

Meyerhoff WL, Kim CG, Paparella MM. Pathology of chronic otitis media. Ann Otol Rhinol Laryngol. 1978;87:74961.

Mutlu C, Costa SS, Paparella MM, et al. Clinical histopathological correlations of pitfalls in middle ear surgery. Eur Arch Otorhinolaryngol. 1998;255:18994.

Rizer FM. Tympanoplasty: a historical review and a comparison of techniques. Laryngoscope (suppl). 1997;107:1–36.

Shambaugh GE, Glasscock ME. Tympanoplasty. In: Surgery of the ear. 3rd ed. Philadelphia: WB Saunders; 1980.

Sheehy JL, Benecke JE. Middle ear reconstruction: current status. Adv Otolaryngol Head Neck Surg. 1987;1:143–70.

Sheehy JL, Glasscock ME. Tympanic membrane grafting with temporalis fascia. Arch Otolaryngol. 1967;86:57–68.

Tympanoplasty: The Inlay Technique Step by Step

51

José Faibes Lubianca Neto, João Pedro Neves Lubianca, Marcelo Neves Lubianca, and Roland Douglas Eavey

Introduction

Tympanoplasty is the term that describes reconstructive surgeries in the tympanic cleft, including tympanic membrane and ossicles. When exclusively tympanic membrane perforation is closed, the correct term is myringoplasty. Since the original description of tympanoplasty by Zollner [1] and Wullstein [2], numerous techniques were developed. Common approaches to tympanoplasty involve the endomeatal, endaural, or postauricular route. Three main techniques are used to insert the graft according to tympanic annulus (TA): overlay (TA is not elevated and graft lies lateral to it) [3], underlay (TA is elevated and graft is inserted under it and lies medially to it) [4], and inlay (the graft is inserted through the tympanic membrane perforation and lies on it) [5]. The first two approaches need creation of tympanomeatal flap. There are a few techniques, however, that cannot be classified based on these criteria, as the palisade technique [6], for example, and other that are mixed, like over-under technique [7, 8].

Tympanoplasty can be done using different types of grafts, including temporalis fascia, fascia lata, perichondrium, cartilage, vein, periosteum, skin, amniotic membrane, dura mater, adipose tissue, artificial tissues [9], cornea, peritoneum, pericardium, and others. Placental tissues, meninges, and other not mentioned allografts and xenografts are not used anymore in majority of places due to biological concerns with some viral disease, like acquired immune deficiency syndrome, hepatitis, and Creutzfeldt–Jakob's disease [10]. Temporalis muscle fascia is the most used graft and is often the material chosen for primary cases. Cartilage (tragal or conchal) is gaining popularity more recently for primary cases, but it is classically the option for revision cases [11].

The butterfly tympanoplasty is an endomeatal (transcanal) inlay technique that uses cartilage as graft. This technique was called by different names in the literature: butterfly tympanoplasty, butterfly myringoplasty, butterfly wing tympanoplasty, butterfly cartilage graft inlay tympanoplasty, transcanal butterfly cartilage tympanoplasty, transcanal cartilage butterfly inlay technic, transcanal endoscopic tympanoplasty with inlay cartilage graft, inlay butterfly cartilage tympanoplasty, inlay cartilage tympanoplasty, minimally invasive inlay tympanoplasty, inlay butterfly myringoplasty, inlay diabolo myringoplasty, bivalve cartilage inlay myringoplasty, plug cartilage tympanoplasty, and cartilage button tympanoplasty and collar button myringoplasty.

The Original Eavey Technique: From the Conception and Description of the Technique Step by Step to the First Results

Although today the technique is known all over the world, what very few people know is that this this was created by a challenge proposed by a single patient. He was an Argentine child who used to consult in Boston and the next day he took a plane to go to Disney and in a few days to return to his country. So, a technique was needed that was proof of pressure changes in flight and that uses a resistant graft. At the same time, postoperative dressings should be dispensable. That is why cartilage was chosen and this technique developed. A description and illustrations of each step of the surgical technique are presented below:

J. F. Lubianca Neto (✉)
Federal University of Health Sciences of Porto Alegre (UFCSPA), Santo Antonio Children's Hospital, Porto Alegre, RS, Brazil
e-mail: lubianca@otorrinospoa.com.br

J. P. N. Lubianca
Federal University of Rio Grande do Sul (UFRGS), Porto Alegre, RS, Brazil

M. N. Lubianca
Pontifical Catholic University of Rio Grande do Sul (PUCRS), Porto Alegre, RS, Brazil

R. D. Eavey
Department of Otolaryngology-Head and Neck Surgery, Vanderbilt University Medical Center, Nashville, TN, USA

M. V. Goycoolea et al. (eds.), *Textbook of Otitis Media*, https://doi.org/10.1007/978-3-031-40949-3_51

1. The patient is anesthetized, prepped, and draped for a sterile procedure. Lidocaine and epinephrine 1:100,000 are used for skin injection into the meatal surface of the tragus. Originally, this technique was described to be performed under microscope, but the endoscope is an interesting alternative [12]. The patient is positioned, and the tympanic membrane perforation is viewed in a transcanal fashion.
2. If the middle ear mucosa appears healthy and no unexpected pathology is encountered, a straight pick is used to circumferentially puncture the perimeter of the perforation; a microcups instrument is used to grasp the narrow punctured circular strip to freshen the perforation margin. Squamous epithelium is swept or suctioned away from the new perimeter of the perforation (Fig. 51.1). Importantly, in the original description, this technique could proceed only if all aspects of the newly enlarged perforation were still seen transcanally and if a sufficient tympanic membrane remainder existed circumferentially to provide an edge against which to secure the graft. As we will see in other section of this chapter, the indications have been expanded to large and even marginal perforations [13].
3. The dimensions and shape of the perforation are measured with right-angled hooks, 1–4 mm in length (Fig. 51.2).
4. The tragus is approached and with a #15 blade and an incision is made approximately halfway between the lateral extent of the tragal dome and the meatus (Fig. 51.3). The incision is carried through skin, subcutaneous tissue, and cartilage in one sweep. The lateral tragal dome is retracted with a skin hook; a forceps grasps the medial tragal cartilage. A small, sharply pointed scissors is used to spread the soft tissues. Importantly, the perichondrium on both sides of the cartilage is included in the graft. Scissor cuts are created cephalad, caudad, and deep to remove the cartilage. The small incision is closed with 6-0 mild chromic suture. Some authors do not suture the incision, allowing it to close spontaneously.
5. Because the dimensions and the shape of the perforation will have been measured previously, the same hook is

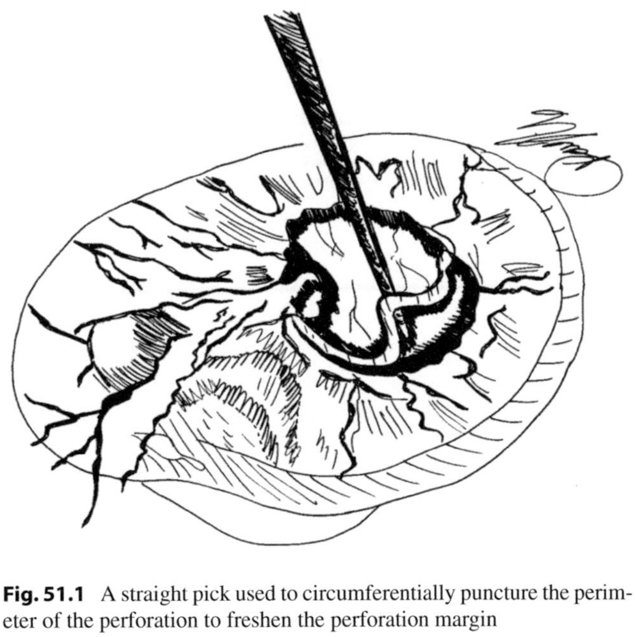

Fig. 51.1 A straight pick used to circumferentially puncture the perimeter of the perforation to freshen the perforation margin

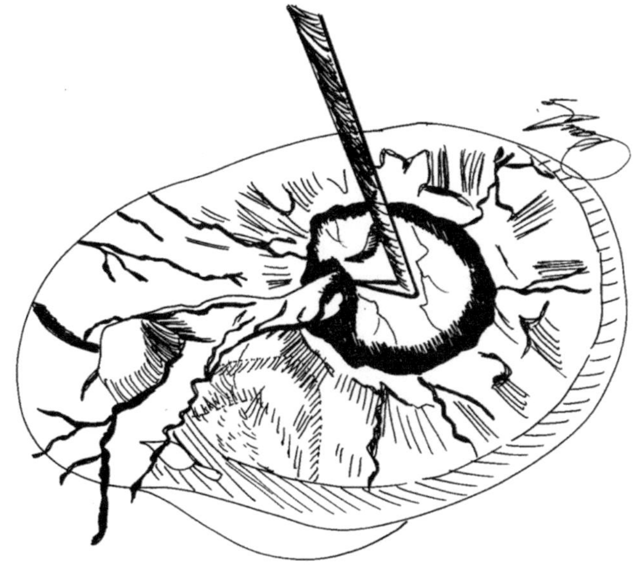

Fig. 51.2 A right-angled hook measuring the dimensions of the perforation

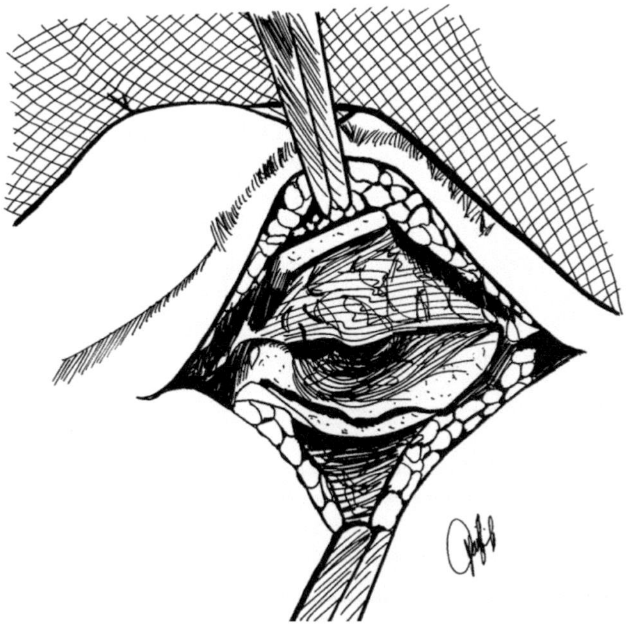

Fig. 51.3 Incision made approximately halfway between the lateral extent of the tragal dome and the meatus, saving the domus to prevent esthetic sequela

used to estimate the size and shape of the perforation on the harvested cartilage, which has been placed on a cutting surface and is viewed with the microscope. The piece of cartilage that will become the inlay is created in the same shape but must be slightly larger than the actual size of the perforation. For example, a perforation approximately 4 × 5 mm in area would require a cartilage graft approximately 6 × 7 mm in area. Once the approximate shape and size have been estimated with the right-angled hook, a Beaver #6700 mini-blade or even a # 15 or #11 standard blade is used to cut out the graft from the larger piece of tragal cartilage. The graft cartilage is then turned to 90″ so that the surgeon views the edge of the cartilage, still via the microscope. The blade is used to score the thin edge, parallel between the two sheets of perichondrium. The graft must be rotated in order to score circumferentially around the entire perimeter. The surgeon will note that the retained perichondrium causes the thin cartilage edges to curl apart from the incision line made by the blade. The spreading of the two cartilage surfaces, on edge, resembles the wings of a butterfly The scoring depth should be sufficient (Fig. 51.4). The exposed malleus and tympanosclerotic plaques serve to interlock with the graft. Note the remaining rim of the tympanic membrane that must be present circumferentially to interlock with the graft. A right-angled hook is used to estimate the size of the perforation (approximately 1–2 mm) so that the edge of tympanic membrane will be able to penetrate into this circumferential groove to secure the cartilage graft.

6. The surgeon again microscopically or endoscopically views the perforation. Superficial squamous epithelium near the edge of the perforation should have been swept away previously using a #5 instrument and a #20 suction. Should any residual suspicious shreds of epithelium be noted, complete removal should be performed. The butterfly cartilage graft is grasped with a toothless alligator forceps and inserted in a transcanal fashion. The leading edge of the graft initially gains a purchase on the anterior edge of the perforation. Usually, the graft will nestle in so that one butterfly wing remains lateral to the edge of the perforation and the other wing is on the medial side of the tympanic membrane. It is necessary to inspect and to instrument the entire perimeter to make certain that the graft is anchored into the perforation correctly. The time of actual graft placement can vary from a few seconds to about 2 min. At times, the graft convincingly will "pop" into the perforation, at other times the graft will appear to lie against the surface and will require perimeter inspection to discern that only the lateral butterfly wing is superficial to the drum (Fig. 51.5). Should the graft be slightly large, the situation is easily remedied. Either a small incision at the perimeter of the perforation can be made to slightly enlarge the opening or the graft can be removed, and the circumferential scoring can be deepened. Should the graft be too small, a new graft can be created from the remaining tragal cartilage. At this point, Eavey's preference is to place a split-thickness skin graft over the perichondrium of the cartilage graft. One of the Lubianca's modifications of the original technique is not to use the skin graft, with similar results [14]. When used, the skin will have been harvested from the inner aspect of the arm and placed on silk impregnated with water-based gel. The silk is removed immediately after placement of the skin graft into the ear. No packing is placed in the ear. Antibiotic drops may be used. Only a cotton ball is inserted at the meatus, the ball can be removed later on the day of surgery.

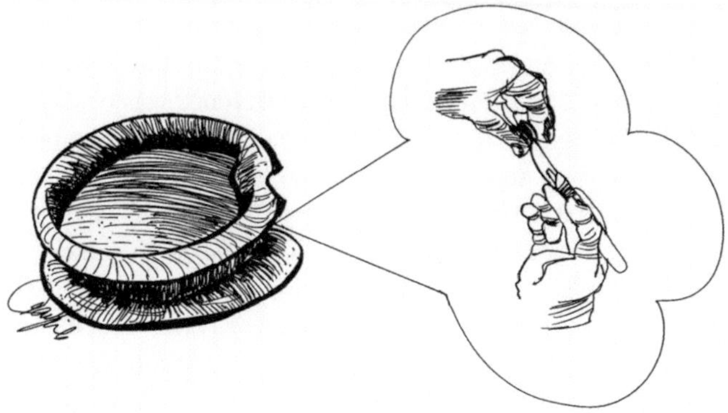

Fig. 51.4 Cartilage edges curling apart from the incision line made between the two sheets of perichondrium circumferentially, resembling the wings of a butterfly

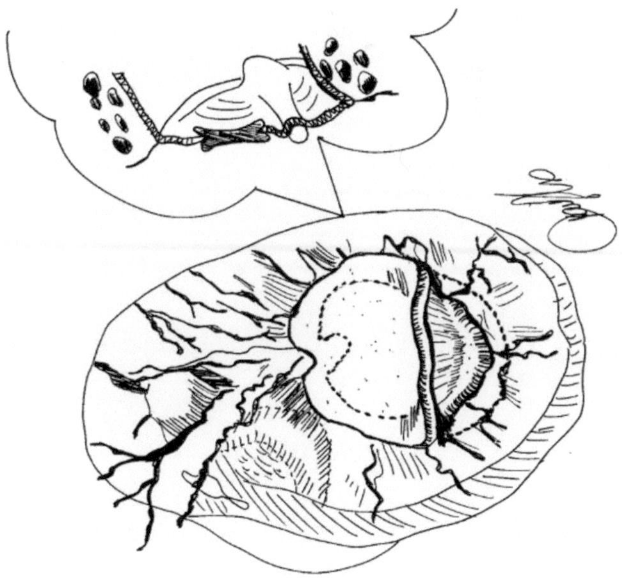

Fig. 51.5 The graft was then inserted, and one wing was placed on the lateral side and the other wing remained on the medial side of the TM. The graft was inserted per-aurally mounted on crocodile fórceps. The procedure is similar to inserting a grommet

Eavey's inlay butterfly cartilage tympanoplasty was first used in 1994. Four years later, it was published at Laryngoscope appearing in the cover photo of the edition (Fig. 51.6).

The results in nine cases were described, with a 100% take rate of the graft and pure-tone averages increased for all ten ears from 5 to 20 dB, with an average of 12 dB [5]. In Fig. 51.7, successful cases at different follow-up times are shown.

From the Original Technique First Results to the Replication, Modifications, and Finally to the Randomized Clinical Trial

Returning to Brazil, after fellowship at the Massachusetts Eye and Ear Infirmary Pediatric Otorhinolaryngology Division, at that time (1997) headed by Dr. Roland Eavey, one of the authors (JFLN) started to replicate the results. However, few modifications have been introduced, such as the fact that the skin graft is not used, the surgery was performed in adults and under local anesthesia. In 2000, we published a series of 20 patients, achieving a graft take rate of 90% and good hearing results [14].

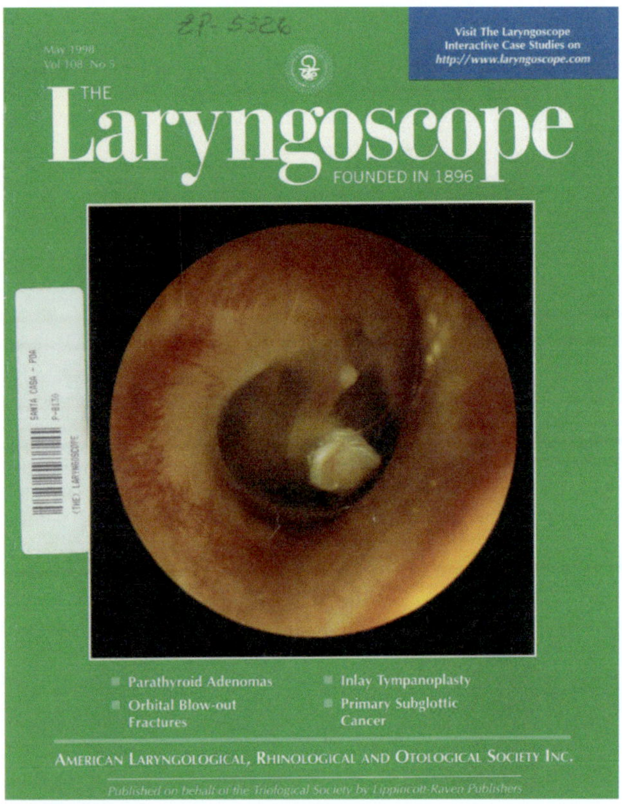

Fig. 51.6 Cover of the May 1998 edition of laryngoscope with the endoscopic image of a late postoperative result of a butterfly cartilage inlay tympanoplasty

Even the processes of conception, publication of the first results and replication in another center were finished, there was still no comparison with the traditional technique. This motivated a randomized clinical trial, published in 2001 [15], that was the first randomized clinical trial published in the field of tympanoplasty comparing surgical techniques. The next clinical trials appear in 2006 and evaluated the necessity of ventilatory tube in cartilage tympanoplasties and the effect of the use of dry or wet temporal fascia graft on tympanoplasty [16, 17]. It was not until 9 years after our publication that the first clinical trials appeared comparing different techniques of tympanoplasties themselves [18–20]. There are other randomized clinical trials published before 2001, but they deal with anesthetic drugs, use of hyaluronic acid, and prophylactic antibiotics.

The purpose of our clinical trial was to evaluate the efficacy of modified-cartilage inlay tympanoplasty in adults compared with underlay tympanoplasty with a temporalis fascia graft by assessing the "take rate" and postoperative audiometric results. A total of 70 patients aged 15–65 years who had nonmarginal TM perforations that could be seen entirely through a transcanal view and which were smaller than 50% of the total surface of the TM were potentially eligible. Patients who had an ear infection at least in the 2 preceding months, who required exploration of the middle ear or possible cholesteatoma were excluded. A stratified randomization for tympanosclerosis (a positive prognostic factor for the take rate with inlay technique) with random permuted blocks for each stratum was done.

The "take rate" did not differ between groups on the 30th postoperative day (88.2% in the inlay tympanoplasty group vs 86.1% in the underlay tympanoplasty group; $P < 0.8$). After a mean follow-up of 7.5 ± 3.8 months (range, 3–16 months), the "take rate" was 85.3% in the inlay tympanoplasty group and 83.3% in the underlay tympanoplasty group ($P = 0.8$). In the inlay tympanoplasty group, there was closure of the air-bone gap (ABG) to within 10 dB in 64.7% and to within 20 dB in 94.1%. The corresponding numbers to underlay tympanoplasty were 75% and 97.2%. In only 2 cases (5.9%) in the inlay tympanoplasty group and in 1 case (2.8%) in the underlay tympanoplasty group, the ABG was greater than 20 dB. No audiometric difference was observed between groups ($P = 0.6$). Most patients in the inlay tympanoplasty group reported immediate improvement in their hearing ($P < 0.0001$). Pain was reported by 10 patients in the inlay tympanoplasty group and by 30 patients in the underlay tympanoplasty group on the first postoperative day ($P < 0.0001$). The duration of the surgery (mean ± standard deviation) was 33.6 ± 7.8 min for the inlay tympanoplasty group and 62.9 ± 12.7 min for the underlay tympanoplasty group ($P < 0.001$). The estimated charge for inlay tympanoplasty at our institution was 65% less expensive than underlay tympanoplasty [15].

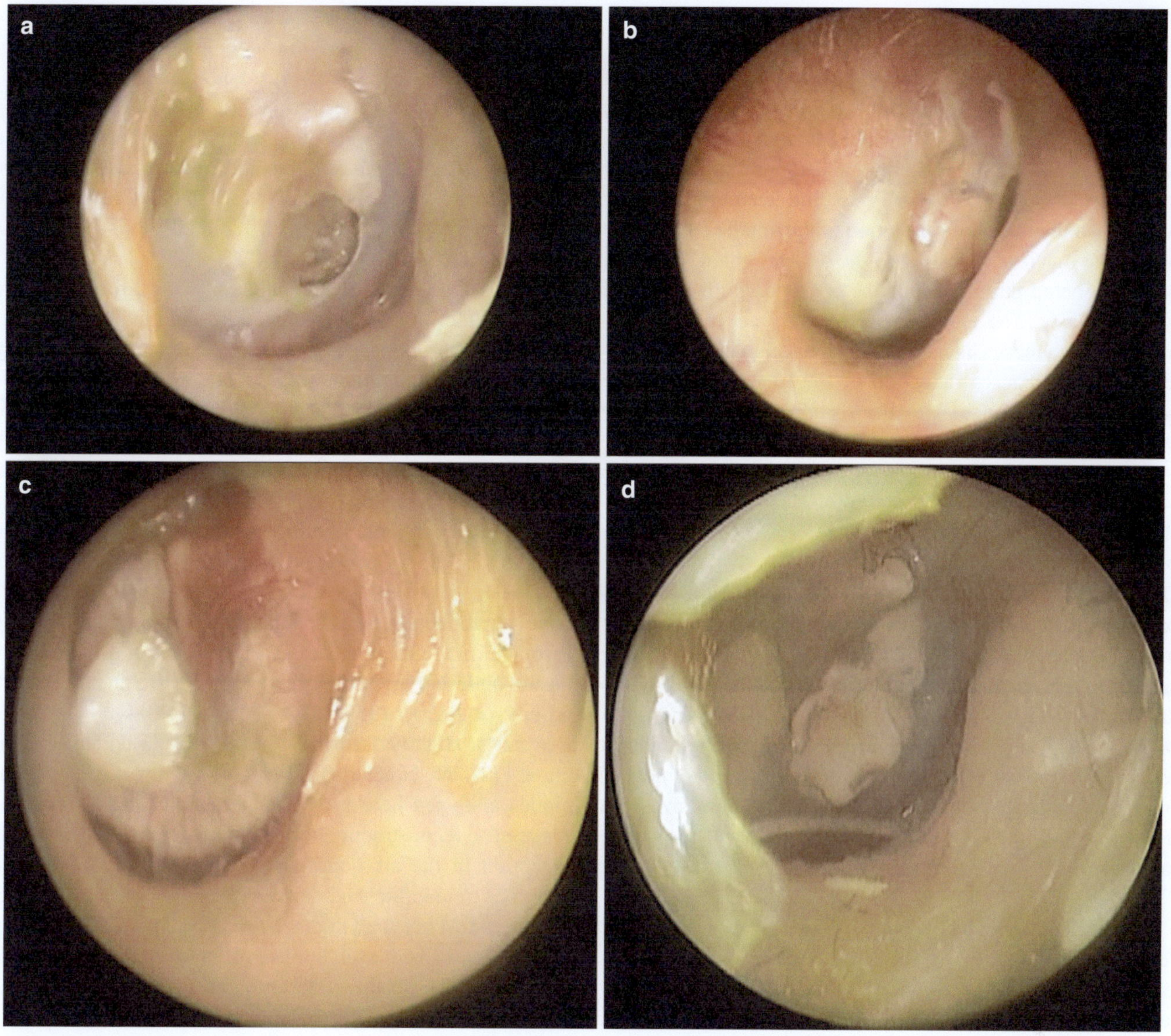

Fig. 51.7 (**a–c**) The same case with preoperative anterior perforation in the right tympanic membrane and 3 years after the operation, and the contralateral side showing a good graft take at the third postoperative month; (**d**) another patient with 1 year of follow-up

In conclusion, according to Gertrude Stein (1920), "for a difference to be a difference it has to make a difference". Although the take rate and audiometric results following inlay cartilage tympanoplasty or underlay tympanoplasty were similar, inlay butterfly cartilage tympanoplasty did not require general anesthesia in patients greater than 15 years, was less expensive, and more comfortable to the patient.

Advantages and Limitations

The inlay technique provides several practical advantages. The surgeon can insert the cartilage graft even into a myringosclerotic tympanic membrane setting; no external canal packing or middle ear support is necessary because the graft stabilizes instantly at insertion; patient postoperative comfort is enhanced; and the procedure is less expensive because of diminished operative and recovery room time.

The technique has three main limitations. Theoretically, it may predispose to cholesteatoma, similarly to the placement of ventilation tubes. However, if it happens, it should be very uncommon and no case has been reported in the literature so far, even in children or adults [21, 22]. At least two explanations are plausible for this finding. The first one is the theory that the healing process of the tympanic membrane perforation starts from the fusion of the graft with the lamina propria layer of the tympanic membrane remnant [23]. In addition, is our experience that the excess perichondrium and the cartilage part of the chondroperichondrial graft lateral to the tympanic membrane remnant became necrotic in a short period of time (between the second week and 1 month) postoperatively and the complete epithelization over the cartilage graft is ready in 3 months in the great majority of cases. After epithelization is complete, there is no longer the risk of pearl formation or even cholesteatoma development. Other disadvantage of the technique is that it does not allow to explore the tympanic cavity to find membranous diaphragms in the routes of ventilation of the middle ear, pathology of the mucosa, or lesions to the ossicles chain. It should be remembered that the technique is a myringoplasty, not a tympanoplasty. The endoscope, however, can at least partially obviate these diagnostic problems. Finally, the cartilaginous graft causes reduction of the transparency of the tympanic membrane, making the visualization of the tympanum more difficult.

Results over the World

One of the most frequently asked questions from the surprised audience after the first conferences on the butterfly inlay tympanoplasty was "do medical insurance pay the same for this technique as for the traditional one?". The answer was an absolute "yes". Probably due to the simplicity of the surgical steps and the shorter time of surgery, the butterfly technique had a tremendous receptivity in the midst of otology in different countries. Table 51.1 summarizes the articles already published on the technique. Their respective take rates and audiometric improvements are presented at Table 51.2.

There are five metanalysis [6, 72–75] and one systematic review [76] comparing cartilage and fascia as grafts for tympanoplasties. Only three of them included the cartilage butterfly inlay technique [72, 73, 74]. In general, they showed a certain degree of superiority in the cartilage group in terms of successful closure of the perforation and no difference regarding to audiometric results. Unfortunately, they analyze the cartilage group, not discriminating results among different techniques. Another metanalysis, dealing only with myringoplasty without tympanomeatal flap elevation in children, compared the take rate and audiometric results with different sizes of perforation, using microscope or endoscope. In the butterfly cartilage inlay group closure of the tympanic perforation was achieved in 246/299 patients (82.3% overall: 93.3% and 75.8% for endoscopic and microscopic procedures, respectively), with a mean follow-up of 12 months. Overall, the normalized postoperative hearing was achieved in 85.5% of the sample, and there was not a difference between microscopic and endoscopic procedures. The mean postoperative GAP was 8.5 dB. Only 3 out 10 studies reviewed reported the differential in air–bone gaps, with a mean reduction of 9.2 dB [21].

Finally, two recent meta-analyses by our group compare anatomical (closure of the perforation) and functional (reduction of the air–bone gap) outcomes between the butterfly inlay cartilage and temporal fascia underlay techniques [77] and between the endoscopic and microscopic approaches for performing the butterfly inlay cartilage tympanoplasty [78]. In the first one comparing techniques, 577 patients from 10 studies were included. The graft take rate was 82.8% in the butterfly cartilage inlay tympanoplasty group and 85.2% in the temporal fascia underlay tympanoplasty group (relative risk, 1.01; 95% CI, 0.93–1.11; $I^2 = 42\%$, $P = 0.08$). The air–bone gap reduction ranged from 6.1 to 11.28 in the butterfly cartilage inlay group and from 5.2 to 12.66 in the temporal fascia underlay group, with a mean difference between groups of −2.08 (95% CI, −3.23 to −0.94; $I^2 = 58\%$, $P = 0.04$), slightly favoring temporal fascia underlay technique [77]. We concluded that the two tympanoplasty techniques analyzed here produced similar results in terms of successful reconstruction of the tympanic membrane and reduction in the air–bone gap. Neither age nor follow-up length of time influenced outcomes. In the last one, comparing the endoscopic and microscopic approaches, 318 patients were included from a total of five different studies. Graft take rate was 91.3% in the endoscopic group and 93.6% in the microscopic group (RR 0.98; 95% CI 0.93–1.03; I^2 0%; $P = 0.68$). Four studies provided data about the auditory results, all showing significant reductions in air–bone gap, ranging from 5.7 to 11.0 in the endoscope group and from 5.8 to 11.6 in the microscope group, with a mean difference between groups of 0.85 (95% CI = 0.79–2.48). We concluded that endoscopic and microscopic butterfly cartilage graft inlay tympanoplasties have similar results on anatomical and hearing outcomes, making the selection between such approaches an individual choice for the surgeon.

Table 51.1 First author and provenance of the study, type of surgical approach, sample size, age of the participants, study design, follow-up, size and location of the perforations, and take rate. Studies are shown according to the year of publication

First author (year)	Country	Technique	N (ears)	Age in years Mean ± SD (range)	Study design	Follow-up in months Mean ± SD (range)	Perforation size	Position #	Take rate
Eavey RD (1998) [5]	USA	MBT	9 (11)	11.9 (6–19)	Retrospective	10–40	ND	A: 36.3%, AI: 9.1%, I: 9.1%, PI: 9.1%, C: 36.3%	100%
Lubianca Neto JF (2000) [14]	Brazil	MBT	20	(15–64)	Retrospective	7.25 (2–13)	2–4 mm	ND	90%
Mauri M (2001) [15]	Brazil	MBT	34 (range, 15–65)	7.5 ± 3.8 (3–16)	Prospective (RCT)	7.5 ± 3.8 (3–16)	2–5 mm (50%)	ND	85.3%
Anand TS (2002) [24]	India	MBT	2 0	9–50	Retrospective	6	3–6 mm	ND	90%
Effat KG (2005) [25]	Egypt	MBT	21 (28)	24.5 (8–58)	Retrospective	8	ND	ND	43%
Couloigner V (2005) [26]	France	MBT	59	9.9 ± 3.4 (3–17)	Retrospective	26.6 ± 19.9	<25%: 64.5% 25–50%: 32% >50%: 3.5%	A: 47.5% C: 37.3% P: 13.6% I: 1.7%	71.2%
Karakullukçu B (2006) [27]	Turkey	MBT	11	30 (21–45)	Retrospective	9.5 (1–18)	2–6 mm	ND	90.9%
Monfared A (2008) [28]	USA	MBT	145	49.2 ± 17.3	Retrospective	13.9 (1–78)	Mean 3.65 ± 1.19 (range, 1–7 mm)	C 50.34%, AI 26.21%, PI 11.03%, PS 5.52%, AS 4.14%	67.6%
Neto JAM (2008) [29]	Brazil	MBT	23	10.3 (3–15)	Retrospective	9 (2–12)	15–90% (mean 38.64%)	ND	82.6%
Rourke T (2010) [30]	UK	MBT	36	35 (5–86)	Retrospective	6 ± 5.2	Mean 2.4 mm (±1.0 mm): 1 mm (11.1%) 2 mm (44.4%) 3 mm (27.8%) 4 mm (5.6%) 6 mm (27.8%)	A + AI = 90%	94%
Yu MS (2010) [31]	Korea	MBT	17	40.12 (9–64)	Retrospective	13 (6–43)	Small to moderate	AI, PI, C	100%
Lin YC (2011) [32]	Taiwan	MBT	62 (72)	31–87 (mean [SD] age, 61.2 [12.9] years)	Retrospective	>6 months 21.19 ± 9.49	–	ND	87.3%
Belhossine I (2012) [33]	France	MBT	26	38 (9–73)	Retrospective	20	<20%: 65.4% >20% to <50%: 34.6%	A: 69.23% P: 7.69% C: 23.08%	92.3%
Hod R (2013) [34]	Israel	MBT	42	27 (14–75)	Retrospective	24 (3–36)	<33%: 23.8% 33–66%: 64.3% >66%: 11.9%	ND	92%
Ciuman R (2014) [35]	Germany	MBT	10	12–71	Prospective	6	<6 mm	ND	100%
Eren SB (2014) [36]	Turkey	MBT	25	30.1	Prospective	6	3 ± 0.6 mm	ND	88.2%
Haksever M (2014) [37]	Turkey	MBT	29	(15–65)	Retrospective	12	4–6 mm	ND	96.5%
Kim HJ (2014) [38]	Korea	MBT	56	56.5 ± 13.8	Retrospective	10.6 ± 3.1	Small: 35.7% Medium: 35.7% Large: 28.6%	ND	96.4%

(continued)

Table 51.1 (continued)

First author (year)	Country	Technique	N (ears)	Age in years Mean ± SD (range)	Study design	Follow-up in months Mean ± SD (range)	Perforation size	Position #	Take rate
Dorlodot C (2015) [39]	Belgium	EBT or MBT	40	18.5 ± 16.1 (5–53)	Retrospective	5.2 ± 5.7	ND	ND	85%
Eren SB (2015) [40]	Turkey	EBT	22	33.5 ± 12.4	Retrospective	11.8 ± 3.7	3.7 ± 1 mm (2.5–5.5)	A: 100%	95.5%
Wu PW (2015) [41]	Taiwan	MBT	25 (27)	60.3 (42–76)	Retrospective	18.86 (12.30–35.83)	Small, large	ND	84%
Callioglu EE (2016) [42]	Turkey	MBT	25	37 ± 15.8	Retrospective	31	<50 (2–5 mm)	C, P	92%
Alain H (2016) [43]	Israel	MBT	33	34 (19–76)	Retrospective	14.5	ND	ND	94%
Özgür A (2016) [44]	Turkey	EBT	42 (45)	31 (9–56)	Retrospective	14.4 ± 5.4 (6–25)	Small 46.7% Medium 53.3%	A: 66.7%, P: 24.4%, AI:8.9%	95.6%
Riss JC (2016) [45]	France	MCT	26	7.7 (2–12)	Retrospective	25 (10–96)	11.1–36.4% (mean, 26.3%)	I and AI: 50%, AS: 31.1%, A: 17.9%	85.7%
Akyigit (2017) [46]	Turkey	EBT	32	13.9 ± 2.3 (8–17)	Retrospective	23.37 ± 9.55	<3 mm: 37.5% 3–6 mm: 72.5%	A: 28.1% P: 18.8% AP: 53.1%	93.7%
Isaacson G (2017) [47]	USA	EBT	30	6 (3.5–17)	Retrospective	3	ND	ND	55%
Kaya (2017) [48]	Turkey	EBT	18	39 (18–58)	Prospective	6	Up to 7 mm	A, I	100%
Jumaily M (2018) [49]	USA	EBT or MBT	23	(5–17)	Retrospective	13.4 (1–85)	ND	ND	69.6%
Karabulut B (2018) [50]	Turkey	EBT	56	35 (17–58)	Retrospective	29.2 (24–39)	<3 mm: 41.1% 3–6 mm: 58.9%	A: 35.7% P: 32.1% C: 32.1%	94.6%
Karataş M (2018) [51]	Turkey	MBT or EBT	Overall: 66. MBT: 10, EBT: 56	29.2 ± 15.2 (5–63)	Retrospective	Overall: 20.21 ± 6.09 (10–30). M: 27.20 ± 6.53. E: 18.96 ± 5.20	Small: 39.4% Medium: 43.9% Large: 16.7%	C: 65.15% A: 31.82% P: 3.03%	Overall 86.33%; BT: 90%; EBT: 85.71%
Kaya (2018) [23]	Turkey	EBT	93	40.3	Retrospective	Mean 41.8 months (range, 24–105 moths)	Small: 43.01%. Medium: 56.9%	A—Small 22.5%, medium 24.5% P—Small 27.5%, Medium 35.9% C—Small 50.0%, Medium 39.6%	94.6%
Mourya A (2018) [52]	India	MBT	100	28.3	Prospective	24	Small to medium (<5 mm)	I: 52.67%, C: 24.34%	97%
Toro PC (2018) [53]	Spain	MBT	32	21.1 (4–59)	Retrospective	12–59 (mean 28.75)	2–8 (2 mm: 6.3%; 3 mm: 43.8%; 4 mm: 28.1%; 5 mm: 9.4%; 6 mm: 3.1%; 7 mm: 3.1%; 8 mm: 3.1%)	AI: 50%, AS: 3.1%, PS: 3.1%, PI: 7.5%, ST: 6.25%	84%
Ulku CH (2018) [54]	Turkey	MBT	25	32.0 (11–73)	Retrospective	27.4	ND	-ND	92%
Wang H (2018) [55]	China	MBT	12	39.5 (23–53)	Retrospective	2–24	5 (small), 7 (média)	ND	83.3%
Pontes-Madruga (2019) [56]	Brazil	EBT	83	37.5 ± 13.8 (13–69)	Retrospective	6 months	≤25%	ND	76%%

Table 51.1 (continued)

First author (year)	Country	Technique	N (ears)	Age in years Mean ± SD (range)	Study design	Follow-up in months Mean ± SD (range)	Perforation size	Position #	Take rate
Bartel R (2019) [57]	Spain	EBT	29	10.7 ± 2.9 (7–16)	Prospective	6	ND	ND	92.6%
Dave VC (2019) [58]	India	MBT	5	33 ± 9.7	Retrospective	15.6	Small (3) medium (2)	ND	80%
Demir E (2019) [59]	Turkey	EBT	26	35.4 ± 15.2 (13–64)	Retrospective	13.3 ± 7.1 (6–32)	ND	ND	96%
Karataş M (2019) [60]	Turkey	MBTor EBT	MBT: 21 EBT: 58	MBT: 12.6 ± 3.3. EBT: 13.3 ± 3.30	Retrospective	M: 23.19 ± 9.40 E: 21.40 ± 9.15	MBT—Small: 9.5%; Medium: 42.9%; Large: 47.6; EBT—Small: 27.6%; Medium: 32.8%; Large: 39.7%	MBT—C: 85.71%, A: 0, P: 14.3%; MBE—C: 77.7%, A: 20.7%, P: 1.72%	MBT: 85.7%. EBT: 91.4%
Khoza-Shangase K, (2019) [61]	South Africa	MBT	38	39.4 (18–63)	Retrospective	6	–	ND	ND
Kim MB (2019) [62]	Korea	MBT	22 (23)	47.9 ± 15.7	Retrospective	10.0 ± 7.3	3–7 mm	ND	91.3%
Lee SA (2019) [63]	Korea	MBT or EBT	MBT: 24. EBT: 39	MBT: 53.0 ± 16.3 EBT: 55.1 ± 16.2	Retrospective	6 months	MBT—2 mm: 45.8%, 3 mm: 37.5%, 4 mm: 16.8% Endoscopic—2 mm: 51.3% 3 mm: 35.9% 4 mm: 12.8%	MBT—Cl: 66.7%, A: 33.3%; EBT—C: 48.7% A: 51.3%	MBT: 95.8% EBT: 92.3%
Leonard JA (2019) [64]	USA	MBT	21	13.4	Retrospective	>6	30.6%	AI: 28.6%, AS: 9.5%, A: 23.8%, PI: 4.8%, PS: 4.8%, I: 23.8%	85.7%
Li Y (2020) [65]	China	EBT	38	34.5 ± 14.2	Retrospective	9.4 ± 3.1 (6–18 months)	Small	AI, AS	94.7%
Gülşen S (2020) [66]	Turkey	EBT	34	31.6 ± 10.8 (21–47)	Prospective	8.2	4.9 ± 1.7 mm (range, 3–5.5 mm)	A	94.1%
Hashim ND (2020) [67]	Malaysia	EBT or MBT	60	57.9	Retrospective	12.58	Small: 27.3% Medium: 66.7% Large: 6%	C: 100%	98.4%
Özdemir D (2020) [68]	Turkey	EBT	54	33.2 ± 16.4	Retrospective	6	Small: 48.2% Medium: 40.7% Large: 11.1%	A: 59.3% P: 22.2% AP: 18.5%	98.1%
Buck LS (2021) [69]	USA	EBT or MBT	52	<16	Retrospective	4 mml: 28.9%, 5 mm: 18.8%, 6 mm: 19.2%	4–6 mm	ND	Mean: 92%, 4 mm: 94%, 5 mm: 96% 6 mm: 67%
Demir E (2021) [70]	Turkey	EBT	17		Retrospective			A: 10, I: 6, P: 1	100%
Ravi N (2021) [71]	India	MBT or EBT	50	(18–60)	Prospective (ECR)	3 months	Small to medium	ND	EBT: 96 ± 4% MBT: 92 ± 8%

MBT microscopic butterfly technique; *EBT* endoscopic butterfly technique; *A* anterior; *P* posterior; *AI* antero-inferior; *PI* postero-inferior; *PS* postero-superior; *AS* antero-superior; *I* inferior; *C* central; *ST* subtotal; *ND* no data

Table 51.2 Main audiological results of the inlay butterfly cartilage tympanoplasty according to the year of publication

First author (year)	Follow-up in months mean ± SD (range)	PostOp ABG[a] in decibel (dB)	ABG variation in decibel			Improvement in four-PTA in decibel		
Eavey RD (1998) [5]	(10–40)	ND	ND				Preop	Postop
						Mean PTA	19.7	10
Lubianca Neto JF (2000) [14]	7.25	ND	ND				Preop	Postop
						Mean PTA	52.7 ± 19.3	46.6 ± 21.7
Mauri M (2001) [15]	7.61 ± 4.1			Preop	Postop	ND		
		0–10 dB: 64.7%	0–10	17.6%	64.7%			
		11–20 dB: 29.4%	11–20	38.2%	29.4%			
		>20 dB: 5.9%	>20	44.1%	5.9%			
			Mean ABG closure:					
			<0	8.8%				
			0–10	50.0%				
			11–20	26.5%				
			>21	14.7%				
Anand TS (2002) [24]	6	ND	ND			5–10 dB: 20%		
						4–15 dB: 30%		
						16-20 dB:20%		
						21-25 dB:15%		
						26-30 dB:5%		
						No improvement: 10%		
Effat KG (2005) [25]	(12–41)	ND	ND			ND		
Couloigner V (2005) [26]	26.6 ± 19.9	ND	ND				Preop	Postop
						500 Hz	24 ± 12	19 ± 14
						1 KHz	21 ± 11	15 ± 11
						2 KHz	19 ± 9	14 ± 10
						4 KHz	20 ± 11	20 ± 13
Karakullukçu B (2006) [27]	9.5	6.5		Preop	Postop			
			ABG	18 (10–25)	6.5 (5–15)			
Monfared A (2008) [28]	(1–78)	ND	ND				Preop	Postop
						Mean PTA	36.8	28.2
Neto JAM (2008) [29]	–	ND		Preop	Postop	ND		
			01–10 years/old	16.3 (5–30)	5.0 (0–15)			
			11–15 years/old	26.6 (5–50)	12.4 (0–30)			
Rourke T (2010) [30]	1.5	12.7 ± 11.5	ABG	Preop (%)	Postop (%)	ND		
			<0	3	0			
			0–10	7	52			
			11–20	52	31			
			21–30	24	4			
			31–40	10	4			
			41–50	0	7			
			>50	4	0			
				Preop	Postop dB			
			Mean ABG	19.7 ± 10.6	12.7 ± 11.5			
			Mean decrease ABG	7.0 dB ± 6.4				
Yu MS (2010) [31]	13.0	8.4	Mean ABG				Preop	Postop
			Preop	Postop		Mean PTA	29.2	21.4
			15.8	8.4				
			Mean ABG	Preop	Postop			
			0–10	29.4%	70.6%			
			11–20	47.1%	17.6%			
			21–30	11.8%	11.8%			
			31–40	1.8%	0.0%			

Table 51.2 (continued)

First author (year)	Follow-up in months mean ± SD (range)	PostOp ABG[a] in decibel (dB)	ABG variation in decibel			Improvement in four-PTA in decibel		
Lin YC (2011) [32]	21.19 ± 9.49 (10–41)	12.6 ± 12.9	Mean ABG	Preop	Postop		Preop	Postop
				19.8 ± 10.3	12.6 ± 12.9	Mean SRT	52.7 ± 19.3	46.6 ± 21.7
			ABG < 10 dB: 75%					
Belhossine I (2012) [33]	20	(3.5–15.2)	Range ABG	Preop	Postop	ND		
				7.5–20.5	3.5–15.2			
			27.8 to 20.1 (mean gain 7.5 dB)					
Hod R (2013)[a] [34]	24 (3–36)	ND	Mean ABG	Preop	Postop	ND		
				49.6	26.2			
Ciuman R (2014) [35]	6	6.5 ± 3.9	ABG	Preop	Postop	ND		
				11.7 ± 10.1	6.5 ± 3.9			
			0–10	50%	70%			
			11–20	20%	20%			
			21–30	20%	–			
			>30	–	–			
Eren SB (2014) [36]	6	With OC[b]: 9.2 ± 2.8 Without OC: 9.4 ± 2.4	ABG	Preop	Postop	ND		
			WOC	17.5 ± 1.3	9.2 ± 2.8			
			W/O OC	18.2 ± 2.8	9.4 ± 2.4			
			Improvement in ABG: 9.0 ± 1.5					
			Improvement in ABG: 7.9 ± 2.6					
Haksever M (2014) [37]	1.5	0–10: 58.6% 11–20: 31.0% 21–40: 10.3%	ABG	Preop	Postop	ND		
			s0–10	20.7%	58.6%			
			11–20	37.9%	31.0%			
			21–40	41.4%	10.3%			
			Improvement in mean ABG: 18.8 ± 8.09—11.9 ± 7.12					
Kim HJ (2014) [38]	10.4 ± 3.4 (9–18)	0–10: 51.8% 11–20: 37.5% >20: 10.7%		Preop	Postop	ND		
			0–10 dB	17.9%	51.8%			
			11–20 dB	44.6%	37.5%			
			>20 dB	37.5%	10.7%			
			Mean ABG closure: 7.9 ± 2.2					
Dorlodot C (2015) [39]	5.2 ± 5.7	<10: 85%	Mean ABG within 10 dB: 85%			ND		
Eren SB (2015) [40]	11.8 ± 3.7	10.8 ± 4.5	ABG	Preop	Postop	ND		
				19.3 ± 3.3	10.8 ± 4.5			
Wu PW (2015) [41]	18.9 (12.3–35.8)	Small perforation: 10.1 ± 10.6 Large Perforation: 11.5 ± 21.9	Mean ABG closure: Small perforations: 2.3 ± 11.6 Large perforations: 16.3 ± 6.01			Small perforation: Pre-operative 47.3 ± 14.5 Postoperative 49.1 ± 19.1 Average hearing gain: −1.8 ± 13.19 Large perforation: Pre-operative: 59.7 ± 15.6 Postoperative: 44. 9 ± 22.0 Average hearing gain: 14.77 ± 9.35		
Callioglu EE (2016) [42]	31	10.9 ± 5.8	ABG	Preop	Postop	ND		
				16.4 ± 5.4	10.9 ± 5.8			

(continued)

Table 51.2 (continued)

First author (year)	Follow-up in months mean ± SD (range)	PostOp ABG[a] in decibel (dB)	ABG variation in decibel			Improvement in four-PTA in decibel		
Alain H (2016) [43]	12	11.3	ABG	Preop	Postop	37.7–10.6		
				29.7	11.3			
Özgür A (2016) [44]	6	9.1 ± 2.5		Preop	Postop		Preop	Postop
			Mean ABG	18.5 ± 6.4	9.1 ± 2.5	Mean PTA	28.4 ± 11.6	17.4 ± 7.2
			ABG reduction: 9.4 ± 5.6					
Riss JC (2016) [45]	25 (10–96)	ND	ABG	Preop	Postop	ND		
			0–10	3.6%	42.9%			
			11–20	53.6%	42.9%			
			21–30	35.7%	10.7%			
			31–40	7.1%	3.5%			
			Mean ABG	20.2 (10–31.3)	14 (5–31.3)			
Akyigit (2017) [46]	12	7.9 ± 3.3	ABG	Preop	Postop	ND		
			0–10	12.5%	78.1%			
			11–20	50%	21.9%			
			21–30	37.5%	–			
Isaacson G (2017) [47]	3	ND	**ND**			**ND**		
Kaya (2017) [48]	6	ND	ND				Preop	Postop
						Mean PTA	27.7	10.5
Jumaily M (2018) [49]	13.4	Successful 0–10: 73.7%; 11–20: 21.1% 21–30: 5.3% >30: 0 Unsuccessful 0–10: 50.0% 11–20: 40.0% 21–30: 0 >30: 10.0%	Decrease in mean Air-bone GAP			ND		
			Preop ABG	Successful	Unsuccessful			
			0–10	28.6%	54.5%			
			11–20	57.1%	27.3%			
			21–30	4.8%	9.1%			
			>30	9.6%	9.1%			
			Post ABG	Successful	Unsuccessful			
			0–10	73.7%	50.0%			
			11–20	21.1%	40.0%			
			21–30	5.3%	0			
			>30	0	10.0%			
			Overall (13.4 dB to 6.9 dB)					
Karabulut B (2018) [50]	24	12.4 ± 3.1	Mean ABG	Preop	Postop		Preop	Postop
				24.2 ± 3.8	12.4 ± 3.1	Mean PTA	35.2 ± 3.9	20.4 ± 3.2
Karataş M (2018) [51]	6	10.4 ± 4.8	Mean ABG	Preop	Postop	ND		
				23.1 ± 8.6	10.4 ± 4.8			
			ABG improvement: 13.55 ± 8.17					
Kaya (2018) [23]	24	11.9 ± 5.5		Preop	Postop		Preop	Postop
			Mean ABG	22.1 ± 7.1	11.9 ± 5.5	Mean PTA	36.4 ± 15.1	24.9 ± 14.1
Mourya A (2018) [52]	6	ND	ND				Preop	Postop
						Mean SRT	32.3 ± 12.9	28.3 ± 8.2
Toro PC (2018) [53]	12–59	ND	Mean ABG	Preop	Postop		Pre-op	Postop
				17 (6–25)	7 (0–17)	Mean PTA	35.2 (22–65)	24.0 (15–55)
Ulku CH (2018) [54]	27.4	ND	Mean ABG	Preop	Postop	ND		
				17.1 ± 8.8	5.8 ± 2.3			
			Mean ABG gain: 11.28					
Wang H (2018) [55]	(2–24)	5.2 (range 0–11.2)	Mean ABG	Preop	Postop	ND		
				13.0 (3.7–20)	5.2 (0–11.2)			
			Mean ABG gain: 7.77					
Pontes-Madruga (2019) [56]	6	11.1 ± 1.0		Preop	Postop		Preop	Postop
			Mean ABG	17.9 ± 8.9	11.1 ± 1.0	Mean PTA	33.5 ± 14.3	24.4 ± 15.0

Table 51.2 (continued)

First author (year)	Follow-up in months mean ± SD (range)	PostOp ABG[a] in decibel (dB)	ABG variation in decibel			Improvement in four-PTA in decibel		
Bartel R (2019) [57]	6	6.9	Mean ABG	Preop	Postop[c]	Mean PTA (24.6–16.3)		
				15.5	6.9			
			Mean ABG Postop decrease 8.5 ± 6.3					
Dave VC (2019) [58]	12	18.8 ± 8.1	ABG	Preop	Postop	ND		
				25.5 ± 3.67	18.75 ± 8.12			
			Difference in mean pre and postop ABG: 6.75 ± 5.24					
Demir E (2019) [59]	13.3 ± 7.1 (6–32)	14.4 (2.5–35)	ABG	Preop	Postop	ND		
				21.4	14.4 (2.5–35)			
			Mean Postoperative hearing gain 6.5 ± 4.5 (3–16)					
Karataş M (2019) [60]	6	MBT: 9.8 ± 4.31 EBT: 9.3 ± 3.5	Mean ABG	Preop	Postop		Preop	Postop
			MBT:	22.0 ± 7.1	9.8 ± 4.3	MBT:	33.2 ± 9.3	20.1 ± 6.0
			EBT:	20.9 ± 4.78	9.3 ± 3.5	EBT:	30.3 ± 5.6	18.7 ± 3.45
			ABG Gain MBT: 12.0 ± 7.3 EBT: 11.6 ± 5.5					
Khoza-Shangase K (2019) [61]	(3–6)	ND	ND			Mean Difference Pre minus Postop		
						500 Hz 1 KHz 2 KHz 4 KHz	18.1 ± 22.7 14.4 ± 21 12.0 ± 21.1 9.2 ± 24.83	
Kim MB (2019) [62]	10.9 ± 9.4	13.8 ± 11.3	Mean ABG	Preop	Postop	ND		
				19.9 ± 12.6	13.8 ± 11.3			
			ABG improvement: 6.1 ± 8.2					
Lee AS (2019) [63]	6	MBT: 3.3 ± 4.7 EBT: 3.1 ± 3.8	Mean ABG	Preop	Postop	ND		
			MBT:	8.6 ± 8.0	3.3 ± 4.7			
			EBT:	8.8 ± 4.6	3.1 ± 3.8			
			Mean ABG Improvement: MBT: 5.3 ± 6.9 EBT: 5.7 ± 5.4					
Leonard JA (2019) [64]	>6	500 Hz: 10.6 1 KHz: 8.8 2 KHz: 4.7		Preop	Postop	ND		
			500 Hz 1 KHz 2 KHz	31.7 22.7 17.9	10.6 8.8 4.7			
			Reduction in ABG: 500 Hz: 19.2 1 KHz: 11.7 2 KHz: 13.2					
Li Y (2020) [65]	9.4 ± 3.1 (6–18)	10.8 ± 6.0	Mean ABG	Preop	Postop		Preop	Postop
				18.4 ± 6.3	10.8 ± 6.0	Mean PTA	30.9 ± 8.9	21.4 ± 7.7
			Mean ABG improvement: 8.3 ± 1.5					
Gülşen S (2020) [66]	6	5.2 ± 4.1 (0–11)	Mean ABG	Preop	Postop	ND		
				16.8 ± 3.7 (12–20)	5.2 ± 4.1 (0–11)			
			ABG improvement: 11.7 ± 2.7					
Hashim ND (2020) [67]	ND	MBT: 13.2 ± 6.8 EBT: 9.4 ± 6.0	Improvement in ABG: MBT: 6.5 ± 4.5 EBT: 9.1 ± 5.7			ND		
Özdemir D (2020) [68]	14.2 ± 6.1	8.5 ± 2.3	Mean ABG	Preop	Postop	ND		
				17.4 ± 5.2	8.5 ± 2.3			

(continued)

Table 51.2 (continued)

First author (year)	Follow-up in months mean ± SD (range)	PostOp ABG[a] in decibel (dB)	ABG variation in decibel			Improvement in four-PTA in decibel		
Buck LS (2021) [69]	4 mm; 28.9 (6–64) 5 mm: 18.8 (6–72) 6 mm: 19.2 (9–60)	4 mm:5.7 ± 3.5 5 mm:5.7 ± 6.9 6 mm:5.8 ± 6.3	Mean ABG			Mean PTA		
				Preop	Postop		Preop	Postop
			4 mm:	13.9 ± 5.8	5.7 ± 3.5	4 mm:	22.0 ± 10.3	11.2 ± 5.5
			5 mm:	15.2 ± 6.5	5.7 ± 6.9	5 mm:	21.8 ± 10.7	12.4 ± 8.2
			6 mm:	15.6 ± 4.6	5.8 ± 6.3	6 mm:	21.1 ± 9.5	13.4 ± 7.7
Demir E (2021) [70]	>6	11.1 ± 7.8 (5–35)		Preop	Postop	Mean PTA	Preop	Postop
			Mean ABG	12.5 ± 8.1 (5–35)	11.1 ± 7.8 (5–35)		19.7 ± 9.6 (10–45)	18.2 ± 9.3 (10–45)
Ravi N (2021) [71]	ND	3	ABG improvement: EBT: 11.0 ± 7.2 MBT: 10.8 ± 7.69 Overall mean ABG improvement: 10.9 ± 7.33			ND		

PTA pure tone average

[a] ABG—Air–bone gap

[b] OC—Otologic compass (the study is a randomized clinical trial comparing the results with using or not an otologic compass to measure the perforation and the tragal graft)

[c] These results apply only for the 32 out of 42 patients in whom there were a significant decrease in the mean air–bone gap from the preoperative period to the last follow-up

New Applications and Further Modifications

Some theoretical limitations initially were described for this method because the original operation was not designed for patients with (1) a perforation that could not be seen entirely by way of transcanal view, (2) conditions requiring exploration of the middle ear, (3) a perforation that abutted the annulus, or (4) a tympanic membrane with extensive granular myringitis [5]. With further experience, however, such theoretical limitations of use of the butterfly cartilage inlay graft have been transcended so that the graft can be advantageously used for more extensive ear surgery.

In 2006, Ron Eavey's group published the first paper about the use of inlay butterfly cartilage technique for larger (medium and large) perforations [13]. The butterfly cartilage inlay graft resulted in a 92% "take rate" with an intact repair. The mean preoperative to postoperative four-tone air–bone gap improved from 23 to 21 dB, a mean gain of 2 dB, which was not statistically significant ($P = 0.109$). The number of ears that demonstrated preoperative to postoperative hearing in the 0–10 dB range doubled from 16 to 32 ears ($P = 0.008$); the majority of postoperative patients (52%) heard in the 0–20 dB range, despite most having disease requiring mastoidectomy. Large perforations, annular perforations, and perforations in conjunction with middle ear exploration and mastoidectomy could be repaired with quite satisfactory results. The same technique of cartilage edge scoring that creates the handy butterfly perimeter to engage residual tympanic membrane also engages the bony annulus or malleus to provide an immediately stable cartilaginous repair [13].

An Israeli study by Alain H et al. (2016), evaluating the efficacy of butterfly tympanoplasty for subtotal and total perforations in 33 adult patients have shown, 1 month after surgery, two patients having a residual perforation (94% success rate). In terms of audiological results, they have demonstrated that the mean SRT was improved by 14 dB, whereas PTA was significantly improved by 27.1 dB. Furthermore, the ABG was closed up to 11.3 dB. Most patients with residual perforation also had improved hearing [43].

A more recent study by Demir et al. (2019) showed graft success rate of 96%, postoperative mean ABG of 14.4 dB and hearing gain of 6.5 dB. This study is the first to present the results of the patient series using the endoscopic tool to perform butterfly inlay myringoplasty procedure for large perforations [59].

Besides the use for large perforations and the introduction of the endoscope, there are other minimal technique modifications introduced. Some authors removed the inner perichondrium of the tragal cartilage and prepared a graft with an outer perichondrium [41, 44, 56], as Ron Eavey had already mention indirectly, when wrote that there is no problem if the inner perichondrium could not be preserved. Kaya et al. left one side of the cartilage placed in anterior–inferior perforations longer to increase graft success [48]. Özdemir et al. aimed to increase the success of the grafts by preparing a larger perichondrium than the cartilage on the cartilage graft and overlay the perichondrium after the cartilage graft was inlaid on the membrane [68]. Finally, at least one Turkish and another German study proposed the total removal of the perichondrium on both sides of the cartilage and placement of the pure cartilaginous graft. Their logical is that perichondrium could be the cause of myringitis found in few patients in the postoperative period in some previous studies. They achieved 94.6 and 100% of success in terms of closure of the perforation, respectively [22, 35]. These four modifications introduced have maintained a take rate over 97%.

In 2008, Monfared e cols. described another modification of the original technique in which they made an 1 cm incision on the posterior conchal bowl skin and carried a dissection bluntly to the perichondrium. With the use of dermal punches, a cartilage graft with both anterior and posterior perichondrium measuring 1 mm larger in diameter than the size of the perforation was harvested. The graft was prepared and placed in the perforation as originally described. Their success rate was 75% [28]. Some other authors use a dermatologic punch with standard sizes to take the graft in loco once the tragus is exposed and other cut the tragal cartilage after is excised from the donor site [30, 33].

Different ways to measuring the perforations were introduced. Some surgeons measure the size of perforation by taking imprint of methylene blue painted over margins of the perforation on a gel-foam sheet and measured with the help of a scale [52]. Others have used a matching paper template [43, 56] or a disposable paper ruler [66]. There is also a description of estimation of the diameter of the freshened perforation by comparing it with a green suction tip (2.0 mm diameter) [30]. Finally, even an otologic compass has been used to measure the size of perforation, showing encouraging results when compared to the measurement made by a Fisch elevator in a randomized clinical trial [36].

Future

Tissue engineering is the field of knowledge that applies the principles of engineering and the life sciences toward the development of biological substitutes that restore, maintain, or improve tissue function. It can be applied to repair damaged or lost tissue of the tympanic membrane, through the laboratory creation of grafts. Hott et al. [79] showed that it is possible to get precisely shaped bovine articular chondrocyte-seeded calcium alginate structures using computer-aided design and injection molding technologies that maintain their shape during at least 10 weeks in culture. At the final of the experiment, the patches could be separated and removed from the mold. The obtained butterfly "plugs," however, seem a little different in structure to the natural hand-made ones during surgery, what can make them difficult to maintaining in position. Another limitation is that plugs are not covered by perichondrium, important in vivo to give vascular supply to them (Ciuman and Dost paper [35], however, has shown the opposite). Finally, to use autologous tragal or conchal cartilage does not obviate the need of a previous surgical procedure. To our knowledge this technique has not been tested in vivo until now, but even with the initial limitations, it has the potential to provide a minimally invasive alternative to traditional methods for the repair of tympanic membrane perforations in the future.

Acknowledgments We are grateful to Dr. Daniela Boeira da Silva, an excellent otorhinolaryngologist and illustrator.

References

1. Zollner F. The principles of plastic surgery of the sound-conducting apparatus. J Laryngol Otol. 1955;69:637–52.
2. Wullstein H. Theory and practice of myringoplasty. Laryngoscope. 1956;66:1076–93.
3. House LR. Clinical experiences in tympanoplasty: results in sixty-one cases. Laryngoscope. 1958;68:1481–9.
4. Austin FD, Shea JJ. A new system of tympanoplasty using vein graft. Laryngoscope. 1961;71:596–611.
5. Eavey RD. Inlay tympanoplasty: cartilage butterfly technique. Laryngoscope. 1998;108:657–61.
6. Jeffery CC, Shillington C, Andrews C, Ho A. The palisade cartilage tympanoplasty technique: a systematic review and meta-analysis. J Otolaryngol Head Neck Surg. 2017;46:48–54.
7. Ciger E, Balci MK, Islek A, Önal K. The wheel-shaped composite cartilage graft (WsCCG) and temporalis fascia for type 1 tympanoplasty: a prospective, randomized study. Eur Arch Otorhinolaryngol. 2018;275:2975–81.
8. Babu S, Luryi AL, Schutt CA. Over-under versus medial tympanoplasty: comparison of benefit, success, and hearing results. Laryngoscope. 2019;129:1206–10.
9. Ghanad I, Polanik D, Trakimas DR, Knoll RM, Castillo-Bustamante M, Black NL, et al. A systematic review of nonautologous graft materials used in human tympanoplasty. Laryngoscope. 2021;131:392–400.
10. Rompaey VV, Farr MRB, Hamans E, Mudry A, Vande Heyning PH. Allograft tympanoplasty: a historical perspective. Otol Neurotol. 2012;34:180–8.
11. Bayram A, Muluk NB, Cingi C, Bafaqeeh SA. Success rates for various graft materials in tympanoplasty—a review. J Otol. 2020;15:107–11.
12. Anzola JF, Nogueira JF. Endoscopic techniques in tympanoplasty. Otolaryngol Clin N Am. 2016;49:1253–64.
13. Ghanem MA, Monroy A, Alizadeh FS, Nicolau Y, Eavey RD. Butterfly cartilage graft inlay tympanoplasty for large perforations. Laryngoscope. 2006;116:1813–6.
14. Lubianca Neto JF. Inlay butterfly cartilage tympanoplasty (Eavey technique) modified for adults. Otolaryngol Head Neck Surg. 2000;123:492–4.
15. Mauri M, Lubianca Neto JF, Fuchs SC. Evaluation of inlay butterfly cartilage tympanoplasty: a randomized clinical trial. Laryngoscope. 2001;111:1479–85.

16. Elsheikh MN, Elsherief HS, Elsherief SG. Cartilage tympanoplasty for management of tympanic membrane atelectasis: is ventilatory tube necessary? Otol Neurotol. 2006;27:859–64.
17. Alkan S, Baylancicek S, Sözen E, Basak T, Dadas B. Effect of the use of dry (rigid) or wet (soft) temporal fascia graft on tympanoplasty. J Otolaryngol Head Neck Surg. 2009;38:126–32.
18. Wafaie MM, Elsherif AM, Bakr MS. Comparative study of the clinical and audiological outcome of myringoplasty using temporalis fascia graft versus tragal cartilage graft. AAMJ. 2010:8.
19. Cabra J, Moñux A. Efficacy of cartilage palisade tympanoplasty: randomized controlled trial. Otol Neurotol. 2010;31:589–95.
20. Alzoubi FQ, Tarifi AA, Khader Y, de Carpentier J. Comparison between transtymapnic and elevation of tympanomeatal flap approaches in tympanoplaty. Otol Neurotol. 2010;31:773–5.
21. Chatelet F, Leboulanger N, Achard S, Couloigner V, Denoyelle F, Simon F. Myringoplasty without tympanomeatal flap elevation in children: a systemic review. Eur Ann Otorhinolaryngol Head Neck Dis. 2021;138:92–9.
22. Kaya I, Benzer M, Uslu M, et al. Butterfly cartilage tympanoplasty long-term results: excellent treatment method in small and medium sized perforations. Clin Exp Otorhinolaryngol. 2018;11:23-9.
23. Zahnert T, Hüttenbrink KB, Mürbe D, Bornitz M. Experimental investigations of the use of cartilage in tympanic membrane reconstruction. Am J Otol. 2000;21:332–8.
24. Anand TS, Kathuria G, Kumar S, Wadhwa V, Pradhan T. Butterfly inlay tympanoplasty: a study in Indian scenario. Indian J Otolaryngol Head Neck Surg. 2002;54:11–3.
25. Effat KG. Results of inlay cartilage myringoplasty in terms of closure of central tympanic membrane perforations. J Laryngol Otol. 2005;119:611–3.
26. Couloigner V, Baculard F, El Bakkouri W, Viala P, François M, Narcy P, et al. Inlay butterfly cartilage tympanoplasty in children. Otol Neurotol. 2005;26:247–51.
27. Karakullukçu B, Acioglu E, Pamukçy M. Transcanal butterfly cartilage tympanoplasty. Kulak Burun Bogaz Ihtis Derg. 2006;16:160–3.
28. Monfared A, Bergeron CM, Ortiz J, Lee H, Kamine K, Dray T, Gunsalus R. Bivalve cartilage inlay myringoplasty: an office-based procedure for closing small to medium-sized tympanic membrane perforations. Otolaryngol Head Neck Surg. 2008;139:630–4.
29. Neto JAM, Neiva FC, Brodskyn F, Palumbo MN, Bittar ACV, Petrilli RNB, et al. Plug cartilage tympanoplasty in children. Rev Bras Otorrinolaringol. 2008;74:890–5.
30. Rourke T, Snelling JD, Aldren C. Cartilage graft butterfly myringoplasty: how we do it. Clin Otolaryngol. 2010;35:135–46.
31. Yu MS, Yoon TH. Bilateral same-day surgery for bilateral perforated chronic otitis media: inlay butterfly cartilage myringoplasty. Otolaryngol Head and Neck Surg. 2010;143:669–72.
32. Lin YC, Wang WH, Weng HH, Lin YC. Predictors of surgical and hearing long-term results for inlay cartilage tympanoplasty. Arch Otolaryngol Head Neck Surg. 2011;137:215–9.
33. Belhossine I, Pezzettigotta S, Genty E, Erminy M, Lecanu JB. Modified butterfly cartilage tympanoplasty: retrospective study on 26 patients. Rev Laryngol Otol Rhinol (Bord). 2012;133:77–80.
34. Hod R, Buda I, Hazan A, Nageris BI. Inlay "butterfly" cartilage tympanoplasty. Am J Otolaryngol–Head Neck Med Surg. 2013;34:41–3.
35. Ciuman RR, Dost P. Tips & tricks—collar button technique: safe and patient friendly myringoplasty technique. Laryngorhinootologie. 2014;93:442–5.
36. Eren SB, Tugrul S, Ozucer B, Dogan R, Ozturan O. A randomized prospective trial of a novel device for measuring perforation size during inlay "butterfly" myringoplasty. Am J Otolaryngol Head Neck Med Surg. 2014;35:305–8.
37. Haksever M, Akduman D, Solmaz F, Gündoğdu E. Inlay butterfly cartilage tympanoplasty in the treatment of dry central perforated chronic otitis media as an effective and time-saving procedure. Eur Arch Otorhinolaryngol. 2015;272:867–72.
38. Kim HJ, Kim MJ, Jeon JH, Kim JM, Moon IS, Lee WS. Functional and practical outcomes of inlay butterfly cartilage tympanoplasty. Otol Neurotol. 2014;35:145–6.
39. de Dorlodot C, De Bie G, Deggouj N, Decat M, Gérard JM. Are bovine pericardium underlay xenograft and butterfly inlay autograft efficient for transcanal tympanoplasty? Eur Arch Otorhinolaryngol. 2015;272:327–31.
40. Eren SB, Tugrul S, Ozucer B, Veyseller B, Aksoy F, Ozturan O. Endoscopic transcanal inlay myringoplasty: alternative approach for anterior perforations. Otolaryngol Head Neck Surg. 2015;153:891–3.
41. Wu PW, Wang WH, Huang CC, Lee TJ, Huang CC. Comparison of short-o and long-term hearing outcomes of successful inlay cartilage tympanoplasty between small and large eardrum perforations. Clin Exp Otorhinolaryngol. 2015;8:359–63.
42. Callioglu EE, Tuzuner A, Demirci S, Bercin AS, Oguzhan T, Korkmaz MH. The effect of inlay butterfly cartilage tympanoplasty technique on compliance. Acta Otolaryngol. 2016;136:669–72.
43. Alain H, Esmat NH, Ohad H, Yona V, Nageris BI. Butterfly myringoplasty for Total, subtotal, and annular perforations. Laryngoscope. 2016;126:2565–8.
44. Özgür A, Dursun E, Terzi S, Erdivanlı ÖÇ, Coşkun ZÖ, Oğurlu M, Demirci M. Endoscopic butterfly cartilage myringoplasty. Acta Otolaryngol. 2016;136:144–8.
45. Riss JC, Roman S, Morredu E, Farinetti A, Nicollas R, Triglia JM. Butterfly-cartilage tympanoplasty in children: a 28-case series and literature review. Otorhinolaryngol Head Neck Dis. 2016;133:179–82.
46. Akyigit A, Karlidag T, Keles E, Kaygusuz I, Yalcın S, Polat C, Eroglu O. Endoscopic cartilage butterfly myringoplasty in children. Auris Nasus Larynx. 2017;44:152–5.
47. Isaacson G, Harounian JA. Results of pediatric endoscopic and endoscopically assisted tympanoplasty. World J Otorhinolaryngol Head Neck Surg. 2017;3:136–41.
48. Kaya I, Benzer M, Gode S, et al. Butterfly cartilage tympanoplasty: an alternative new technique instead of conventional surgery method. Eur Arch Otorhinolaryngol. 2017;274:3311–4.
49. Jumaily M, Franco J, Gallogly JA, Hentzelman JL, Costa DJ, Wild APK, Mikulec AA. Butterfly cartilage tympanoplasty outcomes: a single-institution experience and literature review. Am J Otolaryngol. 2018;39:396–400.
50. Karabulut B, Mutlu F, Sahin S, Cirik AA. Anatomical and functional long-term results of endoscopic butterfly inlay myringoplasty. Eur Arch Otorhinolaryngol. 2018;275:2653–8.
51. Karataş M, Kaskalan E. Simultaneous bilateral butterfly tympanoplasty using tragal cartilage from one ear. Auris Nasus Larynx. 2018;46:324–9.
52. Mourya A, Jain L, Jadia S, Qureshi S. A comparative study of various office procedures for the management of small to medium size tympanic membrane perforations. Indian J Otolaryngol Head Neck Surg. 2018;70:351–4.
53. Toro PC, Castillo AC, Martínez RM, Juan ID. Inlay butterfly miringoplasty. Our experience. Acta Otorrinolaringol Esp. 2018;69:30–4.
54. Ulku CH. Inlay butterfly cartilage tympanoplasty: anatomica and functional results. Indian J Otolaryngol Head Neck Surg. 2018;70:235–9.
55. Wang H. Initial observations of inlay "butterfly" cartilage tympanoplasty. Lin Chung Er Bi Yan Hou Tou Jing Wai Ke Za Zhi. 2018;32:69–70.
56. Pontes-Madruga TC, Neto FBN, Suzuki FAB, Testa JRG, Onishi ET. Endoscopic tympanoplasty with inlay cartilage graft in a university hospital. Braz J Otorhinolaryngol. 2019;S1808-8694(19):30135–1. https://doi.org/10.1016/j.bjorl.2019.10.002.

57. Bartel R, Levorato M, Adroher M, Cardelus S, Diaz A, Lacima J, et al. Transcanal endoscopic type 1 tympanoplasty in children: cartilage butterfly and fascia temporalis graft. Int J Pediatr Otorhinolaryngol. 2019;121:120–2.
58. Dave V, Sharma S. Comparative analysis of fascia lata and cartilage graft in revision type 1 tympanoplasty. Indian J Otolaryngol Head Neck Surg. 2019;71(Suppl 2):S1232–7.
59. Demir E, Coskun ZO, Celiker M, Terzi S, Erdivanli OC, Balaban GA, Dursun E. Endoscopic butterfly inlay myringoplasty for large perforations. Eur Arch Otorhinolaryngol. 2019;276:2791–5.
60. Karataş M, Doğan S. Endoscopic inlay butterfly cartilage tympanoplasty in pediatric patients. Int J Pediatr Otorhinolaryngol. 2019;121:10–4.
61. Khoza-Shangase K, Ramdin N. Audiological function in a group of adults following myringoplasty: an exploratory study in South Africa. Pan Afr Med J. 2019;34:57–72.
62. Kim MB, Park JA, Suh MJ, Song CI. Comparison of clinical outcomes between butterfly inlay cartilage tympanoplasty and conventional underlay cartilage tympanoplasty. Auris Nasus Larynx. 2019;46:167–71.
63. Lee SA, Kang HT, Lee YJ, Kim BG, Lee JD. Microscopic versus endoscopic inlay butterfly cartilage tympanoplasty. J Audiol Otol. 2019;23:140–4.
64. Ference RS, Leonard JA, Weinstock MS, Bent JP. Evaluating butterfly inlay tympanoplasty. Int J Pediatr Otorhinolaryngol. 2019;127:109684. https://doi.org/10.1016/j.ijporl.2019.109684. Epub 2019 Sep 15
65. Li Y, Liu HQ, Sheng Y, Yan J, Xu YL, Liang JM, Wu BJ, Zhang Q, Ren XY. Clinical study of butterfly cartilage myringoplasty for anterior quadrant tympanic perforation under endoscope. Zhonghua Er Bi Yan Hou Tou Jing Wai Ke Za Zhi. 2020;55:611–4.
66. Gülsen S, Erden B. Comparison of endoscopic butterfly-inlay versus endoscopic push-through myringoplasty in repairing anterior perforations of the tympanic membrane. J Laryngol Otol. 2020:1–7. https://doi.org/10.1017/S0022215120000006.
67. Hashim ND, Lee SA, Jang SH, Moon IS. A comparison of endoscopic and microscopic inlay butterfly cartilage tympanoplasties and their educational utility. PLoS One. 2020;15:e0241152. https://doi.org/10.1371/journal.pone.041152.
68. Özdemir D, Özgür A, Mehel MM, Bedir A, Çelebi M, Aydemir S, Turgut NF. Endoscopic butterfly inlay myringoplasty: new technique extended perichondrium butterfly. Acta Otolaryngol. 2020;140:277–80.
69. Buck LS, Carter EB, Carron CJ, Carron JD. Effect of graft size on air-bone gap closure in cartilage button Tympanoplasty. Otol Neurotol. 2021;42:438–41.
70. Demir E, Terzi S, Celiker M, Erdivanli OC, Coskun ZO, Dursun E. Revision of cartilage tympanoplasty with endoscopic butterfly inlay myringoplasty. Eur Arch Otorhinolaryngol. 2021;279:187. https://doi.org/10.1007/s00405-021-06669-w.
71. Ravi N, Meher R, Rathore PK, Singh I. Comparison of efficacy of endoscopic versus microscopic transcanal inlay butterfly cartilage myringoplasty. Am J Otolaryngol. 2021;42:102978.
72. Iacovou E, Vlastarakos PV, Papacharalampous G, Kyrodimos E, Nikolopoulos TP. Is cartilage better than temporalis muscle fascia in type I tympanoplasty? Implications for current surgical practice. Eur Arch Otorhinolaryngol. 2013;270:2803–13.
73. Jalali MM, Motasaddi M, Kouhi A, Dabiri S, Soleimani R. Comparison of cartilage with temporalis fascia tympanoplasty: a meta-analysis of comparative studies. Laryngoscope. 2017;127:2139–48.
74. Lyons SA, Su T, Vussers LET, Peters JPM, Smit AL, Grolman W. Fascia compared to one-piece composite cartilage-perichondrium grafting for tympanoplasty. Laryngoscope. 2016;126:1662–70.
75. Yang T, Wu X, Peng X, Zhang Y, Xie S, Yong HS. Comparison of cartilage graft and fascia in type 1 tympanoplasty: systematic review and meta-analysis. Acta Otolaryngol. 2016;136:1085–90.
76. Moahamad SH, Khan I, Hussain M. Is cartilage Tympanoplasty more effective than fascia Tympanoplasty? A systematic review. Otol Neurotol. 2002;33:699–705.
77. Lubianca Neto JF, Schuster AK, Lubianca JPN, Eavey RD. Comparison of inlay cartilage butterfly and underlay temporal fascia tympanoplasty. Oto Open. 2022;6:1–7.
78. Lubianca Neto JF, Schuster AK, Fanzini TA, Lubianca JPN, Mostardeiro LR, Eavey RD. Comparison between endoscopic and microscopic butterfly cartilage graft inlay tympanoplasty: a systemic review and metanalysis. Eur Arch Otorhinolaryngol. 2023;280:151–8.
79. Hott ME, Megerian CA, Beane R, Bonassar LJ. Fabrication of tissue engineered tympanic membrane patches using computer-aided design and injection molding. Laryngoscope. 2004;114:1290–5.

Medio-Lateral Graft Tympanoplasty for Anterior or Subtotal Tympanic Membrane Perforation: An Update

52

Timothy T. K. Jung

One of the common sequelae of chronic otitis media is tympanic membrane (TM) perforation, which can cause hearing loss and/or otorrhea. The two classic methods for reconstruction of TM perforation have been medial (underlay) or lateral (overlay) graft technique. In the underlay technique, the graft is placed entirely medial to the remaining TM and malleus. In the overlay technique the graft is placed lateral to the annulus and any remaining fibrous middle layer after the squamous layer has been carefully removed. The anterior canal wall is widened with a drill to minimize blunting, while the graft is placed just medial to the long process of malleus to prevent lateralization. Each of these techniques has its advantages and disadvantages [1, 2].

The anterior or subtotal TM perforation is difficult to repair due to less vascularity than posterior tympanic membrane [3] and the anterior bony overhang which blocks visualization. Because of reduced vascularity in the anterior tympanic membrane, there is a greater risk of necrosis and reabsorption of the fascia graft [3]. When the medial graft technique is used to repair anterior or subtotal TM perforation, the anterior portion of fascia graft may fall away resulting in reperforation and obliteration of anterior part of middle ear cavity [4]. While lateral graft technique has higher success rate for the reconstruction of anterior or subtotal TM perforation, serious lateralization of graft may occur. These problems have been managed by a variety of surgical techniques, such as the use of Williams's microclip [5], sandwich graft tympanoplasty [4], and over-under tympanoplasty [6]. Yet, still better method is needed to repair anterior or subtotal TM perforation.

During the past 27 years, the medio-lateral graft tympanoplasty, an innovative new method for repair of anterior or subtotal tympanic membrane perforation, has been successfully used. In the medio-lateral graft technique, fascia graft is placed medial to the posterior half of the TM perforation and lateral to the anterior half of the perforation [7, 8]. This method is a hybrid between medial and lateral graft technique taking advantage of both methods. The purpose of this study is to describe and evaluate the medio-lateral graft tympanoplasty for the reconstruction of anterior or subtotal TM perforation.

Materials and Methods

Patients

The charts of 100 patients who underwent the medio-lateral tympanoplasty for reconstruction of anterior or subtotal TM perforation during the years 1995–2001 were retrospectively reviewed. The main outcome measure was intact TM without lateralization or anterior blunting. All patients underwent preoperative and postoperative audiograms. Concomitant mastoidectomy was performed in 86% of the patients. In addition, ossiculoplasty was also done as needed. The choice of prosthesis was made according to the condition and anatomy of the middle ear cleft at the time of the surgery. Prostheses used were various type made of either hydroxyappetite (Applebaum, Weird, or Rosenberg design) or titanium.

Patients with less than 6 months follow-up were excluded.

Surgical Technique

The procedure is usually performed under general anesthesia. Transcanal, endaural, or postauricular approaches are used depending on the clinical situation. Temporalis fascia or tragal perichondrium is harvested, pressed, and air-dried. A rim of tissue is removed from the perforation edge to de-epithelialize and encourage migration of the mucosal layer and epithelium. Vertical canal incisions are made at 12 and 6 o'clock position. The 6 o'clock incision can be extended

T. T. K. Jung (✉)
Department of Otolaryngology-Head & Neck Surgery, Loma Linda University School of Medicine, Jerry L. Pettis Memorial Veterans Medical Center and Inland Ear Head & Neck Clinic, Loma Linda, CA, USA

M. V. Goycoolea et al. (eds.), *Textbook of Otitis Media*, https://doi.org/10.1007/978-3-031-40949-3_52

right up to the annulus. The 12 o'clock incision is made down to a few millimeters above the annulus to preserve blood supply when anterior canal skin is used as the superiorly based flap. A posterior tympanomeatal flap is elevated and ossicles evaluated (Fig. 52.1a). Mastoidectomy and/or ossiculoplasty are performed at the appropriate time if needed. Using a curved round knife, horizontal incision is made in the anterior canal skin. The distance of anterior–horizontal canal incision from the anterior annulus should be about the same as the diameter of the perforation. After the incision, the anterior canal skin is elevated laterally and medially. As the anterior canal skin is elevated, canalplasty is performed by drilling anterior bony overhang using diamond burrs and suction irrigator until a full view of anterior annulus is possible. Antero-medial canal skin flap is elevated up to the annulus or margin of the TM. At the annulus, only squamous epithelial layer of TM is carefully elevated to the anterior half of the perforation edge leaving the anterior annulus intact (Fig. 52.1b). The middle ear cavity is packed with Gelfoam soaked in non-ototoxic fluoroquinolone antibiotic otic drops. Unlike in the case of usual medial graft technique, the middle ear packing does not have to be tight. The temporalis fascia or tragal perichondrium is grafted medially for the posterior half of the perforation and laterally over the annulus anterior half of the perforation (Fig. 52.1c). To avoid anterior blunting, the fascia graft is brought only to the anterior sulcus on the annulus and not above the annulus. As a second layer of closure, antero-medial canal skin is rotated to cover perforation and fascia as a superiorly based flap (Fig. 52.1d). Antero-lateral canal skin is replaced, and packings are placed. Traditional "rose-bud" packing is inserted using otosilk strips with small- to medium-sized cotton ball inside soaked in the antibiotic otic drops. Rest of the ear canal is packed with a gauze strip of Xeroform gauze. The incision site is closed in the usual manner.

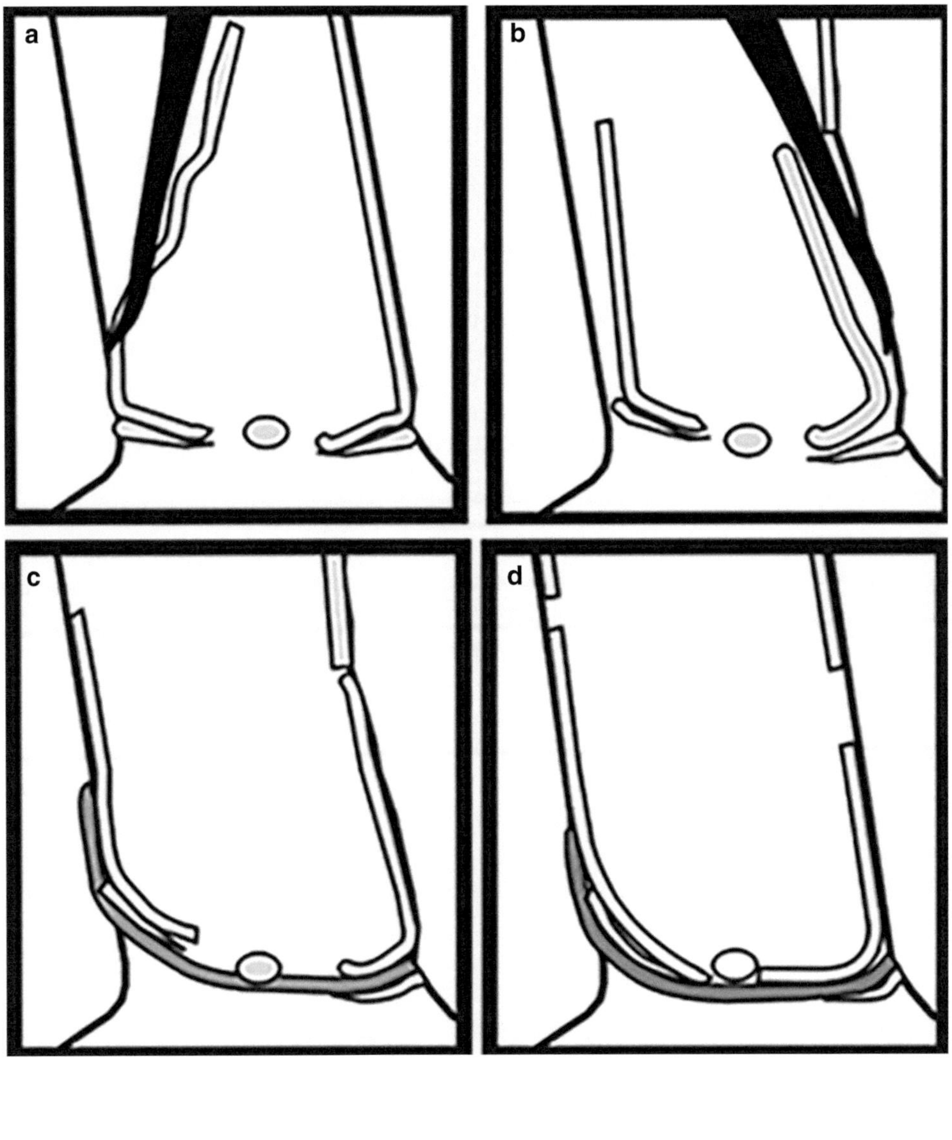

Fig. 52.1 Surgical steps of medio-lateral graft tympanoplasty. (**a**) A posterior tympanomeatal flap is elevated and ossicles are evaluated. (**b**) Anteromedial canal skin is elevated along with epithelial layer of TM up to anterior half of the perforation. (**c**) The temporalis fascia is placed medially (underlay) posterior half of the perforation and laterally (overlay) anterior half of the perforation up to the annulus. (**d**) Antero-medial canal skin is rotated as a superiorly based flap to cover perforation and fascia as a second layer. Posterior canal skin can be rotated and used also for the subtotal TM perforation

Results

There were five complications such as TM pearl (2 cases), re-perforation of TM (postoperative infection; 1 case, recurrent cholesteatoma; 1 case), and anterior blunting (1 case). There were no lateralization and anterior fall away of fascia. Two of epithelial pearls on the tympanic membrane were removed easily in the office setting. There were three failures (97% success rate) due to a postoperative infection, recurrent cholesteatoma, and anterior blunting. It was noted that healing of the reconstructed TM took place much faster with medio-lateral graft method compared to traditional medial or lateral graft technique.

Results of postoperative audiogram showed no significant hearing loss compared to the preoperative hearing. Over 60% of the operated ears had hearing improvement of 0–20 dB (0–10 dB in 19% of ears, and 11–20 dB in 44%) even without ossiculoplasty. With ossiculoplasty using either partial ossicular replacement prosthesis (PORP, 15%) or total ossicular replacement prosthesis (TORP, 11%), there were various degrees of hearing improvement from 11 to 30 dB.

Discussion

Over the years, various techniques have been attempted to improve tympanoplasty results. These include overlay tympanoplasty [9], underlay tympanoplasty [10], gelfilm sandwich tympanoplasty [11], Crowncork tympanoplasty [12], swinging door tympanoplasty [13], sandwich graft tympanoplasty [4], laser-assisted spot welding technique [14], fascia pegging [15], microclip techniques [16], and over-under tympanoplasty [6]. Among them underlay and overlay techniques are most commonly used. The advantages of medial (underlay) graft include ease of learning the technique, avoidance of the risk of lateralization and blunting of the anterior sulcus, and high success rate especially for the posterior perforation. The disadvantages of medial graft are inadequate visualization of anterior middle ear, possible anterior graft fall away, reduction of middle ear space with consequent increased risk of adhesions, and less suitable for reconstruction of anterior perforation [1, 2]. The lateral (overlay) graft provides superior exposure, suitable for all perforations, and minimizes reduction of the middle ear space. This technique has a high success rate and has been particularly effective for large, anterior perforations. The disadvantages of lateral graft include anterior blunting, possible lateralization of graft, tendency to create more epithelial pearls, need for malleus manipulation, longer healing time, increased operation time, and complexity for repair of small posterior perforations [1, 2].

One of the most serious complications of the graft techniques is lateralization of TM. Lateralization of the TM is a condition in which the visible surface of the TM is located to the bony annular ring and loses contact with the conducting mechanism of the middle ear. Lateralization of TM may be associated with considerable morbidity, including hearing loss and cholesteatoma. Surgical repair is often necessary for significant underlying disease, but reestablishment of a normal TM can be challenging [17]. Medio-lateral graft tympanoplasty avoids lateralization of the graft by placing fascia medial to the posterior half of the TM. Also, lateralization of graft is prevented by placing graft under the manubrium. In our study, there was no lateralization of graft.

This method is a hybrid between medial and lateral graft method and taking advantage of both methods. The medio-lateral graft tympanoplasty has many advantages over traditional medial or lateral graft: (1) prevent anterior fall away of fascia; (2) graft is stable like "a button in the button hole"; (3) no need for tight gelfoam packing to support the graft; (4) prevention of lateralization of graft; (5) better blood supply because anterior canal skin is rotated as a rotational flap rather than free graft; (6) easier because epithelial layer of only anterior half of the TM remnant is elevated rather than entire TM; and (7) less malleus manipulation. In our study, there were five complications such as TM pearl (2 cases), re-perforation of TM (postoperative infection; 1 case, recurrent cholesteatoma; 1 case) and anterior blunting (1 case). There were no lateralization and anterior fall away of fascia. Two of epithelial pearls on the tympanic membrane were easily removed in the office setting. There were three failures (97% success rate) due to a postoperative infection, anterior blunting, and recurrent cholesteatoma.

Conclusion

The medio-lateral graft method is easier and superior to the traditional medial or lateral graft technique for the large anterior or subtotal TM perforation. It takes advantage of both medial and lateral grafting method while avoiding their pitfalls.

Acknowledgments I gratefully acknowledge John Jenkins in the Media Development Service at the Jerry L. Pettis Memorial Veterans Medical Center, Loma Linda, California for producing computer graphic figures used in this paper.

References

1. Rizer FM. Overlay versus underlay tympanoplasty. Part I: Historical review of the literature; part II; the study. Laryngoscope. 1997;107:26–36.

2. Kriskovich M, Shelton C. Surgical treatment of chronic otitis media & cholesteatoma. In: Canalis RF, Lambert PR, editors. The ear: comprehensive otology. Philadelphia: Lipponcott Williams & Wilkins; 2000.
3. Applebaum EL, Deutsch EC. An endoscopic method of tympanic membrane fluorescein angiography. Ann Otol Rhinol Laryngol. 1986;95:439–43.
4. Farrior JB. Sandwich graft tympanoplasty: experience, results, and complications. Laryngoscope. 1989;99:213–7.
5. Weider DJ. Use of the Williams microclip in various aspect of tympanoplastic surgery. Laryngoscope. 1981;91:2106–25.
6. Kartush JM, Michaelides EM, Becvarovski Z, et al. Over-under tympanolasty. Laryngoscope. 2002;112:802–7.
7. Jung T, Park S. Mediolateral graft tympanoplasty for anterior or subtotal tympanic membrane perforation. Otolaryngol Head Neck Surg. 2005;132:532–6.
8. Jung T, Youhyun K, Yoonhwan K, Park S, Martin D. Medial or medio-lateral graft tympanoplasty for repair of tympanic membrane perforation. Int J Ped Otorrhinolaryngo. 2009;73:941–3.
9. House WF. Myringoplasty. Arch Otolaryngol. 1960;71:399–404.
10. Shea JJ Jr. Vein graft closure of eardrum perforations. J Laryngol Otol. 1960;74:358–62.
11. Karlan MS. Gelatin film sandwich in tympanlasty. Otolaryngol Head Neck Surg. 1979;87:84–6.
12. Hartwein J, Leuwer RM, Kehrl W. The total reconstruction of the tympanic membrane by the 'Crowncork' technique. Am J Otolaryngol. 1992;13:172–5.
13. Schwaber MK. Postauricular undersurface tympanic membrane grafting: some modifications of the 'swinging door' technique. Otolaryngol Head Neck Surg. 1986;95:182–7.
14. Escudero LH, Castro AO, Drumond M, et al. Argon laser in human tympanoplasty. Arch Otolaryngol. 1979;105:252–3.
15. Goodman WS, Wallace IR. Tympanoplasty: 25 years later. J Otolaryngol. 1980;9:155–64.
16. Willians JD. Microclip application in tympanoplasty. Ann Otol Rhinol Laryngol. 1977;86:223–6.
17. Sperling NM, Kay D. Diagnosis and management of the lateralized tympanic membrane. Laryngoscope. 2000;110:1987–93.

53 Flexible Approach Tympanoplasty/Mastoidectomy: A Pathology-Guided, Pathogenesis—Oriented Surgery for the Middle Ear

Sady Selaimen da Costa, Michael M. Paparella, and Rochane Figini Maciel

Preoperative evaluation remains the cornerstone in the determination of an appropriate surgical procedure for patients with otologic disease. Clinical microscopic examination, sophisticated audiometric evaluation, and CT scanning and MRI techniques all suggest the exact dimensions of pathologic conditions in the ear. As every surgeon understands from experience, surgical exposure of pathologic tissue usually provides a better, more thorough understanding and more information than preoperative estimation of disease. Surgical techniques should fit the pathology, as it is understood intraoperatively. The flexible approach has been found to be adaptable to many and various forms of pathologic conditions found in the temporal bone. These include inflammation or infection, congenital stenosis, benign and malignant tumors, and traumatic injuries. Through experience, surgeons have observed that some routinely used procedures are not always readily adaptable to an unexpected intraoperative pathologic finding. The flexible approach was designed to use a stepwise protocol to assess pathologic findings or abnormal anatomy as actually encountered and to treat conservatively what is found.

Among all pathologic findings in temporal bone, this approach finds its best indication in the surgical treatment of otitis media (OM) and its sequel. OM is a multifaceted disease, and many of these facets are not completely understood. For example, many questions about the classification and pathogenesis of OM await answers. Researchers at the authors' institutions have shown that even when human and animal temporal bones with OM are studied through the powerful lenses of last-generation microscopes by the most talented otopathologists, the histopathologic boundaries between one form and another are thin, if not intersecting, suggesting that we are not dealing with specific and isolated diseases but with one single condition evolving through progressive stages. This progression may not be linear, being influenced by cofactors generally linked to the aggressor, the subject, and facilitating or moderating circumstances. This diagnostic difficulty is not limited to being an academic issue but is also intrinsic to daily work, with deep clinical implications. In some patients it is difficult defining precisely which form of otitis we are dealing with, according to Bluestone. This difficulty is the result of the constant dynamic behavior through which that pathologic process has been verified to go [1].

A procedure conceived to treat this dynamic process should be tailored to confront and manage unexpected provocative situations. The flexible tympanoplasty is a stepwise approach designed to explore methodically the contents of the middle ear and in the process to disclose, confirm, and often treat the disease encountered. The authors strongly believe that the flexible approach is a modem way, guided by pathology and oriented toward pathogenesis, to treat patients with OM. In the next paragraphs, we will describe our method in detail. For the sake of convenience, we will cover all the possible steps involved in the procedure: from the approach to an open inside-out tympanomastoidectomy (which is frequently combined to the flexible approach). It should be stressed that the extension of the procedure will be intrinsically related to the magnitude and location of the pathology encountered and very often operation is abbreviated after the first steps. It is also important to point out that the flexible approach may be combined with any mastoidectomy technique. Still, in those cases associated with cholesteatomas (especially those involving the posterior recesses), our preference is for an open cavity, which is carried out subcortically. Frequently, after a careful analysis of the patient (signs and symptoms, imaging examinations, and other features), we may decide preoperatively for a CWD technique.

S. S. da Costa (✉)
Hospital de Clínicas de Porto Alegre, Universidade Federal do Rio Grande do Sul, Porto Alegre, Brazil

M. M. Paparella
Department of Otolaryngology, University of Minnesota and Paparella Clinic, Minneapolis, MM, USA

R. F. Maciel
Chronic Otitis Media Study Group, School of Medicine, Federal University of Rio Grande do Sul (UFRGS), Porto Alegre, RS, Brazil

M. V. Goycoolea et al. (eds.), *Textbook of Otitis Media*, https://doi.org/10.1007/978-3-031-40949-3_53

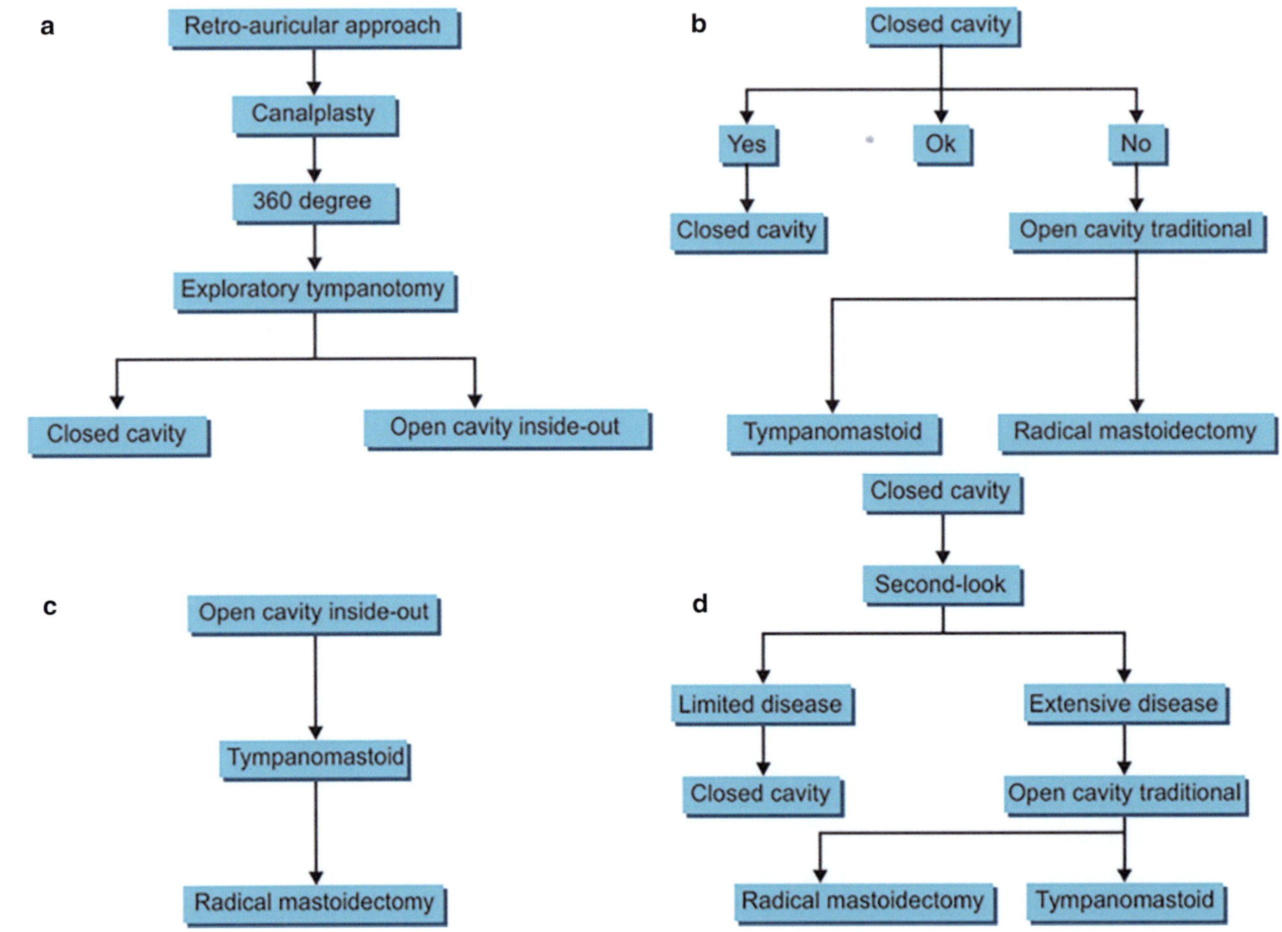

Fig. 53.1 (**a**–**d**) Surgical decision-making algorithm. (**a**) Retroauricular approach is followed by an ample canalplasty with a 360° view of the tympanic membrane. The exploratory tympanotomy will dictate the further steps: closed or open technique. (**b**) If the option was a closed technique during the procedure, it may be converted to a traditional open cavity (radical or not). (**c**) If the preoperative decision was for a canal wall-down technique, the inside-out technique is employed and the middle ear reconstruction will depend on the surgical findings. (**d**) After a canal wall-up procedure, the findings during the second look will dictate whether the posterior wall will be lowered or not

In such circumstances, we perform from the very beginning the inside-out technique. The final result may be very similar to the traditional open cavities, but there is one big difference: the technique includes a wide canalplasty and the removal of the posterosuperior aspect of the wall as an early step. In the other hand, when we decide for a CWU procedure, depending on the surgical findings, we may have to reorient the procedure converting a close into an open cavity. We try to avoid this situation because whenever it happens the final result is a bigger cavity since a complete mastoidectomy has already been created at this stage. As a rule, the CWU involves an ample drilling of the mastoid in order to identify important landmarks. To avoid a constricted dissection that prevents adequate angular visualization of deep-lying structures (and to safely accomplish further steps of the dissection, i.e., the facial recess opening), a wide cortical removal should be first completed. The cortex in unroofed from the posterior canal back and beyond the sigmoid sinus and at an adequate distance into the mastoid tip [2]. In the process, the surgeon may eventually open areas in the mastoid (i.e., the tip) that are not involved by disease. The confluence of these "innocent" spaces and other areas where pathology was actually encountered may result in an undesired larger cavity. Figure 53.1a–d summarizes our surgical decision-making algorithm.

Surgical Technique

The Patient

The hair is shaved up to 3 cm above and behind the ear. The skin is cleansed with an iodine-based soap, rinsed with water, and spayed with tincture of benzoin. A sterile plastic adhesive drape is applied. The patient is placed on the table with his/her head at the foot of the operating table. He/she must be securely taped to the table to prevent slipping when it is tipped from side to side. The patient's head should be as near the surgeon as possible, and the table is usually placed in a few degrees of Trendelenburg and rolled slightly toward the surgeon [3].

Anesthesia

Some of these surgeries can be performed as outpatient procedure under local anesthesia. The authors systematically use general anesthesia in small children, extremely anxious patients, or when a great deal of bone work is anticipated.

Infiltration

The key to success in otologic surgery is to operate on a wide, clean, clear, dry field. In this regard, selection of the approach and good, effective hemostasis are mandatory. A local anesthetic with vasoconstrictor is used, usually 2% lidocaine with 1:100,000 epinephrine. A syringe that affords easy injection is preferred (carpule or an insulin syringe). A 27-gauge or 30-gauge needle is used. A nasal or Lempert speculum is used for initial injections in the inferior, superior, and posterior quadrants. The infiltration should be done slowly to avoid formation of blebs or maceration of the canal skin. When it is well accomplished, the surgeon can see anesthetic blanching and "dissecting" in the skin of the external canal, from the point of injection to the tympanic annulus. Additional injections are performed along the postauricular sulcus and the incisura auris, with care not to inject too anteroinferiorly or too deeply, to avoid anesthesia of the facial nerve.

Postauricular Incision and Cortical Exposure

The incision spans from the helical rim to the mastoid tip and is well hidden in the postauricular region. It rarely causes any visible scarring. The incision should be about 1 cm behind the postauricular crease to avoid unsightly deepening of the sulcus, which can occur when the incisions are placed directly in the crease. The incision is more posterior in young children to avoid a superficial facial nerve near the mastoid tip. The incision is made through the skin with a scalpel. An avascular plane is elevated anteriorly toward the external auditory canal just below the subdermal fat, leaving a layer of loose areolar tissue on the temporalis fascia. This plane is developed down to the mastoid tip. The attachments of the sternocleidomastoid muscle can be separated from the mastoid tip for increased exposure [4]. This dissection can be accomplished with the unipolar cautery leaving the periosteum in place and delineating the posterior semicircle of the external auditory canal. A periosteal flap is then customized to fit the surgical planning. Initial steps are summarized on Fig. 53.2.

Exposure and Removal of the Temporalis Fascia

The postauricular incision extends up into the region of the temporalis fascia. A self-retaining retractor is inserted, and by lifting it up, one can lift the scalp off the temporalis muscle. The loose areolar tissue is then set apart from the true fascia through sharp and blunt dissection. Local anesthetic is injected under the fascia to elevate it from the muscle, and with the scalpel the fascia is sectioned in a roughly ovoid shape and harvested. After being harvested, the fascia is spread on a polytetrafluoroethylene (PTFE) block, with the undersurface upward, and any adherent muscle is removed.

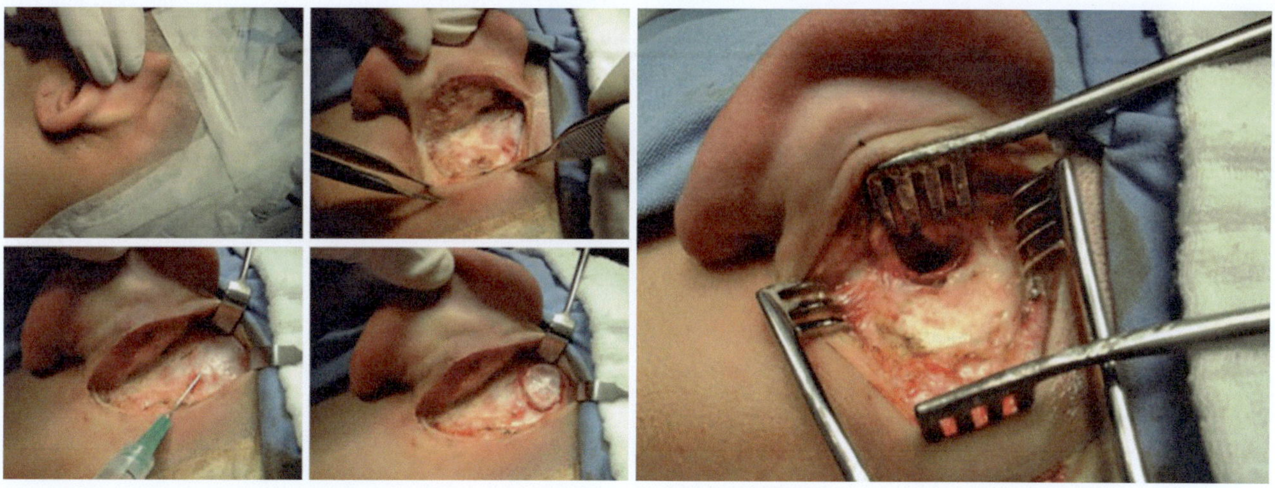

Fig. 53.2 Initial steps of postauricular tympanoplasty

The PTFE block is placed under an electric lamp, and after approximately 10 min, the fascia is dry.

Incisions in the Canal

After the elevation of the periosteal flap, the bony landmarks of the mastoid cortex (spine of Henle, *linea temporalis*, and cribriform area) are identified. Attention is directed to the posterior margin of the external auditory canal, and the skin is gently elevated loose for a few millimeters. Here lays a difference between the underlay and overlay techniques. If the overlay technique is being performed, the anterior dissection will eventually meet the previously executed horizontal TC incisions and the vascular strip (describe later). In the other hand, whenever deciding for an underlay technique, we consider the initial TC steps a waste of time. All the incisions (including the EAC skin) are performed from behind. In this is the case, a number 11-blade knife is used in a straight angle to incise the skin from behind entering the lumen of the canal. A small Koerner flap is created and the self-retaining retractor repositioned. At this point, the canal is extended superiorly, inferiorly, and anteriorly around the 360° of the bony canal (Fig. 53.3).

Vertical Incisions in the Canal

A sickle knife is used for the first vertical incision at 12 o'clock in a direction straight toward the surgeon. A second vertical incision is made at 6 o'clock, curving toward the first vertical incision (Fig. 53.4). As we have approached from behind the horizontal incision has been already performed completing the rectangular tympanomeatal flap. The length

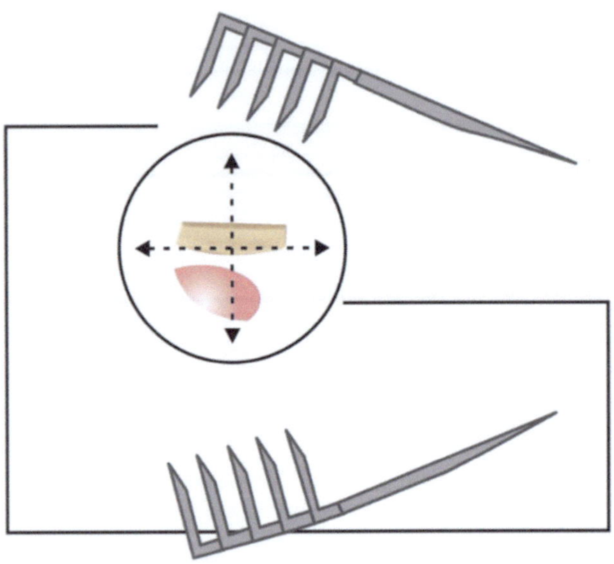

Fig. 53.3 After repositioning of the self-retaining retractors the complete circumference of the external canal comes into view

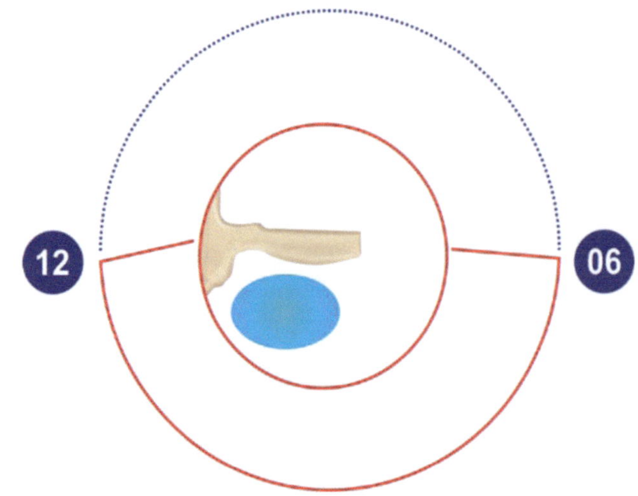

Fig. 53.4 Vertical incisions in external auditory canal (EAC)

of this flap can vary according to the anticipated pathological condition. In a routine tympanoplasty, a 6 mm flap should suffice, whereas a more extensive bony canal is to be removed, an 8 mm flap might be necessary [5]. When making the incisions, the underlying bone should be "felt" with an instrument, even to the point of producing a sound, to make certain the skin is completely sectioned. The junction of the skin with the annulus, at 12 o'clock is usually thicker and richer in connective tissue. Complete sectioning of this area is very important; a Bellucci scissor is very helpful for this purpose. No attempt to lift flaps or gain entrance into the middle ear should be made until the incisions are completed and the skin flaps are free [5].

Elevation of the Flaps and Entering the Middle Ear

With the skin edges free, the surgeon uses a duckbill elevator or even the Rosen knife to gently separate the skin flap from the underlying bone. Dissection should be slow and careful in order to preserve the flap intact. The suction tip (finger off the hole) should be used against the elevator blade in order to keep the field clean from blood. Care should be taken to avoid suctioning and damaging the flap. The skin is elevated evenly, avoiding tunneling until it reaches the annulus. At this point, greater magnification can be used (10× or 16×) in the microscope. The annulus is positively identified and elevated with the elevator working always against the bone. Once the annulus is lifted away from the bony annulus, a needle or the sickle knife can be used to open the mucosa and entering the middle ear always beneath the annulus and, if possible, inferiorly toward the round window. At this point, the duckbill can be passed through this initial hole, pressed firmly against the bony annulus, and moved downward in order to liberate completely the posteroinferior TM. Upward a needle or the sickle knife can be used gently to liberate the posterosuperior TM taking care to not disturb the ossicles. The *chorda tympani nerve* should be identified and carefully moved out of the vision field. If this would stretch it, the best course is simply to cut it with a Bellucci scissor. The chorda tympani should never be grasped and pulled inferosuperiorly in order to avoid a traction lesion on the mastoid segment of the facial nerve [5].

Canalplasty (Optional)

After the flap has been elevated and the osseous canal exposed, the canal is drilled lateral to the annulus in a way that allows better exposure of the annulus and associated mesotympanum. When an anterior bump is present, the anterior osseous canal may be drilled, allowing better exposure of the anterior mesotympanum. Attention must be exercised to avoid entering the temporomandibular joint anteriorly or damaging the skin flap with the burr. For such, after the elevation of the flap, it is carefully folded and protected from the rotating burrs with a round shield fashioned previously with the external packing of the catgut suture. The shield is interposed between the flap and the burr protecting the first of being accidentally detached from the sulcus by the action of the high-speed burr. An extraprotection is to switch to a diamond burr when the drilling gets close to the flap and the residual TM. During the posterior canalplasty, the surgeon should watch for an anterior and more laterally located descendent portion of the mastoid segment of the facial nerve. During the course of posterior canalplasty, very often a few mastoid cells are opened, thus allowing a first glimpse of pathologic conditions in the mastoid. In fact, we always over drill the posterosuperior aspect of the canal opening the cells located lateral to the antrum. A prominent tympanosquamous and tympanomastoid suture lines are also taken off at this point to increase exposure of the pars flaccida [6]. When the drilling is complete, the field should be rinsed with saline solution to wash out bone chips and so that the surgeon will have a panoramic 360° view of the tympanic membrane (Figs. 53.5 and 53.6).

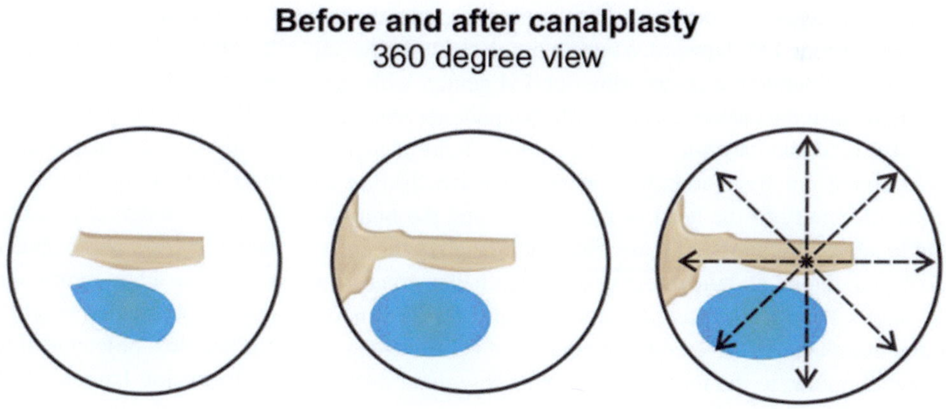

Fig. 53.5 Middle ear visualization improvement after canalplasty

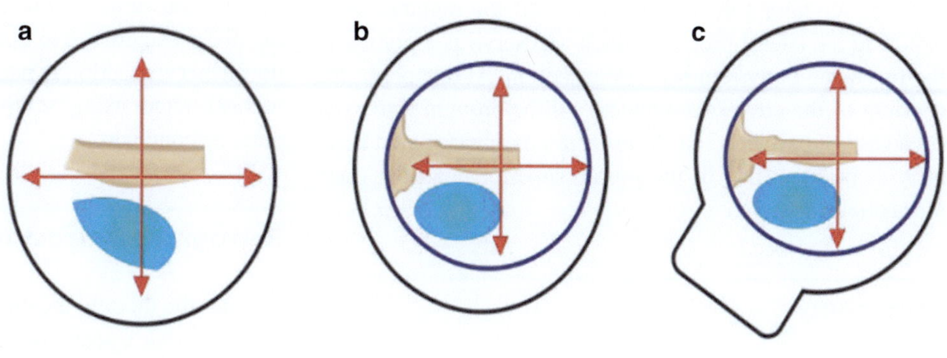

Fig. 53.6 (**a**) Tympanic membrane view before the canalplasty. (**b**) After the canalplasty, a 360° view of the tympanic membrane with one position of the microscope. (**c**) During the canalplasty, a preliminary notch is created in the posterosuperior aspect of the canal, opening the cells located lateral to the antrum

Freshening the Perforation Margins

After the canal has been straightened, the whole TM comes into view and the dimensions of the perforation can be fully appreciated. At this point with a sickle knife or a needle, the fibrous ring at the edges of the perforation is first separated off the healthy drum and then with an alligator forceps completely removed. At the end of this step, the borders of the drum remnant should be oozing.

Entering the Middle Ear

After the canalplasty is complete, the tympanomeatal flap is further elevated to the annulus. At this point, greater magnification can be used (10× or 16×) in the microscope. The annulus is positively identified and elevated with the elevator, working always against the bone. After the annulus is lifted away from the bony sulcus, a needle or the sickle knife can be used to open the mucosa, entering the middle ear always beneath the annulus and, if possible, inferiorly toward the round window. At this point, the duckbill can be passed through this initial hole, pressed firmly against the bony annulus, and moved downward to liberate completely the posteroinferior TM. Upward, a needle or the sickle knife can be used to liberate the posterosuperior TM gently, with care not to disturb the ossicles. The chorda tympani nerve should be identified and carefully moved out of the field of vision. As pointed out by Dornhoffer, when extensive drilling in close proximity to the head of the malleus and the body of the incus is anticipated, it is necessary to visualize the incudostapedial joint and the integrity of the lenticular process of the incus as an initial step. Except in cases of very limited retraction pockets, the incudostapedial joint is disarticulated to avoid trauma to the inner ear from the subsequent drilling [7]. The TM elevated up to the malleus. It is then grasped with the alligator forceps and peeled off the malleus neck, exposing the lateral process, which will serve as a pointer to the following bony removal of the scutum. At this point, the opening of the cholesteatoma sac will be brought into view (in a case of pars flaccida cholesteatoma) or exfoliated keratin will be identified in the posterosuperior quadrant (pars tensa cholesteatoma).

Atticotomy

The superior aspect of the bony canal is carefully removed with the drill. The atticotomy or amount of bone removed can be small, medium, or large to facilitate exposure of the pathologic conditions at hand. This may be done to allow better exposure of the ossicles (i.e., the neck and head of the malleus and the incudomallear joint) or to follow mesotympanic disease extending toward the aditus ad antrum. Anatomic dimensions of the attic and its parts vary, and pathologic conditions certainly can exist in the attic, contributing to obstruction at this site. Anatomic or pathologic obstruction of the attic or aditus ad antrum results in pathologic tissues that can occupy the mastoid, even with preservation of normal or near-normal findings in the middle ear. This is particularly true for pars flaccida cholesteatomas. When disease extends to the attic, the authors initially follow it, increasing the size of the atticotomy in an attempt to reach the end of the pathologic tissue. Working laterally to the ossicular chain, the bony removal continues until the incudomallear joint is perfectly visualized. The next structure to be positively identified is the *tegmen tympani* or middle cranial fossa dural plate. It is important to know that the *tegmen* at the lateral external canal frequently is more inferior than the medial *tegmen* at the level of the epitympanum, so care must be taken to avoid injury to the dura laterally. Preoperative CT helps to predict the height of the tegmen on the coronal view [8]. The final objective of the atticotomy is to bring into view the following landmarks: head of the malleus, the body of the incus, and the *tegmen* (Fig. 53.7a and b). The matrix of the cholesteatoma frequently covers these structures. When the disease is limited to this area and can peel off the ossicles no further dissection is necessary; the surgical defect can be reconstructed using sculptured cortical bone chips, bone pate, or bone wax.

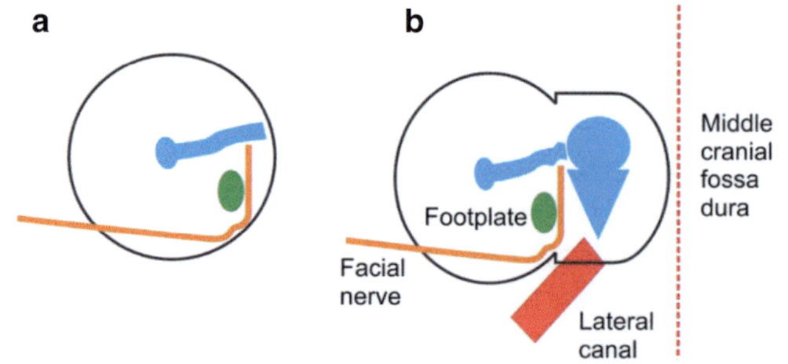

Fig. 53.7 (**a**) The mesotympanic view before the atticotomy. (**b**) The final objective of the atticotomy has been achieved: identification of the head of the malleus, the body of the incus and the tegmen tympani

Retrograde Antrostomy

Frequently, though, the cholesteatoma penetrates posteriorly from Prussak's space (following the embryologic course of the *saccus medius*), passing through the superior incudal space, and then traversing the *aditus ad antrum* to enter deeply into the mastoid. In this situation, the fundus of the cyst cannot be reached through atticotomy. An inside-out antrostomy in sclerotic bones is the next step in the procedure. For that, the dissection should proceed backward later-

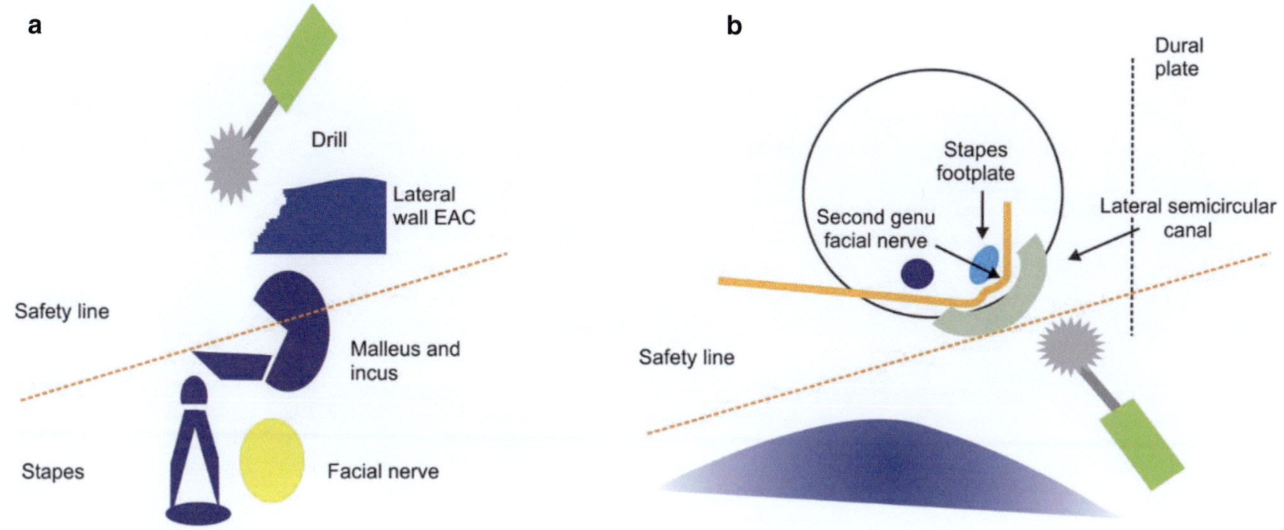

Fig. 53.8 (**a** and **b**) The inside-out mastoidectomy offers protection to the facial nerve. (**a**) Coronal section showing the interposition of the ossicular mass between the burr and the tympanic segment of the facial nerve. (**b**) Axial section of the antrostomy with the lateral semicircular shielding the second genu of the facial nerve from the rotating burr

ally to the ossicular chain, following the dural plate. The next landmarks to be identified are the short process of the incus medially and a few millimeters below the solid bone of the dome of the lateral semicircular canal (Fig. 53.8a). After opening a few more cells, the final objective of the antrostomy has been achieved: the identification of the antrum itself (filled with cholesteatoma), the lateral semicircular canal, and the dural plate. It should be emphasized that the inside-out technique offers a very safe approach to the antrum. It immediately exposes and thereby allows protection of important structures that may otherwise be subject to injury. First, the drilling is carried out lateral to the ossicular chain interposing the head of the malleus and the body of the incus between the burr and the facial nerve (the possibility of an acoustic trauma is minimized since the incudostapedial joint has already been disarticulated as an earlier step). Second, the most flagrant landmark of the antrum is the dome of the lateral semicircular canal, which protects the second genu of the facial nerve (located slightly medially and inferiorly) from an inadvertent and catastrophic drilling accident (Fig. 53.8b).

As the antrum is widely opened, the extent of the cholesteatoma can be appreciated. The goal is to remove only the bone necessary to expose the back edge of the sac, and many times a complete mastoidectomy is not necessary. In a sclerotic mastoid, the surgeon may frequently find the cholesteatoma extending only to the antrum, so minimal drilling is needed. After drilling the bony bridge over the aditus, the three upper compartments of the middle ear are completely identified: the attic (with the incudomallear joint), the transitional aditus, and the antrum (with the lateral semicircular canal). The lateral and posterior wall of the epitympanum must be removed until the *tegmen* mastoid and *tegmen tympani* are continuous. The transition between the middle ear and mastoid must be smooth and uninterrupted.

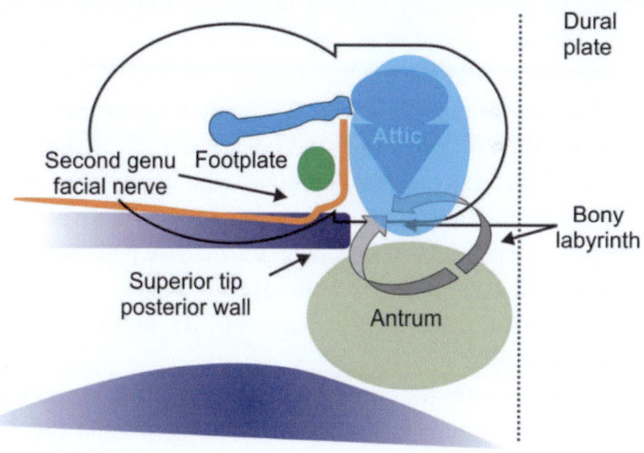

Fig. 53.9 The three upper compartments of the middle ear are completely identified: the attic (with the incudomallear joint), the transitional aditus and the antrum (with the lateral semicircular canal). The tip of the posterior wall is still high blocking a better view of the tympanic facial nerve

At this point, the tip of the posterior wall is still high (with the malleus and incus remnants in place), preventing a better view of the tympanic segment of the facial nerve (Fig. 53.9).

Mastoidectomy

Once this step is accomplished, it opens a large and safe two-way avenue. The first way goes (straight) all the way to the sinodural (Citelli's) angle; the second makes a right angle turn toward the bottom of the mastoid (Fig. 53.10a and b). The cholesteatoma sac is followed back as posteriorly and

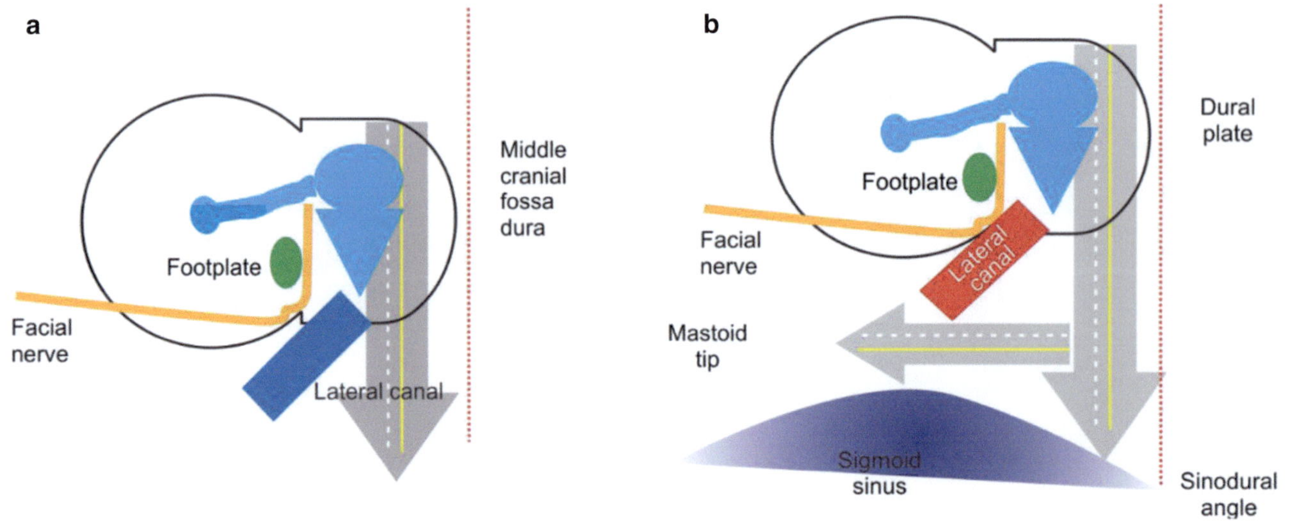

Fig. 53.10 (**a**) After opening the antrum two landmarks are identified: the lateral semicircular canal and the dural plate. (**b**) The lateral canal shields de second genu of the facial nerve and with the dural plate opens a two-arm avenue: the first leads to the sinodural angle; and the second contours the lateral canal and continues toward the tip of the mastoid

inferiorly as necessary or until normal air cells are encountered [8]. Along the way, any cell filled with cholesterol granuloma should be explored and suctioned. Granulation tissue is also frequently found at this point either around the cholesteatoma or infiltrating the posterior wall. It should be also removed from the irregular bone, which is then smoothed with the diamond burr. The amount of bone removal in the mastoid is dependent of how deep the disease penetrates into the bone. Conceptually, we classify the degree of mastoid exenterating in three levels: I: antrum; II: midmastoid, and III: tip (Fig. 53.11).

When the pathology in the mastoid has been completely delineated, attention is directed back to the middle ear: first the incus is disarticulated from the malleus and removed. With the malleus nipper, the head of the malleus is also removed gaining access to the medial wall of the attic (frequently lined by the cholesteatoma matrix). After drilling anteriorly and parallel to the dural plate, the anterior attic (supratubal recess) is widely exposed and cleaned of any residual disease. It is important to dissect the dural plate all the way to the confluence of the anterior wall of the external auditory canal where a 90° angle is created and then rounded off (Fig. 53.12).

During this step, the tegmen tympani should be checked for areas of bony defects. Small or large dehiscence are common findings and may be either congenital or consequence of the bone erosion power of cholesteatoma and/or granulation tissue. Most of them are not clinically relevant and should be left alone. Larger areas especially when associated with dural herniation should be immediately corrected. As we have mentioned before, the roof of the middle ear and the mastoid must be smooth and uninterrupted.

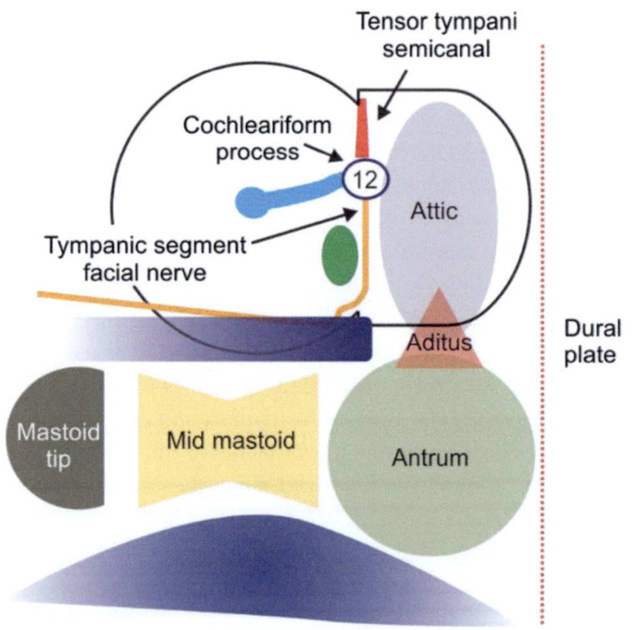

Fig. 53.11 The three upper compartments of the middle ear are completely identified: the attic (with the incudomallear joint), the transitional adits and the antrum (with the lateral semicircular canal). The tip of the posterior wall is still high blocking a better view of the tympanic facial nerve

The bottom of the cholesteatoma sac is then identified and dissected with the aid of a Rosen knife and a cotton ball impregnated with saline solution. The dissection progresses cautiously from posterior to anterior with the removal of the matrix. Any sign of a perilymphatic fistula should be explored, especially in lateral semicircular canal, and, if positively identified, gently handled. In this circumstance,

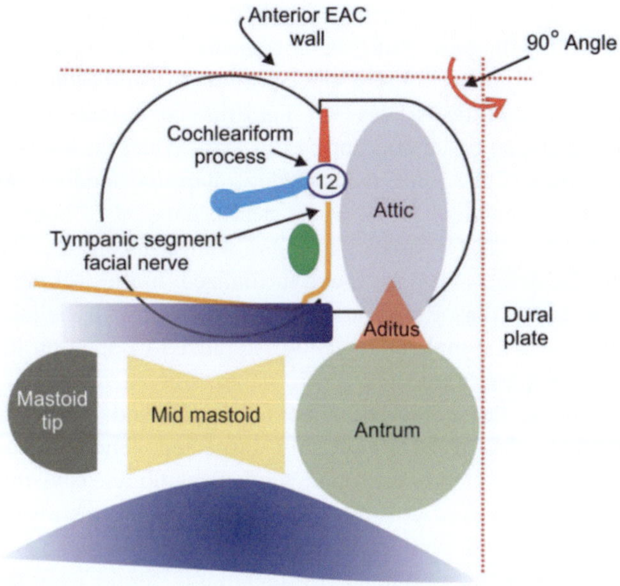

Fig. 53.12 Dural plate is dissected all the way to the confluence of the anterior wall of the external auditory canal, where a 90° angle is created and then rounded off. The roof of the middle ear and the mastoid must follow a smooth and uninterrupted plane

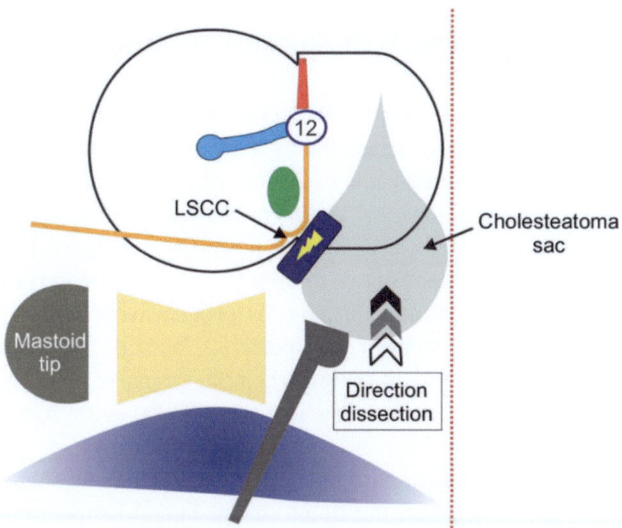

Fig. 53.13 During the removal of the cholesteatoma, the medial wall of the sac should be palpated to detect any bony erosion especially on the dome of the lateral semicircular canal. In this circumstance, matrix should be left over the site to protect (even if eventual removal is planned), while the remainder of the ear is cleared of disease.

matrix should be left over the site to protect (even if eventual removal is planned) while the remainder of the ear is cleared of disease. This protects the area from subsequent bone dust and saline irrigation. If the removal of the matrix is planned at that operative setting, it should be the last maneuver performed prior to completing the operation and closing the ear. When a fistula is inadvertently exposed, it should be quickly covered with a tissue seal (Fig. 53.13).

Exploratory Tympanotomy

Next, attention is directed to the most superior aspect of the posterior wall. Bone is drilled partially decreasing its height only to make possible an angled vision of the mesotympanum. The dissection is then directed toward the middle ear, beginning along the superoanterior mesotympanum by exposing the semicanal of the tensor tympani muscle, the remaining malleus, and the cochleariform process. Among all the anatomical landmarks of the middle ear, the authors consider the cochleariform process of utmost importance. Its resistance to pathologic aggression, its relationship with the malleus, and its central position in the middle ear cleft makes it a readily identifiable structure. When the cochleariform process is spotted, one can determine the position of the geniculate ganglion (just medial to the cochleariform process) and, through a cranio-caudal line, divide the middle ear into anterior and posterior compartments. The anterior compartment is related to the promontory (anteroinferiorly) and with the protympanum and, some millimeters ahead, with the tympanic orifice of the ET. The carotid canal is found more anteriorly at a minimum distance of 6.6 mm. The posterior compartment is related to the tympanic portion of the facial nerve, pointing to the path to its second genu and, posteroinferiorly, to the area of the windows (Fig. 53.14).

The facial nerve should be approached with extreme care because it is one of the most vulnerable structures of the temporal bone, especially when there is a dehiscence of the facial canal on the side toward the middle ear. The reported incidence of dehiscence of the facial canal seen surgically is 7.0–11.4 [9] and seen histologically is from 15 to 74% [10,

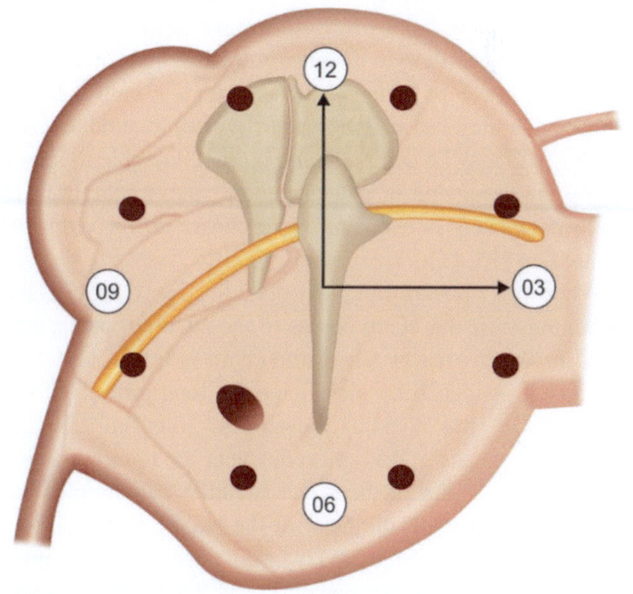

Fig. 53.14 Anatomic landmarks showed after identifying cochleariform process at 12 o'clock

11]. The most common site of dehiscence is the area near the oval window, where the nerve may prolapse over the stapedial footplate. As pointed out by Mutlu et al. [12], in these not-so-rare circumstances, a cholesteatoma or a mass of granulation tissue can distort the normal anatomy of the nerve. Careless manipulation of the disease can elevate the nerve out of its normal bed and produce additional stretching injuries. From the cochleariform process, the dissection is carried along the promontory and toward the protympanum in a sheetlike fashion, dissecting toward the hypotympanum and ultimately ending at the posterior tympanum and the superior mesotympanum near the stapes [13]. The protympanum is carefully examined, and sites of obstructions are looked for. These may include bony prominences in various regions of the middle ear, thickened mucosa, or granulation tissue in the middle ear and disease of the anterior TM or anterior mesotympanum, such as tympanosclerosis. The contour of the promontory is observed for obstruction at this level of the mesotympanum. The round window, sinus tympani, and facial recess are also assessed. Any loculated collection of fluid should be suctioned, and granulation tissue strategically located within the middle ear cleft must be approached with care and, if possible, removed. Care should be exercised while removing disease from the protympanum and the area nears the orifice of the ET because they are in close relationship to the carotid canal. Costa and colleagues [14] showed that the artery may be exposed in this segment, either congenitally or secondary to disease. Even when not exposed, the minimal mean thickness of the bony canal has been measured at 0.18 mm [14]. To avoid this major catastrophe, the area near the canal should always be approached with anticipation, and erosions should be searched for through gentle palpation with a blunt instrument. This recommendation also holds true during exploration of the hypotympanum. According to Overton and Ritter [15] and Mutlu et al. [12], in 6% of temporal bones, a jugular bulb is found lying above the level of the inferior tympanic annulus. The jugular bulb may be dehiscent and more vulnerable to injury during the dissection of cholesteatoma from hypotympanic or retrofacial cells or even during the elevation of a tympanomeatal flap [16, 17].

When the posterosuperior quadrant is reached, the remaining ossicular chain comes to the attention of the surgeon. In the few cases where the chain is intact, ossicular mobility is evaluated by mobilizing the long process of the malleus with the duckbill elevator or joint knife while observing changes in the light reflex near the round window. Testing the mobility of the stapes includes palpation of the incudostapedial joint, the head of the stapes, and the footplate. The curette is employed over the posterosuperior margin of the canal to enhance exposure of the stapes joint and the oval window. For such a procedure, a sharp curette should be used, with gentle but firm movements from inside to outside and from the 12 to 6 o'clock position to avoid accidental dislocation of the ossicles [18]. The drill with a small cutting burr can also be helpful during this step. When the surgeon can identify the joint, oval window, stapedial tendon, and tympanic segment of the facial nerve, removal of bone is complete. After long-standing OM with effusion, the TM and the malleus may be found medialized. In these circumstances, the tensor tympani tendon is severed with the joint knife, and the malleus is gently lateralized to open up the mesotympanic space.

During this exploration, both the oval and the round window should be thoroughly inspected. The surgeon should note whether the round window membrane is visible or is in a covered position in the niche, as well as distinguish the membrane from mucosal folds in the niche (so-called false membrane). Any pathologic tissue over the windows should be meticulously addressed and, if possible, removed. The integrity of the round window membrane and the footplate should never be jeopardized during a first-stage procedure [15].

Lowering the Facial Ridge and Posterior Wall

The next step after the perfect identification of the middle ear key landmarks (the stapes, the tympanic segment of the VII nerve, and the lateral canal in the antrum), the facial ridge is lowered under direct view. At this point, there will be a bump between the facial canal and the posterior wall since both structures are located in two different levels. A diamond burr is now employed, and the bone is progressively removed from the lateral, anterior, and posterior faces of the ridge. The ideal situation is achieved when the tympanic segment, the genu, and the vertical segment of the facial nerve follow a smooth course from the middle ear to the mastoid. The final aspect of the superior pole of the posterior canal should never be higher than the dome of the lateral semicircular canal. A careful and meticulous bone removal in this region makes possible the inspection and cleaning of the so-called posterior compartments of the middle ear: (a) facial recess, (b) sinus tympani, and (c) round window niche (Fig. 53.15). Patience should be highly exercised during this step since the three most dreaded complications of the surgery lay within a distance of only 4.5 mm! (Fig. 53.16).

The facial nerve should be followed initially from the genu to the beginning of its descending portion (Fig. 53.17).

Depending on the size of the mastoid defect that has been created, the posterior wall will be lowered as far as the level II (midmastoid) or III (tip) nerve. It is mandatory to fine-

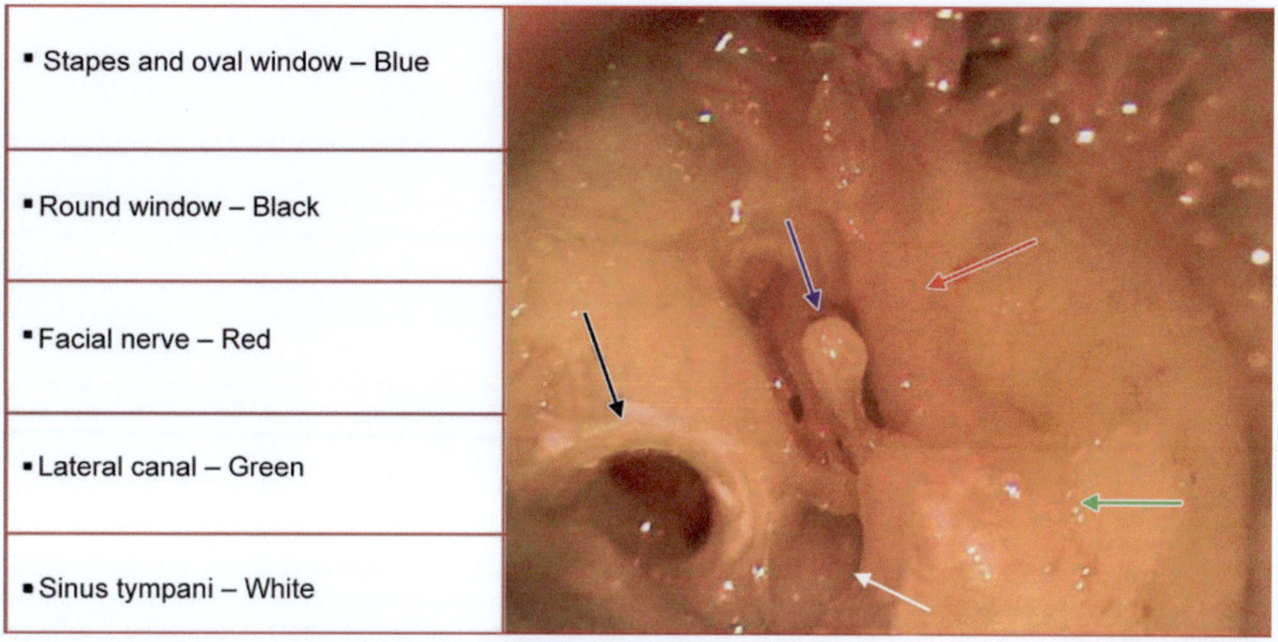

Fig. 53.15 Photograph of the so-called posterior recesses of the mesotympanum

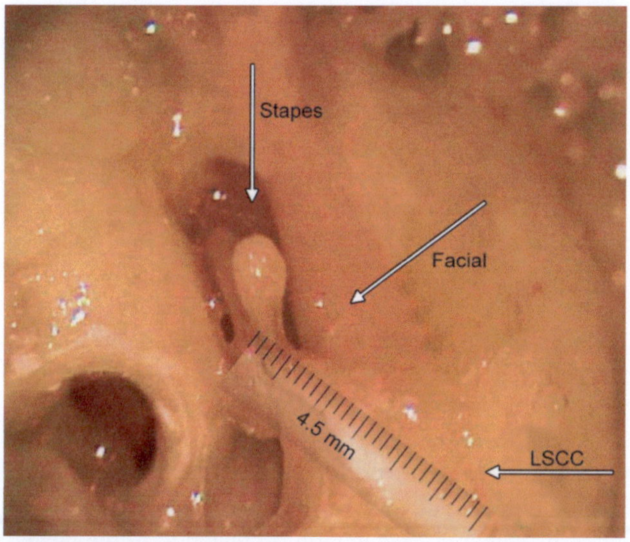

Fig. 53.16 Along a linear distance of 4.5 mm the three components of the "critical triad": (1) lateral semicircular canal; (2) facial nerve; (3) stapes and oval window. Source: Paparella MM, personal communication

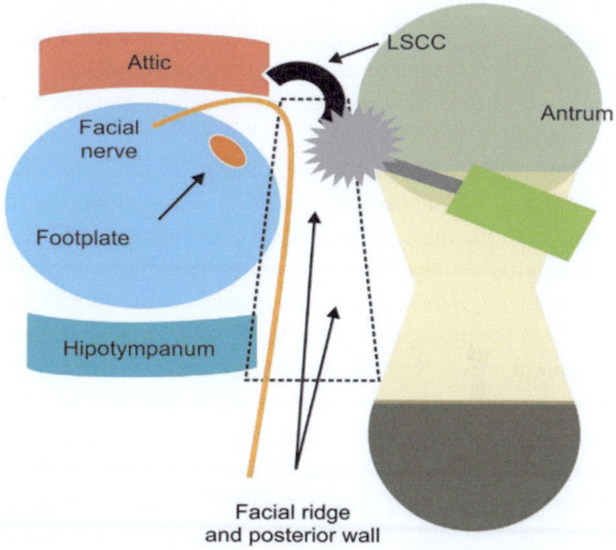

Fig. 53.17 The superior pole of the wall will be completely lowered only after the perfect identification of the stapes (or the footplate), the facial nerve, and its second genu

tune the drilling of the posterior wall according to the final size of the mastoidectomy. When only the antrum has been opened, the work is limited to the superior pole of the posterior wall and the beginning of the vertical segment. The midmastoid level pushes the dissection inferiorly and bone should be removed all around the wall. A smooth continuity must be maintained with the proximal segment. Whenever the level III (mastoid tip) has been reached, some extra details should be observed. First, the vertical segment of the facial nerve must be totally exposed (Fig. 53.18). Care should be used to preserve a thin layer of bone over the nerve. The posterior semicircular canal, the exit of the chorda tympani nerve, and the digastric ridge can be used as valuable additional landmarks during the dissection. Second,

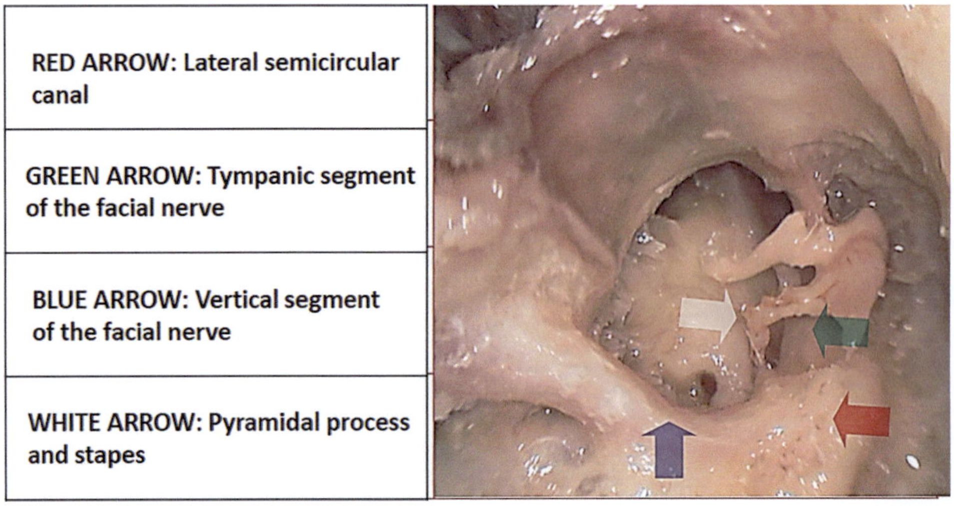

Fig. 53.18 The final landmarks after a wide-open mastoidectomy. Notice that the posterior wall has been reduced in all dimensions: the tympanic facial nerve, the genu, and the vertical segment follow a smooth course, and the hypotympanum and the anterior aspect of the wall have also been drilled

the medial floor of the external auditory canal needs to be lowered as close to the inferior level of the hypotympanum as possible. This makes the inferior floor of the middle ear accessible for routine office cleaning. Again bone has to be removed from the lateral, anterior, and posterior aspects of the most caudal segment of the posterior wall and its junction with the EAC. There, the mastoid tip must be addressed. In our opinion, there are two alternatives to manage the tip: (a) it may be cleaned of all cells and then amputated. This can be performed by stripping the periostium from the mastoid tip and amputating it using a Gigli saw, or alternatively, the bone can simply be removed as part of the mastoidectomy using a combination of cutting and diamond burrs. Removal of the mastoid tip and the bone inferior and lateral to the sigmoid sinus allows soft tissue to collapse medially toward the sigmoid sinus. This removes a substantial volume from the postoperative mastoid cavity in an area that is difficult to access through even a large meatus [18]. (b) The tip of the mastoid and part of the midmastoid may be obliterated with the periosteal flap when it is returned to its original position. It is important to clean all epithelial remnants off the tip before repositioning the flap. To decrease the final size of the mastoid bowl, it is also necessary to remove all the sharp edges around the surgical defect. Saucerization should be preferably performed at the beginning of the mastoidectomy because the enlarged cavity permits more light to penetrate to the depths of the cavity and creates more working room [18].

Ossiculoplasty

After pathologic tissue in the middle ear has been eradicated, thorough attention is directed to assessment and reconstruction of the ossicular chain. Three prerequisites to obtaining good functional restoration in cases of COM exist: (1) an intact TM; (2) an air-containing, mucosa-lined middle ear space; and (3) a precise connection between the eardrum and fluids in the ear [19]. Materials often used for ossiculoplasty are grouped as autografts, homografts, or synthetic prostheses. Each material has advantages and disadvantages, and no universal agreement exists concerning the most suitable prosthesis for ossiculoplasty [10].

Bone and cartilage came into use in the 1960s and continues to be used alone or in combination with other materials. The authors believe that using the patient's own tissue (sculptured incus, malleus, or cortical bone) is the best option. When these are not available, or when interpositioning of an ossicle is not reasonable, we employ synthetic materials (hydroxyapatite or titanium). In cases in which the incus is absent, the stapes is normal, and the wall has been taken down, decreasing the size of the middle ear cleft, the authors have used an autograft bony disc to bridge the gap between the stapes and eardrum. This disc is sculptured in situ using the drill and a small cutting burr in the mastoid cortex. The disc has a mean diameter of 3.5 mm, and in its center an acetabulum is created to fit the head of the stapes. It is then carefully detached from the cortex using a small chisel, trimmed to its final form, and positioned over the head of the stapes (Fig. 53.20a and b). When only the footplate is remaining, we also have used cortical bone. The only difference is that in this circumstance, a T-shaped TORP is sculptured in the cortex of the mastoid. The window is lined with fascia or perichondrium, the prostheses is trimmed to its final size, inserted in the niche, and held in place with small pledges of Gelfoam (Fig. 53.19a and b).

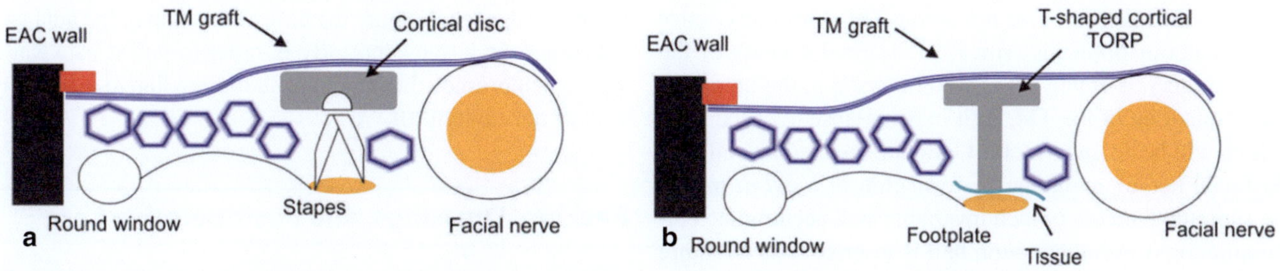

Fig. 53.19 (**a** and **b**) Ossiculoplasty with cortical bone: (**a**) A PORP (sculptured disc of cortical bone) has been interposed between the tympanic membrane and the head of stapes. (**b**) A TORP replaces the chain (also sculptured with cortical bone). The footplate has been line with tissue (fascia, perichondrium, or periosteum)

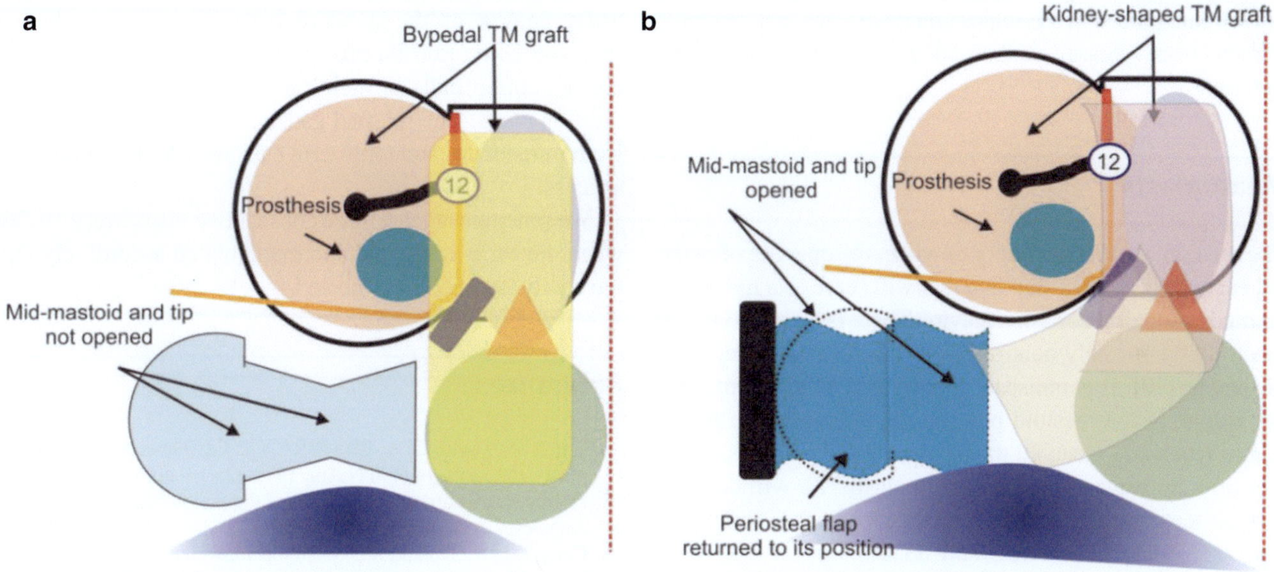

Fig. 53.20 (**a**) A bipedal graft is employed, covering the middle ear and wrapping the attic, the lateral semicircular canal and the medial wall of the antrum-mastoid opening level I. (**b**) When a level II or III defect has been created, a kidney-shaped graft is fashioned, covering the middle ear and lining the attic, antrum, and the partially the mastoid (the tip has been removed or obliterated by the periosteal flap)

Grafting the TM

After final inspection and irrigation of the middle ear, the flap is folded fully anteriorly. Any debris or bone dust should be meticulously cleaned away. The dried temporalis fascia is removed from the block of PTFE and trimmed to fit medial to the remnant of the eardrum, the manubrium, and the tympanomeatal flap. The graft is tailored to its final shape according to the surgical defect. When only the antrum has been exposed, a bipedal graft is employed covering the middle ear and wrapping the attic, the lateral semicircular canal, and the medial wall of the antrum (Fig. 53.20a). When a level II or III defect has been created, kidney-shaped graft is fashioned, covering the middle ear and lining the attic, antrum, and partially the mastoid (the tip has been removed or obliterated (Fig. 53.20b). Gelfoam soaked in saline solution is placed in the middle ear and the orifice of the ET to occlude the tube temporarily and to offer support for the graft anteriorly. Enough Gelfoam should be used to create a true cushion in the middle ear to support the graft. Care should be used, though, to respect the limits of the fibrous and bony annulus because the um, moistened Gelfoam tends to absorb liquid and expand. After the cushion is completed, a cotton ball is pressed against it, any solution or drops of blood are suctioned, and the cotton is gently removed. The graft is grasped with an alligator forceps, rehydrated briefly with saline solution, and placed as far anteriorly in the middle ear as possible and medial to the manubrium. The remaining base of the graft is spread over the Gelfoam cushion and the mastoid walls contouring the dome of the lateral canal. The flap is returned to its original position with a duckbill, and the surgeon's attention is directed to tucking the graft carefully into the margins of the remaining TM. Absolute control of the anterior border is critical to the final success of the entire surgery. A small, slit should be made in the anterosuperior quadrant of the TM, so it may collapse over the graft (which will be resting over the Gelfoam, the medial wall, and the facial nerve), avoiding the formation of a *cul-de-sac* in the supratubal recess (which invariably will accumulate epithelial debris). Another cotton ball is inserted, and moisture or blood is gently suctioned through the cotton. After its removal, the graft and flap are checked. After the flap has been meticulously returned to its original position, the cavity is packed firmly with Gelfoam pledgets. The first piece of packing is a small, dry, rolled-up, tightly compressed piece of Gelfoam placed in the sulcus anteriorly. The self-retaining retractors are released, and an adequate meatoplasty is carried out.

Meatoplasty

The meatoplasty is mandatory to widen the opening of external ear and to create a skin flap that will serve as a matrix for epithelization of the mastoid cavity. There is no question that meatoplasty strongly contributes to the functional recovery of the ear [20]. It is indispensable in OCTM to monitor the conditions of the mastoid bowl in the postoperative period and to reach and clean all the newly created recesses. There are different ways to perform meatoplasty. We will describe a basic technique, most used in our experience, which is a simple five-step procedure (Table 53.1).

The first step of meatoplasty is the initial incision of skin made in the beginning of the surgery. Thereafter, as mentioned before, two vertical incisions are done at 1 and 5 o'clock to prepare a Köerner's flap. Next step consists in dissection soft tissues of Köerner's flap, leaving only skin. A smooth pressure with middle finger can support and guide this moment. It is important to remove a slice of conchal cartilage for the purpose of increasing the mobility of this skin flap.

After this, vertical incisions are prolonged. The higher they extend toward the free skin of the pinna, the greater the amplitude of meatus. A good parameter is the point when external meatus freely accepts the introduction of the index finger. Last stage is suture the base of this flap in the adjacent subcutaneous tissue superiorly in order to pull it backward, which will promote healing tension forcing flap to meet bony wall of the cavity [20].

Table 53.1 Meatoplasty: a five-step procedure

Incisions in the skin of the auditory canal
Dissection of subcutaneous tissue
Identification, release, and partial resection of the pinna cartilage
Vertical incisions in the skin of the pinna (Köerner's flap)
Flap sutures

Packing, Dressings, and Postoperative Care

After the meatoplasty, the self-retaining retractors are released and the ear is returned to its original position and sutured in place. Gauze impregnated in antibiotic ointment is used to line the cavity to prevent infection and to minimize adhesions of raw surface areas. Postoperative dressings generally consist of the standard mastoid dressing, which is removed 24 h after the procedure. Patients are instructed to change cotton balls in their ear and keep the postauricular incision clean. The internal gauze is left in place for 7 days. Both immediate- and long-term care are vital for the surgical success.

We schedule at least three consecutive visits every 10 days when the ear is inspected and manipulated accordingly until the cavity is completely healed.

References

1. Costa SS, Souza LCA, Piza MRT. The flexible endaural tympanoplasty. Otolaryngol Clin N Am. 1999;32:413–40.
2. Nelson RA. Temporal bone surgical dissection manual. 2nd ed. Los Angeles, CA: House Ear Inst; 1991.
3. Cody DT, McDonald TJ. Mastoidectomy for acquired cholesteatoma: follow-up to 20 years. Laryngoscope. 1984;94(8):1027–30.
4. Bennett M, Warren F, Haynes D. Indications and technique in mastoidectomy. Otolaryngol Clin N Am. 2006;39:1095–113.
5. Costa SS, Silva MNL, Silva DP. Mastoidectomia aberta e fechada: indicações e técnicas. Pró-ORL. 2009;4-1:65–88.
6. Schuknecht HF. Surgical pathology. In: Pathology of the ear. Cambridge, MA: Harvard University Press; 1993. p. 564–7.
7. Sourdille M. New techniques in the surgical treatment of severe and progressive deafness from otosclerosis. Bull NY Acad Med. 1937:13673–91.
8. Dornhoffer JL. Retrograde mastoidectomy. Otolaryngol Clin N Am. 2006;39:1115–27.
9. Hough JVD. Malformation and anatomical variations seen in the middle ear during the operation for mobilization of the stapes. Laryngoscope. 1958;68:1337–79.
10. Chole RA, Kim HJ. Ossiculoplasty with presculpted banked cartilage. Operative techniques. Otolaryngol Head Neck Surg. 1996;7:38–44.
11. Moreano E, Paparella MM, Zelterman D, et al. Prevalence of facial canal dehiscence and of persistent stapedial artery in human middle ear: a report of 1000 temporal bones. Laryngoscope. 1994;104:309–20.
12. Mutlu C, Costa SS, Paparella MM, et al. Clinical histopathological correlations of pitfalls in middle ear surgery. Eur Arch Otorhinolaryngol. 1998;255:189–94.

13. Meyerhoff WL, Kim CG, Paparella MM. Pathology of chronic otitis media. Ann Otol Rhinol Laryngol. 1978;87:749–61.
14. Costa SS, Cruz OM. Exploratory tympanotomy. Operative techniques. Otolaryngol Head Neck Surg. 1996;7:20–5.
15. Overton SB, Ritter FN. A high placed jugular bulb in the middle ear: a clinical and temporal bone study. Laryngoscope. 1973;83:1986–93.
16. Costa SS, Colli BO, Fonseca N, et al. Anatomia cirurgica da arteria carotida intrapetrosa. J Bras Neurocirurgia. 1996;7:730–43.
17. Neely JG. Tympanoplasty. In: Pillsbury HC, Goldsmith MM, editors. Operative challenges in otolaryngology head and neck surgery. Chicago, IL: Year Book Medical Publisher; 1990. p. 24–32.
18. Moore PJ. The high jugular bulb in the ear: three case reports and a review of the literature. J Laryngol Otol. 1994;108:772–5.
19. Costa SS, Paparella MM, Schachern PA, et al. Temporal bone histopathology in chronically infected ears with intact and perforated tympanic membranes. Laryngoscope. 1992;102:1229–36.
20. Graham MD. The jugular bulb: its anatomical and clinical considerations in contemporary otology. Laryngoscope. 1997;87:105–25.

Principles of Surgical Management of Cholesteatoma

54

Adam C. Kaufman and Peter L. Santa Maria

Introduction

Cholesteatoma was first described in the literature in 1683 by Guichard Duverney as a temporal bone lesion [1]. However the term cholesteatoma was not coined until 1838 by Johannes Muller [2]. It was believed, at that time, incorrectly, to be a tumor and to be associated with cholesterin leading to the name [1]. It would be many decades before there was a general consensus that cholesteatoma was the progressive growth of keratinizing stratified squamous epithelium into the middle ear or the pneumatized temporal bone [3]. As cholesteatomas are expansile and locally destructive, they usually require intervention [4].

Management Overview

Although the existence of cholesteatomas has been known for hundreds of years, there is still ongoing debate about the best management options [1]. Surgery is the definitive curative treatment however there are a number of different surgical options and techniques available [5]. A hierarchy of goals has been established to help determine the choices made in surgery [6]. The primary goal of surgery is to establish a "safe ear" as untreated cholesteatoma can lead to significant complications including cranial nerve palsies, inner ear invasion causing permanent sensory hearing loss, intracranial infection, venous thrombosis and otic hydrocephalus [7–9]. These patients have a tendency for recurrent episodes of otorrhea often exacerbated by water exposure [10]. Therefore, for patient comfort and to potentially reduce risk of recurrence, the next goal of surgery is to achieve a dry and safe ear. Cholesteatoma patients often present with conductive hearing loss and in some instances with sensorineural hearing loss [11, 12]. The final goal is to stop further progression of hearing loss and creating conditions in the middle ear that maximize hearing. Complete restoration of hearing cannot always be achieved when trying to achieve the earlier goals [13].

In addition to surgery, there are few medical interventions for consideration. Smoking cessation and management of uncontrolled allergies should be attempted. Smokers have an increased rate of recurrence and higher rates of needing ossicular chain reconstruction [14, 15]. Additionally, smokers have an increased rate of Eustachian tube dysfunction which impairs middle ear mechanics [16, 17]. Uncontrolled allergies can also lead to Eustachian tube dysfunction mirroring what is seen in smokers [18]. Of course, once cholesteatoma is established neither of these interventions will reverse the process. Patients that are too medically fragile to undergo surgery and with limited disease can potentially be managed with frequent in-office debridement to help control further growth of the cholesteatoma and prevent additional complications [19].

Pre-operative Evaluation

All patients who have a cholesteatoma should receive a pure-tone audiogram [20]. Large air-bone gaps can indicate the presence of ossicular destruction which will guide the reconstructive plan intraoperatively [21]. Moreover, understanding the contralateral ear's hearing status can help guide surgical decision making. If there is cholesteatoma in an only hearing ear, traditionally, surgeons have erred on performing more aggressive surgery in an attempt to protect that ear from further auditory decline although that philosophy is

A. C. Kaufman
Otorhinolaryngology – Head & Neck Surgery, University of Maryland, Baltimore, Baltimore, MD, USA
e-mail: Adam.Kaufman@som.umaryland.edu

P. L. Santa Maria (✉)
Otolaryngology, Head & Neck Surgery, Stanford University, Stanford, CA, USA
e-mail: petersantamaria@stanford.edu

M. V. Goycoolea et al. (eds.), *Textbook of Otitis Media*, https://doi.org/10.1007/978-3-031-40949-3_54

slowly changing [22]. Unexpected sensorineural hearing loss can alert the surgeon to an inner ear fistula. Sometimes these can also present with third window features on the audiogram with elevation of the bone thresholds [23].

Imaging with computer tomography (CT) imaging to help define the extent of disease, identify potential areas of danger for disease complications and help the surgeon prepare for the anatomy they will encounter such as a low-lying or dehiscent tegmen, dehiscent facial nerve, labyrinthine fistula, or an anterior sigmoid sinus [24, 25]. The CT hallmarks of cholesteatoma included opacification in Prussak's space with scutal erosion and ossicular destruction [24, 26] (Fig. 54.1).

Although magnetic resonance imaging (MRI) does not delineate bony anatomy well, it plays a role in the workup of some patients with cholesteatoma. Cholesteatoma appears as a hypointense lesion on T1 sequences, hyperintense lesion on T2 sequences, and can have rim enhancement with contrast administration [27]. MRI is also useful to help delineate other pathology within the mastoid such as meningoceles, encephaloceles, or dural involvement [28]. It can also be used to investigate areas that are difficult to access surgically, such as the petrous apex. Diffusion weighted imaging (DWI) is particularly useful for distinguishing cholesteatoma from granulation tissue, scar tissue, and cholesterol granulomas [29]. It is for this reason that DWI has become more prominent in recent years. Non-echo planar DWI has excellent sensitivity and specificity of 89% and 93% respectively for detecting cholesteatoma. Studies report detecting all cholesteatomas greater than 2mm in one study and 5 mm in another [30, 31]. It has been reported that it is not reliable in discriminating cholesteatoma smaller than 3 mm [30, 32]. There is continued work on novel imaging sequences that will continue to improve the resolution and diagnostic capabilities [33, 34].

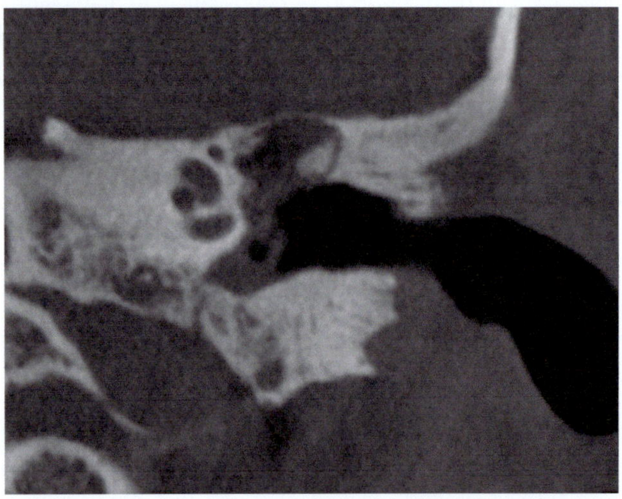

Fig. 54.1 Coronal CT scan demonstrating the classical features of cholesteatoma. There is opacification of the attic and Prussak's space, scutal erosion, and ossicular destruction in a left ear

Surgical Management Options

As previously alluded to, there are a number of surgeries available to manage cholesteatoma. There are pros and cons to each surgical options and therefore the choice of which to perform will depend on the extent of disease and patient characteristics. Herein we describe broadly the different variations that exist however subsequent chapters will cover each in significantly more depth.

For limited disease that is located entirely within the mesotympanum, a tympanoplasty can be performed to remove the cholesteatoma and repair any defects in the tympanic membrane. If the disease extends into the epitympanum, a scutectomy can be considered to gain access to the attic and this is formally called an atticotomy [35] (Fig. 54.2).

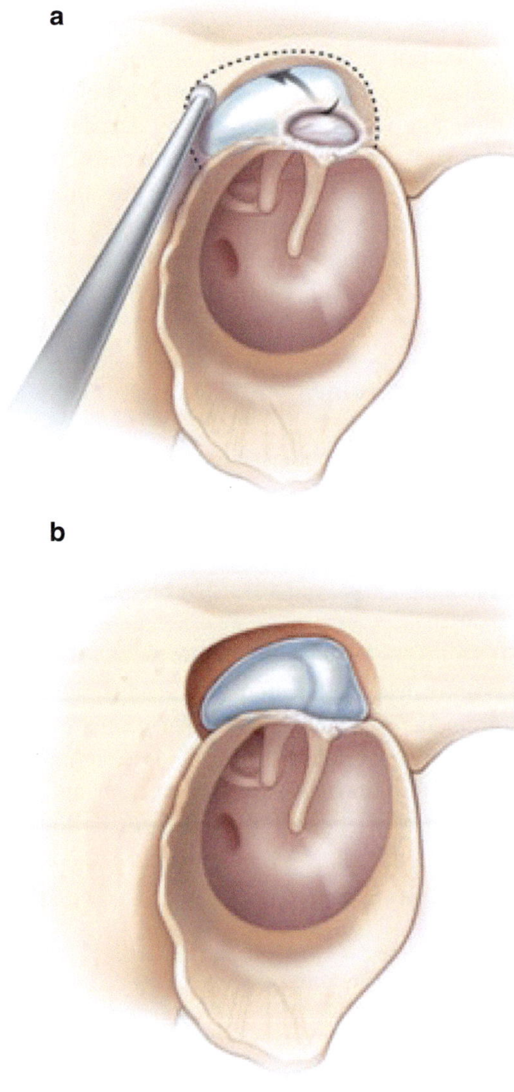

Fig. 54.2 (**a**) Hash marks demonstrating the area of bone within the epitympanum that should be removed for an atticotomy. (**b**) The fully exposed cholesteatoma after the bony removal of an atticotomy. (© Robert Jackler, Chris Gralapp 2023. All Rights Reserved)

If there is extension further into the antrum, an atticoantrostomy can be performed. These procedures are generally not recommended if there is disease anterior to the head of the malleus, medial to any of the ossicles, or significant extension into the mastoid.

If there is more extensive disease within the mastoid, a mastoidectomy is likely required to fully eliminate the cholesteatoma [35]. A cortical mastoidectomy, which is the removal of the lateral cortex of air cells within the temporal bone, is often insufficient. At a minimum, a canal wall-up tympanomastoidectomy is required. This is a complete exenteration of all the air cells within the temporal bone and a tympanoplasty while leaving the posterior wall of the external auditory canal intact (Fig. 54.3). An additional variant is where the posterior wall is removed creating a common cavity with mastoid and the external auditory canal (Fig. 54.4). This is termed a canal wall-down tympanomastoidectomy, which is also known as the modified radical mastoidectomy [36].

The Bondy mastoidectomy is a modification to the canal wall-down mastoidectomy, when there is a relatively normal middle ear, where the epitympanum is exteriorized so that the mastoid, epitympanum and external canal become a common cavity [37] (Fig. 54.5). The pars tensa and ossicular chain are left intact; however, the cholesteatoma sac is externalized with the aim to become self-cleaning. The final option for control of cholesteatoma is a radical mastoidectomy which is a canal wall-down mastoidectomy with removal of the ossicles and the tympanic membrane with complete obliteration of the Eustachian tube.

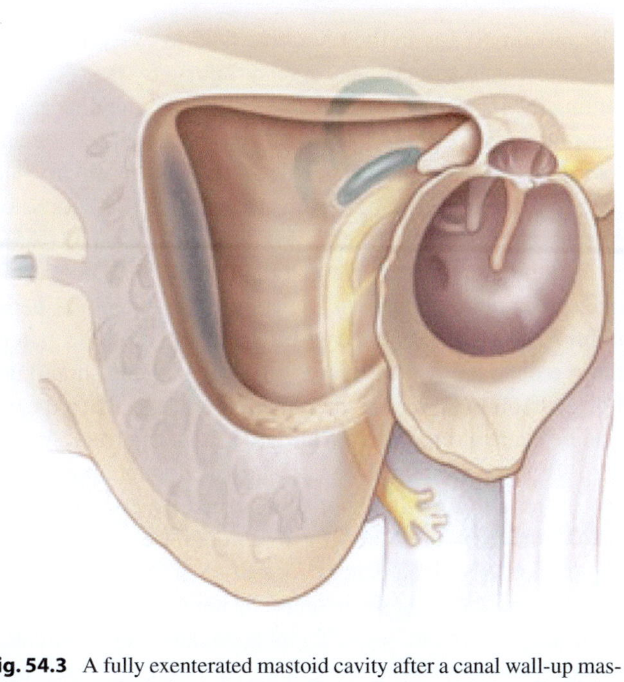

Fig. 54.3 A fully exenterated mastoid cavity after a canal wall-up mastoidectomy. (© Robert Jackler, Chris Gralapp 2023. All Rights Reserved)

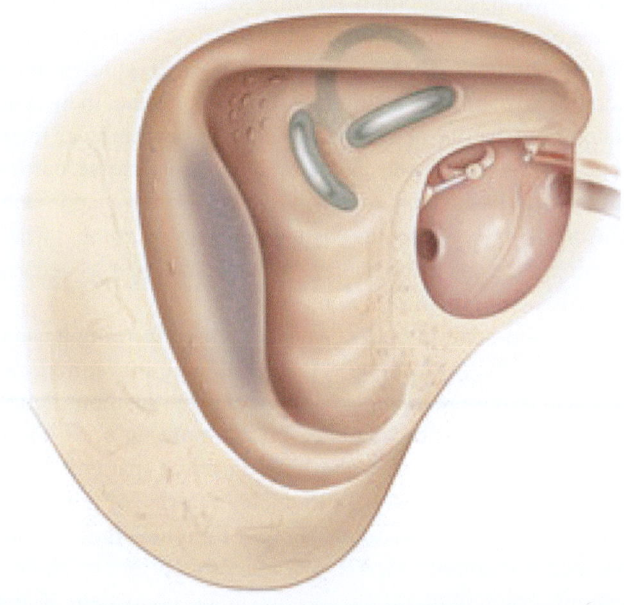

Fig. 54.4 A fully exenterated mastoid cavity with the posterior external auditory canal removed as seen in a canal wall-down mastoidectomy. (© Robert Jackler, Chris Gralapp 2023. All Rights Reserved)

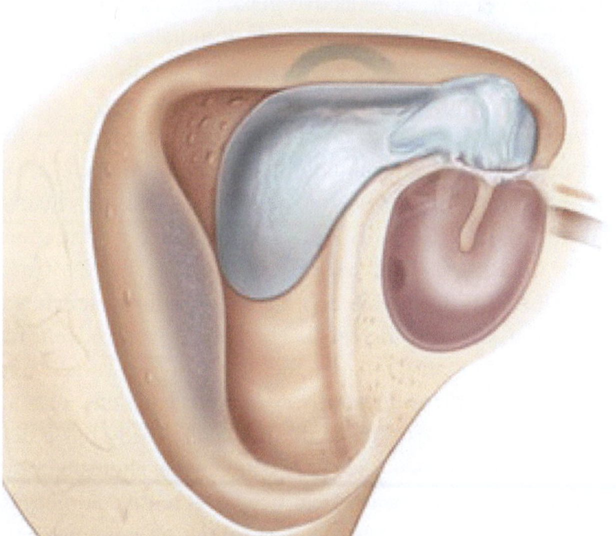

Fig. 54.5 The creation of a common cavity between the epitympanum and the mastoid cavity as seen in a Bondy mastoidectomy with cholesteatoma enveloping the ossicles in the attic and extending through the antrum. (© Robert Jackler, Chris Gralapp 2023. All Rights Reserved)

At its core, the fundamental question in cholesteatoma surgery is whether the canal wall should remain or be taken down. The major advantage of a canal wall-down mastoidectomy is the ability to more fully, but not completely, visualize the sinus tympani and the anterior epitympanum. This improved visualization is the likely cause of the lower rate of recurrence [38, 39]. Historically, it was thought that the canal wall-down mastoidectomy had inferior hearing outcomes, in terms of air bone gap closure, which has been seen in a number of studies [40–42]. However, not all studies have consistently shown this difference [43]. Of course, there is an inherent difficulty in comparing hearing outcomes in these two surgical approaches as more significant disease burden often necessitates a canal wall-down approach. Unsurprisingly, there are better hearing outcomes when some portion of the ossicular chain remains just as seen in other ossicular reconstructions [44, 45].

An additional thing to consider when performing a canal wall-down mastoidectomy is the creation of a mastoid bowl that will require regular cleaning to remove squamous debris as well as dry ear precautions. Furthermore, in order to be able to adequately clean the bowl in clinic, patients often need a meatoplasty as well. Reducing the size of the cavity through mastoid obliteration can help limit how much maintenance is required [46, 47]. The rate of recurrent of cholesteatoma after obliteration appears to be equivalent if not lower than in non-obliterative procedures [48]. If recurrence does occur, it is likely to be it the mesotympanum or the ear canal [49]. A variety of material can be used to fill the cavity including bone dust, cartilage, fascia, vascularized soft tissue flaps, bone cement, or bioactive glass [50–53]. Obliterating the cavity with any material can help eliminate a persistently draining cavity; however, vascularized tissue flaps are particularly useful for this [54].

While institutions and surgeons have their preferences for each approach, the debate continues. However, there are a some scenarios where it is often desirable to consider a canal wall-down mastoidectomy, which is described by the mnemonic "FUSION." The patient with a semicircular canal *Fistula* benefits from this approach as it allows leaving a matrix of tissue over the canal. The patient who is *Unfit* for second look surgery reduces their risk of recurrence and thereby the need for any further surgery. A patient with an *Involved* posterior external auditory canal already has a disease induced canal wall down. A patient with cholesteatoma involving their *O*nly hearing ear needs aggressive surgery to protect any remaining hearing. The follow-up *noncompliant* patient benefits from this by reducing their risk of undetected recurrence although they do have a mastoid cavity that would require cleaning.

See Chaps. 23, 25, 26 and 29 for a further discussion regarding when to employ each of these operations.

Visualization

As cholesteatoma has a tendency to insinuate itself into small crevices within the bone, complete visualization of the lesion is essential for adequate removal. Contemporary approaches involve open cavity techniques with saucerization of the bony edges to allow direct visualization and light from the operating microscope. When performing non-open cavity approaches such as a transcanal tympanoplasty or a canal wall-up mastoidectomy, the natural anatomy can preclude seeing the edges of the cholesteatoma. There is continuing debate regarding the utility of endoscopes versus the microscope to perform these dissections [55]. The endoscope may provide an advantage particularly in clearing cholesteatoma around the crura of the stapes or in the sinus tympani due to the ability to use angled lenses while the microscope requires direct line of sight [56]. However, one hand must hold the endoscope taking away the ability to perform bimanual surgery and the images are limited by the two-dimensional quality of the endoscope. Conversely, the microscope provides three-dimensional images and allows for two handed surgery. A number of trials have shown similar outcomes in the ability to clear cholesteatoma between the two [56, 57]. As the technology has continued to improve the most recent studies suggest improved rates of clearance with lower rates of recurrence when using an endoscope [58, 59]. The exoscope is an upcoming technology that combines the three-dimensional images and hands-free nature of a microscope with the "heads-up" surgeon positioning and angled views of an endoscope that has been used effectively for cholesteatoma surgery [60–62]. The need for a large access corridor to get the exoscope in place and the limited image quality are the current major limitations to widespread adoption [61].

Protecting the Facial Nerve

The facial nerve is in the operative field in every variant of cholesteatoma surgery. Iatrogenic injury to the nerve is among the most devastating complications in middle ear and mastoid surgery. Injury has been linked with depression and loss of self-esteem [63]. Rates of injury during primary surgery are reported to range from 0.6 to 3.7% [64]. Revision surgery carries an even higher risk of injury at 4–10% [65].

It is therefore imperative that the surgeon take all reasonable precautions to protect the nerve. Intraoperative nerve monitoring (IONM) is a cost-effective technique to potentially reduce the risk of injury [66]. The surgeon should use IONM in otologic cases where there is a reasonable expectation of encountering the facial nerve. It is important for the surgeon to be familiar with this and develop an understanding on how to trouble shoot monitoring issues. The use of IONM should not lull the surgeon into a false sense of security particularly given that the lack of an alarm does not necessarily imply that the facial nerve is not at risk.

A deep understanding of facial nerve anatomy is essential to safely perform these operations. The tympanic and mastoid segments of the facial nerve are the portions mostly at risk [65]. The tympanic (horizontal) segment runs inferior to the cog and superior to the cochleariform process [67]. It continues just superior to the oval window before turning at the second genu and going posterior to the pyramidal eminence within the curve of the lateral semicircular canal. It then descends as the mastoid (vertical) segment traveling posterior to the facial recess [68]. The short process of the incus and the digastric ridge are additional landmarks that can be utilized to find the mastoid segment [69].

While drilling near the facial nerve, one must be cognizant to use plenty of irrigation to avoid thermal injury [70]. Meticulous hemostasis is necessary to maintain visualization of the nerve at all times. Further, the surgeon should avoid drilling or dissecting underneath any bony overhangs that can block their vision [71, 72].

In the event of an injury, one should stay calm and, if possible, reach out to a colleague for additional help. If the nerve appears to be grossly intact and able to be stimulated proximal to the site of injury, the nerve should be given time to recover spontaneously [73]. If the nerve is transected, one should attempt a neurorrhaphy and can decompress the nerve near the injury to allow for additional length if needed. If a tension-free anastomosis cannot be achieved a nerve graft can utilized. The great auricular nerve, which is near the surgical field although a sensory nerve, or the sural nerve, which is further away but is a motor nerve, is a commonly used option [74, 75]. An unexpected complete facial palsy postoperatively that lasts longer than the length of local anesthetic effects is an indication to promptly remove the ear canal packing and re-explore the surgical site to identify any sites of unknown nerve injury [76].

Areas Requiring Special Attention

Cholesteatoma involving the stapes crura, the footplate, and the oval window can make for a difficult dissection. Dissection may involve delicately removing the stapes superstructure to gain access to this area. Alternatively, some surgeons recommend leaving the cholesteatoma matrix down over the footplate during the initial resection and only during the second look surgery addressing the remnant [77]. There are advocates for the use of otologic lasers to help dissect cholesteatoma from mobile ossicles [78]. If using a laser, the surgeon must be mindful of the close proximity of the facial nerve to the oval window, any possible dehiscences and the potential for local heat generation as there is a reported rate of 0.6% for injury in this setting [79].

The sinus tympani is another area of difficult dissection related to poor direct visualization available in this space. The sinus tympani is located deep to the facial nerve between the ponticulus and subiculum [80]. It is the among the most common places for residual cholesteatoma to be left [81]. The space has a variable degree of pneumatization, which affects the difficulty in fully clearing the area of cholesteatoma [82] (Fig. 54.6). Cholesteatoma can potentially be removed by approaching it anteriorly and attempting to pull it out as a single piece although this is a blind maneuver when the sinus tympani is not shallow. Afterward, a curved instrument can be used to palpate the walls of the space to check for any residual disease. An angled endoscope can allow for further confirmation of complete removal. A deeper sinus tympani may require lowering the facial ridge toward the facial nerve, the bone just anterior to the facial

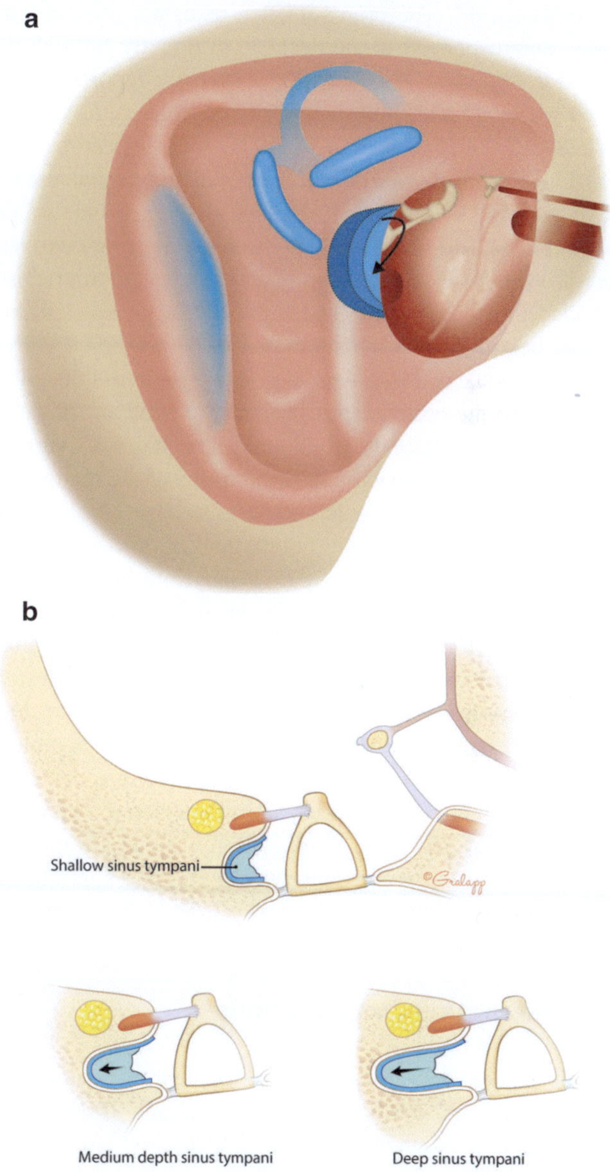

Fig. 54.6 (**a** and **b**) The differing degrees of pneumatization of the sinus tympani and its relationship to the facial nerve. Disease within a deep sinus tympani can be difficult to clear entirely. Even with a canal wall down mastoidectomy, the facial nerve limits the ability to directly visualize this area. (© Robert Jackler, Chris Gralapp 2023. All Rights Reserved)

nerve, to allow for adequate clearance. Alternatively, it may require conversion to a canal wall-down mastoidectomy, allowing the operative microscope to be directed from an anterior angle, to fully eliminate disease. Lastly, an extremely deep sinus tympani may be approached retrofacially; however, this space is limited by the anatomy of the patient's facial nerve, jugular bulb, and posterior semicircular canal [83, 84].

Cholesteatoma involving the petrous apex is problematic from a technical standpoint as well as a decision-making one particularly in the hearing ear [85]. Cholesteatoma often gains access to this area from extension from the middle ear or mastoid [86]. The routes it often takes are infralabyrinthine, anterosuperior to the cochlea, or directly through the superior semicircular canal [86]. There are reports of isolated petrous apex cholesteatomas and congenital variants [87, 88]. Typically, these patients have cholesteatoma that has invaded the labyrinth by the time of diagnosis and already have reduced hearing [89]. The most direct routes to the petrous apex, translabyrinthine or transcochlear, are destructive procedures leading to loss of function so are not recommended in a hearing ear. In the event that patient still has usable hearing, it can be attempted to be preserved with a middle fossa, infracochlear, or even a transsphenoidal approach to the petrous apex [89, 90]. As with all operative decisions in cholesteatoma surgery, the choice of surgery will depend on the specific location of the cholesteatoma as well as the nearby anatomic structures specifically the internal carotid artery, the jugular bulb, the geniculate ganglion, and the otic capsule [91]. A partial labyrinthectomy can be performed if there is extensive disease in the petrous apex in a hearing ear [92, 93]. This has been reported to be at times a hearing preservation procedure [94]. After the cholesteatoma is removed from the petrous apex, a large and deep cavity will be created which can be difficult to keep clean and maintain in the office afterward. Therefore, ear canal closure and blind sac creation can be considered. The major limitation to this though is the inability to directly monitor for future recurrence and consequently requires surveillance with DWI MRI [95].

Cholesteatoma Complications

Cholesteatoma can lead to the development of a number of intracranial and extracranial complications (Fig. 54.7). Subdural and parenchymal infection/abscess, otic hydrocephalus, CSF leak, and sigmoid sinus thrombosis are all among the possible problems that can develop from an uncontrolled cholesteatoma [96]. Cholesteatoma can also lead to semicircular canal fistula, mastoiditis, and conductive hearing loss [97].

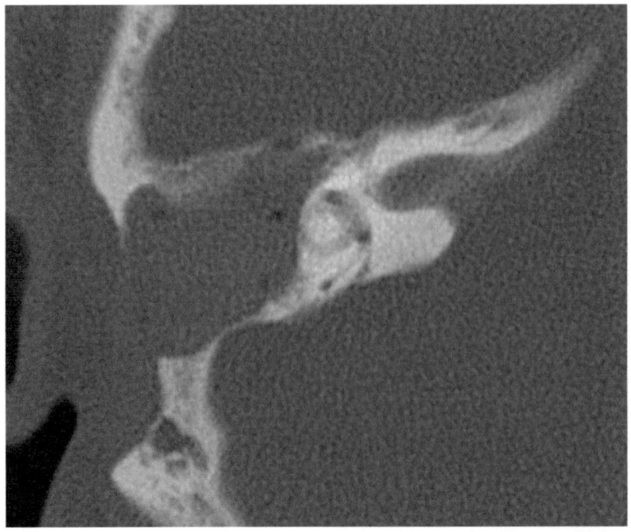

Fig. 54.7 Axial CT scan demonstrating lateral semicircular canal fistula and tegmen dehiscences in the setting of an uncontrolled cholesteatoma

Cholesteatoma can erode the tegmen leading to exposure of the dura [98]. Once a defect is created, an meningocele, encephalocele, or a frank CSF leak can occur [99]. If the defect is relatively small and there is no herniation of dura or brain, then it does not necessarily have to be repaired [100]. Conversely, if too large, the defect should be closed with cartilage, fascia, or bone depending on surgeon preference and size of the defect [101, 102].

Semicircular canal fistulas secondary to cholesteatoma growth is a relatively common occurrence [103]. Depending on how destructive the cholesteatoma is, it may have eroded through the periosteal, endochondral, or endosteal layers [104]. The ideal management of these fistulae remains unclear. There is significant debate over whether to remove or leave the cholesteatoma matrix over the fistula [105]. A recent meta-analysis showed no statistical difference in hearing outcomes between matrix removal and exteriorization [106]. However, when analyzing outcomes based on fistula size, there was an apparent difference in hearing outcomes. Fistulae smaller than 3 mm had significantly better hearing preservation (97%) when the matrix was removed while larger fistulae did much worse (71%) [107]. Understanding that, it is reasonable to leave the matrix over large fistulae especially in an only hearing ear. A canal wall-down mastoidectomy can be performed to allow for exteriorization of the matrix and in office monitoring and debridement [108]. Alternatively, a second look procedure can be planned for if a canal wall-up mastoidectomy is completed. That will give ample time for the matrix to develop an epithelial pearl or to spontaneously disappear [109, 110].

Until proven otherwise, the surgeon should always presume that a semicircular canal fistula is present. Dissection of this area should be left until the end of the case to reduce the risk of exposing the inner ear to bone dust or blood products as well as to lessen the chance of disrupting the repair. Methodical and careful dissection are essential to avoiding damage. One should avoid suctioning directly into the fistula and should immediately cover the fistula after removal of the cholesteatoma sac.

Antibiotics and surgery are the mainstay treatments for the management of sigmoid sinus thrombosis secondary to cholesteatoma [111]. Surgically, the sigmoid sinus should be decompressed via mastoidectomy [112]. It remains unclear whether there is a need to open the sinus and remove the thrombus. The majority of patients will recanalize the sinus without direct intervention [113]. Furthermore, the resolution of symptoms does not appear to be correlate with this recanalization [114]. The evidence currently does not support routine anticoagulation for these patients as it does not lead to improved outcomes and can be associated with harm as related to hemorrhagic stroke [115–117] Classically, ligation of the internal jugular vein was considered to potentially limit embolization and spread of the infection. Recent literature has moved away from this intervention due to ligation not limiting spread through collateral vessels and the risk of retrograde spread intracranially [118, 119]. It can still be considered if there is propagation of thrombus after mastoidectomy with adequate antibiotic coverage.

Recidivism

Residual cholesteatoma after surgery is a common occurrence [120]. Further, the underlying factors leading to the initiation of the disease are not always resolved leading to recurrent disease, despite clearance of the original disease. Recidivism, encompassing both residual disease and recurrent disease, is reported at rates ranging from 10 to 40% [121–123]. The variability between studies is likely related to the length of follow-up and which operation was performed. Risk factors associated with residual disease are age younger than 15, cholesteatoma localized to the mastoid, incus erosion, stapes erosion, and large canal defects [124, 125]. Long follow-up is essential as recurrence often appears years later [126]. Regular office evaluations for recidivism are crucial to finding the disease at its earliest stage. Canal wall-up mastoidectomies have a higher rate of recidivism than canal wall-down mastoidectomies [127]. A sequential surgery months afterward is often performed to check for residual disease after canal wall-up mastoidectomies. This second look surgery is able to keep the rate of recidivism between the two types of mastoidectomies roughly equivalent [128]. Many otolaryngologists use DWI MRI to help monitor for recidivism. It has not yet obviated the need for second look surgeries, but it has reduced the frequency and has been found to be cost effective [129].

References

1. Soldati D, Mudry A. Knowledge about cholesteatoma, from the first description to the modern histopathology. Otol Neurotol. 2001;22(6):723–30.
2. Ferlito A. A review of the definition, terminology and pathology of aural cholesteatoma. J Laryngol Otol. 1993;107(6):483–8.
3. Aslier M, et al. Analysis of histopathological aspects and bone destruction characteristics in acquired middle ear cholesteatoma of pediatric and adult patients. Int J Pediatr Otorhinolaryngol. 2016;82:73–7.
4. Schmerber S, et al. Surgical treatment of cholesteatomatous labyrinthine fistula by hydrodissection. Eur Ann Otorhinolaryngol Head Neck Dis. 2020;138:279.
5. Ajalloueyan M. Experience with surgical management of cholesteatomas. Arch Otolaryngol Head Neck Surg. 2006;132(9):931–3.
6. Fischer JL, Nesbitt NB, Littlefield PD. Bone pate obliteration in canal wall down mastoidectomy: modifications of an established technique. Otol Neurotol. 2020;41(3):352–8.
7. Nadol JB Jr. Causes of failure of mastoidectomy for chronic otitis media. Laryngoscope. 1985;95(4):410–3.
8. Dongol K, Rayamajhi P, Gurung U. Complications of acute and chronic otitis Media in a Tertiary Referral Center in Nepal. Turk Arch Otorhinolaryngol. 2020;58(4):234–40.
9. Prasad SC, et al. Current trends in the management of the complications of chronic otitis media with cholesteatoma. Curr Opin Otolaryngol Head Neck Surg. 2013;21(5):446–54.
10. Patil S, et al. Secondary obliteration surgery for troublesome mastoid cavities: a prospective series of 228 pediatric and adult cases. Otol Neurotol. 2021;Publish Ahead of Print:e881.
11. Holt JJ. Cholesteatoma and otosclerosis: two slowly progressive causes of hearing loss treatable through corrective surgery. Clin Med Res. 2003;1(2):151–4.
12. Gulustan F, et al. Evaluation of the presence of sensorineural hearing loss and the relationship with intraoperative findings in cholesteatoma. Ear Nose Throat J. 2021;100(3_suppl):249S–52S.
13. Leonard CG, et al. Measurement properties of the hearing environments and reflection of quality of life (HEAR-QL) 28-item questionnaire in cholesteatoma. Otol Neurotol. 2021;42(3):e304–10.
14. Kaylie DM, et al. Effects of smoking on otologic surgery outcomes. Laryngoscope. 2009;119(7):1384–90.
15. Patel S, Wooles N, Martin T. A systematic review of the impact of cigarettes and electronic cigarettes in otology. J Laryngol Otol. 2020;134:1–6.
16. Patel MA, et al. Tobacco smoke exposure and Eustachian tube disorders in US children and adolescents. PLoS One. 2016;11(10):e0163926.
17. Seibert JW, Danner CJ. Eustachian tube function and the middle ear. Otolaryngol Clin N Am. 2006;39(6):1221–35.
18. Juszczak HM, Loftus PA. Role of allergy in eustachian tube dysfunction. Curr Allergy Asthma Rep. 2020;20(10):54.
19. Pusalkar AG. Cholesteatoma and its management. Indian J Otolaryngol Head Neck Surg. 2015;67(3):201–4.
20. Ardic FN, et al. Correlation between surgical outcome and stage of acquired middle ear cholesteatoma: revalidation of the EAONO/JOS staging system. J Int Adv Otol. 2020;16(1):34–9.
21. Martins O, Victor J, Selesnick S. The relationship between individual ossicular status and conductive hearing loss in cholesteatoma. Otol Neurotol. 2012;33(3):387–92.

22. Carlson ML, et al. Evolving considerations in the surgical management of cholesteatoma in the only hearing ear. Otol Neurotol. 2014;35(1):84–90.
23. Ho ML, et al. Spectrum of third window abnormalities: semicircular canal dehiscence and beyond. AJNR Am J Neuroradiol. 2017;38(1):2–9.
24. Gulati M, et al. HRCT imaging of acquired cholesteatoma: a pictorial review. Insights Imaging. 2019;10(1):92.
25. Visvanathan V, Morrissey MS. Anatomical variations of the temporal bone on high-resolution computed tomography imaging: how common are they? J Laryngol Otol. 2015;129(7):634–7.
26. Bae MR, Kang WS, Chung JW. Comparison of the clinical results of attic cholesteatoma treatment: endoscopic versus microscopic ear surgery. Clin Exp Otorhinolaryngol. 2019;12(2):156–62.
27. Barath K, et al. Neuroradiology of cholesteatomas. AJNR Am J Neuroradiol. 2011;32(2):221–9.
28. Papanikolaou V, et al. Idiopathic temporal bone encephalocele. Skull Base. 2007;17(5):311–6.
29. Pisaneschi MJ, Langer B. Congenital cholesteatoma and cholesterol granuloma of the temporal bone: role of magnetic resonance imaging. Top Magn Reson Imaging. 2000;11(2):87–97.
30. Bazzi K, et al. Diffusion-weighted magnetic resonance imaging in the detection of residual and recurrent cholesteatoma in children: a systematic review and meta-analysis. Int J Pediatr Otorhinolaryngol. 2019;118:90–6.
31. Muzaffar J, et al. Diffusion-weighted magnetic resonance imaging for residual and recurrent cholesteatoma: a systematic review and meta-analysis. Clin Otolaryngol. 2017;42(3):536–43.
32. Jindal M, et al. A systematic review of diffusion-weighted magnetic resonance imaging in the assessment of postoperative cholesteatoma. Otol Neurotol. 2011;32(8):1243–9.
33. Benson JC, et al. Cholesteatoma localization using fused diffusion-weighted images and thin-slice T2 weighted images. Laryngoscope. 2021;131(5):E1662–7.
34. Corrales CE, Blevins NH. Imaging for evaluation of cholesteatoma: current concepts and future directions. Curr Opin Otolaryngol Head Neck Surg. 2013;21(5):461–7.
35. Abdelaziz AA. The role of preoperative computed tomography of temporal bone in atticotomy as a new tool for determining the approach. Indian J Otolaryngol Head Neck Surg. 2019;71(Suppl 2):1272–5.
36. Conway RM, et al. Perioperative cost evaluation of canal wall down mastoidectomy. Am J Otolaryngol. 2020;41(6):102733.
37. Shaan M, et al. Modified Bondy technique. Am J Otol. 1995;16(5):695–7.
38. Wilkie MD, et al. Canal wall down mastoidectomy with obliteration versus canal wall up mastoidectomy in primary cholesteatoma surgery. J Laryngol Otol. 2019;133(12):1074–8.
39. Tomlin J, et al. Surgical technique and recurrence in cholesteatoma: a meta-analysis. Audiol Neurootol. 2013;18(3):135–42.
40. Olmedo Martinez J, Ropero Romero F, Sanchez Gomez S. Cholesteatoma: influence of surgical technique and EAONO/JOS stage on audiological results. Acta Otorrinolaringol Esp. 2021;73:184.
41. Berenholz LP, et al. Ossiculoplasty in canal wall down mastoidectomy. Otolaryngol Head Neck Surg. 2000;123(1 Pt 1):30–3.
42. Tos M, Lau T. Hearing after surgery for cholesteatoma using various techniques. Auris Nasus Larynx. 1989;16(2):61–73.
43. Kim MB, et al. Hearing outcomes according to the types of mastoidectomy: a comparison between canal wall up and canal wall down mastoidectomy. Clin Exp Otorhinolaryngol. 2010;3(4):203–6.
44. Babighian G, Albu S. Stabilising total ossicular replacement prosthesis for ossiculoplasty with an absent malleus in canal wall down tympanomastoidectomy—a randomised controlled study. Clin Otolaryngol. 2011;36(6):543–9.
45. Cook JA, Krishnan S, Fagan PA. Hearing results following modified radical versus canal-up mastoidectomy. Ann Otol Rhinol Laryngol. 1996;105(5):379–83.
46. Mehta RP, Harris JP. Mastoid obliteration. Otolaryngol Clin N Am. 2006;39(6):1129–42.
47. Lee WS, et al. Mastoid and epitympanic obliteration in canal wall up mastoidectomy for prevention of retraction pocket. Otol Neurotol. 2005;26(6):1107–11.
48. van der Toom HFE, van der Schroeff MP, Pauw RJ. Single-stage mastoid obliteration in cholesteatoma surgery and recurrent and residual disease rates: a systematic review. JAMA Otolaryngol Head Neck Surg. 2018;144(5):440–6.
49. Vercruysse JP, et al. Mastoid and epitympanic bony obliteration in pediatric cholesteatoma. Otol Neurotol. 2008;29(7):953–60.
50. Sioshansi PC, Alyono JC, Blevins NH. Mastoid obliteration using autologous bone dust following canal wall down mastoidectomy. Otol Neurotol. 2021;42(1):68–75.
51. Maniu A, Cosgarea M. Mastoid obliteration with concha cartilage graft and temporal muscle fascia. ORL J Otorhinolaryngol Relat Spec. 2012;74(3):141–5.
52. Singh V, Atlas M. Obliteration of the persistently discharging mastoid cavity using the middle temporal artery flap. Otolaryngol Head Neck Surg. 2007;137(3):433–8.
53. Ezzat AE, Eid MI. Evaluation of using bioglass((R)) in obliteration of mastoid cavity. Curr Sci Int. 2014;3(2):87–94.
54. Harun A, et al. The role of obliteration in the achievement of a dry mastoid bowl. Otol Neurotol. 2015;36(9):1510–7.
55. Bennett ML, et al. Comparison of middle ear visualization with endoscopy and microscopy. Otol Neurotol. 2016;37(4):362–6.
56. Verma B, Dabholkar YG. Role of endoscopy in surgical management of cholesteatoma: a systematic review. J Otol. 2020;15(4):166–70.
57. Presutti L, et al. Results of endoscopic middle ear surgery for cholesteatoma treatment: a systematic review. Acta Otorhinolaryngol Ital. 2014;34(3):153–7.
58. Das A, et al. Endoscopic versus microscopic management of attic cholesteatoma: a randomized controlled trial. Laryngoscope. 2020;130(10):2461–6.
59. Li B, et al. Endoscopic versus microscopic surgery for treatment of middle ear cholesteatoma: a systematic review and meta-analysis. Am J Otolaryngol. 2021;42(2):102451.
60. Wierzbicka M, et al. Otosurgery with the high-definition three-dimensional (3D) exoscope: advantages and disadvantages. J Clin Med. 2021;10(4).
61. Colombo G, et al. Introducing the high-definition 3D exoscope in ear surgery: preliminary analysis of advantages and limits compared with operative microscope. Eur Arch Otorhinolaryngol. 2021;278:4217.
62. Minoda R, Miwa T. Non-microscopic middle ear cholesteatoma surgery: a case report of a novel head-up approach. Otol Neurotol. 2019;40(6):777–81.
63. Misra BK. Facial nerve monitoring during surgery of cerebellopontine angle and skull base surgery. World Neurosurg. 2013;80(6):e195–6.
64. Wilson L, Lin E, Lalwani A. Cost-effectiveness of intraoperative facial nerve monitoring in middle ear or mastoid surgery. Laryngoscope. 2003;113(10):1736–45.
65. Ryu NG, Kim J. How to avoid facial nerve injury in mastoidectomy? J Audiol Otol. 2016;20(2):68–72.
66. Heman-Ackah SE, Gupta S, Lalwani AK. Is facial nerve integrity monitoring of value in chronic ear surgery? Laryngoscope. 2013;123(1):2–3.

67. Nikolaidis V, et al. The tympanic segment of the facial nerve: anatomical study. Clin Anat. 2009;22(3):307–10.
68. Merati M, et al. Radiologic evaluation of the mastoid segment of the facial nerve tract in the intact temporal bone. Surg Radiol Anat. 2021;43(2):145–51.
69. Wetmore SJ. Surgical landmarks for the facial nerve. Otolaryngol Clin N Am. 1991;24(3):505–30.
70. Abbas GM, Jones RO. Measurements of drill-induced temperature change in the facial nerve during mastoid surgery: a cadaveric model using diamond burs. Ann Otol Rhinol Laryngol. 2001;110(9):867–70.
71. Hohman MH, Bhama PK, Hadlock TA. Epidemiology of iatrogenic facial nerve injury: a decade of experience. Laryngoscope. 2014;124(1):260–5.
72. Green JD Jr, Shelton C, Brackmann DE. Surgical management of iatrogenic facial nerve injuries. Otolaryngol Head Neck Surg. 1994;111(5):606–10.
73. Green JD Jr, Shelton C, Brackmann DE. Iatrogenic facial nerve injury during otologic surgery. Laryngoscope. 1994;104(8 Pt 1):922–6.
74. Alberti PW. The greater auricular nerve. Donor for facial nerve grafts: a note on its topographical anatomy. Arch Otolaryngol. 1962;76:422–4.
75. Leonetti JP, et al. Intratemporal grafting of the facial nerve following lateral skull base tumor resection. Skull Base. 2007;17(3):181–6.
76. Asma A, et al. Iatrogenic facial nerve palsy: lessons to learn. Singap Med J. 2009;50(12):1154–7.
77. Savic D, Djeric D. Cholesteatoma in the oval window niche. Eur Arch Otorhinolaryngol. 1990;247(2):81–3.
78. Hamilton JW. Efficacy of the KTP laser in the treatment of middle ear cholesteatoma. Otol Neurotol. 2005;26(2):135–9.
79. Lau K, et al. Lasers in cholesteatoma surgery: a systematic review. Ear Nose Throat J. 2021;100(1_suppl):94S–9S.
80. Donaldson JA, et al. The surgical anatomy of the sinus tympani. Arch Otolaryngol. 1970;91(3):219–27.
81. Volgger V, et al. Identification of risk factors for residual cholesteatoma in children and adults: a retrospective study on 110 cases of revision surgery. Braz J Otorhinolaryngol. 2020;86(2):201–8.
82. Leonetti JP, Buckingham RA, Marzo SJ. Retraction cholesteatoma of the sinus tympani. Am J Otol. 1996;17(6):823–6.
83. Ozturan O, et al. Dimensions of the sinus tympani and its surgical access via a retrofacial approach. Ann Otol Rhinol Laryngol. 1996;105(10):776–83.
84. Pulec JL. Sinus tympani: retrofacial approach for the removal of cholesteatomas. Ear Nose Throat J. 1996;75(2):77, 81–3, 86–8.
85. Atlas MD, Moffat DA, Hardy DG. Petrous apex cholesteatoma: diagnostic and treatment dilemmas. Laryngoscope. 1992;102(12 Pt 1):1363–8.
86. Robert Y, et al. Petrous bone extension of middle-ear acquired cholesteatoma. Acta Radiol. 1996;37(2):166–70.
87. Maxwell AK, Muelleman T, Brackmann DE. Congenital cholesteatoma of the sphenoid, occipital, and temporal bones: 54-year follow up. Otol Neurotol. 2020;41(5):e593–6.
88. Pradhan S, et al. Exclusive endoscopic transcanal approach to lateral skull base lesions: institutional experience of 3 cases. J Otol. 2021;16(1):55–60.
89. Moffat D, Jones S, Smith W. Petrous temporal bone cholesteatoma: a new classification and long-term surgical outcomes. Skull Base. 2008;18(2):107–15.
90. Morino T, et al. Management of Intractable Petrous Bone Cholesteatoma with a combined Translabyrinthine-Transsphenoidal approach. Otol Neurotol. 2021;42(3):e311–6.
91. Li KL, et al. Surgical approaches to the petrous apex. World J Otorhinolaryngol Head Neck Surg. 2020;6(2):106–14.
92. Magliulo G, et al. Partial labyrinthectomy in the treatment of labyrinthine fistula: how we do it. Clin Otolaryngol. 2008;33(6):607–10.
93. Vashishth A, et al. Extensive intratemporal cholesteatomas: presentation, complications and surgical outcomes. Eur Arch Otorhinolaryngol. 2015;272(2):289–95.
94. Taplin MA, et al. Transmastoid partial labyrinthectomy for brainstem vascular lesions: clinical outcomes and assessment of postoperative cochleovestibular function. Skull Base. 2006;16(3):133–43.
95. Isaacson B, Kutz JW, Roland PS. Lesions of the petrous apex: diagnosis and management. Otolaryngol Clin N Am. 2007;40(3):479–519. viii
96. Sharma N, et al. Complications of chronic suppurative otitis media and their management: a single institution 12 years experience. Indian J Otolaryngol Head Neck Surg. 2015;67(4):353–60.
97. Osma U, Cureoglu S, Hosoglu S. The complications of chronic otitis media: report of 93 cases. J Laryngol Otol. 2000;114(2):97–100.
98. Chiat H, Kittredge RD. Cholesteatoma of the temporal bone. Radiology. 1958;71(4):559–62.
99. Keseroglu K, et al. Is septal cartilage graft via transmastoid approach safe enough in the repair of large Tegmen defects? ORL J Otorhinolaryngol Relat Spec. 2021;83(2):112–8.
100. Schwarz D, et al. Analysis of the dura involvement in cholesteatoma surgery. Auris Nasus Larynx. 2018;45(1):51–6.
101. Marchioni D, et al. Combined approach for tegmen defects repair in patients with cerebrospinal fluid otorrhea or herniations: our experience. J Neurol Surg B Skull Base. 2014;75(4):279–87.
102. Kari E, Mattox DE. Transtemporal management of temporal bone encephaloceles and CSF leaks: review of 56 consecutive patients. Acta Otolaryngol. 2011;131(4):391–4.
103. Rosito LPS, et al. Cholesteatoma labyrinthine fistula: prevalence and impact. Braz J Otorhinolaryngol. 2019;85(2):222–7.
104. Mafee MF, et al. Large vestibular aqueduct and congenital sensorineural hearing loss. AJNR Am J Neuroradiol. 1992;13(2):805–19.
105. Sagar P, et al. Cholesteatoma induced labyrinthine fistula: is aggressiveness in removing disease justified? Indian J Otolaryngol Head Neck Surg. 2017;69(2):204–9.
106. Lim J, Gangal A, Gluth MB. Surgery for Cholesteatomatous labyrinthine fistula. Ann Otol Rhinol Laryngol. 2017;126(3):205–15.
107. Ikeda R, et al. Risk factors for deterioration of bone conduction hearing in cases of labyrinthine fistula caused by middle ear cholesteatoma. Ann Otol Rhinol Laryngol. 2012;121(3):162–7.
108. Castle JT. Cholesteatoma pearls: practical points and update. Head Neck Pathol. 2018;12(3):419–29.
109. Geerse S, et al. Management of labyrinthine fistula: hearing preservation versus prevention of residual disease. Eur Arch Otorhinolaryngol. 2017;274(10):3605–12.
110. Sanna M, et al. Management of the labyrinthine fistula in cholesteatoma surgery. ORL J Otorhinolaryngol Relat Spec. 1984;46(3):165–72.
111. Viswanatha B, Naseeruddin K. Lateral sinus thrombosis in otology: a review. Mediterr J Hematol Infect Dis. 2010;2(3):e2010027.
112. Raja K, et al. Otogenic lateral sinus thrombosis: a review of fifteen patients and changing trends in the management. Int Arch Otorhinolaryngol. 2018;22(3):208–13.
113. Neilan RE, et al. Pediatric otogenic lateral sinus thrombosis recanalization. Int J Pediatr Otorhinolaryngol. 2011;75(6):850–3.
114. Aguiar de Sousa D, et al. Recanalization in cerebral venous thrombosis. Stroke. 2018;49(8):1828–35.
115. Mather M, Musgrave K, Dawe N. Is anticoagulation beneficial in acute mastoiditis complicated by sigmoid sinus thrombosis? Laryngoscope. 2018;128(11):2435–6.
116. Rosenberg JD, Parikh SR. Anticoagulation therapy as a supplement to recanalization for the treatment of sigmoid sinus thrombosis: a case report. Ear Nose Throat J. 2011;90(9):418–22.

117. Cundiff DK. Anticoagulants for cerebral venous thrombosis: harmful to patients? Stroke. 2014;45(1):298–304.
118. Manolidis S, Kutz JW Jr. Diagnosis and management of lateral sinus thrombosis. Otol Neurotol. 2005;26(5):1045–51.
119. Bradley DT, Hashisaki GT, Mason JC. Otogenic sigmoid sinus thrombosis: what is the role of anticoagulation? Laryngoscope. 2002;112(10):1726–9.
120. Gaillardin L, et al. Residual cholesteatoma: prevalence and location. Follow-up strategy in adults. Eur Ann Otorhinolaryngol Head Neck Dis. 2012;129(3):136–40.
121. Haginomori S, et al. Residual cholesteatoma: incidence and localization in canal wall down tympanoplasty with soft-wall reconstruction. Arch Otolaryngol Head Neck Surg. 2008;134(6):652–7.
122. Barakate M, Bottrill I. Combined approach tympanoplasty for cholesteatoma: impact of middle-ear endoscopy. J Laryngol Otol. 2008;122(2):120–4.
123. Kennedy KL, et al. Postoperative recurrent cholesteatoma in rural versus urban populations. Otol Neurotol. 2021;42(4):e459–63.
124. Britze A, Moller ML, Ovesen T. Incidence, 10-year recidivism rate and prognostic factors for cholesteatoma. J Laryngol Otol. 2017;131(4):319–28.
125. Angeli S, et al. Predicting recidivism for acquired cholesteatoma: evaluation of a current staging system. Otol Neurotol. 2020;41(10):1391–6.
126. Mishiro Y, et al. The investigation of the recurrence rate of cholesteatoma using Kaplan-Meier survival analysis. Otol Neurotol. 2008;29(6):803–6.
127. Neudert M, et al. Cholesteatoma recidivism: comparison of three different surgical techniques. Otol Neurotol. 2014;35(10):1801–8.
128. Keeler JA, Kaylie DM. Cholesteatoma: is a second stage necessary? Laryngoscope. 2016;126(7):1499–500.
129. Henninger B, Kremser C. Diffusion weighted imaging for the detection and evaluation of cholesteatoma. World J Radiol. 2017;9(5):217–22.

Canal Wall Down v/s Canal Wall Up

55

Jorge Caro, Jai-sen F. Leung, and Phoebe H. Ramos

To be, or not to be, that is the question:
Whether 'tis nobler in the mind to suffer
The slings and arrows of outrageous fortune,
Or to take Arms against a Sea of troubles,
And by opposing end them: to die, to sleep;
No more; and by a sleep, to say we end
The heart-ache, and the thousand natural shocks
That Flesh is heir to? 'Tis a consummation
Devoutly to be wished. To die, to sleep,
To sleep, perchance to Dream; aye, there's the rub,
For in that sleep of death, what dreams may come,
When we have shuffled off this mortal coil,
Must give us pause.

A dilemma is a situation in which one must choose between two similarly good or bad options. It is also defined as an argument formed by two contrary propositions, in such a way that, denied or accepted, a conclusion must be stated. This was prince Hamlet's dilemma, described in this article as a difficult question to solve. In medicine, we can find several examples of dilemmas, particularly in otology clinical practice. Mastoidectomy is a surgical procedure used in patients suffering from chronic cholesteatomatous otitis media. There are two types of mastoidectomy, canal wall down (CWD) and canal wall up (CWU). Choosing between performing a CWD versus CWU surgery represents a medical dilemma which scientific and medical evidence must be able to resolve in our current modern times. This dilemma has been extensively discussed in the literature and is still a source of controversy. Different clinical practical guidelines and authors and otologists with vast experience have referred to the subject and most likely will continue to, without reaching clear consensus. Powerful arguments justify choosing performing CWD (wide cavity open to the external canal wall) as well as, other not less powerful arguments justify choosing preforming CWU (closed cavity) especially when considering the presence of cholesteatoma.

The main objective in these cases is the complete eradication of the disease and to prevent recurrence, as well as preserving the greatest amount of healthy mucosa to restore middle ear physiology. In addition to prevent future severe complications depending on the cholesteatoma characteristics, avoid infections, residual presence of cholesteatoma, improve hearing and last but not less important, to achieve a better quality of life [1]. Although this debate is still present in our current clinical practice, there is a marked tendency to perform CWU especially in young patients. In most cases, mastoidectomy surgical technique decision is made by the surgeon, and his or her personal experience and patients characteristics. Intraoperative extension of the disease, mastoid pneumatization, tegmen height, sigmoid sinus prominence, posterior wall external auditory canal (EAC) condition, middle ear mucosa and indemnity of the ossicular chain, and the Eustaquian Tube function are all findings that should be taken into consideration [2, 3]. In Table 55.1, we describe the main advantages and disadvantages that both surgeries present, characteristics which will be described during this chapter.

J. Caro (✉) · J.-s. F. Leung · P. H. Ramos
Pontificia Universidad Católica de Chile, Santiago, Chile
e-mail: jfleung@uc.cl; phramos@uc.cl

M. V. Goycoolea et al. (eds.), *Textbook of Otitis Media*, https://doi.org/10.1007/978-3-031-40949-3_55

Table 55.1 Comparison of advantages and disadvantages of canal wall down and canal wall-up surgical techniques

	CWD	CWU
Advantages	• Great visualization for complete resection of the cholesteatoma • Lower risk of recurrence (2–18%) • Reconstruction during the same procedure • Preferred in patients with difficult follow-up	• Faster healing period • Less chance of infection post-surgery • External auditory canal maintains its normal shape, allowing normal epithelial migration and a preserved self-cleaning mechanism • The most important advantage is the improvement in hearing outcome
Disadvantages	• Delayed healing, chronic otorrhea, accumulation of wax and keratin (which leads to a greater number of bacterial and fungal infections). • Difficulty with the use of hearing aid • The inability to get the operated ear wet • Cosmetic problems • Studies have shown that they present a greater number of complications and more visits to the ENT after surgery	• Higher recurrence than CWD (11–34%) recurrence combines both residual and recurrent disease • Greater recurrence due to increased formation of retraction pockets.

Canal Wall Down (CWD)

CWD surgery or open mastoidectomy (Fig. 55.1) consists in a more aggressive surgery by performing a complete mastoidectomy with resection of the posterior wall of the EAC as well as resection of the lateral portion of the attic, leaving a vast exposed cavity to the ear canal [4, 5]. The classical surgical approach is a post auricular incision approximately 0.5–1 cm posterior to the pinna implantation. This incision must be posterosuperior to the root of the helix, separating skin from muscle. This incision must be wide to expose the beginning of the zygomatic apophysis reaching the tip of the mastoid bone. Then, the muscular incision must expose the mastoid cortex dissecting the periosteum throughout the temporal line to continue to expose the EAC recognizing anatomical landmarks that will guide the mastoidectomy such as Henle spine and the cribriform area. The initial milling over the mastoid cortex must form a triangle. One must mill through the mastoid cortex, exposing mastoid cells identifying the Koerner septum. If one continues milling toward the deepest portion of the mastoid bone, one will find the mastoid antrum that must be identified to avoid injury to the facial nerve. Important anatomical landmarks are the tegmen antri (superior landmark), where pink color can be seen because of small blood vessels in the dura; sigmoid sinus as a posterior landmark can be seen in a blue color. Lateral semicircular canal and the short process of the incus if present must be recognized. Bone covering the Fallopian aqueduct must be identified especially in its tympanic portion and throughout its second turn to be able to lower the facial nerve wall and to obtain a better visualization in postoperative controls. Subsequently, one proceeds to remove the posterior wall of the EAC drilling the tympanosquoamosal suture and the lateral epitypamic wall, as well as the bone bridge that communicates it with the facial nerve's wall. Depending on the magnitude and compromise of the disease some elements in the middle ear can be conserved or removed, if the latter is

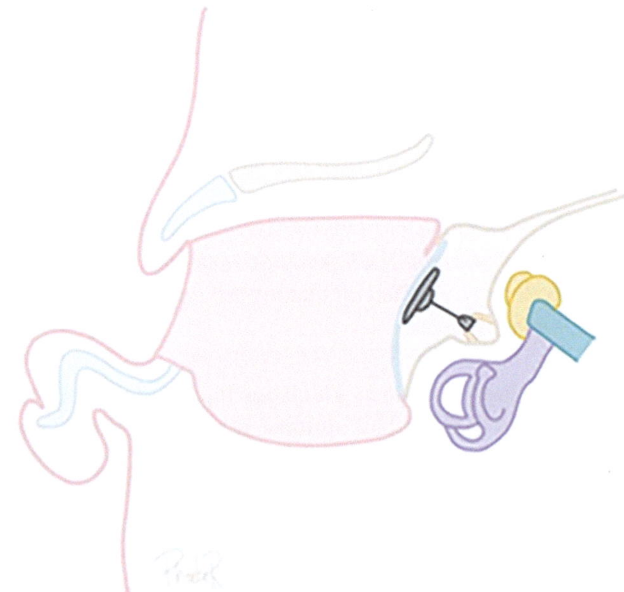

Fig. 55.1 Canal wall-down surgical technique and reconstruction technique with a partial ossicular replacement prosthesis

needed to be done, surgical reconstruction of the ossicles with or without prothesis, tympanic membrane repair with fascia or tragal/auricular cartilage graft must be attempted. Reconstruction of the middle ear must consider the importance of epithelization of the tympanomastoid cavity with skin from the ear canal; therefore, the surgical zone must be covered with some graft. Usually, one uses temporal muscle fascia, and, in cases in which the mastoid cavity is too vast, one could reduce its size using temporal muscle, bone wax, or bone dust from mastoid milling and over this filling, covering it with temporal fascia. It is important to point out that this surgery requires a wide meatoplasty for a better access to the mastoid cavity for postoperative in box procedures. International publications suggest preforming wide meatoplasties because of high rates of scaring and stenosis. Several surgical techniques have been described for meatoplasty. One of the most recognized techniques consist in exposing and resecting the conchal cartilage.

As CWD technique is more aggressive, in most cases, this surgical technique limits auditory reconstruction, it also requires more postoperative visits and constant debriding because of detritus accumulation. As well as worst quality of life due to inability to get the ear wet, intermittent otorrhea, even induced vertigo due to sudden temperature changes (air or water) [6].

Nevertheless, this is considered the most effective technique when it comes to eradication outcomes of cholesteatoma because it allows a better mastoid and middle ear structure visualization, achieving less recurrence and relapse rates, with a higher probability of complete disease eradication [4, 7].

In the literature there have been authors that describe CWD surgery with posterior EAC wall reconstruction associated with mastoid cavity obliteration (using in most cases autologous materials such as fascia or bone wax) [4]. This technique offers better exposition and visualization during the surgery with less recurrence, especially if the epitympanic cavity is obliterated; nevertheless, one must consider that this is a more complex surgery, associated with a greater surgical time, although some authors state that its benefits overpass surgical difficulty [2].

Mastoid Cavity Filling Materials

Over the last period, there has been great development on synthetic filling materials to obliterate the mastoid cavity such as bioactive glass, hydroxyapatite, silicone, and titanium. The mastoid cavity filling can be performed in primary or during revision surgery, as well as in unstable cavities. Bioactive glass is the most used synthetic material to obliterate the mastoid cavity. There are different types, being the most studied and used number S53P4 and 45S5 [8]. S53P4 is called because of its composition (53% SiO_2 and 4% of P_2O_5) it has the advantage that it does not reabsorb until the present of new bone formation. In the same way, 45S5 presents greater reabsorption, being even faster than S53P4. Antibacterial, osteoconductive, and angiogenic associated effects have been described with the use of S53P4, which has led to a more frequent use of this material.

On the other hand, hydroxyapatite ($Ca_{10}(PO_4)_6(OH)_2$) is the second most used material to fill the mastoid cavity, it has a similar composition to bone and is characterized by its great biocompatibility, osteoconductive capacity and chemical bound formation with surrounding tissues [8, 9]. This material can be found in granule forms, cement, or other types of bone implants. Nevertheless, this material has been associated with complications such as infections, osteitis, delayed consolidation, and foreign body reactions. Therefore, some studies suggest that using granules of hydroxyapatite is safer, it allows angiogenesis reducing associated cement complications [10]. Other hydroxyapatite derivatives such as β-tricalcium phosphate with poliphosphate (β-TPP or polibone) have been used in animals with promising results regarding osteoblastic stimulation and successful material integration, although there are not any studies in humans. Silicone use has been widely described in other otologic surgeries, such as ventilation tubes and cochlear implants, being a safe material with low immunogenicity. An advantage of this material is its great flexibility and adaptation capacity to fill the mastoid cavity, as well as its low cost. There has been description of foreign body reactions [11].

Finally, titanium is a synthetic material that has also been used to fill mastoid cavities, proven to be biocompatible and to have great osteointegration within the bone.

Comparing effectiveness of these materials, weighing their possible complications and extrusion rates, S53P4 has shown great results, achieving dry ears up to 96% of the cases [12] with low risks of extrusion (0.5%) [12, 13]. No foreign body reaction has been described, and up to 92% of cases manage to obliterate completely the mastoid cavity or to make it smaller [14]. On the other side, 15% may present with otorrhea, and in 10% of the cases, there has been reports of residual cholesteatoma [15]. Hydroxyapatite presents up to 16% of extrusion risk, requiring in some cases revision surgery if being used in its cement form [10]. With silicone no extrusion cases have been reported, only improvement in 95% of cases of tympanic perforations is associated with possible improvement in auditory capacity [11]. Finally, titanium use, no complications have been reported.

Canal Wall Up (CWU)

CWU surgical technique or closed mastoidectomy consists in performing a complete mastoidectomy (described previously) without compromising the posterior EAC wall (Fig. 55.2). Milling must be thoroughly done throughout the whole mastoid resecting every compromised mastoid cell up to the aditus ad antrum, identifying key anatomical landmarks such as the external canal or lateral wall, short process of the incus (if present). Through the EAC, after performing a wide timpanomeatal flap, the atical region and in occasions the epitympanum must be exposed. While completing the atticoantrotomy complete resection of cholesteatoma must be reassured, checking the atic and its content, with special emphasis in the epytimpanic anterior region and possible projection of the cholesteatoma to the meso and hypotympanum. The main objective is to achieve a clear endocanal and retrograde vision through the mastoidectomy, maintaining the posterosuperior wall of the EAC intact. This brings difficulty in visualizing two critical areas where residual cholesteatoma can be found if not fully explored, one of them is

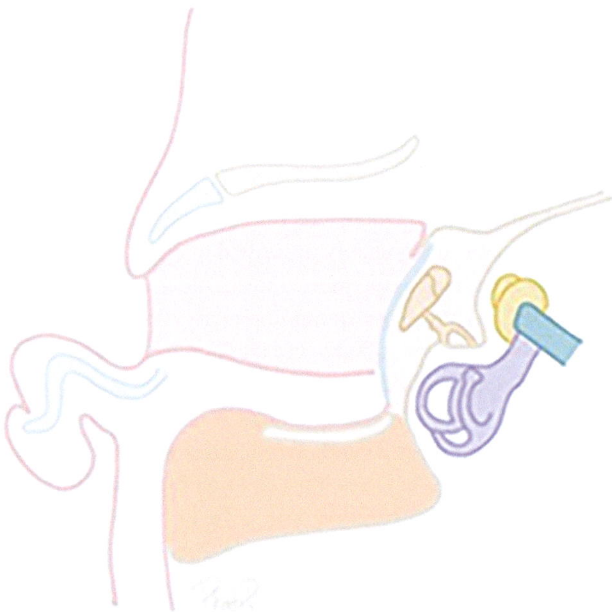

Fig. 55.2 Canal wall-up surgical technique

the sinus tympani and the other one is the facial recess. Therefore, it is important to have previous tomographic study as well as endoscopic image support during surgery. Authors suggest performing a posterior tympanotomy to be able to completely visualize both areas and ensure complete extraction of cholesteatoma. With both surgical techniques, ossicular chain repair must be achieved, and in CWU repair of epitympanic, eventual damages must be fixed.

In CWU technique, the main objective is to maintain the posterosuperior wall of the EAC intact, achieving a less aggressive and destructive surgery, allowing to keep original anatomy, hence achieving better hearing results [6, 7]. The downside of this surgery is that it presents a higher rate of recurrence of disease. Being a close cavity makes it difficult to be able to look for recurrences in postoperative visits [4–7, 16]. Therefore, it is necessary to request diffusion brain magnetic resonance imaging (MRI) or a second look surgery to monitor and determine the presence of recurrent or residual disease [7]. Most frequent recurrence location is the sinus tympani [7]. Other recurrent or residual areas are the anterior portion of the attic and facial nerve recess when not fully explored in the surgical act.

Some studies suggest the use of ear endoscopy [4] associated or not to performing posterior tympanotomy to be able to visualize this zones, reduce recurrence, and/or residual rates [7].

Brain diffusion MRI is the safest radiologic exam to confirm recurrent and/or residual cholesteatoma when physical exam and computerized tomography (CT) are not enough. It is preferred before second look surgery. It has high sensitivity and specificity, as well as a high predictive negative value as a screening method to residual cholesteatoma after CWU surgery. This exam is able to detect the presence of small residual cholesteatoma, selecting patients that are candidate to revision surgery avoiding unnecessary second look surgeries [7].

Karamert et al. [7] performed a 25-month average follow-up of 40 patients who went through CWU surgery (28 patients were also submitted to posterior tympanotomy and 12 without the latter), and 36 patients who went through CWD surgery. Auditive reconstruction was performed in both groups (cartilage graft or titanium prothesis). Achieving auditory success in 75% of patients in CWU group and 47.2% of patients in CWD group [7]. Cholesteatoma recurrence rate was of 8.3% in patients with CWU associated with posterior tympanotomy [7], while 10.7% in patients with CWU alone and 19.4% in patients with CWD [7].

Wilson et al. [2] performed a retrospective study with a total of 148 operated patients with CWU, in most cases, they performed a two-stage surgery (cholesteatoma resection and auditory reconstruction in the revision surgery). Most frequent recurrence localization was the mesotympani, 42% surrounding oval window and/or stapes; 29% sinus tympani; followed by 41% of cases in the epytimpani and mastoid in 24% of the cases [2].

Hanna et al. [17] performed a retrospective study that evaluated patients who presented compromise that extended beyond the mesotympani, who were submitted to minimally invasive surgery. They divided these patients into three groups, transcanal approach, retroauricular approach, and CWU. They point out that recurrence rates with these three surgical minimally invasive techniques are quite similar to those reported in patients with CWD, this is because the use of ear endoscopy reduces the need to perform large mastoidectomies in 35% of the cases without needing to sacrifice disease resection. Reinforcing the need of graft cartilage and ventilation tubes to reduce the possibility of pockets of retraction and disease recurrence [17].

Respecting studies published in the literature, we believe, there is bias associated regarding follow-up of these patients, studies describe different follow-up criteria [5]. Most studies are retrospective; therefore, prospective controlled randomized studies are needed to obtain better conclusions.

Use of Endoscopy in Cholesteatoma Surgery

Endoscopic surgery in pediatric and adult patients has presented important growth in the last years, being widely used worldwide [18, 19]. Closed surgeries such as CWU preserve more anatomy at the expense of increased risk of residual disease and possible need of revision surgery [20, 21]. Nevertheless, multiple studies have demonstrated that performing endoscopic surgery for cholesteatoma or microscopic surgery assisted with endoscopic instruments reduce residual lesions and recurrence rates significatively [22–24]. Reports have described that the use of endoscope as an additional tool has reduced the rate of residual disease from 0 to 10% with the sole use of microscope to 10–43% in CWU surgery [20]. In the same way, the risk of recurrence disease for CWU ranges between 16 and 61%, being significantly reduced using endoscope as a complementary tool to 0–10% [20]. Studies suggest that recurrence may be secondary to constant negative pressure in the tympanic cavity due to Eustaquian tube disfunction and loss of support of the tympanic membrane due to scutum defect. Therefore, reconstruction of a defected scutum is very important in CWU surgery [20].

The use of endoscope provides a better visualization through the camaras by being able to capture difficult angles in areas which are challenging to completely visualize with the sole use of the microscope such as the epytimpanic anterior recess, sinus tympani, and the inferior scutum surface [20, 22, 24, 25]. This is due to the limited straight vision given by the microscope to these areas that can hold residual disease and therefore be one of the main reasons of higher residual cholesteatoma or recurrence of disease in these patients [25].

In this way, it is widely supported in the literature to complement microscopic approach with the use of endoscope in cholesteatoma surgeries, the latter allows to have a wider view of corners of the tympanic and mastoid cavity [26], reducing residual disease and recurrence [27–30], as well as higher possibilities to preserve the ossicular chain, and/or being able to perform a primary ossiculoplasty [29–32]. As well as reducing mucose damage during the surgical procedure [33] is by reducing surgical time and patient postoperative recovery [27, 34]. Nevertheless, this may not be a possibility in every center where this type of disease is managed.

Subtotal Petrosectomy

This is a derivative surgical technique from the total petrosectomy. Subtotal petrosectomy consists in resecting all mastoid cells, middle ear structures, and the aired projections that are compromised in the petrose region. It consists in the resection of the retrosigmoid, retro facial, antral, and retrolabyrinthe, supratubal, and pericarotid cells. The otic capsule may or may not be resected. The EAC must be closed in a blind sac form, and the cavity must be obliterated with fat (abdominal fat is preferred), and finally covering it with a wide temporal muscle flap. Surgical indications for this technique are rare and may be applied in special cases such as chronic otitis media without any chance of hearing recovery, and in patients in whom a failed CWD mastoidectomy was previously performed. Other indications are tumors, osteoradionecrosis tumor treatment complications, cerebrospinal fluid fistula, and in combination with other neuro otologic procedures. Special indication is seen in patients with open cavities that require cochlear implant [35, 36].

Expert Opinion

Fifteen otolaryngology experts, well renowned in otology, were summit from different clinical centers in our country. They were given a 25-question survey on different aspects of this dilemma (Table 55.2). The participating experts have an average of 28.2 years practicing this specialty. Likert scale was used for this evaluation, and answers were grouped in three groups, agree, partially agree, and disagree.

Table 55.2 Survey results on expert otologists' preferences for canal wall down and canal wall up

Questions	Answers				
	1. Strongly disagree	2. Disagree	3. Partially agree	4. Agree	5. Strongly agree
1. When performing a CWU mastoidectomy I usually perform a meatoplasty	60%	33.3%	6.7%		
2. When performing a CWD mastoidectomy, I usually perform a meatoplasty					100%
3. CWU technique needs detritus cleaning on a regular basis	46.7%	53.3%			
4. CWD technique needs detritus cleaning on a regular basis				6.7%	93.3%
5. Lesion recurrence with the CWD technique is low		6.7%	20%	33.3%	40%
6. Lesion recurrence with the CWU technique is higher than with the CWD technique	6.7%	13.3%	6.7%	26.7%	46.7%
7. One of the problems with the CWD technique is the inability to get the operated ear wet		6.7%	26.7%	26.7%	40%
8. After a CWU technique with high suspicion of recurrence after 1 year, you prefer as a first diagnostic alternative:	**Perform diffusion MRI:** 66.7%		**Diffusion MRI or surgery (either):** 13.4%	**Surgery:** 20%	
9. CWU surgery provides a better quality of life than CWD		6.7%	6.7%	26.7%	60%

(continued)

Table 55.2 (continued)

Questions	Answers 1. Strongly disagree	2. Disagree	3. Partially agree	4. Agree	5. Strongly agree
10. CWD surgery requires obliteration of the radical cavity unlike CWU	6.7%	6.7%	53.3%	26.7%	6.7%
11. CWU surgery is more laborious and therefore requires more surgical experience than CWD.		6.7%	13.3%	33.3%	46.7%
12. CWD surgery requires less surgical time than CWU.		6.7%	33.3%	26.7%	33.3%
13. CWU surgery has better hearing outcomes than CWD		6.7%	13.7%	40%	40%
14. In my opinion, the CWU technique makes the use of hearing aids more complicated.	73.3%	20%	6.7%		
15. In my opinion, the CWD technique makes the use of hearing aids more complicated.	13.3%	13.3%	20%	46.7%	6.7%
16. The choice of the technique for radical ear surgery should be made considering the socioeconomic condition of each patient.	13.3%	20%	40%	20%	6.7%
17. CWD is a more aggressive surgical approach when deciding surgical technique		20%	40%	26.7%	13.3%
18. CWU is a more conservative surgical approach when deciding surgical technique	6.7%	20%	40%	13.3%	20%
19. CWD surgery would be preferred in older patients		20%	33.3%	33.3%	13.3%
20. CWU surgery would be preferred in younger patients	6.7%	26.7%	26.7%	26.7%	13.3%
21. CWD surgery requires only the use of a microscope, unlike CWU, where endoscopic vision is also required to rule out the presence of residual disease.		33.3%	26.7%	20%	20%
22. CWD surgery eliminates the functional state of the middle ear mucosa, unlike CWU, which preserves it.		33.3%	20%	33.3%	13.3%
23. Do you agree with the exposed characteristics of each technique?	**Yes:** 60%		**No:** 40%		
24. Finally, which technique do you prefer to use in most cases?	**CWU:** 53.3%		**CWD:** 46.7%		

Surgical Technique

Regarding surgical technique, different surgical characteristics were evaluated such as aggressiveness of the technique, use of microscope and/or endoscope, meatoplasty performance, mastoid cavity obliteration, surgical complexity, middle ear mucosa impact, and total surgical time.

Concerning technical characteristics, taking into consideration that a more aggressive surgical technique is defined as one which main objective is to definitively eradicate the disease, without respecting the anatomy. Although a more conservative surgery aims for the same first objective, it intends to preserve as much of the anatomy as possible. Most experts consider that CWD is a more aggressive technique against a cholesteatoma, while CWU corresponds to the conservative alternative against this disease.

Similarly, the preference in the use of microscope/endoscope in these surgeries was evaluated, noting that most consider that both CWD and CWU techniques require the use of an associated endoscope to be able to rule out the presence of residual disease during surgical procedure. While a not lesser percentage of expert otologists consider performing these surgeries only with the use of a microscope, probably due to the comfort and experience associated with its use. In relation to performing a meatoplasty, all experts agree the need to perform a wide meatoplasty in CWD surgery, to allow a secure post-operative mastoid cavity control. Similarly, the need to perform a meatoplasty in CWU is rejected almost unanimously, since there is no need to expand the visual field within the ear canal as there is no cavity. Additionally, those who are in favor of choosing CWU to the detriment of CWD find that performing a meatoplasty in the latter is fundamental, being a point of advantage in choosing close cavity surgery. Regarding the perception of difficulty between these two surgical techniques, most participants stated that CWU is more laborious and requires more surgical experience. Only one expert states that CWD is more laborious and difficult that CWU.

Considering that CWD technique frees que mucosa of the mastoid and eventually of the tympanic cavity, consideration on the impact on the middle ear mucosa of both surgeries was evaluated. When evaluating the responses of our experts, it is a very controversial issue, since although the majority considers that CWD surgery defunctionalizes the mucosa of the mastoid cavity, there is a not lesser proportion of experts who consider that CWD would not have a worse impact on the mucosa. To the best of our knowledge, there are no recent studies addressing this subject, or that compare this aspect between both surgical techniques. In CWU technique, the idea of a close cavity is that the middle ear mucosa must return to its original placing. In CWD technique, the mastoid cavity is supposed to epithelize with new skin. What does this mean, does this have specific repercussions or how important is this subject, we still do not know.

Finally, comparing total surgical time between both techniques, a wide majority considers that CWD surgery is associated with shorter total surgical time probably due to the greater ease of its technique, unlike CWU which is more laborious. Only one expert considers that CWU would have less total surgical time compared to CWD.

Postoperative Results

One of the most important requirements after surgery and crucial difference between both surgical techniques is the postoperative evaluations. In CWD, the need of frequent postoperative periodic evaluations to achieve a correct cleaning of detritus and evaluate surgical result is a reality, reflected in the unanimous opinion of the experts consulted. CWU frequent postoperative evaluations can be dispensed. However, in the latter, patients are not exempt from spaced postoperative evaluations because of higher risk of residual or recurrent disease.

Most experts agree that disease recurrence in CWD is low. Nevertheless, when comparing both surgical techniques we found greater dispersion in the responses. The great majority affirms that CWU presents higher rates of relapse and/or recurrence than CWD, and a minority states that the rates between both techniques are rather similar.

On the other hand, follow-up post-operative clinical decision regarding relapses and/or recurrences was evaluated. Most experts are inclined to request imaging studies, specifically diffusion brain MRI. A minority proposes performing revision surgery without a prior imaging study, also known as "second look" surgery, and an even smaller percentage of the participants state that both options would be equally valid.

Outcome

In the literature, it is described that CWU technique would have better hearing postoperative results compared to CWD technique [7, 37]. Most of the experts surveyed agree with this affirmation and only a minority disagrees with it. Regarding the use of hearing aids after these surgeries, experts state that CWU technique does not complicate the use of these devices. However, there is greater dispersion when evaluating the use of a hearing aids associated with CWD surgical technique, where half of the surveyed participants agree with the fact that this surgical technique complicates the use of these devices, while the other half states that neither technique affects the ease of wearing hearing aids.

On the other hand, as previously described in this chapter, the literature suggests that CWU surgery provides a better quality of life compared to CWD. When evaluating the opinion of our expert panel on this subject, it is observed that the majority agree that CWU would have a lesser impact on quality of life by reducing restrictions and reducing the need of frequent postoperative evaluations. While only one expert suggests that CWD technique would not have greater impact in quality of life than CWU. Quality of life is associated with both hearing capacity and the possibility of exposing the ear to water, most experts consider that one of the main problems of the CWD surgery is its restriction to submerge under water.

Surgical Indications

Due to the implications of each surgical technique previously exposed in this chapter, one would think that there is a predilection for any of them depending on the type of patient and sociodemographic conditions. However, to our knowledge, there is no data published in the literature to support this position. In this way, we evaluated whether our panel of experts had any preference according to patients age, observing that the majority would be inclined to perform an open technique such as CWD in an elderly patient, if possible, while a minority would seek to perform CWU in these group of patients. In younger patients, most experts would perform CWU surgery, although up to a third of the participants would not agree to perform this technique just because of a younger age.

In the same way, given the need for frequent postoperative check-ups, radiological exams or revision surgeries that mean higher expenses for patients, we sought to assess whether there would be any preference in the surgical technique according to socioeconomic level. Most experts agree that there is flexibility when choosing one surgical technique or another considering the patient socioeconomic level, without detriment to achieving the treatments' main objective, to eradicate disease.

Preference on Surgical Technique

Considering every aspect described previously, preference toward choosing surgical technique is still controversial, this can be verified by analyzing the preferences stated by the experts that participated in this evaluation, were by a low percentage CWU is apparently the preferred technique.

Discussion

The discussion refers especially to the mastoid approach for cholesteatoma, it does not contemplate smaller cholesteatoma located lateral o medial to the attic region. After a thorough analysis of different national and international publications, the dilemma will continue and it will be difficult to reach consensus given the dissimilar experiences and results of different otologist and their centers.

Following our methodology and analysis, regarding surgical technique, we believe that CWD surgery is certainly more aggressive than CWU as it alters ear anatomy to a greater extent with the result of larger cavities and more frequent postoperative care. The growing use of endoscopes in ear surgery improves the visualization of lesions during surgery in both surgical techniques. This has been a significant advance, and it also allows excellent quality audiovisual documentation. In CWD surgery, the performance of a meatoplasty is fundamental, thus we suggest the resection of great part of the conchal cartilage. Frequently in postoperative care of patients with CWD meatoplasties tend to scar and close being insufficient for the mastoid cavity and EAC to self-clean. Both CWD and CWU surgeries are complex, and to be successful one must be very thorough. CWU surgery requires more advanced surgical training, especially in relation to the sinus tympani and the facial nerve recess exploration. The latter can mean more surgical time in CWU surgery. Finally, this last technique preserves the natural state of the mucosa, which would eventually be more suitable for a closed technique.

Considering postoperative care, there are significant differences between both techniques. After the normal immediate postoperative period, CWD surgery will need more frequent controls, in many cases for life, a different situation for CWU surgery. Nevertheless, in nearly every revised bibliography, CWU presents higher recurrence and relapse of cholesteatoma than CWD. Therefore, in these cases, the need of image with diffusion brain MRI and/or surgical revision is crucial. In the last reports, the difference between both surgical techniques has been shortened significantly, probably due to the contribution of optical endoscope.

When analyzing hearing outcomes, CWU technique undoubtedly presents better results than CWD [7, 37]. This is an important point to consider in experts that incline mostly toward CWU especially in younger patients. The same previous considerations refer to the possible use of hearing aids, which is an advantage for the CWU technique. In addition to the considerations already stated, there is no doubt that the quality of life is better in CWU surgery.

Age as a surgical indication between both surgical techniques is also a point of discussion, seeming to be higher preference for choosing CWU in young patients and CWD in older patients. Other consideration in relation to surgical indication refers to the possibility of systematic control considering the patients socioeconomic background and access to specialists, therefore we believe that this is an important point to considerate when indicating these surgeries.

Conclusion

The dilemma of the ideal surgical technique in the management of chronic cholesteatomatose otitis media is no doubt a controversial subject. However, based on the data published in the literature, as well as our experience and preferences reported by the expert otologists of our country, it seems that the balance underlying the CWD and CWU technique would tilt in favor of the latter. Therefore, the authors share the idea that the ideal treatment cannon in modern times should be choosing CWU over CWD when possible, especially in pediatric population and younger patients. Being able, within the surgeons' skills to provide a lesser rate of cholesteatoma recurrence or relapse than what is published for CWD technique. To this end, the authors agree that perfecting surgical technique is fundamental, including the implementation of endoscopic image and instruments during surgery. Despite this, the limitations and requirements of the conservative technique must be considered, such as the need to perform a diffusion brain MRI and/or revision surgery to rule out recurrences or residual lesions. On the other hand, CWD technique must not be seen as an obsolete technique, but rather an alternative that has greater limitations than CWU technique, including aspects from the quality of life of patients to difficulty in corroborating absence of disease in sites that are difficult to access with otomicroscopy such as the mastoid tip. Despite this, CWD is still a very useful technique when CWU cannot be performed safely, such as in cases of little experience of the surgeon, very large and/or extensive middle ear cholesteatomas. Although surgical indications for CWD could be more restricted in current times, it is crucial that at the time of performing these surgeries, an acceptable functional result is achieved together with ensuring complete eradication of the disease and safe control in the future. To this end, reconstruction of the ossicular chain should be performed whenever possible, as well as obliteration of the mastoid tip to facilitate subsequent examination of the cavity.

Finally, for the reasons previously stated and the evolution and focus of the surgical treatment approach toward one that causes less deterioration in quality of life, CWU surgery will be increasingly frequent, requiring training and familiarization of the specialist with this technique to achieve an optimal, safe result, according to the patients need.

References

1. Dutta M. Canal wall up versus canal wall down mastoidectomy: considerations for the new-age otologists. J Int Adv Otol. 2018;14(3):506–8.
2. Wilson KF, Hoggan RN, Shelton C. Tympanoplasty with intact canal wall mastoidectomy for cholesteatoma: long-term surgical outcomes. Otolaryngol Head Neck Surg. 2013;149(2):292–5.
3. Sergi B, Galli J, Battista M, De Corso E, Paludetti G. Dealing with paediatric cholesteatoma: how we changed our management. Acta Otorhinolaryngol Ital. 2014;34(2):138–43.
4. Roux A, Bakhos D, Lescanne E, Cottier J-P, Robier A. Canal wall reconstruction in cholesteatoma surgeries: rate of residual. Eur Arch Otorhinolaryngol. 2015;272(10):2791–7.
5. Kerckhoffs KGP, Kommer MBJ, van Strien THL, Visscher SJA, Bruijnzeel H, Smit AL, et al. The disease recurrence rate after the canal wall up or canal wall down technique in adults. Laryngoscope. 2016;126(4):980–7.
6. Wilkie MD, Chudek D, Webb CJ, Panarese A, Banhegyi G. Canal wall down mastoidectomy with obliteration versus canal wall up mastoidectomy in primary cholesteatoma surgery. J Laryngol Otol. 2019;133(12):1074–8.
7. Karamert R, Eravcı FC, Cebeci S, Düzlü M, Zorlu ME, Gülhan N, et al. Canal wall down versus canal wall up surgeries in the treatment of middle ear cholesteatoma. Turk J Med Sci. 2019;49(5):1426–32.
8. Della Santina CC, Lee SC. Ceravital reconstruction of canal wall down mastoidectomy: long-term results. Arch Otolaryngol Head Neck Surg. 2006;132(6):617–23.
9. Hydroxyapatite granules for mastoid cavity obliteration: a study of 25 cases. Internet J Otorhinolaryngol. 2005;3. https://doi.org/10.5580/2727.
10. Ridenour JS, Poe DS, Roberson DW. Complications with hydroxyapatite cement in mastoid cavity obliteration. Otolaryngol Head Neck Surg. 2008;139(5):641–5.
11. Cho SW, Cho Y-B, Cho H-H. Mastoid obliteration with silicone blocks after canal wall down mastoidectomy. Clin Exp Otorhinolaryngol. 2012;5(1):23–7.
12. Silvola JT. Mastoidectomy cavity obliteration with bioactive glass. Otolaryngol Head Neck Surg. 2012;147:119–26. https://doi.org/10.1177/0194599812438168.
13. Sorour S, Sorour SS, Mohamed NN, Abdel Fattah MM, Elbary ME-SA, El-Anwar MW. Bioglass reconstruction of posterior meatal wall after canal wall down mastoidectomy. Am J Otolaryngol. 2018;39:282–5. https://doi.org/10.1016/j.amjoto.2018.03.007.
14. Stoor P, Pulkkinen J, Grénman R. Bioactive glass S53P4 in the filling of cavities in the mastoid cell area in surgery for chronic otitis media. Ann Otol Rhinol Laryngol. 2010;119:377–82. https://doi.org/10.1177/000348941011900603.
15. Ezzat AEM, Eid MI. Evaluation of using bioglass in obliteration of mastoid cavity. Curr Sci Int. 2014;3(2):87–94.
16. de Azevedo AF, de Soares AB, Garchet HQC, de Sousa NJA. Tympanomastoidectomy: comparison between canal wall-down and canal wall-up techniques in surgery for chronic otitis media. Int Arch Otorhinolaryngol. 2013;17(3):242–5.
17. Hanna BM, Kivekäs I, Wu Y-H, Guo LJ, Lin H, Guidi J, et al. Minimally invasive functional approach for cholesteatoma surgery. Laryngoscope. 2014;124(10):2386–92.
18. Glikson E, Feinmesser G, Sagiv D, Wolf M, Migirov L, Shapira Y. Trans-canal endoscopic ear surgery and canal wall-up tympanomastoidectomy for pediatric middle ear cholesteatoma. Eur Arch Otorhinolaryngol. 2019;276(11):3021–6.
19. Kapadiya M, Tarabichi M. An overview of endoscopic ear surgery in 2018. Laryngoscope Investig Otolaryngol. 2019;4(3):365–73.
20. Wu N, Zuo W, Wang F, Hou K, Yang S, Hou Z. Scutum reconstruction technique and classification in endoscopic middle ear cholesteatoma surgery. Acta Otolaryngol. 2020;140(11):904–8.
21. Chiao W, Chieffe D, Fina M. Endoscopic Management of Primary Acquired Cholesteatoma. Otolaryngol Clin N Am. 2021;54(1):129–45.
22. Li B, Zhou L, Wang M, Wang Y, Zou J. Endoscopic versus microscopic surgery for treatment of middle ear cholesteatoma: a systematic review and meta-analysis. Am J Otolaryngol. 2021;42(2):102451.
23. Dixon PR, James AL. Evaluation of residual disease following transcanal totally endoscopic vs postauricular surgery among children with middle ear and attic cholesteatoma. JAMA Otolaryngol Head Neck Surg. 2020;146(5):408–13.
24. Pollak N. Endoscopic and minimally-invasive ear surgery: a path to better outcomes. World J Otorhinolaryngol Head Neck Surg. 2017;3(3):129–35.
25. Bennett M, Wanna G, Francis D, Murfee J, O'Connell B, Haynes D. Clinical and cost utility of an intraoperative endoscopic second look in cholesteatoma surgery. Laryngoscope. 2018;128(12):2867–71.
26. Tarabichi M, Nogueira JF, Marchioni D, Presutti L, Pothier DD, Ayache S. Transcanal endoscopic management of cholesteatoma. Otolaryngol Clin N Am. 2013;46(2):107–30.
27. Bae MR, Kang WS, Chung JW. Comparison of the clinical results of attic cholesteatoma treatment: endoscopic versus microscopic ear surgery. Clin Exp Otorhinolaryngol. 2019;12(2):156–62.
28. Glikson E, Yousovich R, Mansour J, Wolf M, Migirov L, Shapira Y. Transcanal endoscopic ear surgery for middle ear cholesteatoma. Otol Neurotol. 2017;38(5):e41–5.
29. Marchioni D, Mattioli F, Alicandri-Ciufelli M, Presutti L. Endoscopic approach to tensor fold in patients with attic cholesteatoma. Acta Otolaryngol. 2009;129(9):946–54.
30. Imai T, Nishiike S, Oshima K, Tanaka H, Tsuruta Y, Tomiyama Y. The resected area of the posterior wall of the external auditory canal during transcanal endoscopic ear surgery for cholesteatoma. Auris Nasus Larynx. 2017;44(2):141–6.
31. Tarabichi M. Endoscopic management of limited attic cholesteatoma. Laryngoscope. 2004;114:1157–62. https://doi.org/10.1097/00005537-200407000-00005.
32. Marchioni D, Villari D, Mattioli F, Alicandri-Ciufelli M, Piccinini A, Presutti L. Endoscopic management of attic cholesteatoma: a single-institution experience. Otolaryngol Clin N Am. 2013;46(2):201–9.
33. Presutti L, Anschuetz L, Rubini A, Ruberto M, Alicandri-Ciufelli M, Dematte M, et al. The impact of the Transcanal endoscopic approach and mastoid preservation on recurrence of primary acquired attic cholesteatoma. Otol Neurotol. 2018;39(4):445–50.
34. Magliulo G, Iannella G. Endoscopic versus microscopic approach in attic cholesteatoma surgery. Am J Otolaryngol. 2018;39:25–30. https://doi.org/10.1016/j.amjoto.2017.10.003.
35. Fisch U, Mattox DE. Microsurgery of the skull base. Thieme; 1988.
36. Linder T, Schlegel C, DeMin N, van der Westhuizen S. Active middle ear implants in patients undergoing subtotal petrosectomy. Otol Neurotol. 2009;30:41–7. https://doi.org/10.1097/mao.0b013e31818be812.
37. Şevik Eliçora S, Erdem D, Dinç AE, Damar M, Bişkin S. The effects of surgery type and different ossiculoplasty materials on the hearing results in cholesteatoma surgery. Eur Arch Otorhinolaryngol. 2017;274(2):773–80.

Simple Mastoidectomy: Indications and Techniques

56

Jefferson André Bauer and Felipe da Costa Huve

Simple Mastoidectomy

Simple mastoidectomy comprises total exenteration of the mastoid cell system, without interfering with the middle ear content and preserving the posterior wall of the external auditory canal.

The idea for this procedure was born from the need for a *life-saving procedure* in cases of severe complications from inflammatory processes of the temporal bone. The first description of draining a mastoid abscess is by the French physician Ambroise Paré, who performed the procedure on King François II of France in 1560. His mother, Catherine de Medici, did not authorize him to undergo surgery. The young monarch died shortly afterward [1].

In 1671, Johannes Riolanus, an anatomist at the University of Paris, indicated the procedure in cases where the benefit outweighed the harm, which was very high until then. Over the years, at the end of the nineteenth century, still in the pre-antibiotic era, this surgery already enjoyed general acceptance and was proclaimed as an unsurpassable measure in saving lives [2].

In 1873, Schwartze and Eysell published the first article describing and systematizing the procedure of mastoidectomy. In the twentieth century, with the advent of penicillin, the number of inflammatory complications of the temporal bone declined sharply. Nevertheless, there is a need for otorhinolaryngologists to master the technique of this procedure, which, in addition to saving lives and mitigating complications, has expanded its indications [3].

Years of experience in accessing the auditory cleft through mastoidectomy have made it possible for this procedure to represent an alternative access to other surgeries. The main indications for simple mastoidectomy are

- Surgical treatment of coalescent mastoiditis (Fig. 56.1)
- Exposure of the endolymphatic sac (decompression)
- Access to trans-labyrinthine and peri-labyrinthine procedures
- Access for performing a posterior tympanotomy (cochlear implant)

However, considering that simple mastoidectomy does not allow exploring the middle ear and the attic-antral region, it is not indicated for the surgical treatment of chronic otitis media, given that the pathophysiology of this disease necessarily involves the mesotympanum and/or epitympanum.

Surgical Technique

Before starting surgery, it is necessary to check the conditions of the operating room and the availability of adequate material, which includes:

- Comfortable, stable chair positioned at a distance from the surgical field where the surgeon's arm can rest safely
- Surgical table that allows rotation in the lateral axis and with space for the surgeon's legs below the headboard
- Surgeon arm support
- Surgical drill and high-speed motor
- Microscope with extra auxiliary output—always check its operation
- Drill irrigation system (coupled or via syringe)
- Specific surgical material and in adequate conditions

The preoperative study of tomographic and/or magnetic resonance images is essential, in order to facilitate the location of anatomical landmarks, better surgical control of the

J. A. Bauer · F. da Costa Huve (✉)
Hospital de Clinicas de Porto Alegre, Porto Alegre, Brazil

Hospital Mãe de Deus, Porto Alegre, Brazil

Universidade Federal do Rio Grande do Sul, Porto Alegre, Brazil

Instituto Gaúcho de Otorrinolaringologia, Porto Alegre, Brazil

M. V. Goycoolea et al. (eds.), *Textbook of Otitis Media*, https://doi.org/10.1007/978-3-031-40949-3_56

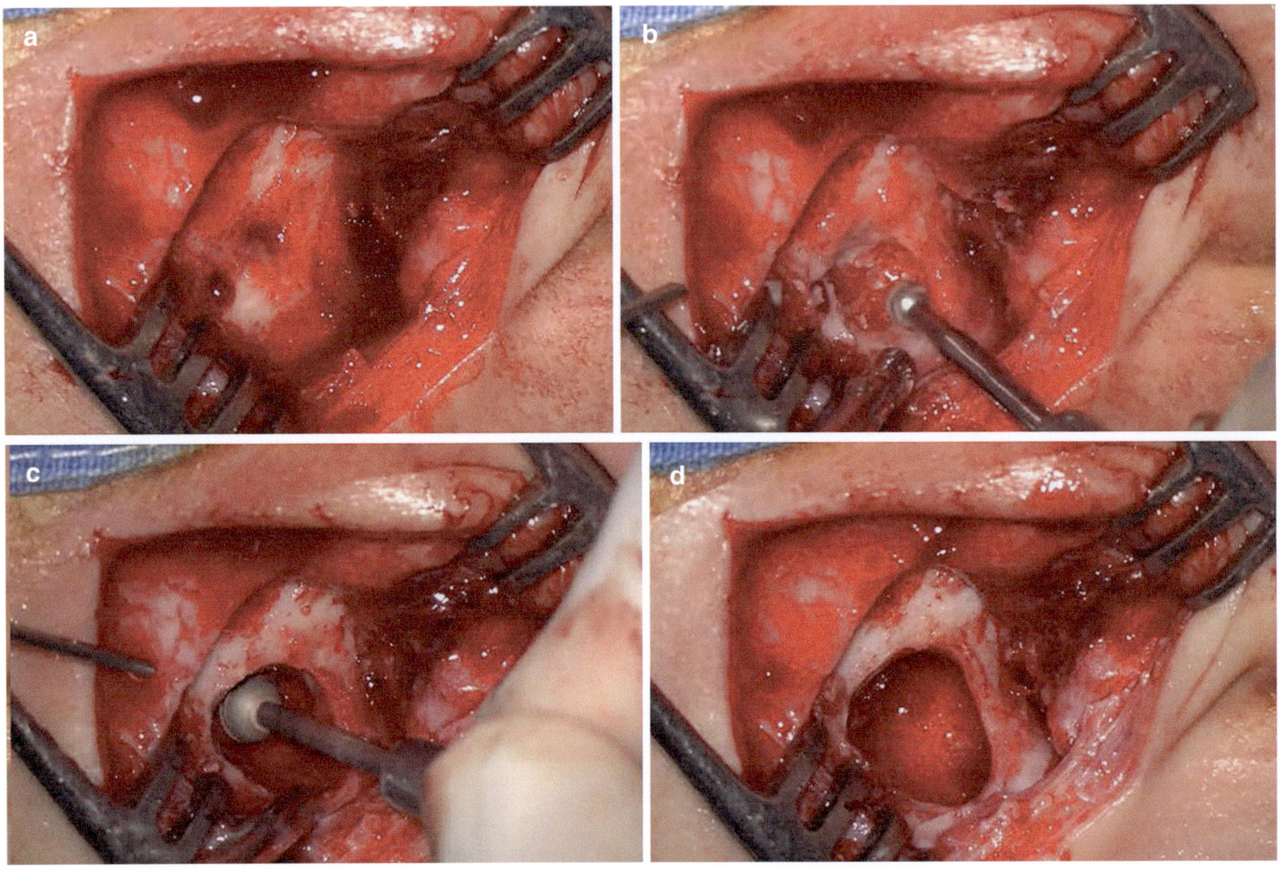

Fig. 56.1 Acute mastoiditis in the right ear of a 1-year-old child; (**a**) exposition of the mastoid cortical bone (with active suppuration); (**b**) removal of superficial mastoid cells; (**c**) removal of deep mastoid cells; (**d**) final aspect of the simple mastoidectomy

disease, and reduce the risk of complications. These exams should be available in the operating room during the procedure [4, 5].

Preparation and Positioning

Simple mastoidectomy is performed with the patient in the supine position on the operating table, with the head elevated at 20° and rotated 45–60° in the opposite direction to the operated side. Excessive rotation should be avoided, especially in older patients or those with reduced cervical mobility. When a greater rotation of the head is necessary, this must be done using the rotation system of the lateral axis of the stretcher. The head must rest in this position without the aid of fixation, and an occipital band may be used. The 20–30° inclination of the head of the table in the horizontal axis facilitates venous return and contributes to hemostasis of the surgical field.

After intubation and monitoring of the patient, all anesthetic equipment and monitors should be positioned below the patient's waistline, thus allowing the patient's cephalic and thoracic space to have free access for the surgical team.

Trichotomy of the hair close to the ear is performed, up to three centimeters above and behind the pavilion, sparing the region of the whiskers. A cap is then made to remove the hair and isolate the surgical field. This can be done with micropore and adhesive tape, wrapping the entire head or simply around the shaved area.

After hand antisepsis and gowning, the surgical field is antisepsis with non-ototoxic substances, such as aqueous iodine. Local infiltration is performed with a topical anesthetic solution and adrenaline (1:1,000,000), waiting 5 min until the incision is made for it to take effect. Infiltration can also occur during patient preparation, after intubation.

The surgeon must position himself in front of the ear to be operated on, with the assistant on the patient's head. The auxiliary microscope display must always be positioned on the contralateral side to the operated ear, so that the auxiliary surgeon can use it when sitting at the head of the ear. The scrub nurse is positioned opposite the surgeon, on the side of the contralateral ear. The microscope base is behind the assistant, continuous with the headboard [4, 7].

Surgical Technique

The reference points used in performing simple mastoidectomy are those corresponding to levels I, II, III, V, and VI (see Chap. 19).

Levels I and II of the dissection correspond to the retroauricular access, also specified in Chap. 19. As it is a closed mastoidectomy technique, the simple mastoidectomy flap is pedicled posteriorly. This facilitates that at the end of the surgery it is sutured in its original position and allows the closure to take place in two planes—periosteal and cutaneous. In this way, the risk of skin retractions and unfavorable esthetic-functional results is reduced.

Removal of mastoid cells has the final objective of identifying the mastoid antrum (anterior-superiorly), the tympanic tegmen (cranially), and the sigmoid sinus (posteriorly), with a complete exposure of the anatomical landmarks and removal of the disease, when necessary case. Safety in dissection with a drill will be achieved by the stability of the surgeon's hand, which must remain supported and with a "pen" grip [6].

The cut is always made by the side of the drill and not by its tip. Thus, the drilling must proceed parallel to the anatomical landmarks. The largest possible drill bit is always used, thus reducing the risk of injury to the structures and the formation of small recesses. The drill is always used at maximum speed (50–60 k rotations/min) to maintain dissection stability. Exceptions are made for dissection close to areas of potential acoustic trauma, such as the inner ear.

The importance of constant drill irrigation is highlighted, reducing the risk of thermal injury to structures (especially the facial nerve) and bone necrosis. Irrigation also acts by removing bone debris, thus improving the exposure of the surgical field.

Whenever possible, the drill is used in side-to-side movements (preferably from right to left) and *inside-out*, that is, with the tip of the drill starting the dissection from the most medial to the most lateral position. The tip of the drill must always be visible in these movements. The efficiency of the dissection depends on the time the drill will be in contact with the area to be removed, so one should avoid quickly manipulating it from one point to another.

The amplitude of movements must also be controlled: the deeper we are in the dissection, the greater the proximity and delicacy of the structures, requiring increasingly shorter movements. The drill must never be pressed excessively against the bone, and it is desirable to reduce the pressure exerted during the dissection of noble structures [4, 7].

In simple mastoidectomy, detachment of the tympanomeatal flap and exploration of the middle ear are not performed (thus, level IV anatomical landmarks are excluded). The first step after retroauricular access is exposure of the cribriform area and removal of the soft tissues. The region of the zygomatic process of the temporal must be adequately exposed using a retractor in an anterior direction. This movement facilitates identification of McEwen's triangle and Henle's spine [8].

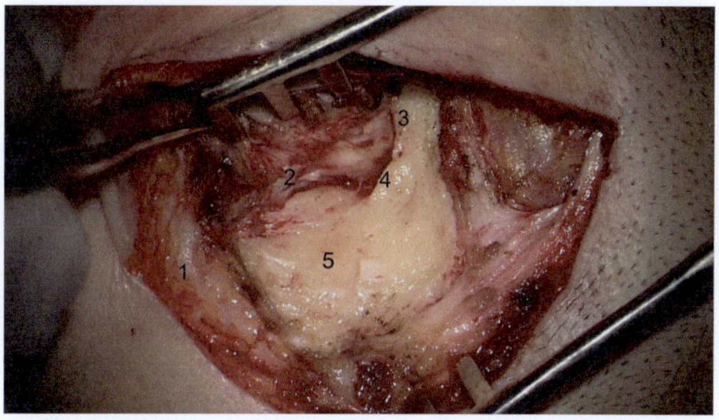

Fig. 56.2 Surgical access image in the left ear: mastoid process (1), EAC (2), zygomatic process (3), spine of Henle (4), and cribriform area (5)

Next, the retractors are positioned, identifying the anatomical references of level III (Fig. 56.2):

- posterior wall and skin of EAC
- Temporal line
- Henle's spine
- cribriform area and MacEwen's triangle
- mastoid process

The removal of the cortical bone must be done in a wide way, never in a funnel, with the intention of obtaining the best possible exposure of the anatomical landmarks. Remember: the more light that enters your surgical field, the better your visualization will be. Thus, at the beginning of the mastoidectomy, cutting burs are used [9].

Drilling of the mastoid cortex begins in the cribriform area, having as limits the temporal lines (superiorly), the posterior wall of the EAC (anteriorly) and by an imaginary line corresponding to the sigmoid sinus (posteriorly). These three lines form the so-called "attack triangle". The less pneumatized the mastoid, the more important the definition of the attack triangle.

Removal of the mastoid cortical bone begins along the temporal line, which is an approximate marker of the height of the tegmen tympani and, consequently, of the middle cerebral fossa. When close to the dura mater, a change in tissue color is observed, from the pearly white of the bone to a salmon pink. Also, the sound generated by the drilling starts to have a more acute tone, easily perceptible to the most trained ears. Also, there is a greater amount of bleeding, due to the dura mater being much more vascularized than the bone cells of the mastoid. Therefore, these three signs must be constantly evaluated when dissecting the tegmen. Its height, its variations and possible dehiscence must be evaluated in preoperative imaging exams.

Drilling the posterior wall of the EAC must maintain a constant bone thickness throughout the entire dissection up to the antrum, and with minimal support so that it does not fracture. In the tympanomastoidectomies, when canaloplasty is necessary, this must be done before mastoid drilling, so that the external conduit has its final shape at the beginning of the mastoidectomy.

The mastoid antrum, an area of fundamental interest for the mastoidectomy, will be found in a medial (deep) point to the perpendicular crossing of the superior and posterior lines of the EAC.

Subsequently, the sigmoid sinus will be identified after removal of presigmoid cells, paying attention to its position as assessed on CT. After the complete drilling of the superficial mastoid cells, we then identified the anatomical landmarks of level V (Fig. 56.3):

- posterior wall of EAC and root of zygoma
- tympanic tegmen and middle fossa dura mater
- sigmoid sinus
- sinodural or Citelli angle
- Koerner septum
- mastoid process

The triangular dissection now follows the same landmarks in its deep (medial) projection: cranially, the dura mater of the middle fossa in the tegmen, extending anteriorly to the root of the zygoma; the EAC anteriorly; the sigmoid sinus and the bony walls of the mastoid posteroinferiorly. The medial boundary of the level V dissection is Koerner's septum, also known as the petrosquamous lamina or false antrum.

Koerner's septum is best identified in well-pneumatized mastoids, and can be easily confused with the lateral canal or the mastoid antrum. When in doubt, the surgeon can be guided by other anatomical landmarks and use a curette to dissect the septum. Once removed, the deep mastoid cells appear medially to it, showing the next level of dissection.

The last step of simple mastoidectomy is level VI dissection (Fig. 56.4):

- posterior wall of EAC
- tympanic tegmen and middle fossa dura mater
- sigmoid sinus
- Sinodural or Citelli's angle
- mastoid antrum
- lateral and posterior semicircular canals
- digastric ridge

Medially to Koerner's septal lamina, we removed the remaining mastoid cells until we found the aditus ad antrum and the mastoid antrum, the angle of Citelli (between the

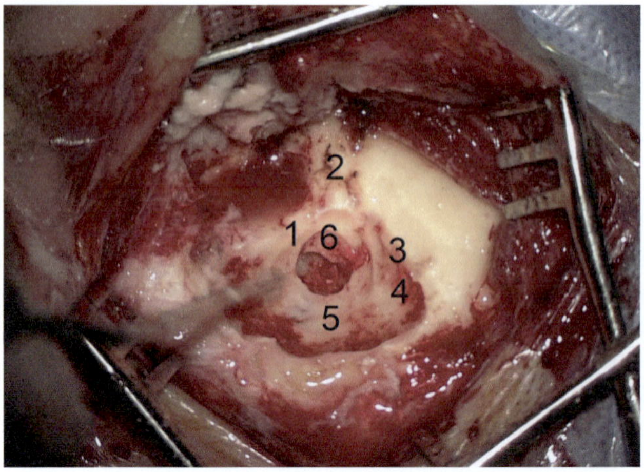

Fig. 56.3 Left ear, level V. EAC (1), root of zygoma (2), tegmen tympani (3), sinodural angle (4), sigmoid sinus (after partial removal of mastoid cells) (5), and partially opened Koerner's septum (6)

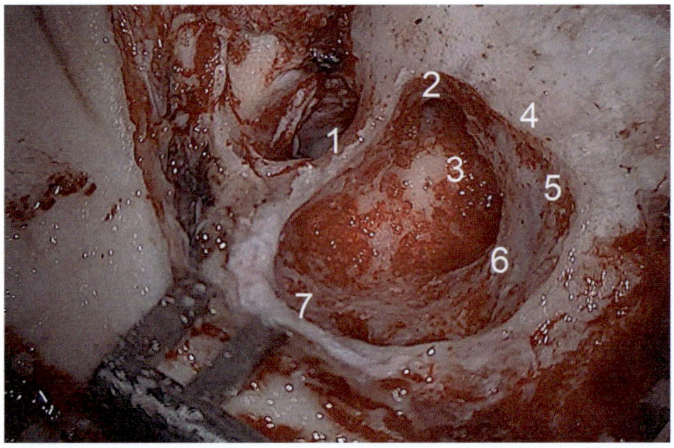

Fig. 56.4 Left ear, level VI. EAC (1), mastoid antrum (2), lateral semicircular canal (3), tympanic tegmen (4), sinodural or Citelli's angle (5), sigmoid sinus (6), digastric ridge (7)

dura of the middle fossa and the sigmoid sinus) and the lateral semicircular canal, the final medial limit of the simple mastoidectomy.

It is also possible to identify other structures at this level, depending on the surgery to be performed: the posterior semicircular canal, the endolymphatic sac in Trautmann's Triangle, the incudal fossa and the short process of the incus and the digastric groove at the tip of the mastoid. Trautmann's triangle is the region between the posterior semicircular canal, the tympanic tegmen and the sigmoid sinus, serving as a reference for accessing the endolymphatic sac.

The mastoid antrum is perhaps the main point of interest in this step, since it connects the two cavities of the auditory cleft (middle ear and mastoid). It is often blocked by inflammatory processes and injuries and should be treated with care due to its physiopathogenic importance. The antrum is the largest and most constant mastoid cell, present even in sclerotic mastoids. In these cases, the safest route to the antrum is dissection based on the position of the tegmen and the posterior wall of the EAC, deep to the antrum, and from there to the other anatomical landmarks.

Medially to the antrum, it is possible to verify that the bone of the labyrinthine block has a much higher density than the bone of the cells. This serves as a guide for anterior and posterior dissections and for identifying the lateral and posterior semicircular canals. The lateral canal forms part of the bottom of the antrum and serves as a reference for identifying the tympanic segment of the facial nerve, immediately inferior to it.

Drilling is continued anteriorly to the antrum and at a height that is already posterosuperior to the EAC, with a delicate or diamond cutting bur, always in a direction parallel to the tegmen and the zygomatic process, superiorly, and respecting the circumference of the EAC, inferiorly. This process is called "anterior tympanotomy."

The incudal fossa is then identified, where the body of the incus and its short branch are located. Sometimes, it may be necessary to rotate the patient on the stretcher (in the opposite direction to that of the surgeon). Again, the use of a curette can help remove small bone fragments and ensure safe dissection close to the ossicular chain.

One can test the permeability of the antrum by irrigating saline toward the middle ear. If the liquid passes easily, we can infer that ventilation of the mastoid will be guaranteed in the postoperative period, reducing the risk of recurrence of inflammatory diseases. If communication is still impaired, the anterior tympanotomy should be expanded. It is also recommended to clean the antrum and the incudal fossa through blunt dissection with a small piece of cotton, gently pushed anteriorly to remove any adhesions and tissue remains (Fig. 56.5).

Once the mastoid antrum and the structures related to it have been identified, the dissection proceeds posteriorly and inferiorly: the sigmoid sinus and the sinusoidal angle are dissected and the last cells are removed. Inferiorly, the digastric groove is identified at the tip of the mastoid process, corresponding to the external insertion of the digastric muscle.

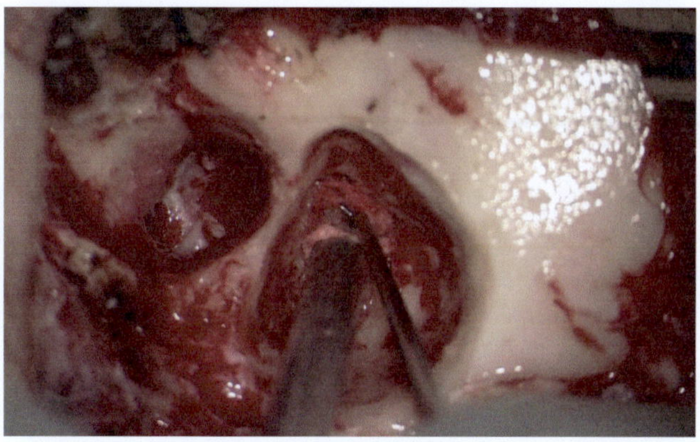

Fig. 56.5 Left mastoidectomy, removal of tissue remains in the additus-antrum using cotton and blunt instruments

The last cells to be removed should be the retrofacial ones. With the other landmarks already under control, the cells close to the mastoid segment of the facial nerve are then removed in the posteroinferior portion of the EAC. The nerve must never be exposed.

After removing most of the cells, the cutting bur is replaced by a diamond bur (as an option, the cutting bur can be used in reverse mode). Due to its ability to "sand" the bone and its consequent lower destructive potential, the diamond bur is useful in defining the edges of the cavity and in the dissection close to noble structures.

The more completely the cells and their mucosa are removed, the less the chance of residual disease and the less granulation process in the postoperative period, guaranteeing a recovery free of recurrence and with fewer complications. Residual inflammatory tissue can increase exudation and facilitate secondary infections, as well as hinder the incorporation of eventual grafts (which, in the case of simple mastoidectomy, are normally not necessary) [4, 10–12].

References

1. Bento RF, Fonseca AC d O. A brief history of mastoidectomy. International. Arch Otorhinolaryngol. 2013;17(2):168–78.
2. Cruz OLM, da Costa SS. Otologia clinica e cirúrgica. Chapter 15. Rio de Janeiro: Revinter; 2000. p. 472.
3. Schwartze HH, Eysell CG. Uber die Kunstliche Eröffnung des Warzenfortsatzes. Arch Ohrenh. 1983;7:157–62.
4. Fisch U. Tympanoplasty, mastoidectomy and stapes surgery. 2nd ed; 2008.
5. Bennett M, Warren F, Haynes D. Indications and technique in mastoidectomy. Otolaryngol Clin N Am. 2006;39(6):1095–113.
6. Singh A, Thakur R, Kumar R, Verma H, Irugu DVK. Grading of the position of the mastoid tegmen in human temporal bones—a surgeon's perspective. J Int Adv Otol. 2020;16(1):63–6.
7. Arnoldner C, et al. Manual of otologic surgery. 2015.
8. Goycoolea MV. Mastoid and tympanomastoid procedures in otitis media: classic mastoidectomy (simple, modified, and radical) and current adaptations; open-cavity, closed-cavity, and intact-bridge tympanomastoidectomy. Otolaryngol Clin N Am. 1999;32(3):513–23.
9. Piromchai P, Wijewickrema S, Smeds H, Kennedy G, O'Leary S. Correlations of external landmarks with internal structures of the temporal bone. Otol Neurotol. 2015;36(8):1366–73.
10. Ozaki A, Haginomori SI, Ayani Y, Ichihara T, Inui T, Jin-Nin T, Inaka Y, Kawata R. Facial nerve course in the temporal bone: anatomical relationship between the tympanic and mastoid portions for safe ear surgery. Auris Nasus Larynx. 2020;47(5):800–6.
11. Nadol JB Jr. Revision mastoidectomy. Otolaryngol Clin N Am. 2006;39(4):723–40, vi–vii.
12. Luers JC, Hüttenbrink KB. Surgical anatomy and pathology of the middle ear. J Anat. 2016;228(2):338–53.

Canal Wall Up Tympanomastoidectomy

57

Alex Joseph Fejta Tampio and Douglas Backous

Middle Ear and Mastoid Physiology

Gas and fluid exchange in the middle ear mucosa is similar to the process seen in lung alveoli [1]. The mucosa in the anterior-inferior middle ear is similar to respiratory epithelium. Posteriorly and superiorly the mucosa transitions to cuboidal epithelium toward the mastoid antrum where the majority of the gas exchange occurs in the middle ear [2]. Healthy mucosa absorbs oxygen and nitrogen at the same rate that carbon dioxide is expelled. With inflammation, the vascularity to the middle ear and mastoid mucosa increases and results in oxygen and nitrogen being more rapidly than carbon dioxide is diffused which resulting in a negative pressure [1]. A well functioning eustachian tube resets the middle ear to ambient atmospheric pressure. Without the pressure resetting function of the Eustachian tube, inflammation in the middle ear and mastoid can generate negative pressure resulting in tympanic membrane retraction, cholesteatoma formation, serous effusion or perforation. Boyle's law states that at a constant temperature, pressure multiped by volume equals a constant. Pressure and volume are inversely related [1]. Mastoid volume that acts as a buffer against pressure changes in the ear. A poorly developed mastoid houses a smaller volume and is less resistant to pressure changes, which may explain the trend where patients with sclerotic or poor mastoid development represent a large proportion of patients who suffer from chronic ear disease [3].

A. J. F. Tampio · D. Backous (✉)
Department of Neurotology, Proliance Surgeons, Puget Sound ENT, Edmonds, WA, USA
e-mail: A.Tampio@proliancesurgeons.com; D.Backous@proliancesurgeons.com

Indications for Canal Wall Up Tympanomastoidectomy

Chronic Otitis Media Without Cholesteatoma

The etiology of chronic otitis media is multifactorial with an association in patients with poor middle ear aeration, poor mastoid pneumatization and chronic middle ear and mastoid inflammation. In a cohort of 72 patients, Sade reported secretory otitis media occurred in roughly 52% of patients with poorly pneumatized mastoid cavities compared to 20% of those with well-aerated mastoid spaces. Tympanic membrane atelectasis occurred in 37.3% of patients of with poor mastoid aeration vs. 5.7% in those ho were well-aerated [3]. Though chronic inflammation is one important factor in the pathogenesis of chronic otitis media without cholesteatoma, the source of inflammation is not well understood. There are many hypotheses regarding the etiology of chronic inflammation that include an acute infection developing into a chronic infection, a chronic infection via a tympanic membrane perforation and perhaps patient factors that allow chronic inflammation (i.e. immunological pathology, smoking, untreated acute and chronic otitis media). Overall, the definition of chronic otitis media is chronic and irreversible changes in the mucosa of the middle ear cleft [4].

Chronic inflammation can affect the middle ear and mastoid by impeding the function of the Eustachian tube. Hadas et al. reported the impaired mucocilliary clearance of non-soluble saccharin through the Eustachian tube in patients with chronic otitis media that was worse in patients with wet/draining ears and those with atelectasis when compared to patients wit normal ear function [5]. Granulation tissue in the aditus ad antrum can prevent communication between the middle ear and mastoid impeding gas exchange. Proctor described two anatomic pathways from the middle ear to the antrum: the first is between the tensor tympani tendon and the stapes, and the second between the short process of the incus and the stapedius muscle [6]. Blockage to the antrum functionally decreases the volume of the middle ear by cut-

M. V. Goycoolea et al. (eds.), *Textbook of Otitis Media*, https://doi.org/10.1007/978-3-031-40949-3_57

ting access to the mastoid, making the middle ear less resistant to changes in pressure and more susceptible to retraction and atelectasis. In our practice, we have a low threshold for mastoidectomy for the purposes of removing an attic block that is commonly found in patients with chronic otitis media without cholesteatoma. Indications to strongly consider a mastoidectomy are chronic or frequent otorrhea, middle ear inflammation, failed tympanoplasty, and evidence of opacified mastoid air cells on imaging.

Atelectasis

Atelectasis is defined as severe tympanic membrane retraction as the result of a reduced or absent collagenous layer within the tympanic membrane. A normal pars tensa has three layers: an outer epidermal layer, a middle collagenous layer, and an internal mucosal layer. A normal pars flaccida has only two, as it lacks the middle collagenous layer. Patients with atelectatic tympanic membranes have a attenuated or absent fibrous layer, which results in increased susceptibility to retraction of the pars tensa. Sade and collogues categorized four stages of tympanic membrane retraction. Stage IV is classified as adhesive otitis media where the epithelial layer of the tympanic membrane fuses with the mucosa of the medial middle ear. Sade went on to show that the inflammatory process in the middle ear led to the reduction of the collagenous layer which in turn lead to greater of tympanic membrane retraction [7].

With an atrophic tympanic membrane, sound conduction is reduced resulting in conductive hearing loss. Retraction on the incudostapedial joint can cause erosion resulting in a more pronounced conductive hearing loss. The weakened tympanic membrane may also lead to cholesteatoma formation with mesotympanic spread of the pars tensa into the facial recess and sinus tympani, spreading posteriorly and medial to the head of the malleus and body of the incus. Surgery is indicated to create a safe ear, reinforce the structure of tympanic membrane, and improve a conductive hearing loss. Patients with no evidence of cholesteatoma and a minimal conductive hearing loss may be followed clinically.

Cholesteatoma

A cholesteatoma is an epithelial inclusion cyst consisting of a matrix of keratinizing squamous epithelium and keratin debris that can generate inflammation and osteoclastic activity through release of inflammatory cytokines. Jackler described five different theories of acquired cholesteatoma formation that include retraction of the tympanic membrane due to negative middle ear pressure, squamous metaplasia, squamous immigration (through a perforation), squamous basal cell hyperplasia, and the mucosal traction theory [8].

Jackler also described three middle ear growth pathways for cholesteatoma. The first and most common is posterior epitympanic retraction of the pars flaccida which travels lateral to the malleus and the incus into the antrum. The second most common is a mesotympanic retraction of the pars tensa onto facial recess, incudostapedial joint, and sinus tympani with retraction medial to the malleus and incus before extending to the antrum. The third is an anterior retraction pocket of the pars flaccida toward the supratubal recess [9]. Identification of a specific growth pattern has implications for operative planning. For example, an inside out mastoidectomy may be all that is required to address an early posterior epitympanic cholesteatoma, which would avoid the need for a postauricular incision. A surgeon may more strongly consider a postauricular approach for a mastoidectomy for a mesotympanic retraction cholesteatoma with an intact ossicular chain. The goal of treating a cholesteatoma is to first create a safe nondraining ear while. A canal wall-intact mastoidectomy is useful for increased visualization of the disease process to foster complete removal. In cases where there is extensive disease a canal wall down mastoidectomy may be indicated in order to exteriorize disease and create a safe ear.

Other Indications

There are many other conditions that are managed well with a canal wall intact mastoidectomy with or without tympnoplasty Glomus tympanicum/jugulare may involve the entirety of the middle ear, necessitating a posterior approach through a mastoidectomy. The facial recess or a retrofacial aircell tracts in combination with a tympanoplasty may be needed to fully remove or debulk a glomus tumor. Eosinophilic granulomas, cholesterol granulomas, and other miscellaneous middle ear tumors are all etiologies that may benefit from the increased exposure a canal wall intact mastoidectomy.

Surgical Technique

Introduction

Perfroming a mastoidectomy and tympanoplsty consists of basic steps to create safe surgery and consistent results. This phioosophy of ear surgery allows less tie spent on essential yet routine steps and preserves more for addressing the more delicate or unique surgical situations or presentations.

Postauricular Tympanoplasty

One percent lidocaine 1/100,000 epinephrine (local) is injected prior to prepping and draping the patient. A complete auricular block is performed (injection of the superiorly around the superficial temporal artery, postauricular, conchal bowl, and tragus). A posterior cervical local block can be used for added pain control. The external auditory canal is irrigated with 30 mL of saline prior to ear canal injections in all four quadrants of the ear canal skin.

A postauricular incision is made with monopolar cautery on cut roughly 2 mm posterior to the postauricular crease. The superior limit of the incision is the point which intersects with an imaginary line 30° superior to the plane of the porion. The inferior limit of the incision extends to the level of the antihelix. A double-pronged skin hook is used while dissecting the auricle anteriorly and generating a Palva flap. Superiorly, the temporal parietal fascia (also termed fools fascia) is identified. Using tenotomy scissors, a plane is developed superficial to the temporalis fascia, but deep to the temporal parietal fascia and a graft slightly larger than 1 × 1 cm^2 is taken, pressed with a fascia press and set on the back table to dry. In cases of revision surgery, temporalis fascia may be used.

Periosteal incisions are made with monopolar cautery making the shape of a lazy S from the level of the zygoma inferior to the temporalis muscle to an area 1 cm superior to the mastoid tip. A Lempert elevator is used to lift the periosteum. A number 11 blade is used to make the canal skin cuts. We prefer using a Perkins retractor retract both the ear and the posterior external auditory canal skin.

External auditory canal incisions are made the same way for every surgery. For a right ear with a clock laying on its back and 12 o'clock corresponding to the lateral process of the malleus, lateral incisions are made along the 1 o'clock and 5 o'clock reference points with a roller knife or a sickle knife and are connected to the transcanal cuts making the tympanomeatal flap (Fig. 57.1). The length of the tympanomeatal flap is roughly 15 mm. The flap is elevated with a round knife using every effort to preserve the tympanic annulus and the corda tympani. If visualization of the annulus is difficult given the anatomy of the canal, a canaloplasty is preformed protecting the tympanomeatal flap. If the anterior canal is prominent obstructing the view of the annulus for graft placement, a round knife is used to back elevate the anterior canal skin from medial to lateral starting just lateral to the annulus. A number 3 diamond burr is used to complete the canaloplasty circumferentially with irrigation so that the entirety of the annulus is viewed for exact graft placement. The perforation (if present), round window, ossicular chain and the course of the facial nerve (to evaluate for dehissence) are inspected. We often longitudinally split the tympanomeatal flap to improve visualization of the perforation and the middle ear to bead the perforation and to remove any skin ingrowth beneath the drum. The perforation is freshened with Bellucci scissors.

Repair of the perforation is used with either free grafts of temporal parietal fascia, temporalis fascia, or cartilage, depending on the specific needs of the case. A cartilage graft harvested from the tragus or posterior cymba concha is used for added structure for reconstruction of the scutum, resist-

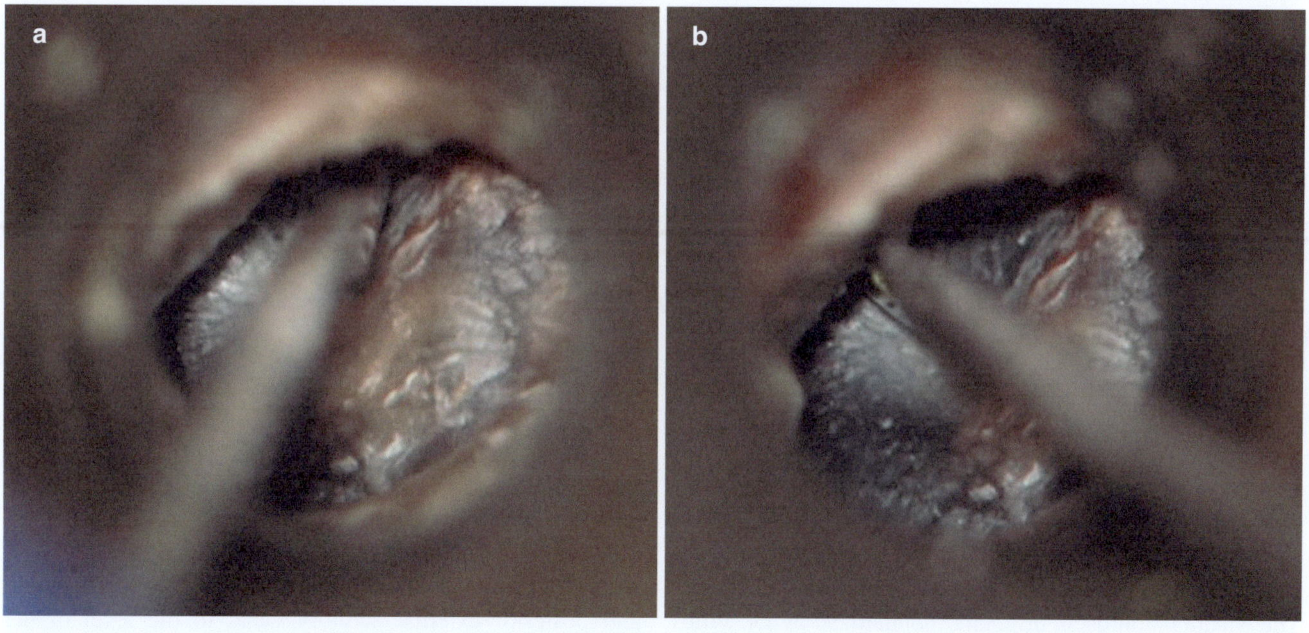

Fig. 57.1 With the lateral process of the malleus defined as 12 o'clock in a left ear, lateral cuts are made with a sickle knife in the 11 o'clock (**a**) and 7 o'clock (**b**) position (1 o'clock and 5 o'clock in a right ear)

ing posterior mesotympanic retraction reformation in cholesteatoma cases or in revision cases where there is limited temporalis or temporal parietal fascia.

Mastoidectomy

Patients needing revisions, have chronic/frequent otorrhea, or have evidence of chronic inflammation/adhesions in the middle ear area are all patients who may require mastoidectomy with the goal to remove an attic block. The cortex is removed down to Koerner's septum without a microscope. This allows for a full view of the surgical field for establishing landmarks. We also tend to minimize the number drill burrs for each mastoidectomy; a 5 mm cutting burr and if needed, a 3 or 2 mm coarse diamond burr. Smaller burrs have a greater potential to cause damage to critical structures, while the larger surface area burrs allows for better identification and protection of structures.

Without the use of a microscope, we begin using a number 5 cutting burr making our initial cuts in a line tangential to a line 30° superior from the level of the root of the zygoma, along the posterior external auditory canal to the spine of Henle and connecting it posteriorly and identify the sinodural angle to establish the level of the tegmen. The posterior external auditory canal is then thinned to 1–2 mm which allows for better identification of the facial neve and facial recess later. It is important to follow the posterior external auditory canal superiorly and into the root of the zygoma, which will allow for easier identification of the horizontal canal and the incus. We then proceed through Korner's septum into the antrum and identify the horizontal semicircular canal. We continue anteriorly using the same number 5 cutting burr drilling in the root of the zygoma from medial to lateral until the incus is identified. In the vast majority of cases, a number 5 cutting burr is sufficient to perform a mastoidectomy to evaluate for and remove attic block. If the attic block is extensive, the facial nerve is identified with copious irrigating using a number 5 cutting burr with long strokes in the direction of the facial nerve. Then, a 3 mm coarse diamond burr is used to expose the facial recess for increased ventilation between the middle ear and mastoid. Opening the facial recess provides an additional ventilation pathway in cases of extensive attic block. In cases where the incus is removed or eroded by disease, the facial recess is drilled open by removing the incus buttress.

Endaural Approach

The endaural approach, originally popularized by Dr. Julius Lempert, provides adequate visualization for a tympanoplasty and can be extended to accommodate a mastoidectomy. If needed while avoiding a postauricular incision. A postauricular incision, which can be associated with postoperative neurogenic pain, numbness, and asymmetry of the auricles, can be avoided in select cases.

After tympanomeatal flap incisions are made (described above) (Fig. 57.1), an incision along the tympanosquamous suture line is made with a number 11 blade down to the bone medially and through the cartilage laterally making a medial triangular shaped tympanomeatal flap that is wider superiorly (Fig. 57.2). Bleeding laterally is controlled by using monopolar or bipolar cautery. The incision can be extended from the incision in the external auditory canal, superior to the tragus and along the anterior aspect of the root of the helix as needed for visualization. Self-retaining retractors are used to open the canal to provide visualization. Often, a canaloplasty is required to visualize the entirety of the annulus for accurate graft placement. The anterior canal is often prominent. A round knife is used to back elevate the anterior external auditory canal skin. While protecting the tympanomeatal flap, a 3 mm coarse diamond is used to drill away the anterior canal until the entire tympanic annulus is visualized (Fig. 57.3). Care should be taken to avoid entering the capsule of the temporomandibular joint located in the anterior external auditory canal. An inside-out mastoidectomy (described below) (Fig. 57.4) to evaluate the antrum can be performed with a number 3 diamond burr or a complete mastoidectomy can be performed after extending the endaural incision. If graft material is required for reconstruction, tragal cartilage is harvested and used. Incisions visible in the lateral external auditory canal are closed primarily with a 4-0 monocryl suture.

Inside-Out Mastoidectomy

An inside-out mastoidectomy can provide adequate transcanal access for accessing an attic block in the case of chronic otitis media without cholesteatoma or an attic retraction cholesteatoma extending toward the antrum from the posterior pars flaccida. In some cases, a patient's external auditory canal is wide enough to accommodate an inside-out mastoidectomy. This technique is often used in combination with an endaural incision to improve visualization.

After the tympanomeatal flap is elevated and protected with metal foil cut from a suture packet and the endaural incision is made to allow adequate visualization, 3 mm diamond burr is used. Keeping within the boundaries of the lateral process of the malleus anteriorly, the incus buttress posteriorly and the head of the malleus/body of the incus medially, the 3 mm diamond is used to drill away the scutum and posterior external auditory canal to the level of the antrum (Fig. 57.4). We commonly utilize a 30° endoscope to better visualize into the antrum for a complete assessment. If

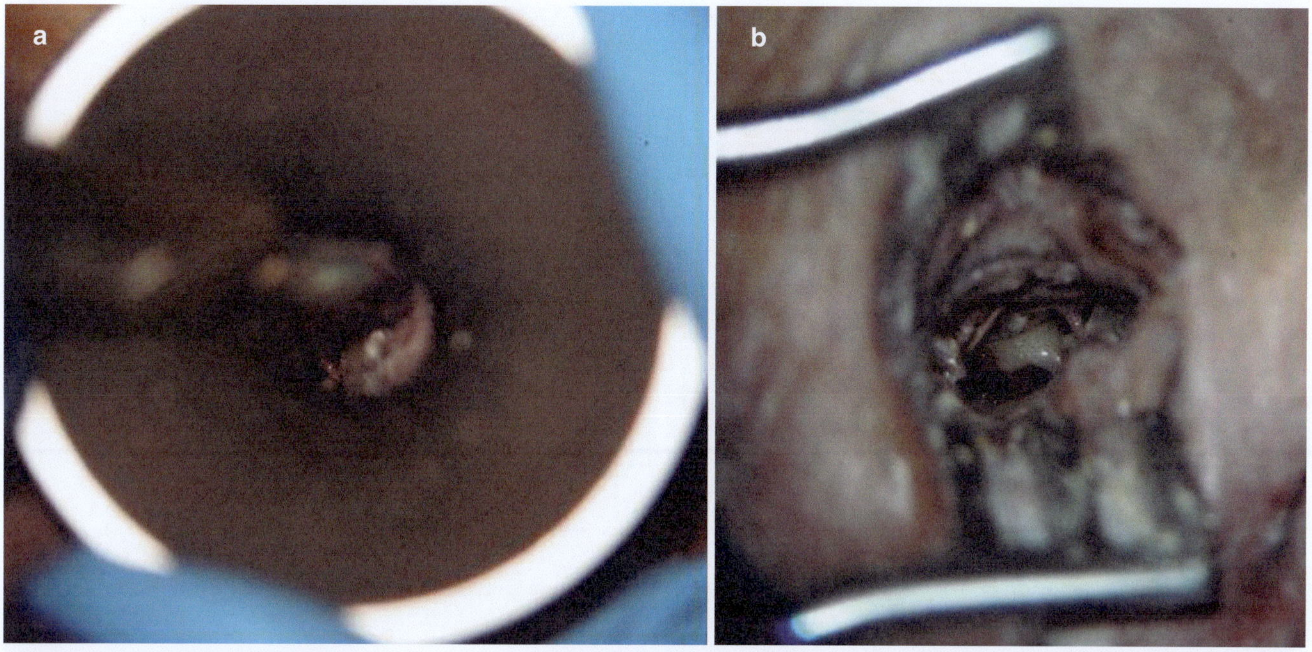

Fig. 57.2 Using a #15 blade, an incision along the tympanosquamous suture line is made toward the anterior helical fold (**a**). The speculum is removed, and a self-retaining retractor is placed for visualization (**b**)

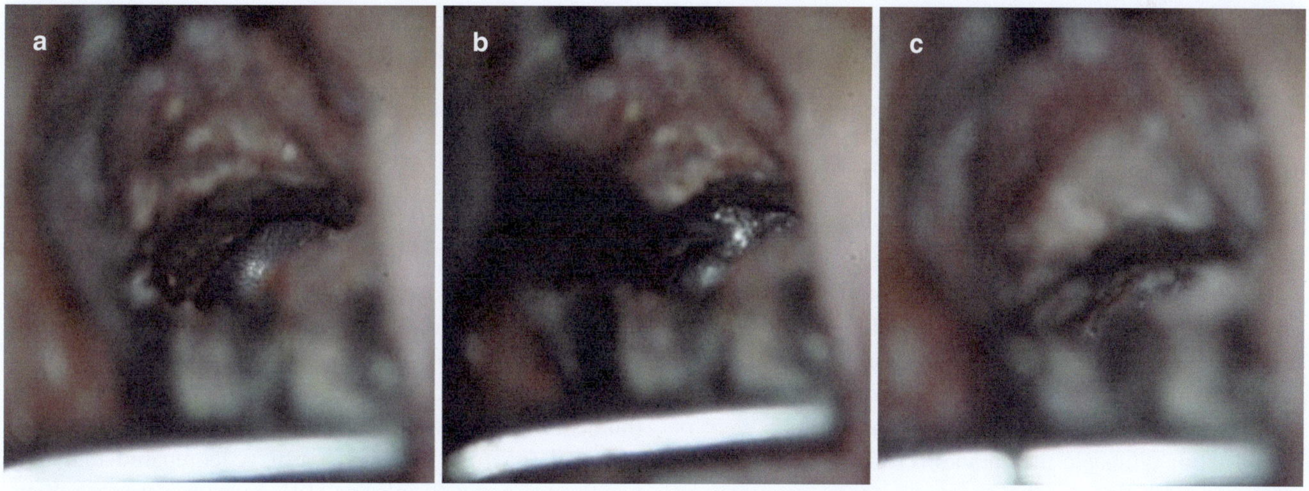

Fig. 57.3 The anterior canal wall obscures visualization of the annulus (**a**). A #3 coarse diamond burr is used to perform a canaloplasty (**b**) until the annulus is easily seen (**c**)

present, attic block or cholesteatoma are removed using various elevators. The posterior wall of the external auditory canal is then reconstructed with a tragal cartilage graft.

Role of Cartilage

The traditional teaching was that cartilage and fascia showed similar rates of success in tympanic membrane perforation repair. In pooled studies and metanalyses, cartilage grafts used to repair tympanic membrane perforations appear to have a modest benefit over fascia. One metanalysis suggested that cartilage grafts showed a 2.8% improved success over fascia [10], while another metanalysis of 11 prospective and 26 retrospective studies suggested that cartilage grafts used to repair a tympanic membrane perforation benefited from 92% success in perforation closure compared to 82% when fascia alone was used ($p < 0.001$) [11].

In our experience with the aforementioned surgical technique, we do not clinically see any significant difference between fascia and cartilage for perforation repair. In our experience, success of tympanic membrane repair depends

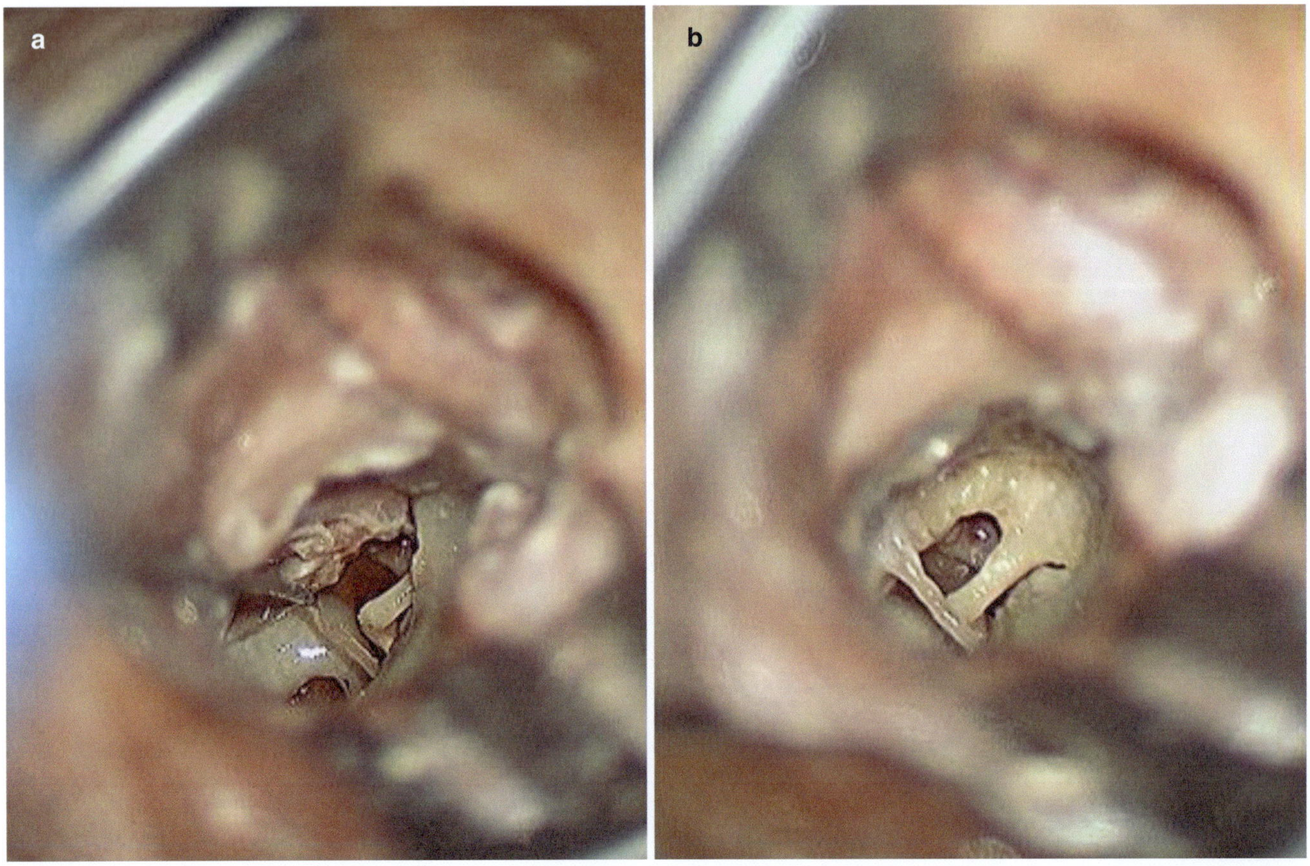

Fig. 57.4 The tympanomeatal flap has been elevated exposing the incudostapedial joint, the chorda tympani, and the round window (**a**). A #3 coarse diamond burr is used along the tympanosquamous suture line to expose the head of the malleus and the body of the incus (**b**). This can be expanded to expose visualization into the aditus ad antrum

more on adequate graft placement rather than the type of graft used. It is for this reason that we preform canaloplasties often to visualize the entirety of the annulus. Our indications for harvesting and using cartilage are very specific. We use cartilage for reconstruction of the posterior external auditory canal after an inside-out mastoidectomy, reinforcement of the posterior tympanic membrane to resist posterior mesotympanic retraction in cholesteatoma cases, repairing an atelectatic tympanic membrane, providing a barrier between an ossicular prosthesis and the tympanic membrane, and for repairing a tympanic membrane perforation in transcanal tympanoplasties.

When a postauricular approach is used, we use cartilage from the cymba concha by making an incision with monopolar cautery followed by removal of the necessary amount of cartilage with a number 10 blade. The perichondrium is then sutured together with a 4-0 monocryl. This avoids an additional incision into the tragus when cartilage is freely available postauricularly.

In cases where a transcanal tympanoplasty and inside-out mastoidectomy is preformed, tragal cartilage is used. An incision is made medial the tragal cap with a 10 blade, suprapericho ndrial pockets are made on either side of the cartilage with tenotomy scissors and the necessary amount of cartilage is removed. The skin incision is approximated primarily with a 4-0 monocryl suture.

After harvesting the cartilage, it is then prepared and thinned. Previous studies have shown similar vibratory properties of 0.5 mm thickness cartilage compared that of a healthy tympanic membrane [12]. As such, we use a thickness of 0.5 mm when incorporating a cartilage graft into the tympanic membrane repair.

Cartilage Embedded Tympanosotomy Tube

Some patients require long-term middle ear ventilation. In cases of middle ear atelectasis, this can be challenging given the flaccidity of the tympanic membrane. Cartilage provides a rigid structure that can help reinforce a flaccid tympanic membrane and prevent premature extrusion. A T-tube can be incorporated within the cartilage to provide long-term ventilation while reducing the incidence of persistent tympanic membrane perorations commonly associated with T-tubes

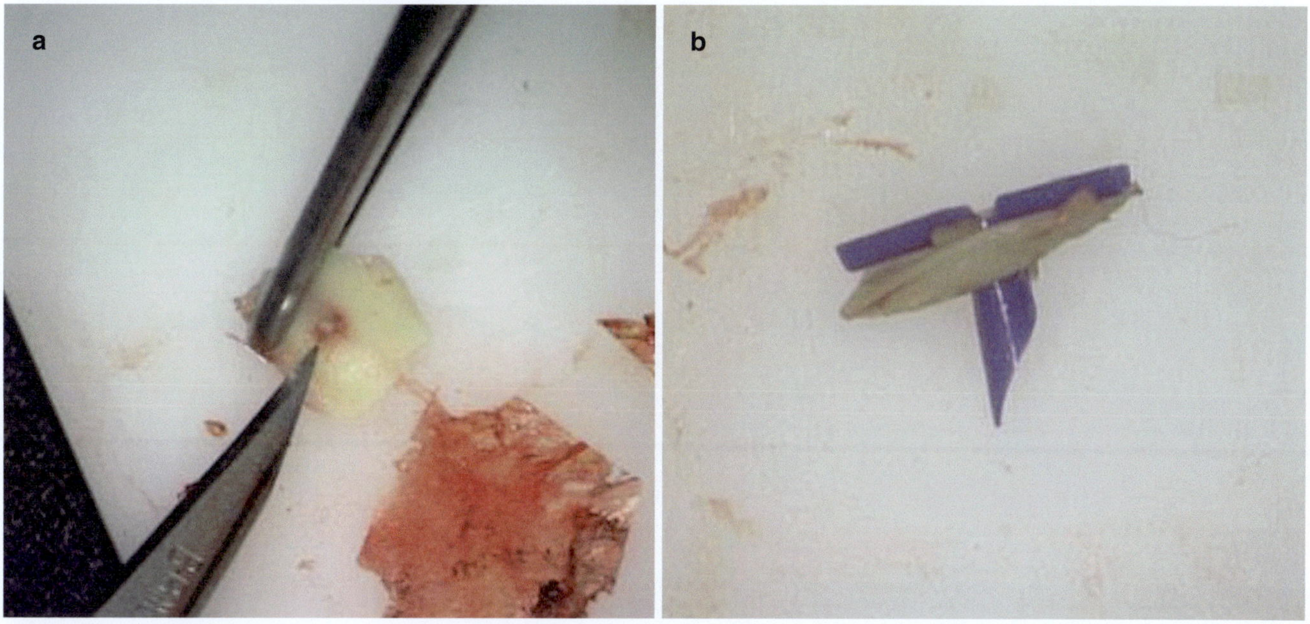

Fig. 57.5 A #11 blade is used to create a 1.5 mm square in the center of a cartilage graft (**a**). A T-tube is then introduced through the cartilage with an alligator forceps until the flanges are against the cartilage and a bevel is cut into the T-tube with a knife (**b**)

[13]. If otorrhea from a biofilm build up occurs or if the patient's physical exam improves, the T-tube can be removed in clinic and replaced in clinic as needed through the cartilage. A cartilage embedded tympanostomy tube is a useful addition to any otologist's took kit in managing chronic ear disease.

After harvesting cartilage, removing the perichondrium, and reducing the thickness to 0.5 mm, a small 1.5 mm box of cartilage is removed from the center of the cartilage using a number 11 blade to accommodate a T-tube (Fig. 57.5). We use a modified Richards T-tube with an inner diameter of 1.32 mm and place the shaft of the tube through the cartilage. The flanges of the tube are cut to the width of the cartilage shield. The length of the tube is trimmed to a length of roughly 4 mm to reduce the flow resistance as flow resistance is directly proportional to the tube's length (Poiseuille's Law: $R = 8\ \text{nL}/\pi r^4$). Flanges are shorted to 2–3 mm. A myringotomy is made in the anterior inferior quadrant of the tympanic membrane, a tympanomeatal flap is elevated, and the cartilage embedded T tube is placed in the middle ear (Fig. 57.6). The T-tube is then pulled from medial to lateral through the myringotomy until the cartilage is flush with the tympanic membrane.

Extended Approaches

Occasionally variations in the extent and location of disease will require the extended exposure in the mastoid.

As described previously, some patients with chronic otitis media without cholesteatoma have a large degree of attic block. In cases where attic block from tenacious adhesions are encountered, which prevents aeration into the mastoid, the facial recess is drilled to provide an additional ventilation pathway between the middle ear and mastoid. In cases where the facial recess is drilled and the incus is eroded or removed, the incus buttress should be removed in order to maximize ventilation.

Although rare, cholesteatoma can track inferiorly into the hypotympanum and petrous apex and anteriorly toward the eustachian tube and suprtubal air-cell tracts. Access to the hypotympanum can be achieved by drilling the air cells posterior to the facial nerve via a retrofacial approach. One must be cautions of the posterior semicircular canal and cochlear aqueduct at the superior aspect of the retrofacial recess and the jugular bulb inferiorly. This provides adequate visualization inferiorly and medially up to the supratubal recess.

Not infrequently, residual cholesteatoma can be left or iatrogenically placed in air cells extending into the zygoma that may extend toward the capsule of the temporomandibular joint. Care must be taken to identify the extent anteriorly and whether or not dura is exposed on preoperative imaging (Fig. 57.7). While completing or revising a mastoidectomy, the root of the zygoma is exposed using a cutting burr. Superiorly one must be careful of potential dura exposure. Anteriorly, one must be mindful of the temporomandibular joint. If dura is exposed after disease removal, a vascularized muscle flap form the temporalis muscle can be used to protect it prior to closure.

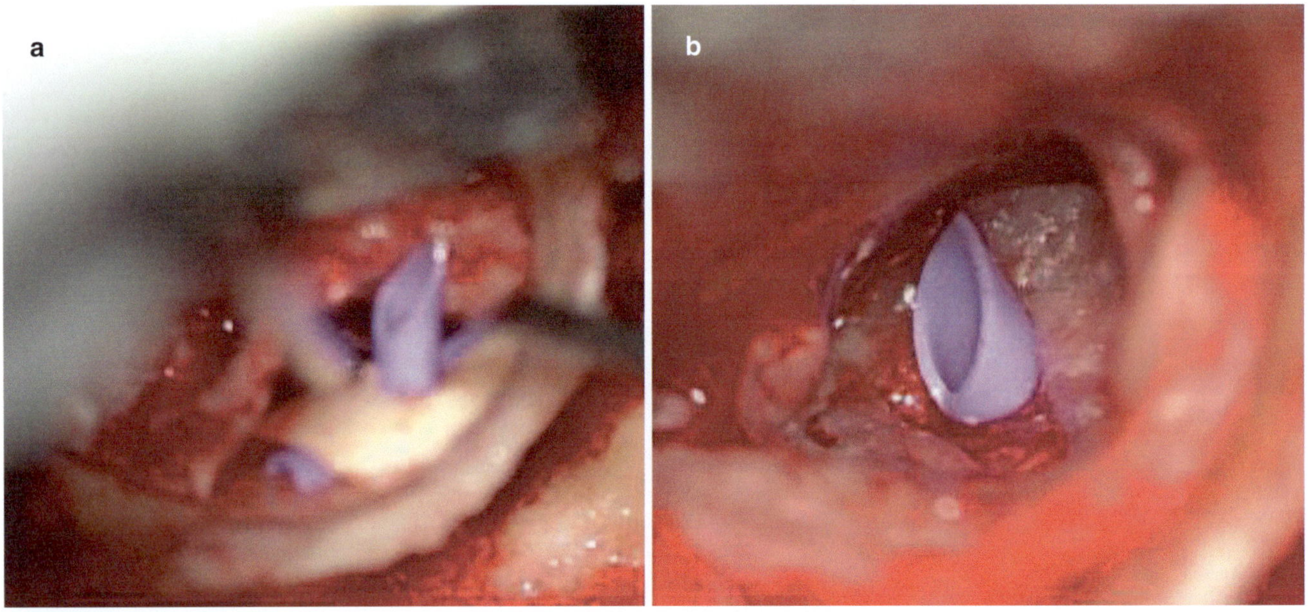

Fig. 57.6 A myringotomy is made and the cartilage embedded tympanostomy tube is placed in the middle ear under the tympanomeatal flap (**a**). The flange of the T-tube is introduced through the myringotomy with the bevel facing inferiorly (**b**)

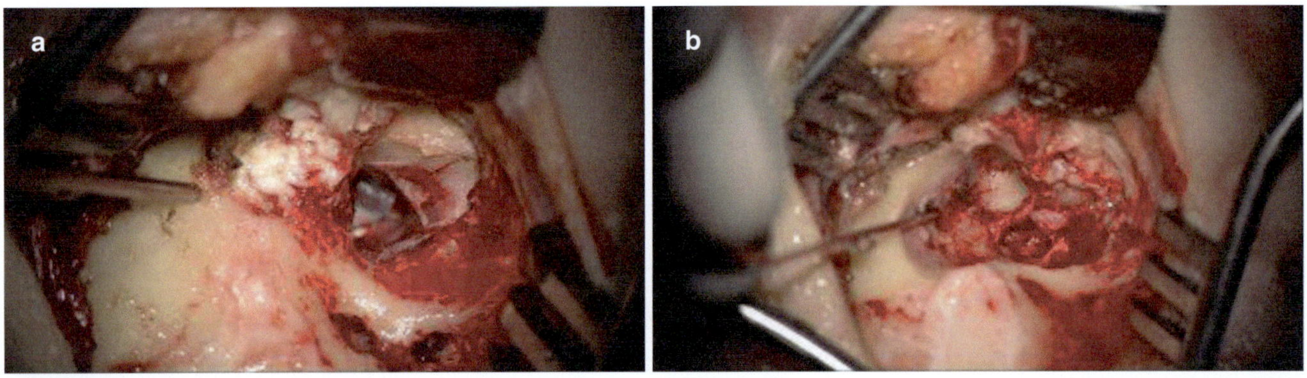

Fig. 57.7 A right ear with a cholesteatoma that is eroding into the root of the zygoma (**a**). The suction is pointing to exposed dura in after removal of disease and drill out of the zygomatic root (**b**)

Controversial Topics

Aerating Mastoidectomy

The concept of an aerating mastoidectomy in the setting of chronic otitis media is a controversial topic. We perform a mastoidectomy in patients with chronic otitis media is to evaluate for an attic block to reestablish physiologic communication between the middle ear and antrum. One retrospective study by Rhul et al. found in their cohort of 135 patients with chronic otitis media, 73% of patients had a sclerotic or poorly pneumatized mastoid and 82.6% of them had evidence of mastoid opacification. Intraoperatively, 93% of them had evidence of mucosal inflammation and attic block. They had a 90% success rate in performing a tympanoplasty and mastoidectomy in repairing tympanic membrane perforations [14]. Additionally, Boyle's law suggests that increased volume of the mastoid cavity should provide increased resistance to pressure changes. Sade reported secretory otitis media occurred in roughly 52% of patients with poorly pneumatized mastoids, compared to 20% of well aerated mastoids and that atelectasis occurred in 37.3% of poorly aerated mastoids vs. 5.7% in well-aerated mastoids.

These findings support the notion that the mastoid acts as a buffer against pressure changes [3].

Some studies argue that preforming a mastoidectomy in patients with chronic otitis media without cholesteatoma does not improve successful repair of a perforation. One retrospective study by Balyan et al. compared three groups: group I (tympanoplasty only in dry ears), group II (tympanoplasty and mastoidectomy in dry ears), and group III (tympanoplasty with active otorrhea). The success rates of tympanic membrane repair were 90.5%, 85.5%, and 89.2% respectively [15] with no significant difference in success among the three groups. It should be noted that the potential for selection bias is present as the authors did not state why they chose to perform a mastoidectomy at the time of surgery. Another retrospective study by Mishiro et al. 2001 [15] compared two groups: group A (tympanoplasty and mastoidectomy) and group B (tympanoplasty only) with success in 90.5% and 93.3% respectively [16]. It should be noted that neither of these two studies included revision cases. There is only one randomized controlled study that we are aware of comparing tympanoplasty with mastoidectomy to tympanoplasty alone (respectively the rate of success was 82.8% and 76% ($p = 0.15$)) [17]. While the trend showed higher success in the tympanoplasty and mastoidectomy group, it did not reach statistical significance. Unfortunately, this study did not perform a sub analysis between these two groups for revision cases, chronic otorrhea, middle ear inflammation, or presence of opacified air cells on CT.

We prefer to do a mastoidectomy in cases with chronic or frequent otorrhea, middle ear inflammation, and in revision cases with failed previous tympanoplasty. We typically do not perform a mastoidectomy are first-time surgery for, dry, traumatic perforations with no evidence of chronic inflammation in the middle ear. Our patient population represents a subset of patients who have some of the most challenging pathology on the disease spectrum who have failed multiple tympanoplasties in the past. The current literature does not stratify the patient population who suffer from chronic otitis media without cholesteatoma and may not be sensitive enough to discriminate differences in success rates in the cohort of patients with the most severe disease.

References

1. Buch NH, Jorgensen MB. Eustachian tube and middle ear. Embryology and pathology. Arch Otolaryngol. 1964;79:472–80.
2. Danner CJ. Middle ear atelectasis: what causes it and how is it corrected? Otolaryngol Clin N Am. 2006;39(6):1211–9.
3. Sadé J, Fuchs C. Secretory otitis media in adults: II. The role of mastoid pneumatization as a prognostic factor. Ann Otol Rhinol Laryngol. 1997;106(1):37–40.
4. da Costa SS, Paparella MM, Schachern PA, Yoon TH, Kimberley BP. Temporal bone histopathology in chronically infected ears with intact and perforated tympanic membranes. Laryngoscope. 1992;102(11):1229–36.
5. Hadas E, Sadé J. Clearance by the mucociliary system in 'simple chronic otitis media'. J Laryngol Otol. 1979;93(8):781–3.
6. Proctor B. The development of the middle ear spaces and their surgical significance. J Laryngol Otol. 1964;78:631–48.
7. Sadé J, Berco E. Atelectasis and secretory otitis media. Ann Otol Rhinol Laryngol. 1976;85(2 Suppl 25 Pt 2):66–72.
8. Jackler RK, Santa Maria PL, Varsak YK, Nguyen A, Blevins NH. A new theory on the pathogenesis of acquired cholesteatoma: mucosal traction. Laryngoscope. 2015;125(Suppl 4):S1–S14.
9. Growth patterns of cholesteatoma. In: Jackler R, editor. Ear surgery illustrated: a comprehensive atlas of otologic microsurgical techniques. 1st ed. New York: Thieme; 2019.
10. Tan HE, Santa Maria PL, Eikelboom RH, Anandacoomaraswamy KS, Atlas MD. Type I tympanoplasty meta-analysis: a single variable analysis. Otol Neurotol. 2016;37(7):838–46.
11. Jalali MM, Motasaddi M, Kouhi A, Dabiri S, Soleimani R. Comparison of cartilage with temporalis fascia tympanoplasty: a meta-analysis of comparative studies. Laryngoscope. 2017;127(9):2139–48.
12. Mürbe D, Zahnert T, Bornitz M, Hüttenbrink KB. Acoustic properties of different cartilage reconstruction techniques of the tympanic membrane. Laryngoscope. 2002;112(10):1769–76.
13. Zuniga SA Jr, Larner S, Souza DM, Khan A, Hillman TA, Chen DA. Long-term outcomes of cartilage-buttressed T-tube tympanoplasty for prolonged middle ear ventilation. Laryngoscope. 2019;129(1):203–8.
14. Ruhl CM, Pensak ML. Role of aerating mastoidectomy in noncholesteatomatous chronic otitis media. Laryngoscope. 1999;109(12):1924–7.
15. Balyan FR, Celikkanat S, Aslan A, Taibah A, Russo A, Sanna M. Mastoidectomy in noncholesteatomatous chronic suppurative otitis media: is it necessary? Otolaryngol Head Neck Surg. 1997;117(6):592–5.
16. Mishiro Y, Sakagami M, Takahashi Y, Kitahara T, Kajikawa H, Kubo T. Tympanoplasty with and without mastoidectomy for noncholesteatomatous chronic otitis media. Eur Arch Otorhinolaryngol. 2001;258(1):13–5.
17. Albu S, Trabalzini F, Amadori M. Usefulness of cortical mastoidectomy in myringoplasty. Otol Neurotol. 2012;33(4):604–9.

Canal Wall-Down Tympanomastoidectomy

58

Sady Selaimen da Costa, Mauricio Noschang Lopes da Silva, Jefferson André Bauer, Fábio André Selaimen, and Letícia Petersen Schmidt Rosito

Introduction and Hystorical Remarks

"One who ignores history would do so at his peril, to be condemned to repeat the same mistakes".
George Santayana

Otologic surgery has gone through a gradual evolution to reach the state of art at which is practiced today. Early contributors promoted surgical techniques which were appropriate for the then available instrumentation and understanding of pathology. Through continued investigation and research as well the introduction of new technologies, the modern otologic surgeon now has many options in choosing a surgical approach [1].

The surgical treatment of chronic otitis media (COM), particularly the cholesteatoma, illustrates like any other this fascinating march. The first recorded mastoid operation for ear drainage was by Jean Petit in the late eighteenth century. In 1853, Sir William Wilde introduced the postauricular incision for drainage of an aural abscess. According to Shambaugh, although Wilde advised opening the bone in far advanced cases, he, apparently, never carried out a mastoidectomy. It remained to Schwartze in 1873 to described the simple mastoid operation. This procedure was first described by Riolanus in 1649, but it remained for Schwartze and Eysell in 1873 to depict thoroughly its surgical technique and proper indications. Simple mastoidectomy indicates the exenteration of the air cell system in the mastoid aspect of the temporal bone, 'consolidating separate air cell cavities into a continuous structure without disturbing the contents of the middle ear'. The procedure had such a tremendous positive impact on the natural history of otitis media that by the end of the nineteenth century, the medical textbooks could not stress enough its importance and stated that as a lifesaving measure few surgical procedures equal and none surpass the efficiency of the modern mastoid operation.

In 1873, von Trolsch suggested a modification of the Schwartze simple mastoid operation for chronic otorrhea caused by cholesteatomas at the attic, antrum, or mastoid. In these situations, cholesteatoma remnants or "left over's" would invariably cause recurrence of the disease. Von Bergmann named this procedure radical mastoid operation which was described in detail by Zaufal in 1890 with the removal of the posterior and superior canal walls, the tympanic membrane, and the malleus and incus, thus converting all the compartments of the middle ear, mastoid, and external auditory canal into a wide, ample common cavity. Usually, the Eustachian tube (ET) is obstructed with tissue and to improve the self-cleansing properties of this cavity, the meatoplasty was introduced 1 year later by Stacke. The radical mastoid operation accomplished most of its planned objectives to control ear infections.

On the other hand, this technique was intrinsically related to the complete sacrifice of the middle ear function. Korner in 1899 was the first to notice that the extreme aggressiveness of the radical operation was, sometimes, unnecessary and could be avoided suggesting that in some special situations the tympanic membrane and the ossicles could be

S. S. da Costa (✉)
Department of Otolaryngology, Head & Neck Surgery, School of Medicine, Universidade Federal do Rio Grande do Sul, Porto Alegre, Brazil

Otology and Neurotology Division, Sistema Hospitalar Mãe de Deus, Porto Alegre, Brazil

M. N. L. da Silva · L. P. S. Rosito
Otology and Neurotology Division, Sistema Hospitalar Mãe de Deus, Porto Alegre, Brazil

Service of Otolaryngology, Head & Neck Surgery, Hospital de Clínicas de Porto Alegre, Porto Alegre, Brazil

J. A. Bauer
Hospital de Clinicas de Porto Alegre, Porto Alegre, Brazil

Hospital Mãe de Deus, Porto Alegre, Brazil

Universidade Federal do Rio Grande do Sul, Porto Alegre, Brazil

Instituto Gaúcho de Otorrinolaringologia, Porto Alegre, Brazil

F. A. Selaimen
Department of Otolaryngology, Head & Neck Surgery, School of Medicine, Universidade Federal do Rio Grande do Sul, Porto Alegre, Brazil

M. V. Goycoolea et al. (eds.), *Textbook of Otitis Media*, https://doi.org/10.1007/978-3-031-40949-3_58

spared. A classic modification of the radical mastoidectomy was first described by Bondy around 1910 and is still sometimes referred to as a *Bondy mastoidectomy* [2]. It is also sometimes referred to as *modified radical mastoidectomy*. This procedure requires removal of the posterior canal wall and creation of an open mastoidectomy cavity without an associated tympanotomy or tympanoplasty. In the classic procedure, the middle ear space is never entered, and the cholesteatoma matrix serves as the lining of the mastoid defect.

The Bondy-modified radical operation must be acknowledged as the first significant step toward to the surgical control of middle ear suppuration with simultaneous consideration for hearing preservation. Subsequent to Bondy's description, surgical innovations to prevent or ameliorate deafness came on a steady and continuous stream. Holmgren showed that the labyrinth could be opened safely provided rigid aseptic techniques were observed. Sourdille [3], in France, described his multistage tympanolabyrinthopexy, which was later modified by Lempert [4] into a more practical one-stage fenestration. About the same time, sulfanilamide was introduced in the form of Prontosil and rapidly became part of the therapeutic arsenal either to control established infections and as a powerful tool in the prophylaxis of suppurative postoperative complications. The success of Lempert's one-stage fenestration was such that otologists from all over the world were attracted to New York to learn his revolutionary techniques. According to Shambaugh & Glasscock [5], thanks to Lempert the climate of otologic thought became definitively hearing oriented. The rebirth of these procedures brought a new interest in the physiology of the ear. Landmarks studies were conducted by Békesy, Juers, Davis, and Walsh shedding lights on very important questions on how the normal and pathological middle ear work. From these studies, the two basic principles of tympanoplasty were defined: sound protection to the round window and sound pressure transformation to the oval window [2].

These concepts offered the necessary ammunition for Fritz Zollner (1951) and Horst Wullstein (1952) to trigger off the next stage in the evolution of the middle ear surgery launching the basis of the modern tympanoplasty [2]. The next logical step was the combination of the radical mastoidectomy with the instrumentation of the middle ear. The end result was the birth of the so-called canal wall down tympanomastoidectomy. The new procedure was essentially the radical operation with a careful preservation of the remaining tympanic membrane (TM) and healthy ossicles. After the conclusion of the bony work, tympanoplasty techniques were employed to reconstruct the tympanossicular system: the TM was grafted with autologous tissue (fascia, periostium, or pericondrium); and the ossicular chain was reconstructed with sculptured bone or cartilage. These concepts were adopted, modified, and developed worldwide. In fact, during the 1950s and 1960s (and by many to date), the wall-down tympanomastoidectomy (also known as open-cavity tympanomastoidectomy—OCTM) became the procedure of choice in the treatment of COM with cholesteatoma and its complications. In 1958, Jansen described the posterior tympanotomy (a triangular area bounded by the fossa incudis, the chorda tympani, and facial nerves) making possible for the surgeon to fully access the facial recess area without removing the posterior wall. The technique includes a thorough simple mastoidectomy, but the posterior canal wall is left intact, and pathologic tissue from the middle ear is exposed through the opening of the facial (suprapyramidal) recess. As a consequence, the wall-up tympanomastoidectomy (closed-cavity tympanomastoidectomy—CCTM—or combined approach) became very popular in the following years. Other otologic surgeons have described this technique as well, including Sheehy and Patterson, Smyth, and Glasscock and Miller. This operation is often planned as a two-stage procedure that includes a second operation (the so-called second look) a year after the initial surgery to check residual disease and hearing restoration [2].

As pointed out before, during the 1950s and 1960s, open-cavity tympanomastoidectomy (OCTM) was generally practiced by all otologists treating COM and mastoiditis with pathologic findings such as cholesteatoma or granulation tissue. Because of problems with the mastoid cavity, and because of the original contribution by Jansen' in the late 1950s, closed-cavity tympanomastoidectomy was enthusiastically practiced by many leading otologists worldwide during the 1970s. A review of the current literature revealed that although many continue to practice CCTM, many former enthusiasts have returned to OCTM because CCTM resulted in (1) multistage operations, (2) higher incidence of recurrent disease, and (3) increased difficulty and risk of complication.

Objectives

A closer analysis of this evolution shows that otologic surgery for the treatment of otitis media and its complications gradually evolved during this last century with at least three different phases: preservation of life, anatomic restoration, and hearing improvement. Interestingly, these three phases bring us to current concepts, which can be perfectly summarized under the contemporary objectives of chronic ear surgery: elimination of infection; preservation of the normal anatomical contours of the ear and, whenever possible, restoration of hearing function. Translating these concepts into practice regardless the technique employed the ultimate goals of surgery for COM is (1) the removal of all diseased tissues of the middle ear cleft, with a complete evacuation of the inflammation/infection process; (2) preservation or reconstruction of the middle/external ear complex; and (3) restoration of the sound-conducting mechanism. These objectives can be achieved in an one-stage procedure or in a planned two-stages procedure when the first operation is aimed to control infection, and the second stage is directed to the reconstruction of the hearing apparatus.

Indications

Even nowadays, the main indication for a mastoidectomy is to treat COM particularly when associated with a cholesteatoma. COM without cholesteatoma but with refractory drainage, immature granulation tissue and/or cholesterol granuloma filling the mastoid, silent COM and previous tympanoplasty failure may also ensure mastoidectomy. Although there are some absolute and relative indications for a mastoidectomy, the type of mastoidectomy is based on the extent of disease, the destruction already present in the ear, the residual hearing, the status and the hearing of the contralateral ear (CLE), the general health conditions, and the social status of the patient. Of paramount importance is the surgeon's skills and familiarity with the techniques and, of course, the patient's preference. The surgical techniques and the main indications of the procedures on the mastoid are summarized in Table 58.1.

Table 58.1 Surgical options in temporal bone

Surgical treatment of chronic otits media
• Closed cavity tympanomastoidectomy (wall up—intact wall—combined approach)
• Open cavity tympanomastoidectomy (wall down)
• Intact bridge tympanostoidectomy
• Modified radical mastoidectomy (bondy operation)
• Radical mastoidectomy
Intratemporal lesions of the facial nerve
• Decompression
• Rerouting
• Anastomosis
Tumors of the temporal bone
• Tympanic or tympanomastoid paragangliomas
• Jugular paragangliomas
• Carcinomas of the external ear
• Carcinomas of the middle ear
Approachs to the posterior cranial fossa
• Translabyrinthine approach
• Pre and retro sigmoid approach to the IAC and CPA
• Transpetrous approach to the clivus
• Transcoclear approach
• Subtotal petrosectomy

Principles of Temporal Bone Surgery

The principle of temporal bone surgery is to move from one known landmark to the next,
guided by the relationships between each.
Only in this way can the temporal bone surgeon avoid the danger of being lost
within a nebulous network off vital structures."
Ralph Nelson (1982)

To operate on an ear is probably one of the most delicate medical acts. Here the limits between success and failure are very thin leaving no room for mistakes. The final outcome will be a summary of a series of small, but important, details that must be observed during the pre, intra-, and postoperative periods. These details, all equally important, sometimes are inappropriately simplified into just "operative technique". It is quite obvious that the control of the operative technique is vital to the success of any surgery. It is also clear that this "domain" does not represent a magic gift nor a "congenital trait" of a talented surgeon. It is actually the end result of a long and difficult period of theoretical and practical training with five major rules:

(a) Complete clinical background in otologic pathology.
(b) Complete and detailed knowledge of the temporal bone anatomy.
(c) A diligent experience at the dissection bench in the temporal bone lab.
(d) Close and astute observation of experienced and skilled otologic surgeons.
(e) Continuing medical education.

These are all sine qua non conditions before any otologic surgeon will take the responsibility for a case. The experience and the skills will be then mastered case by case, day by day and, unfortunately, after a series of failures [2].

Preoperative Evaluation and Workup

A systematic and thorough preoperative evaluation is mandatory in every patient with COM before any surgical decision. This evaluation is carried out on an outpatient basis and involves a six-step approach (1) analysis of symptoms and signs, (2) otologic examination, (3) complete otolaryngologic clinical examination, (4) audiologic evaluation, (5) radiologic evaluation, and (6) preoperative preparation.

Analysis of Symptoms and Signs

A careful analysis of the symptoms and signs allows physicians to determine the need for surgery, its urgency, and the anticipated results. We always discuss with our fellows, residents, and medical student that the art of taking a good medical history can never be overemphasized. Especially when dealing with a disease that has the possibility to recur as one of its trademarks (like the cholesteatoma). It is mandatory to conduct a careful interview with the patient and/or his family focusing three key periods along the timeline: today (the present), yesterday (the past), and tomorrow (the future). The ideal preoperative workup encompasses the art of history taking, a complete ENT physical exam and important ancillary tests (audiology, imaging, etc.). The workup should guide the physician to three distinct temporal moments equally important:

1. TODAY: The diagnosis
2. YESTERDAY: The etiology
3. TOMORROW: The prognosis

This information will permit the clinician to design a rational therapeutic plan which will make possible:

1. TODAY: Treat established disease
2. YESTERDAY: Manage etiologic factors trying to avoid recurrences
3. TOMORROW: Abort the natural history and future complications.

Otorrhea

This most common manifestation of COM should be noted: What is its duration, frequency, character, and odor? Long-lasting, constant, purulent, or bloody malodorous otorrhea is always associated with significant disease in the middle ear and mastoid. Mucoid discharge of short duration, on and off, usually denotes a simple perforation with no major pathologic findings.

Hearing Loss

This second most common complaint is closely related to the amount of damage in the middle ear; thus, in the absence of cholesteatoma, a conductive loss of 20 dB usually indicates integrity of the ossicular chain. Erosion of the ossicles (particularly the long process of the incus) or fixation raises the hearing loss to 30 dB or more. Interestingly, some cholesteatomas can destroy the ossicular chain but still preserve good hearing. In these situations, the cholesteatoma can transmit the sound from the external ear to the oval window in a so-called "columellar effect" (Fig. 58.1).

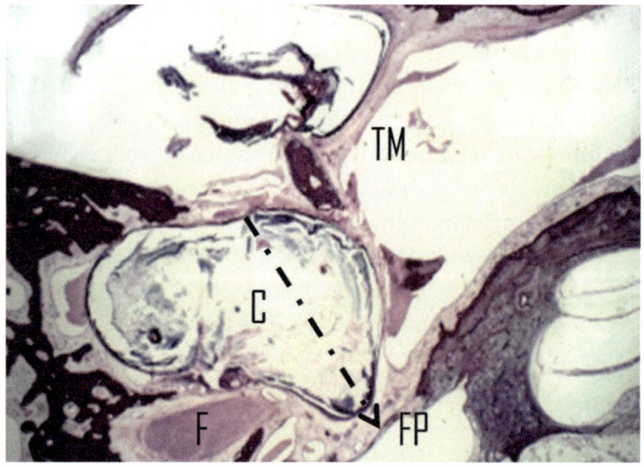

Fig. 58.1 Collumelar effect: a cyst of cholesteatoma (C) bridges the gap between the tympanic membrane (TM) and the footplate of the stapes (FP). Facial nerve (F). (HP section belongs to the collection of the Otopathology Lab – University of Minnesota)

Pain

Pain is not a common complaint, so, when present, it should be approached carefully. An associated external otitis, an expanding mass of cholesteatoma, or a suppurative complication must be ruled out.

Vertigo

Continuous true vertigo in the presence of a cholesteatoma represents a labyrinthine irritation or a fistula in a semicircular canal until proven otherwise.

Paralysis or Paresis of the Facial Nerve

Currently, these are uncommon complications of COM. Whenever present, a cholesteatoma, a tumor, or an acute aggressive infection should be considered, and prompt exploration of the middle ear cleft and mastoid is indicated.

Otologic Examination

Careful inspection of the ear includes at least an otoscopic and physical examination under magnification with the surgical microscope. An otoendoscope can be helpful in reaching hidden recesses of the temporal bone in follow-up of an open cavity. This tool is of particular importance in cases presenting a pars flaccida cholesteatoma. Sometimes even the otomicroscopy may overlook a silent erosion of the scutum due to the straight field of vision of the microscope. The endoscope penetrating deeper in the ear canal will never miss a finding like this. The whole 360° of the tympanic membrane should be inspected, but special care is dedicated to the pars flacida, the area near the attic, and the posterosuperior quadrant. Besides discharge (discussed earlier), one should note the pattern of perforation and the status of mucosa in the middle ear. A test for fistula should be used when vertigo or dizziness is present. A patch test and a test of the ET, with rare exceptions, are excluded from the authors' workup.

Perforation

Perforations of the drumhead can be classified into two types: (1) central and (2) marginal. Central perforations may vary in size but always have a margin of drum remnant surrounding them. Marginal perforations extend to the tympanic sulcus and fail to have a surrounding drum remnant. Marginal perforations can be classified into three subtypes: (1) attic (when the pars flaccida is involved), (2) posterosuperior (below the malleolar ligament), and (3) total. Marginal perforations are by far more frequently associated with cholestatomas (according to the migratory theory). During otomicroscopy, the canal should be meticulously cleansed of all secretions, debris, and cerumen. Special attention should be paid to the pars flaccida, where, not rarely, small perforations may be covered by dried crusts. As the authors often say, "never trust an attic cerumen."

Status of Mucosa of the Middle Ear

The status of the mucosa is a good indicator regarding the outcome of surgery. The presence of a normal or near normal mucosa is favorable for prognosis. Squamous epithelium in the middle ear or a large mass of granulation tissue there represents more aggressive disease. Ossicular disruption is often encountered. In these situations, the long process of the incus is the first to be involved. When the stapedial superstructure is absent, the prognosis for restoration of hearing is less favorable. If the handle of the malleus is absent, a two-staged operation may be required to reconstruct the ossicular chain. The presence of tympanosclerosis must be adequately addressed. Tympanosclerosis refers to a hyalinization of the subepithelial space and often represents a final stage of COM. According to Friedmann [6], two types of tympanosclerosis exist: (1) sclerosing mucositis (more superficial and amenable to total surgical removal) and (2) osteoclastic mucoperiostitis (an invasive form that often completely involves the ossicles and the areas near the windows and defies or prevents complete surgical removal).

Complete Otolaryngologic Clinical Examination

According to the old concept of "anatomophysiologic solidarity" of the upper aero digestive tract, any unsolved problem in the head and neck increases the risk for a poor surgical outcome. Before surgery, a complete examination of the head and neck is mandatory. Gross abnormalities, suppurative sinus diseases, and allergies should be brought under control before the operation is carried out.

Audiologic Evaluation

Careful audiometric tests should be performed routinely. These findings must be compared with those of the basic tests with tuning forks performed by the otologist. The audiometric battery should include pure-tone bone/air-conduction thresholds, speech-reception levels, and speech discrimination scores. Results of these more sophisticated tests must always coincide with results of the tuning fork test. Because the authors rarely order a test of ET function in their routine, tympanometry and tests of acoustic reflex are performed only in the presence of an intact tympanic membrane.

Radiologic Evaluation

The imaging evaluation of patients with COM is not always necessary and should be adapted according to clinical findings. In the authors' routine, they dispense with further investigations in patients who present with dry, central perforations and good hearing. Patients with marginal perforations, small cholesteatomas, or an air-bone gap of more than 25 dB and who have no signs of complications are requested to get at least a screening lateral (Schiiller) plain view of the mastoid. This simple radiograph affords valuable information on the size and degree of pneumatization of the mastoid from which the surgeon can assess how much room exists between the external auditory meatus, the middle cranial fossa above, and the lateral sinus behind [7].

These pieces of information are helpful when the surgeon makes a decision to approach the antrum, either through the mastoid (outside-in) or through the attic (inside-out). Gross bony destruction can also be seen on films as rounded radiolucent osseous defects [7]. Large cholesteatomas, gross bony erosions, exuberant granulation tissue filling the external canal and preventing visualization of structures within the middle ear, chronic silent otitis media, unilateral marked hearing loss, suspicion of malignancy of the temporal bone, or presence of complications demand full radiologic assessment. For such conditions, CT scanning or MR imaging should be ordered. High-resolution CT scans are preferred to assess bony pathologic conditions, and this is the authors' most frequent choice. Granulation tissue, probably the most common cause of debris in the middle ear, is diagnosed on CT by its lack of bony erosion or ossicular displacement. Granulation tissue enhances intensely with gadolinium on T1-weighted images, thus differentiating it from cholesteatoma, which does not enhance with gadolinium.

Attic cholesteatomas are better appreciated through a coronal CT scan, where erosion of the lateral wall is almost pathognomonic of this condition. Acquired cholesteatomas arising from posterosuperior retraction pockets extend to the facial recess and are best seen on axial CT scans.

Regardless of the site of origin or etiologic basis, cholesteatomas do not enhance with gadolinium unless infiltrated by granulation tissue. This is a helpful differential diagnostic point that distinguishes these pathologic conditions from other retrotympanic masses, such as paragangliomas or schwannomas [8]. Cholesterol granuloma is a specific subtype of granulation tissue lined by fibrous connective tissue that can be present in any location in the temporal bone. The appearance on CT scanning of cholesterol granuloma in the tympanic cavity is nonspecific and similar to that of typical granulation tissue. MR imaging is diagnostic because extracellular methamoglobin within the lesion results in a bright signal in all spin-echo pulse sequence [8].

In practice, we always order a CT scan in cases associated with a cholesteatoma. It is important to develop a protocol while analyzing the sections otherwise the exam will be useless. Our checklist including at least nine steps is illustrated in Fig. 58.2.

Life-threatening complications of OM may develop inside or outside the limits of the temporal bone. Each complication follows a typical clinical course and should be addressed accordingly.

Preoperative Preparation

Almost every patient with COM presents at one time or another with purulent discharge and active infection in the ear. To maximize the rates of "take" for a graft, the infection should be brought under control at least 30 days before surgery is performed. This ideal situation is sometimes never achieved, even though the authors' clinic follows a preoperative protocol that contemplates every possible circumstance in an attempt to improve general conditions in the ear as much as possible before scheduling a case. Our protocols are summarized in Figs. 58.3 and 58.4.

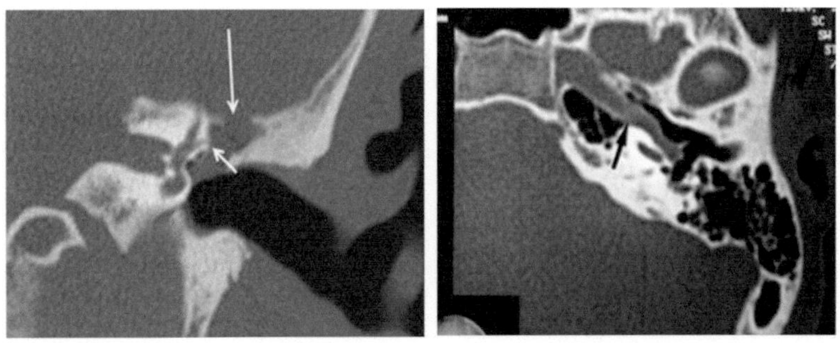

- ✓ Pneumatization of mastoid
- ✓ Course of the Facial nerve
- ✓ Ossicular chain status
- ✓ Tegmen Timpani & Dural deiscences
- ✓ Anatomical Variations
- ✓ Labyrinthine fistulas
- ✓ Carotid artery
- ✓ Jugular bulb
- ✓ Sigmois sinus
- ✓ Aeration of the protympanum
- ✓ Bone spur of Chaussé

Fig. 58.2 CT scan checklist in COM

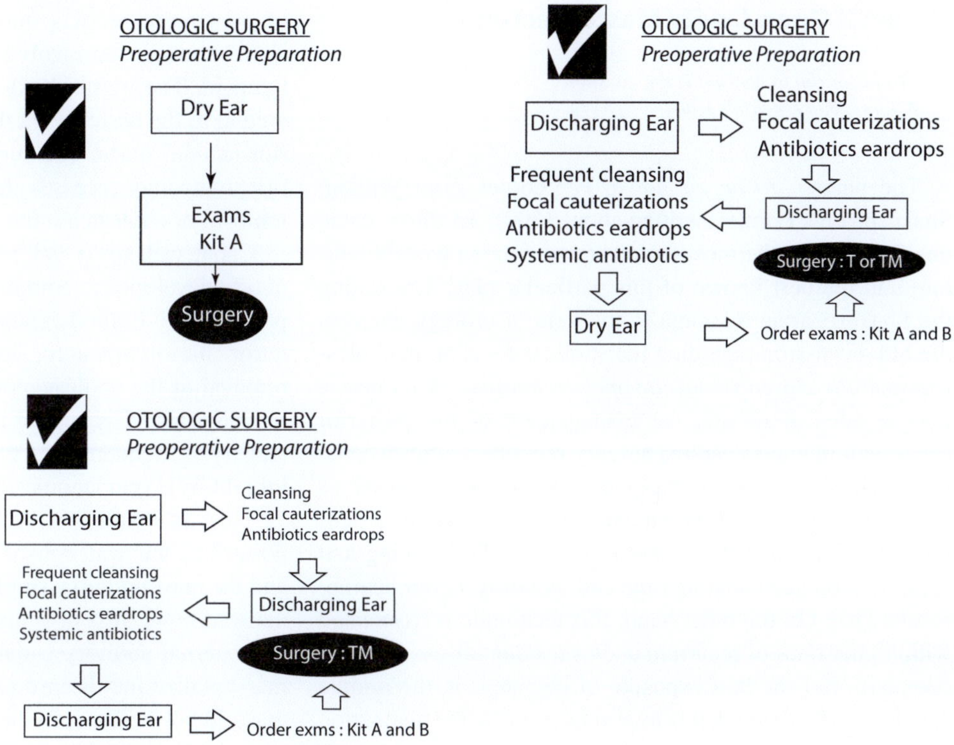

Fig. 58.3 Preoperative preparation of a dry ear, a discharging ear and a discharging ear refractory to treatment. (Adapted from Goycoolea MV, Paparella MM, Nissen RL: Atlas of Otologic Surgery. Philadelphia, WB Saunders, 1989) [9]

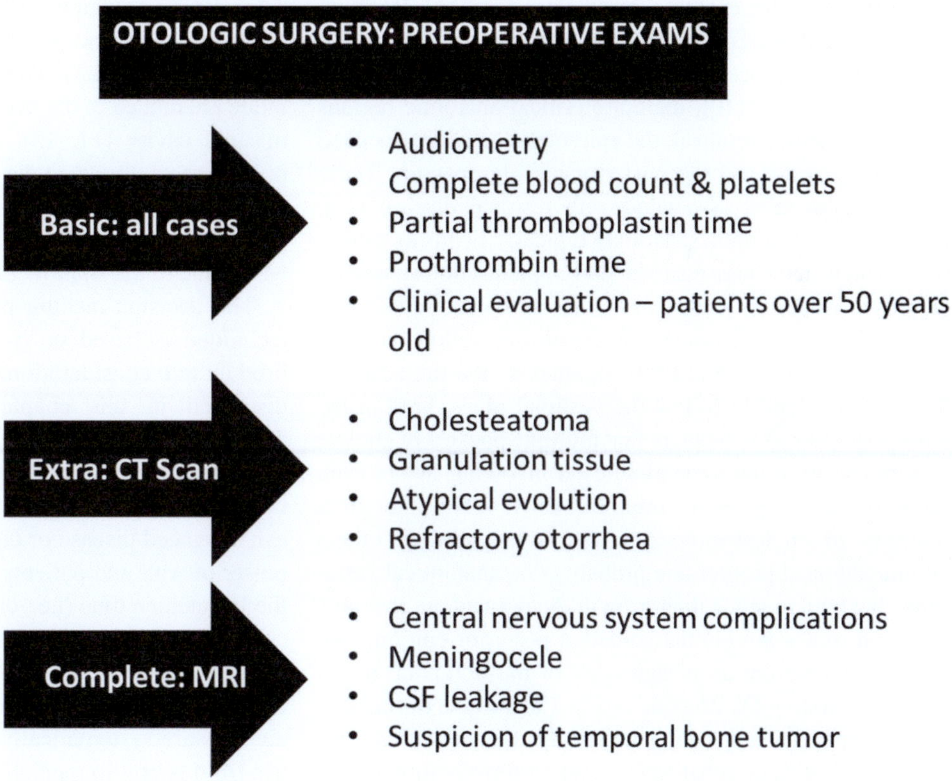

Fig. 58.4 Preoperative complementary exam—Kit A for all patients and Kit B for selected patients. (Adapted from Goycoolea MV, Paparella MM, Nissen RL: Atlas of Otologic Surgery. Philadelphia, WB Saunders, 1989) [9]

Closed X Open Cavity Mastoidectomy

"To be, or not to be-That is the question"
William Shakespeare's Hamlet

The phrase "*to be, or not to be*" comes from William Shakespeare's Hamlet (written about 1600), act three, scene one. It is one of the most famous quotations in world literature and the best known of this particular play. Translating the Shakespearian dilemma to the field of otology emerges the old discussion regarding the surgical decision in cholesteatoma: *the closed* versus *the open techniques!* After nearly five decades of debate, the management of the posterior canal wall in cholesteatoma surgery remains a controversial issue. The canal wall-up tympanomastoidectomy preserves the normal anatomy of the ear canal, thus avoiding the risk of bowl problems and the necessity for periodic cleaning and leading to reduced healing time and, possibly, better hearing results [10]. On the other hand, this technique is associated with higher rates of recurrent and/or residual disease since it does not offer the best exposure of key areas in the middle ear cleft. In this regard, it is important to make the distinction between recurrent and residual disease. The first situation is due to what we call uncontrolled pathogenesis (or not correctly managing the factors responsible for the development of the disease—for example, middle ear aeration). Residual pathology means basically that some disease was left behind during the first procedure (incomplete removal). As pointed out by Dornhoffer [10], there are critical anatomic regions for cholesteatoma removal: the epitympanum and associated supratubal recess and the posterior mesotympanum. These are the areas most associated with residual disease [11]. Primary acquired cholesteatomas typically begin as retraction pockets in the pars flaccida (epitympanic cholesteatoma) or posterosuperior pars tensa (mesotympanic cholesteatoma). The cholesteatomas in expansion follow sinuous routes, between mucosal folds, ligaments, and the ossicles. These routes tend to follow the vestigial plans, bred in the embryogenesis. It is frequent that multiple pockets of cholesteatoma occur in the same middle ear involving two or even three routes of growth simultaneously. While the great majority of cholesteatomas follows one pathway, others assume atypical progression probably due anatomical variations that tend to guide their growth. As pointed out the most common routes are (1) the so-called posterior epitympanic route initiates from an invagination of the Shrapnell membrane penetrating the Prussak's space (laterally to the neck of the malleus) and expanding anteriorly toward the anterior epitympanum (supratubal recess) and posteriorly through the aditus to the antrum and mastoid. It can also reach the posterior mesotympanum by descending through the floor of the Prussak's space into the posterior space of Von Tröeltsch; (2) posterior mesotympanic route: the postero-superior portion of *pars tensa* retracts into the mesotympanum, forming a cholesteatoma sac involving the facial recess and the sinus tympani. The mastoid extension of these cholesteatomas is medial to the ossicles via the posterior isthmus and the inferior incudal space. The surgical inaccessibility of the posterior tympanic recesses frequently hinders the complete removal of cholesteatomas located in these spaces [12].

Canal wall-up (CWU) surgery, especially in cases with poorly developed zygomatic root cells and a low tegmen, can provide very limited exposure of the epitympanum and posterior mesotympanum, leading to blind and piecemeal removal of the cholesteatoma which contributes to the high recitative rate. Because of these short comings, second-stage surgery is frequently recommended 9–12 months after the initial CWU tympanomastoidectomy [10].

The canal wall-down (CWD) technique remove the bony posterior canal wall consolidating the external auditory canal and the mastoid into a single common cavity often known as mastoid bowl. It is also necessary to expand the opening of the external auditory canal (meatoplasty) in order to better marsupialize the disease allowing the full inspection of the mastoid bowl. The epitympanum, cog, and supratubal recess are widely exposed, facilitating complete removal of the cholesteatoma sac and lowering the recurrence rate to 5–10% [11, 13]. Taking the canal wall down to the level of the facial ridge deals adequately with facial recess disease and affords improved, but by no means complete, view of the sinus tympani [10] (Fig. 58.5). The main disadvantages of this technique are related to the necessity for periodic cleaning of the mastoid cavity [11, 13]. Subsequent bowl infections can occur, especially when the cavity becomes wet, causing significant lifestyle changes, particularly in the pediatric age group [13]. In addition, the hearing results are frequently worse due to the shallow middle ear cleft [11, 13].

The decision-making process of choosing one or other technique is based on a series of issues which must be brought into consideration. Some of them have already been discussed in this chapter and can be summarized in Table 58.2.

In our clinical routine, we almost always decide for the open technique in cases with sclerotic mastoid, only hearing ear, advanced disease or complications, gross erosion of the posterior wall and patients with well-known malfunction of the Eustachian tube (i.e., cleft palate, Down syndrome).

An open-cavity mastoidectomy can be performed beginning either laterally or medially. The classic simple mastoidectomy begins by removing the lateral mastoid cortex. The air cells are systematically removed, and dissection continues from lateral to medial. First, the sigmoid sinus is identified and skeletonized, then Körner's septum is removed, the mastoid antrum is entered, and the short process of the incus (when present) and horizontal semicircular canal are located. Because it begins laterally at the cortex, such operations are

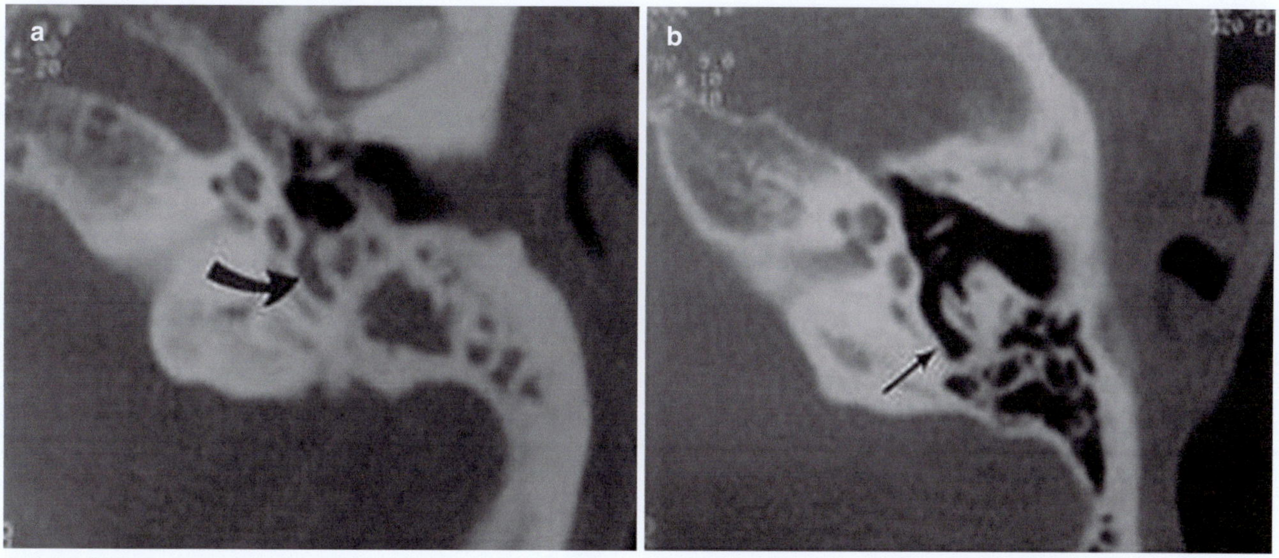

Fig. 58.5 Axial CT section showing (**a**) a very deep sinus tympani filled with pathologic tissue (bolded arrow) and (**b**) a clean sinus tympani (arrow). It should be noticed that in both sections, the sinus tympani penetrates deep below the vertical segment of the facial nerve precluding a the surgical view through conventional techniques. (The CT sections belong to Dr. Silvio Caldas' collection – Recife/Brazil.)

Table 58.2 Decision-making chart for choosing the surgical approach in COM

	CWD	CWU
Aggressive disease—complications	++++	–
Pars tensa cholesteatoma	+++	+
COM without cholesteatoma	–	++++
Recurrent disease	+++	+
Children	+++	++
Bad general health	++++	–
Access to medical care	?	?
Possibility of second stage	+	+++
Sclerotic mastoid on CT	+++	+
Pneumatized mastoid (CT)	+	+++
Dead ear	++++	++
Low or dehiscent tegmen tympani	+++	+
Cholesteatoma contralateral ear	+++	+
Atelectasis	+++	+
Risk group (cleft palate, down)	+++	+
Only hearing ear	+++	+
Water sports	+	+++
Profession depending on hearing	+	+++
Surgeon experience	?	?

Adapted from Costa SS, Silva MNL, Silva DP. Mastoidectomia Aberta e Fechada: Indicações e Técnicas. Pró-ORL 4(1):123–150 [14]

often referred to as *cortical mastoidectomies*, *outside-in mastoidectomies*, or *lateral-to-medial-mastoidectomies*.

Mastoidectomies can also be performed from medial to lateral. After elevating the tympanic membrane, the lateral process of the malleus is identified and used as a landmark. The bone is progressively removed in the attic. The incudomallear joint and the dural plate are identified and dissection progresses sequentially toward the aditus, antrum, and mastoid. This approach can be referred to as an *inside-out mastoidectomy, subcortical mastoidectomy*, or *medial-to-lateral mastoidectomy*.

Once we have decided in the preoperative evaluation that the best option for a particular patient is the open technique, we always employ the inside-out or subcortical mastoidectomy (which will be described in detail in the next paragraphs).

Surgical Decision

Preoperative evaluation remains the cornerstone in the determination of an appropriate surgical procedure for patients with otologic disease. Still, as every surgeon understands from experience, surgical exposure of pathologic tissue usually provides a better and more complete understanding about the extension of the disease.

It is extremely important to point out that once we have decided preoperatively for a CWD, we perform *from the very beginning* the inside-out technique. The final result may be very similar to the traditional open cavities, but there is one big difference: the technique includes a wide canalplasty and the removal of the postero-superior aspect of the wall as an early step. In the other hand, when we decide for a CWU procedure, depending on the surgical findings, we may have to reorient the procedure converting a closed into an open cavity. We try to avoid this situation because whenever it happens the final result is a bigger cavity since a complete mastoidectomy has already been created at this stage. As a rule, the CWU involves an ample drilling of the mastoid in order to identify important landmarks. To avoid a constricted dissection that prevents adequate angular visualization of

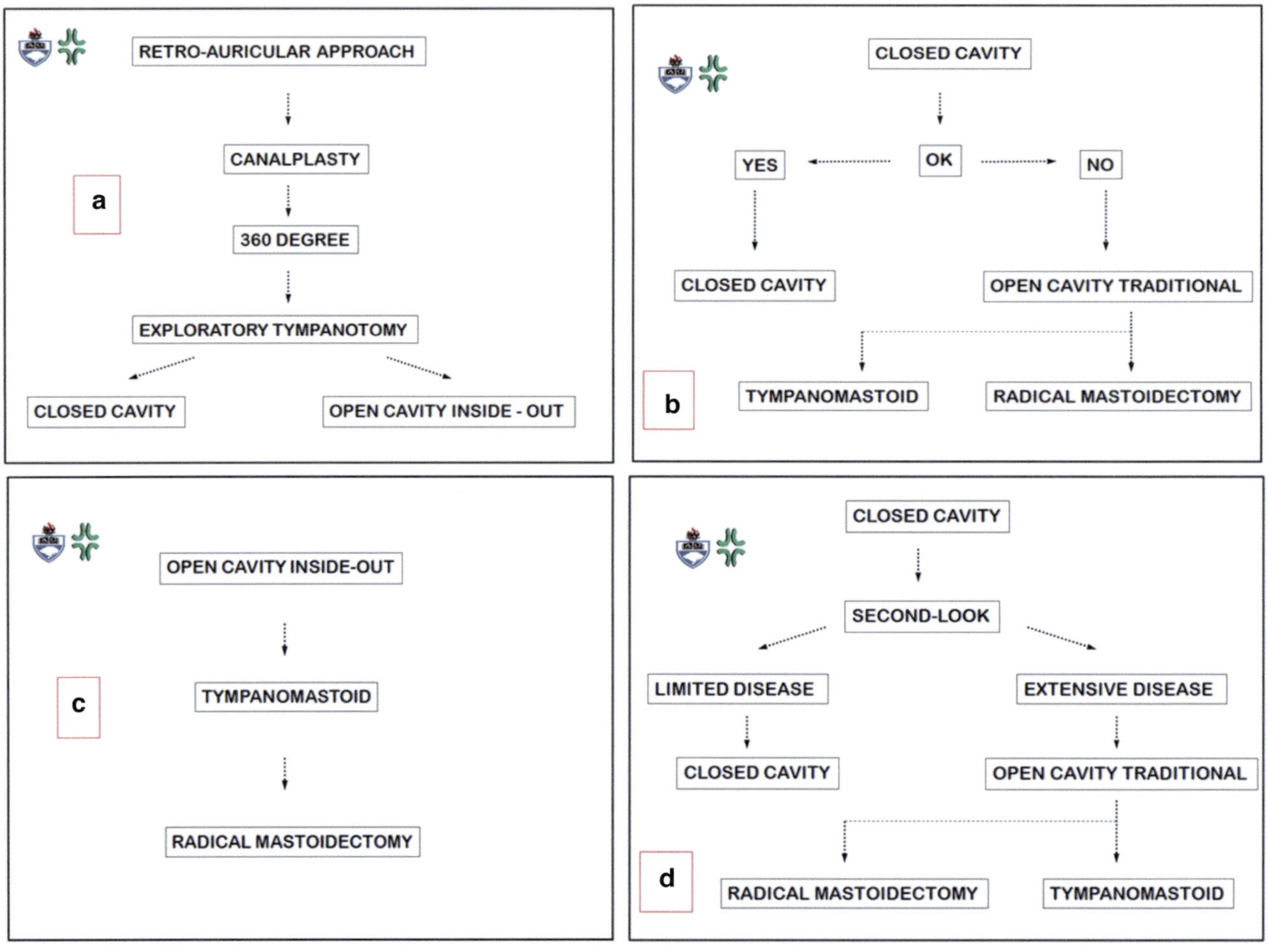

Fig. 58.6 Surgical decision-making algorithm: (**a**) Retroauricular approach is followed by an ample canaplasty with a 360° view of the TM. The exploratory tympanotomy will dictate the further steps: closed or open technique. (**b**) If the option was a closed technique during the procedure it may be converted to an traditional open cavity (radical or not). (**c**) If the preoperative decision was for a CWD, the inside-out technique is employed and the middle ear reconstruction will depend on the surgical findings. (**d**) After a CWU, the findings during the second-look will dictate whether the posterior wall will be lowered or not

deep-lying structures (and to safely accomplish further steps of the dissection, i.e., the facial recess opening) a wide cortical removal should be first completed. The cortex in unroofed from the posterior canal back and beyond the sigmoid sinus and at an adequate distance into the mastoid tip [15]. In the process, the surgeon may eventually open areas in the mastoid (i.e. the tip) that are not involved by disease. The confluence of these "innocent" spaces and other areas where pathology was actually encountered may result in an undesired larger cavity. Figure 58.6 summarizes our surgical decision-making algorithm.

Surgical Technique

Patient

The hair may be shaved, depending on the approach, up to 3 cm above and behind the ear. The skin is cleansed with an iodine-based soap, rinsed with water, and sprayed with tincture of benzoin. A sterile plastic adhesive drape is applied. The patient is placed on the table with his or her head at the foot of the operating table. He or she must be securely taped to the table to prevent slipping when the table is tipped from side to side. The patient's head should be as near to the surgeon as possible, and the table is usually placed in a few degrees of Trendelenburg and rolled slightly toward the surgeon. It is very useful to prepare a side table where the surgeon may rest his arm during the drilling.

Anesthesia

Some of these surgeries can be performed as outpatient procedures with the patient under local anesthesia. The authors systematically use general anesthesia in small children, extremely anxious patients, or when a great deal of work on bone is anticipated.

Selection of the Approach and Infiltration

The key to success in otologic surgery is to operate on a wide, clean, clear, dry field. In this regard, selection of the approach and good, effective hemostasis is mandatory. A local anesthetic with vasoconstrictor is used, usually 2% lidocaine with 1:100,000 epinephrine. A syringe that affords easy injection is preferred (carpule or an insulin syringe). A 27-gauge or 30-gauge needle is used. A nasal or Lempert speculum is used for initial injections in the inferior, superior, and posterior quadrants.

The infiltration should be done slowly to avoid formation of blebs or maceration of the canal skin. When it is well accomplished, the surgeon can see anesthetic blanching and "dissecting" in the skin of the external canal, from the point of injection to the tympanic annulus. Additional injections are performed along the postauricular sulcus and the incisura auris, with care not to inject too anteroinferiorly or too deeply, to avoid anesthesia of the facial nerve Three approaches to the middle ear and mastoid can be used: (1) transcanal, (2) endaural, and (3) post auricular. Among them, the authors consider the post auricular approach the most eclectic and comfortable because, with only one or two adaptations, it can fit any unexpected situation encountered during an exploration of the middle ear. The incision spans from the helical rim to the mastoid tip and is well hidden in the post auricular region. It rarely causes any visible scarring. The incision should be about 1 cm behind the post auricular crease to avoid unsightly deepening of the sulcus, which can occur when incisions are placed directly in the crease. The incision is more posterior in young children to avoid a superficial facial nerve near the mastoid tip. The incision is made through the skin with a scalpel. An avascular plane is elevated anteriorly toward the external auditory canal just below the subdermal fat, leaving a layer of loose areolar tissue on the temporalis fascia. This plane is developed down to the mastoid tip. The attachments of the sternocleidomastoid muscle can be separated from the mastoid tip for increased exposure [16]. This dissection can be accomplished with the unipolar cautery leaving the periostium in place and delineating the posterior semicircle of the external auditory canal. A periosteal flap is then tailored to fit the surgical plan: if the CT scan have revealed an esclerotic mastoid, the flap may be triangular and anteriorly based. In those cases where the mastoid is expected to be drilled down to the tip, the flap is rectangular and inferiorly based. The reason for this modification is that at the end of the procedure the flap is returned to its original position filling in partially the surgical defect and decreasing the final size of the mastoid bowl (Fig. 58.7).

Exposure and Removal of the Temporalis Fascia

The post-auricular incision extends up into the region of the temporalis fascia. A self-retaining retractor is inserted, and by lifting it up, one can lift the scalp off the temporalis muscle. The loose areolar tissue is then set apart from the true fascia through sharp and blunt dissection. Local anesthetic is injected under the fascia to elevate it from the muscle, and with the scalpel the fascia is sectioned in a roughly ovoid shape and harvested. After being harvested, the fascia is spread on a polytetrafluoroethylene (PTFE) block, with the undersurface upward, and any adherent muscle is removed. The PTFE block is placed under an electric lamp, and after approximately 10 min, the fascia is dry.

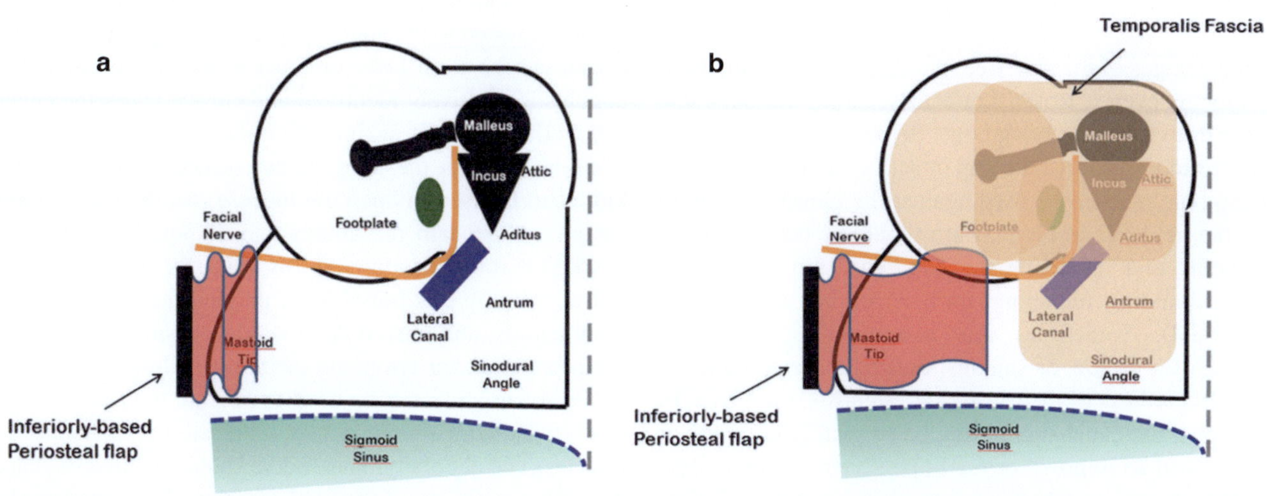

Fig. 58.7 (**a**) The periostium of the mastoid cortex is elevated as an inferiorly based flap and held in position by the self-retaining retractors. (**b**) At the end of the procedure, the flap returns to its original position filling in partially the surgical defect and decreasing the size of the mastoid bowl

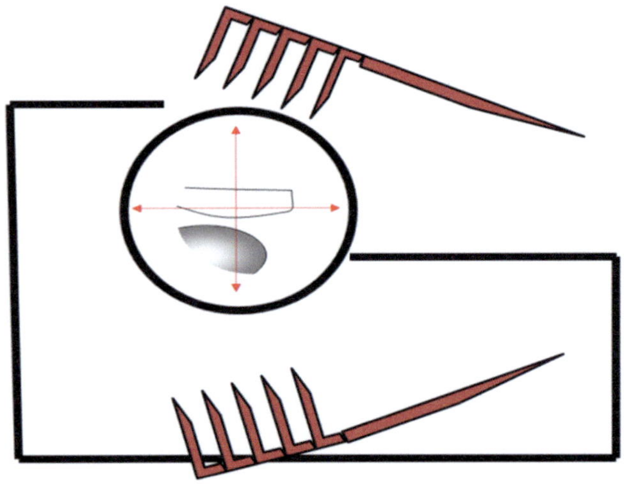

Fig. 58.8 After repositioning of the self-retaining retractors the complete circumference of the external canal comes into view

Incisions in the Canal

After the elevation of the periosteal flap, the bony landmarks of the mastoid cortex (spine of Henle, *linea temporalis,* and cribiform area) are identified. Attention is directed to the posterior margin of the external auditory canal, and the skin is gently elevated loose for a few millimeters. A number 11 blade knife is used in a straight angle to incise the skin from behind entering the lumen of the canal. A small Köerner flap is created and the self-retaining retractor repositioned. At this point, the canal will become completely into view, and the first incision is extended superiorly, inferioly, and anteriorly around the 360° of the bony canal (Fig. 58.8).

Elevation of the Meatal Flap

With the edges of the skin free, the surgeon uses a duckbill elevator or even a Rosen knife to separate the skin flap gently from the underlying bone. Separation must be slow and careful to preserve the flap intact. A suction tip (finger off the hole) should be used against the elevator blade to keep the field free of blood. Care should be taken to avoid suctioning and damaging the flap. The skin is elevated evenly, avoiding tunneling, until it reaches the annulus (Fig. 58.8). Sometimes this dissection is obstructed because of a narrow or sinuous, twisted external auditory canal. Regardless of the cause (e.g., stenosis, exostosis, or osteomas), the canal should first be surgically enlarged or straightened to improve or facilitate access to the middle ear. We always prefer to perform the canalplasty before entering the middle ear.

Canalplasty

After the flap has been elevated and the osseous canal exposed, the canal is drilled lateral to the annulus in a way that allows better exposure of the annulus and associated mesotympanum. When an anterior bump is present, the anterior osseous canal may be drilled, allowing better exposure of the anterior mesotympanum. Attention must be exercised to avoid entering the temporomandibular joint anteriorly or damaging the skin flap with the burr. For such, after the elevation of the flap, it is carefully folded and protected from the rotating burrs with a round shield fashioned previously with the external packing of the catgut suture. The shield is interposed between the flap and the burr protecting the first of being accidentally ripped off from the sulcus by the action of the high-speed burr. An extraprotection is to switch to a diamond burr when the drilling gets close to the flap and the residual TM. During the posterior canalplasty, the surgeon should watch for an anterior and more laterally located descendent portion of the mastoid segment of the facial nerve. During the course of posterior canalplasty, very often a few mastoid cells are opened, thus allowing a first glimpse of pathologic conditions in the mastoid. In fact we always over drill the postero-superior aspect of the canal opening the cells located lateral to the antrum. A prominent tympanosquamous and tympanomastoid suture lines are also taken off at this point to increase exposure of the pars flaccida [10].

When the drilling is complete, the field should be rinsed with saline solution to wash out bone chips and so that the surgeon will have a panoramic 360° view of the tympanic membrane (Fig. 58.9).

Entering the Middle Ear

After the canalplasty is complete, the tympanomeatal flap is further elevated to the anulus. At this point, greater magnification can be used (10× or 16×) in the microscope. The annulus is positively identified and elevated with the elevator, working always against the bone. After the annulus is lifted away from the bony sulcus, a needle or the sickle knife can be used to open the mucosa, entering the middle ear always beneath the anulus and, if possible, inferiorly toward the round window. At this point, the duckbill can be passed through this initial hole, pressed firmly against the bony anulus, and moved downward to liberate completely the posteroinferior tympanic membrane. Upward, a needle or the sickle knife can be used to liberate the posterosuperior tympanic membrane gently, with care not to disturb the ossicles. The chorda tympani nerve should be identified and carefully moved out of the field of vision. As pointed out by Dornhoffer, this technique involves extensive drilling in

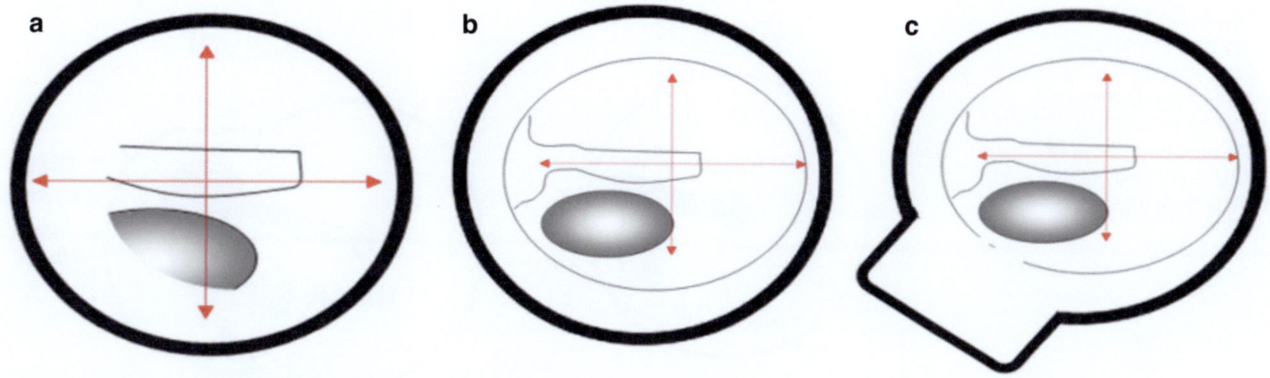

Fig. 58.9 (**a**) TM view before the canalplasty. (**b**) After the canalplasty a 360° view of the tympanic membrane with one position of the microscope. (**c**) During the canalplasty, a preliminar notch is created in the postero-superior aspect of the canal opening the cells located lateral to the antrum

close proximity and just lateral to the head of the malleus and the body of the incus, it is necessary to visualize the incudostapedial joint and the integrity of the lenticular process of the incus as an initial step. Except in cases of very limited retraction pockets, the incudostapedial joint is disarticulated to avoid trauma to the inner ear from the subsequent drilling [10]. The TM elevated up to the malleus. It is then grasped with the alligator forceps and peeled off the malleus neck exposing the lateral process, which will serve as a pointer to the following bony removal of the scutum. At this point, the opening of the cholesteatoma sac will be brought into view (in a case of pars flaccida cholesteatoma) or exfoliated keratin will be identified in the posterosuperior quadrant (pars tensa cholesteatoma).

Atticotomy

The superior aspect of the bony canal is carefully removed with the drill. The atticotomy or amount of bone removed can be small, medium, or large to facilitate exposure of the pathologic conditions at hand. This may be done to allow better exposure of the ossicles (i.e., the neck and head of the malleus and the incudomalleolar joint) or to follow mesotympanic disease extending toward the aditus ad antrum. Anatomic dimensions of the attic and its parts vary, and pathologic conditions certainly can exist in the attic, contributing to obstruction at this site. Anatomic or pathologic obstruction of the attic or aditus ad antrum results in pathologic tissues that can occupy the mastoid, even with preservation of normal or near-normal findings in the middle ear. This is particularly true for pars flaccida cholesteatomas. When disease extends to the attic, the authors initially follow it, increasing the size of the atticotomy in an attempt to reach the end of the pathologic tissue. Working laterally to the ossicular chain, the bony removal continues until the incudomallear joint is perfectly visualize.

The next structure to be positively identified is the tegmen tympani or middle cranial fossa dural plate. It is important to know is that the tegmen at the lateral external canal frequently is more inferior than the more medial tegmen at the level of the epitympanum, so care must be taken to avoid injury to the dura laterally. Preoperative CT helps to predict the height of the tegmen on the coronal view [10]. The final objective of the atticotomy is to bring into view the following landmarks: head of the malleus, the body of the incus, and the tegmen (Figs. 58.10 and 58.11). These structures are frequently covered by the matrix of the cholesteatoma. When the disease is limited in this area and can be peel off the ossicles no further dissection is necessary, the surgical defect can be reconstructed using sculptured cortical bone chips, bone pate, or bone wax.

Retrograde Antrostomy

Frequently, though, the cholesteatoma penetrates posteriorly from Prussak's space (following the embryologic course of the saccus medius), passing through the superior incudal space, and then traversing the aditus ad antrum to enter deeply into the mastoid. In this situation, the fundus of the cyst cannot be reached through atticotomy. An inside-out antrostomy in sclerotic bones is the next step in the procedure. For such, the dissection should proceed backward laterally to the ossicular chain and following and in close contact with the dural plate. The next landmarks to be identified are the short process of the incus medially and a few millimeters bellow it the solid bone of the dome of the lateral semicircular canal (Fig. 58.12a). After opening a few more cells the final objective of the antrostomy has been achieved: the identification of the antrum itself (filled with cholesteatoma) the lateral semicircular canal and the dural plate. It should be emphasized that the inside-out technique offers a very safe approach to the antrum. It immediately exposes

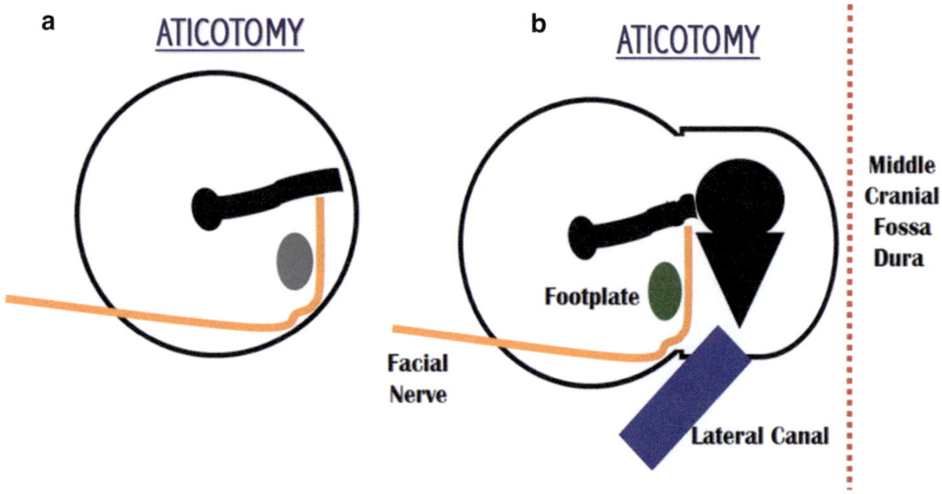

Fig. 58.10 (**a**) The mesotympanic view before the atticotomy. (**b**) The final objective of the atticotomy has been achieved: identification of the head of the malleus, the body of the incus, and the tegmen tympani

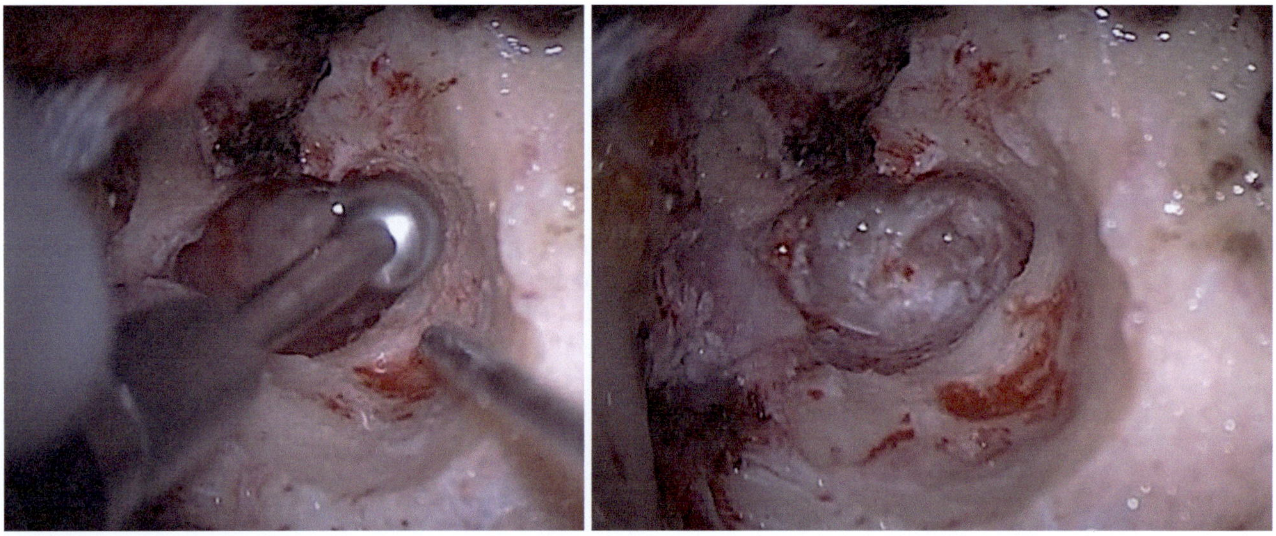

Fig. 58.11 Surgical view. Left picture: Drilling Chaussé spur bone. Right picture: Atticotomy was performed

and thereby allows protection of important structures that may otherwise be subject to injury. First, the drilling is carried out lateral to the ossicular chain interposing the head of the malleus and the body off the incus between the burrs and the facial nerve (the possibility of an acoustic trauma is minimized since the incudostapedial joint has already been disarticulated as an earlier step). Second, the most flagrant landmark of the antrum is the dome of the lateral semicircular canal which protects the second genu of the facial nerve (located slightly medially and inferiorly) from an inadvertent and catastrophic drilling accident (Figs. 58.12b and 58.13).

As the antrum is widely opened, the extent of the cholesteatoma can be appreciated. The goal is to remove only the bone necessary to expose the back edge of the sac, and many times a complete mastoidectomy is not necessary. In a sclerotic mastoid, the surgeon may frequently find the cholesteatoma extending only to the antrum, so minimal drilling is needed. After drilling the bony bridge over the aditus, the three upper compartments of the middle ear are completely identified: the attic (with the incudo-mallear joint), the transitional aditus, and the antrum (with the lateral semi-circular canal). The lateral and posterior wall of the epitympanum must be removed until the tegmen mastoid or tegmen tympani are continuous. The transition between the middle ear and mastoid must be smooth and uninterrupted.

At this point the tip of the posterior wall is still high and with the malleus and incus in place prevent a better view of the tympanic segment of the facial nerve (Fig. 58.14).

Mastoidectomy

Once this step is accomplished, it opens a large and safe two-way avenue. The first way goes (straight) all the way to the sino-dural (Citelli's) angle; the second makes a right angle turn toward the bottom of the mastoid (Fig. 58.15). The cho-

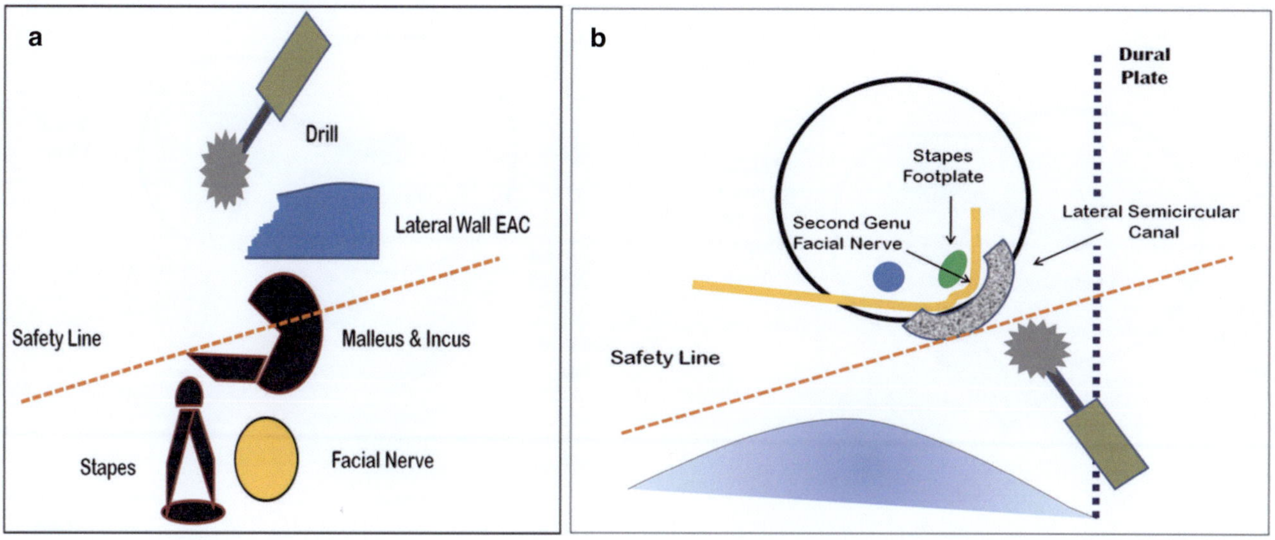

Fig. 58.12 The inside-out mastoidectomy offers protection to the facial nerve. (**a**) Coronal section showing the interposition of the ossicular mass between the burr and the tympanic segment of the facial nerve. (**b**) Axial section of the antrostomy with the lateral semicircular shielding the second genu of the facial nerve from the rotating burr

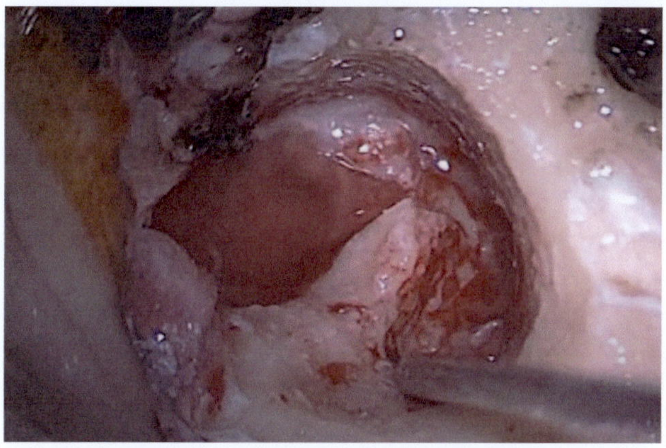

Fig. 58.13 Drilling aditus until reach the antrum

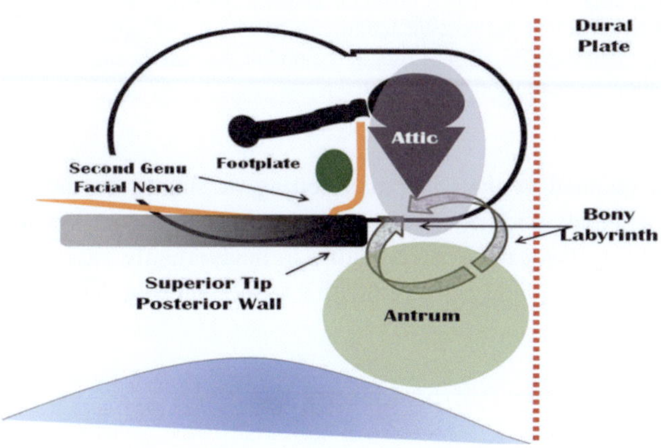

Fig. 58.14 The three upper compartments of the middle ear are completely identified: the attic (with the incudo-mallear joint), the transitional aditus, and the antrum (with the lateral semi-circular canal). The tip of the posterior wall is still high blocking a better view of the tympanic facial nerve

lesteatoma sac is followed back as posteriorly and inferiorly as necessary or until normal air cells are encountered [10]. Along the way, any cell filled with cholesterol granuloma should be explored and suctioned. Granulation tissue is also frequently found at this point either around the cholesteatoma or infiltrating the posterior wall. It should be also removed from the irregular bone which is then smoothed with the diamond burr. The amount of bone removal in the mastoid is dependent of how deep the disease penetrates into the bone: Conceptually, we classify the degree of mastoid exenteration in three levels: I: antrum; II: mid-mastoid; and III: tip (Fig. 58.16).

When the pathology in the mastoid has been completely delineated attention is directed back to the middle ear: first, the incus is disarticulated from the malleus and removed. With the malleus nippler, the head of the malleus is also removed gaining access to the medial wall of the attic (frequently lined by the cholesteatoma matrix). After drilling anteriorly and parallel to the dural plate, the anterior attic (supratubal recess) is widely exposed and cleaned of any residual disease. It is important to dissect the dural plate all the way to the confluence of the anterior wall of the external auditory canal where a 90° angle is created and then rounded off (Figs. 58.17 and 58.18). During this step, the tegmen tympani should be checked for areas of bony defects. Small or large dehiscence is a common finding and may be either congenital or consequence of the bone erosion power of cholesteatoma and/or granulation tissue. Most of them are not clinically relevant and should be left alone. Larger areas especially when associated with dural herniation should be immediately corrected. As we have mentioned before, the roof of the middle ear and the mastoid must be smooth and uninterrupted.

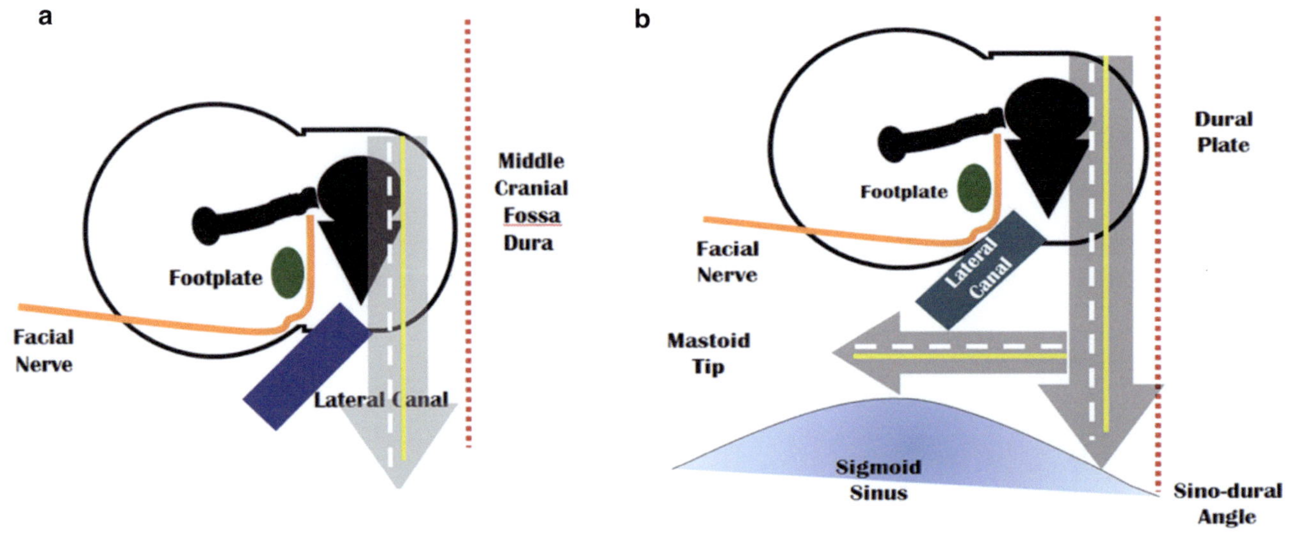

Fig. 58.15 (**a**) After opening the antrum two landmarks are identified: the lateral semicircular canal and the dural plate. (**b**) The lateral canal shields de second genu of the facial nerve and with the dural plate opens an two-arms avenue: the first leads to the sino-dural angle; and the second contours the lateral canal and continues toward the tip of the mastoid

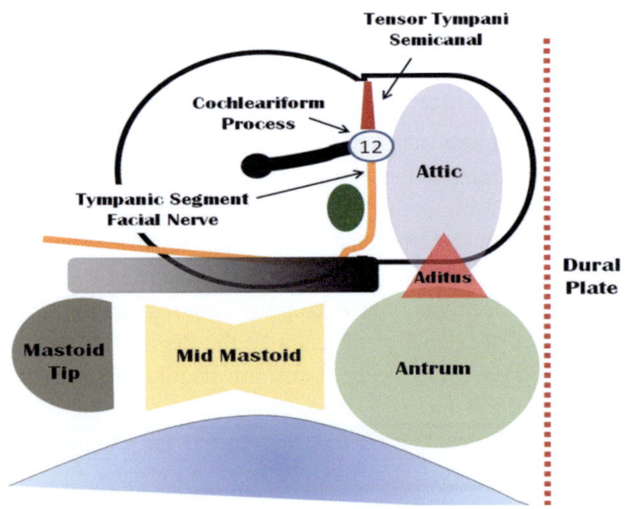

Fig. 58.16 The three upper compartments of the middle ear are completely identified: the attic (with the incudo-mallear joint), the transitional aditus and the antrum (with the lateral semi-circular canal). The tip of the posterior wall is still high blocking a better view of the tympanic facial nerve

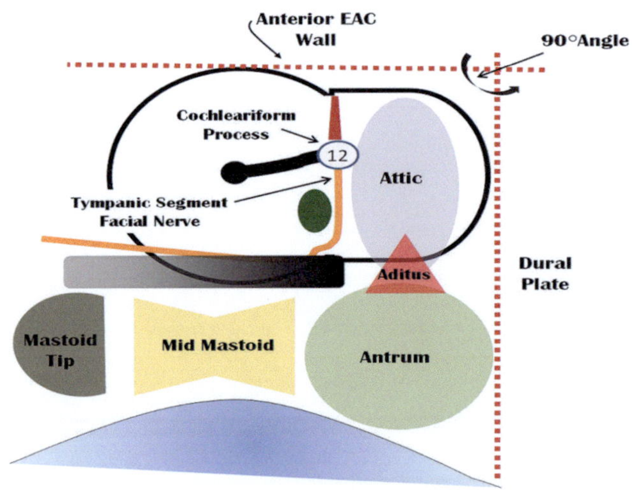

Fig. 58.17 Dural plate is dissected all the way to the confluence of the anterior wall of the external auditory canal where a 90° angle is created and then rounded off. The roof of the middle ear and the mastoid must follow a smooth and uninterrupted plane

The bottom of the cholesteatoma sac is then identified, and dissected with the aid of a Rosen knife and a cotton ball impregnated with saline solution. The dissection progresses cautiously from posterior to anterior with the removal of the matrix. Any sign of a perilymphatic fistula in one the semicircular canals (especially the lateral one) should be searched for and, if positively identified, gently handle. In this circumstance, matrix should be left over the site to protect (even if eventual removal is planned) while the remainder of the ear is cleared of disease. This protects the area from subsequent bone dust and saline irrigation. If the removal of the matrix is planned at that operative setting, it should be the last maneuver performed prior completing the operation and closing the ear. When a fistula is inadvertently exposed it should be quickly covered with a tissue seal (Fig. 58.19).

Exploratory Tympanotomy

Next, attention is directed to the most superior aspect of the posterior wall. Bone is drilled partially decreasing its height only to make possible an angled vision of the mesotympanum.

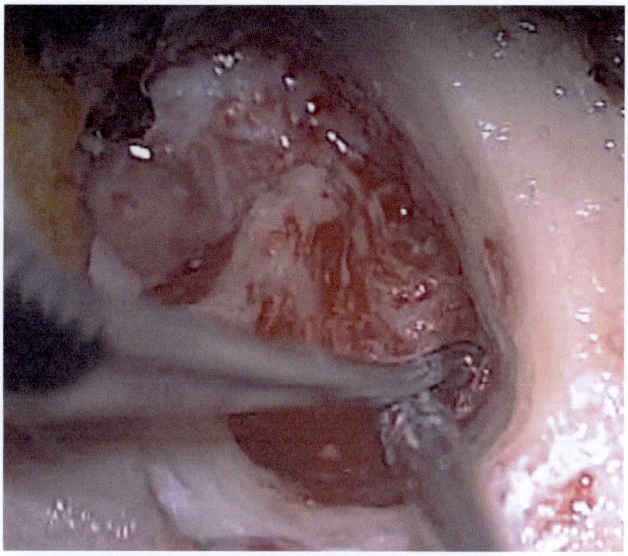

Fig. 58.18 Surgical view—mastoidectomy was performed

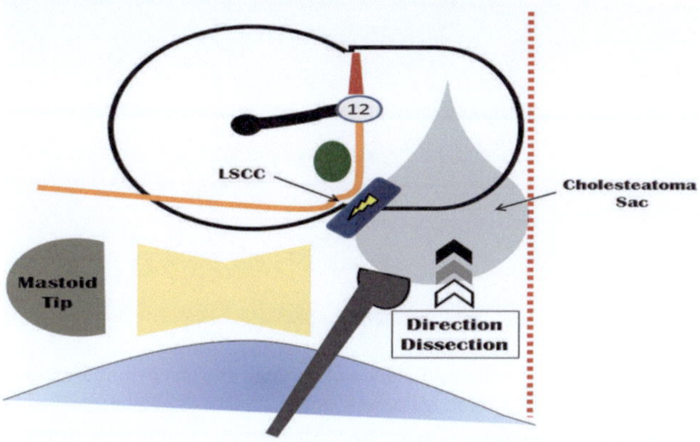

Fig. 58.19 During the removal of the cholesteatoma, the medial wall of the sac should be palpated to detect any bony erosion especially on the dome of the lateral semicircular canal. In this circumstance, matrix should be left over the site to protect (even if eventual removal is planned,) while the remainder of the ear is cleared of disease

The dissection is then directed toward the middle ear, beginning along the superoanterior mesotympanum by exposing the semicanal of the tensor tympani muscle, the remaining malleus and the cochleariform process. Among all the anatomical landmarks of the middle ear, the authors consider the cochleariform process of utmost importance. Its resistance to pathologic aggression, its relationship with the malleus, and its central position in the middle ear cleft makes it a readily identifiable structure. When the cochleariform process is spotted, one can determine the position of the geniculate ganglion (just medial to the cochleariform process) and, through a craniocaudal line, divide the middle ear into anterior and posterior compartments. The anterior compartment is related to the promontory (anteroinferiorly) and with the protympanum and, some millimeters ahead, with the tympanic orifice of the Eustachian Tube. The carotid canal is found more anteriorly at a minimum distance of 6.6 mm. The posterior compartment is related to the tympanic portion of the facial nerve, pointing to the path to its second genu and, posteroinferiorly, to the area of the windows.

The facial nerve should be approached with extreme care because it is one of the most vulnerable structures of the temporal bone, especially when there is a dehiscence of the facial canal on the side toward the middle ear. The reported incidence of dehiscence of the facial canal seen surgically is 7.0–11.4% [17] and seen histologically is from 15 to 74% [18, 19]. The most common site of dehiscence is the area near the oval window, where the nerve may prolapse over the stapedial footplate. As pointed out by Mutlu et al. [20] in these not-so-rare circumstances, a cholesteatoma or a mass of granulation tissue can distort the normal anatomy of the nerve. Careless manipulation of the disease can elevate the nerve out of its normal bed and produces additional stretching injuries. From the cochleariform process, the dissection is carried along the promontory and toward the protympanum in a sheetlike fashion, dissecting toward the hypotympanum and ultimately ending at the posterior tympanum and the superior mesotympanum near the stapes [21]. The protympanum is carefully examined, and sites of obstructions are looked for. These may include bony prominences in various regions of the middle ear, thickened mucosa or granulation tissue in the middle ear, and disease of the anterior tympanic membrane or anterior mesotympanum, such as tympanosclerosis. The contour of the promontory is observed for obstruction at this level of the mesotympanum. The round window, sinus tympani, and facial recess are also assessed. Any loculated collection of fluid should be suctioned, and granulation tissue strategically located within the middle ear cleft must be approached with care and, if possible, removed. Care should be exercised while removing disease from the protympanum and area near the orifice of the ET because they are in close relationship to the carotid canal. Costa and colleagues [22] showed that the artery may be exposed in this segment, either congenitally or secondary to disease. Even when not exposed, the mean thickness of the bony canal has been measured at 0.18 mm [22]. To avoid this major catastrophe, the area near the canal should always be approached with anticipation, and erosions should be searched for through gentle palpation with a blunt instrument. This recommendation also holds true during exploration of the hypotympanum. According to Overton and Ritte [23]' and Mutlu et al. [20], in 6% of temporal bones, a jugular bulb is found lying above the level of the inferior tympanic anulus. The jugular bulb may be dehiscent and more vulnerable to injury during the dissection of cholesteatoma from hypotympanic or retrofacial cells or even during the elevation of a tympanomeatal flap [24, 25].

Fig. 58.20 Photo of the so-called posterior recesses of the mesotympanum

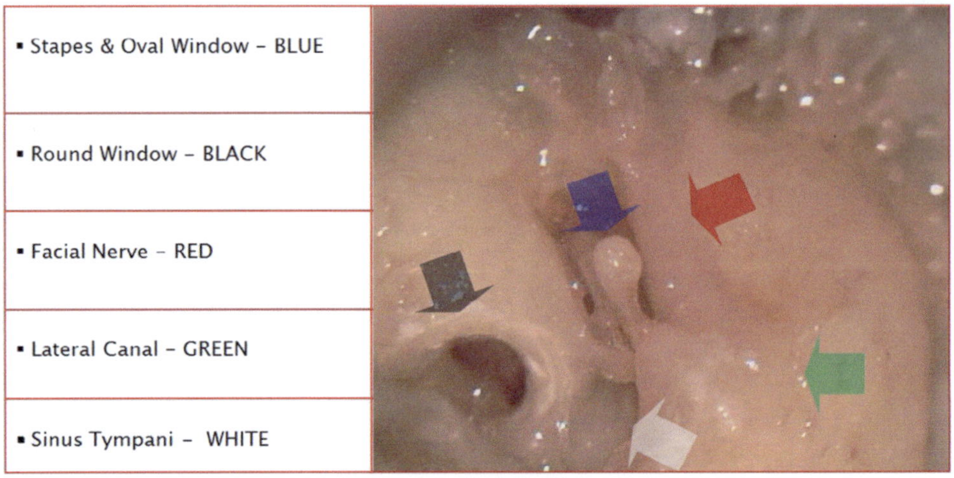

When the posterosuperior quadrant is reached, the remaining ossicular chain comes to the attention of the surgeon. In the few cases where the chain is intact, ossicular mobility is evaluated by mobilizing the long process of the malleus with the duckbill elevator or joint knife while observing changes in the light reflex near the round window. Testing the mobility of the stapes includes palpation of the incudostapedial joint, the head of the stapes, and the footplate. The curet is employed over the posterosuperior margin of the canal to enhance exposure of the stapes joint and the oval window. For such a procedure, a sharp curet should be used, with gentle but firm movements from inside to outside and from the 12 to 6 o'clock position to avoid accidental dislocation of the ossicles [9, 26]. The drill with a small cutting burr can also be helpful during this step. When the surgeon can identify the joint, oval window, stapedial tendon, and tympanic segment of the facial nerve, removal of bone is complete. After longstanding OM with effusion, the tympanic membrane and the malleus is medialized. In these circumstances, the tensor tympani tendon is severed with the joint knife, and the malleus is gently lateralized to open up the mesotympanic space (Fig. 58.6a and b).

During this exploration, both the oval and the round window should be thoroughly inspected. The surgeon should note whether the round window membrane is visible or is in a covered position in the niche, as well as distinguish the membrane from mucosal folds in the niche (so-called "false membrane). Any pathologic tissue over the windows should be meticulously addressed and, if possible, removed. The integrity of the round window membrane and the footplate should never be jeopardized during a first-stage procedure [9, 26].

Lowering the Facial Ridge and Posterior Wall

The next step after the perfect identification of the middle ear key landmarks (the stapes, the tympanic segment of the VII nerve and the lateral canal in the antrum) the facial ridge is lowered under direct view. At this point, there will be a bump between the facial canal and the posterior wall since both structures are located in two different levels. A diamond burr is now employed, and the bone is progressively removed from the lateral, anterior, and posterior faces of the ridge. The ideal situation is achieved when the tympanic segment, the genu, and the vertical segment of the facial nerve follow a smooth course from the middle ear to the mastoid. The final aspect of the superior pole of the posterior canal should never be higher than the dome of the lateral semicircular canal. A careful and meticulous bone removal in this region makes possible the inspection and cleaning of the so-called posterior compartments of the middle ear: (a) facial recess; (b) sinus tympani; and (c) round window niche (Fig. 58.17). Patience should be highly exercised during this step since the three most dreaded complications of the surgery lay within a distance of only 4.5 mm! (Figs. 58.20 and 58.21).

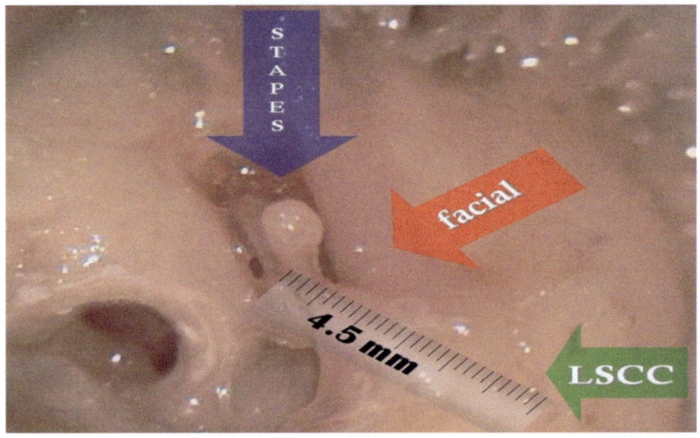

Fig. 58.21 Along a linear distance of 4.5 mm the three components of the "critical triad": (1) lateral semicircular canal; (2) facial nerve; (3) stapes and oval window. (Paparella MM: Personal Communication)

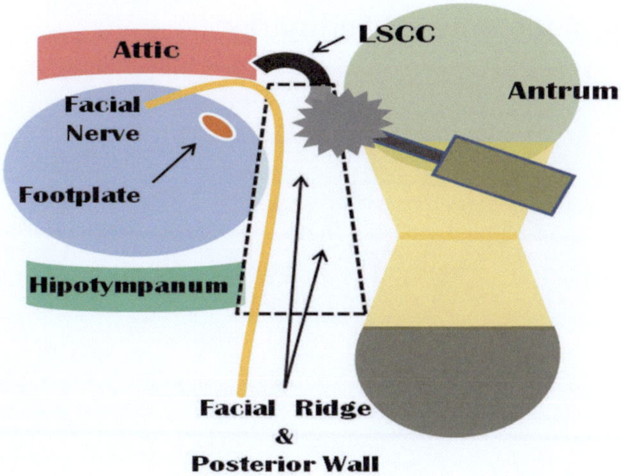

Fig. 58.22 The superior pole of the wall will be completely lowered only after the perfect identification of the stapes (or the footplate), the facial nerve, and its second genu

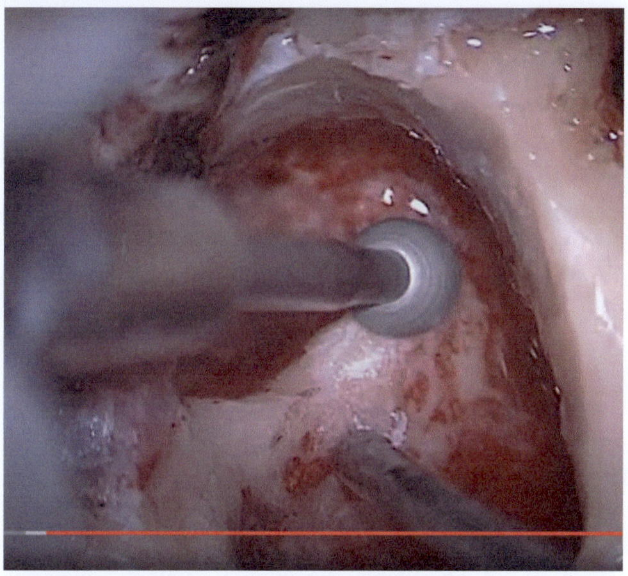

Fig. 58.23 Surgical view—lowering the facial ridge

The facial nerve should be followed initially from the genu to the beginning of its descending portion (Figs. 58.22 and 58.23).

Depending on the size of the mastoid defect that has been created, the posterior wall will be lowered as far as the level II (mid-mastoid) or III (tip) nerve. It is mandatory to fine-tune the drilling of the posterior wall according to the final size of the mastoidectomy: When only the antrum has been opened, the work is limited to the superior pole of the posterior wall and the beginning of the vertical segment. The mid-mastoid level pushes the dissection inferiorly and bone should be removed all around the wall. A smooth continuity must be maintained with the proximal segment. Whenever the level III (mastoid tip) has been reached, some extra details should be observed: First, the vertical segment of the facial nerve must be totally exposed (Fig. 58.24). Care should be used to preserve a thin layer of bone over the nerve. The posterior semicircular canal, the exit of the chorda tympani nerve, and the digastric ridge can be used as valuable additional landmarks during the dissection. Second, the medial floor of the external auditory canal needs to be lowered as close to the inferior level of the hypotympanum as possible. This makes the inferior floor of the middle ear accessible for routine office cleaning. Again, bone has to be removed from the lateral, anterior, and posterior aspects of the most caudal segment of the posterior wall and its junction with the EAC. Three, the mastoid tip must be addressed. In our opinion, there are two alternatives to manage the tip: (a) it may be cleaned of all cells and then amputated. This can be performed by stripping the periostium from the mastoid tip and amputating it using a Gigli saw, or alternatively, the bone can simply be removed as part of the mastoidectomy using a combination of cutting and diamond burrs. Removal of the mastoid tip and the bone inferior and lateral to the signroid sinus allows soft tissue to collapse medially toward the sigmoid sinus. This removes a substantial volume from the postoperative mastoid cavity in an area that is difficult to access through even a large meatus [27]. (b) The tip of the mastoid and part of the mid-mastoid may be obliterated with the periosteal flap when it is returned to its original position (Figs. 58.7b and 58.22b). It is important to clean all epithelial remnants off the tip before repositioning the flap. To decrease the final size of the mastoid bowl, it is also necessary to remove all the sharp edges around the surgical defect. Saucerization should be preferably performed at the beginning of the mastoidectomy because the enlarged cavity permits lighter to penetrate to the depths of the cavity and creates more working room [27].

Conventional Canal Wall Down Tympanomastodectomy

Although the authors prefer to perform CWD as previously described using the inside-out technique, there are cases in which it can be performed after a simple mastoidectomy using the conventional technique. The main indications are in patients with very pneumatized mastoids and in those who have previously undergone CWU.

In these cases, the technique follows the same steps already described up to the item "ENTERING MIDDLE EAR". At this point, the mastoid cortex is drilled following the traditional references, such as temporal line, posterior wall of the EAC, and sigmoid sinus line. When progressing medially, Koerner's septum can be identified and after removing it, the lateral semicircular canal (LSC) must be

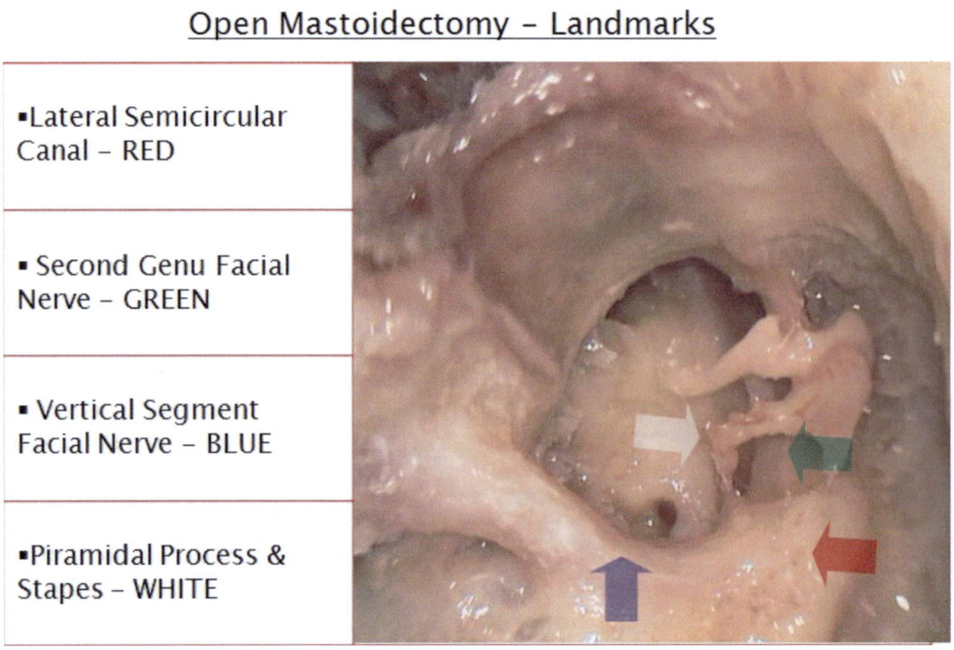

Fig. 58.24 The final landmarks after a wide-open mastoidectomy. Notice that the posterior wall has been reduced in all dimensions, the tympanic facial nerve, the genu and the vertical segment follow a smooth course and the hipotympanum, and the anterior aspect of the wall have also been drilled

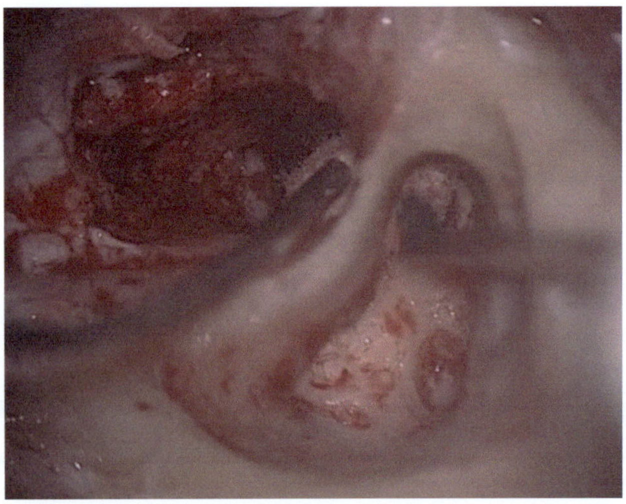

Fig. 58.25 Surgical view—conventional mastoidectomy before lowering facial ridge

sought (Fig. 58.25). It is important complete exenteration of mastoid cells and skeletonize the tegmen and sigmoid sinus. Then, the thinning of the posterior wall of the EAC is performed. In this CWD technique, after completing the mastoidectomy and exploring the ME, the lowering of the posterior wall of the EAC begins to reach the level of the LSC. From this point, the surgery follows the same steps described below.

Ossiculoplasty

After pathologic tissue in the middle ear has been eradicated, thorough attention is directed to assessment and reconstruction of the ossicular chain. Three prerequisites to obtaining good functional restoration in cases of COM exist: (1) an intact tympanic membrane; (2) an air-containing, mucosa-lined middle ear space; and (3) a precise connection between the eardrum and fluids in the ear. Thirty-two materials often used for ossiculoplasty are grouped as autografts, homografts, or synthetic prostheses. Each material has advantages and disadvantages, and no universal agreement exists concerning the most suitable prosthesis for ossiculoplasty [19].

Bone and cartilage came into use in the 1960s and continues to be used alone or in combination with other materials. The authors believe that using the patient's own tissue (sculptured incus, malleus, or cortical bone) is the best option. When these are not available, or when interpositioning of an ossicle is not reasonable we employ synthetic materials (hydroxyapatite or titanium). In cases in which the incus is absent, the stapes is normal, and the wall has been taken down, decreasing the size of the middle ear cleft, the authors have used an autograft bony disc to bridge the gap between the stapes and eardrum. This disc is sculptured in situ using the drill and a small cutting burr in the mastoid cortex. The disc has a mean diameter of 3.5 mm, and in its center an acetabulum is created to fit the head of the stapes. It is then carefully detached from the cortex using a small chisel, trimmed to its final form, and positioned over the head of the stapes (Fig. 58.26). When only the footplate is remaining we also have used cortical bone. The only difference is that in this circumstance a T shaped TORP is sculptured in the cortex of the mastoid. The window is lined with fascia or perichondrium, the prostheses is trimmed to its final size, inserted in the niche, and held in place with small pledges of gelfoam (Fig. 58.26).

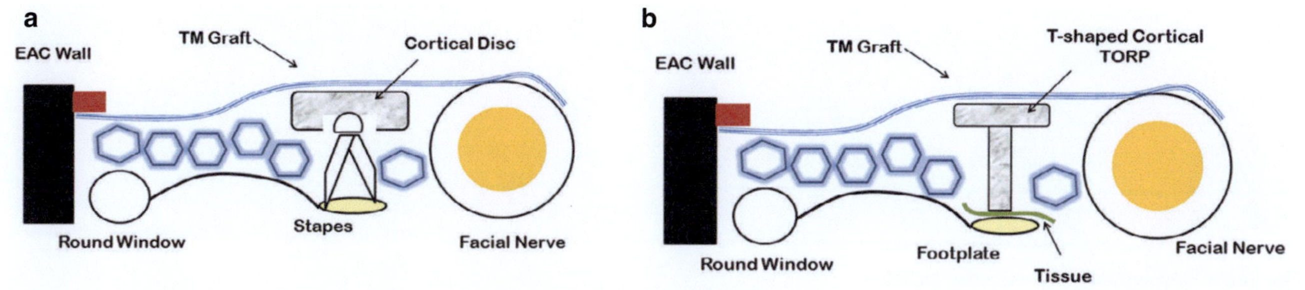

Fig. 58.26 Ossiculoplasty with cortical bone: (**a**) A PORP (sculptured disc of cortical bone) has been interposed between the TM and the head of stapes. (**b**) A TORP replaces the chain (also sculptured with cortical bone). The footplate has been line with tissue (fascia, pericondrium, or periosteum)

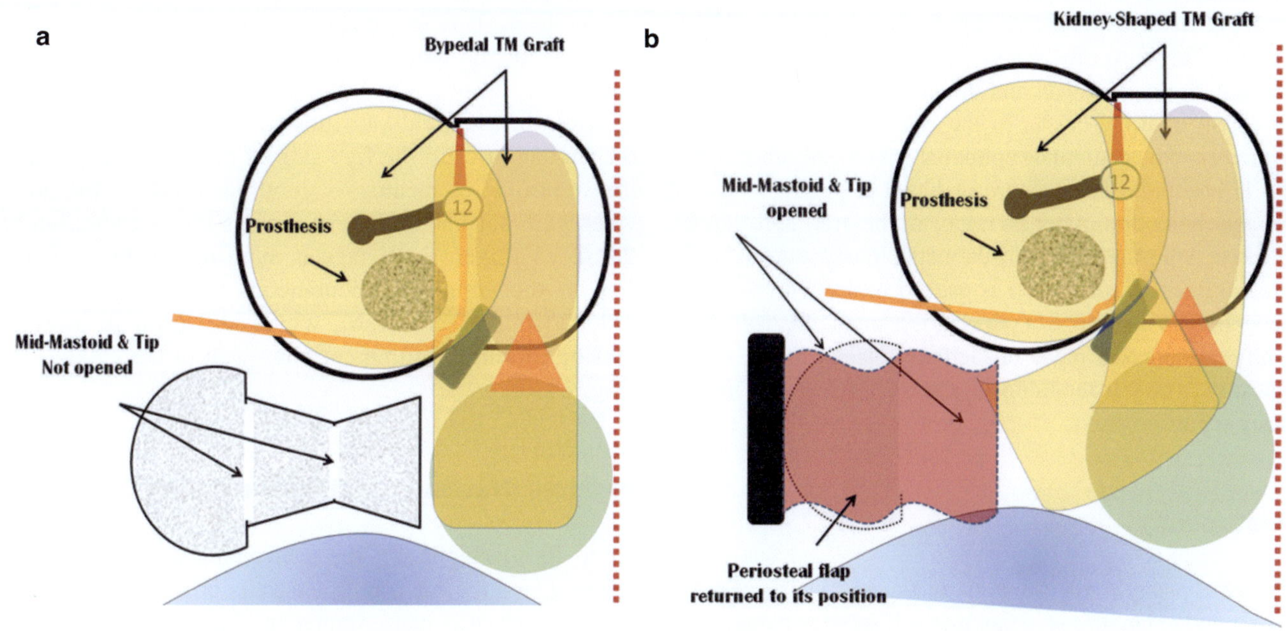

Fig. 58.27 (**a**) A bipedal graft is employed covering the middle ear and wrapping the attic, the lateral semicircular canal, and the medial wall of the antrum—Mastoid opening level I. (**b**) When a level II or III defect has been created a kidney-shaped graft is fashioned covering the middle ear and lining the attic, antrum, and the partially the mastoid (the tip has been removed or obliterated by the periosteal flap)

Grafting the Tympanic Membrane

After final inspection and irrigation of the middle ear, the flap is folded fully anteriorly. Any debris or bone dust should be meticulously cleaned away. The dried temporalis fascia is removed from the block of PTFE and trimmed to fit medial to the remnant of the eardrum, the manubrium, and the tympanomeatal flap. The graft is tailored to its final shape according to the surgical defect. When only the antrum has been exposed, a bipedal graft is employed covering the middle ear and wrapping the attic, the lateral semicircular canal, and the medial wall of the antrum (Fig. 58.27a). When a level II or III defect has been created, a kidney-shaped graft is fashioned covering the middle ear and lining the attic, antrum, and the partially the mastoid (the tip has been removed or obliterated) (Fig. 58.27b). Gelfoam soaked in saline solution is placed in the middle ear and the orifice of the ET to occlude the tube temporarily and to offer support for the graft anteriorly. Enough Gelfoam should be used to create a true cushion in the middle ear to support the graft. Care should be used, though, to respect the limits of the fibrous and bony annulus because the moistened Gelfoam tends to absorb liquid and expand. After the cushion is completed, a cotton ball is pressed against it, any solution or drops of blood are suctioned, and the cotton is gently removed. The graft is grasped with an alligator forceps, rehydrated briefly with saline solution, and placed as far anteriorly in the middle ear as possible and medial to the manubrium. The remaining base of the graft is spread over the Gelfoam cushion and the mastoid walls contouring the dome of the lateral canal. The flap is returned to its original position with a duckbill, and the surgeon's attention is

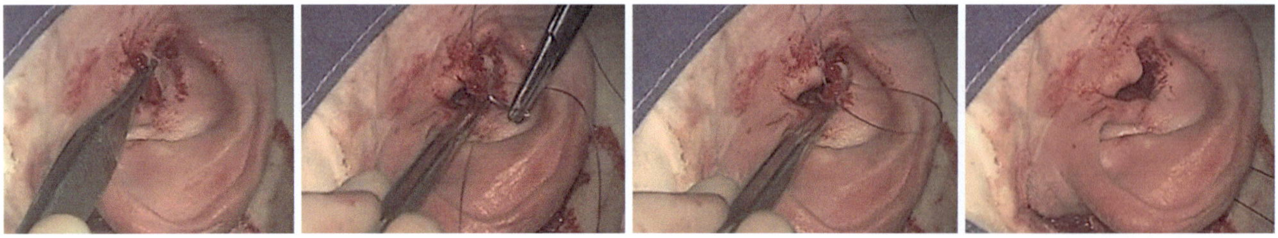

Fig. 58.28 Meatoplasty—Köerner flap technique

directed to tucking the graft carefully into the margins of the remaining TM. Absolute control of the anterior border is critical to the final success of the entire surgery. A small, slit should be made in the antero-superior quadrant of the TM so it may collapse over the graft (which will be resting over the gelfoam, the medial wall and the facial nerve) avoiding the formation of a cul-de-sac in the supratubal recess (which invariably will accumulate epithelial debris). Another cotton ball is inserted, and moisture or blood is gently suctioned through the cotton. After its removal, the graft and flap are checked. After the flap has been meticulously returned to its original position, the cavity is packed firmly with Gelfoam pledgets. The first piece of packing is a small, dry, rolled-up, tightly compressed piece of Gelfoam placed in the sulcus anteriorly. The self-retaining retractors are released, a meatoplasty is carried out.

Meatoplasty

The meatoplasty is mandatory to widen the opening of external ear and to create a skin flap that will serve as a matrix for epithelization of the mastoid cavity. There is no question that meatoplasty strongly contributes to the functional recovery of the ear [28]. It is indispensable in open-cavity tympanomastoidectomy to monitor the conditions of the mastoid bowl in the postoperative period and to reach and clean all the newly created recesses. There are different ways to perform meatoplasty. We will describe a basic technique, most used in our experience which is a simple five steps procedure.

Steps:

1. Incisions in the skin of the auditory canal
2. Dissection of subcutaneous tissue
3. Identification, release, and partial ressection of the pinnal cartilage
4. Vertical incisions in the skin of the pinna (Köerner's flap)
5. Flap sutures

First step of meatoplasty is the initial incision of skin made in the beginning of the surgery. Thereafter, as mentioned before, two vertical incisions are done at 1 and 5 o'clock to prepare a Köerner's flap. Next step consists in dissection soft tissues of Köerner's flap, leaving only skin. A smooth pressure with middle finger can support and guide this moment. It is important to remove a slice of conchal cartilage for the purpose of increase mobility of this skin flap.

After this, vertical incisions are prolonged. The higher they extend toward the free skin of the pinna, the greater the amplitude of meatus. A good parameter is the point when external meatus freely accepts the introduction of the index finger. Last stage is suturing the base of this flap in the adjacent subcutaneous tissue superiorly in order to pull it backward, which will promote healing tension forcing flap to meet bony wall of the cavity [28] (Fig. 58.28).

Packing, Dressings, and Postoperative Care

After the meatoplasty the self-retaining retractors are released, and the ear is returned to its original position and sutured in place. A gauze impregnated in antibiotic ointment is used to line the cavity to prevent infection and to minimize adhesions of raw surface areas. Postoperative dressings generally consist of the standard mastoid dressing which is removed 24 h after the procedure. Patients are instructed to change cotton balls in their ear and keep the postauricular incision clean. The internal gauze is left in place for 7 days. Both immediate and long-term care are vital for the surgical success.

We schedule at least three consecutive visits every 10 day when the ear is inspected and manipulated accordingly until the cavity is completely healed.

Advantages of the Inside-Out Tympanomastoidectomy and Rules of the Thumb

Our accumulated experience in the last years with chronic ear surgery allow us to conclude that the inside-out tympanomastoidectomy has several advantages over the traditional OCTM:

- Low rate of recurrences and residual disease
- Similar hearing results
- Small postoperative cavities due to the hipopneumatization
- Post-operative otorrhea is rare if:
  - Cavity is well designed
  - No recesses
  - Eustachian tube is properly managed
  - Adequate meatoplasty
  - Rigid postoperative care

Finally the inside-out technique is

- Safer
- Faster
- Follow cholesteatoma natural pathways
- More physiological
- Smaller cavities
- Customized meatus

Acknowledgments The first author wishes to dedicate this chapter to the inspirational work of Dr. Michael M. Paparella (Minneapolis, USA), Dr. Octacílio Lopes Filho (São Paulo, Brazil), Dr. Rudolf Lang (Porto Alegre, Brazil), and Dr. Nelson Rêgo Caldas (Recife, Brazil).

References

1. Alleva M, Paparella MM, Morris MS, et al. The flexible/intact bridge tympanomastoidectomy technique. Otolaryngol Clin N Am. 1989;22:41–9.
2. Costa SS, Souza LCA, Piza MRT. The flexible endaural tympanoplasty. Otolaryngol Clin N Am. 1999;32:413–40.
3. Sourdille M. New techniques in the surgical treatment of severe and progressive deafness from otosclerosis. Bull NY Acad Med. 1937:13673–91.
4. Lempert J. Improvement of hearing in cases of otosclerosis. Arch Otolaryngol. 1938;28:42–97.
5. Shambaugh GE, Glasscock ME. Tympanoplasty. In: Surgery of the ear. 3rd ed. Philadelphia: WB Saunders; 1980.
6. Friedmann I. Tympanosclerosis. Ann Otol Rhinol Laryngol. 1971;80:411–3.
7. Desai SB, Mehta PS. Imaging of the temporal bone. In: Souza SD, Claussen C, editors. Modem concepts of neurotology. Mumbai, India: Prajakta; 1997. p. 13–66.
8. Swartz JD, Hamsberger R, Mukherji SK. The temporal bone: contemporary diagnostic dilemmas. Radiol Clin North Am. 1998;36:819–53.
9. Goycoolea MV, Paparella MM, Nissen RL. Atlas of otologic surgery. Philadelphia: WB Saunders; 1989.
10. Dornhoffer JL. Retrograde Mastoidectomy. Otolaryngol Clin N Am. 2006;39:1115–27.
11. Smith JA, Christopher JD. Complications of chronic otitis media and cholesteatoma. Otolaryngol Clin N Am. 2006;39:1237–5.
12. Jackler RK. The surgical anatomy of cholesteatoma. Otolaryngol Clin N Am. 1989;22:883–96.
13. Cody DT, McDonald TJ. Mastoidectomy for acquired cholesteatoma: follow-up to 20 years. Laryngoscope. 1984;94(8):1027–30.
14. Costa SS, Silva MNL, Silva DP. Mastoidectomia Aberta e Fechada: Indicações e Técnicas. Pró-ORL. 2012;4(1):123–50.
15. Nelson RA. Temporal bone Surgical dissection manual. 2nd ed. Los Angeles, CA: House Ear Ins; 1991.
16. Bennett M, Warren F, Haynes D. Indications and technique in mastoidectomy. Otolaryngol Clin N Am. 2006;39:1095–113.
17. Hough JVD. Malformation and anatomical variations seen in the middle ear during the operation for mobilization of the stapes. Laryngoscope. 1958;68:1337–79.
18. Moreano E, Paparella MM, Zelterman D, et al. Prevalence of facial canal dehiscence and of persistent stapedial artery in human middle ear: a report of 1000 temporal bones. Laryngoscope. 1994;104:309–20.
19. Chole RA, Kim HJ. Ossiculoplasty with presculpted banked cartilage. Operative techniques. Otolaryngol Head and Neck Surg. 1996;7:38–44.
20. Mutlu C, Costa SS, Paparella MM, et al. Clinical histopathological correlations of pitfalls in middle ear surgery. Eur Arch Otorhinolaryngol. 1998;255:189–94.
21. Neely JG. Tympanoplasty. In: Pillsbury III HC, Goldsmith III MM, editors. Operative challenges in otolaryngology head and neck surgery. Chicago: Year Book Medical Publisher; 1990. p. 24–32.
22. Costa SS, Colli BO, Fonseca N, et al. Anatomia cirurgica da arteria carotida intrapetrosa. J Bras Neurocirurgia. 1996:730–43.
23. Overton SB, Ritter FN. A high placed jugular bulb in the middle ear: a clinical and temporal bone study. Laryngoscope. 1973;83:1986–93.
24. Moore PJ. The high jugular bulb in the ear: three case reports and a review of the literature. J Laryngol Otol. 1994;l08:772–5.
25. Graham MD. The jugular bulb: its anatomical and clinical considerations in contemporary otology. Laryngoscope. 1977;87:105–25.
26. Costa SS, Cruz OM. Exploratory tympanotomy. Operative techniques. Otolaryngol Head and Neck Surg. 1996;7:20–5.
27. Meyerhoff WL, Kim CG, Paparella MM: Pathology of chronic otitis media. Ann Otol Rhinol Laryngo l87:749–761, 1978.
28. Sousa LCA, Meatoplasty. Operative techniques in otolaryngology. Head Neck Surg. 1996;7:78–81.

59 Endoscopic Assisted Canal Wall Up Tmpanomastoidectomy: The Combined Approach Redefined

Mauricio Noschang Lopes da Silva, Sady Selaimen da Costa, and Fábio André Selaimen

Although it seems that the use of optical fibers in the middle ear is a modern topic, it has been developing for decades. The first publication of endoscopy in middle ear (ME) dates back to 1967. Mer SB developed an endoscopy system to improve preoperative diagnosis, at a time when temporal bone radiology was still incipient. His instrument was formed from parts of a microscope, an external tungsten light source, lenses for angled vision, and optical fibers (Fig. 59.1).

Conceptually very similar to current endoscopes. Obviously, the quality of the image obtained was much lower, but with technological advances, especially with powerful light sources and high-resolution cameras, there has been an enormous improvement. Kiringoda, Kozin, and Lee demonstrated the expressive development in image generation (Fig. 59.2).

Mer's project was the embryo for this instrument to enter the diagnostic armamentarium in otorhinolaryngological offices and later become part of the therapy in surgical centers. In the early 1990s, Poe DS described the introduction of a very small-bore endoscope to assess the ME through a minute tympanotomy. In 1999, Tarabichi M already published a series of 165 cases operated exclusively with endoscopes.

More recently, there has been a wide dissemination of endoscopic procedures in the middle ear. The main justification would be the possibility of better visualization of the structures than using only the microscope. As the microscope gives the surgeon a straight view, with a beam of light perpendicular to the structures, those located in deeper and more angulated recesses could not be approached properly. Optical fibers have several possible angulations and allow viewing any region of the middle ear.

The first use of endoscopy was to complement the microscope. When the surgeon cannot see an area, he makes use of the optics that can be angled to check, for example, the total removal of the pathology. Then, endoscopic techniques evolved and part of the surgery began to be performed without the use of a microscope. Currently, there are surgeons who advocate fully endoscopic middle ear surgery.

It should be noted that there are marked differences in the operative technique of microsurgery and endoscopic surgery. The use of the endoscope gives the surgeon a view in only two dimensions and can reduce his or her perception of depth. In addition, the fact of having to hold the optical fiber with one hand adds the limitation of operating using only the other hand. Finally, there is still the difficulty of introducing the optical fiber and one more instrument through the external auditory canal, which can be narrow and make the procedure very complicated.

The advantages of the routine use of endoscopes in ear surgery are better visualization of all middle ear and mastoid recesses; certainty of removal of the pathology involved; and possibility of less invasive surgeries, since less bone drilling is required for surgical access. It is postulated that the use of both tools, microscope and endoscope, can add their advantages. Figure 59.3 demonstrates the arrangement of instruments in the room in combined endoscopic surgery.

Endoscopic surgery of the middle ear must follow a routine to achieve its objectives. It is essential to meticulously inspect the main anatomical landmarks of the middle ear in all surgeries. A protocol described by Costa SS, Lavinsky M, and Smith MM is suggested, where, like the hours on the clock, we find regularly located structures in the middle ear that are of vital importance for controlling the disease. Table 59.1 describes the 12 o'clock structures, considering a right ear.

The location, visualization, and manipulation of these tiny structures can be systematically performed with the endoscope. Anschuetz, Presutti, and Marchioni thoroughly described how to visualize each microstructure of the ME in an endoscopic anatomical study on cadavers. The main anatomical landmarks are shown in Fig. 59.4.

M. N. L. da Silva (✉) · F. A. Selaimen
Hospital de Clínicas de Porto Alegre, Porto Alegre, Brazil

S. S. da Costa
Department of Otolaryngology, Head & Neck Surgery, School of Medicine, Universidade Federal do Rio Grande do Sul, Porto Alegre, Brazil

M. V. Goycoolea et al. (eds.), *Textbook of Otitis Media*, https://doi.org/10.1007/978-3-031-40949-3_59

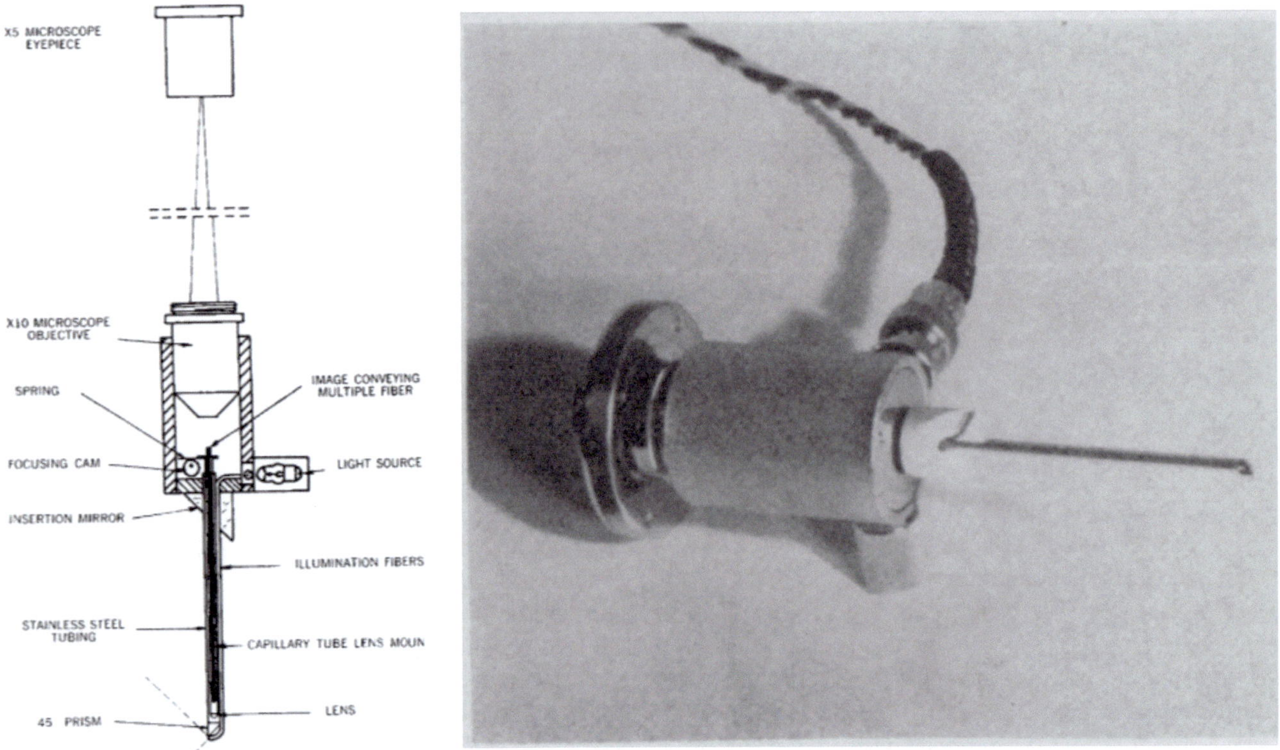

Fig. 59.1 Photo and schematic drawing of the endoscope developed by Mer in 1967 [1]

Fig. 59.2 Incudostapedial joint seen endoscopically over the years. Taken from Kiringoda et al. [2]

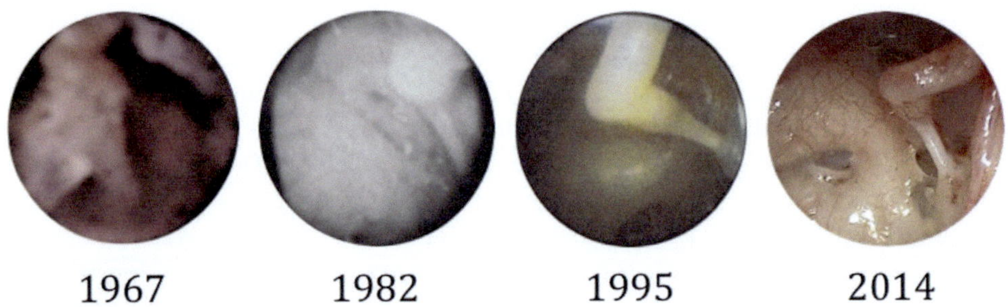

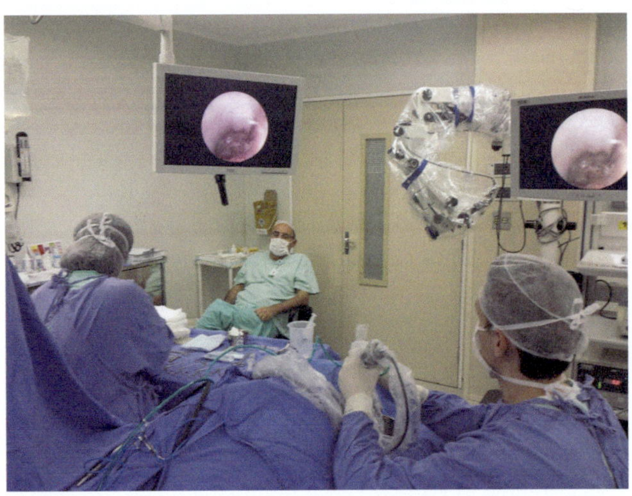

Fig. 59.3 Arrangement of resources in the operating room. Endoscopic time being performed and microscope prepared for use

Table 59.1 Routine inspection of middle ear structures (right ear)

12 h	In the center of the clock, there is the cochleariform process and the tensor tympani tendon
1 h	Anterior epitympanum
2 h	Tensor tympani fold, semi-channel of the tensor tympani muscle
3 h	Opening of the Eustachian tube ostium
4 h	Lower lip of the Eustachian tube
5 h	Cells of the infracochlear tract and vertical segment of the internal carotid artery
6 h	Hypotympanic cells
7 h	Round window niche
8 h	Subiculum
9 h	Facial recess and sinus timpanii
10 h	Critical triad: second genu of facial nerve, stapes/oval window, lateral semicircular canal
11 h	Tympanic segment of the facial nerve

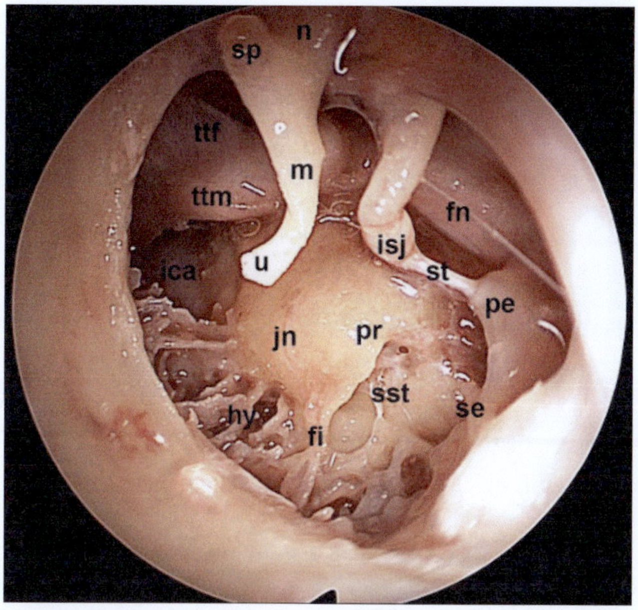

Fig. 59.4 Left ear, 0° endoscope: View of the tympanic cavity after elevation of the tympanic-meatal flap. The meso and hypotympanum as well as parts of the epi-, retro- and protympanum are visualized. *pr* promontory; *jn* Jacobson's nerve; *hy* hypotympanic; *fi* finiculus; *sst* subtympanic sinus; *se* styloid eminence; *pe* pyramidal eminence; *ts* stapedial tendon; *isj* incudostapedial joint; *fn* facial nerve; *u* umbo; *m* manubrium; *sp* short process; *n* neck of malleus; *ttm* tensor tympani muscle; *ttf* tensor tympani fold; *ica* internal carotid artery. Taken from: Anschuetz L et al. [3]

Evidently, some anatomical landmarks are more important, but every turn of the clock is fulfilled. In Proctor's anatomical descriptions in the 60 s, it was already clear that the aeration of the auditory slit followed certain routes. Therefore, it is essential to inspect and manipulate *"key microspots"* that interfere and may be obstructing these predetermined routes. In order to correct possible anatomical alterations or inflammatory sequelae that interfere in the pathogenesis of chronic otitis media, it is always important to ensure that the tympanic isthmus, anterior and posterior von Tröltsch pouches, Prussak space, and inferior incudal recess are patent. We can divide the hours on the clock into two groups: those that are fundamental to remove the disease and avoid a residual cholesteatoma and those that have the purpose of optimizing the physiology and aeration of the auditory cleft compartments. The structures located at positions 1 o'clock, 5 o'clock, 6 o'clock, 7 o'clock, 8 o'clock, 9 o'clock, 10 o'clock, and 11 o'clock are clearly related to sites where incomplete removal of cholesteatomas occurs more frequently, therefore, at these points, fragments of keratin left behind are incessantly sought. The structures described above are obviously those located in the retrotympanum. These compartments are the most inaccessible in conventional microscopic surgery. Marchioni systematized the endoscopic evaluation of this region, as can be seen in Fig. 59.5.

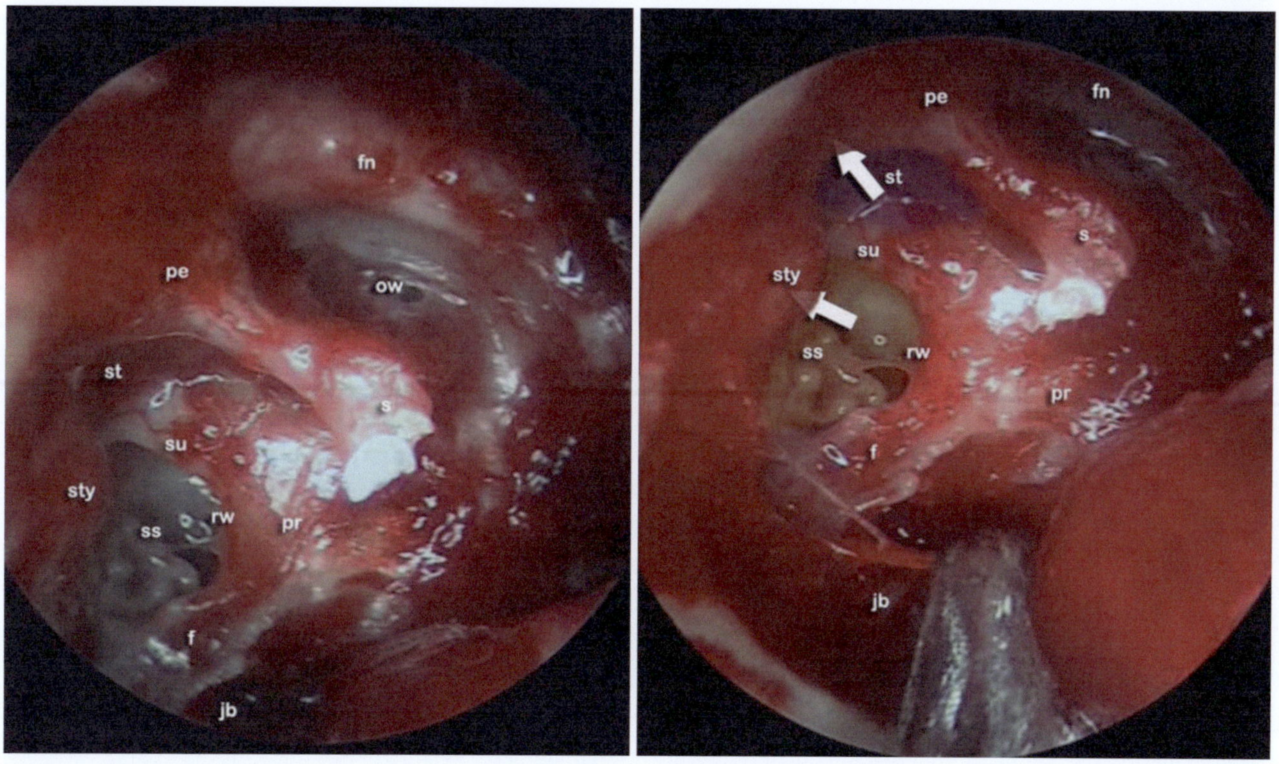

Fig. 59.5 The arrows indicate the posterior extension of the subtympanic sinus and tympanic sinus. Right side. *fn* facial nerve; *pe* pyramidal space; *ow* oval window; *st* tympanic sinus; *s* stirrup; *su* subiculum; *sty* styloid complex; *ss* subtympanic sinus; *rw* round window; *pr* headland; *f* finiculus; *jb* jugular bulb. Taken from Marchioni D et al. [4]

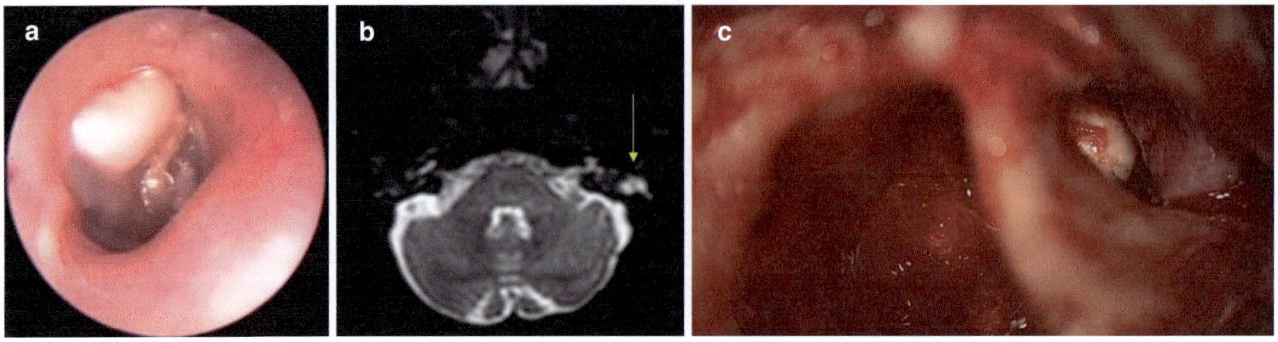

Fig. 59.6 (**a**) Residual cholesteatoma diagnosed on otoendoscopy. (**b**) Residual cholesteatoma diagnosed on DW-MRI (arrow). (**c**) Residual cholesteatoma diagnosed in revision surgery

The reference points located in the most anterior positions (2 o'clock, 3 o'clock, 4 o'clock, and 12 o'clock) need careful manipulation to improve gas exchange between the compartments of the middle ear/mastoid complex and, thus, try to avoid the formation of a new retraction pocket.

Several existing studies point to good results in the effectiveness of endoscopic surgery and envision a change in the surgical routine of the middle ear. In a retrospective cohort study, James AL et al. compared the results of a group of patients operated with endoscopes and another with the conventional technique and demonstrated a reduction in recurrence in the first group with NNT = 9. Arindam Das et al. conducted a randomized clinical trial and described a smaller area of bone drilling and shorter surgical time in attic cholesteatomas. In this study, recurrence was not evaluated and only initial *pars flaccida* cholesteatomas were included.

Cholesteatoma is characterized by a high incidence of recurrence. Marchioni D et al. compared their results of the totally endoscopic technique in early cholesteatomas with the Canal Wall Up technique in mastoid cholesteatomas and found an incidence of residual disease of 19% vs. 34%, respectively. Neudert M et al. reported 6.5% residual disease with endoscopic surgery.

Cholesteatoma Recidivism

The concept of cholesteatoma recidivism is divided into (1) recurrence of pathogenesis and (2) development of residual disease. Recurrence is defined when, after surgery, the growth pattern is repeated and a new cholesteatoma is formed. This situation shows that the first surgery, despite completely removing the cholesteatoma, was not able to resolve the causal factors that trigger the pathogenesis of the disease. The main examples of surgical acts with this purpose are clearing the ostium of the tube, lateralization of the malleus, and/or section of the tendon of the tympanic tendon, opening of the tympanic isthmus, section of the tympanic tensor fold to aerate the anterior epitympanum, and removal of hyperplastic mucosa involving the ossicular chain and blocking ventilation of the additus.

The concept of recidivism due to the presence of residual disease is more simplistic. It consists of detecting a cholesteatoma that developed from fragments of squamous epithelium that were not completely removed in the primary surgery. It is pathology left behind. The gold standard of diagnosis is revision surgery. However, it can be performed through otoscopy, when it is possible to observe keratin pearls under an intact tympanic membrane (TM). Another method based on the literature is through the use of DW-MRI (Fig. 59.6).

The difference between residual and recurrent disease is extremely important in the chapter of the surgical treatment of acquired cholesteatoma. When we discuss congenital cholesteatoma, the pathogenesis is well known (rests of epithelial cells resting in some areas of the temporal bone) and once completely removed the recurrence is almost impossible. Recurrences, on the other hand, are common when the primary mechanism of cholesteatoma formation follows the progressive retraction model. Expanding a little bit this subject, residual disease can be left (1) on purpose, as those cases when some matrix of the cholesteatoma is left over a perilymphatic fistula on the lateral canal or the stapes footplate or (2) inadvertently in the facial recess or the sinus tympani. So, it brings us to the second question: what is the definition of second look, revision surgery or staged procedure.

Second-Look, Revision Surgery, or Second-Stage

Second-look refers to those situations where you have attempted to completely remove the disease in the first operation and have accomplished this objective (surgeon's interpretation) but according to the nature of the pathology and the limited extension of the surgery, you cannot assure the complete removal. So, you will wait some time for a regrowth of possible remnants and schedule a second procedure in order to check this possibility.

If you clearly identify a cholesteatoma during the follow-up of a close or open cavity, you will carry out a revision surgery or reoperation. During this second procedure, you have already figured out previously what is the dimensions of the disease and the extension of the new procedure. The same concept holds true when you find residual disease during the DW-MRI follow-up after a close cavity.

On the other hand, whenever we intentionally stage the procedure from the very beginning (for example, as we have mentioned before, leaving matrix in key areas of the middle ear for the sake of safety) or deciding for an ossiculoplasty only after assuring the final position of the tympanic membrane) the second surgery is planned assuming that recurrent or residual disease are not expected and the procedure is best defined as a second-stage operation.

Choosing Endoscopic-Assisted Tympanomastoidectomy

One of the major paradigms in cholesteatoma surgery is the option for open tympanomastoidectomy versus the closed technique. The first confers high rates of resolution and low recidivism. However, it has the inconvenience of needing cavity toilets, limiting water sports and worse hearing results. On the other hand, Canal Wall Up technique preserves the posterior wall of the EAC, maintains the anatomy of the middle ear and TM. It enables more successful ossicular chain reconstruction techniques and ultimately promotes a more satisfactory hearing result. Another advantage for patients is being able to wet their ears without protection. However, the Closed-cavities have the disadvantage of high recidivism.

Endoscopic ear surgery is gaining ground in the treatment of cholesteatoma, especially because it allows better visualization of the most inaccessible compartments, such as the facial nerve recess and tympanic sinus. It is possible to remove completely hidden epithelial fragments. In addition, it allows manipulation of the tiny structures that influence the aeration routes of ME. The use of optical fibers proposes to reduce the incidence of recidivism in cholesteatoma surgery. Endoscopic surgery may be the link between more conservative techniques, such as canal wall up, and more effective results like open techniques.

Silva MNL and Costa SS conducted a randomized clinical trial comparing endoscopic-assisted tympanomastoidectomy (EAT) versus the classical microscopic *Canal Wall Up technique* to determine efficacy in reducing recidivism secondary to the presence of residual disease. The group that underwent EAT technique had half the incidence of recidivism due to residual disease. When analyzing the subgroup of *pars tensa* cholesteatomas, the difference was much greater, reaching 25% ($p < 0.05$) and NNT of four. This study showed that for every four patients in whom the endoscopic technique is used, we can avoid one residual cholesteatoma when compared to the conventional wall up technique (Fig. 59.7).

Surgical Technique

There are several techniques of endoscopic ear surgery. Silva MNL et al. described the combined technique that we believe is the most rational way to treat cholesteatomas. Instead of arguing which tool is better, microscope or endoscope, we use both. During the surgical act, we keep the microscope and endoscope prepared and use it according to the needs of each case, maintaining a routine as described below:

1. Retroauricular incision

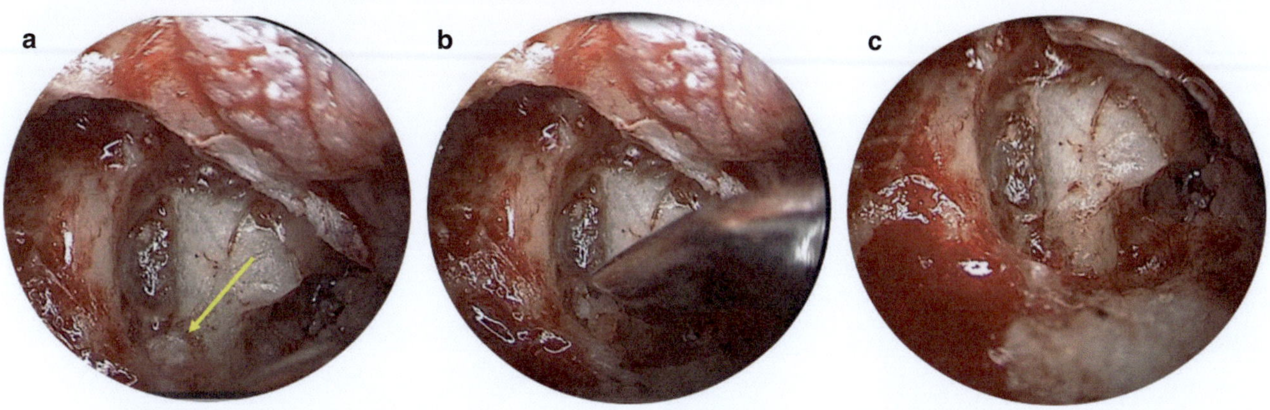

Fig. 59.7 (**a**) Presence of cholesteatoma residues in the retrotympanum (arrow). (**b**) Suction of the cholestestoma endoscopically. (**c**) Completely disease-free posterior recesses

Microscopic Phase

2. Drilling of the mastoid and opening of the facial recess in all patients (Fig. 59.8)
3. Preservation of the posterior wall of the external auditory channel (EAC)
4. Removal of any visible cholesteatoma (Fig. 59.9). A thorough routine review of all middle ear compartments is performed. Careful observation of the main structures of the middle ear, such as the protympanum, eustachian tube, supratubary recess, anterior and posterior epitympanum, facial recess, oval and round window niche, and hypotympanum, was performed. In the mastoid region, the aditus, antrum, and tip were also examined.

Endoscopic Phase

5. Thorough removal of any covert disease. It followed a routine of endoscopic revision of the middle ear and mastoid to identify possible foci of residual disease and improve the aeration routes. Mesotympanum, ossicular chain, and mastoid were visualized with a 0° endoscope. Protympanum, eustachian tube, supratubal recess, and tensor fold were inspected with a 30° endoscope angled forward (Fig. 59.10). When the endoscope is motioned up, the tegmen, epitympanum, and aditum can be observed. A 30° pivot of the endoscope aims to visualize the facial recess, tympanic sinus, and oval and round windows (Fig. 59.11).
6. Tympanoplasty with temporal fascia and/or cartilage (endoscopic or microscopic)
7. Suturing

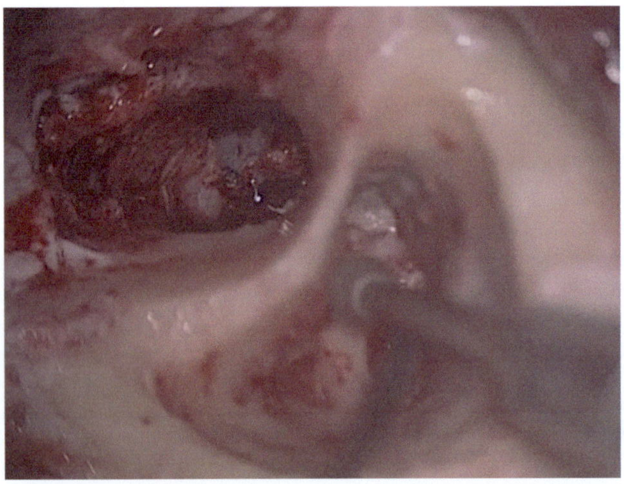

Fig. 59.8 Microscopic drilling of mastoid

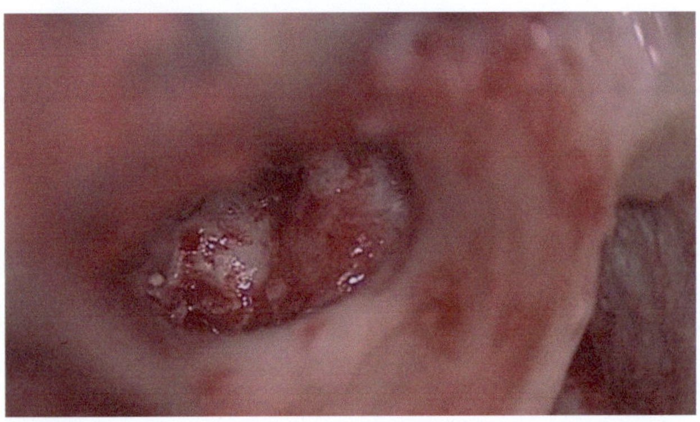

Fig. 59.9 End of microscopic phase without visible cholesteatoma

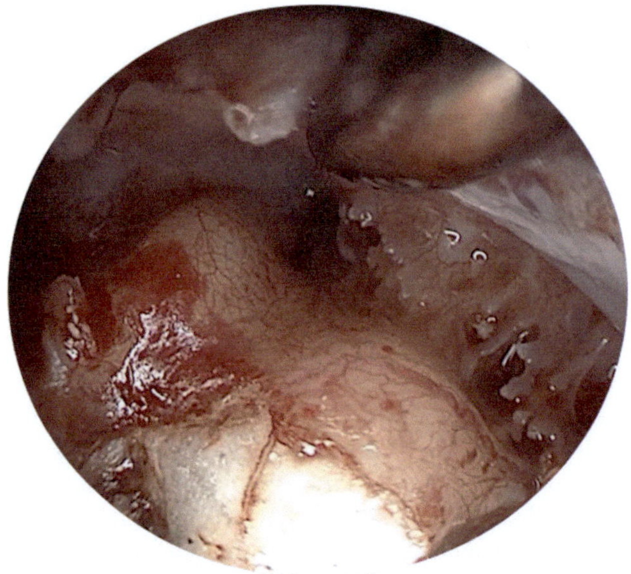

Fig. 59.10 Visualization of Eustachian tube

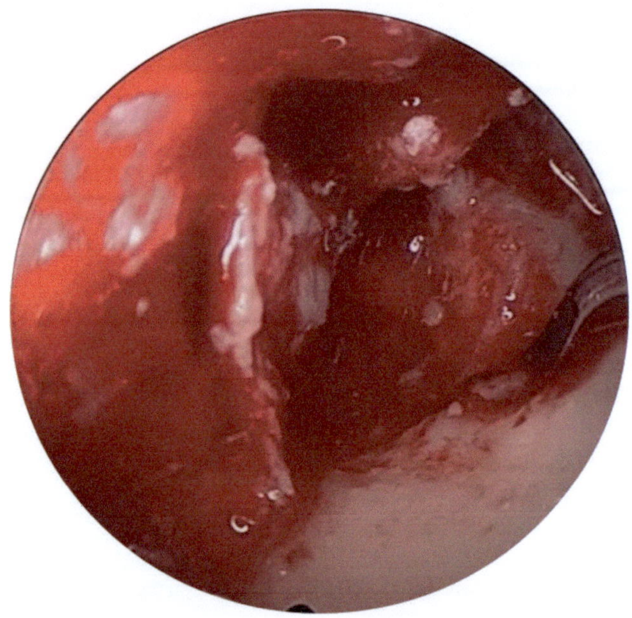

Fig. 59.11 Removal of hidden cholesteatoma in the retrotympanum

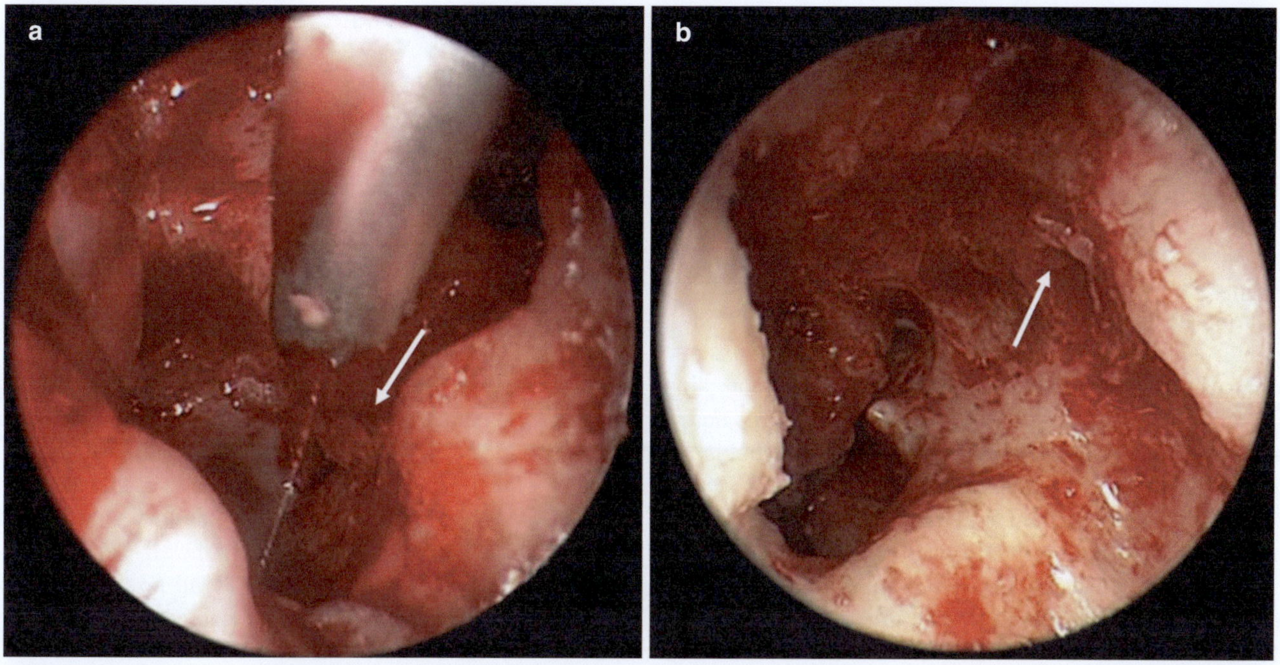

Fig. 59.12 Endoscopic view: residual cholesteatoma (arrows) after microscopic phase. (**a**) posterior recesses. (**b**) *tegmen timpani*

When performing this technique routinely, we could observe that the use of endoscopes in cholesteatoma surgery favors better visualization of covert disease. Cholesteatomas of the *pars tensa* present more hidden disease and they were significantly more common in the posterior recesses and tegmen tympani (Fig. 59.12).

Complications of Endoscopic Ear Surgery

Microscopic ear surgery adds the risk of several complications. The main ones are sensorineural hearing loss, disarticulation of the ossicular chain, postoperative tympanic perforation, perilymphatic fistula, damage to the dura mater, dysgeusia, and facial paralysis. When a new surgical technique is proposed, it is important assess whether the learning curve can increase these risks. It should also be noted that in endoscopic surgery there are some factors that may rise the incidence of complications.

The first condition to be considered is that traditional microscopic surgery allows the surgeon to use both hands. In endoscopic surgery, the limitation of using only one hand is undoubtedly a difficulty to be overcome. It becomes more evident when manipulating delicate structures such as the stapes or the facial nerve.

A second important aspect concerns the visualized image. Unlike the microscope, which confers a 3-dimensional image, the endoscope only generates images in 2 dimensions. This difference could lead to incorrect judgments of depth and even cause damage to structures with the tip of the endoscope.

A third and important factor to be taken into account is the temperature. The heat from the light source used by the optical fibers can greatly raise the temperature in the ME, in the labyrinthine fluids and cause nerve damage. Temperatures seem to be more intense when using a *Xenon* source than a *light-emitting diode* (LED) source. Ito et al., in an experimental study, demonstrated that the temperature of the ME is 31 °C during the surgical procedure and, using a *Xenon source* with 100% intensity and a 4 mm optical fiber, the temperature reached 44 °C. They concluded that it would be safer to use a 2.7 mm endoscope and an LED source. Kozin et al., in another experimental study in temporal bones, described that the temperature of the ME quickly rises to 46 °C when the tip of the endoscope is 1 mm away for 30–124 s, but it also cools down soon after using the aspirator and turning it off periodically the light source.

Finally, there is still a fourth element to be taken care of. Some surgeons use anti-fog solutions. It is prudent not to choose ototoxic substances and to avoid soaking the optical fiber excessively so that these solutions do not fall into the tympanic cavity.

Several studies have evaluated the auditory safety of endoscopic surgery. Marchioni and Presutti presented their case series of complications in 2018. They described 825 surgeries for cholesteatoma, chronic otitis media, and otosclerosis. They had no major complications and 34 (4%) minor complications: 16 (1.9%) chorda tympani nerve damage, 10 (1.2%) sensorineural hearing loss (no anacusis), 2 (0.2%) perilymphatic *gushers*, 2 (0.2%) traumatic TM perforations, 1 (0.1%) accidental ossicular chain disarticulation, and 1 (0.1%) stapes footplate fracture (no cochlear damage). Bianconi et al. analyzed 150 endoscopic stapedotomies. They presented results of closing the air–bone gap similar to microscopic surgery and absence of major complications. They had one case of sensorineural hearing loss. Iannella et al. presented 40 cases of endoscopic ossicular reconstruction using the techniques of TORP, PORP, incus interposition, and cartilage ossiculoplasty. There were no cases of complications, and the hearing results were satisfactory. Tolisano et al. compared the auditory results of 22 endoscopic pediatric stapedial surgeries versus 52 microscopic ones in a retrospective study. They found no major complications or anacusis in the endoscopic group and had two anacusis in the microscopic group. Postoperative thresholds and air–bone *gap* were slightly better in microscopic surgery with no statistical difference. Fernandes et al. performed 34 endoscopic revisional stapedotomies and obtained 89.8% of air–bone *gap* < *20 dB*. Sproat presented his comparative series of 34 endoscopic and 47 microscopic stapedotomies. He achieved 79% air–bone *gap closure* and no inner ear complications. The auditory result did not vary between techniques. An Indian study randomized 64 patients with tympanic perforation who underwent endoscopic myringoplasty to use *Xenon light* vs LED. The group that was operated on with *Xenon* showed greater deterioration of auditory thresholds at high frequencies (4.6 and 8 KHz).

Silva MNL and Costa SS, in a randomized clinical trial, demonstrated that the use of endoscopes did not increase the risk of intraoperative complications in relation to microscopic closed tympanomastoidectomy in patients with cholesteatoma. Hearing thresholds, especially in the bone conduction, are not worse when endoscopic time is added to conventional surgery, which demonstrates safety for inner ear function.

Endoscopic techniques have been used in different diseases and procedures in ME. As it may increase some additional risks, it is essential to adopt a care routine to obtain hearing results similar to conventional microscopic techniques. Mitchell and Coulson summarized a list of strategies for reducing risk:

- Choose the smallest possible endoscope as long as it provides adequate sharpness (e.g., 3 mm)
- Prefer LED light sources
- If choosing a *Xenon* source, do not adjust the intensity to 100% (select the minimum intensity necessary for adequate lighting)
- Endoscopes should not be left in the middle ear for long periods (less than 5 min)
- Take regular breaks and irrigation of the endoscope tip
- Endoscope tip should not come into direct contact with tissues
- Maintain a distance of 8 mm between the optical fiber and the structures

Final Considerations

The association of endoscopic surgery with conventional microscopic techniques has gained space, since most institutions already have the necessary instruments and technological resources. The literature is becoming robust regarding the effectiveness and safety of endoscopic surgery in cholesteatomas.

The authors of this chapter conducted a clinical trial providing level I evidence showing a real benefit in employing this technique. Residual disease incidence really can be modified with a surgical technique that more completely removes the pathology. We believe that the use of the endoscope has a great impact on this type of recidivism.

As for the hearing results, we could observe that the endoscopic surgery proved to be safe. The auditory thresholds of bone and air conduction, in addition to the air–bone *gap,* are similar to those of microscopic canal wall up tympanomastoidectomy. There is no auditory damage when manipulating the ME with the endoscope using only one hand.

We believe that there is sufficient support for the routine use of endoscopic surgery in the treatment of cholesteatomas. The association of optical fibers to the conventional microscopic technique reduces the incidence of residual disease, does not increase costs to the system, and does not add additional risks to the patient. We recommend the use of the endoscope, especially in cases with indication for closed tympanomastoidectomy.

References

1. Mer SB, Derbyshire AJ, Brushenko AB, Pontarelli DA. Fiberoptic endotoscopes for examining the middle ear. Arch Otolaryngol. 1967;85(4):387–93.
2. Kiringoda R, Kozin ED, Lee DJ. Outcomes in endoscopic ear surgery. Otolaryngol Clin N Am. 2016;49:1271–90.
3. Anschuetz L, Presutti L, Marchioni D, Bonali M, Wimmer W, Villari D, Caversaccio M. Discovering middle ear anatomy by transcanal endoscopic ear surgery: a dissection manual. J Vis Exp. 2018;131:56390. https://doi.org/10.3791/56390.
4. Marchioni D, Alicandri-Ciufelli M, Piccinini A, Genovese E, Presutti L. Inferior retrotympanum revisited: an endoscopic anatomic study. Laryngoscope. 2010;120(9):1880–6. https://doi.org/10.1002/lary.20995.

Suggested Reading

Paparella MM. Current concepts in otitis media. Henry Ford Hosp Med J. 1983;31(1):30–6.

Silva MNL, Selaimen da Costa S, André Selaimen F, da Costa Huve F, Lang Silva A, Dias Toshiaki Koga F, Martins-Costa LL, Bernard Rosa Nery M, Zanardini M, Sperling N. Residual cholesteatoma after endoscopic-assisted canal wall-up tympanomastoidectomy: a randomized controlled trial. Otol Neurotol. 2022;43(7):803–7. https://doi.org/10.1097/MAO.0000000000003575.

Silva MNL, Selaimen FA, Huve FDC, Koga FDT, Martins-Costa LL, Bergamaschi JAP, Silva AL, da Costa SS. Endoscopic-assisted canal wall-up tympanomastoidectomy for reduction of residual cholesteatoma. Int Arch Otorhinolaryngol. 2021;26(2):e260–4. https://doi.org/10.1055/s-0041-1730455.

Coast SS. Contribution to the study of chronic otitis media. Masters dissertation. USP School of Medicine – Ribeirão Preto; 1991.

Bluestone CD. In: Vanghan VC, Mckay RJ, Behrman RE, editors. Nelson's textbook of pediatrics. Philadelphia: WB Saunders; 1997.

Costa SS, Cruz OLM, Oliveira JAA. Otorhinolaryngology: principles and practice. 2nd ed. Artmed; 2006.

Ferlito A, Devaney KO, Rinaldo A, Milroy CM, Wenig BM, Iurato S, McCabe BF. Ann Clinicopathological consultation. Ear cholesteatoma versus cholesterol granuloma. Otol Rhinol Laryngol. 1997;106(1):79–85.

Rosito LS, Netto LS, Teixeira AR, da Costa SS. Sensorineural hearing loss in cholesteatoma. Otol Neurotol. 2016;37(3):214–7.

Stangerup SE, Drozdziewicz D, Tos M. Cholesteatoma in children, predictors and calculation of recurrence rates. Int J Pediatr Otorhinolaryngol. 1999;49(Suppl 1):S69–73.

Jackler RK, Santa Maria PL, Varsak YK, Nguyen A, Blevins NH. A new theory on the pathogenesis of acquired cholesteatoma: mucosal traction. Laryngoscope. 2015;125(Suppl 4):S1–S14.

Paparella MM, Hiraide F, Juhn SK, Kaneco J. Cellular events involved in middle ear fluid production. Ann Rhinol Otol Laryngol. 1970;79(4):766–79.

Jackler RK. The surgical anatomy of cholesteatoma. Otolaryngol Clin North Am. 1989;22(5):883–96.

Rosito LS, Netto LF, Teixeira AR, da Costa SS. Classification of cholesteatoma according to growth patterns. JAMA Otolaryngol Head Neck Surg. 2016;142(2):168–72.

Rosito LP, Teixeira AR, Netto LS, Selaimen FA, da Costa SS. Cholesteatoma growth patterns: are there audiometric differences between posterior epitympanic and posterior mesotympanic cholesteatoma? Eur Arch Otorhinolaryngol. 2016;273(10):3093–9.

Yoon TH, Paparella MM, Schachern PA, Lindgren BR. Morphometric studies of the continuum of otitis media. Ann Otol Laryngol. 1990;99:23–7.

June SK, Paparella MM, Kim LS, Goycoolea MV, Giebink S. Pathogenesis of otitis media. Ann Othol Rhinol Laryngol. 1977;86(4):481–93.

Goycoolea MV, Paparella MM, Carpenter AM. Ovaland roundwindow changes in otitis media. An experimental study in the cat. Surg Forum. 1978;29:598–80.

Meyerhoff WL, Kim CG, Paparella MM. Pathology of chronic otitis media. Ann Othol Rhinol Laryngol. 1978;87(6):749–61.

Costa SS, et al. Histopathology of chronic otitis media with perforated and non-perforated tympanic membrane. Presented at the Midwinter Meetingof the Association for Research in Otolaryngology. Clearwater; 1989.

Costa SS, et al. Laboratóriosof histopathology of theosso temporal: passado, presenteand futuro. Revista Brasileirafrom Otorrinolaringologia. 1990;56(1):15–8.

Costa SS, et al. Temporalbones in chronically infected ears with intact and perforated tympanic membranes. Laryngoscope. 1992;102(11):1229–36.

Costa SS, et al. Otitesaverages-aspectos gerais. In: Cruz OLM, Costa SS, editors. Otology clínicaand surgery. 1st ed. Riofrom Janeiro: Revinter; 1999. p. 137–61.

Casebrant M, Brostoff LM, et al. Otitis media with effusion in preschool children. Laryngoscope. 1985;95:428–36.

Chalton R, Stearns M. The incidence of bilateralchronic otitis media. J Laryngol Otol. 1984;98:337–9.

Vartiainen E, Kansanen M, Vartiainen J. The contralateral ear in patients with chronic otitis media. Am J Otol. 1996;17:190–2.

Rosito LPS, Costa SS, Schachern PA, Dornelles C, Cureoglu S, Paparella MM. Contralateral ear in chronic otitis media: a histologic study. Laryngoscope. 2007;117(10):1809–14.

Costa SS, Smith MM, Dornelles C, Sperling N. The contralateral ear in chronic otitis media: a series of 500 patients. Arch Otolaryngol Head Neck Surg. 2008;134(3):290–3.

Costa SS, Teixeira AR, Rosito LPS. The contralateral ear in cholesteatoma. Eur Arch Otorhinolaryngol. 2016;273(7): 1717–21.

Netto LF, Costa SS, Sleifer P, Braga ME. The impact of chronic suppurative otitis media on children's and teenagers' hearing. Int J Pediatr Otorhinolaryngol. 2009;73(12):1751–6.

Silva MN, Muller JS, Selaimen FA, Oliveira DS, Rosito LP, Costa SS. Tomographic evaluation of the contralateral ear in patients with severe chronic otitis media. Braz J Otorhinolaryngol. 2013;79(4):475–9.

Costa SS, Souza LCA, Andrade MI. Temporal procedures: reviewing the nomenclature. BJORL. 57:170–179.

Costa SS. New concepts in chronic otitis media. Presented at the IX Amrigs Congress. Porto Alegre; 1989.

Petit JL. Traité des Maladies Chirugicales. Paris; 1774.

Ballance CA. Essays on the surgery of the temporal bone. London: Macmillan; 1919.

Schwartze HH, Eysell CG. Uber die Kunstfche Eröffnung des Warzenfodsatzes. Arch Ohrenh. 1983;7:157.

Von Trölsch AF. Lehrbuch der Ohrenheilktunde mit Einschluss der Anatomie des Ohres. Leipzig: Fogel; 1873.

Von Bergmann E. Die Chirurgische Behandlung Von Hirnknurkheiten. Berlin; 1889.

Miglets A, Paparella MM, Saunders WH. Atlas of ear surgery. 4th ed. St. Louis: The CV Mosby Company; 9, 1986.

Kömer O. Die Eitrigen Erkrakungen des Schläfenbeins. Wiesbaden: Bergmann; 1899.

Bondy G. Totalaufmeisselun mit. Erhaltung von Trommelfell und Gehörknöchelchen. Monatsschr. 1910;44:15.

Shambaugh GE Jr, Glasscock ME III. Surgery of the ear. 3rd ed. Philadelphia: WB Saunders Company; 1980. p. 267–88.

Jansen C. über Radikaloperation und Tympanoplastik. Sitz ber Fortbild Aritekamm Ob. 1958;18:2–7.

Sheehy JL, Patterson ME. Intact Canal wall Tympanoplasty with Mastoidectomy. Laryngoscope. 1967;77:1502.

Glasseock ME, Miller GW. Intact canal wall tympanoplasty in the management of cholesteatoma. Laryngoscope. 1976;86:1639.

Paparella MM, Jung TTK. Intact bridge tympanomastoidectomy (IBM): combined essentials features of open vs. closed procedures. J Laryngol Otol. 1983;97(7):575–85.

Zöllner F. Die Radikal-Operation mit Besonderem Bezug Auf die Hörfunktion. Ztschr Laryng Rhin Otol. 1951;30:104.

Wullstein H. Funktionelle Operationem im Mittelohr mit Hilfe des Freien Spaltlappen-Transplantates. Arch Ohren-Nasen-u Kehlkopth. 1951;161:422.

Paparella MM, Morris MS, Costa SS. A one stage compromise of the open vs. closed method-the IBM procedure, Proceedings of the third international conference on cholesteatoma and mastoid surgery. Amsterdam: Kluger Publications; 1988.

Poe DS, Rebeiz EE, Pankratov MM, Shapshay SM. Transtympanic endoscopy of the middle ear. Laryngoscope. 1992;102(9):993–6. https://doi.org/10.1288/00005537-199209000-00007.

Tarabichi M. Endoscopic middle ear surgery. Ann Otol Rhinol Laryngol. 1999;108:39.

Ghaffar S, Ikram M, Zia S, Raza A. Incorporating the endoscope into middle ear surgery. Ear Nose Throat J. 2006;85(9):593–6.

Lima Tde O, Araújo TF, Soares LC, Testa JR. The impact of endoscopy on the treatment of cholesteatomas. Braz J Otorhinolaryngol. 2013;79(4):505–8.

Tarabichi M, Ayache S, Nogueira JF, Al Qahtani M, Pothier DD. Endoscopic management of chronic otitis media and tympanoplasty. Otolaryngol Clin N Am. 2013;46(2):155–63. https://doi.org/10.1016/j.otc.2012.12.002. Epub 2013 Feb 5.

Costa SS, Lavinsky M, Smith MM. Rock around the clock in the middle ear cleft. Laryngoscope. 2002;112(6):1122–5.

Proctor B. The development of the middle ear spaces and their surgical significance. J Laryngol Otol. 1964;78:631–48. https://doi.org/10.1017/s002221510006254x.

Proctor B. Surgical anatomy and embryology of the middle ear. Trans Am Acad Ophthalmol Otolaryngol. 1963;67:801–14.

Proctor B. Chronic middle ear disease: its surgical exploration with interpretation of pathology. Arch Otolaryngol. 1963;78:276–83. https://doi.org/10.1001/archotol.1963.00750020286008.

Marchioni D, Soloperto D, Rubini A, Villari D, Genovese E, Artioli F, Presutti L. Endoscopic exclusive transcanal approach to the tympanic cavity cholesteatoma in pediatric patients: our experience. Int J Pediatr Otorhinolaryngol. 2015;79(3):316–22.

Badr-El-Dine M, James AL, Panetti G, Marchioni D, Presutti L, Nogueira JF. Instrumentation and technologies in endoscopic ear surgery. Otolaryngol Clin N Am. 2013;46(2):211–25. https://doi.org/10.1016/j.otc.2012.10.005.

James AL, Cushing S, Papsin BC. Residual cholesteatoma after endoscope-guided surgery in children. Otol Neurotol. 2016;37(2):196–201.

Arindam Das MS, Sandipta Mitra MS, Debasish Ghosh MS, Arunabha Sengupta MS. Endoscopic versus microscopic management of attic cholesteatoma: a randomized controlled trial. Laryngoscope. 2019;00:1–6.

Neudert M, Lailach S, Lasurashvili N, Kemper M, Beleites T, Zahnert T. Cholesteatoma recidivism: comparison of three different surgical techniques. Otol Neurotol. 2014;35(10):1801–8.

De Foer B, Vercruysse JP, Bernaerts A, Deckers F, Pouillon M, Somers T, Casselman J, Offeciers E. Detection of postoperative residual cholesteatoma with non-echo-planar diffusion-weighted magnetic resonance imaging. Otol Neurotol. 2008;29(4):513–7. https://doi.org/10.1097/MAO.0b013e31816c7c3b.

Marchioni D, Rubini A, Gazzini L, Alicandri-Ciufelli M, Molinari G, Reale M, Presutti L. Complications in endoscopic ear surgery. Otol Neurotol. 2018;39(8):1012–7. https://doi.org/10.1097/MAO.0000000000001933.

Ito T, Kubota T, Takagi A, et al. Safety of heat generated by endoscope light sources in simulated transcanal endoscopic ear surgery. Auris Nasus Larynx. 2016;43:501–6.

Kozin ED, Lehmann A, Carter M, et al. Thermal effects of endoscopy in a human temporal bone model: implications for endoscopic ear surgery. Laryngoscope. 2014;124:E332–9.

Hunter JB, Rivas A. Outcomes following endoscopic stapes surgery. Otolaryngol Clin N Am. 2016;49(5):1215–25. https://doi.org/10.1016/j.otc.2016.05.012.

Bianconi L, Gazzini L, Laura E, De Rossi S, Conti A, Marchioni D. Endoscopic stapedotomy: safety and audiological results in 150 patients. Eur Arch Otorhinolaryngol. 2020;277(1):85–92. https://doi.org/10.1007/s00405-019-05688-y. Epub 2019 Oct 17.

Iannella G, De Vincentiis M, Greco A, Vicini C, De Vito A, Meccariello G, Cammaroto G, Pelucchi S, Magliulo G. Endoscopic approach in second stage ossicular chain reconstruction. Am J Otolaryngol. 2019;40(5):735–42. https://doi.org/10.1016/j.amjoto.2019.07.004. Epub 2019 Jul 3.

Tolisano AM, Fontenot MR, Nassiri AM, Hunter JB, Kutz JW Jr, Rivas A, Isaacson B. Pediatric stapes surgery: hearing and surgical outcomes in endoscopic vs microscopic approaches. Otolaryngol Head Neck Surg. 2019;161(1):150–6. https://doi.org/10.1177/0194599819836679. Epub 2019 Mar 12.

Fernandez IJ, Villari D, Botti C, Presutti L. Endoscopic revision stapes surgery: surgical findings and outcomes. Eur Arch Otorhinolaryngol. 2019;276(3):703–10. https://doi.org/10.1007/s00405-019-05280-4. Epub 2019 Jan 11.

Sproat R, Yiannakis C, Iyer A. Endoscopic stapes surgery: a comparison with microscopic surgery. Otol Neurotol. 2017;38(5):662–6. https://doi.org/10.1097/MAO.0000000000001371.

Das A, Mitra S, Agarwal P, Sengupta A. Prolonged intra-operative thermal exposure in endoscopic ear surgery: is it really safe? J Laryngol Otol. 2020;134(8):727–31. https://doi.org/10.1017/S0022215120001449. Epub 2020 Aug 24.

Mitchell S, Coulson C. Endoscopic ear surgery: a hot topic? J Laryngol Otol. 2017;131(2):117–22. https://doi.org/10.1017/S0022215116009828. Epub 2017 Jan 10.

Intact-Bridge Mastoidectomy

60

Rafael da Costa Monsanto, Henrique Furlan Pauna, and Michael M. Paparella

Introduction

There is a long-standing debate over open cavity and closed cavity tympanomastoidectomies, as both have their specific advantages and disadvantages [1]. In all patients with chronic otitis media and mastoiditis with intractable tissue pathology, the primary objective is total eradication of disease with the achievement of a dry safe ear while a concomitant, but secondary objective is maintenance of the patient hearing, and even hearing restoration in certain cases [2]. The major advantages of closed cavity tympanomatoidectomies are to minimize postoperative care, preserve the external auditory canal, achieve optimal auditory results, and provide sufficient mastoid space to simulate physiological conditions [3]. Open-cavity tympanomastoidectomies, on the other hand, provide better visualization of the middle ear structures and allow better space to work and eradicate tissue pathology during surgery [4]. However, open-cavity procedures result in loss of the normal external ear anatomy, worse hearing results, and require frequent postoperative care [5]. Although the use of intact wall procedures would be mostly warranted as they would preserve normal anatomy and increase chances of achieving optimal hearing results, a cases series showed a high rate of recurrent or residual cholesteatoma associated with intact-wall procedures, indicating that open-cavity techniques would be safer at the infection resolution standpoint [6].

In 1977, Paparella and Kim had reported that most patients with chronic otitis media (COM) and mastoiditis have sclerotic and hypocellular mastoids [7]. Paparella and Jung then developed, in 1983, the intact bridge mastoidectomy (IBM) technique, which has provided excellent results through the past four decades [4]. The most critical advantages of the IBM technique are that it combines the most important features of both open-cavity (intact canal wall) and closed-cavity (canal wall down) techniques, allowing eradication of disease and reconstruction of hearing mechanisms in a single-stage procedure; allows better reconstruction of the middle ear and ossicles and enhances tympanoplastic methods; and enhances obliteration of the mastoid, when that is indicated.

R. da Costa Monsanto (✉) · M. M. Paparella
Department of Otolaryngology, Head & Neck Surgery, University of Minnesota, Minneapolis, MN, USA
e-mail: rdacosta@umn.edu

H. F. Pauna
Hospital IPO, Curitiba, Paraná, Brazil

Department of Otolaryngology, Hospital Universitario Cajuru, Curitiba, Paraná, Brazil

The "Intact Bridge Mastoidectomy"

The IBM procedure is frequently preceded by a stepwise exploratory procedure called "flexible approach" [8]. These techniques have been designed in such a way to providing a step-by-step manner dedicated to uncovering and eradicating the tissue abnormalities and allowing adaptation of the surgical steps depending on the specific type of pathologic changes found during the procedure [9]. The flexible approach will be described in detail in a different chapter. In brief, the surgical flexible approach procedure includes endaural incisions, canalplasty, exploratory tympanotomy, reconstruction of the middle ear, atticotomy, mastoidotomy, mastoidectomy either open- or closed-cavities, depending on the development and pneumatization of the mastoid), and finally development of the mastoid bridge. The size of the endaural incision can vary from small, to allow placement of retractors for bimanual surgery, to large enough to allowing complete exposure of the mastoid cortex for a mastoidectomy. The endaural incisions can be made small to allow placement of retractors for bimanual surgery or large to completely expose the mastoid cortex for mastoidectomy. In the case of an endaural approach, the canalplasty is critical to allowing proper visualization of the middle ear during surgery. If few mastoid cells are opened during the canalplasty, this would allow the surgeon to evaluate whether there is presence of tissue abnormalities in the mastoid. After elevation of the tympanomeatal flap, the middle ear must be evalu-

M. V. Goycoolea et al. (eds.), *Textbook of Otitis Media*, https://doi.org/10.1007/978-3-031-40949-3_60

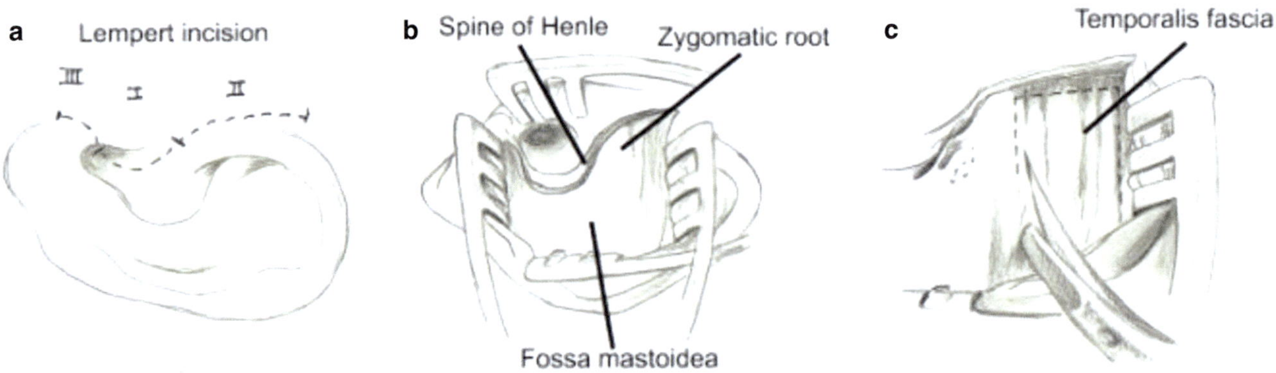

Fig. 60.1 Intact bridge mastoidectomy for chronic otitis media and chronic mastoiditis. (**a**) An endaural incision is routinely used (most frequently II). (**b**) A large tympanomeatal flap is shaped, fascia removed, and the mastoid cortex exposed. (**c**) Harvesting of the temporalis fascia for grafting

ated meticulously for the presence of tissue abnormalities. When necessary, an atticotomy could be performed to provide sufficient exposure to evaluate and clean the tissue pathology in the epitympanum and aditus ad antrum. In patients who have a well-pneumatized mastoid, it is possible to proceed with a posterior mastoidotomy via the fossa mastoideum. This step would provide the means necessary for the examination of the mastoid antrum and some mastoid cells. Whenever necessary, the mastoidectomy can be made as a final stage.

The IBM procedure is indicated for chronic otitis media and chronic mastoiditis with intractable tissue disease such as cholesteatoma, granulation tissue, or cholesterol granulomas in the mastoid and middle ear. Intact canal wall tympanomastoidectomy, Bondy's modified mastoidectomy, and classical open-cavity mastoidectomy are historical predecessors. The IBM operation is a modern-day terminology that replaces the classical modified operation. We advocate that the IBM should be indicated as the first procedure for patients who do have the posterior wall of the external auditory canal intact (Fig. 60.1). The IBM procedure steps are:

1. Incision: an endaural incision is necessary in all cases. It is important that the mastoid cortex is exposed in its entirety. The surgery proceeds with the external ear canal incisions necessary for a large tympanomeatal flap. The fascia temporalis graft is harvested (Fig. 60.1a–c).
2. Meatoplasty: It is important that a wide meatoplasty is performed, and it may include removal of a large piece of the conchal cartilage. When necessary, the harvested conchal cartilage might be preserved and used for ossiculoplasty in a later stage of the surgery.
3. Canalplasty: Following the incisions and the meatoplasty, the tympanomeatal flap is elevated, and the canalplasty is performed by drilling the posterior wall of the external ear canal (Fig. 60.2a–c). In some cases, the posterior drilling might result in the opening a few mastoid cells, providing the opportunity to glance at the presence of pathological tissue changes in the mastoid. In selected cases, elevation of the skin and drilling of the anterior wall of the canal are necessary to provide adequate middle ear exposure (Fig. 60.2d and e). In these cases, it is important that the temporomandibular joint is not inadvertently opened, as this could lead to postoperative pain and stenosis of the external ear canal. To provide optimal exposure of the middle ear structures and the epitympanum, the posterior bony meatus and part of the bony attic wall must be removed. Any pathologic tissue in the middle ear or affecting the ossicles can be removed at this point. Canalplasty enhances visualization of the TM (and thus the middle ear) during the procedure and also during follow-up in the clinic.
4. Mastoidotomy (optional): In cases where the surgeon is unsure of the presence of pathologic tissue in the mastoid is unknown, a mastoidotomy opening can be made through the fossa mastoideum of Macewen's triangle. This step allows for adequate exposition of the antrum and mastoid cells. In cases where the presence of pathologic changes is seen, a mastoidectomy is warranted (Figs. 60.2c and 60.3a).
5. Mastoidectomy and sculpture of the bridge: a thorough open mastoidectomy is done, preserving the bridge. The height and sculpturing of the bridge will depend upon the presence of disease in the region. The height of the bridge should be enough to provide an increase of the posterior mesotympanic space and allowing adequate removal of pathologic tissue in the mastoid. The aditus is also enlarged to remove diseased tissue in the epitympanic space. In cases presenting with extensive disease affecting the attic, an atticotomy should be added to the procedure. The facial or suprapyramidal recess is cleaned but not drilled open. The mastoidectomy should extend to the point where all pathologic tissue is removed, and the bony walls seen are free from disease

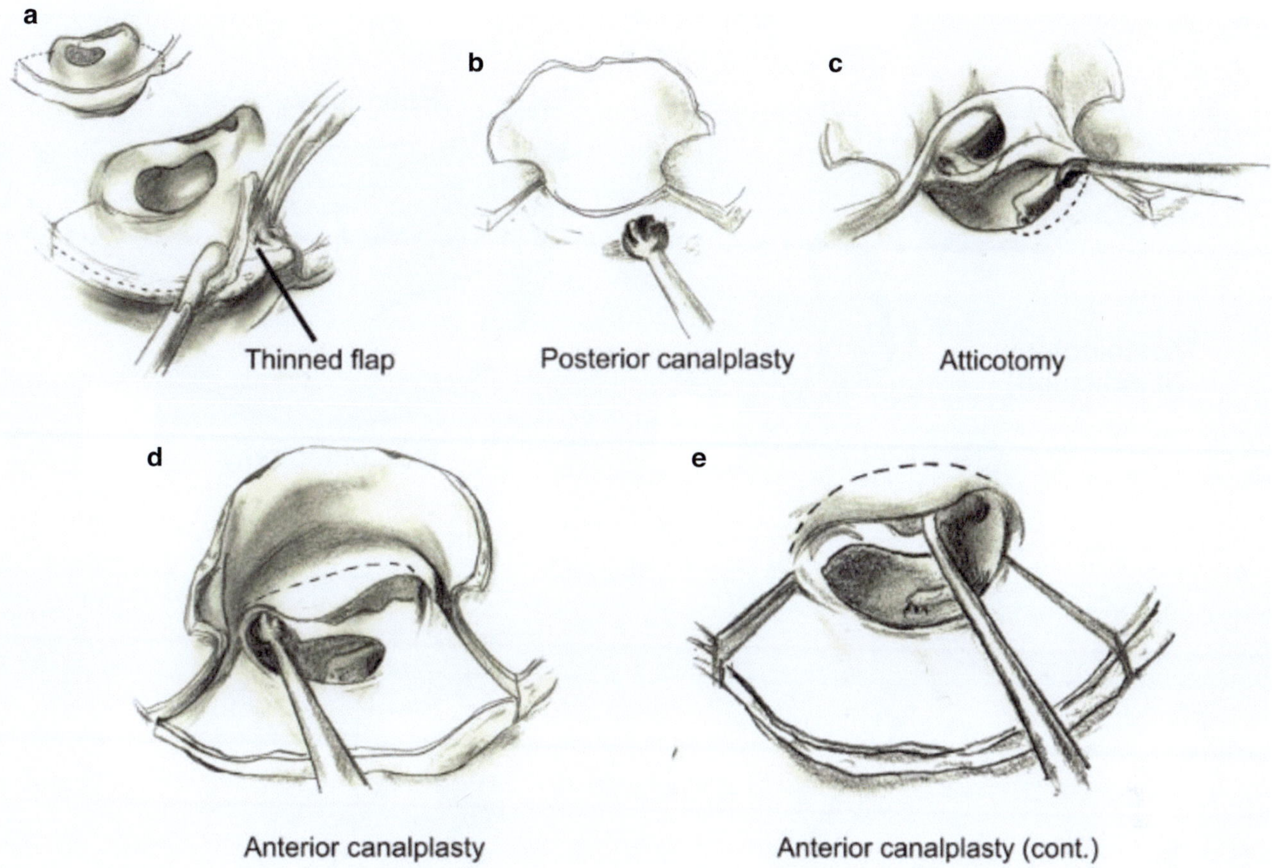

Fig. 60.2 (**a**–**c**) The flap is thinned, the posterior canalplasty is done by drilling the posterior canal wall, and then the atticotomy is performed. Anterior canalplasty might be performed as well if needed (**d** and **e**)

(Figs. 60.3b–d and 60.4a–c). Through this technique, the middle ear is enlarged in depths and diameter, which facilitates tympanoplasty and ossiculoplasty, as well as removal of pathology. The atticus and the shape and location of the bridge are important to accomplish the goal through improved visualization.

6. Ossiculoplasty: After complete removal of the pathologic tissue from the middle ear and mastoid, the surgeon must carefully inspect the ossicular chain. The tensor tympani tendon is cut, and the manubrium lateralized to increase the mesotympanum. A ventilation tube is placed in the anterior denuded drumhead to compensate for Eustachian tube dysfunction in selected cases. In cases of ossicular chain erosion, total and partial ossicular replacement prostheses can be used, as well as cartilage or periosteum (Figs. 60.4d, e and 60.5a–c).
7. Closure of aditus. Gelfilm is softened in Ringer's solution and placed over the aditus. In the past, cartilage and/or a paté of bone have been used to obliterate the aditus, but currently we use periosteum removed from the mastoid cortex for the same purpose (Fig. 60.6c and d).
8. Grafting: The fascial graft is positioned in such a way to cover the drumhead anteriorly and the middle ear. It extends over the bridge-buttress and covers the aditus, reflecting into the mastoid cavity. Underplanted and/or overplanted grafts are used, preferably with skin from an overlying regional pedicle (double- or ripple-layered closure) (Figs. 60.5d, 60.6a, b, and 60.7).
9. Mastoid obliteration (optional): If the resulting mastoid cavity is too large, mastoid obliteration can be performed by using the Palva flap or other methods.
10. Thiersch grafting (optional): In cases where the patient presents with raw surfaces after 3 or 4 weeks of careful postoperative care, a Thiersch graft is applied in the office or as an ambulatory procedure. A thin, transparent skin is removed from the upper medial arm and placed on all exposed surfaces, preserving a thin, granular layer; the tympanoplastic graft can also be trimmed and debridement done or the meatoplasty enlarged, if indicated.

A summary of the surgical steps is seen in Fig. 60.7.

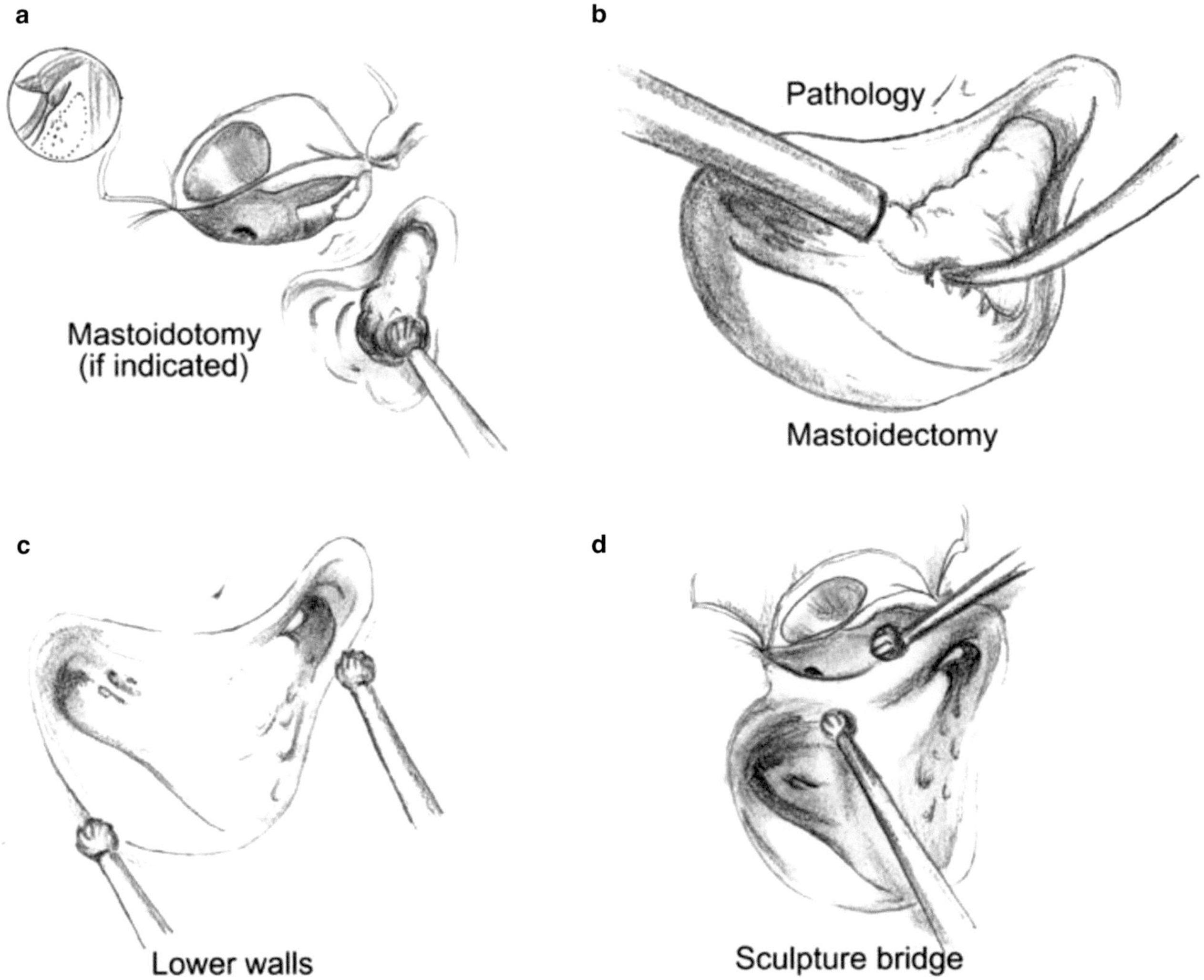

Fig. 60.3 (**a** and **b**) If intractable pathology in the mastoid is known, proceed to mastoidectomy. If mastoid pathology is uncertain, an opening is made in the fossa mastoideum (in cases of adequate pneumatization), and the anterior and regional cells are explored. (**c** and **d**) A thorough open mastoidectomy is done, preserving the bridge. The bridge should be high enough to increase the mesotympanic space adequately

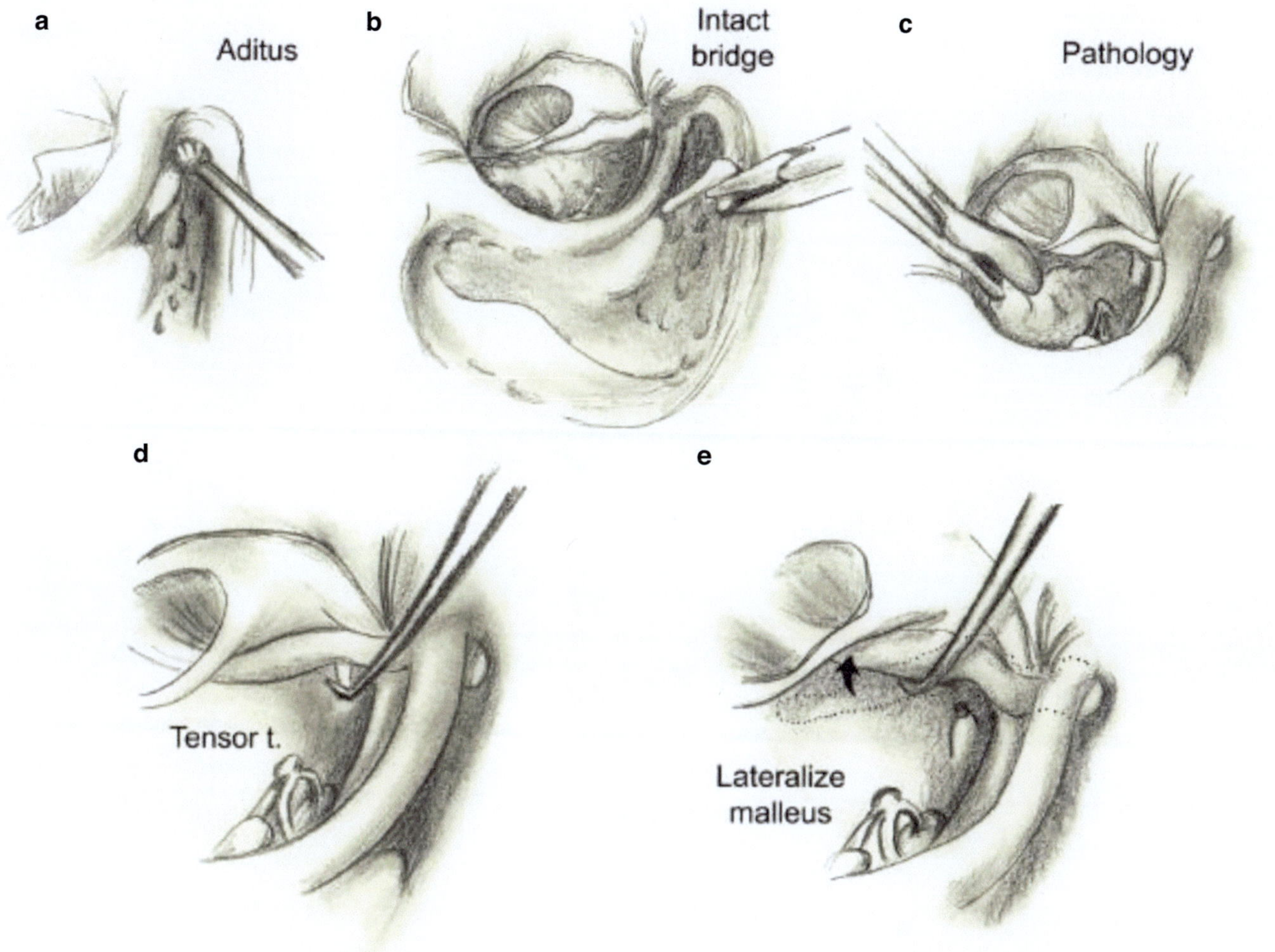

Fig. 60.4 (**a**) The aditus is enlarged to remove diseased tissue, and atticotomy is combined if attic pathology is extensive. After removal of pathology (**b**), ossiculoplasty and middle ear reconstruction are carried out as necessary. (**c**) Pathologic tissue is then carefully removed. The tensor tympani is cut (**d**) to increase the mesotympanum and enhance PORP and TORP placement when indicated (**e**). Sometimes malleus is too far forward but usually PORPs and TORPs can be placed under the malleus manubrium

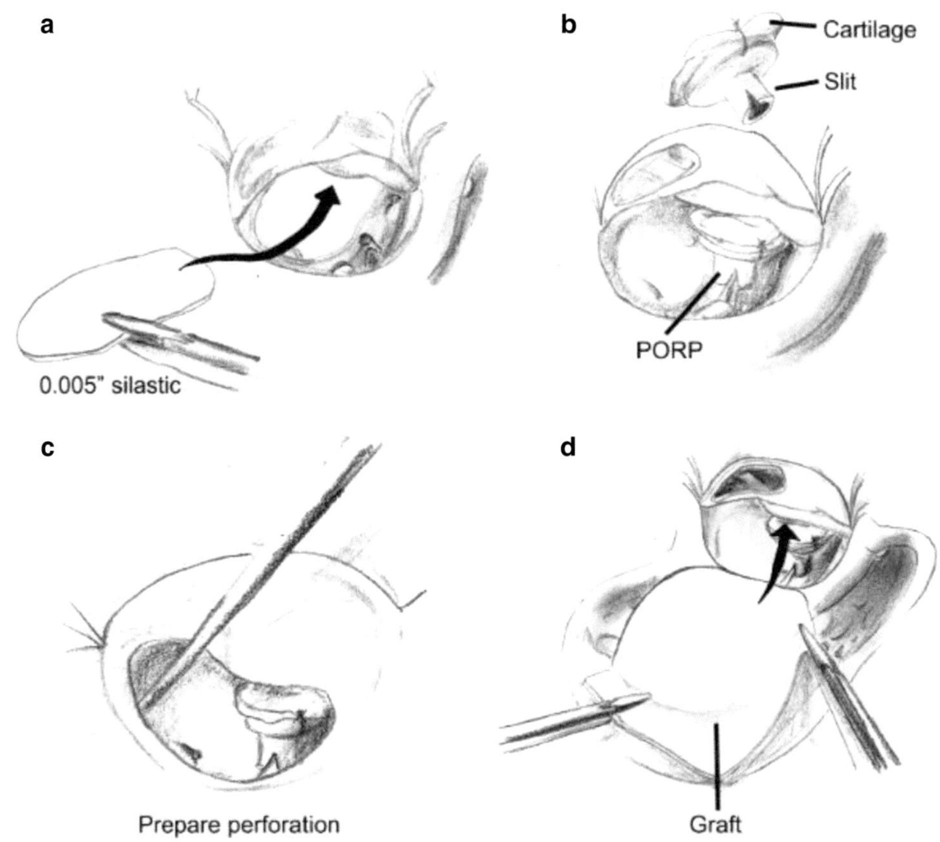

Fig. 60.5 (**a**) A crescent-shaped Silastic sheet is cut and placed between the eustachian tube and round window. A total ossicular reconstructive prosthesis (TORP) or partial ossicular reconstructive prosthesis (PORT) is used as needed (**b** and **c**). The fascial graft is then applied (**d**)

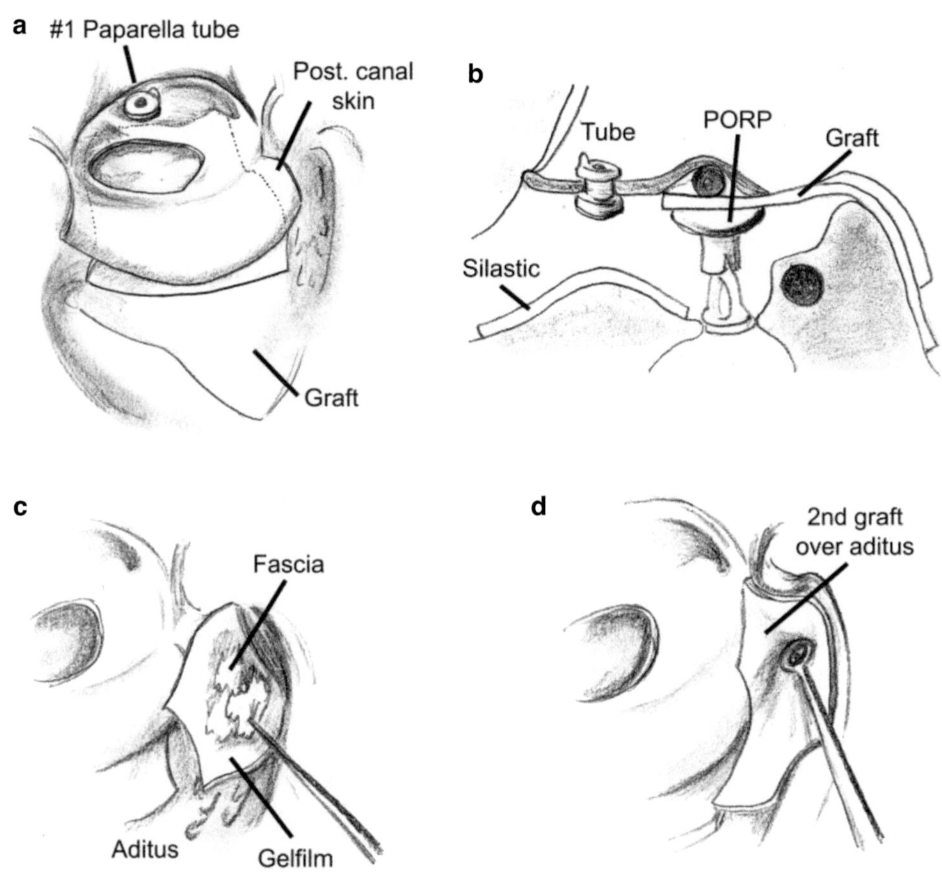

Fig. 60.6 A small no. 1 ventilation tube is placed in the anterior denuded drumhead (**a**). It is not considered wise to place the tube through the graft. (**b**–**d**) Gelfilm is then placed over the aditus, and periosteum is removed from the mastoid cortex to obliterate the aditus. The fascial graft is placed to cover the drumhead anteriorly and the middle ear extending over the bridge buttress and covering the attic

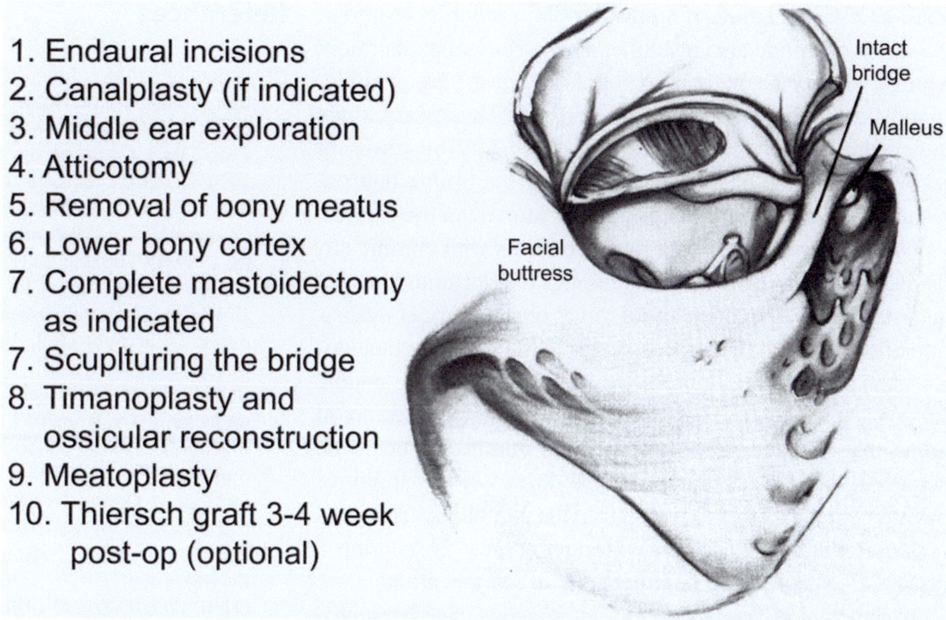

Fig. 60.7 Steps of the IBM and the final aspect. Note increase in mesotympanic space, which enhances ossiculoplasty (e.g., partial ossicular reconstructive prosthesis)

Follow-Up Studies

We studied the results obtained in 47 ears from patients who underwent the IBM technique within the period of 3 years [5]. The patients ranged in age from 10 to 80 years (average = 41 years). There were 21 women and 19 men. Most of them underwent a Thiersch graft from the upper medial arm to the mastoid cavity 3–4 weeks after the IBM procedure on an outpatient basis.

The most common type of tympanoplastic reconstruction was type I, performed on 19 ears. Partial ossicular reconstruction was performed 15 ears, and total ossicular reconstruction prosthesis in ten ears. The average follow-up was 13 months, and the preoperative and postoperative audiograms were assessed. In 48% of the ears the air-bone gap was 10 dB or less. An air-bone gap of 20 dB or less was achieved in 70% of the ears and 30 dB or less in 83%.

The most common abnormality found in the postoperative care was granulomatous otomastoiditis (53% of the cases). The ears became dry within 4–12 weeks, with an average of 5.2 weeks. No revisions to date have been necessary for recurrent or residual disease, and only three patients underwent minor revisions, one for a Thiersch graft revision that was not done adequately the first time, followed by two patients for subsequent tympanoplasty revision to help improve hearing.

Comparison Between Mastoidectomy Techniques

The closed-cavity tympanomastoidectomy allows preservation of the normal architecture of the external ear canal and middle ear, preventing some of the most frequent issues observed in open-cavity procedures [5, 10]. As this approach results in preservation of the normal anatomy, it usually results in better auditory functional results as well. However, as the closed cavities do not allow for adequate postoperative care, the recurrence rate of cholesteatoma is higher as compared with the open-cavity procedures [5]. Some authors advocate that the closed-cavity tympanomastoidectomy must be followed by a subsequent "second-look" procedure a few months after the surgery [11].

The open-cavity procedures have been shown to reduce the risks of recurrent disease. The open-cavity procedure also results in better visualization of the middle ear structures and allow for a more extensive removal of pathologic tissue, which reduces the chances of residual cholesteatoma. The disadvantages associated with open-cavities frequently include a cavity that requires periodic cleaning and may result in frequent otorrhea. Also, it makes adaptation with conventional hearing aids challenging, as it may result in accumulation of debri in the mastoid cavity and reverberation of sound.

The IBM procedure seems to provide adequate visualization of the mastoid and middle ear, while preserving most of the normal anatomy. Prof. Michael Paparella has operated thousands of patients by using this technique in the past four decades: in his experience, these procedures resulted in dry, safe ear usually with little or no need for revisional surgery. Furthermore, as a one-stage operation, the IBM procedure is advantageous as compared with other strategies that require second- and third-stage planned surgeries, which result in additional cost, discomfort, and inconvenience for the patient.

The main advantages of closed-cavity procedures (preservation of the architecture and optimal hearing results) seem to be met by the IBM procedure. Also, considering the opening of the mastoid, it also would provide the advantages of an open-cavity procedure. If a mastoid obliteration is required, the IBM technique also results in a posterior-canal abutment against which placement of materials and grafts are possible. In most cases, however, obliteration is rarely necessary, since the method of reducing the size of the cavity by lowering cortical walls and preserving or shaping the bridge-buttress results in a small cavity that is not problematic in most cases.

One frequent feature observed in patients with chronic otitis media and mastoiditis is the presence of a tortuous external auditory canal. A tortuous canal might prevent proper evaluation of some middle ear spaces. As the IBM procedure includes a wide canalplasty to improve the visualization of the middle ear space through the external ear canal. Although some could argue that a better visualization of the middle ear could be achieved with the use an endoscope; however, the ability of having both hands free to manipulate the pathologic tissue and ossicular chain might be an important asset it is securing a disease-free cavity with minimum risk of complications.

In conclusion, many different approaches have been proposed for the treatment of chronic otitis media and mastoiditis. The surgeon must weight many variables in the decision-making process on what would be the optimal technique for each specific patient, one of which is the experience of the surgeon in each of these techniques. The IBM procedure is a safe procedure that combines the most prominent advantages of the open- and closed-cavity mastoidectomies, being one among the procedures used to treat chronic otitis media. The IBM, when executed with sufficient expertise, provides a clean and dry middle ear and mastoid while also preserving and enhancing hearing.

References

1. Paparella MM, Jung TT. Intact-bridge tympanomastoidectomy. Otolaryngol Head Neck Surg. 1984;92:334–8. https://doi.org/10.1177/019459988409200317.
2. Cole JM. Conservative tympanomastoidectomy. Laryngoscope. 1974;84:783–92. https://doi.org/10.1288/00005537-197405000-00009.
3. Smyth G. Combined approach tympanoplasty. Arch Otolaryngol. 1969;89:250–1. https://doi.org/10.1001/archotol.1969.00770020252007.
4. Paparella MM, Jung TTK. Intact bridge tympanomastoidectomy (I.B.M.)—combining essential features of open vs. closed procedures. J Laryngol Otol. 1983;97:579–85. https://doi.org/10.1017/S0022215100094639.
5. Sajjadi H. A one-stage, versatile procedure: intact-bridge mastoidectomy. Otolaryngol Clin N Am. 1999;32:555–65. https://doi.org/10.1016/s0030-6665(05)70152-3.
6. Sajjadi H, Paparella MM. Intact-bridge mastoidectomy: operative techniques. Operat Tech Otolaryngol Head Neck Surg. 1996;7:55–61. https://doi.org/10.1016/S1043-1810(96)80063-7.
7. Paparella MM, Kim CS. Mastoidectomy update. Laryngoscope. 1977;87:1977–88. https://doi.org/10.1288/00005537-197712000-00001.
8. da Costa SS, de Souza LCA, Piza MRD. The flexible endaural tympanoplasty—pathology-guided, pathogenesis-oriented surgery for the middle ear. Otolaryngol Clin N Am. 1999;32:413. https://doi.org/10.1016/S0030-6665(05)70143-2.
9. Paparella MM, Jung TT. Experience with tympanoplasty for atelectatic ears. Laryngoscope. 1981;91:1472–7.
10. Holmquist J, Bergström B. The mastoid air cell system in ear surgery. Arch Otolaryngol. 1978;104:127–9. https://doi.org/10.1001/archotol.1978.00790030013003.
11. Ho SY, Kveton JF. Efficacy of the 2-staged procedure in the management of cholesteatoma. Arch Otolaryngol - Head Neck Surg. 2003;129:541–5. https://doi.org/10.1001/archotol.129.5.541.

Radical Mastoidectomy

61

Francisco Tocornal J.

Introduction

Before the introduction of tympanoplasty and its various modifications in the mid-1950s, mastoid cholesteatoma was treated by radical mastoidectomy (RM) or modified Radical Mastoidectomy. The RM is a procedure that consists of the complete resection of the mastoid cells associated with the removal of the sound transmission system (except the stapes footplate) and the obliteration of the Eustachian tube. The "modified RM" initially referred to the conservation of the ossicular chain and the structures of the middle ear, after a mastoidectomy, without conservation of the posterior wall of the canal (Canal wall Down: CWD) in cases in which the cholesteatoma did not compromise the middle ear (Bondi surgery) [1]. The subsequent introduction of the CWD technique associated with a tympanoplasty led to confusion regarding the nomenclature, since the latter technique is sometimes referred to as modified radical surgery [2–4].

Initially indicated for the management of chronic suppuration of the ear, usually cholesteatoma, as well as for the surgical management of some mastoid lesions or of the tympanic cavity (cholesterol granulomas, glomus tympanicum, etc.). With the development of microsurgery of ear, this technique was reserved for pathologies in which it was not possible to preserve the posterior wall of the bony external auditory canal, which forced to communicate the mastoid space with the middle ear.

Currently, its indication also includes te surgery in elderly patients with severe to profound sensorineural hearing loss, in whom dry and safe ear is sought.

It is also indicated in some perilymph fistulas, cholesteatomas in locations that are very difficult to manage, such as a deep sinus tympani, intracranial complications of cholesteatoma, benign tumors of the middle ear, and mastoids with severe neurosensory compromise [2, 4].

F. Tocornal J. (✉)
Department of Otolaryngology, Clínica Universidad de Los Andes, Santiago, Chile
e-mail: ftocornal@clinicauandes.cl

The patient must be informed about the loss of functionality of the ear, the objective of eradicating the pathology, the time of postoperative care, and of the possibility of transient or permanent alterations in the function of the facial nerve. They should also be informed of long-term follow-up and the possibility of recurrence.

This procedure is considered by most otologists to be a safe surgery to eradicate the infectious pathology of the ear associated with cholesteatoma, which makes impossible the physiological transmission of sound to the stapes footplate. For this reason, in certain clinical circumstances, it is proposed as a safe treatment, in a patient who may not have adequate follow-up or in whom other previous surgical attempts have not eradicated the pathology of the middle-mastoid ear and achieved a dry ear.

Soft Tissue Management

At the beginning of the procedure, an otoscopy is performed to examine the ear canal and tympanic membrane under anesthesia, which will allow a clearer idea of the characteristics of the retraction pockets and the presence or absence of epithelial sheets. At that stage, it can be useful to ask the anesthetist to use protoxide in order to raise the retraction pockets that are ventilated.

Two longitudinal incisions are then made in the duct, at the level of the tympanomastoid and tympanosquamous suture lines, then connecting them through an arcuate incision parallel to the tympanic annulus, lateral to the diseased tissue (Fig. 61.1).

Another incision is made in the skin at the retroauricular groove or slightly posterior to it, from the upper end of the insertion of the auricle to the level of the lower edge of the external auditory canal (Fig. 61.2).

In the posteroinferior aspect of the external auditory canal, the posterior auricular artery and vein are located, which must be controlled to avoid bleeding.

M. V. Goycoolea et al. (eds.), *Textbook of Otitis Media*, https://doi.org/10.1007/978-3-031-40949-3_61

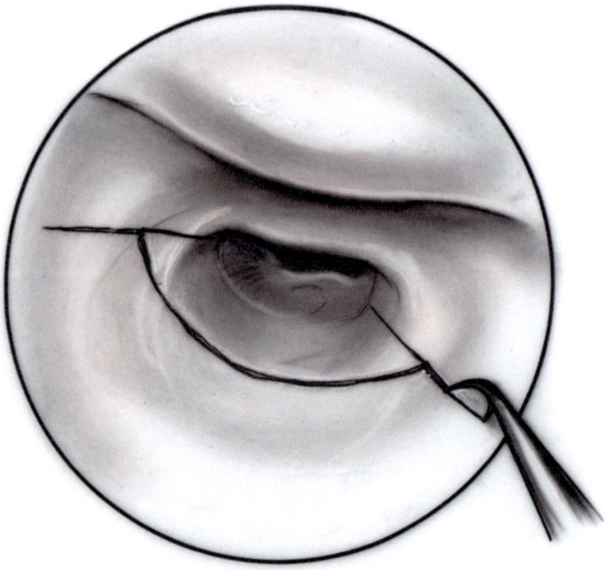

Fig. 61.1 Ear canal incisions. (Reproduced with permission of the author [7])

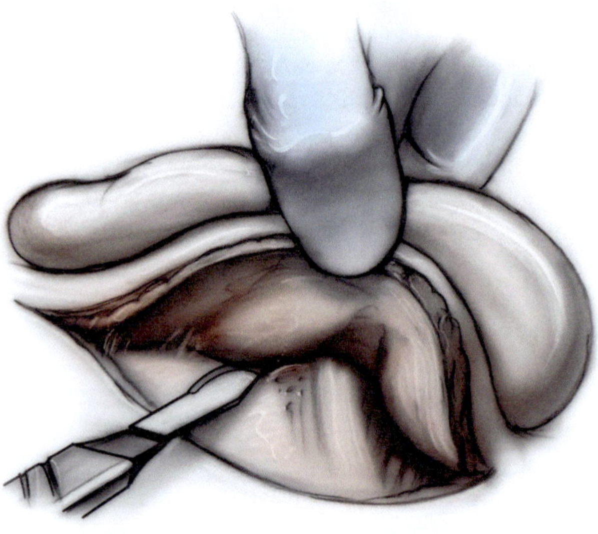

Fig. 61.2 Retroauricular incision. (Reproduced with permission of the author [7])

Upon reaching the muscular plane, it is recommended to take a wide graft of fascia from the temporalis muscle, which can be used at the time of closure to cover some of the structures exposed during surgery or in the case of a modification of the technique, to perform a tympanoplasty.

The incision in the muscular plane must consider the type of closure that will be performed, for a wide meatoplasty. Part of the postauricular soft tissue, attached to the cartilaginous external auditory canal, can be preserved to facilitate the fixation of the sutures to the meatoplasty flaps, or to use part of this tissue in the obliteration of the cavity with the Palva technique [5].

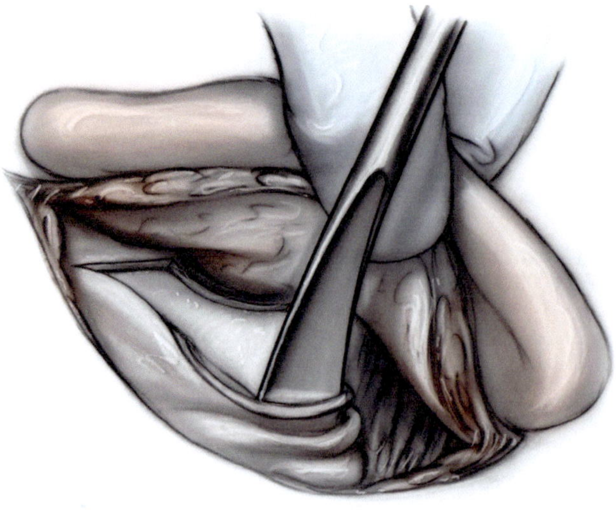

Fig. 61.3 Elevation of the soft tissue. (Reproduced with permission of the author [7])

The periosteum is usually incised together with the muscle plane, and a retraction is performed with a periosteal elevator of all the soft tissues in a radial direction from the external auditory canal in order to disinsert the most superior fibers of the sternocleidomastoid muscle to the mastoid (Fig. 61.3), with the aim of clear the bone plane in the entire projection of the mastoid cavity, taking as limits the temporal line superiorly, the ear canal anteriorly, the tip of the mastoid as the inferior limit, and the projection of the sigmoid sinus as the posteroinferior limit. At this point, it may be necessary to control bleeding from the mastoid emissary vein by drilling with a large diamond drill (without irrigation) or with bone wax.

In the anterior limit, the incision will meet the external auditory canal by raising the flap that was previously prepared through the canal, once it has been raised and the incision is communicated to the canal, the retractors are placed, first at the level of the duct by gently grasping anteriorly the skin flap of the ear canal. At the posterior aspect of the incision, the retractor should rest against the posterior edge of the wound. Using a tape across the ear canal can help pull the soft tissues of the ear canal forward (Fig. 61.4).

A second retractor can be supported to retract the temporalis muscle fibers and the soft tissues surrounding the tip of the mastoid (Fig. 61.5).

After delimiting the field, the exposure of the area to be drilled is improved, separating the soft tissue toward the top of the spine of Henle which, once exposed, will allow an adequate view of the cribriform area, which is the external projection area of the mastoid antrum and the area immediately anterosuperior where the attic exposure will be made.

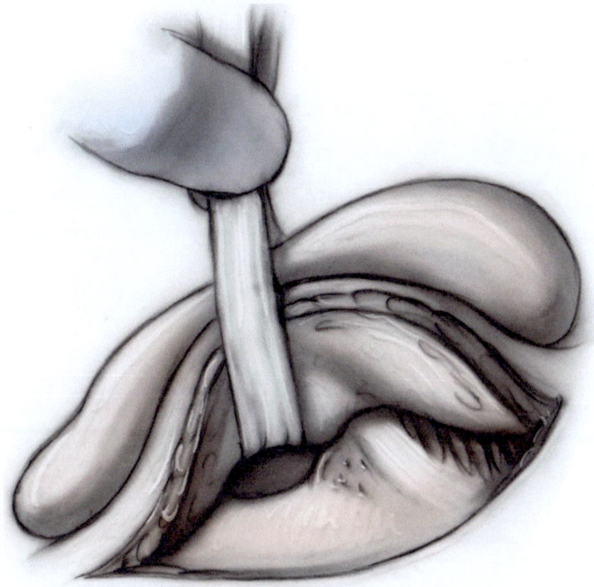

Fig. 61.4 The tape across the ear canal. (Reproduced with permission of the author [7])

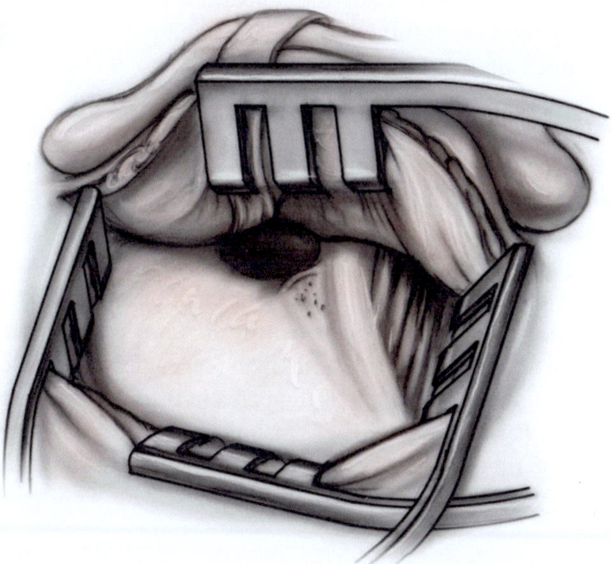

Fig. 61.5 The position of the retractors. (Reproduced with permission of the author [7])

Mastoid Drilling

The safest place to start mastoid drilling is the cribriform area, posterior to the spine of Henle. This last structure can be kept as a reference until the lateral semicircular canal is exposed.

It is convenient to mark a triangle whose limits are superiorly, a line inferior and parallel to the zygomatic line that determines the approximate location of the plane of the meninges in the middle fossa, anteriorly, a slightly arched line, immediately posterior to the posterior wall of the ear canal and a posteroinferior line that remains anterior and superior to the projection of the sigmoid sinus. This form of entry, similar to a simple mastoidectomy, will be comfortable for most surgeons who perform Canal Wall Up (CWU) surgeries more frequently. Although the posterior wall of the external bony canal can also be drilled directly, if you have previously decided to do a CWD technique.

Once the cells of the antrum have been opened and this structure has been recognized, the superior plane immediately inferior to the meninges can be defined, which can be recognized by the progressive decrease in mastoid cells, the transparency of the meningeal vessels through the thinned bone layer and a particularly high-pitched sound emitted by the bur when approaching the meningeal limit [4].

With the meningeal plane identified, an antrostomy is completed until the lateral semicircular canal is seen medially and the short process of the incus is identified anteriorly.

In case of finding attical cholesteatoma, it may be necessary to mobilize it anteriorly, pushing with a cotton soaked in saline solution, in order to identify the lateral semicircular canal, and anterior and inferior to it, the facial nerve will be found in its second portion, which can be identified with the nerve stimulator.

The semicircular canal is an important anatomical landmark because it provides the depth level at which the facial nerve can be encountered and must be positively identified before proceeding.

To perform the atticotomy, look for the incudis fossa that contains the short process of the incus, a very useful anatomical landmark because it points directly to the second bend of the facial nerve, at the level of the pyramidal eminence. When extending the dissection forward, the incudomalleolar joint will be found in the epitympanum. In case of confirming an extensive cholesteatoma that does not allow its eradication with a closed technique, at this point, it is possible to go through the external auditory canal by lifting the tympanic membrane, disinserting the annulus from its bony groove, to expose the chain of ossicles in the middle ear and perform an incudo-stapedial disarticulation, in order to avoid unnecessary stimulation of the inner ear when manipulating the ossicular chain. The stapes suprastructure, if possible, will be kept in place at this stage of the surgery [1].

With the chain disarticulated, it is possible to return to the attic to remove the incus and cut the head of the malleus, which will give ample access to the attic by drilling its lateral wall and will allow all attical cholesteatoma, to be resected and expose the upper aspect of the tympanic cavity, the cochleariform process, anterior to the point where the second portion of the facial (tympanic segment) ends in its reflection

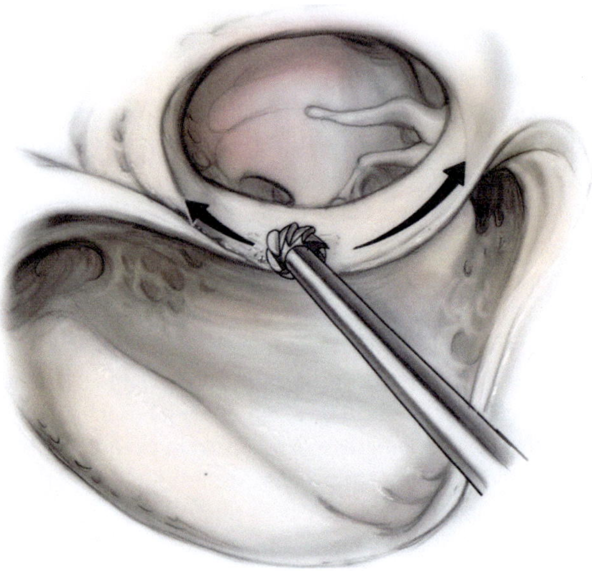

Fig. 61.6 Correct direction of the bur in the facial ridge drilling. (Reproduced with permission of the author [7])

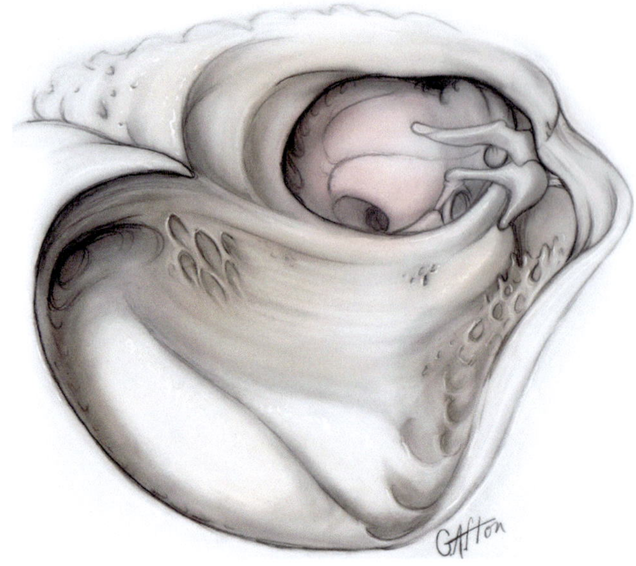

Fig. 61.7 The canal wall is completely lowered and the facial ridge exposed. (Reproduced with permission of the author [7])

towards the geniculate ganglion. Once this point has been identified, the posterior wall of the supratubal cell can be drilled (the medial insertion of this bone lamella marks the projection zone of the geniculate), whose lower limit is the malleus muscle on the superior aspect of the Eustaquian tube.

Once the attical dissection is finished, we return to drilling the mastoid region, extending the cavity downward, taking as a reference the second bend of the facial, already identified, to drill the posterior wall of ear canal, eliminating the cells lateral to the labyrinthine block to the level of the facial nerve. In this way, the posterior wall of the bony auditory canal will be lowered until the facial recess is completely exposed, with a large diamond bur, in the axis of the projection of the third portion of the nerve, under generous irrigation (Fig. 61.6). A pink color can be progressively identified, and the characteristic longitudinal vessels of the Fallopian duct in the third portion can be seen. The facial ridge level, preserving a thin layer of bone as protection, is critical to achieve a dry cavity in the postoperative period, and this dissection will extend from the second bend to the anterior limit of the digastric ridge, that marks the position of the stylomastoid foramen. Although a positive identification of the facial nerve can be achieved taking into account only the anatomical landmarks described, the use of a nerve stimulator is very convenient, considering that many times the inflammatory pathology can modify the appearance of the tissue or erode the bony canal of the facial nerve (Fig. 61.7).

Once the fascial nerve has been identified in its second and third portions, the mastoidectomy is completed by identifying the sigmoid sinus posteriorly, which will allow to drill all the cells until the sinodural angle is cleared, leaving the labyrinthine block medial and posterior to the meninges of the fossa posterior, medial to the sigmoid sinus.

The extension of the drilling downward and anteriorly, following the sigmoid sinus, allows us to identify the curvature of the sinus anteriorly to go toward the jugular bulb.

At this stage, all the cells of the mastoid tip must be lowered, identifying the projection area of the insertion of the digastric muscle on the medial aspect of the mastoid tip (digastric ridge). It is convenient in this dissection to preserve the cortical of the mastoid tip to prevent the collapse of the soft tissues toward the drilling area in the mastoid. Once these cells have been drilled, in highly pneumatized mastoids, the tip of the mastoid lateral to the digastric ridge can be cut, which will allow finally a smaller cavity with fewer complications.

The anterior end of the digastric ridge is at the level of the stylomastoid foramen, an important reference to be able to reduce all of the bone that is lateral to the third portion of the facial nerve. The drilling will continue anteriorly, to reduce the tympanal bone, to regularize the cavity in the posteroinferior part of the canal toward the hypotympanum, where special attention should be paid to the jugular bulb, which will have been previously evaluated in the CT images of the patient. This structure is sometimes exposed in the hypotympanum, and it is very important to avoid injuring it due to the difficulties involved in controlling bleeding at that level (Fig. 61.8).

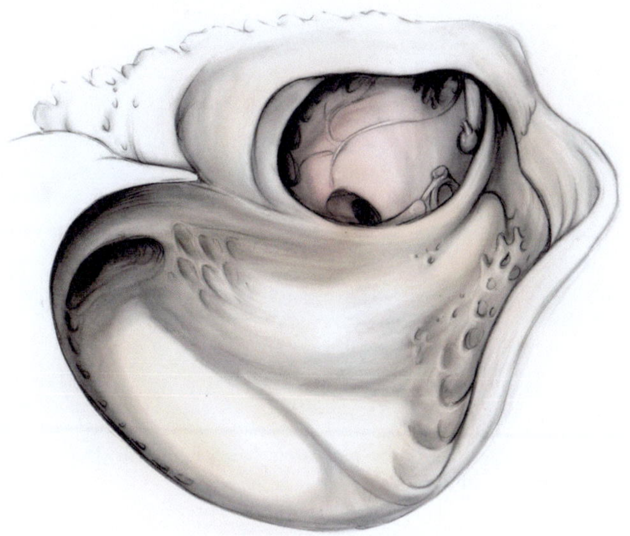

Fig. 61.8 The mastoid cavity is communicated with the middle ear and the ossicular chain has been resected. (Reproduced with permission of the author [7])

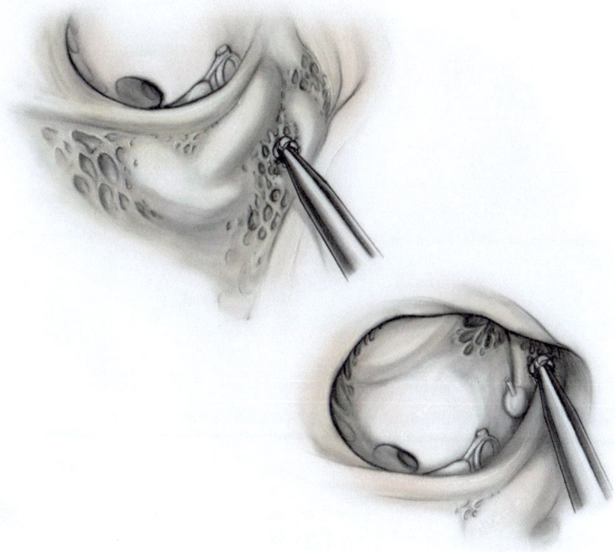

Fig. 61.9 The cavity is been regularized with a drill. (Reproduced with permission of the author [7])

Management of Bleeding from the Venous Sinuses

In RM, the venous sinuses should not be injured, but the surgeon who performs this technique must have surgical tools to manage these complications. In the event of bleeding of this nature, one must remain calm, since venous bleeding will generally stop with slight compression and patience, a gelatinous sponge or Surgicel[R] can be used and if necessary, cover it with a cottonoid while waiting for the spontaneous hemostasis. If the injury is small and there is bone around it, bone wax or a diamond bur can be used. If bleeding cannot be stopped by these means, consider external compression with bone wax in the jugular bulb or in cases of extensive injury, including ligation of the internal jugular vein in the neck and intraluminal and/or extraluminal tamponade of the damaged sinus [3, 4].

Resection of the Tympanic Membrane

Once the mastoidectomy is completed, you must return to the ear canal where an incision is made in its skin, lateral to the anterior edge of the tympanic annulus, which will allow the annulus to be disinserted and the tympanic membrane to be completely resected, taking care to cut the malleus tendon, if this has not already been done.

The resection of the membrane will give adequate access to regularize the limit between the attic and the Eustachian tube, where special care will be taken not to leave cholesteatomatous disease, removing any bone spicule that prevents adequate control of the cavity.

Finally, the entire mastoid cavity must be regularized in the anteroinferior aspect, leaving a drilled bed between the lowered facial in its third distal portion and the floor of the bony canal and the projection zone of the temporomandibular joint, whose soft tissues can be exposed in a limited extension, which is not a problem for our dissection. In the inferior aspect of the external auditory canal, there may be annoying bleeding due to perforating branches of the anterior tympanic artery that will be controlled with a diamond bur (without using irrigation), or with bone wax.

Finally, a final check is made with a large diamond bur of any irregularity that may have been left in the entire cavity during the dissection, obtaining a cavity with smooth walls (Fig. 61.9).

Obliteration of the Eustachian Tube

Once the cholesteatoma has been eradicated and a smooth cavity has been achieved, that includes the entire mastoid cavity and the middle ear, and once any remaining inflamed mucosa has been resected from the cavity and the fallopian tube mucosa has been resected, as far as possible, you have to obliterate the Eustachian tube with soft tissue, which can be done with cartilage, muscle and/or fascia, which is inserted under pressure into the lumen of the tube to prevent respiratory secretions from escaping into the cavity (Fig. 61.10).

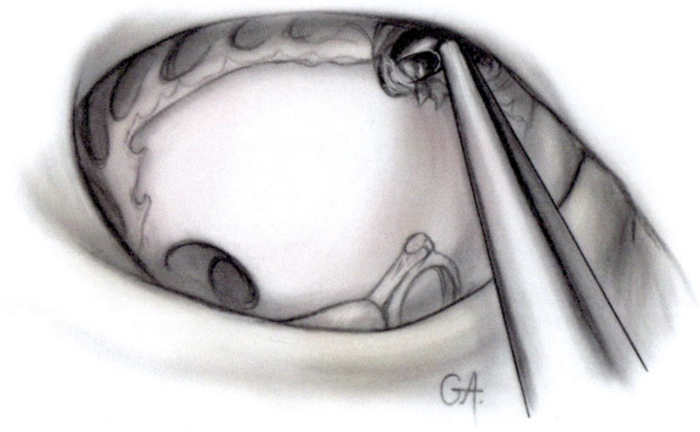

Fig. 61.10 The Eustaquian tube is been obliterated. (Reproduced with permission of the author [7])

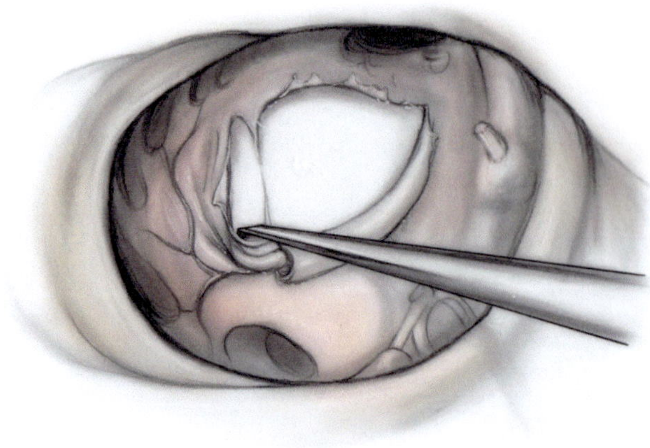

Fig. 61.11 The middle ear mucosa is being removed. (Reproduced with permission of the author [7])

Final Handling of the Cavity

Finally, once the drilling of the cavity is finished, all the mucosa of the tympanic cavity that persists should be removed as far as possible (Fig. 61.11).

Then, considering that the bone bed usually produces a difficult epithelialization and sometimes of poor quality, many surgeons use the temporal fascia to cover the exposed bone areas, paying special attention to blocking cells that could not be drilled, for example, perilabyrinthine cells that go toward the tip of the mastoid, retrofacial or you can use the fascia to give additional protection to the facial nerve.

A radical cavity is a large space connected to the ear canal and through it to the outside, which is susceptible to infection and recurrent or chronic moisture. To maintain a dry cavity, it is important to have a cavity with smooth edges, with a good obliteration of the mastoid tip, an adequate seal and closure of the tube, a facial ridge lowered to the level of the nerve and a wide meatoplasty to allow a good ventilation and cavity control in the office.

Various cavity obliteration techniques have been described for highly pneumatized mastoids, although there is no consensus on their use, such as the one proposed by Palva [5] with retromeatal muscle-periosteum, or different techniques described for making a temporal muscle and/or muscle-periosteal flap and posterior periosteum, for a partial obliteration of the radical mastoid cavity [6], in order to finally have a smaller mastoid cavity that would facilitate a small and dry cavity.

Meatoplasty

Meatoplasty is a technique that aims to achieve an external auditory meatus proportional in size to the cavity that has been achieved with mastoid dissection. To achieve this goal, different ways have been described, but the element common to all of them is the resection of the cartilage of the posterior wall of the external auditory canal and of the medial and posterior portion of the auricular concha.

The meatoplasty begins by extending the longitudinal incisions that were made in the duct at the beginning of the surgery to the auricular concha, then the cartilage that remains adhered to the posterior skin flap of the ear canal is removed (Fig. 61.12). If cartilage is exposed at the remaining flap at the lateral skin edges on the side of both incisions, it will also be resected. In this way, when the ear is restored to its anatomical position, the posterior flap can rest on the posterior portion of the mastoid cavity that has been made and its skin will be the starting point for epithelialization of the cavity. This flap can be fixed by means of sutures to the immediately posterior soft tissues to ensure its position.

The opposite edges of the posterior flap will be sutured to the soft tissue around the mastoid cavity in order to keep the meatus obtained in an open position (Fig. 61.13), whose limits are anterior to the posterior aspect of the tragus, superior to the skin of the original external auditory canal and posteriorly the edge of the incision made in the canal, posteriorly the skin flap posterior to the canal and inferiorly the inferior

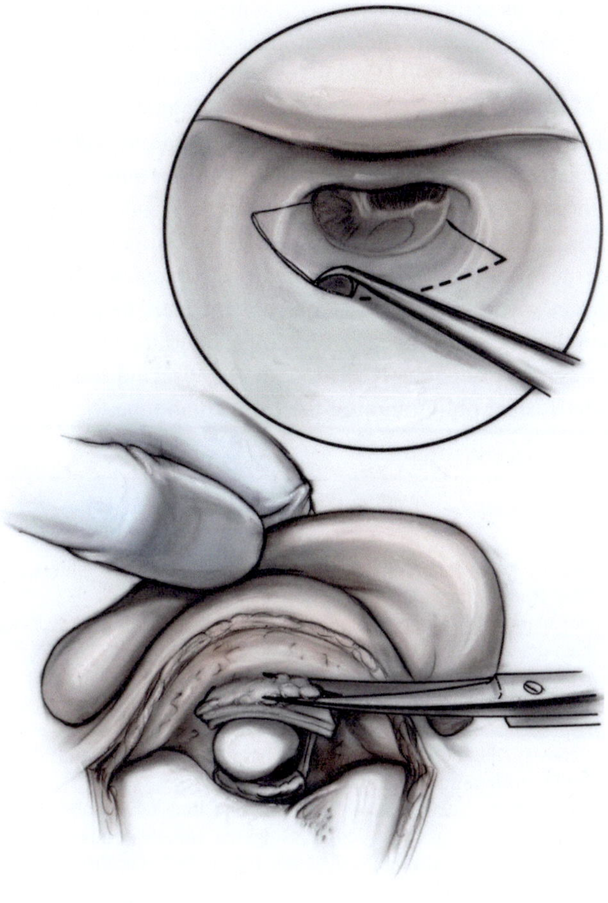

Fig. 61.12 Incisions to perform the meatoplasty. (Reproduced with permission of the author [7])

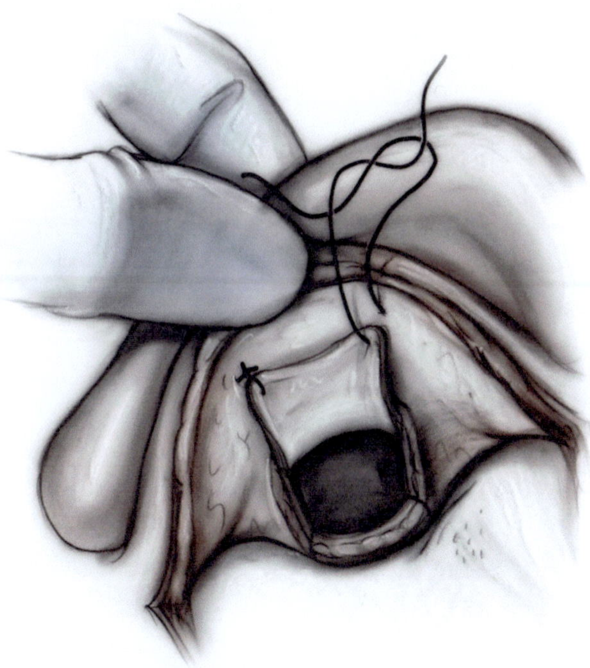

Fig. 61.13 The meatoplasty flap sutured to the soft tissue. (Reproduced with permission of the author [7])

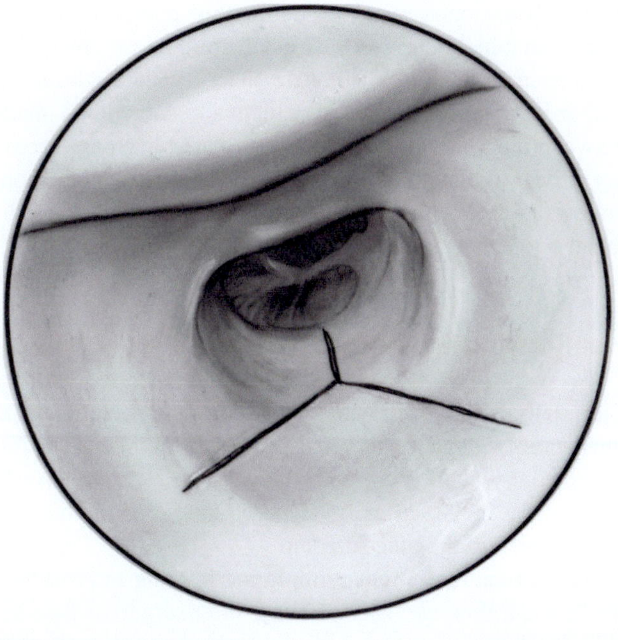

Fig. 61.14 Alternative incision to the meatoplasty. (Reproduced with permission of the author [7])

edge of the canal wound in the posterior part and the original skin of the inferior wall of the external auditory canal in the anterior part. A round drilling of the edges or "saucerization" of the entire contour of the mastoid cavity and resection of the mastoid tip will contribute to a significant reduction in the volume of the cavity achieved at the end of surgery [3].

Another meatoplasty design alternative can be done by making a longitudinal incision in the cartilaginous external auditory canal, in its posterior wall, ending in a Y in its most lateral aspect. The cartilage of the edges is resected and in this case it will be the skin of the canal in two upper and lower flaps with a wide base, which will carry the epithelialization to the cavity. The small posterior triangle will be supported in the most posterior part of the cavity (Fig. 61.14) [7].

Functional Management Alternatives

In certain circumstances, a functional time can be associated with radical surgery, which is achieved by avoiding the obliteration of the Eustachian tube, placing a graft of fascia or perichondrium and a columella of cartilage or bone on the remnant of the stapes. This graft rests anteriorly on the preserved anterior tympanic membrane remnant and posteriorly on the facial ridge and towards the attic it rests on soft tissues that have been used to obliterate the attic. A similar technique can be used to reconstruct a previous operated radical cavity, in which hearing has been defunctionalized, but in which eustachian tube patency is observed, which can be confirmed by an air gap seen on the anterior aspect of the cavity. Brackmann suggests doing this operation in two stages, an initial one to reconstruct the middle ear cavity that is allowed to heal with a silastic sheet to avoid adhesions, and then a second stage in which a columella is made between the graft and the stapes footplate to achieve recovery of hearing function. One must be very careful when reoperate a radical cavity, due to the possible exposed areas of the facial nerve that could be hidden under the soft tissues [3].

Healing and Post-operative Care

The cavity is stabilized with a gelatin sponge packing and at the meatus with gauze soaked in antibiotic ointment. The retroauricular wound is closed in layers with separate absorbable sutures in the musculoperiosteal plane and with the skin closure preferred by the surgeon.

The patient is left with a simple ear dressing and is scheduled for a follow-up visit 7–10 days after surgery, where the skin stitches are removed, if applicable, and the gauze is removed from the duct, then you start the use of antibiotic drops that the patient will use until the cavity is dry. The patient will be controlled every 4 weeks until a dry cavity is achieved, which in most of our patients is obtained between 3 to 6 months after surgery.

Final Considerations

Radical mastoidectomy, which was once the treatment for most cholesteatomas, is now considered a technique limited to certain specific indications. The ear surgeon must be familiar with this technique because in some occasions, during surgery to remove a cholesteatoma, circumstances will be encountered that will lead him to indicate radical surgery.

On the other hand, there are cases of patients previously operated with this technique, who for different reasons, did not achieve the eradication of the cholesteatoma or persist with humidity and suppuration, which will lead to indicating a surgical revision and that is where the surgery has to be oriented to the basic factors that allow a dry cavity that are: a correct meatoplasty, an adequately lowered facial (ideally maintaining a thin bone coverage), a smooth cavity without recesses, an adequately drilled and/or resected mastoid tip and a correct obliteration of the Eustachian tube.

References

1. Sheehy J. Cholesteatoma surgery: canal wall down procedures. Ann Otol Rhinol Laryngol. 1988;97:30–5.
2. Portmann M. Traité de Technique Chirurgicale O.R.L et Cervico-Faciale. 1st ed. Masson & Cie; 1975.
3. Brackmann et al. Otologic surgery. 2nd ed. Saunders;2001.
4. Sanna, et al. The temporal bone: anatomical dissection and surgical approaches. 1st ed. Stuttgart: Thieme; 2018.
5. Palva T, Mäkinen J. The meatally based Musculoperiostial flap in cavity obliteration. Arch Otolaryngol. 1979;105:377–80.
6. Tan AD, et al. Post-operativehealing and long-term stability after mastoid cavity reconstruction using the middle temporal artery and inferior musculoperiosteal flaps. Eur Arch Otorhinolaryngol. 2022;279:639–44.
7. Goycoolea M. Atlas of otologic surgery and magic otology. 1st ed. Jaypee; 2012.

62 Local Management of the Mastoidectomy Cavity

Leandro Rodríguez, Raimundo José García-Matte, and Marcos V. Goycoolea

Introduction

Canal wall down mastoidectomy (CWD) has been used for the treatment of cholesteatoma for a long time. It roughly consists of removing the mastoid air cells, aggressive saucerization of the cortical edges of the mastoid and tip, complete removal of the superior and posterior canal walls, and a meatoplasty. Tympanic membrane reconstruction can also be part of the surgery.

The described CWD advantages lie in the improved visualization of the mesotympanum and epitympanum. As a result, cholesteatoma removal is made more accessible, which results in a significantly decreased incidence of residual disease. The CWD cholesteatoma recidivism rate of 6–20% is lower than the canal wall-up technique (up to 45%) [1–5]. Also, it is much easier to detect any residual disease at the follow-ups because the only area inaccessible to direct visualization in the clinic setting is the mesotympanum.

Nevertheless, the CWD technique has its own disadvantages and challenges caused by the loss of self-cleaning capacity of the ear and the anatomical changes involved. The main ones are chronic discharge and infection of the mastoid cavity (MC), hearing loss, caloric-induced dizziness after temperature or pressure changes, precautionary water avoidance measures, and difficulty fitting hearing aids [6–10]. In addition, the need for frequent visits to the outpatient clinic is also something to consider when deciding on this surgery, as nearly 60% of CWD patients require long-term outpatient care [11].

L. Rodríguez (✉)
Department of Otolaryngology, Clínica Universidad de Los Andes, and Hospital del Salvador, Santiago, Chile

R. J. García-Matte · M. V. Goycoolea
Department of Otolaryngology, Clínica Universidad de Los Andes, Santiago, Chile

Follow-Up Care

Follow-up care aims to assess the cavity for the remote chance of a recurrence or complication developing and to maintain the cavity's lining as healthy as possible. Therefore, the patient's ear status will determine how frequent these postoperative visits need to be. A good microscope, various ear tweezers, and a sound suction system are paramount to proper management.

A healthy ear, cholesteatoma recidivism signs, or a discharging MC are the main options to encounter during outpatient visits.

Healthy Ear

Some MC re-epithelialize rapidly and, within a year or so, have a clean, dry lining that requires little cleaning. These are the ideal patients as the disease is treated and no further treatment is needed.

Cholesteatoma Recidivism

Residual/recurrent cholesteatoma is a possible finding that warrants prompt management most times with revision surgery and is outside the scope of this chapter.

Discharging MC

A chronic or recurrent discharging ear is another possible finding during the outpatient assessment. It is also referred to as active, problematic, or unstable MC and will be the focus of this chapter.

M. V. Goycoolea et al. (eds.), *Textbook of Otitis Media*, https://doi.org/10.1007/978-3-031-40949-3_62

The Active MC

The hallmark of an active MC is chronic otorrhea, which often can be pretty foul smelling. Worsened hearing, otic fullness, and pain are possible but less common symptoms [12]. Vertigo may also be present but less frequently. Sometimes when the meatoplasty is too wide, temperature changes can generate heating effects and cause vertigo, even in a stable cavity. As long as an MC remains unstable, it will be impossible to fit hearing aids.

Merchant et al. developed a four-point rating scale that grades the signs and symptoms of the active MC, such as otorrhea and the presence of granulation tissue. It goes from a dry, healed ear (grade 0) to grade 3, defined as daily constant purulent otorrhea, or otologic exam showing extensive granulation tissue or need for a revision procedure to control infection [13].

A review of the literature projects a variable rate of open MC instability ranging from 10% to 60% over the long term [9, 12, 14–16], significantly affecting the quality of life [12, 17].

Factors that Influence an Active MC

A high facial ridge, an open Eustachian tube, a small external auditory meatus, and a large volume cavity are some of the traditionally cited factors causing MC instability [9]. In the classic paper by Sade, the presence of all of those simultaneously had a 100% likelihood of cavity instability. Furthermore, the prospective study by Wormald and Nilssen reported that the facial ridge height, the contour of the junction between the inferior canal wall and the mastoid cavity, the integrity of the tympanic membrane, and the size of the external auditory meatus all correlated with stability [15].

Residual mastoid air cells with persistent disease are also to be considered since they might require removal by revision surgery.

Preventing the Active MC

The phrase "prevention is better than cure" is often attributed to the Dutch philosopher Desiderius Erasmus around 1500 and applies here as prevention is the most critical measure for MC instability.

Meatoplasty

There should be an excellent, wide, and cosmetically acceptable meatoplasty. The adequacy of the calibre of the eternal auditory meatus is judged against the dimensions of the underlying cavity. As such, there are no absolute size requirements for a meatus to be satisfactory. As a rule, the entirety of the MC should be easily viewed and manipulated as needed. The most common area that cannot be adequately assessed is the posterior sulcus of the cavity, which is located adjacent to the sigmoid sinus and sinodural angle [18, 19].

Facial Ridge

A high facial ridge is defined as having >2 mm of bone overlying the mastoid segment of the facial nerve, and it should be lowered at least to the level of the chorda tympani–facial nerve junction [15]. The recommendation is to lower the facial ridge as much as possible, allowing a better epithelialization of the cavity and a better cleaning under a microscope.

Cavity Irregularities

Whereas some minor cavity irregularities may be unavoidable, especially in the perilabyrinthine area, excessive undrilled air cells cause widespread dimpling of the resultant cavity that may tend to retain debris. Drilling down to the smooth bone of the middle and posterior fossa dural plates and the sigmoid sinus should minimize this. When inspected, a note is made whether these irregularities are involved with retention. Additionally, a severely atelectatic tympanic membrane may act in a similar matter [18].

Kidney Shape

The so-called kidney shape refers to the contour of the cavity as defined by the junction between the inferior tympanic bone and its transition into the mastoid cavity. If not adequately lowered, there is a prominent convex corner in this area that can be perceived to define the hilum of an imaginary kidney. Similar to a high facial ridge, this will prevent epithelial migration from the inferior aspect of the mastoid cavity into the native external auditory canal [18].

Open Eustachian Tube

An intact barrier must be separating the epithelialized mastoid cavity and the mucosalized middle ear or Eustachian tube. An open Eustachian tube most commonly will take the form of a tympanic membrane perforation. However, if the epitympanum has been exteriorized without closure of the anterior communication to the mesotympanum and protympanum, a similarly acting pseudoperforation will occur.

Likewise, if radical mastoidectomy has been performed and the tympanic membrane is thus absent, failure to plug the Eustachian tube orifice will have the same effect.

Non-saucerized Cavity

Suppose the periphery of the cavity has not been widely beveled or saucerized. In that case, steep edges may prevent the inward collapse of soft tissue that will otherwise act to auto-obliterate some of the cavity volume. The former is particularly important concerning the removal of bone in the retrosigmoid region, which, when performed in combination with mastoid tip amputation, will have the effect of collapsing the lateral soft tissue in a way that establishes the anterior edge of the sigmoid sinus as the posterior boundary of the cavity [19].

Fascia over the Mastoid Cavity After a CWD Mastoidectomy

Applying fascia temporalis in the mastoid cavity has been shown to reduce re-epithelialization time in the first 3 months after surgery, according to studies by Bongale, Bhat, and Shetty [20]. They also achieved a dry cavity in less time, in addition to protecting the lateral semicircular canal that can be stimulated during cavity cleans and temperature changes and protecting possible exposure when had some dehiscence in the facial nerve.

Managing the MC in the Office

Examination and Evaluation of a Mastoid Cavity

Microscopic examination of the ear should include inspection for pus, fungal elements, granulation tissue, aural polyp, cholesteatoma, and myringitis. In addition, a careful note is made of the status of the neotympanic membrane.

Treatment in the Office and at Home

One of the most important and relevant factors in maintaining a dry cavity is carrying out a proper and meticulous cleaning before applying topical drops or other antibiotics, as this can be very painful. It is also imperative to have the necessary instruments and be very careful in the procedure.

When performing cavity debridement, it is crucial to systematically examine each region of the exteriorized tympanomastoid space in a stepwise manner, including the neotympanic membrane, epitympanum, tegmen, sinodural angle, and mastoid tip. In addition, it is also essential to identify the facial nerve and the lateral semicircular canal and, when suctioning, to consider the possibility of underlying dehiscence or fistula, respectively.

When granulation tissue or myringitis is found, application of a cauterizing agent is helpful, typically silver nitrate or phenol. When doing so, extreme care must be taken to avoid application onto the facial nerve and to prevent chemical access into the mesotympanum through a nonintact tympanic membrane. An aural polyp can usually be successfully debrided in the office with cupped forceps. Silver nitrate application over granulation tissue and polypoidal formations often works wonderful. If the tympanic membrane is intact, the ongoing application of drying and acidifying agents at home, such as a combination of boric or acetic acid in ethanol, is advocated [18].

Antimicrobial Therapy and Microbiology

It is helpful to routinely obtain bacterial and fungal cultures specimens to direct antimicrobial therapy properly. Although the same pathogens that affect any ear with chronic suppurative otitis media may be present, namely *Pseudomonas aeruginosa*, the most commonly encountered pathogen in an unstable MC is *Staphylococcus aureus* [21]. Fungus infections are also common, especially when antibiotics and steroid-containing otic drops have been long standing. The primary treatment of the MC with otorrhea is fluoroquinolone-containing drops with or without a steroid, especially if there is a tympanic membrane perforation. However, there are a few unique aspects to consider when dealing with an open cavity compared to an intact ear. In particular, the distribution of otic drops to reach the entire cavity may be problematic, mainly if prescribed according to usual dosing for an intact canal wall. In general, at least 8–10 drops per application will be required to have any chance of reaching the entire surface area of a mastoid cavity. Also, chronic overuse of fluoroquinolone drops often leads to developing a secondary fungal infection, especially if debris remains within the cavity. One-percent clotrimazole solution is also safe to apply in the middle ear as an antifungal, but it tends to burn severely and can cause pain in the application.

Alternative preparations, such as ointment or powder, may be preferred in refractory cases. Powders have the advantage of potential custom compounding to include various combinations of antibiotic, antifungal, acidifying, and corticosteroid agents per a particular patient's needs. Patients can easily self-administered these at home using a powder insufflation applicator. There are a number of antibiotic powders that are very efficient such as ciprofloxacin and chloramphenicol. Chloramphenicol currently has very little resistance topically since systemically it is no longer indicated because of secondary effects. Topical rifampicin is also very efficient, however, since it is effective for tuberculosis, its use for other purposes is restricted. Ointments have the advantage of completely filling an MC and coating its entire surface area over a long time. These are usually applied in the office through a syringe and a large angiocath, with the expectation that it will take 1–2 weeks for the ointment to fully clear. Mupirocin ointment is particularly beneficial in treating drug-resistant *S. aureus* infection in an open mastoid cavity. As needed, this can be mixed in the office with steroid (triamcinolone) or antifungal (nystatin) ointments. A nonantibiotic solution such as Burow's solution (aqueous solution of aluminum acetate), which is astringent and has antibacterial and antifungal properties can be efficient in many cases. Topical gentian violet is also efficient in fungal and in bacterial infections and can be at times quite useful.

Decision-Making for Revision Surgery

When the cumulative burden of negative symptoms, frequent office visits, medication application, and hearing aid intolerance overwhelm a given patient's tolerance or suspected disease recurrence, revision surgery should be considered.

Conclusion

Managing an MC is a challenge for the ENT specialist, and keeping it dry depends on several factors that begin in the surgical room. With good management of these factors, it will be easier to maintain a stable cavity. In the office follow-up, it is imperative to maintain cleanliness with a microscope and against repeated infections, perform cultures, and use adequate antibiotic therapy.

References

1. Glasscock ME, Miller GW. Intact canal wall tympanoplasty in the management of cholesteatoma. Laryngoscope. 1976;86:1639–57.
2. Sade J, Berco E, Brown M. Results of mastoid operations in various chronic ear diseases. Am J Otol. 1981;3:11–20.
3. Sheehy JL, Brackmann DE, Graham MD. Cholesteatoma surgery: residual and recurrent disease. A review of 1,024 cases. Ann Otol Rhinol Laryngol. 1977;86:451–62.
4. Smyth GD. Postoperative cholesteatoma in combined approach tympanoplasty. Fifteen year report on tympanoplasty. Part I. J Laryngol Otol. 1976;90:597–621.
5. Nadol JB Jr. Revision mastoidectomy. Otolaryngol Clin N Am. 2006;39(723–740):vi–vii.
6. Uluyol S, Ugur O, Arslan IB, Yagiz O, Gumussoy M, Cukurova I. Effects of cavity reconstruction on morbidity and quality of life after canal wall down tympanomastoidectomy. Braz J Otorhinolaryngol. 2018;84(5):608–13.
7. Mehta RP, Harris JP. Mastoid obliteration. Otolaryngol Clin N Am. 2006;39(6):1129–42.
8. Palva T. Operative technique in mastoid obliteration. Acta Otolaryngol. 1973;75(4):289–90.
9. Sade J, Weinberg J, Berco E, Brown M, Halevy A. The marsupialized (radical) mastoid. J Laryngol Otol. 1982;96(10): 869–75.
10. Vercruysse JP, van Dinther JJ, De Foer B, et al. Long-term results of troublesome CWD cavity reconstruction by mastoid and epitympanic bony obliteration (CWR-BOT) in adults. Otol Neurotol. 2016;37(6):698–703.
11. Khalil HS, Windle-Taylor PC. Canal wall down mastoidectomy: a long term commitment to the outpatients? BMC Ear Nose Throat Disord. 2003;3(1):1.
12. Males AG, Gray RF. Mastoid misery: quantifying the distress in a radical cavity. Clin Otolaryngol Allied Sci. 1991;16:12Y4.
13. Merchant SN, Wang P, Jang CH, et al. Efficacy of tympanomastoid surgery for control of infection in active chronic otitis media. Laryngoscope. 1997;107:872Y7.
14. Smyth GD. Canal wall for cholesteatoma: up or down? Long-term results. Am J Otol. 1985;6(1):1–2.
15. Wormald PJ, Nilssen EL. The facial ridge and the discharging mastoid cavity. Laryngoscope. 1998;108(1 Pt 1):92–6.
16. Youngs R. The histopathology of mastoidectomy cavities, with particular reference to persistent disease leading to chronic otorrhoea. Clin Otolaryngol Allied Sci. 1992;17(6):505–10.
17. Dornhoffer JL, Smith J, Richter G, Boeckmann J. Impact on quality of life after mastoid obliteration. Laryngoscope. 2008;118:1427Y32.
18. Dornhoffer JL, Gluth MB. Chapter 14: Office evaluation and management of a canal wall-down mastoid. In: The chronic ear. 2016. pp. 106–110.
19. Gluth MB, Metrailer AM, Dornhoffer JL, Moore PC. Patterns of failure in canal wall down mastoidectomy cavity instability. Otol Neurotol. 2012;33(6):998–1001.
20. Bongale KR, Bhat VK, Shetty AM. The effect of fascia and free skin graft on the healing of mastoid cavity after canal wall down mastoidectomy. J Laryngol Otol. 2021;135:1094–9.
21. Gluth MB, Tan BY, Santa Maria PL, Atlas MD. Unique microbiology of chronically unstable canal wall down tympanomastoid cavities: considerations for surgical revision. J Laryngol Otol. 2013;127(5):458–62.

Reconstruction and Obliteration of the Mastoid Cavity

63

Michael B. Gluth and Ryan T. Judd

Introduction

The mastoid air cells comprise part of a network of mucosalized spaces within the pneumatized temporal bone that allow for the free flow of gases between the mastoid and middle ear. Although the exact purpose of these air cells is not definitively understood, it is thought that they play a role in middle ear gas homeostasis and may additionally aid in sound conduction [1, 2]. There is significant variation in the extent of pneumatization of the mastoid between individuals [3], which is likely related to a combination of genetics and the effects of chronic middle ear disease [4, 5]. If obstruction of mastoid ventilation pathways is prominent during childhood, there may be development of a sclerotic and poorly pneumatized temporal bone that is associated with several chronic pathologies, including cholesteatoma, atelectasis of the tympanic membrane, and chronic attico-antral otitis media [6, 7]. Even when mastoid development is normal, obstruction of the aditus ad antrum, which connects the mastoid to the middle ear, will result in chronic inflammatory and/or infectious changes in the mastoid air cells known as mastoiditis.

Mastoidectomy refers to a range of surgical procedures applied to the mastoid and surrounding structures that are utilized either for therapeutic purposes to treat mastoiditis or as a means to provide surgical access to various temporal bone structures, including the lateral skull base, the labyrinth, the sigmoid sinus, the middle ear, or the facial nerve. In virtually all types of mastoidectomy, the mastoid cortex and central air cell tracts are drilled away to create a common cavity. The extent to which the air cells are drilled open and which additional structures are preserved differentiates the types of mastoidectomy [8]. In simple terms, types of mastoidectomy are divided into procedures that preserve the circumferential integrity of the bony external auditory canal (intact canal wall or "canal wall-up" mastoidectomy) versus those that intentionally remove the posterior and superior bony external auditory canal wall (radical or "canal wall-down" mastoidectomy) with intent to exteriorize the mastoid and epitympanic spaces in continuum with the external auditory canal. Although there are anatomic and physiological consequences to both types of mastoidectomy procedures, canal wall-down surgery is clearly associated with far greater negative consequences. The purpose of this chapter is to present various surgical options that are available to minimize the negative impact of mastoidectomy surgery via either reconstructive or obliterative techniques.

M. B. Gluth (✉) · R. T. Judd
University of Chicago Section of Otolaryngology-Head and Neck Surgery, Chicago, IL, USA

Mastoid Cortex Reconstruction (Intact Canal Wall)

Patient Selection

Reconstruction of the mastoid cortex in the context of intact canal wall mastoidectomy is considered either in the primary setting (at the time of mastoidectomy) or when a patient presents with cosmetic deformity and/or pain in the mastoid postoperatively. Usually, during intact canal wall mastoidectomy, the common mastoid cavity is left open, and the overlying skin and soft tissues are sutured closed to generate a lateral soft tissue diaphragm. Over time, the mastoid cavity is filled with fibrous tissue and possibly some degree of new bone formation [2, 9]. It is well established, based on the collective experience of the otologic surgery community of several decades, that the overwhelming majority of intact canal wall mastoidectomy surgeries heal well without the need for any bony reconstruction and without development of any major postoperative sequelae. Nevertheless, certain instances do exist where excessive inward scarring of soft tissue following mastoidectomy will result in an unsightly or painful postauricular divot (Fig. 63.1) [9, 10], and in such instances, it is reasonable to consider secondary revision mastoid cortex reconstruction.

M. V. Goycoolea et al. (eds.), *Textbook of Otitis Media*, https://doi.org/10.1007/978-3-031-40949-3_63

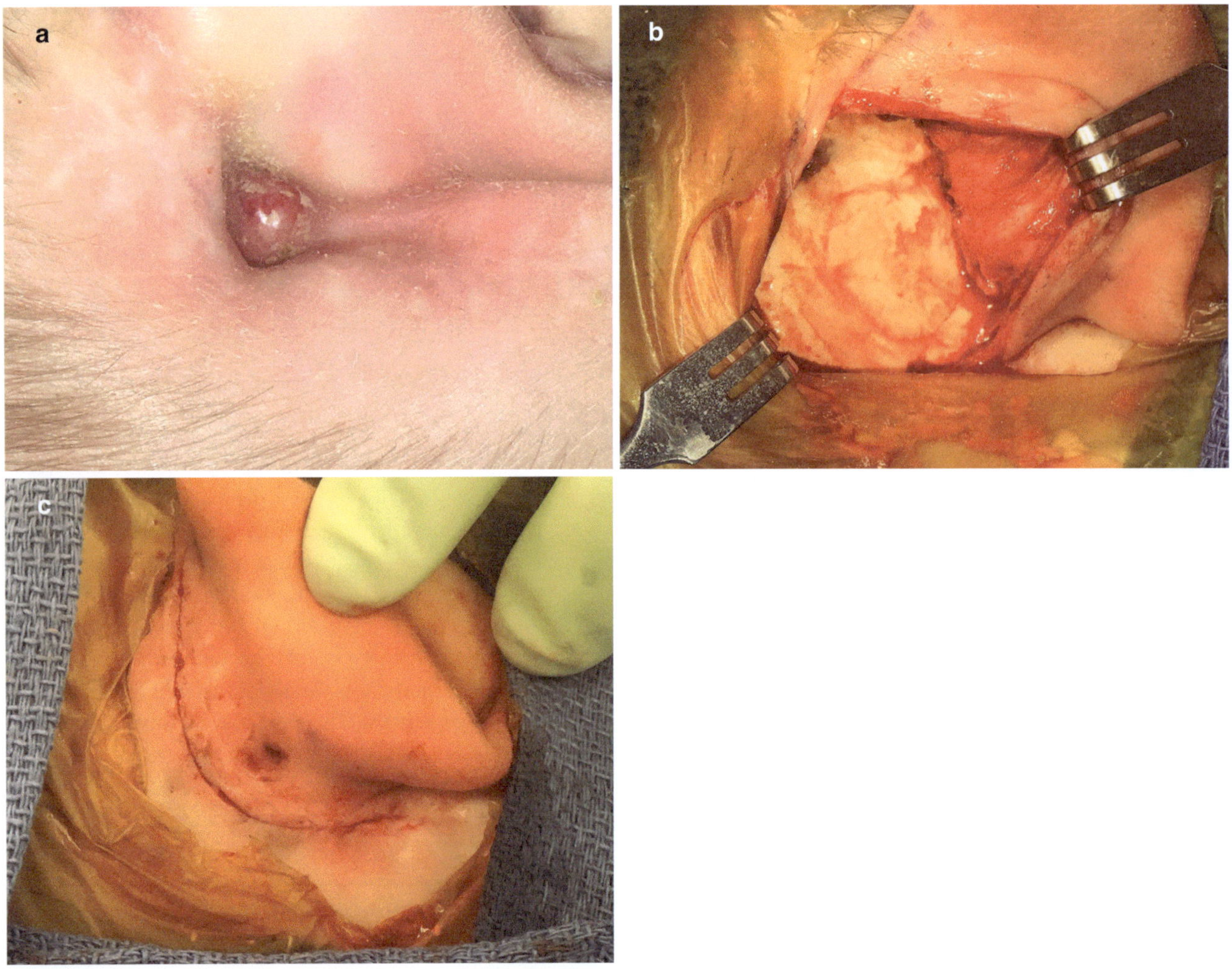

Fig. 63.1 Postauricular retraction and reconstruction. (**a**) Unsightly postauricular retraction that resulted in chronic retention of debris, skin irritation, and pain. (**b**) Following postauricular incision and sharp excision of the soft tissue that had grown into the mastoid cavity, the mastoid cortex was reconstructed using HAC. (**c**) Improvement in the appearance of the postauricular site is immediately evident upon closure of the incision

There may also be certain cases where proactively reconstructing the mastoid cortex upfront at the time of mastoidectomy may be reasonably considered in order to proactively prevent negative sequalae. For example, surgical cases that involve extensive mastoid bone removal, such as is encountered during lateral skull base surgery, may result in a particularly large defect that could benefit from proactive cortex reconstruction. Further, if a patient expresses considerable concern about having a postauricular divot during the preoperative counseling phase, it may also be reasonable to plan upfront cortex reconstruction.

The main contraindications to mastoid cortex reconstruction are active chronic infection or cholesteatoma status with risk of recurrence. Because many mastoid cortex reconstructive techniques involve non-autologous materials such as bone cement or titanium mesh, they should only be applied when infection is definitively absent and unlikely to recur and only when clearance of cholesteatoma has been definitively established.

Surgical Technique

Reconstruction Materials

Synthetic Materials

Both synthetic and autologous reconstructive material have been used for mastoid cortex reconstruction following intact canal wall mastoidectomy. The two most commonly used synthetic materials for this purpose are HAC and titanium mesh. HAC is a calcium-phosphate cement that upon intraoperative preparation sets to become hydroxyapatite, the main component of skeletal bone. It becomes a thick, easily moldable paste that hardens and becomes osteoconductive over time. Infectious complications are rare, especially in the setting of a low preoperative risk of infection [10, 11]. Titanium mesh is screwed directly over the mastoid defect and can be modified to approximate the size of the defect. There is minimal ingrowth of soft tissue beyond the mesh into the mastoid cavity [12]. Titanium mesh can be easily removed and recycled in the setting of a second-look procedure. There is a rare complication of extrusion, so titanium mesh should be used cautiously in the setting of thin overlying skin or if reconstruction of the external canal wall is undertaken concurrently [12].

Autologous Materials

Autologous materials include bone pate and cortical bone cap. Bone pate is collected during mastoid drilling, and the water in the pate is removed by applying pressure with gauze. The pate may be mixed with fibrin glue such that a bone pate plate is created that can be cut to create a roof for the mastoid cavity [2]. Infectious complications are rare, and soft tissue ingrowth has not been reported. Potential disadvantages include that, at second-stage operation, the bone pate is occasionally partially reabsorbed [2] and that bone pate collection can be relatively time consuming. A cortical bone cap can be harvested prior to drilling the mastoid cavity. A triangle of mastoid cortical bone about 2 mm deep is drilled and chiseled to approximate the mastoid cavity defect and is placed atop the defect upon completion of mastoidectomy. While the surgical technique may not be familiar to all surgeons, Sun et al. reported that average reconstructive time was only 3 min [13]. Although this technique has only been used in one case series [13], no infections or extrusions were reported. Of course, the cortical bone cap can be used only in the case of primary mastoid reconstruction.

Surgical Application of Cortex Reconstruction

In the setting of primary mastoid surgery, reconstruction is undertaken just prior to soft tissue closure. For cases involving a combined transmastoid/middle fossa craniotomy, replacement of middle fossa craniotomy bone flap is undertaken prior to reconstruction. In the setting of secondary revision mastoid reconstruction, the soft tissue ingrowth within the mastoid cavity is sharply incised and resected (Fig. 63.1). The technique for reconstruction varies based on the reconstruction material used. The authors prefer the use of hydroxyapatite cranioplastic cement (HAC) [10]. To begin reconstruction, a large, dry piece of absorbable gelatin sponge is cut to fit the mastoid defect and inlayed to serve as a medial diaphragm for the mastoid cavity. The purpose of the sponge is to prevent the inward egress of HAC onto the ossicular chain and to preserve an aerated mastoid cavity medially. HAC is mixed according to the manufacturer's instructions and promptly applied to the mastoid cavity defect lateral to the gelatin sponge and shaped to create a natural cortical contour. The HAC should be allowed to set prior to closure of the soft tissue flap over the reconstructed mastoid cortex.

Mastoid Cavity Obliteration (Canal Wall-Down)

Open (canal wall-down) mastoidectomy approaches have long been considered the gold standard for surgical extirpation of cholesteatoma as they have generally been associated with the lowest rates of disease recidivism—typically in the 10% range. However, removal of the canal wall radically alters the anatomical landscape of the ear in ways that impart significant permanent negative consequences related to the collective burden of chronic otorrhea, lifetime office visits for cleaning, expensive pharmacotherapy, and occasional discomfort [14–17]. In the pediatric population, where tolerance of office examination and aural toilet may be poor, this is a particular dilemma [18]. A review of the literature portrays a long-term postoperative rate of having a period of prolonged mastoid cavity instability in the 10–60% range, with some variation accounted for by the skill and experience of the surgeon in creating a smooth, rounded mastoid bowl and sufficient meatoplasty. Even in the best cases, a stable cavity can still cause caloric-effect vertigo, and impede optimal hearing aid fitting. These challenging realities have driven surgeons to develop techniques that obliterate the mastoid space in order to avoid some of these undesirable aspects [19–24]. Because performing canal wall-down mastoid surgery or encountering an unstable cavity in the clinic are common aspects of otologic practice, familiarity with cavity obliteration techniques should be viewed as a valuable tool within an otologic surgeon's skill set.

Patient Selection

Candidates for mastoid cavity obliteration include both adults and children undergoing either primary or revision canal wall-down mastoidectomy surgery. The general obliterative scheme utilized and extent of obliteration will vary depending on factors such as the nature of the underlying cholesteatoma, temporal bone pneumatization, and degree of infection. In general, obliterative techniques are frowned upon in areas deemed at high risk of cholesteatoma recurrence; however, such risk often does not particularly apply to the mastoid because cholesteatoma within the mastoid is rarely difficult to expose and definitively remove. This point is highlighted by the fact that recurrent cholesteatoma within the mastoid cavity during second-stage intact canal wall surgery is rare [25].

If temporal bone pneumatization is limited, it is quite common to achieve a small self-cleaning cavity without the need for mastoid obliteration. However, combined mastoid and epitympanic obliteration in these cases may still be deemed advantageous as a means of repositioning the height of the tympanic membrane at the approximate level of the native tympanic ring, thereby preserving normal middle ear volume and facilitating a successful ossiculoplasty. When infection is severe or factors are present that negatively impact healing, such as diabetes, radiation, immunosuppression, or tobacco use, mastoid obliteration is particularly advantageous as patients with these conditions may be at high risk of developing an unstable cavity [14].

Surgical Technique

Obliteration Schemes

The first step made by the surgeon is deciding which areas to obliterate. In the typical situation where the mastoid is deemed to be at low residual cholesteatoma risk, the mastoid cavity is obliterated with application of both a filler and a liner in sequence. When doing so, the purpose of the filler is not only to eliminate cavity volume but also to fill cavity irregularities and to provide a smoothly contoured platform upon which to apply a liner that will subsequently epithelialize. If epitympanic cholesteatoma risk is also deemed low, the obliteration scheme can be expanded to include the epitympanum. In the uncommon situation where the mastoid cavity is felt to be at high risk, such as infiltrative cholesteatosis involving the perilabyrinthine air cells, the obliterative scheme can be limited by partially obliterating a single area such as the tip. Alternatively, the surgeon can achieve safe partial obliteration by applying only a thin soft tissue liner without the use of underlying bulky fillers.

The technique of canal wall-down mastoidectomy may slightly differ in a pneumatized versus a sclerotic temporal bone, which may also impact the approach taken towards obliteration. In a pneumatized bone, the general scheme often will involve lowering the edges of the cavity via wide saucerization and perhaps amputation of the mastoid tip, which results in a broadened shallow cavity that will invite inward soft tissue collapse. Obliteration of these large cavities is often best approached with sensible application of filler materials followed by lining with vascularized soft tissue flaps. In contrast, a sclerotic temporal bone may be reconstructed with simpler techniques as these cases may involve comparatively less drilling of canal wall and solid mastoid tip bone once the cholesteatoma and a limited number of diseased air cells have been eliminated. Mastoid obliteration in a sclerotic temporal bone thus may be completed with less filler and application of a simple pressed tissue soft graft as a liner alongside any preserved native canal wall epithelium.

Obliteration Materials

Bone Pate

Bone pate is a commonly used filler material, but it must be covered by a liner to prevent extrusion and infection. Bone pate is abundantly available, in particular from the squamous temporal bone deep to the temporalis muscle. Harvest of bone pate is undertaken by reflecting the temporalis and drilling cortical bone with a cutting burr, followed by collection either using a commercially available reservoir connected to the suction tubing, or, if plentiful, by simply scooping pate from the surgical field into a specimen cup. A specialized two-fluted cutting bur generates pate with particularly large grain that is ideal for this purpose. It is crucial that bone pate only be harvested from outside of the mastoid so as not to include mucosa or infected material, and this is typically done prior to the actual mastoidectomy drilling.

After harvest, bone pate is soaked in antibiotic solution while the remaining portions of surgery are completed. For placement, it is essential that the pate is applied into the defect and then densely packed utilizing a suction cannula and cotton pledget (Fig. 63.2). In doing so, it is typical to sequentially apply pate several times in one site to achieve the desired tightly packed density. If bone pate is not densely packed, there is a tendency toward reabsorption that can result in eventual formation of "pot-holes" within the obliterated cavity. Bone pate must always be covered by some type of soft tissue liner.

Cartilage Chips

Auricular cartilage chips are harvested either from the tragus or concha. Once large pieces of cartilage have been acquired from these sites, they are stripped of perichondrium and morselized with a scalpel blade. If there is concern for infection, cartilage chips may be soaked in antibiotic solution, similar to soaking bone pate. After application into the mastoid cavity, a liner is typically applied to prevent extrusion (see Fig. 63.3). Compared to bone pate, cartilage is more resistant to reabsorption and infection, but it may be less abundant in cases where extensive tympanic membrane cartilage grafting has been performed. If needed, it is possible to combine the cartilage with bone pate or synthetic filler. Some surgeons will add fibrin glue to bone pate and/or cartilage chips to aid in placement and adherence within the desired areas targeted for obliteration.

Synthetic Materials

Various synthetic materials have been described as fillers in mastoid obliteration, particularly biocompatible ceramics. If use of a synthetic material is desired, porous ceramics in a granular form are favored over cements since the latter seem to bear a higher risk of infection. Also, if an extraordinarily large bone defect requires obliteration, osseo-inductive

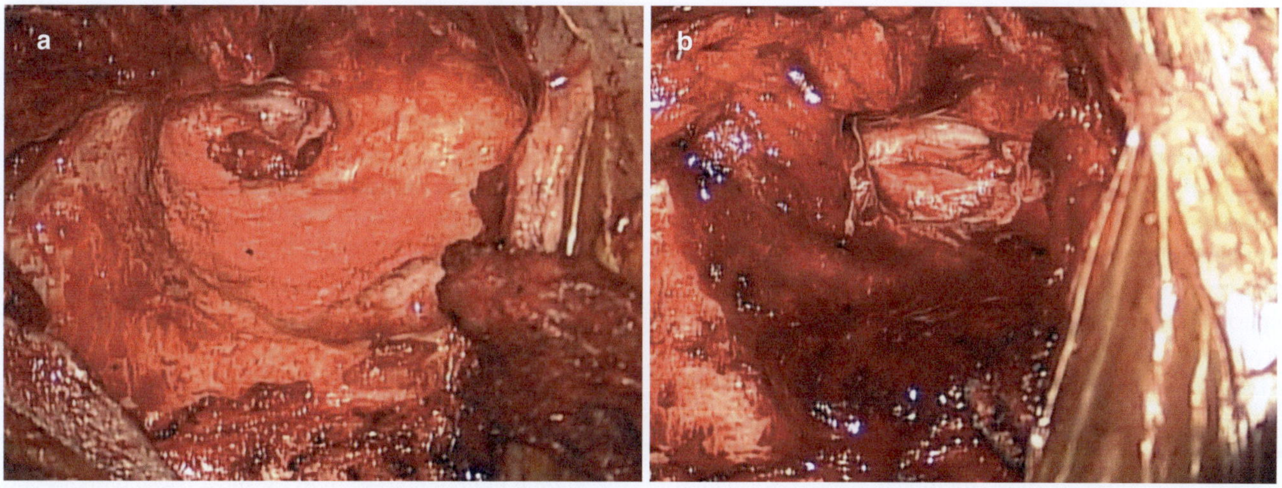

Fig. 63.2 Application of bone pate. (**a**) Bone pate harvested from the outside of the mastoid cavity is densely packed with a suction cannula and cotton pledget, with multiple applications in order to fill cavity irregularities (left ear), reduce cavity volume, and generate a smoothly countered platform upon which to apply a soft tissue liner. (**b**) In this case the middle temporal artery flap and interior musculoperiosteal flap was utilized as a liner and the tympanic membrane is reconstructed with cartilage

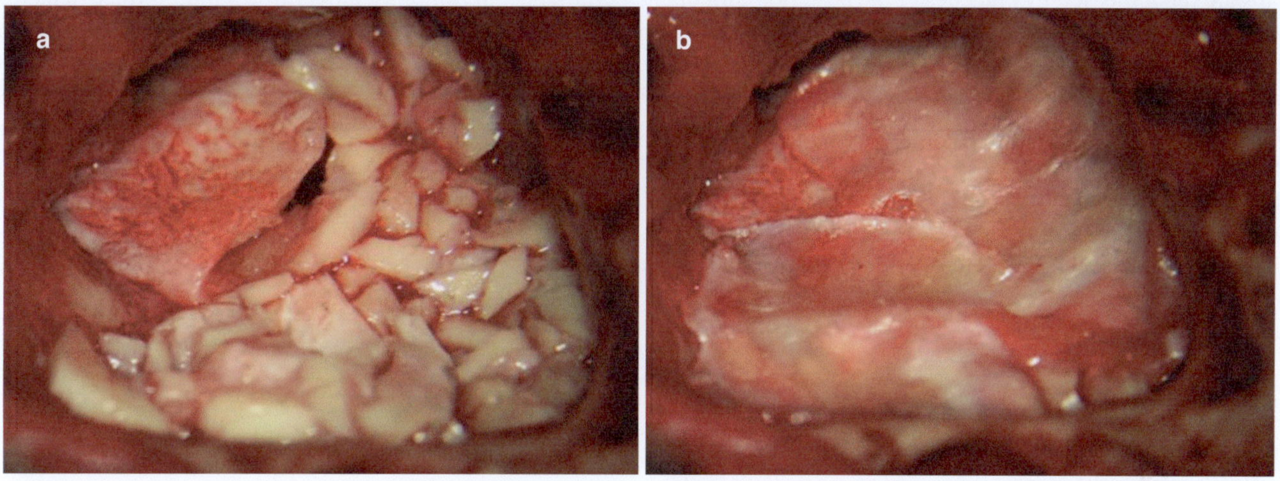

Fig. 63.3 Application of cartilage chips. (**a**) Cartilage chips are harvested from the tragus and/or concha and morselized with a scalpel blade and packed up to the level of the reconstructed tympanic membrane. (**b**) The obliterated mastoid and tympanic membrane are draped with pressed perichondrium

materials, such as bioactive glass (BoneAlive, Boston Medical, Boston, Massachusetts, USA), which are gradually replaced by new bone, may have theoretic advantages. Commercially available xenograft materials, such as demineralized bone matrix (DBX, Osteotech, Inc., Eatontown, NJ, USA), are also an option in small quantities [26].

Although synthetic materials offer the advantage of being readily available in bulk, they generally share a common tendency to extrude or to become infected. As such, it is favorable to avoid use of synthetic materials altogether or to apply them judiciously in limited quantity when overt infection is not present. Often, it is possible to obliterate the areas deep within the mastoid cavity, such as the sinodural angle and opened retrofacial air cell tract, using synthetic materials, and then to cover these with a layer of cartilage or bone pate that will constitute the outer interface. If it is deemed necessary to use synthetic fillers in larger quantities, lining with a vascularized soft tissue flap is recommended.

Fascia, Perichondrium, and Pressed Muscle

Thin autologous connective tissues, such as temporalis fascia, pressed skeletal muscle, and auricular perichondrium, can all be used as liners. Such tissue is readily available and easy to process. When very little filler material is required, when there is a large quantity of intact healthy native canal wall epithelium, and/or when the interface with filler materials is small, such as with a sclerotic mastoid defect, these materials generally work well. However, if extensive coverage of filler material is necessary, particularly if the filler is synthetic, nonvascularized grafts may undergo necrosis, infection, and/or delayed epithelialization.

Soft Tissue Flaps

Rotational soft tissue flaps may variably comprise fascia, periosteum, and/or muscle, having either a distinct or random blood supply. These are pedicled either from a posterior-inferior base or superior-anterior base. In the case of the superior-anterior-based group, thick muscular flaps, such as those composed of temporalis muscle, are best avoided due to the potential for this thick pedicle to obstruct or narrow the external auditory meatus as it enters the tympanomastoid compartment.

Vascular supply to most rotational flaps described for mastoid obliteration is random or variably robust. For example, the commonly used Palva flap does not have a distinct vascular supply, and, therefore, it is prone toward shrinkage and less apt to resist infection. Most posterior-inferior-based flaps are randomly fed by branches of the posterior auricular or occipital arteries proximally but tend to be avascular like the Palva flap at the most superior (distal) aspect.

One notable exception to this trend is the authors' favored middle temporal artery flap [27], a thin pliable anterior-superior-based flap chiefly composed of periosteum, which is based on the axial blood supply of the muscular branch of the superficial temporal artery (Fig. 63.4). The middle temporal artery flap is elevated by releasing the posterior attachment of the temporalis muscle and dissecting in a plane immediately deep to the temporalis muscle. In doing so, the artery is reliably identified by its "train track" appearance (due to the presence of venae comitantes flanking either side). On average, the muscular branch of the middle temporal artery can be identified at a point 9 mm superior and 4 mm posterior to the spine of Henle, where it takes an abrupt turn from its posterior course to then pass towards the vertex of the skull. In comparison to the other rotational flaps, on histologic examination, the middle temporal artery flap is thicker with a more robust blood supply (Fig. 63.5) [27].

Table 63.1 depicts some of the characteristics of various soft tissue flaps that have been described for mastoid obliteration.

The authors' favored usage of soft tissue flaps involves the middle temporal artery flap for most cases with addition of a concurrent inferior musculoperiosteal flap when additional coverage in the tip region is needed [23]. The middle temporal artery is applied as lining for the obliterated sinodural angle as well as coverage for the tegmen and epitympanum. The inferior musculoperiosteal flap, which tends to have more bulk, is applied to fill inferior aspect of the central mastoid defect (Fig. 63.6). The inferior flap is typically held in place with a 3.0 vicryl stay suture that secures the base of the flap to the soft tissue inferior to the native external auditory canal (parotid fascia).

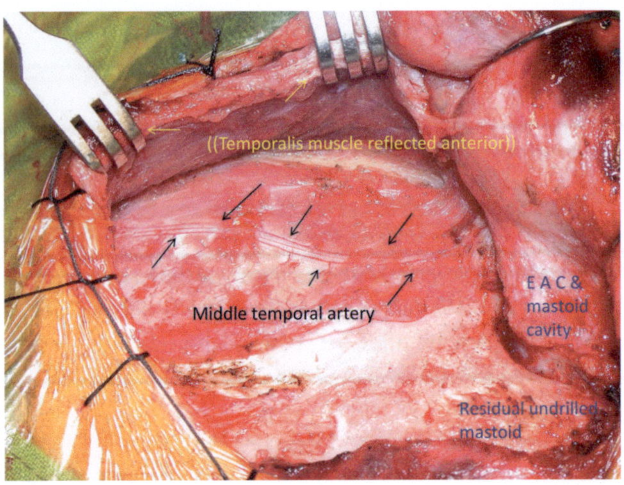

Fig. 63.4 Middle temporal artery flap. The middle temporal artery flap is harvested (right ear) by releasing the posterior attachment of the temporalis muscle, which is reflected anteriorly (yellow arrows). The middle temporal artery is identified in a plane immediately deep to the muscle within the periosteum (black arrows). The artery has a typical "railroad track" appearance running within the periosteum. After identification of the artery, it will provide an axial blood supply to a large anteriorly based flap (3 cm × 6 cm) that is thin and pliable

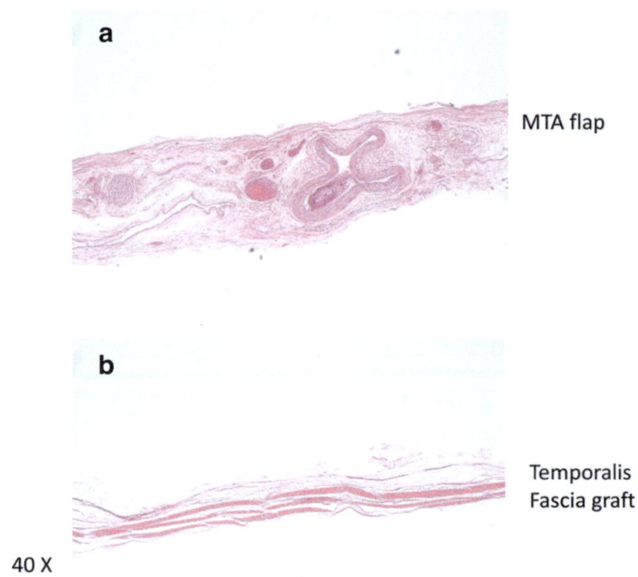

Fig. 63.5 Histology of middle temporal artery flap. (**a**) Hematoxylin and Eosin staining of a middle temporal artery periosteal rotational flap at 40× microscopy shows an approximately 3-mm flap with the middle temporal artery and its venae comitantes. (**b**) Comparison H&E staining of the deep temporalis fascia at 403 microscopy demonstrates that the flap is minimally vascularized and two to three times thinner

Table 63.1 Soft tissue flaps used in mastoid obliteration

Flap	Composition	Blood supply	Advantages	Disadvantages
Palva [33]	Musculo-periosteum, hinged on posterior aspect of pinna	Random	Ease of harvest	Avascular, delayed shrinkage and fibrosis, blind rotation into cavity
Hong Kong [24]	Vascularized temporalis fascia	Middle temporal artery (superficial branch)	Thin and pliable, vascularized, anteriorly based	Lacks bulk, difficulty filling mastoid tip in large cavity, blood supply may be cut during prior surgery
Middle temporal artery [21, 23, 27, 34]	Vascularized periosteum (± thin sheet of muscle)	Middle temporal artery (muscular branch)	Thin and pliable, vascularized, anteriorly based	Difficulty filling mastoid tip in large cavity, blood supply may be cut during prior surgery
Temporalis muscle (Musculoplasty) [35]	Temporalis muscle	Middle temporal artery and deep temporal artery	Ease of harvest, abundance of tissue	Overly bulky, risk of blocking view of epitympanum and risk of meatal stenosis
Temporoparietal fascia [36, 37]	Inferiorly based temporoparietal fascia	Random via superficial temporal and occipital arteries	Thin and pliable, abundance of tissue	Risk of alopecia, scalp numbness, variable blood supply
Inferior musculoperiosteal [22, 23, 38]	Inferiorly based muscle, fascia, and mastoid periosteum	Random via occipital and posterior auricular arteries	Abundance of tissue, useful for inferior aspect of mastoid cavity, ease of harvest	Avascular at distal tip of flap, risk of mastoid bleeding during harvest, scalp numbness

Skin Grafts

Full or split-thickness skin grafts may be used to line the bone of a mastoid cavity in order to promote rapid healing and to slightly reduce cavity irregularities; nevertheless, skin grafts in general do not impart significant obliterative effects. If vascularized soft tissue flaps are utilized, it is possible to apply small split-thickness skin grafts over the vascularized soft tissue of a rotational flap. This is particularly advocated when there is very little residual native canal wall or tympanic membrane epithelium present.

Surgical Application

Through a postauricular skin incision, the contents of the mastoid cavity are elevated and removed—ideally as a single continuous skin flap. Confident removal of all epithelium from the mastoid and epitympanum is critical if obliteration is to be performed; if there is doubt regarding this step, obliteration should be avoided. Drilling and shaping of the mastoid cavity is undertaken according to the desired obliterative scheme. If the epitympanum is deemed safe for obliteration, it may not be necessary to completely lower the posterior canal wall bone and facial ridge as the goal is to "raise" the mastoid and epitympanum up to the level of the natural canal wall and tympanic annulus via obliteration. If the epitympanum is to be exteriorized or if the majority of the canal wall bone has been previously removed, then the facial ridge must be completely lowered.

After middle ear work is completed, tympanoplasty should be completed prior to mastoid obliteration—typically with a large composite perichondrium and cartilage island graft harvested from the tragus. If the epitympanum is to be obliterated, it is useful to perform ossiculoplasty at the primary stage because the prosthesis will act as a spacer to hold the reconstructed eardrum near the natural annulus height. To estimate this height, a 2-mm partial (PORP) or 4-mm total ossicular replacement prosthesis (TORP) is generally used. This newly established tympanic membrane graft height then determines the height boundary of the obliteration materials. Lastly the free end of the tympanoplasty materials are draped overlying the obliteration liner.

Alternatively, for cases where the epitympanum is to remain intentionally exteriorized, the mastoid obliteration will only extend up to the level of the posterior aspect of the reconstructed tympanic membrane near the facial ridge; whereas, the superior free edge of the tympanoplasty graft will be draped onto the medial wall of the epitympanum while covering the tympanic segment of the fallopian canal. In this instance, the middle ear volume has been reduced, so there typically is not adequate space to accommodate a standard full-length ossicular replacement prosthesis; thus, the surgeon has the option of a Type III direct stapes columella reconstruction with tympanic membrane graft placement directly onto the superstructure versus placement of a shortened prosthesis or autograft. Alternatively, the surgeon may wish to place silastic sheeting in the middle ear and stage ossiculoplasty, especially if there is a risk of residual mesotympanic cholesteatoma.

Postoperative Care

After application of obliteration materials, meatoplasty is performed. Silastic sheeting is applied overlying the junction between the reconstructed tympanic membrane and the obliterated mastoid cavity. Ribbon gauze coated in antibiotic ointment is then used to fill any remaining cavity volume as well as to stent the meatoplasty. Patients are treated with oral

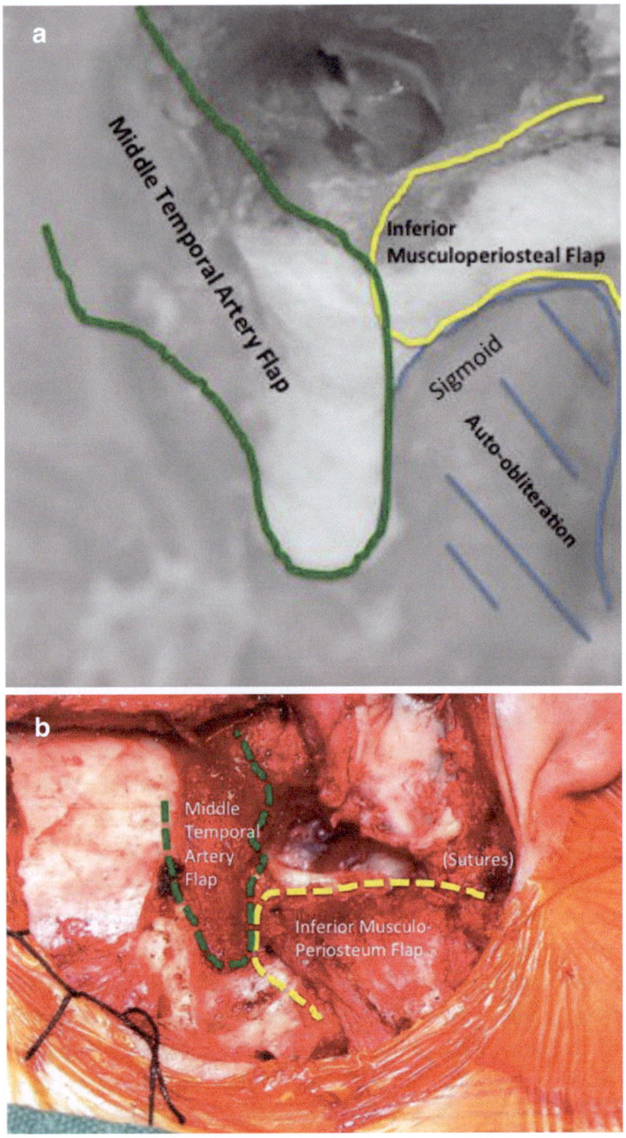

Fig. 63.6 Mastoid obliteration with vascularized soft tissue flaps. (**a**) Scheme of obliteration is depicted in a right ear, which involves application of pressed bone pate that is lined with a combination of the middle temporal artery (green) and inferior musculoperiosteal (yellow) flaps. In this approach, the epitympanum is exteriorized, the mastoid tip is amputated from the digastric muscle, and the retrosigmoid aspect of the cavity is allowed to auto-obliterate (blue). This scheme is ideal for a large cavity from a well-pneumatized mastoid. (**b**) Intraoperative view of the obliterated cavity following rotation of soft tissue flaps. The inferior flap (yellow) is secured in place at its base with a single suture to the adjacent parotid fascia. Suturing is not required to inset the middle temporal artery flap (green)

antibiotics for 10 days and examined in clinic 2–3 weeks later, at which point the ribbon gauze and silastic sheeting are removed and excessive secretions and debris are suctioned. If the obliteration involves a large surface area that must heal, it may be repacked with ribbon gauze on a serial basis every 2 weeks until it reaches near complete epithelialization. If the cavity is small, repacking may be unnecessary and the patient is simply started on a combination antibiotic/steroid-containing otic drop for several days. Patients are advised to adhere to water precautions until complete epithelialization is confirmed. Premature cessation of postoperative care before healing is complete may result in failure to rehabilitate a cavity. When needed, excessive granulation tissue can be cauterized in the office using silver nitrate. Most obliterated cavities should be completely epithelialized by 2–3 months postoperatively.

Outcomes of Mastoid Reconstruction and Obliteration

Mastoid Cortex Reconstruction (Intact Canal Wall)

Generally, outcomes following mastoid cortex reconstruction with intact canal wall mastoidectomy are excellent. Complications include infection and extrusion, but for all reported techniques and material, these complications are quite rare and do not appear to be more common in either the primary or revision setting [2, 10–13]. It should be noted that since a large majority of patients who undergo intact canal wall mastoidectomy do quite well without mastoid reconstruction, most cases in which reconstruction was undertaken in the literature had a low preoperative risk of infection. Reconstruction should generally not be considered as essential in intact canal wall mastoidectomy when infectious complications are more than minimal.

Mastoid Cavity Obliteration (Canal Wall Down)

In the setting of canal wall-down mastoidectomy, if properly executed, mastoid cavity obliteration should result in a smoothly epithelialized surface lacking any fissures that could accumulate debris or infection (see Fig. 63.7). Favorable outcomes following mastoid obliteration using a variety of techniques have been reported, with success rates for creating a stable ear ranging from 70 to 100% [19–24]. Such outcomes should be viewed favorably in light of the fact that many of the cases depicted in these reports had already failed past canal wall-down mastoid surgery and thus represent some of the most difficult chronic ears. By obliterating with soft tissue flaps, O'Sullivan and Atlas reported a reduction in cavity volume to an average of 1.6 mL in 100 patients with postoperative follow-up ranging from 6 months to 4 years [21]. Utilizing a scheme of partial obliteration with bone pate and cartilage plates, Beutner et al. reported an average postoperative cavity volume of 3.1 mL in 26 patients with an average follow-up of 6 years. Additionally, they reported a reduction of caloric-

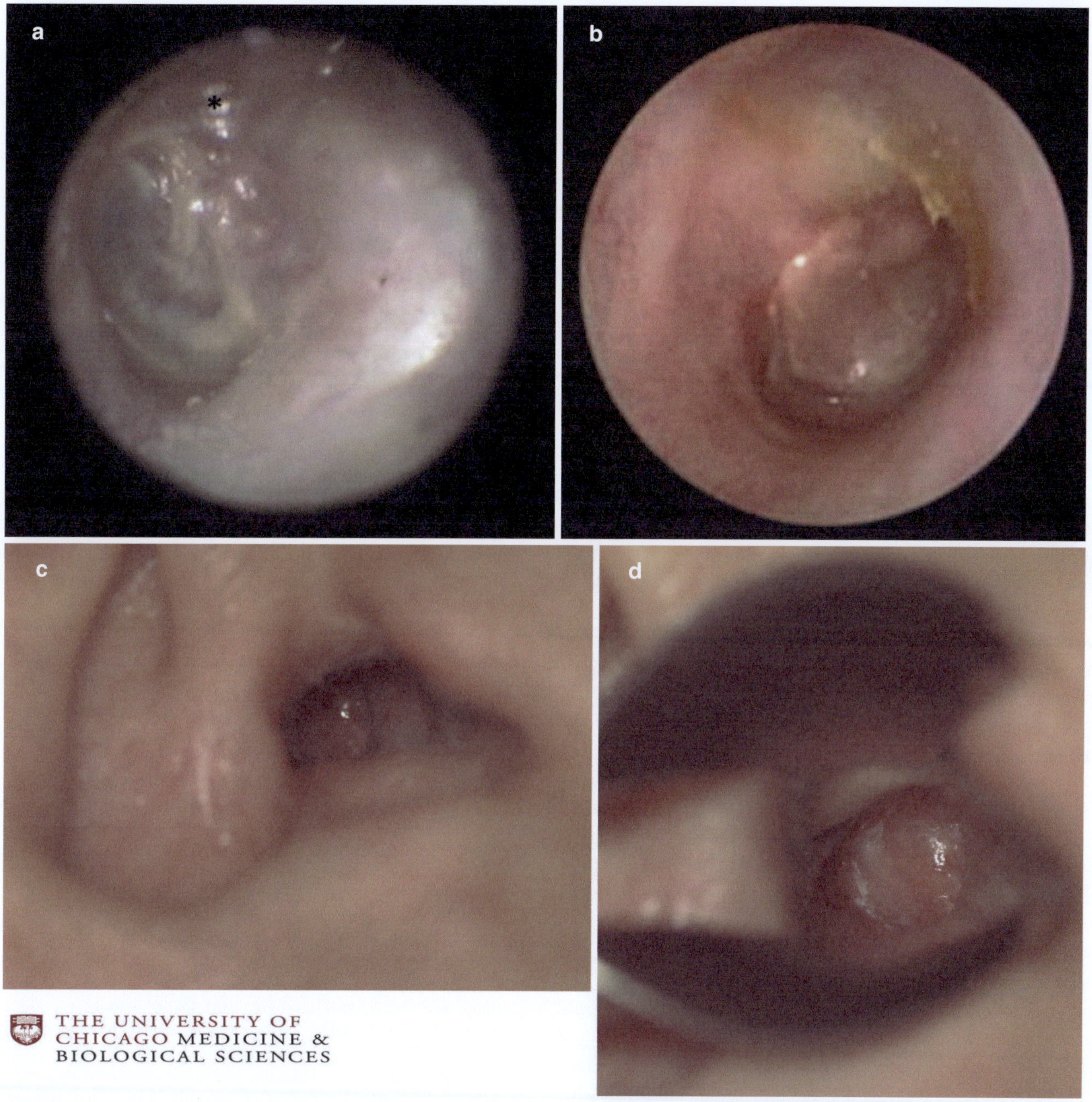

Fig. 63.7 Postoperative view of healed ears following mastoid cavity obliteration. These ears were obliterated using bone pate and vascularized soft tissue flaps. (**a**) Note the presence of an exteriorized epitympanum (asterisk) in a left ear that underwent mastoid cavity obliteration. (**b**) This right ear underwent concurrent obliteration of the mastoid cavity and epitympanum utilizing bone pate and the middle temporal artery flap alongside reconstruction of a subtotal tympanic membrane perforation utilizing a large underlay composite cartilage and perichondrium island graft. (**c**) The small cavity volume means that a conservative Fisch style meatoplasty is adequate. (**d**) With the meatus open with a speculum, the smooth contour of the reconstruction and lack of irregularities is appreciated

effect vertigo in all of the patients (54%) who had been experiencing this preoperatively based on postoperative caloric testing [28].

Dornhoffer et al. reported changes in quality of life following mastoid obliteration as depicted by the Glascow Benefit Inventory [29]. These findings demonstrated a statistically significant improvement in overall quality-of-life scores and improvements within most subcategories. Furthermore, >90% of subjects reported that they would recommend the procedure to a family member. Gluth et al. reported an 85% success rate of attempted conventional hearing aid usage after mastoid cavity revision and obliteration among 20 subjects who had been completely unable to wear a hearing aid preoperatively [30].

Complications of Mastoid Reconstruction and Obliteration

Iatrogenic Cholesteatoma

Perhaps the most feared complication of mastoid reconstruction or obliteration is bulky coverage of residual cholesteatoma, which could potentially go undetected until quite large and even result in an intracranial complication. Although this complication is certainly possible, actual reports of this happening are scarce in the literature, and it must be remembered that similar complications can also occur after standard intact canal wall and canal wall-down mastoid surgeries. In the authors' experience, rare instances of recurrent cholesteatoma within an obliterated mastoid have typically presented in a manner similar to standard cholesteatoma, with granulation tissue, otorrhea, and an expanding cyst. Like all cholesteatoma surgeries, ultimately the safety of mastoid obliteration is dependent upon the wisdom and judgment of the surgeon in determining when and how to proceed. If there is concern for residual cholesteatoma, it may be best to perform staged obliteration, schedule second-look surgery, and/or obtain diffusion-weighted magnetic resonance imaging (MRI) 1–2 years postoperatively [31].

Infection

Infection following mastoid cortex reconstruction obliteration is possible, especially if a large amount of filler is required, synthetic materials are used, or there is an abundance of nonvascularized soft tissue. Although *Pseudomonas aeruginosa* infection is commonplace in a chronic ear, *Staphylococcus aureus* appears to be much more frequently encountered in revision canal wall-down mastoidectomy surgery [32]. When the index of suspicion for infection is high, preoperative culture acquisition is wise and culture-directed antibiotic therapy can be preventative. Some centers advocate perioperative treatment with intravenous antibiotics for several doses following mastoid obliteration.

Extrusion and Delayed Reabsorption of Fillers

In contrast to mastoid cortex reconstruction, bone pate and synthetic materials used for mastoid obliteration are at risk for partial extrusion or delayed reabsorption that can result in defects and irregularities of an obliterated cavity. It has been hypothesized that application of vascularized soft tissue flaps may reduce this occurrence. In the authors' experience, taking care to very densely pack bone pate and/or to combine bone pate or synthetic materials with available cartilage chips will reduce the likelihood and severity of filler loss.

Conclusion

In summary, various mastoid reconstructive and obliterative schemes exist, and these typically involve application of filler and liner materials with the goals of reducing the negative impacts of mastoidectomy. In general, surgeons are advised to avoid bulky obliteration over areas deemed to be at high risk of underlying residual cholesteatoma and are discouraged from excessive application of fillers and nonvascularized soft tissue other than cartilage. Whichever method is used, there appears to be a common trend of achieving dry, stable ears, and in improving a patient's quality of life.

References

1. Mastoid Buffering Properties: I. Gas Partial Pressures | Ovid. 2021. https://oce.ovid.com/article/00000627-199908080-00007.
2. Yanagihara N, Hinohira Y, Sato H. Mastoid cortex plasty using bone pate. Otol Neurotol. 2002;23(4):422–4.
3. Virapongse C, Sarwar M, Bhimani S, Sasaki C, Shapiro R. Computed tomography of temporal bone pneumatization: 1. Normal pattern and morphology. Am J Roentgenol. 1985;145(3):473–81.
4. Schulter-ellis FP. Population differences in cellularity of the mastoid process. Acta Otolaryngol. 1979;87(3–6):461–5.
5. Tos M, Stangerup S-E, Hvid G. Mastoid pneumatization: evidence of the environmental theory. Arch Otolaryngol. 1984;110(8):502–7.
6. Toros SZ, Habesoglu TE, Habesoglu M, Bolukbasi S, Naiboglu B, Karaca CT, et al. Do patients with sclerotic mastoids require aeration to improve success of tympanoplasty? Acta Otolaryngol. 2010;130(8):909–12.
7. Sadé J. The correlation of middle ear aeration with mastoid pneumatization. Eur Arch Otorhinolaryngol. 1992;249(6):301–4.
8. Paparella MM, Kim CS. Mastoidectomy update. Laryngoscope. 1977;87(12):1977–88.
9. Yanagihara N, Komori M, Hinohira Y. Total mastoid obliteration in staged canal-up tympanoplasty for cholesteatoma facilitates tympanic aeration. Otol Neurotol. 2009;30(6):766–70.
10. Thomas JMN, Gluth MB. Reconstruction of mastoid cortex defects with hydroxyapatite cement for negative sequelae of mastoidectomy. Ann Otol Rhinol Laryngol. 2021;130(4):338–42.
11. Kveton JF, Coelho DH. Hydroxyapatite cement in temporal bone surgery: a 10 year experience. Laryngoscope. 2004;114(1):33–7.
12. Kim HH, Wilson DF. Titanium mesh for functional reconstruction of the mastoid cortex after mastoidectomy. Otol Neurotol. 2006;27(1):33–6.
13. Sun J-Q, Sun J-W, Hou X-Y, Bie Y-Z, Chen J-W. Using autogenous mastoid cortical bone cap to cover the mastoidectomy defect during cochlear implantation. Int J Pediatr Otorhinolaryngol. 2015;79(3):419–22.
14. Gluth MB, Metrailer AM, Dornhoffer JL, Moore PC. Patterns of failure in canal wall down mastoidectomy cavity instability. Otol Neurotol. 2012;33(6):998–1001.
15. Males AG, Gray RF. Mastoid misery: quantifying the distress in a radical cavity. Clin Otolaryngol Allied Sci. 1991;16(1):12–4.
16. Sadé J, Weinberg J, Berco E, Brown M, Halevy A. The marsupialized (radical) mastoid. J Laryngol Otol. 1982;96(10):869–75.
17. Wormald PJ, Nilssen ELK. The facial ridge and the discharging mastoid cavity. Laryngoscope. 1998;108(1):92–6.
18. Dornhoffer JL, Friedman AB, Gluth MB. Management of acquired cholesteatoma in the pediatric population. Curr Opin Otolaryngol Head Neck Surg. 2013;21(5):440–5.

19. Dornhoffer JL. Surgical modification of the difficult mastoid cavity. Otolaryngol Head Neck Surg. 1999;120(3):361–7.
20. Hung T, Leung N, Hasselt CA van, Liu KC, Tong M. Long-term outcome of the Hong Kong vascularized, Pedicled temporalis fascia flap in reconstruction of mastoid cavity. Laryngoscope 2007;117(8):1403–1407.
21. O'sullivan PG, Atlas MD. Use of soft tissue vascular flaps for mastoid cavity obliteration. Laryngoscope. 2004;114(5):957–9.
22. Ramsey MJ, Merchant SN, McKenna MJ. Postauricular periosteal-pericranial flap for mastoid obliteration and canal wall down tympanomastoidectomy. Otol Neurotol. 2004;25(6):873–8.
23. Singh V, Atlas M. Obliteration of the persistently discharging mastoid cavity using the middle temporal artery flap. Otolaryngol Head Neck Surg. 2007;137(3):433–8.
24. van Hasselt CA. Mastoid surgery and the Hong Kong flap. J Laryngol Otol. 1994;108(10):825–33.
25. Wilson KF, Hoggan RN, Shelton C. Tympanoplasty with intact canal wall mastoidectomy for cholesteatoma: long-term surgical outcomes. Otolaryngol Head Neck Surg. 2013;149(2):292–5.
26. Leatherman BD, Dornhoffer JL. The use of demineralized bone matrix for mastoid cavity obliteration. Otol Neurotol. 2004;25(1):22–6.
27. Talmage GD, Sunde J, Walker DD, Atlas MD, Gluth MB. Anatomic basis of the middle temporal artery periosteal rotational flap in otologic surgery. Laryngoscope. 2016;126(6):1426–32.
28. Beutner D, Helmstaedter V, Stumpf R, Beleites T, Zahnert T, Luers JC, et al. Impact of partial mastoid obliteration on caloric vestibular function in canal wall down mastoidectomy. Otol Neurotol. 2010;31(9):1399–403.
29. Dornhoffer JL, Smith J, Richter G, Boeckmann J. Impact on quality of life after mastoid obliteration. Laryngoscope. 2008;118(8):1427–32.
30. Gluth MB, Friedman AB, Atcherson SR, Dornhoffer JL. Hearing aid tolerance after revision and obliteration of canal wall down mastoidectomy cavities. Otol Neurotol. 2013;34(4):711–4.
31. Li PMMC, Linos E, Gurgel RK, Fischbein NJ, Blevins NH. Evaluating the utility of non–echo-planar diffusion-weighted imaging in the preoperative evaluation of cholesteatoma: a meta-analysis. Laryngoscope. 2013;123(5):1247–50.
32. Gluth MB, Tan BYB, Santa Maria PL, Atlas MD. Unique microbiology of chronically unstable canal wall down tympanomastoid cavities: considerations for surgical revision. J Laryngol Otol. 2013;127(5):458–62.
33. Palva T. Reconstruction of ear canal in surgery for chronic ear. Arch Otolaryngol. 1962;75(4):329–34.
34. Fagan PA, Rodrigues SJ. Middle temporal artery flap in mastoid surgery. Otol Neurotol. 2004;25(3):242–4.
35. Turner J. Symposium on ear surgery. I. Soft tissue technique in musculoplasty obliteration of mastoidectomy cavities. Laryngoscope. 1972;82(7):1145–59.
36. Cheney ML, Megerian CA, Brown MT, Mckenna MJ. Mastoid obliteration and lining using the temporoparietal fascial flap. Laryngoscope. 1995;105(9):1010–3.
37. East CA, Brough MD, Grant HR. Mastoid obliteration with the temporoparietal fascia flap. J Laryngol Otol. 1991;105(6):417–20.
38. Gibb AG, Tan KK, Sim RST. The Singapore swing. J Laryngol Otol. 1997;111(6):527–30.

Subtotal Petrosectomy

64

Gianluca Piras, Wenlong Tang, Antonio Caruso,
Lorenzo Lauda, Abdelkader Taibah, and Mario Sanna

Introduction

Although this technique was introduced in the late 1950s and 1960s [1, 2], Ugo Fisch introduced the term "subtotal petrosectomy" in 1965 [3]. He described STP as the complete exenteration of all pneumatic tracts in the temporal bone, including retrofacial, retrosigmoid, antral, retrolabyrinthine, supralabyrinthine, infralabyrinthine, peritubal, and pericarotid cell tracts. Although the initial description involved preservation of the otic capsule, it allowed expanding the procedure, when necessary, to exenterate the cochlea, the labyrinth, or the internal auditory canal.

Indications

- Canal wall down cavity with intractable inflammation with no serviceable hearing
- Chronic otitis media with no serviceable hearing with multiple previous surgeries
- Recurrent cholesteatoma with huge mastoid aeration
- Sustained cerebrospinal fluid (CSF) leak with either spontaneous, posttraumatic, or surgical origin
- Large meningoencephalic herniation
- Extensive exposure of middle fossa dura
- Cochlear implants in special cases
- Paragangliomas of Class B3

Surgical Steps (Right Ear)

1. A C-shaped skin incision is made, extending 4–5 cm behind the retroauricular sulcus.
2. The external auditory canal is transected at the bony cartilaginous junction (Fig. 64.1). The skin of the lateral part is dissected free from the cartilage for 1 cm (Fig. 64.2). Two stay sutures are then placed through this skin. Using an artery forceps, the sutures are pulled through the external auditory canal, thus everting the free skin edges. These are then closed with 3-0 Vicryl sutures (Fig. 64.3). The cartilage is then folded and sutured in place to reinforce the blind sac closure (Fig. 64.4).

G. Piras (✉) · W. Tang · A. Caruso · L. Lauda · A. Taibah · M. Sanna
Gruppo Otologico and Mario Sanna Foundation, Piacenza-Rome, Italy

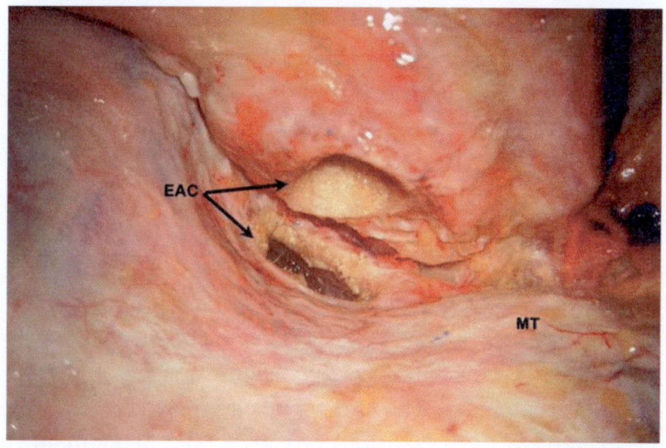

Fig. 64.1 The external auditory canal is transected at the bony cartilaginous junction. *EAC* external auditory canal; *MT* mastoid tip

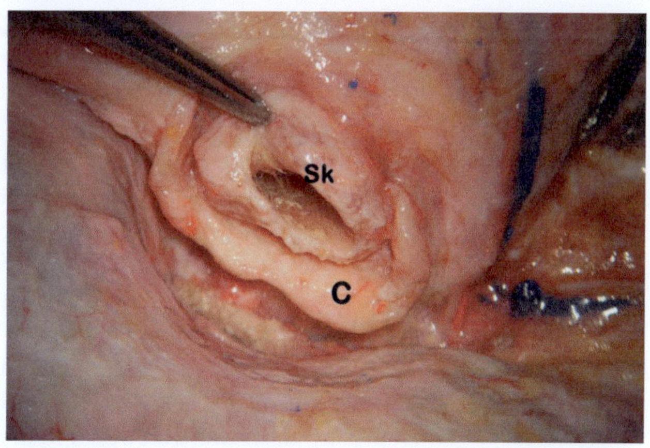

Fig. 64.2 The skin of the lateral part is dissected free from the cartilage. *Sk* skin; *C* cartilage

M. V. Goycoolea et al. (eds.), *Textbook of Otitis Media*, https://doi.org/10.1007/978-3-031-40949-3_64

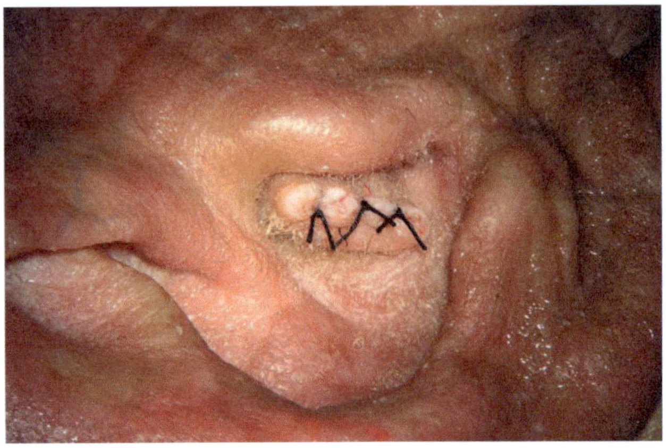

Fig. 64.3 The everted skin is tightly sutured with 3-0 Vicryl sutures

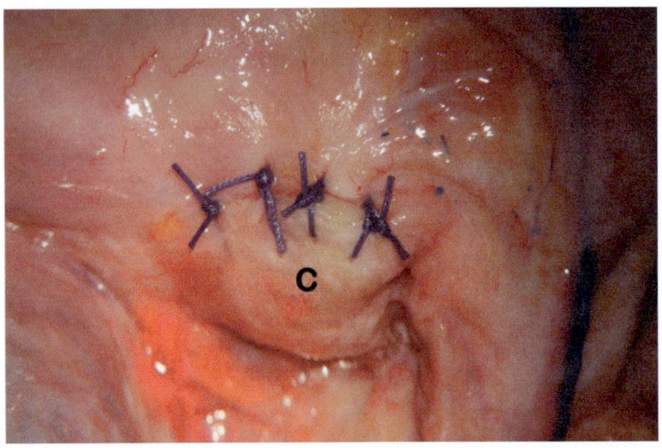

Fig. 64.4 The medial cartilage is then folded and sutured in place to reinforce the blind sac closure. *C* cartilage

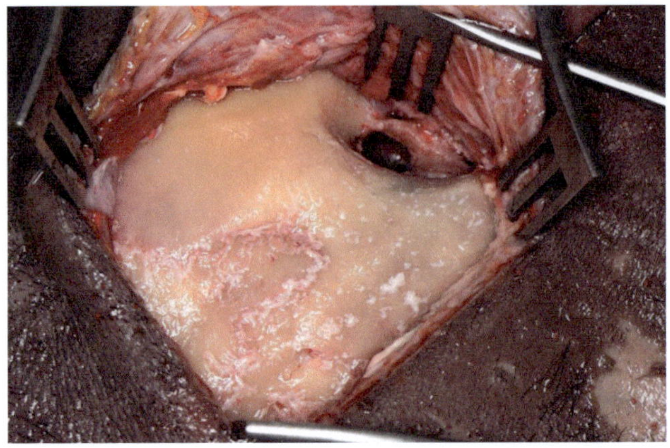

Fig. 64.5 The soft tissues are held with two articulated self-retaining retractors. The sternocleidomastoid muscle is retracted to expose the entire mastoid tip

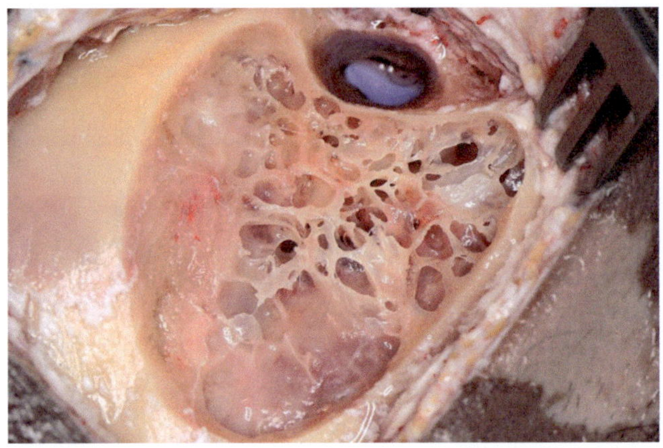

Fig. 64.6 In the early stage of mastoidectomy, drilling is carried out with a large cutting burr. Large cutting burrs allow faster bone removal and easier identification of structures. If drilling is conducted correctly, no important structure in danger is present in the triangle formed by the sigmoid sinus posteriorly, the middle fossa plate superiorly, and the posterior meatal wall anteriorly

3. A T-shaped musculofascial incision is made with monopolar diathermy. The soft tissues are elevated from the mastoid with the mastoid raspatory. The attachment of the sternocleidomastoid muscle is freed from the lateral portion of the mastoid tip. The soft tissues are held with two articulated self-retaining retractors. The sternocleidomastoid muscle is retracted to expose the entire mastoid tip (Fig. 64.5). A microraspatory is used to elevate the remnants of the external auditory canal skin down to the tympanic annulus.
4. The initial stages of the mastoidectomy are done without magnification (Fig. 64.6). Drilling is extended well above the level of the middle fossa dura and behind the sigmoid sinus to facilitate saucerization of the cavity. All pneumatic cells are removed. A thin sheet of bone is left protecting the dura and sigmoid sinus. The middle cranial fossa dura is identified first, followed by the sigmoid sinus, sinodural angle, mastoid tip cells, and the mastoid antrum. The posterior bony canal wall is lowered to the level of the remaining skin margin. Drilling is done with a cutting burr with continuous suction-irrigation. All overhanging edges of bone are removed to allow collapse of the overlying tissues when the wound is closed.
5. All air cell tracts associated with the middle ear and mastoid should be totally removed. The facial nerve is identified at the digastric ridge by following the stylomastoid periosteum which runs medial and anterior to the stylomastoid foramen. The facial bridge is removed with curette to expose the fallopian canal from the oval window to the stylomastoid foramen. The tympanic membrane is now removed in continuity with the cuff of canal skin to expose the ossicular chain (Fig. 64.7).
6. The incudostapedial joint is separated with an angled hook or joint knife (Fig. 64.8). The incus is then removed with forceps. The tympanic segment of the facial nerve is identified inferior to the lateral semicircular canal at the oval

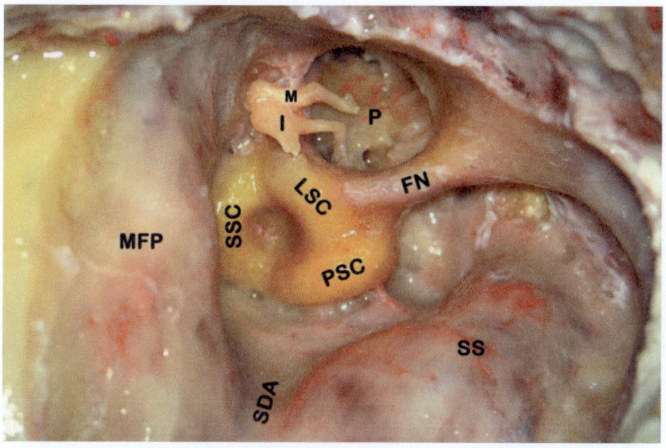

Fig. 64.7 The facial ridge is lowered evenly by drilling the posterior canal wall. All air cell tracts associated with the middle ear and mastoid should be totally removed. The facial bridge is removed with curette. The tympanic membrane is removed in continuity with the cuff of canal skin to expose the ossicular chain. *MFP* middle fossa plate; *SS* sigmoid sinus; *SDA* sinodural angle; *LSC* lateral semicircular canal; *PSC* posterior semicircular canal; *SSC* superior semicircular canal; *FN* facial nerve; *I* incus; *M* malleus; *P* promontory

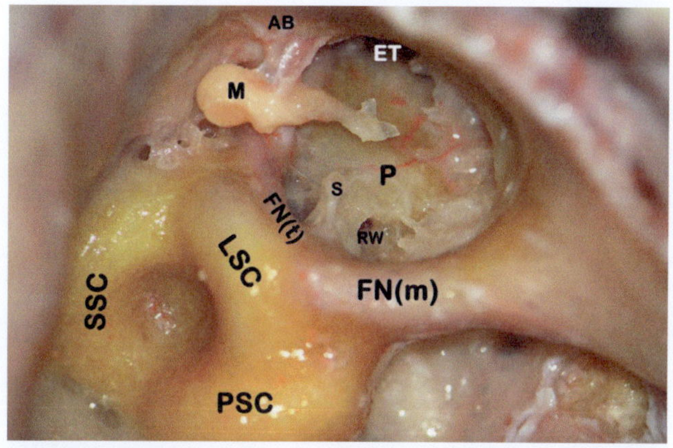

Fig. 64.9 The incus is then removed with forceps to expose the tympanic segment of the facial nerve. *LSC* lateral semicircular canal; *PSC* posterior semicircular canal; *SSC* superior semicircular canal; *FN(t)* tympanic segment of the facial nerve; *FN(m)* mastoid segment of the facial nerve; *M* malleus; *S* stapes; *P* promontory; *RW* round window; *ET* eustachian tube; *AB* anterior buttress

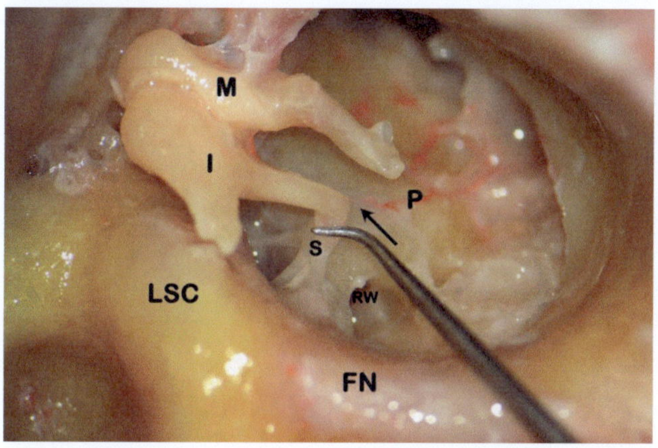

Fig. 64.8 The incudostapedial joint is disarticulated using a small dissector, with movement from posterior to anterior. *LSC* lateral semicircular canal; *FN* facial nerve; *I* incus; *M* malleus; *S* stapes; *P* promontory; *RW* round window

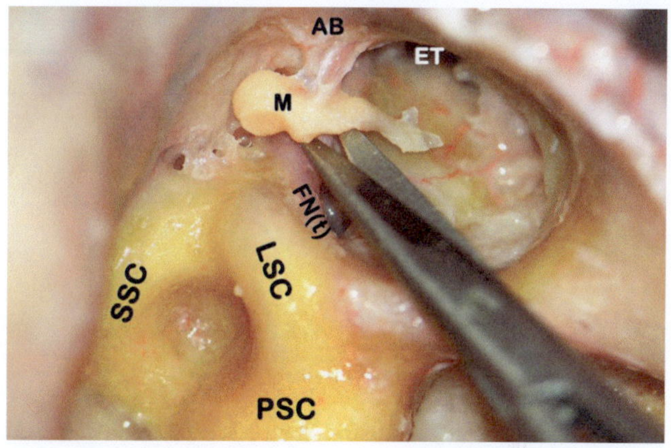

Fig. 64.10 The tensor tympani tendon and anterior malleal ligament are sectioned with microscissors. *LSC* lateral semicircular canal; *PSC* posterior semicircular canal; *SSC* superior semicircular canal; *FN(t)* tympanic segment of the facial nerve; *M* malleus; *ET* eustachian tube; *AB* anterior buttress

window (Fig. 64.9).The tensor tympani tendon and anterior malleal ligament are sectioned with microscissors (Fig. 64.10). The anterior epitympanic space is visualized, in particular the cog and its relationship to the tympanic segment of the facial nerve, cochleariform process, and tensor tympani canal (Fig. 64.11). Cog is removed with a diamond burr to expose the supratubal recess (Fig. 64.12). All bone except for a thin covering is removed from the nerve. The pneumatic cells are exenterated in the following order: retrosigmoid, retrofacial, retrolabyrinthine, supralabyrinthine, infralabyrinthine, pericarotid, and supratubal.

7. The hypotympanic cells are further drilled (Fig. 64.13). Through the subfacial recess tympanotomy, the cells under the carotid artery are opened using the largest possible diamond burr (Figs. 64.13, 64.14, 64.15, and 64.16).
8. The stapes arch is removed to avoid inadvertent luxation of the footplate when the surgeon is working deeper in the temporal bone.
9. The eustachian tube orifice is obliterated with bone wax and pieces of musculofascial graft.
10. The cavity is obliterated with abdominal fat.

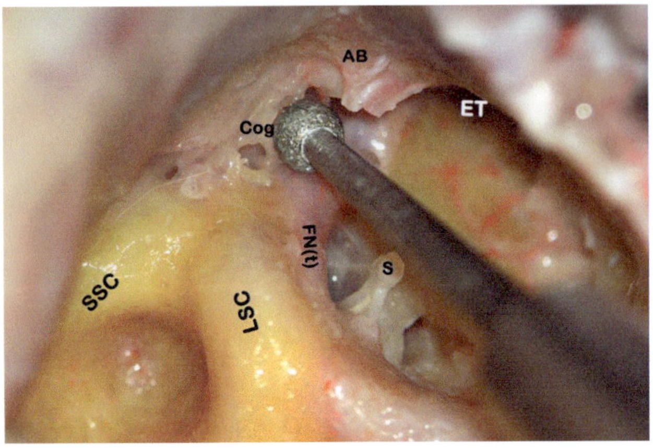

Fig. 64.11 The anterior epitympanic space is visualized, in particular the cog and its relationship to the tympanic segment of the facial nerve, cochleariform process, and tensor tympani canal. The structures around the cochleariform process are shown. *LSC* lateral semicircular canal; *PSC* posterior semicircular canal; *SSC* superior semicircular canal; *FN(t)* tympanic segment of the facial nerve; *FN(m)* mastoid segment of the facial nerve; *ET* eustachian tube; *AB* anterior buttress; *CP* cochleariform process; *P* promontory; *S* stapes; *RW* round window

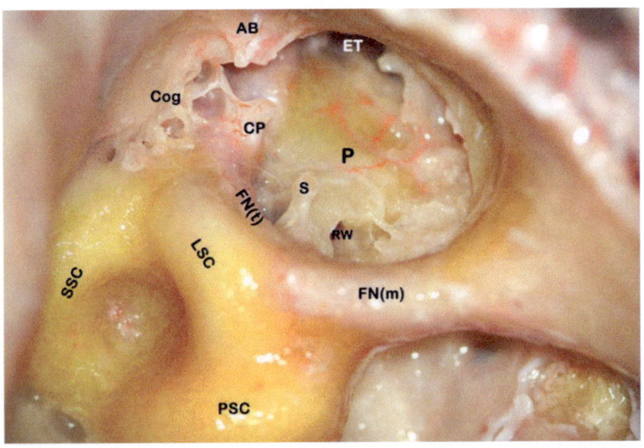

Fig. 64.12 Cog is removed with a diamond burr to expose the supratubal recess. The anterior buttress is removed to make the cavity rounded. *LSC* lateral semicircular canal; *SSC* superior semicircular canal; *FN(t)* tympanic segment of the facial nerve; *ET* eustachian tube; *AB* anterior buttress; *S* stapes

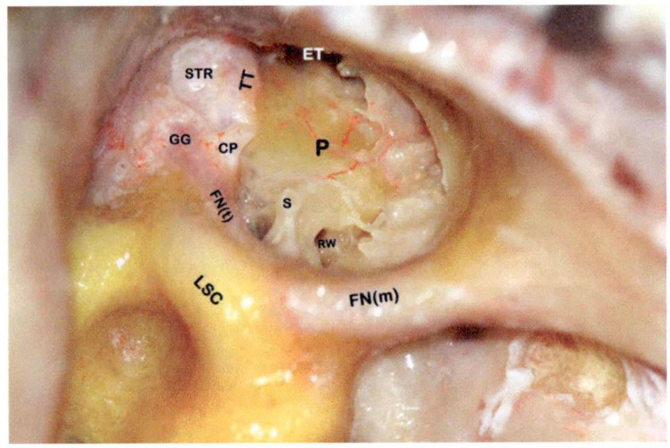

Fig. 64.13 The supratubal recess is completely opened and visualized. *LSC* lateral semicircular canal; *FN(t)* tympanic segment of the facial nerve; *FN(m)* mastoid segment of the facial nerve; *GG* geniculate ganglion; *ET* eustachian tube; *S* stapes; *CP* cochleariform process; *P* promontory; *RW* round window; *TT* tensor tympani muscle; *STR* supratubal recess

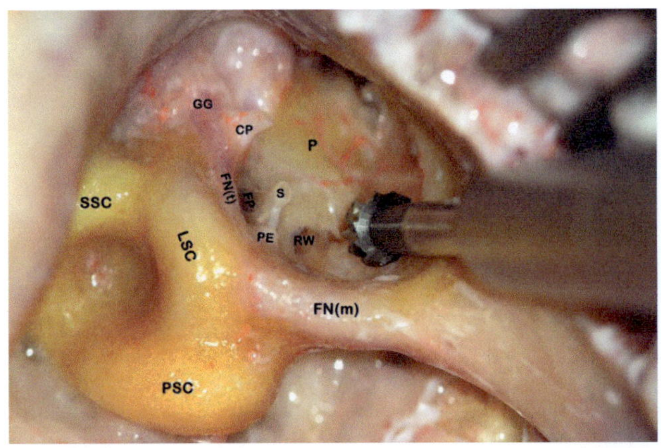

Fig. 64.14 The hypotympanic cells are further drilled. *LSC* lateral semicircular canal; *PSC* posterior semicircular canal; *SSC* superior semicircular canal; *FN(t)* tympanic segment of the facial nerve; *FN(m)* mastoid segment of the facial nerve; *GG* geniculate ganglion; *S* stapes; *CP* cochleariform process; *P* promontory; *RW* round window; *FP* footplate of stapes; *PE* pyramidal eminence

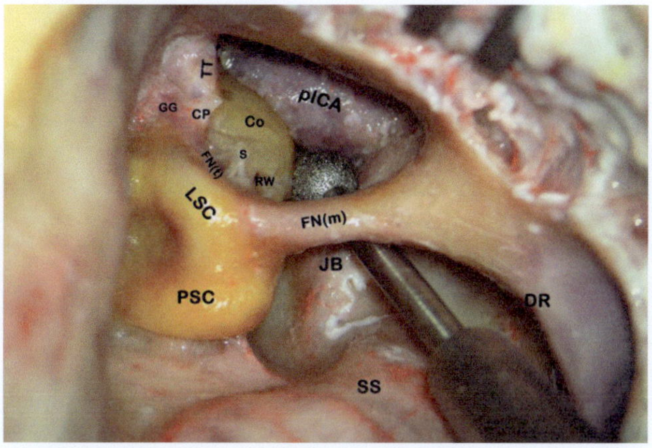

Fig. 64.15 Through the subfacial recess tympanotomy, the cells under the carotid artery are opened using the largest possible diamond burr. *LSC* lateral semicircular canal; *PSC* posterior semicircular canal; *FN(t)* tympanic segment of the facial nerve; *FN(m)* mastoid segment of the facial nerve; *GG* geniculate ganglion; *S* stapes; *CP* cochleariform process; *RW* round window; *Co* cochlea; *TT* tensor tympani muscle; *JB* jugular bulb; *pICA* petrous segment of internal carotid artery; *SS* sigmoid sinus; *DR* digastric ridge

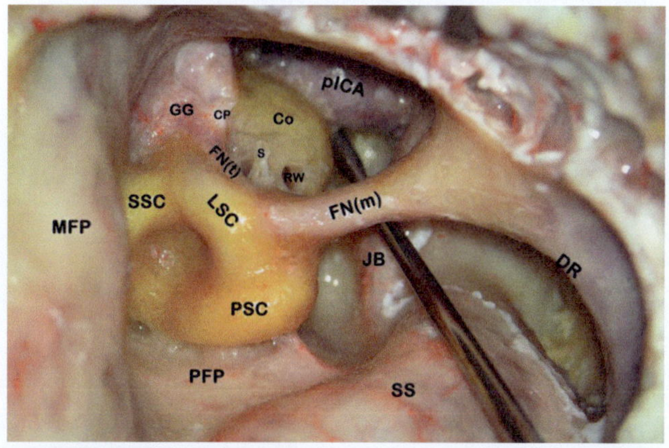

Fig. 64.16 The retrofacial and hypotympanic air cells have been drilled, as shown by the passage of the pointer medial to the mastoid segment of the facial nerve. *LSC* lateral semicircular canal; *PSC* posterior semicircular canal; *SSC* superior semicircular canal; *FN(t)* tympanic segment of the facial nerve; *FN(m)* mastoid segment of the facial nerve; *GG* geniculate ganglion; *S* stapes; *CP* cochleariform process; *RW* round window; *Co* cochlea; *JB* jugular bulb; *pICA* petrous segment of internal carotid artery; *MFP* middle fossa plate; *SS* sigmoid sinus; *PFP* posterior fossa plate; *DR* digastric ridge

Clinical Case

In order to illustrate the role of subtotal petrosotomy in the treatment of chronic otitis media, we will present a clinical case.

The patient underwent middle ear surgery, which was followed by progressive hearing loss complicated by intractable otorrhea. Otoscopic examination showed a pinkish pulsating mass in the external auditory canal. Radiological examination revealed meningoencephalic herniation in the middle ear (Figs. 64.17, 64.18, 64.19, 64.20, 64.21, 64.22, 64.23, 64.24, 64.25, 64.26, 64.27, 64.28, 64.29, 64.30, and 64.31).

Meningoencephalic Herniation with Cholesteatoma

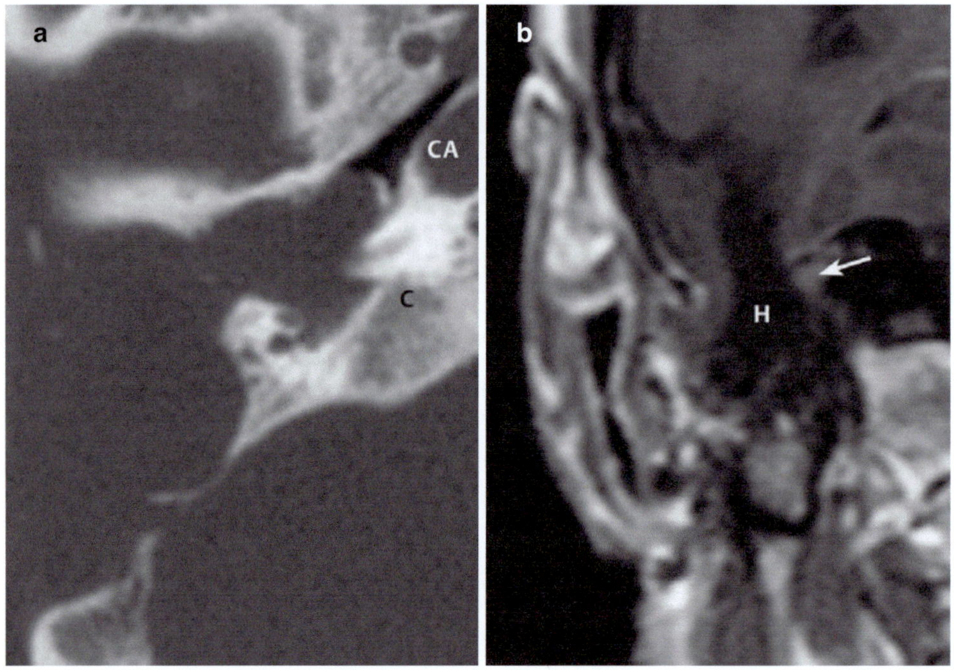

Fig. 64.17 The patient underwent middle ear surgery, which was followed by progressive hearing loss complicated by intractable otorrhea. Otoscopic examination showed a pinkish pulsating mass in the external auditory canal. Radiological examination revealed meningoencephalic herniation in the middle ear. In the axial CT (**a**), a large amount of soft tissue with smooth border is seen. The coronal MRI (**b**) shows herniation of the brain tissue into the middle ear from the defect in the middle fossa plate (arrow). *C* cochlea; *CA* carotid artery; *H* herniated tissue

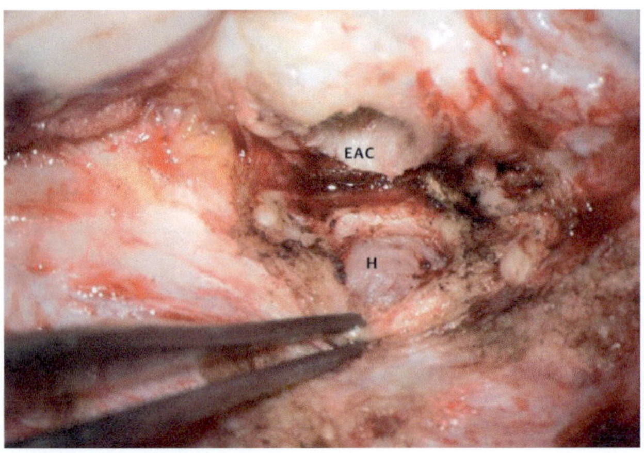

Fig. 64.18 A retroauricular incision is made and the musculoperiosteal layer covering the area of the mastoid is exposed. A circumferential cut at this level exposes meningoencephalic herniation in the external auditory canal. *EAC* external auditory canal; *H* meningoencephalic herniation

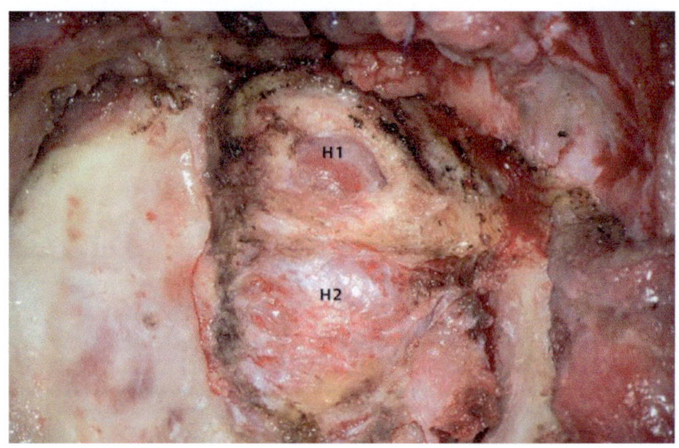

Fig. 64.19 Blind-sac closure of the external auditory canal is conducted, and the musculoperiosteal layer is elevated to expose the large herniated tissue occupying the mastoid cavity. *H1* herniation in the external auditory canal; *H2* herniation in the mastoid

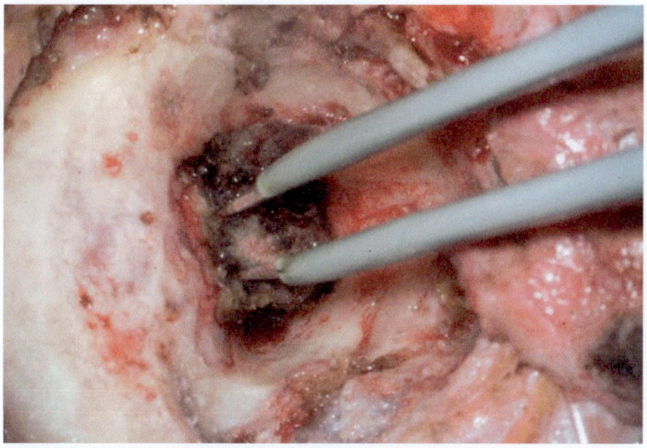

Fig. 64.20 The herniation is coagulated with the bipolar coagulator. The procedure shrinks herniated tissue and facilitates dissection from the surrounding structures

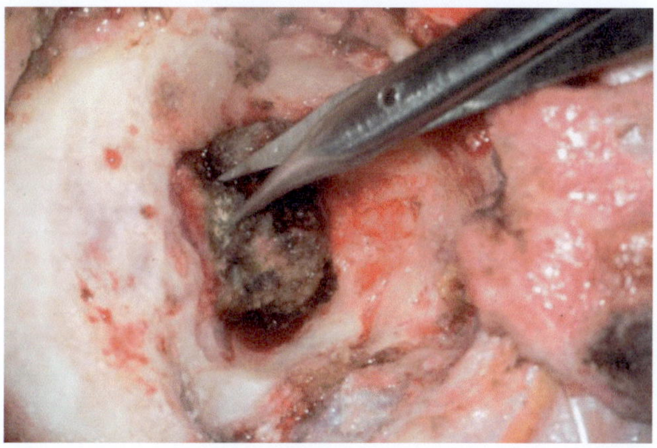

Fig. 64.21 The coagulated tissue is cut with scissors in piecemeal fashion

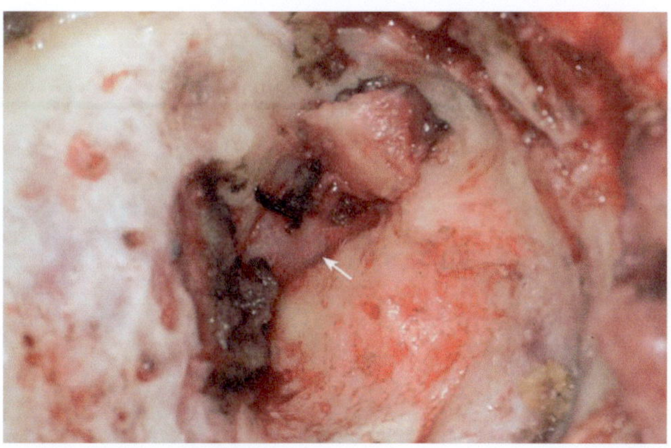

Fig. 64.22 Another herniated tissue mass is seen medially in the external auditory canal (arrow)

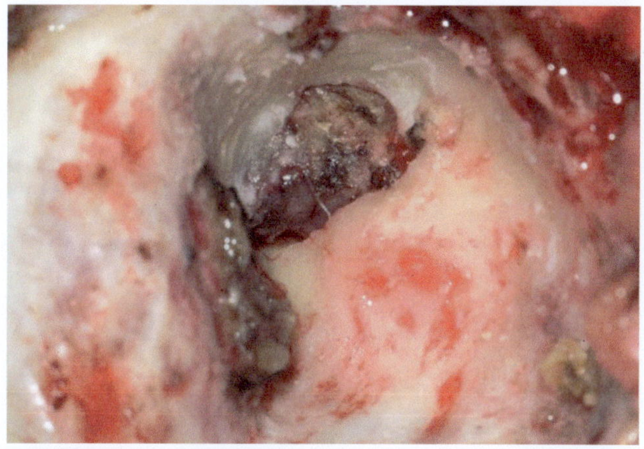

Fig. 64.23 The coagulated tissue has been cut with scissors in piecemeal fashion

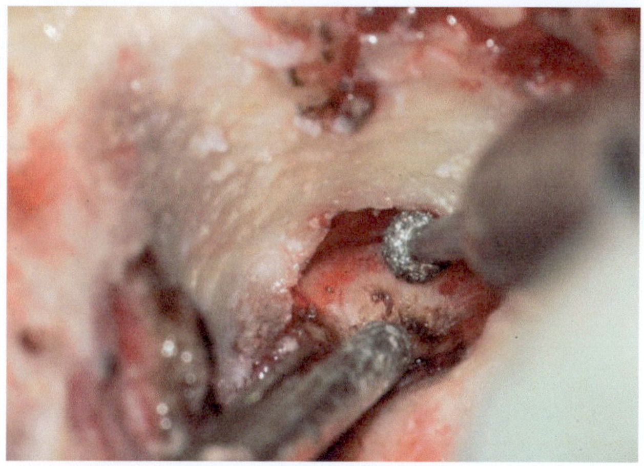

Fig. 64.24 Canalplasty is carried out to sufficiently visualize the herniation in the meatus

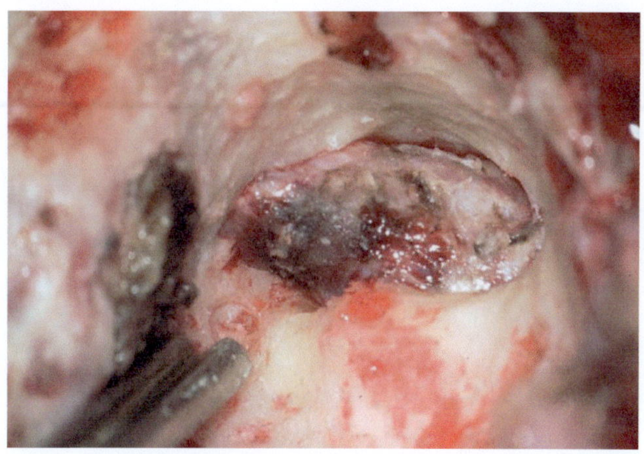

Fig. 64.25 The herniated tissue occupying the tympanic cavity is exposed

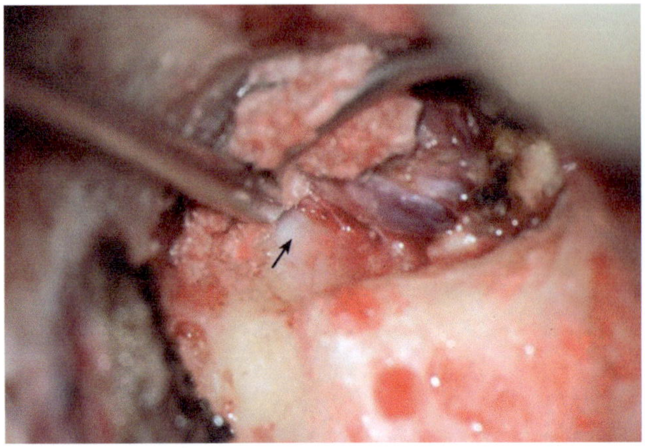

Fig. 64.26 The herniated tissue is dissected from the tympanic segment of the facial nerve (arrow) using a Cottonoid. Note that the nerve is extensively exposed in this area

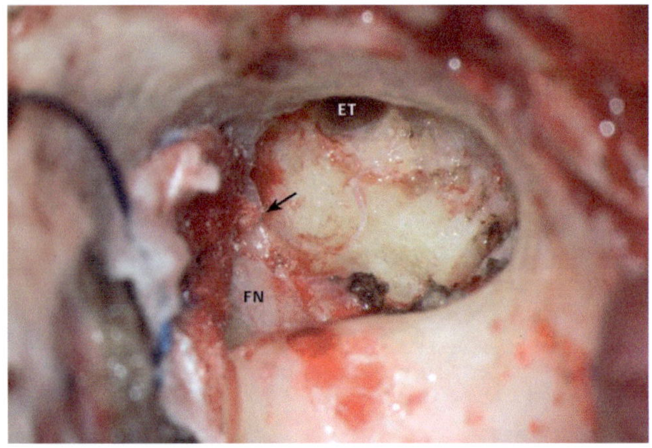

Fig. 64.29 All the skin and herniated tissue have been eradicated from the middle ear. The exposed facial nerve is seen running just superiorly to the cochleariform process (arrow). *ET* eustachian tube; *FN* facial nerve

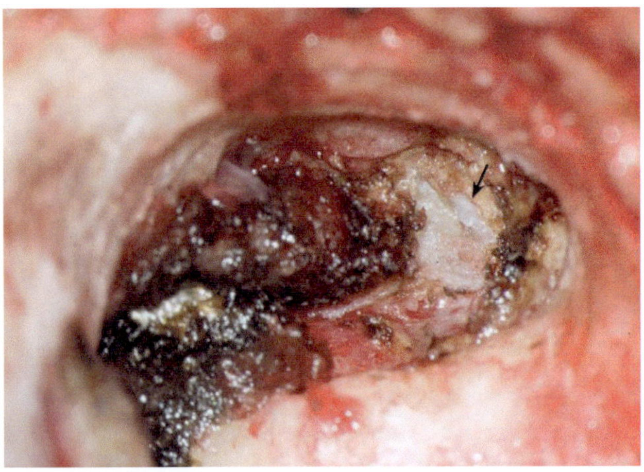

Fig. 64.27 Medially to the herniation, entrapped skin has formed cholesteatoma (arrow)

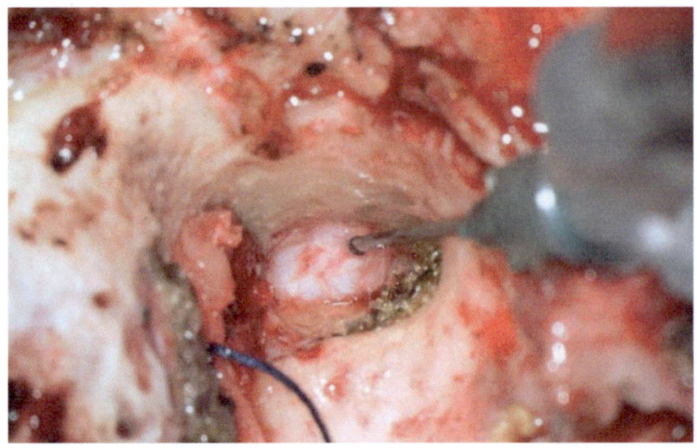

Fig. 64.30 The eustachian tube is obliterated with pieces of periosteum. Fibrin glue is applied to ensure closure in this case

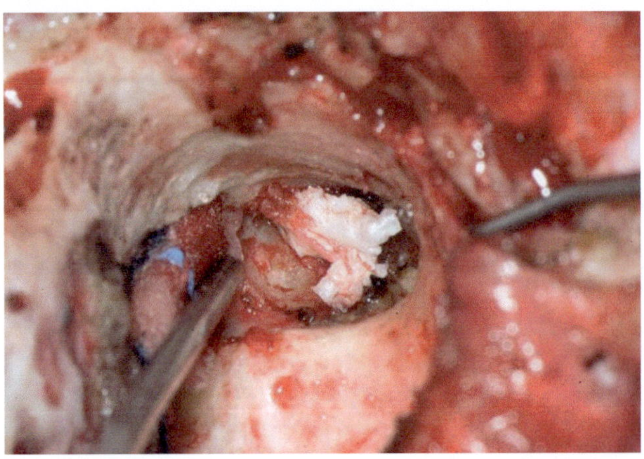

Fig. 64.28 The cholesteatoma is dissected from the tympanic cavity

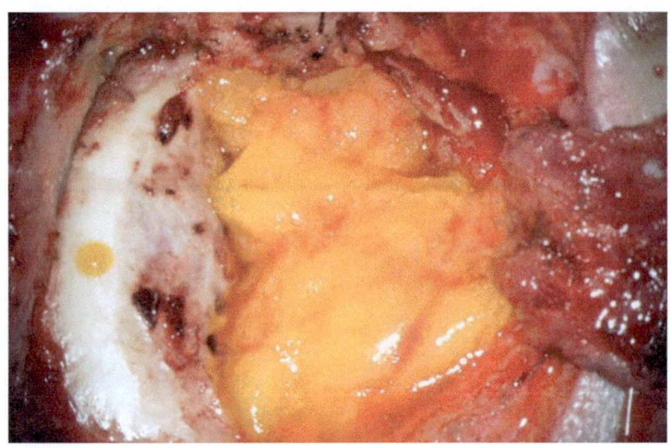

Fig. 64.31 The cavity is packed with abdominal fat

Summary

STP is indicated in any disease primarily in the middle ear and mastoid with limited extensions into deeper parts of the temporal bone that leaves behind a large cavity [4]. In lateral skull base surgery, this procedure is a preliminary step in many approaches such as transotic, transcochlear, the infratemporal fossa approaches, temporal bone resections, and other skull base procedures for particular cases involving middle and posterior fossa tumors. STP is a very useful and effective surgical tool in the management of a variety of problematic situations, it offers excellent exposure, provides middle ear exclusion, and can be combined safely with hearing implantation procedures [5–12].

Hints and Pitfalls

- The postauricular incision must be wide to avoid a fistula that can arise from the friable skin due to previous surgeries.
- In pleuri-operated cases, the tragal cartilage can be brought back posteriorly and sutured to a soft tissue flap as a second layer for external auditory canal closure.
- The skin, annulus, and tympanic membrane with malleus and incus can be removed en bloc to lower the risk of leaving some skin behind.
- While performing the canal wall down mastoidectomy, it is better to remove as many cell tracts as possible to ensure that there is no residual disease.
- The perilabyrinthine, peritubal, and hypotympanic cell tracts are removed routinely except in cases of Cochlear Implant in noninfective cases.
- The stapes superstructure has to be removed, because leaving it behind could allow fat to exert a piston-like pressure on the stapes or frank subluxation, leading to postoperative vertigo.
- Closure of the Eustachian tube must be done meticulously to prevent an opening.
- The wound is closed in two or three layers.
- Follow up is mandatory with high-resolution computed tomography (HRCT) and magnetic resonance imaging (MRI) scans of the temporal bone and skull base, the latter with diffusion weighted sequences (MRI-DWI non-EPI).

References

1. Rambo JH. Musculoplasty: a new operation for suppurative middle ear deafness. Trans Am Acad Ophthalmol Otolaryngol. 1958;62:166–77.
2. Rambo JH. Primary closure of the radical mastoidectomy wound: a technique to eliminate postoperative care. Laryngoscope. 1958;68:1216–27.
3. Fisch U. Microsurgery of the Skull Base. Stuttgart, Germany: Georg Thieme Verlag; 1988.
4. Coker NJ, Jenkins HA, Fisch U. Obliteration of the middle ear and mastoid cleft in subtotal petrosectomy: indications, technique, and results. Ann Otol Rhinol Laryngol. 1986;95:5–11.
5. Gacek RR. Mastoid and middle ear cavity obliteration for control of otitis media. Ann Otol Rhinol Laryngol. 1976;85:305–9.
6. Nadol JB Jr, Schuknecht HF. Obliteration of the mastoid in the treatment of tumors of the temporal bone. Ann Otol Rhinol Laryngol. 1984;93:6–12.
7. Sanna MM, Free RH, Falcioni M. Subtotal petrosectomy in cochlear implantation surgery for cochlear and other auditory implants. Stuttgart, Germany: Georg Thieme Verlag; 2016.
8. Sanna MS, Khrais T, Mancini F, Piazza P, Russo A, Taibah A. Atlas of microsurgery of the lateral skull base. Stuttgart, Germany: Georg Thieme Verlag; 2007.
9. Sanna M, Dispenza F, Flanagan S, De Stefano A, Falcioni M. Management of chronic otitis by middle ear obliteration with blind sac closure of the external auditory canal. Otol Neurotol. 2008;29:19–22.
10. Sanna M, Free R, Merkus P, Falcioni M. Subtotal petrosectomy in cochlear implantation surgery for cochlear and other auditory implants. Stuttgart, Germany: George Thieme Verlag; 2016.
11. Prasad SC, Roustan V, Piras G, Caruso A, Lauda L, Sanna M. Subtotal petrosectomy: surgical technique, indications, outcomes, and comprehensive review of literature. Laryngoscope. 2017;127(12):2833–42.
12. Grinblat G, Vlad D, Caruso A, Sanna M. Evaluation of subtotal Petrosectomy technique in difficult cases of Cochlear implantation. Audiol Neurootol. 2020;25(6):323–35. https://doi.org/10.1159/000507419. Epub 2020 May 29.

Index

M. V. Goycoolea et al. (eds.), *Textbook of Otitis Media*, https://doi.org/10.1007/978-3-031-40949-3

MIX
Papier aus verantwortungsvollen Quellen
Paper from responsible sources
FSC® C105338

If you have any concerns about our products,
you can contact us on
ProductSafety@springernature.com

In case Publisher is established outside the EU,
the EU authorized representative is:
Springer Nature Customer Service Center GmbH
Europaplatz 3, 69115 Heidelberg, Germany

Printed by Libri Plureos GmbH
in Hamburg, Germany